Ultrasound and Carotid Bifurcation Atherosclerosis

Andrew Nicolaides • Kirk W. Beach
Efthyvoulos Kyriacou
Constantinos S. Pattichis
Editors

Ultrasound and Carotid Bifurcation Atherosclerosis

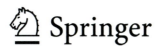

Editors
Andrew Nicolaides, MS, FRCS,
FRCSE, PhD (Hon)
Imperial College and Vascular Screening
and Diagnostic Centre
London, UK

Efthyvoulos Kyriacou, PhD
Department of Computer Science
and Engineering
Frederick University Cyprus
Lemesos, Cyprus

Kirk W. Beach, MD, PhD
Department of Surgery and Bioengineering
University of Washington
Seattle, WA, USA

Constantinos S. Pattichis, PhD
Department of Computer Science
University of Cyprus
Nicosia, Cyprus

ISBN 978-1-84882-687-8   e-ISBN 978-1-84882-688-5
DOI 10.1007/978-1-84882-688-5
Springer London Dordrecht Heidelberg New York

British Library Cataloguing in Publication Data
A catalogue record for this book is available from the British Library

Library of Congress Control Number: 2011942267

© Springer-Verlag London Limited 2012
Apart from any fair dealing for the purposes of research or private study, or criticism or review, as permitted under the Copyright, Designs and Patents Act 1988, this publication may only be reproduced, stored or transmitted, in any form or by any means, with the prior permission in writing of the publishers, or in the case of reprographic reproduction in accordance with the terms of licences issued by the Copyright Licensing Agency. Enquiries concerning reproduction outside those terms should be sent to the publishers.
The use of registered names, trademarks, etc. in this publication does not imply, even in the absence of a specific statement, that such names are exempt from the relevant laws and regulations and therefore free for general use.
Product liability: The publisher can give no guarantee for information about drug dosage and application thereof contained in this book. In every individual case the respective user must check its accuracy by consulting other pharmaceutical literature.

Printed on acid-free paper

Springer is part of Springer Science+Business Media (www.springer.com)

Foreword

Atherosclerotic plaques at the carotid bifurcation are a common problem in individuals over 50 years of age in developed countries. Although most of these plaques produce no ill effects, a small minority produce embolic strokes. Because the carotid bifurcation is easily approached by open surgery and endovascular techniques, invasive treatment of carotid plaques has been widely advocated as a stroke prevention measure. However, whether or not such treatment is justified in asymptomatic patients and how this plaque neutralization should be performed (by carotid endarterectomy or stenting) remain topics of much controversy and debate. Because of the frequency of carotid plaques, these controversies carry enormous financial implications for society and for the physicians performing these procedures.

This gem of a book addresses all the issues surrounding the natural history and management of these carotid plaques. It provides an up-to-date summary of accurate scientific information about the pathophysiology of carotid plaques, their significance, and why they remain quiescent or become active. Most importantly, it provides a current summary of information for imaging techniques using ultrasound, including methods for measuring carotid arterial wall changes such as IMT, plaque thickness, area and volume used as predictors of future cardiovascular events, mainly myocardial infarction, and a means of better selection of individuals for prevention. In addition, it provides cutting edge information on carotid plaque characterization so that those at high risk of producing strokes can be selected for invasive treatment. In that way, information in this valuable text forms the basis for selecting out those patients with high risk plaques so they can be treated invasively while the vast majority of patients with low risk plaques can be treated medically and conservatively. This will avoid the absurd and enormously expensive current practice of invasively treating most asymptomatic plaques, a practice which may benefit the physician specialists performing the procedures but certainly does not benefit most patients.

In this rapidly advancing and controversial field which impacts so many asymptomatic individuals and patients, methods for selecting those at increased risk are sorely needed. Although there are glimmers that some methods have prospects for doing so, none are generally accepted as being dependably effective. So the expensive and risky practice of treating many patients who do not need treatment continues. This volume provides starting points for those interested in seeing this unmet need resolved.

This book also reviews important current information on the most recent developments in monitoring plaque growth and destabilization or stabilization and regression during medical treatment. Enormous advances have been made in this area recently, chiefly because of improvements in ultrasound imaging techniques and the widespread availability of statins. Advances in medical therapy have greatly diminished cardiovascular risk including stroke risk of asymptomatic carotid plaques, raising the real possibility that few if any asymptomatic plaques have to be treated invasively. Of course, this like other future advances in the management of carotid plaque disease will have to be proven by appropriate randomized controlled trials. This volume will be an essential primer, a must read, for those who are designing and interpreting such trials, and for all others interested in the prevention of cardiovascular atherosclerotic disease in general as well as the management of carotid bifurcation plaques.

Frank J. Veith

Preface

Atherosclerosis is a multifactorial and dynamic disease that makes the process of prevention and management highly complex. New methods of ultrasonic imaging have made the noninvasive visualization and assessment of arterial wall changes possible with precise measurements. The latter include the thickness of the intima media complex, estimation of the severity of stenosis due to atherosclerotic plaque, plaque thickness, area and volume, plaque characterization, and evaluation of the hemodynamic effects of the stenosis and forces on the plaque. The ability to assess plaque morphology and hence identify high risk individuals offers the advantage of monitoring plaque stabilization by drug therapies and the development of new therapeutic and prophylactic strategies, contributing toward the reduction of cardiovascular events. During the last two decades, the rapid advancements in imaging technologies, linked with the advancements in information technology, have significantly improved the objective assessment of carotid plaque morphology. This volume is intended to provide a comprehensive overview of the most recent advances in ultrasound image processing and applications on images of carotid plaques, and how these may affect clinical management.

The book consists of 37 chapters, grouped into 5 parts. Part I discusses the pathophysiology of carotid bifurcation atherosclerosis, related symptomatology, and the controversy over the management of patients with asymptomatic stenosis. Part II covers ultrasound image instrumentation and imaging techniques, including despeckling and ultrasound contrast agents. Part III deals with measurements and image analysis. It includes intima-media thickness (IMT), plaque thickness, area and volume measurements, automated classification of plaques, texture feature extraction, elastography, and plaque motion analysis. Part IV discusses the validated and emerging ultrasonic and other biomarkers associated with early atherosclerosis and their value in epidemiological studies and population screening with emphasis on advice for individual persons in terms of prevention. Part V covers late atherosclerosis, grading of internal carotid stenosis, the significance of hypoechoic plaques, and markers associated with the latter. It includes intravascular ultrasound (IVUS), transcranial Doppler (TCD), and carotid plaque characterization with emphasis on clinical applications such as the effect of statin therapy and stroke risk stratification. It indicates how methods described in previous sections can be applied for the benefit of the patient.

The book is intended for all those working in the field of atherosclerosis, ultrasound imaging, and cardiovascular risk, including the clinician, the vascular ultrasonographer, the epidemiologist, the molecular biologist, the biomedical engineer, and the informatics scientist. Furthermore, the book aims to bridge the gap between researchers and clinicians who are keen to incorporate the latest results of research to their daily practice.

It is hoped that this volume will provide a forum for the dissemination of the most recent medical and technological advances in the area of ultrasound and carotid bifurcation atherosclerosis, thus facilitating the development of emerging imaging and informatics technological systems, and medical strategies for the investigation of both asymptomatic individuals and patients.

Contents

Part I Pathophysiology of Atherosclerotic Plaques

1 **Stable and Vulnerable Atherosclerotic Plaques** 3
Alkystis Phinikaridou, Ye Qiao, and James A. Hamilton

2 **Pathophysiology of Carotid Atherosclerosis** 27
Heather A. Hall and Hisham S. Bassiouny

3 **Vascular Hemodynamics of the Carotid Bifurcation
and Its Relation to Arterial Disease** 41
Andreas Anayiotos and Yannis Papaharilaou

4 **The Problem with Asymptomatic Carotid Stenosis** 53
A. Ross Naylor

Part II Imaging Techniques

5 **Principles of Ultrasonic Imaging and Instrumentation** 67
Kirk W. Beach

6 **Despeckling** 97
Christos P. Loizou and Constantinos S. Pattichis

7 **Vascular Ultrasound Imaging with Contrast Agents:
Carotid Plaque Neovascularization and the Hyperplastic
Vasa Vasorum Network** 121
Michalakis A. Averkiou, Christophoros Mannaris,
and Andrew Nicolaides

8 **Nonlinear Contrast Intravascular Ultrasound** 137
David E. Goertz, Martijn E. Frijlink, Nico de Jong,
and Antonius F.W. van der Steen

9 Molecular Imaging of Carotid Plaque with Targeted Ultrasound Contrast 153
Joshua J. Rychak and Alexander L. Klibanov

Part III Measurement and Image Analysis

10 Methodological Considerations of Ultrasound Measurement of Carotid Artery Intima-Media Thickness and Lumen Diameter 165
John C.M. Wikstrand

11 Automated Measurement of Carotid Artery Intima-Media Thickness 177
Filippo Molinari and Jasjit S. Suri

12 Image Normalization, Plaque Typing, and Texture Feature Extraction 193
Maura Griffin, Efthyvoulos Kyriacou, Stavros K. Kakkos, Kirk W. Beach, and Andrew Nicolaides

13 Automated Classification of Plaques 213
Göran ML. Bergström, Ulrica Prahl, and Peter Holdfeldt

14 Plaque Feature Extraction 223
Christodoulos I. Christodoulou, Efthyvoulos Kyriacou, Marios S. Pattichis, and Constantinos S. Pattichis

15 Plaque Classification 247
Efthyvoulos Kyriacou, Christodoulos I. Christodoulou, Marios S. Pattichis, Constantinos S. Pattichis, and Stavros K. Kakkos

16 Volumetric Evaluation of Carotid Atherosclerosis Using 3-Dimensional Ultrasonic Imaging 263
Grace Parraga, Andrew A. House, Adam Krasinski, J. David Spence, and Aaron Fenster

17 Carotid Plaque Surface Irregularity 279
Bernard Chiu, Vadim Beletsky, J. David Spence, Grace Parraga, and Aaron Fenster

18 Carotid Plaque Texture Analysis Using 3-Dimensional Volume Ultrasonic Imaging 299
Andrew Nicolaides, Maura Griffin, Gregory C. Makris, George Geroulakos, Dawn Bond, Efthyvoulos Kyriacou, Antonios A. Polydorou, and Victoria Polydorou

19 Wall Motion Analysis 325
Peter R. Hoskins and Andrew W. Bradbury

20	**Noninvasive Carotid Elastography**	341
	Hendrik H.G. Hansen and Chris L. de Korte	
21	**Motion Estimation of Carotid Artery Plaques**	355
	Sergio E. Murillo Amaya and Marios S. Pattichis	

Part IV Early Atherosclerosis

22	**Carotid Intima-Media Thickness Measurement: A Suitable Alternative for Cardiovascular Risk?**	379
	Michiel L. Bots, Sanne A.E. Peters, and Diederick E. Grobbee	
23	**Intima-Media Thickness and Carotid Plaques in Cardiovascular Risk Assessment**	397
	Thomas-Duythuc To and Tasneem Z. Naqvi	
24	**Plaque Size, Growth, Echogenicity and Cardiovascular Risk: The Tromsø Study**	419
	Ellisiv B. Mathiesen and Stein H. Johnsen	
25	**Toward Clinical Applications of Carotid Ultrasound: Intima-Media Thickness, Plaque Area, and Three-Dimensional Phenotypes**	431
	J. David Spence and Tatjana Rundek	
26	**Arterial Wall, Plaque Measurements, Biomarkers, and Metabolic Syndrome: Results from the Gothenburg Studies**	449
	Björn O. Fagerberg	
27	**Novel Biomarkers and Subclinical Atherosclerosis**	461
	Andrie G. Panayiotou, Debra Ann Hoppensteadt, Andrew Nicolaides, and Jawed Fareed	
28	**Subclinical Atherosclerosis, Markers of Inflammation, and Oxidative Stress**	487
	Stefan Kiechl, Philipp Werner, Michael Knoflach, and Johann Willeit	
29	**Screening for Cardiovascular Risk Using Ultrasound: A Practical Approach**	511
	Andrew Nicolaides, Maura Griffin, Andrie G. Panayiotou, and Dawn Bond	

Part V Late Atherosclerosis

30	**Grading Internal Carotid Artery Stenosis**	521
	Kimon Bekelis, Nicos Labropoulos, Maura Griffin, and Andrew Nicolaides	

31	The Significance of Echolucent Plaques: Past and Future Perspectives	543
	Martin Græbe and Henrik Sillesen	
32	Intravascular Ultrasound: Plaque Characterization	551
	Donald B. Reid, Carol Watson, Barun Majumder, and Khalid Irshad	
33	Grayscale-Based Stratified Color Mapping of Carotid Plaque	563
	Roman Felix Sztajzel	
34	Transcranial Doppler and Cerebrovascular Risk Stratification in Patients with Internal Carotid Artery Atherosclerosis	571
	Anne L. Abbott	
35	Effect of Statin Therapy on Carotid Plaque Morphology	595
	Gregory C. Makris, Andrew Nicolaides, Anthi Lavida, and George Geroulakos	
36	Image Analysis of Carotid Plaques and Risk Stratification	601
	Andrew Nicolaides, Efthyvoulos Kyriacou, Maura Griffin, Stavros K. Kakkos, and George Geroulakos	
37	Ultrasonic Plaque Characterization: Results from the Asymptomatic Carotid Stenosis and Risk of Stroke (ACSRS) Study	613
	Andrew Nicolaides, Stavros K. Kakkos, Efthyvoulos Kyriacou, Maura Griffin, George Geroulakos, and Constantinos S. Pattichis	
Index		633

Contributors

Anne L. Abbott Department of Preventative Health, Baker IDI Heart and Diabetes Institute, Melbourne, VIC, Australia

Andreas Anayiotos Department of Mechanical and Materials Engineering, Cyprus University of Technology, Limassol, Cyprus

Michalakis A. Averkiou Department of Mechanical and Manufacturing Engineering, University of Cyprus, Nicosia, Cyprus

Hisham S. Bassiouny Department of Surgery, University of Chicago, Chicago, IL, USA

Kirk W. Beach Department of Surgery and Bioengineering, University of Washington, Seattle, WA, USA

Kimon Bekelis Department of Neurosurgery, Dartmouth-Hitchcock Medical Center, Hanover, NH, USA

Vadim Beletsky Department of Clinical Neurosciences, LHSC, University of Western Ontario, London, ON, Canada

Göran ML. Bergström Wallenberg Laboratory for Cardiovascular Research, and Center for Cardiovascular and Metabolic Research, Sahlgrenska Academy, Institute of Medicine, University of Gothenburg, Gothenburg, Sweden

Dawn Bond Vascular Screening and Diagnostic Centre, London, UK

Michiel L. Bots Julius Center for Health Sciences and Primary Care, University Medical Center Utrecht, Utrecht, The Netherlands

Andrew W. Bradbury Department of Vascular Surgery, University of Birmingham, Birmingham, UK

Bernard Chiu Imaging Research Laboratories, Robarts Research Institute, London, ON, Canada

Christodoulos I. Christodoulou Department of Computer Science, University of Cyprus, Nicosia, Cyprus

Björn O. Fagerberg Wallenberg Laboratory for Cardiovascular Research, Department of Molecular and Clinical Medicine, Institute of Medicine, Sahlgrenska University Hospital, Gothenburg, Sweden

Jawed Fareed Department of Pathology and Pharmacology, Loyola University Medical Center, Maywood, IL, USA

Aaron Fenster Imaging Research Laboratories, Robarts Research Institute, The University of Western Ontario, London, ON, Canada

Martijn E. Frijlink Department of Probe Research & Development, Esaote Europe BV, Maastricht, The Netherlands

George Geroulakos Department of Surgery, Charing Cross Hospital, London, UK

David E. Goertz Department of Imaging Research, Sunnybrook Health Sciences Centre, Toronto, ON, Canada

Martin Græbe Department of Vascular Surgery, Rigshospitalet, University of Copenhagen, Copenhagen, Denmark

Maura Griffin Vascular Screening and Diagnostic Centre, London, UK

Diederick E. Grobbee Julius Center for Health Sciences and Primary Care, University Medical Center Utrecht, Utrecht, The Netherlands

Heather A. Hall Section of Vascular Surgery, University of Chicago, Chicago, IL, USA

James A. Hamilton Department of Physiology and Biophysics, Boston University School of Medicine, Boston, MA, USA

Hendrik H.G. Hansen Clinical Physics Laboratory, Department of Pediatrics, Radboud University Nijmegen Medical Centre, Njimegen, The Netherlands

Peter Holdfeldt Wallenberg Laboratory for Cardiovascular Research, and Center for Cardiovascular and Metabolic Research, Sahlgrenska Academy, Institute of Medicine, University of Gothenburg, Gothenburg, Sweden

Debra Ann Hoppensteadt Department of Pathology, Loyola University Chicago, Maywood, IL, USA

Peter R. Hoskins Department of Medical Physics, University of Edinburgh, Edinburgh, UK

Andrew A. House Division of Nephrology, London Health Sciences Centre, London, ON, Canada

Khalid Irshad Department of Vascular Surgery, Wishaw General Surgery, Wishaw, Lanarkshire, UK

Stein H. Johnsen Department of Neurology, University Hospital of North Norway, Tromsø, Norway

Nico de Jong Department of Biomedical Engineering, Erasmus MC and University of Twente, Rotterdam, The Netherlands

Stavros K. Kakkos Department of Vascular Surgery, University of Patras Medical School, Patras, Achaia, Greece

Stefan Kiechl Department of Neurology, Medical University Innsbruck, Innsbruck, Tyrol, Austria

Alexander L. Klibanov Department of Medicine, Cardiovascular Division, University of Virginia, Charlottesville, VA, USA

Michael Knoflach Department of Neurology, Medical University Innsbruck, Innsbruck, Tyrol, Austria

Chris L. de Korte Clinical Physics Laboratory, Department of Pediatrics, Radboud University Nijmegen Medical Centre, Njimegen, The Netherlands

Adam Krasinski Stroke Prevention & Atherosclerosis Research Centre, Robarts Research Institute, University of Western Ontario, London, ON, Canada

Efthyvoulos Kyriacou Department of Computer Science and Engineering, Frederick University Cyprus, Lemesos, Cyprus

Nicos Labropoulos Department of Surgery, Stony Brook University Medical Center, Stony Brook, NY, USA

Anthi Lavida Department of Vascular Surgery, Ealing Hospital/Imperial College London, Southall, Middlesex, UK

Christos P. Loizou Department of Computer Science, School of Sciences, Intercollege, Limassol, Cyprus

Barun Majumder Department of Vascular Surgery, Wishaw General Surgery, Wishaw, Lanarkshire, UK

Gregory C. Makris Division of Vascular Surgery, Imperial College of London, London, UK

Christophoros Mannaris Department of Mechanical and Manufacturing Engineering, University of Cyprus, Nicosia, Cyprus

Ellisiv B. Mathiesen Department of Clinical Medicine, University of Tromsø, Tromsø, Norway

Filippo Molinari BioLab, Department of Electronics, Politecnico di Torino, Torino, Italy

Sergio E. Murillo Amaya Department of Electrical and Computer Engineering, University of New Mexico, Albuquerque, NM, USA

Tasneem Z. Naqvi Department of Cardiology, University of Southern California, Los Angeles, CA, USA

A. Ross Naylor Vascular Surgery Group, Division of Cardiovascular Sciences, Leicester Royal Infirmary, Leicester, Leicestershire, UK

Andrew Nicolaides Imperial College and Vascular Screening and Diagnostic Centre, London, UK

Andrie G. Panayiotou Cyprus International institute of Environmental and Public Health, Cyprus University of Technology, Limassol

Yannis Papaharilaou Institute of Applied and Computational Mathematics, Foundation for Research and Technology Hellas, Heraklion, Crete, Greece

Grace Parraga Imaging Research Laboratories, Robarts Research Institute, The University of Western Ontario, London, ON, Canada

Constantinos S. Pattichis Department of Computer Science, University of Cyprus, Nicosia, Cyprus

Marios S. Pattichis Department of Electrical and Computer Engineering, The University of New Mexico, Albuquerque, NM, USA

Sanne A.E. Peters Julius Center for Health Sciences and Primary Care, University Medical Center Utrecht, Utrecht, The Netherlands

Alkystis Phinikaridou Department of Physiology and Biophysics, Boston University School of Medicine, Boston, MA, USA

Antonios A. Polydorou Interventional Cardiac and Peripheral Department, General Hospital of Athens "Evangelismos", Athens, Greece

Victoria Polydorou Department of Internal Medicine, General Airforce Hospital, Athens, Greece

Ulrica Prahl Wallenberg Laboratory for Cardiovascular Research, and Center for Cardiovascular and Metabolic Research, Sahlgrenska Academy, Institute of Medicine, University of Gothenburg, Gothenburg, Sweden

Ye Qiao Department of Radiology, Johns Hopkins University School of Medicine, Baltimore, MD, USA

Donald B. Reid Department of Vascular Surgery, Wishaw General Surgery, Wishaw, Lanarkshire, UK

Tatjana Rundek Department of Neurology, Miller School of Medicine, University of Miami, Miami, FL, USA

Joshua J. Rychak Department of Research, Targeson Inc., San Diego, CA, USA

Henrik Sillesen Department of Vascular Surgery, Rigshospitalet, University of Copenhagen, Copenhagen, Denmark

J. David Spence Stroke Prevention & Atherosclerosis Research Centre, Robarts Research Institute, University of Western Ontario, London, ON, Canada

Antonius F.W. van der Steen Department of Biomedical Engineering, Erasmus MC, Rotterdam, The Netherlands

Jasjit S. Suri Global Biomedical Technologies Inc. (Affiliated with Idaho State University), Roseville, CA, USA

Roman Felix Sztajzel Department of Neurology, University Hospital Geneva/ Switzerland, Geneva, Switzerland

Thomas-Duythuc To Department of Internal Medicine, University of Southern California, Los Angeles, CA, USA

Carol Watson Department of Vascular Surgery, Wishaw General Surgery, Wishaw, Lanarkshire, UK

Philipp Werner Neurovascular Disease and Stroke Center, State Hospital, Feldkirch, Vorarlberg, Austria

John C.M. Wikstrand Wallenberg Laboratory for Cardiovascular Research, Sahlgrenska Academy, Gothenburg University, Gothenburg, Sweden

Johann Willeit Department of Neurology, Medical University Innsbruck, Innsbruck, Tyrol, Austria

Part I

Pathophysiology of Atherosclerotic Plaques

Stable and Vulnerable Atherosclerotic Plaques

Alkystis Phinikaridou, Ye Qiao, and James A. Hamilton

1.1 Introduction

Atherosclerosis is a chronic, systemic, inflammatory disease of the medium and large arteries such as the coronary, carotid and peripheral arteries, and the aorta. It is currently considered a major contributor to the development of cardiovascular disease, the leading cause of death in the United States[1] and worldwide.[2] Atherosclerotic plaques are characterized by intimal thickening from the progressive accumulation of lipids (mainly cholesteryl ester and cholesterol)[3,4] together with numerous cellular and molecular components such as smooth muscle cells (SMC), lipid-filled macrophages, monocytes, T and B lymphocytes, erythrocytes, and platelets.[5–7] Vasoconstricting, which covers the luminal side of the vessel wall, has anti-atherogenic properties and plays an essential role in maintaining vascular homeostasis through the balanced secretion of vasodilating and vasocontricting molecules such as nitric oxide and endothelin-1.[8]

More than 180 years ago, Virchow[9] was the first to suggest that injury of the arterial wall induces an inflammatory response which may be considered the initiating event in the development of atherosclerosis. Later on, this idea was supported by the "response-to-injury" hypothesis proposed in 1976 by Ross et al.,[10,11] who suggested that endothelial denudation/injury caused either by mechanical removal or by cardiovascular risk factors such as hypercholesterolemia, high shear stress, and hypertension dramatically increases the formation of lesions. Furthermore, in 1986, Ludmer et al.[12] showed that endothelial dysfunction occurs early as well as late in the course of coronary atherosclerosis and may play an important role in the pathogenesis of coronary vasospasm. Currently, the term "endothelial dysfunction," which was introduced in 1989 by Gimbrone,[13] is probably the best descriptor of the initiating event in the development of atherosclerosis.

1.2 Progression of Atherosclerosis and Classification of Human Plaques

1.2.1 Histological Structure of a Normal Artery in Humans

The arterial wall consists of three morphologically distinct layers: the intima, media, and adventitia (Fig. 1.1). The normal intima is a very thin region (size exaggerated in the figure) consisting of endothelial cells with a basal lamina covering its luminal side, a subendothelial zone of SMC and extracellular matrix (mainly collagen and proteoglycans), and a layer of elastic fibers (internal elastic lamina). SMC are responsible for the production of collagen and elastic material.[15] The endothelial cells are connected with tight junctions and together with the basal lamina form a barrier to various blood substances. The media consists of layers of elastic lamellae surrounded by

A. Phinikaridou (✉) • J.A. Hamilton
Department of Physiology and Biophysics, Boston University School of Medicine, Boston, MA, USA

Y. Qiao
Department of Radiology, Johns Hopkins University School of Medicine, Baltimore, MD, USA

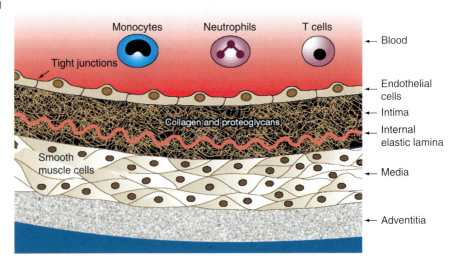

Fig. 1.1 Structure of a normal large artery (Reprinted by permission from Lusis,[14] copyright 2000)

SMC, collagen and elastic fibers, and ground substance. The adventitia consists of connective tissue with interspersed fibroblasts and SMC.

1.2.2 Formation of Atherosclerotic Plaques

Histologic studies of human vessels, mainly coronary and aortic arteries obtained at autopsy, provided a database that was used by the American Heart Association (AHA) Committee on Vascular Lesions to divide plaques into six stages (type I to type VI), on the basis of plaque composition and morphology.[16-18] Later on, Virmani et al.[19] proposed a modified classification system because of additional data regarding the types of plaques that could lead to coronary thrombotic events (Table 1.1). The stages involved in the natural progression of atherosclerosis are presented below and are classified using the AHA nomenclature.

1.2.3 Early Lesions (Types I and II)

Type I and II plaques appear during the first decades of life but do not cause substantial luminal stenosis. Type I plaques, in which histological changes are minimal, consist of isolated groups of lipid-filled macrophages (foam cells) that are visible only with microscopic examination (Fig. 1.2a). In contrast, type II plaques or fatty streaks are visible on gross examination and contain increased numbers of foamy macrophages which become stratified into layers together with some foamy smooth muscle cells (Fig. 1.2b).

The strong similarity between the chemical composition of the low-density lipoprotein (LDL) particles and plaque lipids suggested that the main source of plaque lipids is circulating LDL particles that become entrapped within the subendothelial layer.[22,23] Although endothelial cells act as a selective barrier between the blood and the underlying vessel wall, LDL particles can appear within the vessel wall either by passive diffusion through the endothelium or by receptor-mediated endocytosis. Subsequently, retention of LDL particles within the vessel wall is achieved through ionic interactions between the apolipoprotein-B of the LDL particle and matrix proteoglycans, collagen fibers, and fibronectin found in the vessel wall.[24] Trapped LDL particles undergo extensive modifications such as oxidation, proteolysis, aggregation, and lipolysis. Minimally oxidized LDL particles (mmLDL) are recognized by the LDL receptor,[25] and their accumulation stimulates endothelial cells to express selectins[26] and adhesion molecules,[27] which promote recruitment of monocytes and lymphocytes to the vessel wall. In contrast, severely oxidized LDL particles (oxLDL) are recognized only by scavenger receptors such as SR-A and CD-36 expressed on macrophages and vascular SMC.[28,29] Uptake of oxLDL leads to the formation of foam cells (Fig. 1.3). Physicochemical studies have shown that the cholesteryl esters in fatty streaks exist in a liquid-crystalline

Table 1.1 Classification of atherosclerotic plaque

	Traditional classification	Stary et al.[16,17]	Virmani et al.[19]	Progression
Early plaques		Type I: microscopic detection of lipid droplets in intima and small groups of macrophage foam cells	Intimal thickening	None
	Fatty streak	Type II: fatty streaks visible on gross inspection, layers of foam cells, occasional lymphocytes and mast cells	Intima xanthoma	None
		Type III (intermediate): extracellular lipid pools present among layers of smooth muscle cells	Pathologic thickening	Thrombus (erosion)
Intermediate plaque	Atheroma	Type IV: well-defined lipid core, may develop surface disruption (fissure)	Fibrous cap atheroma	Thrombus (erosion)[c]
Late lesions			Thin fibrous cap atheroma	Thrombus (rupture); hemorrhage/fibrin[d]
		Type Va: new fibrous tissue overlying lipid core (multilayered fibroatheroma)[a]	Healed plaque rupture; erosion	Repeated rupture or erosion with or without total occlusion
		Type Vb: calcification[b]	Fibrocalcific plaque (with or without necrotic core)	
	Fibrous plaque	Type Vc: fibrotic lesion with minimal lipid (could be result of organized thrombi)		
Miscellaneous/ complicated features	Complicated/ advanced plaques	Type VIa: surface disruption		
		Type VIb: intraplaque hemorrhage		
		Type VIc: thrombosis		
			Calcified nodule	Thrombus (usually non-occlusive)

Source: Reprinted from the Burke et al.,[20] copyright 2003, with permission from Elsevier
[a]May overlap with healed plaque ruptures
[b]Occasionally referred to as type VII lesion
[c]May progress further with healing (healed erosion)
[d]May progress further with healing (healed rupture)

or an isotropic liquid phase at body temperature,[31,32] similar to the phases found in LDL particles.

1.2.4 Preatheroma/Intermediate Lesions (Type III)

Type III plaques have a histological appearance that is intermediate between the early fatty streaks and the first advanced lesion type (atheroma), although it is not known whether all plaques progress linearly from one stage to the other. Organized histological layers are seen for the first time in type III plaques; foamy cells are present at the luminal side, a tissue degeneration region in the middle layer, and scattered extracellular lipids at the base of the plaque[33] (Fig. 1.2c). Type III plaques contain more free cholesterol, fatty acids, triglycerides, sphingomyelin, and lysolecithin than fatty streaks.[4] Although the clinical significance of type III lesions has not been clarified, Virmani et al.[19] have proposed that plaques with pathologic intimal thickening, the equivalent of type III plaques, may develop into eroded plaques. In this way, an intermediate type of plaque can directly transform into an advanced, complicated lesion.

1.2.5 Advanced Atherosclerotic Plaques (Atheroma-IV, Fibroatheroma-Va, Calcific-Vb and Fibrotic-Vc)

The transition from plaques at early stages to the more advanced type IV or atheroma (Fig. 1.2d) involves

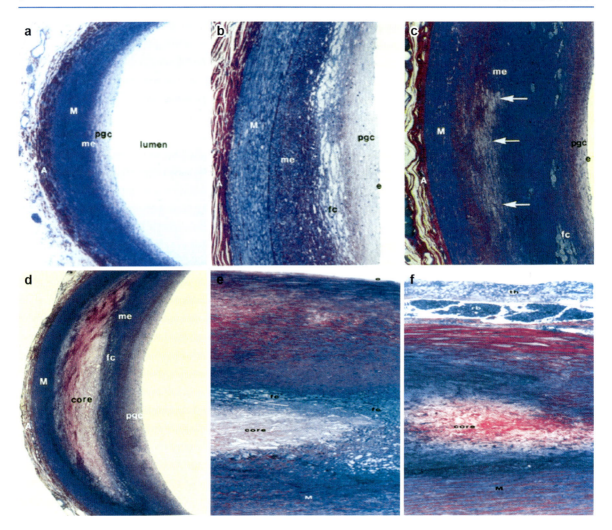

Fig. 1.2 Histological examples of atherosclerotic plaque types classified according to the American Heart Association criteria. (**a**) A crescent-shaped (eccentric) adaptive intimal thickening in the left anterior descending coronary artery at the level of the main bifurcation, *pgc* proteoglycan intima layer, *me* musculoelastic intima layer, *M* media, *A* adventitia, *lumen* lumen of the artery. From a 6-month-old boy. Homicide was the cause of death. Case no. 949 (P-1949). The artery was fixed by perfusion with glutaraldehyde under pressure, tissue was embedded in Maraglas, and the one-micron section was stained with toluidine blue and basic fuchsin. Magnification about ×90. (**b**) A type IIa (progression-prone fatty streak) lesion colocalized with an adaptive thickening in the proximal part of the left anterior descending coronary artery. Macrophage foam cells (*fc*) occupy the intima at the junction of the proteoglycan (*pgc*) and musculoelastic (*me*) intima layers, *e* endothelial cells at the artery lumen, *M* media, *A* adventitia. From a 25-year-old woman. A traffic accident was the cause of death. Case no. 775 (P-1775). Fixation by pressure-perfusion with glutaraldehyde. Maraglas embedding. One-micron section stained with toluidine blue and basic fuchsin. About ×140. (**c**) A type III (preatheroma) lesion colocalized with an adaptive thickening in the left main coronary artery just proximal to the main bifurcation. Extracellular lipid (*arrows*) is pooled in the musculoelastic layer (*me*). Smooth muscle cells, normally closely packed, are separated, compressed, and attenuated by the extracellular lipid. Macrophage foam cells (*fc*) are some distance above the pooled extracellular lipid, *e* endothelial cells at the artery lumen, *pgc* proteoglycan intima, *M* media, *A* adventitia. From a 25-year-old man who died in a traffic accident. Case no. 372 (P-1372). The artery was fixed by perfusion with glutaraldehyde under pressure, tissue was embedded in Maraglas, and the one-micron thick section was stained with toluidine blue and basic fuchsin. About ×95. (**d**) A type IV (atheroma) lesion in the most proximal part of the left anterior descending coronary artery. In addition to all the changes seen in type IIa and III lesions, a massive aggregate of extracellular lipid (lipid core) occupies the musculoelastic layer (*me*). Macrophage foam cells (*fc*) are above the lipid core. *pgc* proteoglycan intima layer, *M* media, *A* adventitia. From a 23-year-old man. Homicide was the cause of death. Case no. 917 (P-1917). Fixation by pressure-perfusion with glutaraldehyde. Maraglas embedding. One-micron thick section was stained with toluidine blue and basic fuchsin. Magnification about ×40. (**e**) A type V (fibroatheroma) lesion in the distal part of the abdominal aorta. The part of the lesion above the lipid core and above the layer of

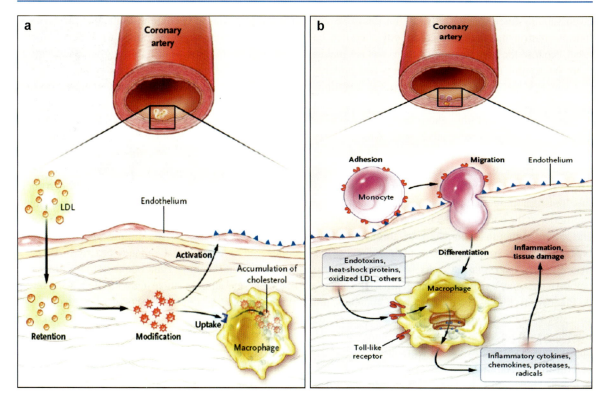

Fig. 1.3 (**a**) Activating effect of LDL infiltration on inflammation in the artery. In patients with hypercholesterolemia, excess LDL infiltrates the artery and is retained in the intima, particularly at sites of hemodynamic strain. Oxidative and enzymatic modifications lead to the release of inflammatory lipids that induce endothelial cells to express leukocyte adhesion molecules. The modified LDL particles are taken up by scavenger receptors of macrophages, which evolve into foam cells. (**b**) Role of macrophage inflammation of the artery. Monocytes recruited through the activated endothelium differentiate into macrophages. Several endogenous and microbial molecules can ligate pattern-recognition receptors (toll-like receptors) on these cells, inducing activation and leading to the release of inflammatory cytokines, chemokines, oxygen and nitrogen radicals, and other inflammatory molecules and, ultimately, to inflammation and tissue damage (Reprinted with permission from Hansson.[30] Copyright © 2005 Massachusetts Medical Society. All rights reserved)

accumulation of abundant extracellular lipids that form a consolidated lipid core located deeply within the intima, and which disorganizes the extracellular matrix. Small capillaries, mainly grown from the adventitia, usually surround the lipid core. The region of the thickened intima between the lipid core and the endothelial surface contains SMC, macrophages with and without lipid droplets, T lymphocytes,[34] and mast cells. SMC in this region proliferate, and also secrete proteoglycans and a few collagen fibers that may gradually thicken the region above the lipid core. Cell death and formation of a necrotic core occurs at the base of the atheroma; the necrotic core is enriched in cellular debris and crystalline cholesterol.

Fig. 1.2 (Continued) macrophage foam cells (*fc*) consists of dense bands of collagen and RER-rich smooth muscle cells, *e* endothelial cells at the artery lumen, *M* media, from a 40-year-old man who died suddenly and unexpectedly from myocardial infarction because of Type VI lesions in the coronary arteries. Case no. 1349 (P-2349). The aorta had been opened and fixed flat by immersion in formalin, tissue was embedded in Maraglas, and the one-micron thick section was stained with toluidine blue and basic fuchsin. Magnification about ×140. (**f**) A type VI (complicated) lesion in the distal part of the abdominal aorta. A recent thrombotic deposit (*th*) is at the luminal surface of the lesion and a small hemorrhage (red blood cells = *rb*) is in the uppermost part of the lesion, *core* lipid core of the lesion, *M* media. From a 37-year-old woman who died of intracerebral hemorrhage. Case no. 1280 (P-2280). The aorta had been opened and fixed flat by immersion in formalin, tissue was embedded in Maraglas, and the one-micron thick section was stained with toluidine blue and basic fuchsin. Magnification about ×140 (Reprinted with permission from Stary[21])

Even though atheromas usually do not cause severe luminal narrowing, their clinical significance can be great because the composition of their surface makes them susceptible to formation of fissures and ruptures that can suddenly transform an atheroma to a complicated plaque.[17]

Type Va plaques or fibroatheromas (Fig. 1.2e) have a thick layer of fibrous connective tissue, which mainly contains collagen fibers and rough endoplasmic reticulum–rich SMC, at the luminal side of the intima. This structure is called the fibrous cap and separates the lipid core from circulating blood constituents. The capillaries at the borders of the lipid core may be larger and more numerous compared to those found in type IV plaques and may also contain lymphocytes, macrophages, and plasma cells. Moreover, microhemorrhages may exist around the capillaries.

Plaques in which mineralization is abundant are subcategorized as type Vb or calcified plaques. Bone morphogenic proteins are expressed in human plaques and stimulate SMC to express osteopontin.[35] Although calcification is common and increases with age, its role in plaque vulnerability remains unclear.[36] In type Vc or fibrotic lesions, intima thickening is primarily caused by the accumulation of collagen fibers whereas lipid accumulation is minimal. Fibrotic lesions could represent extensions of the fibrous component of an adjacent fibroatheroma, through the process of plaque regression. Highly stenotic type Vb and Vc coronary artery plaques may cause angina unless enough collateral circulation is present, which prevents tissue ischemia and helps to maintain such lesions clinically silent. However, surface defects like erosions, fissures, and ruptures can lead to sudden transformation of type V plaques into type VI or complicated plaques with formation of hematomas and thrombi (Fig. 1.2f).

1.3 Definitions of Stable and Vulnerable Plaques

Atherosclerotic plaques that remain clinically silent are termed "stable." However, it is now well documented that most acute coronary syndromes such as unstable angina pectoris and myocardial infarction are caused by transformation of stable plaques into vulnerable plaques.[37-40] In 1990, Little[6] originally used the term "vulnerable" plaque to describe atherosclerotic coronary artery lesions that had the potential to become thrombogenic if exposed to the appropriate triggering stimulus in patients with myocardial infarction or unstable angina. Such lesions need not be obstructive to become thrombogenic, nor do all obstructive lesions have thrombogenic potential. In 1994, Muller et al.[41] proposed a functional definition of plaque vulnerability suggesting that the term "vulnerable plaque should be used to prospectively denote plaques which, by becoming disrupted, have a high likelihood of starting an adverse cascade." Although this definition does not take under consideration the histological characteristics of a vulnerable plaque, it suggests that vulnerable plaques are those with a higher risk of causing thrombosis, which could either lead to asymptomatic plaque progression or to a clinical event. In the "Handbook of the Vulnerable Plaque"[42] the authors suggested that the related terms "high-risk plaque" and "thrombosis-prone plaque" can be used as synonyms of "vulnerable plaque." In contrast, because the term "unstable" is frequently used to describe clinical conditions such as unstable angina pectoris, the term "unstable" plaque should be avoided to eliminate confusions. In addition to the functional definition of plaque vulnerability, Falk and Libby defined the morphology of the "vulnerable" plaque from histologic characteristics as an eccentric lesion composed of a lipid-rich core and an overlying cap rich in macrophages.[43,44] Moreover, Kolodgie et al. defined plaque vulnerability based on the actual thickness of the fibrous cap as measured from histologic sections of coronary ruptured plaques.[45] The "vulnerable" plaque was defined as a lesion with a fibrous cap <65 μm thick, which was infiltrated by macrophages (>25 cells per 0.3 mm diameter field). A thickness of 65 μm was chosen as the threshold because in ruptured plaques, the mean cap thickness was 23 ± 19 μm and 95% of ruptured fibrous caps measured less than 64 μm $\pm$ 2 standard deviations. Kolodgie et al.[45] demonstrated that thin-cap atheromas were most frequently found in patients dying with acute myocardial infarction (the mean number of thin-cap atheromas was ≥ 1.5 per heart), followed by patients dying with stable plaque (mean 1.1 ± 1.3 per heart). However, thin-cap atheromas were less common in patients without acute rupture (0.9 ± 1.2), healed rupture (0.5 ± 0.8) or plaque erosion (0.2 ± 0.5). Interestingly, thin-cap atheromas are more frequent in men compared to women dying of acute myocardial infarction and sudden death.

1.4 Mechanisms of Thrombosis and the Histological Characteristics of the Plaques That Can Lead to Acute Coronary Syndromes

The initial mechanism leading to thrombosis was reported for the first time in 1844, when Fraergeman stated that "the vessel wall contained several atheromatous plaques, one of which quite clearly had ulcerated, pouring the atheromatous mass into the arterial lumen".[46] In 1934, Leary[47] provided additional data supporting the idea that coronary spasm is a possible factor in producing sudden death, but it was the work of Constantinides in 1966 that provided compelling evidence that plaque rupture was the underlying cause of most acute cardiovascular events.[48] In this very meticulous and systematic work, Constantinides et al. studied 22 coronary artery specimens from patients with coronary artery disease, 17 of which had coronary thrombosis. Histology revealed that all of the 17 thrombi were attached to "cracks/fissures" observed at the luminal site of the intima. These observations from autopsy studies of human specimens were further supported by Constantinides' studies using an experimental animal (rabbit) model of atherosclerosis.[49–51]

Finally, the link between plaque rupture and the onset of acute coronary disease was consolidated by the study of Willerson et al. in 1984 showing that altered plaque surfaces act as substrates for platelet adhesion and aggregation.[52] Furthermore, local platelet activation promotes thrombus formation and additional platelet recruitment through the production of cell surface thrombin and the release of several platelet agonists that further sustain the thrombotic process. An example of a vulnerable and a stable carotid atherosclerotic plaque is illustrated in Fig. 1.4.

Rapidly accumulating data from postmortem histologic studies, though limited by their retrospective nature, have provided additional insights into the pathology of the lesions associated with acute coronary events.[39,44,53–60] Currently, three distinct mechanisms, each of which occurs in lesions with distinct histological features (Fig. 1.5), are considered responsible for thrombus formation. It is now well documented that most (65–70%) acute myocardial

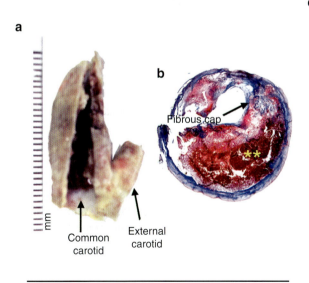

Vulnerable plaque with intraplaque hemorrhage (asterisks)

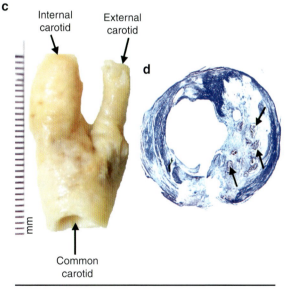

Stable plaque with calcifications (arrows)

Fig. 1.4 Human carotid endarterectomy specimens with corresponding histology (Masson's trichrome staining). (**a, b**) A vulnerable plaque, excised from a symptomatic subject, is characterized by a large intraplaque hemorrhage and a thin fibrous cap. (**c, d**) A stable plaque, excised from a non-symptomatic subject, is rich in collagen with small calcifications (Photo courtesy of Dr. Ye Qiao)

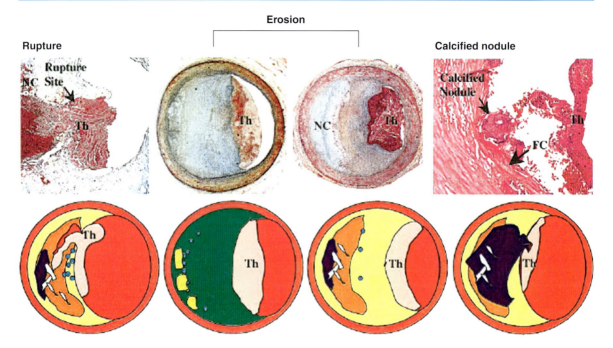

Fig. 1.5 Atherosclerotic lesions with luminal thrombi. Ruptured plaques are thin fibrous cap atheromas with luminal thrombi (*Th*). These lesions usually have an extensive necrotic core (*NC*) containing large numbers of cholesterol crystals and a thin fibrous cap (<65 mm) infiltrated by foamy macrophages and a paucity of T lymphocytes. The fibrous cap is thinnest at the site of rupture and consists of a few collagen bundles and rare smooth muscle cells. The luminal thrombus is in communication with the lipid-rich necrotic core. Erosions occur over lesions rich in smooth muscle cells and proteoglycans. Luminal thrombi overly areas lacking surface endothelium. The deep intima of the eroded plaque often shows extracellular lipid pools, but necrotic cores are uncommon; when present, the necrotic core does not communicate with the luminal thrombus. Inflammatory infiltrate is usually absent, but if present, is sparse and consists of macrophages and lymphocytes. A high-power view of the eroded surface indicated by a box is shown in Fig. 1.6 for comparison with a similar eroded area of a thrombosed region adjacent to a ruptured plaque. Calcified nodules are plaques with luminal thrombi showing calcific nodules protruding into the lumen through a disrupted thin fibrous cap (*FC*). There is absence of an endothelium at the site of the thrombus, and inflammatory cells (macrophages, T lymphocytes) are absent (Reprinted with permission from Virmani et al.[19])

infarctions and sudden deaths are triggered by plaque rupture. Plaque rupture is defined as a discontinuity of the fibrous cap which exposes the thrombogenic material contained within the underlying lipid/necrotic core to circulating blood resulting in luminal thrombosis. Because of the discontinuity of the fibrous cap, the luminal thrombus comes in contact with the underlying lipid core.

Ruptured human plaques typically exhibit: (1) a thin,[40] inflamed[60,62] fibrous cap with increased macrophage content overlaying the rich lipid core, (2) increased neovascularization,[63] (3) medial and adventitial changes,[64] (4) intraplaque hemorrhage,[65] and (5) positive vessel wall remodeling.[66] Because of the histologic combination of thin[45,67] fibrous caps and lipid-rich cores, Kolodgie et al.[45] used the term "thin-cap atheromas" to describe the precursor lesions associated with rupture. Although the role of calcification in plaque vulnerability has yet to be clarified, 80% of ruptured plaques have calcified deposits that appear either speckled or fragmented and infrequently diffuse. Ruptured plaques can be either concentric or eccentric and are more frequent in men and postmenopausal women.[68] Once a plaque becomes disrupted, the thrombogenic material of the core, including extracellular lipids, foamy macrophages, and tissue factor (TF), is exposed to flowing blood constituents. This interaction activates the coagulation cascade and results in the formation of a platelet-rich thrombus and generation of thrombin.[69] Furthermore, the presence of elevated levels of thromboxane A2 in patients with coronary disease suggests the involvement of activated platelets in atherothrombosis. Thromboxane A2 has prothrombotic properties; it not only stimulates activation of new platelets but it also increases platelet aggregation by promoting the expression of the glycoprotein complex IIb/IIIa in the cell membrane of platelets. Circulating fibrinogen binds to these receptors and brings adjacent platelets together that form and further strengthen the thrombus.

The remaining 25–30% of fatal infarctions are caused by superficial plaque erosion in which the thrombus forms over an intima without endothelial cells and a fibrous cap rich in SMC, proteoglycans (hyaluronan and versican), and type III collagen fibers.[70] The underlying plaque appears either as eccentric pathologic intimal thickening (type III lesions) or fibroatheroma with variable degrees of inflammation,[39] rare incidences of necrotic cores[53,60,71,72] and usually speckled calcifications.[73] Plaque erosions most frequently occur in men and women younger than 50 years old and are associated with cigarette smoking, especially in premenopausal women.[74] Since SMC are the major cell type located at the luminal surface of eroded plaques, it has been postulated that they may be the active clotting substrate. However, the thrombogenic nature of SMC remains to be elucidated. To date, studies have demonstrated that growth factors and thrombin in vitro and vascular injury in vivo induce the expression of tissue factor by vascular SMC.[75,76] Furthermore, several studies reported a positive correlation between tissue factor and SMC in coronary plaques from patients with unstable angina.[57,77]

Finally, Virmani et al. found that the remainder (2–5%) of atherothrombi occur as a result of calcified nodules that protrude into the lumen through a disrupted thin fibrous cap lacking endothelial cells.[19] Calcified nodules are frequently found in the mid-right coronary artery of elderly male patients with heavily calcified arteries, where coronary torsion stress is maximal. Although the origin of this lesion is not precisely known, it appears to be associated with previous ruptured and healed plaques. Currently, it is speculated that the disruption of the fibrous cap may be associated with the physical forces exerted by the nodules themselves and/or from the release of proteases from the surrounding cells.

1.5 The Role of Individual Plaque Components in Plaque Vulnerability (Fig. 1.6)

1.5.1 Atheromatous/Lipid Core

Cytotoxic effects of oxLDL, expression of cytokines (e.g., interleukine-1β), and local tissue hypoxia cause breakdown of macrophage foam cells, which release

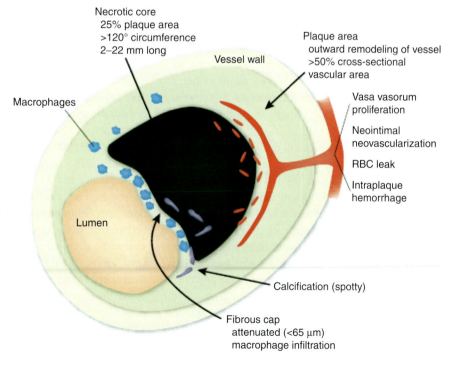

Fig. 1.6 Picturing a popcorn plaque. A large plaque with a large necrotic core is covered by a thin and inflamed cap. Note that even though the plaque is large, the lumen is not significantly obstructed because of the expansive (or outward) remodeling of the vessel. Such plaques are often associated with adventitial proliferation of vasa vasorum and neovascularization of the lesion. RBC leak and intraplaque hemorrhage from newer vasculature contribute to the free cholesterol content of the plaque (Reprinted with permission from Narula and Strauss,[61] copyright 2007)

their intracellular lipids, resulting in the formation of atheromatous lipid cores.[78,79] Although the average stenotic coronary plaque contains much more fibrous tissue than atheromatous cores, a significant atheromatous component is usually present in culprit lesions responsible for acute coronary syndromes.[80] The atheromatous core is rich in extracellular lipids, especially cholesterol and cholesteryl esters.[4,81] It is also avascular, hypocellular, and lacks supporting collagen, resulting in the formation of a soft region which, together with local inflammatory processes, can destabilize the plaque.

The major lipids found in atherosclerotic plaques are phospholipids, cholesteryl esters, and cholesterol whereas triglycerides exist in low amounts ($\leq 6\%$ wt).[4] Physicochemical studies have shown that phospholipids swell in water to form liquid-crystalline bilayers.[82,83] Cholesteryl esters are insoluble in water, and based on the degree of unsaturation of the acyl chains, they can exist in a crystalline, liquid (isotropic), and liquid-crystalline (smectic or cholesteric) phases.[84,85] Free cholesterol is also insoluble in water, but in excess it forms cholesterol monohydrate crystals[86] which incorporate into phospholipids bilayers to a mole ratio of 1:1,[87-89] and the isotropic or crystalline cholesteryl ester phases up to 4 g/100 g of cholesteryl ester. In contrast, cholesteryl esters can be dissolved only up to ~ 2% wt into the phospholipids bilayers. When present in excess amounts of their solubility in the phospholipids, both cholesterol monohydrate crystals and cholesteryl esters phase separate from the bilayers. The interactions between the lipids are considered more important than their interaction with the proteins to determine the physical state of lipids in atherosclerotic plaques.[4,31-33,81,90-92]

The lipids are distributed in different environments and their physical state depends on the relative weight ratio of individual lipids in the local environment. Lipids are usually fluid at room and body temperature. Lipids enriched in cholesteryl esters soften the plaque, whereas crystalline cholesterol has the opposite effect.[4,81] Virmani et al.[93] found that ruptured human coronary plaques had more cholesterol monohydrate crystals and Abela et al.[94] suggested that crystalline cholesterol may compromise the integrity of the fibrous cap as a result of cholesterol crystallization; both the rapid spatial configuration changes and expansion of sharp-edged crystals could damage the fibrous cap.

Postmortem analysis of the composition of plaques from 17 infarct-related arteries (in 5 mm segments) revealed significantly larger atheromatous cores in the 39 segments exhibiting plaque disruption than in the 229 segments with intact surfaces.[95] Similarly, Davies et al.[96] found that the size of the lipid pool positively correlated with the risk of ulceration and thrombosis and they identified that the crucial threshold is 40% of the plaque cross-sectional area in its midpoint (Fig. 1.7). Thus, these authors suggested that intact plaques with a core occupying more than 40% of the plaque area should be considered particularly vulnerable and at high risk of rupture and thrombosis. Moreover, it was shown that the necrotic core occupies approximately 30–50% of the total plaque area in ruptured plaques, whereas in the majority of non-ruptured plaques, it only occupies less than 25% of the plaque area.[20]

The link between increased plaque lipids, matrix metalloproteinases (MMPs), and plaque instability was further supported by studies in rabbits which demonstrated that the pressure required to rupture balloon-induced plaques in rabbit aortas is lower in the lipid-rich plaques of cholesterol-fed rabbits compared to normal chow-fed animals.[97] Furthermore, Fernandez-Ortiz et al.[98] concluded that the lipid core was the most potent substrate for the formation of platelet-rich thrombi in vitro compared to other plaque constituents.

The exact mechanism responsible for the thrombogenic properties of the lipid-rich core still needs to be elucidated. Lipids and/or cellular degradation products in the core were found to activate the hemostatic system.[99] Of all cellular-derived products, tissue factor (TF) was found to play a key role in the initiation of hemostasis.[100] TF forms a high-affinity complex with coagulation factors VII and VIIa and subsequently the TF–VIIa complex activates factors IX and X. This mechanism leads to thrombin generation.[98,100] Immunohistochemical studies of human endarterectomy specimens showed increased expression of TF in the necrotic core surrounding the cholesterol clefts, in monocytes and macrophage-derived foam cells[101] as well as vascular SMC.[102] Furthermore, the expression of TF by human monocytes was shown to be stimulated by oxLDL particles found within the plaque.[103]

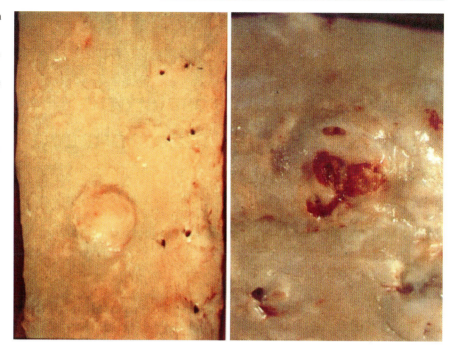

Fig. 1.7 Contrast between an intact advanced aortic plaque (*left*), in which the surface is opaque and smooth, and early ulceration (*right*), in which thrombus has formed over the plaques. A large part of the plaque, however, is not covered by thrombus (Reproduced from Davies et al.,[96] with permission from BMJ Publishing Group Ltd)

1.5.2 Fibrous Cap (Synthesis and Degradation)

Because the majority of coronary thrombi result from rupture of the fibrous cap, extensive studies have attempted to understand the mechanism of fibrous cap rupture by deciphering the metabolism of the macromolecules of the extracellular matrix that comprise the fibrous cap. The fibrous cap contains collagen, elastin, and proteoglycans that are mainly secreted by vascular SMC.[15] Of those, interstitial collagen accounts for most of the tensile strength of the fibrous cap. Ruptured human plaques usually have a thin fibrous cap[40] devoid of SMC and infiltrated by foamy macrophages,[60,104] T lymphocytes,[62] and masts cells,[105] which locally weaken the fibrous cap and reduce its tensile strength.[106] Moreover, reducing the fibrous cap thickness dramatically increases peak circumferential stress in the plaque.[107]

The amount of collagen in the fibrous cap depends on the fine-tuned balance between the rate of its biosynthesis and degradation. Specific factors secreted from degranulating platelets, such as transforming growth factor-beta and platelet-derived growth factor, inhibit SMC proliferation but activate the production of extracellular matrix proteins.[108,109] In contrast, activated T lymphocytes secrete proinflammatory cytokines such as γ-interferon, which inhibits collagen synthesis.[109] Furthermore, interstitial collagen fibrils, especially the triple helical fibrils, can be degraded by proteolytic enzymes, such as matrix metalloproteinases. MMPs consist of 15 members all of which can degrade one or more components of the extracellular matrix. MMPs are divided into collagenases, gelatenases, stromelysins, and membrane type on the basis of their substrate specificity.[110,111] In atherosclerotic plaques, MMPs are secreted by macrophages, SMC, and endothelial cells.[107] Galis et al. showed that MMPs secreted by atheroma macrophages[112] contribute to weakening of the extracellular matrix of rupture-prone atherosclerotic plaques. Moreover, Sukhova et al.[113] demonstrated that all three important interstitial collagenases (MMP–1, –8, –13) are overexpressed in human atheromatous plaques compared to human fibrous plaques, which suggests that atheromatous rather than fibrous plaques might be prone to rupture. Rupture of the fibrous cap usually occurs at the shoulder regions of the fibrous cap where the stress is highest and expression of MMPs is increased.[114] Recent work has also demonstrated that elastases, and cathepsins S and K, are released by macrophages and SMC located in complicated human atherosclerotic plaques.[115]

Histological studies of ruptured human atherosclerotic plaques have defined features additional to the presence of a thin and collagen-poor fibrous cap that might increase the propensity of a plaque to rupture. Geng et al.[78] have proposed that SMC death, either by apoptosis or programmed cell death, may contribute to the lack of SMC in vulnerable plaques. Indeed, some SMC located within the plaque contain fragmented DNA and exhibit other features characteristic of programmed cell death. Because medial SMC determine the elasticity and integrity of the arterial vessel wall, they are essential for maintaining the vasoelastic properties of the vessels. In addition, because SMC are the primary source of plaque connective tissue, their paucity within the plaque may lead to a decreased rate of fibrous cap synthesis, which is associated with plaque instability.

1.5.3 Neovascularization and Intraplaque Hemorrhage

In non-diseased vessels, nourishment of the vessel wall is accomplished mainly by diffusive mechanisms. Diffusion of oxygen is limited to 100 μm from the lumen of the vessel, which in normal arteries is adequate to nourish the inner media and intimal layers. The outer layer of the vessel wall is nourished by oxygen diffusion from the vasa vasorum, and in normal vessels, vasorum-derived microvessels do not extend into the intima but only penetrate the adventitia and outer media regions.[116] However, as the atherosclerotic disease progresses and the intima thickness increases, oxygen diffusion into the vessel wall becomes impaired. Under these circumstances, the vasa vasorum becomes the primary source of oxygen and nutrient supply to the vessel wall. When the thickness of the intima exceeds the effective diffusion distance of oxygen (~500 μm in human aortas[63] and ~350 μm in coronary arteries[117]), local hypoxic conditions[118] trigger the release of hypoxia inducible factor-1 which in turn stimulates the proliferation of the vasa vasorum. Although the newly formed neovessels can deliver oxygen into the vessel wall, they also deliver inflammatory cells and molecules that may induce further plaque progression and instability.

The source of plaque neovessels has been the focus of numerous investigations. Initially, Barger et al.[119] evaluated plaque neovessels in advanced lesions using cinematography and found that neovessels originating from the epicardial fat were distributed into the plaque throughout the vessel wall. Later on, Zhang et al.[120] studied human coronary plaques and reported that the adventitial vasa vasorum were the only source of microvessels, the content of which correlated with intimal thickness and luminal stenosis. Furthermore, Kumamoto et al.[117] showed that microvessels can also originate from the lumen. However, neovessels from the adventitial vasa vasorum were 28 times more abundant compared to those arising from the luminal side. In addition, vasa vasorum–derived microvessels are more frequently found in severely stenotic coronary lesions and correlate with the extent of inflammation and lipid core size. In contrast, luminal neovessels are found in plaques with 40–50% stenosis and are frequently associated with intraplaque hemorrhage or hemosiderin deposits.[117]

Neovascularization has been implicated in plaque progression and vulnerability by extensive investigations. Jeziorska and Woolley[121] reported that neovascularization in early atherosclerotic plaques, including fatty streaks and pre-atheromas, is associated with inflammation and lipid deposition leading to plaque progression into more advanced stages. In these types of plaques, neovascularization was found to be either scattered or widespread but it was closely associated with sites of inflammatory infiltration. Importantly, apolipoproteins A-I and B were located around neovessels suggesting that additional local lipid depositions derive from lipoprotein uptake from the microvasculature. However, extravasation of erythrocytes and intraplaque hemorrhage were not observed in these lesions. Additional studies further illustrated that the neovessels facilitate the recruitment of leukocytes to plaque areas susceptible for disruption including the fibrous cap and shoulders. The recruitment is accomplished through the expression of vascular adhesion molecule-1, intracellular adhesion molecule-1, and E-selectin, which were found be 2–3 times higher on neovessels compared to luminal endothelial cells in human coronary plaques.[122] In addition, Moreno et al.[123] provided histological evidence that plaque neovascularization also serves as a pathway for macrophage infiltration in advanced lipid-rich plaques. Importantly, ruptured plaques exhibit the highest degree of neovascularization (Fig. 1.8) whereas fibrocalcific plaques, which are characterized by the lowest

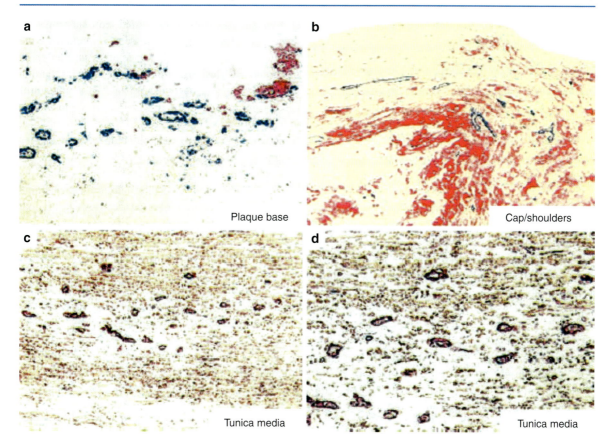

Fig. 1.8 Plaque neovascularization. (**a**) High-power image of microvessels at plaque base, detected with monoclonal endothelial cell marker CD34 linked to blue chromogen, admixed with few CD68/CD3-positive inflammatory cells linked to red chromogen. (**b**) High-power image (×40) from cap and shoulder region of lipid-rich plaque, showing CD34-positive microvessels in blue contrasting sharply with CD68/CD3-positive inflammatory cells linked to red chromogen. (**c**) Medium-power image (×20) of microvessels at tunica media from lipid-rich plaque, demonstrated with monoclonal endothelial cell marker CD34 linked to purple chromogen contrasting with smooth muscle cells of media in brown chromogen stained with α-actin. (**d**) High-power image (×40) of media from same area as in (**c**), showing CD34-positive microvessels in purple chromogen contrasting with smooth muscle cells surrounding neovessels in brown chromogen stained with α-actin (Reprinted with permission from Moreno et al.[124])

content of intimal lipids, exhibit the lowest degree of neovascularization.[124]

Histologic examination of vulnerable lesions has demonstrated that both intraplaque hemorrhage, characterized by the accumulation of erythrocytes as opposed to platelets within the plaque, and plaque rupture are associated with increased neovessel density.[58,125-127] How erythrocytes become incorporated in the plaque remains unclear, but it is generally believed that there are two dominant pathways: (1) erythrocyte extravasation through leaky vasa vasorum,[65] and (2) plaque fissuring, which has also been seen in the coronary vasculature of patients who died from a sudden coronary event.[37] Kolodgie et al.[65] demonstrated that intraplaque hemorrhage plays a crucial role in the progression of asymptomatic human coronary plaques into vulnerable high-risk lesions. This study showed that coronary atherosclerotic lesions prone to rupture had a higher frequency of previous hemorrhages (as detected by glycophorin A) compared to lesions with early necrotic cores or plaques with pathological intimal thickening. Because erythrocyte membranes are rich in phospholipids and free cholesterol (approximately 40% of their weight[128]), it has been postulated that their accumulation within plaques contributes to the expansion of the lipid core and plaque instability. Furthermore, it was recently shown that the total cholesterol content of erythrocyte membranes was significantly higher in patients who experienced acute coronary syndromes.[129] In addition to the contribution of erythrocytes in the progression of the lipid core, extravasated erythrocytes might further accelerate atherosclerosis through macrophage activation. Lysed erythrocytes released free hemoglobin which can induce oxidative tissue damage through its heme iron.[130] Subsequently, production of reactive oxygen species activates the proinflammatory transcription factor NF-kB, leading to further inflammation and angiogenesis.

Neovascularization and intraplaque hemorrhage play a crucial role in the progression of atherosclerosis and the formation of vulnerable lesions, as documented by numerous studies. Histological studies have established that ruptured human plaques have increased neovascularization,[124] which was associated with the presence of intraplaque hemorrhage.[65,131] Arterial neovascularization and inflammation are significantly greater in patients with signs of symptomatic than asymptomatic atherosclerotic disease in iliac, carotid, and renal arteries. Finally, vasa vasorum correlated with intimal macrophage content and they were found to be 2- to 4-fold higher in individuals with previous cardiovascular events than those without clinical history.[127]

1.5.4 Vascular Remodeling

An emerging area of interest in the development of vulnerable plaques involves the role of vascular wall remodeling. Crawford and Levene[132] were the first to report in 1953 that "ordinary atheromatous plaques do not project into the lumen but lie in a depression in the media, which may bulge outwards," based on their observations of pressure-distended or un-distended aortic wall specimens. Thirty years later, arterial expansion at sites of coronary atherosclerotic lesions was confirmed in animal models of coronary disease.[133,134] Armstrong et al.[133] demonstrated that the coronary arteries of cynomolgus monkeys fed on atherogenic diet enlarged in response to plaque formation and that the luminal size was initially unaffected by plaque growth. In an autopsy study of 136 human coronary arteries, Glagov et al.[135] verified that human coronary arteries also undergo "compensatory" enlargement in the presence of atherosclerotic disease. This study showed a significant correlation between the area circumscribed by the internal elastic lamina and plaque area suggesting that coronary arteries enlarge as lesion area increases. Importantly, the lumen area did not decrease in relation to the degree of stenosis (lesion area/internal elastic lamina area*100) for values between 0% and 40% but significantly diminished when the degree of stenosis was greater than 40%. On the basis of these observations, the authors concluded that human coronary arteries enlarge in relation to plaque area and that functionally important luminal stenosis may be delayed until the lesion occupies ~ 40% of the internal elastic lamina area. The preservation of a nearly normal luminal cross-sectional area despite the presence of a large plaque illustrates the limitation of X-ray angiography as a diagnostic procedure to evaluate the severity of atherosclerotic disease. In addition to expansive arterial remodeling, histological[136,137] and in vivo intravascular ultrasound[138,139] studies later showed that arteries may also either fail to enlarge or even shrink/constrict in response to plaque formation, thereby causing substantial luminal narrowing. Histological examples of vessel wall remodeling are illustrated in Fig. 1.9.

Although positive remodeling appears to be initially advantageous because it alleviates luminal narrowing, it is also associated with histological markers of plaque vulnerability (i.e., high number of macrophages, T lymphocytes, low number of SMC, decreased collagen staining, large lipid core, medial thinning, and increased expression of MMPs).[66,141-143] Furthermore, recent in vivo intravascular ultrasound studies demonstrated that positive remodeling is frequently associated with ruptured plaques in patients with unstable clinical symptoms compared to patients with a stable clinical presentation.[144-149] These observations could explain the lack of association between plaque size, percent luminal stenosis, and plaque vulnerability often reported in postmortem histological studies[141,150] and support the findings that the majority of vulnerable plaques cause less than 50% luminal narrowing as reported from X-ray angiographic studies.[151,152] In contrast, although shrinkage of the vessel wall (inward or negative remodeling) causes more luminal narrowing, it was found to be associated with a more stable clinical presentation such as stable angina pectoris.[140,145,146,148,153] Despite intense research, the mechanisms involved in arterial wall remodeling remain unclear. Although constrictive and expansive arterial remodeling has been

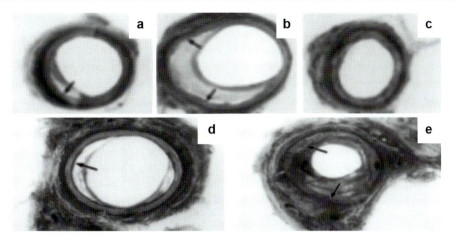

Fig. 1.9 Arterial remodeling. Representative example of compensatory enlargement with luminal overcompensation in a renal artery segment. Arrows indicate the internal elastic lamina. (**a**) Cross-section located proximally to the lesion site, lumen area = 7.2 mm², area encompassed by the internal elastic lamina (IEL area) = 9.0 mm². (**b**) Lesion site, lumen area = 9.0 mm²; IEL area = 15.9 mm². (**c**) Cross-section located distally of the lesion site, lumen area = 8.0 mm²; IEL area = 8.3 mm². Representative example of paradoxical shrinkage in the femoral artery. Arrows indicate the internal elastic lamina. (**d**) Reference segment that contained the least amount of plaque, lumen area = 14.3 mm², area encompassed by the internal elastic lamina (IEL area) = 19.9 mm². (**e**) Lesion site, lumen area = 4.4 mm². IEL area = 14.3 mm², relative IEL area = 72%, percent luminal stenosis = 69% (Reprinted with permission from Pasterkamp et al.[140])

observed in the same arterial segment, it has also been shown that arteries may have a preference to undergo one of the two types of remodeling.[140,154] Several studies have proposed that hemodynamic factors such as the endothelial shear stress, flow and wall stretch as well as cytokines, and vasoactive molecules could play a critical role in arterial wall remodeling.[155,156] In vivo studies of human coronary arteries[157] and of a mouse model in which shear stress alterations were induced in the carotid arteries revealed that low shear stress induced larger lesions with a vulnerable phenotype (positive remodeling, increased inflammation, lipids and MMP activity, and fewer collagen), whereas vortices with oscillatory shear stress induced stable lesions.

1.5.5 Media and Adventitia Changes

In addition to the well-documented intimal changes observed during the progression of atherosclerotic disease, histologic studies have revealed several changes in the media and adventitial layers of the vessel wall that could also be involved in disease progression and plaque vulnerability. One of the first features of advanced atherosclerotic plaques involves rupturing of the internal elastic lamina, which allows growth of the atherosclerotic disease into the tunica media.[132,158] Furthermore, substantial attenuation of the media in human coronary artery segments with advanced atherosclerosis was also observed.[159] Media remodeling depends on complex interactions between growth factors and MMPs and involves both smooth muscle cell movement and degradation of connective tissue. However, whether the decreased medial thickness is caused by tissue degeneration or by inhibition of cell growth is not known. However, the increased MMP activity at the base of the plaque suggests tissue degeneration as a primary contributor to medial thinning.[19]

Adventitial inflammation may also contribute to intimal disease. It has been shown that patients who died due to unstable angina exhibited clustered infiltration of inflammatory cells in the adventitia of their coronary arteries.[160] Thus, the adventitia was considered to be related to the vasospastic component of unstable angina. These findings were further corroborated by the study of Laine et al.[161] in which the infarct-related coronary arteries of patients who died of a myocardial infarction, which included the segments responsible for plaque rupture, contained the greatest numbers of adventitial mast cells. Because these were the only cells that contained histamine, these authors suggested that histamine released from the mast cells may reach the media, where it may locally stimulate coronary spasm and thus contribute to the onset of myocardial infarction. In addition, small numbers of mast cells were also present in the medial layer, and their numbers were greater in segments with plaque rupture.

More recently, Moreno et al.[64] reported that ruptured human aortic plaques were characterized by concurrent changes in the media and adventitia layers of the vessel wall including rupture of the elastic lamina, inflammation, fibrosis, and atrophy. Wolisnky et al.[162] showed that the organization of elastin, collagen, and SMC in the aortic media is responsible for the vasoelastic properties and the compliance of the normal artery wall in mammals. Thus, disorganization and damage of the media and adventitia may promote plaque vulnerability.

1.5.6 Calcification

Calcification is absent in the normal vessel wall and is one of the processes involved in the development of atherosclerosis.[17] Coronary calcification significantly correlates with plaque burden and cardiovascular related deaths. It is first seen in small amounts in early atherosclerotic lesions that appear in the second and third decades of life. Although calcification in diseased vessels is common and increases with age, both in moderate and severely stenotic coronary plaques,[20] its role in plaque vulnerability remains unclear.[36,163] The initial calcium deposits are associated with apoptotic SMC and appear as micro-calcifications bound to membrane vesicles. With plaque progression, the micro-calcifications combine together to form larger calcium deposits that appear as calcium plates which may be interspersed within fibrous tissue. At the later stages, when macrophage-rich cores become calcified, they appear more disordered in decalcified histological sections. These calcification patterns have been described as absent, speckled, fragmented, and diffuse on radiologic and ultrasonographic examination.[164]

In images of coronary arteries obtained by electron beam tomography in initially asymptomatic low- to intermediate-risk individuals, coronary calcification provides incremental prognostic information in addition to age and other risk factors such as hypercholesterolemia, hypertension, diabetes, and cigarette smoking.[165] In addition, Greenland et al.[166] using computer tomography found that high coronary artery calcium scoring can modify the predicted risk obtained from the Framingham risk score alone, especially among patients in the intermediate-risk category in whom clinical decision making is most ambiguous. However, in coronary arteries of patients who died from sudden coronary death, more calcification was seen in healed plaque ruptures, followed by fibroatheroma, thin-cap atheroma, plaque hemorrhage, fibrous plaque, plaque rupture, total occlusion, and finally, plaque erosion.[167] Thus, these data support the idea that plaque calcification may not be related to plaque instability per se. On the other hand, coronary calcification was more extensive in subjects who experienced sudden coronary death than in those dying of acute myocardial infarction or in subjects with unstable angina in vessels with extensive (76–100%) cross-sectional luminal narrowing.[168,169] Interestingly, calcification in coronary atherosclerosis appeared to be delayed in women but was greatest in diabetic women.[73] Although calcification of carotid plaques is similar to that of coronary plaques, in carotid plaques, it usually begins at the luminal site and may lead to the formation of calcific nodules.

1.5.7 Plaque Rupture Without Acute Coronary Syndromes: The Healed Plaques

Although plaque rupture is the most common type of lesion underlying acute coronary syndromes, not all plaque ruptures are associated with cardiovascular symptoms. Histological and imaging studies have shown that some plaque ruptures are silent and become healed without causing any symptoms.[170,171] Healed coronary plaques have been detected histologically by the presence of discontinuities in type I collagen fibers that make up the organized fibrous cap and which are repaired by the deposition of new, type III collagen fibers.[150] The sites of plaque healing are more evident on picrosirius red stained sections viewed under polarized light in which collagen fibers type I appear yellow-red whereas the new collagen fibers at the site of plaque healing appear green. In addition, Movat staining revealed abundant SMC in a proteoglycan-rich matrix at that the site of plaque healing (Fig. 1.10).[172,173]

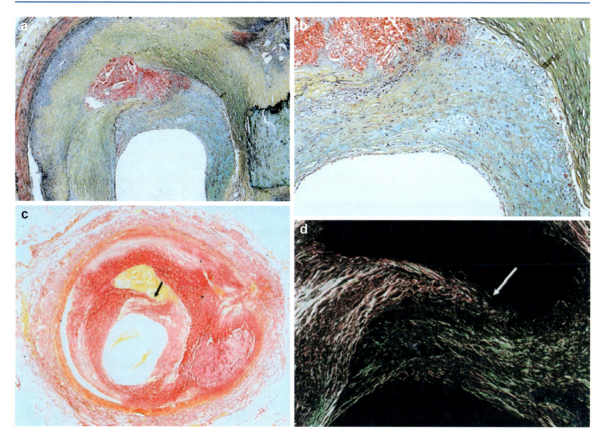

Fig. 1.10 Healed plaque rupture. (**a**) Areas of intraintimal lipid-rich core with hemorrhage and cholesterol clefts. (**b**) Higher magnification of looser SMC formation within collagenous proteoglycan-rich neointima showing clear demarcation, with more fibrous regions of old plaque to right. (**c, d**) Layers of collagen by Sirius red staining. (**c**) Note area of dense, dark-red collagen surrounding lipid hemorrhagic cores seen in corresponding view in (**a**). (**d**) Image taken with polarized light. Dense collagen (type 1) that forms fibrous cap is lighter reddish-yellow and is disrupted (*arrow*), with newer greenish type III collagen on right and above rupture site. (**a**) and (**b**), Movat pentachrome (Reprinted with permission from Burke et al.[172])

Although stenosis is easily identified by angiography, the relationship of plaque progression, vulnerability, and luminal narrowing is currently not well understood. In particular, Mann et al.[150] have shown that the two major determinants of plaque vulnerability, core size and cap thickness, are not statistically related. Furthermore, neither of these two factors was related to the absolute plaque size or to the degree of stenosis. In an effort to understand the mechanisms of plaque progression Burke et al.[172] performed morphometric measurements of plaque burden, luminal stenosis, and smooth muscle cell phenotype in 142 coronary arteries with acute and healed ruptures from men who died of sudden coronary death. This study provided evidence that silent plaque rupture is a form of wound healing that can result in increased percent stenosis. Furthermore, healed ruptures occurred in arteries with lower cross-sectional area luminal narrowing compared to that found in acute plaque ruptures and were frequently found in men who die suddenly with severe coronary atherosclerosis. This mechanism could explain the phasic rather than the linear progression of coronary artery disease observed in angiograms taken annually from patients with chronic ischemic heart disease.[56] However, these conclusions are provisional and need to be validated in vivo provided that an imaging modality could prospectively identify the site of plaque vulnerability and fibrous cap rupture followed by longitudinal studies to monitor the increase in plaque size and luminal narrowing as plaques heal.

1.6 Summary

Histological studies using excised human vessels, collected either postmortem or surgically, and vessels from atherosclerotic animal models have provided indispensable information regarding the pathophysiology of atherosclerotic disease and thrombosis. To date, three distinct histological features – plaque rupture, plaque erosion, and calcified nodule – have been associated with luminal thrombosis. Using the functional definition of plaque vulnerability, which classifies all plaques with a higher risk of thrombosis as "vulnerable," plaques that are prone to rupture, erode, and/or form calcified nodules would be considered vulnerable.

Although histology provides information of morphological features at extremely high resolution, this method has several limitations including its retrospective nature. To overcome some of these limitations and to permit in vivo characterization of plaques, many investigations are exploring both invasive (angiography, angioscopy, intravascular ultrasound, optimal coherence tomography, thermography, Raman spectroscopy, near infra-red spectroscopy) and noninvasive (B-mode ultrasound tomography, computed tomography, positron-emission tomography, magnetic resonance imaging) imaging modalities. In spite of the inherently lower resolution of these imaging modalities, compared to histology, they are providing new insights regarding the progression of atherosclerotic disease and acute cardiovascular events and may permit the prospective detection of vulnerable plaques. In the chapters that follow, the applications of ultrasound imaging to study carotid atherosclerosis are presented in detail.

References

1. Lloyd-Jones D et al. Heart disease and stroke statistics – 2009 update: a report from the American Heart Association Statistics Committee and Stroke Statistics Subcommittee. *Circulation*. 2009;119(3):480–486.
2. Murray CJ, Lopez AD. Global mortality, disability, and the contribution of risk factors: Global Burden of Disease Study. *Lancet*. 1997;349(9063):1436–1442.
3. Anitschkow N. Über die Veränderungen der Kaninchenaorta bei experimenteller Cholesterinsteatose. *Beiträge zur Pathologischen Anatomie und zur Allgemeinen Pathologie*. 1913;56:379–404.
4. Small DM. Progression and regression of atherosclerotic lesions: insights from lipid physical biochemistry. *Atherosclerosis*. 1988;8:103–129.
5. Ross R. Atherosclerosis – an inflammatory disease. *N Engl J Med*. 1999;340(2):115–126.
6. Lusis AJ. Atherosclerosis. *Nature*. 2000;407(6801):233–241.
7. Libby P. Inflammation in atherosclerosis. *Nature*. 2002; 420(6917):868–874.
8. Poredos P. Endothelial dysfunction in the pathogenesis of atherosclerosis. *Clin Appl Thromb Hemost*. 2001;7(4): 276–280.
9. Virchow R. *Phlogose und thrombose im gefassystem. Gesammelte abhandlungen zur wissenschaftlichen medicin*. Frankfurt: Meidinger Sohn and Co; 1856:458.
10. Ross R, Glomset JA. The pathogenesis of atherosclerosis (first of two parts). *N Engl J Med*. 1976;295(7):369–377.
11. Ross R, Glomset JA. The pathogenesis of atherosclerosis (second of two parts). *N Engl J Med*. 1976;295(8): 420–425.
12. Ludmer PL et al. Paradoxical vasoconstriction induced by acetylcholine in atherosclerotic coronary arteries. *N Engl J Med*. 1986;315(17):1046–1051.
13. Gimbrone MA Jr. Endothelial dysfunction and atherosclerosis. *J Card Surg*. 1989;4(2):180–183.
14. Lusis AJ. Stable and vulnerable atherosclerotic plaques. *Nature*. 2000;407(6801):233–241.
15. Shah PK. Pathophysiology of plaque rupture and the concept of plaque stabilization. *Cardiol Clin*. 2003;21(3): 303–314, v.
16. Stary HC et al. A definition of advanced types of atherosclerotic lesions and a histological classification of atherosclerosis. A report from the Committee on Vascular Lesions of the Council on Arteriosclerosis, American Heart Association. *Arterioscler Thromb Vasc Biol*. 1995; 15(9):1512–1531.
17. Stary HC et al. A definition of advanced types of atherosclerotic lesions and a histological classification of atherosclerosis. A report from the Committee on Vascular Lesions of the Council on Arteriosclerosis, American Heart Association. *Circulation*. 1995;92(5):1355–1374.
18. Stary HC. Natural history and histological classification of atherosclerotic lesions: an update. *Arterioscler Thromb Vasc Biol*. 2000;20(5):1177–1178.
19. Virmani R, Kolodgie FD, Burke AP, Farb A, Schwartz SM. Lessons from sudden coronary death: a comprehensive morphological classification scheme for atherosclerotic lesions. *Arterioscler Thromb Vasc Biol*. 2000;20(5): 1262–1275.
20. Burke AP, Virmani R, Galis Z, Haudenschild CC, Muller JE. 34th Bethesda conference: task force #2 – what is the pathologic basis for new atherosclerosis imaging techniques? *J Am Coll Cardiol*. 2003;41(11):1874–1886.
21. Stary HC. Composition and classification of human atherosclerotic lesions. *Virchows Arch A Pathol Anat Histopathol*. 1992;421(4):277–290.
22. Hamilton JA, Cordes EH, Glueck CJ. Lipid dynamics in human low-density lipoproteins and human fibrous plaques: a study by high field 13C NMR. *J Biol Chem*. 1979;254:5435–5441.

23. Napoli C et al. Fatty streak formation occurs in human fetal aortas and is greatly enhanced by maternal hypercholesterolemia. Intimal accumulation of low density lipoprotein and its oxidation precede monocyte recruitment into early atherosclerotic lesions. *J Clin Invest*. 1997;100(11): 2680–2690.
24. Khalil MF, Wagner WD, Goldberg IJ. Molecular interactions leading to lipoprotein retention and the initiation of atherosclerosis. *Arterioscler Thromb Vasc Biol*. 2004;24(12):2211–2218.
25. Navab M et al. The Yin and Yang of oxidation in the development of the fatty streak. A review based on the 1994 George Lyman Duff Memorial Lecture. *Arterioscler Thromb Vasc Biol*. 1996;16(7):831–842.
26. Dong ZM et al. The combined role of P- and E-selectins in atherosclerosis. *J Clin Invest*. 1998;102(1):145–152.
27. Cybulsky MI, Gimbrone MA Jr. Endothelial expression of a mononuclear leukocyte adhesion molecule during atherogenesis. *Science*. 1991;251(4995):788–791.
28. Peiser L, Mukhopadhyay S, Gordon S. Scavenger receptors in innate immunity. *Curr Opin Immunol*. 2002;14(1): 123–128.
29. Podrez EA et al. Macrophage scavenger receptor CD36 is the major receptor for LDL modified by monocyte-generated reactive nitrogen species. *J Clin Invest*. 2000;105(8):1095–1108.
30. Hansson GK. Inflammation, atherosclersosis, and coronary artery disease. *N Engl J Med*. 2005;352(16):1685–1695.
31. Hillman GM, Engelman DM. Compositional mapping of cholesteryl ester droplets in the fatty streaks of human aorta. *J Clin Invest*. 1976;58(4):1008–1018.
32. Engelman DM, Hillman GM. Molecular organization of the cholesteryl ester droplets in the fatty streaks of human aorta. *J Clin Invest*. 1976;58(4):997–1007.
33. Katz SS, Shipley GG, Small DM. Physical chemistry of the lipids of human atherosclerotic lesions. Demonstration of a lesion intermediate between fatty streaks and advanced plaques. *J Clin Invest*. 1976;58(1):200–211.
34. Jonasson L, Holm J, Skalli O, Bondjers G, Hansson GK. Regional accumulations of T cells, macrophages, and smooth muscle cells in the human atherosclerotic plaque. *Arteriosclerosis*. 1986;6(2):131–138.
35. Demer LL, Tintut Y. Osteopontin. Between a rock and a hard plaque. *Circ Res*. 1999;84(2):250–252.
36. Wexler L et al. Coronary artery calcification: pathophysiology, epidemiology, imaging methods, and clinical implications: a statement for health professionals from the American Heart Association. *Circulation*. 1996;94(5): 1175–1192.
37. Davies M, Thomas A. Plaque fissuring – the cause of acute myocardial infarction, sudden ischaemic death, and crescendo angina. *Br Heart J*. 1985;53(4):363–373.
38. Davies MJ. Stability and instability: two faces of coronary atherosclerosis: the Paul Dudley White Lecture 1995. *Circulation*. 1996;94(8):2013–2020.
39. Farb A et al. Coronary plaque erosion without rupture into a lipid core. A frequent cause of coronary thrombosis in sudden coronary death. *Circulation*. 1996;93(7):1354–1363.
40. Burke AP et al. Coronary risk factors and plaque morphology in men with coronary disease who died suddenly. *N Engl J Med*. 1997;336(18):1276–1282.
41. Muller JE, Abela GS, Nesto RW, Tofler GH. Triggers, acute risk factors and vulnerable plaques: the lexicon of a new frontier. *J Am Coll Cardiol*. 1994;23(3):809–813.
42. Muller JE, Moreno PR. Definition of the vulnerable plaque. In: Waksman R, Serruys PW, eds. *Handbook of the Vulnerable Plaque*. 2nd ed. London: Taylor & Francis; 2004:1–13.
43. Falk E. Why do plaques rupture? *Circulation*. 1992;86 (6 suppl):III30-III42.
44. Libby P. Molecular bases of the acute coronary syndromes. *Circulation*. 1995;91(11):2844–2850.
45. Kolodgie FD et al. The thin-cap fibroatheroma: a type of vulnerable plaque: the major precursor lesion to acute coronary syndromes. *Curr Opin Cardiol*. 2001;16(5): 285–292.
46. Fraergeman O. *Coronary Artery Disease: Genes, Drugs and the Agricultural Connection*. New York: Elsevier; 2003:12–13.
47. Leary T. Coronary spasm as a possible factor in producing sudden death. *Am Heart J*. 1934;10:328–337.
48. Constantinides P. Plaque fissures in human coronary thrombosis. *J Atheroscler Res*. 1966;6:1–17.
49. Constantinides P, Booth J, Carlson G. Production of advanced cholesterol atherosclerosis in the rabbit. *Arch Pathol*. 1960;70:80–92.
50. Constantinides P, Chakravarti RN. Rabbit arterial thrombosis production by systemic procedures. *Arch Pathol*. 1961;72:197–208.
51. Constantinides P. *Experimental Atherosclerosis*. New York: Elsevier; 1965.
52. Willerson JT et al. Conversion from chronic to acute coronary artery disease: speculation regarding mechanisms. *Am J Cardiol*. 1984;54(10):1349–1354.
53. Farb A et al. Sudden coronary death. Frequency of active coronary lesions, inactive coronary lesions, and myocardial infarction. *Circulation*. 1995;92(7):1701–1709.
54. Davies MJ. Detecting vulnerable coronary plaques. *Lancet*. 1996;347(9013):1422–1423.
55. Moreno PR, Falk E, Palacios IF, Newell JB, Fuster V, Fallon JT. Macrophage infiltration in acute coronary syndromes. Implications for plaque rupture. *Circulation*. 1994;90(2):775–778.
56. Falk E, Shah PK, Fuster V. Coronary plaque disruption. *Circulation*. 1995;92(3):657–671.
57. Moreno PR et al. Macrophages, smooth muscle cells, and tissue factor in uns angina. Implications for cell-mediated thrombogenicity in acute coronary syndromes. *Circulation*. 1996;94(12):3090–3097.
58. Burke AP et al. Plaque rupture and sudden death related to exertion in men with coronary artery disease. *JAMA*. 1999;281(10):921–926.
59. Pasterkamp G et al. Inflammation of the atherosclerotic cap and shoulder of the plaque is a common and locally observed feature in unruptured plaques of femoral and coronary arteries. *Arterioscler Thromb Vasc Biol*. 1999; 19(1):54–58.
60. van der Wal AC, Becker AE, van der Loos C, Das P. Site of intimal rupture or erosion of thrombosed coronary atherosclerotic plaques is characterized by an inflammatory process irrespective of the dominant plaque morphology. *Circulation*. 1994;89:36–44.

61. Narula J, Strauss W. The popcorn plaques. *Nat Med.* 2007;13(5):532–534.
62. Boyle JJ. Association of coronary plaque rupture and atherosclerotic inflammation. *J Pathol.* 1997;181(1):93–99.
63. Moreno PR, Purushothaman KR, Sirol M, Levy AP, Fuster V. Neovascularization in human atherosclerosis. *Circulation.* 2006;113(18):2245–2252.
64. Moreno PR, Purushothaman KR, Fuster V, O'Connor WN. Intimomedial interface damage and adventitial inflammation is increased beneath disrupted atherosclerosis in the aorta: implications for plaque vulnerability. *Circulation.* 2002;105(21):2504–2511.
65. Kolodgie FD et al. Intraplaque hemorrhage and progression of coronary atheroma. *N Engl J Med.* 2003;349(24): 2316–2325.
66. Pasterkamp G et al. Atherosclerotic arterial remodeling and the localization of macrophages and matrix metalloproteases 1, 2 and 9 in the human coronary artery. *Atherosclerosis.* 2000;150(2):245–253.
67. Virmani R, Burke AP, Kolodgie FD, Farb A. Pathology of the thin-cap fibroatheroma: a type of vulnerable plaque. *J Interv Cardiol.* 2003;16(3):267–272.
68. Burke AP, Farb A, Malcom G, Virmani R. Effect of menopause on plaque morphologic characteristics in coronary atherosclerosis. *Am Heart J.* 2001;141(2 Suppl):S58-S62.
69. Sambola A et al. Role of risk factors in the modulation of tissue factor activity and blood thrombogenicity. *Circulation.* 2003;107(7):973–977.
70. Kolodgie FD et al. Differential accumulation of proteoglycans and hyaluronan in culprit lesions: insights into plaque erosion. *Arterioscler Thromb Vasc Biol.* 2002;22(10):1642–1648.
71. Arbustini E et al. Plaque erosion is a major substrate for coronary thrombosis in acute myocardial infarction. *Heart.* 1999;82(3):269–272.
72. Henriques de Gouveia R, Van der Wal AC, Van der Loos CM, Becker AE. Sudden unexpected death in young adults. Discrepancies between initiation of acute plaque complications and the onset of acute coronary death. *Eur Heart J.* 2002;23(18):1433–1440.
73. Burke AP, Taylor A, Farb A, Malcom GT, Virmani R. Coronary calcification: insights from sudden coronary death victims. *Z Kardiol.* 2000;89(suppl 2):49–53.
74. Burke AP et al. Effect of risk factors on the mechanism of acute thrombosis and sudden coronary death in women. *Circulation.* 1998;97(21):2110–2116.
75. Campeau L. Letter: grading of angina pectoris. *Circulation.* 1976;54(3):522–523.
76. Taubman MB et al. Agonist-mediated tissue factor expression in cultured vascular smooth muscle cells. Role of Ca^{2+} mobilization and protein kinase C activation. *J Clin Invest.* 1993;91(2):547–552.
77. Flugelman MY et al. Smooth muscle cell abundance and fibroblast growth factors in coronary lesions of patients with nonfatal unstable angina. A clue to the mechanism of transformation from the stable to the unstable clinical state. *Circulation.* 1993;88(6):2493–2500.
78. Geng YJ, Libby P. Evidence for apoptosis in advanced human atheroma. Colocalization with interleukin-1 beta-converting enzyme. *Am J Pathol.* 1995;147(2):251–266.
79. Ball RY et al. Evidence that the death of macrophage foam cells contributes to the lipid core of atheroma. *Atherosclerosis.* 1995;114(1):45–54.
80. Falk E. Morphologic features of unstable atherothrombotic plaques underlying acute coronary syndromes. *Am J Cardiol.* 1989;63(10):114E-120E.
81. Lundberg B. Chemical composition and physical state of lipid deposits in atherosclerosis. *Atherosclerosis.* 1985; 56(1):93–110.
82. Small DM. Observations on lecithin. Phase equilibria and structure of dry and hydrated egg lecithin. *J Lipid Res.* 1967;8:551–557.
83. Shipley GG, Avecilla LS, Small DM. Phase behavior and structure of aqueous dispersions of sphingomyelin. *J Lipid Res.* 1974;15(2):124–131.
84. Ginsburg GS, Atkinson D, Small DM. Physical properties of cholesteryl esters. *Prog Lipid Res.* 1984;23(3):135–167.
85. Small DM. The physical state of lipids of biological importance: cholesteryl esters, cholesterol, and triglyceride. In: Blank E, ed. *Surface Chemistry of Biological Systems.* New York: Plenum Press; 1970:55–84.
86. Loomis CR, Shipley GG, Small DM. The phase behavior of hydrated cholesterol. *J Lipid Res.* 1979;20(4):525–535.
87. Bourges M, Small DM, Dervichian DG. Biophysics of lipidic associations. II. The ternary systems: cholesterol-lecithin-water. *Biochim Biophys Acta.* 1967;137(1):157–167.
88. Phillips MC. Cholesterol packing, crystallization and exchange properties in phosphatidylcholine vesicle systems. *Hepatology.* 1990;12(3 pt 2):75S-80S discussion 80S-82S.
89. Peng S, Guo W, Morrisett JD, Johnstone MT, Hamilton JA. Quantification of cholesteryl esters in human and rabbit atherosclerotic plaques by magic-angle spinning (13)C-NMR. *Arterioscler Thromb Vasc Biol.* 2000;20(12): 2682–2688.
90. Small DM, Shipley GG. Physical-chemical basis of lipid deposition in atherosclerosis. *Science.* 1974;185(147): 222-229.
91. Katz SS, Small DM. Isolation and and partial characterization of the lipid phases of human atherosclerotic plaques. *J Biol Chem.* 1980;255(20):9753–9759.
92. Guyton JR, Klemp KF. Development of the lipid-rich core in human atherosclerosis. *Arterioscler Thromb Vasc Biol.* 1996;16(1):4–11.
93. Virmani R, Burke AP, Farb A, Kolodgie FD. Pathology of the vulnerable plaque. *J Am Coll Cardiol.* 2006;47 (8 Suppl):C13-C18.
94. Abela GS, Aziz K. Cholesterol crystals rupture biological membranes and human plaques during acute cardiovascular events – a novel insight into plaque rupture by scanning electron microscopy. *Scanning.* 2006;28(1):1–10.
95. Gertz SD, Roberts WC. Hemodynamic shear force in rupture of coronary arterial atherosclerotic plaques. *Am J Cardiol.* 1990;66(19):1368–1372.
96. Davies MJ, Richardson PD, Woolf N, Katz DR, Mann J. Risk of thrombosis in human atherosclerotic plaques: role of extracellular lipid, macrophage, and smooth muscle cell content. *Br Heart J.* 1993;69(5):377–381.
97. Rekhter MD et al. Hypercholesterolemia causes mechanical weakening of rabbit atheroma: local collagen loss as a

prerequisite of plaque rupture. *Circ Res.* 2000;86(1): 101-108.
98. Fernandez-Ortiz A et al. Characterization of the relative thrombogenicity of atherosclerotic plaque components: implications for consequences of plaque rupture. *J Am Coll Cardiol.* 1994;23(7):1562–1569.
99. Guyton JR, Klemp KF. The lipid-rich core region of human atherosclerotic fibrous plaques. Prevalence of small lipid droplets and vesicles by electron microscopy. *Am J Pathol.* 1989;134(3):705–717.
100. Rapaport SI, Rao LV. Initiation and regulation of tissue factor-dependent blood coagulation. *Arterioscler Thromb.* 1992;12(10):1111–1121.
101. Wilcox JN, Smith KM, Schwartz SM, Gordon D. Localization of tissue factor in the normal vessel wall and in the atherosclerotic plaque. *Proc Natl Acad Sci USA.* 1989;86(8):2839–2843.
102. Schecter AD et al. Release of active tissue factor by human arterial smooth muscle cells. *Circ Res.* 2000;87(2):126-132.
103. Brand K et al. Oxidized LDL enhances lipopolysaccharide-induced tissue factor expression in human adherent monocytes. *Arterioscler Thromb.* 1994;14(5):790–797.
104. Redgrave JN, Lovett JK, Gallagher PJ, Rothwell PM. Histological assessment of 526 symptomatic carotid plaques in relation to the nature and timing of ischemic symptoms: the Oxford plaque study. *Circulation.* 2006;113(19):2320–2328.
105. Kaartinen M et al. Mast cell infiltration in acute coronary syndromes: implications for plaque rupture. *J Am Coll Cardiol.* 1998;32(3):606.
106. Lendon CL, Davies MJ, Born GV, Richardson PD. Atherosclerotic plaque caps are locally weakened when macrophages density is increased. *Atherosclerosis.* 1991;87(1):87–90.
107. Loree HM, Kamm RD, Stringfellow RG, Lee RT. Effects of fibrous cap thickness on peak circumferential stress in model atherosclerotic vessels. *Circ Res.* 1992;71(4):850–858.
108. Libby P. Changing concepts of atherogenesis. *J Intern Med.* 2000;247(3):349–358.
109. Amento EP, Ehsani N, Palmer H, Libby P. Cytokines and growth factors positively and negatively regulate interstitial collagen gene expression in human vascular smooth muscle cells. *Arterioscler Thromb.* 1991;11(5):1223–1230.
110. Loftus IM, Naylor AR, Bell PR, Thompson MM. Matrix metalloproteinases and atherosclerotic plaque instability. *Br J Surg.* 2002;89(6):680–694.
111. Loftus IM, Thompson MM. The role of matrix metalloproteinases in vascular disease. *Vasc Med.* 2002;7(2):117–133.
112. Galis ZS, Sukhova GK, Kranzhofer R, Clark S, Libby P. Macrophage foam cells from experimental atheroma constitutively produce matrix-degrading proteinases. *Proc Natl Acad Sci USA.* 1995;92(2):402–406.
113. Sukhova GK et al. Evidence for increased collagenolysis by interstitial collagenases-1 and -3 in vulnerable human atheromatous plaques. *Circulation.* 1999;99(19):2503–2509.
114. Galis ZS, Sukhova GK, Lark MW, Libby P. Increased expression of matrix metalloproteinases and matrix degrading activity in vulnerable regions of human atherosclerotic plaques. *J Clin Invest.* 1994;94(6):2493–2503.
115. Sukhova GK, Shi GP, Simon DI, Chapman HA, Libby P. Expression of the elastolytic cathepsins S and K in human atheroma and regulation of their production in smooth muscle cells. *J Clin Invest.* 1998;102(3):576–583.
116. Geiringer E. Intimal vascularization and atherosclerosis. *J Pathol Bacteriol.* 1951;63(2):201–211.
117. Kumamoto M, Nakashima Y, Sueishi K. Intimal neovascularization in human coronary atherosclerosis: its origin and pathophysiological significance. *Hum Pathol.* 1995;26(4):450.
118. Carmeliet P. Angiogenesis in health and disease. *Nat Med.* 2003;9(6):653–660.
119. Barger AC, Beeuwkes R 3rd, Lainey LL, Silverman KJ. Hypothesis: vasa vasorum and neovascularization of human coronary arteries. A possible role in the pathophysiology of atherosclerosis. *N Engl J Med.* 1984;310(3):175-177.
120. Zhang Y, Cliff WJ, Schoefl GI, Higgins G. Immunohistochemical study of intimal microvessels in coronary atherosclerosis. *Am J Pathol.* 1993;143(1):164–172.
121. Jeziorska M, Woolley DE. Neovascularization in early atherosclerotic lesions of human carotid arteries: its potential contribution to plaque development. *Hum Pathol.* 1999;30(8):919–925.
122. O'Brien KD, McDonald TO, Chait A, Allen MD, Alpers CE. Neovascular expression of E-selectin, intercellular adhesion molecule-1, and vascular cell adhesion molecule-1 in human atherosclerosis and their relation to intimal leukocyte content. *Circulation.* 1996;93(4):672–682.
123. Moreno PR, Fuster V. New aspects in the pathogenesis of diabetic atherothrombosis. *J Am Coll Cardiol.* 2004;44(12):2293–2300.
124. Moreno PR et al. Plaque neovascularization is increased in ruptured atherosclerotic lesions of human aorta: implications for plaque vulnerability. *Circulation.* 2004;110(14):2032–2038.
125. Jeziorska M, Woolley DE. Local neovascularization and cellular composition within vulnerable regions of atherosclerotic plaques of human carotid arteries. *J Pathol.* 1999;188(2):189–196.
126. Mofidi R et al. Association between plaque instability, angiogenesis and symptomatic carotid occlusive disease. *Br J Surg.* 2001;88(7):945–950.
127. Fleiner M et al. Arterial neovascularization and inflammation in vulnerable patients: early and late signs of symptomatic atherosclerosis. *Circulation.* 2004;110(18):2843–2850.
128. Yeagle PL. Cholesterol and the cell membrane. *Biochim Biophys Acta.* 1985;822(3–4):267–287.
129. Tziakas DN et al. Total cholesterol content of erythrocyte membranes is increased in patients with acute coronary syndrome: a new marker of clinical instability? *J Am Coll Cardiol.* 2007;49(21):2081–2089.
130. Vlodavsky I, Friedmann Y. Molecular properties and involvement of heparanase in cancer metastasis and angiogenesis. *J Clin Invest.* 2001;108(3):341–347.
131. Virmani R et al. Atherosclerotic plaque progression and vulnerability to rupture: angiogenesis as a source of

intraplaque hemorrhage. *Arterioscler Thromb Vasc Biol.* 2005;25(10):2054–2061.
132. Crawford T, Levene CI. Medial thinning in atheroma. *J Pathol Bacteriol.* 1953;66(1):19–23.
133. Armstrong ML, Heistad DD, Marcus ML, Megan MB, Piegors DJ. Structural and hemodynamic response of peripheral arteries of macaque monkeys to atherogenic diet. *Arteriosclerosis.* 1985;5(4):336–346.
134. Bond MG, Adams MR, Bullock BC. Complicating factors in evaluating coronary artery atherosclerosis. *Artery.* 1981;9(1):21–29.
135. Glagov S, Weisenberg E, Zarins CK, Stankunavicius R, Kolettis GJ. Compensatory enlargement of human atherosclerotic coronary arteries. *N Engl J Med.* 1987;316(22):1371–1375.
136. Pasterkamp G et al. Paradoxical arterial wall shrinkage may contribute to luminal narrowing of human atherosclerotic femoral arteries. *Circulation.* 1995;91(5):1444–1449.
137. Pasterkamp G et al. Atherosclerotic arterial remodeling in the superficial femoral artery. Individual variation in local compensatory enlargement response. *Circulation.* 1996;93(10):1818–1825.
138. Nishioka T et al. Contribution of inadequate compensatory enlargement to development of human coronary artery stenosis: an in vivo intravascular ultrasound study. *J Am Coll Cardiol.* 1996;27(7):1571–1576.
139. Mintz GS et al. Contribution of inadequate arterial remodeling to the development of focal coronary artery stenoses. An intravascular ultrasound study. *Circulation.* 1997;95(7):1791–1798.
140. Pasterkamp G et al. The impact of atherosclerotic arterial remodeling on percentage of luminal stenosis varies widely within the arterial system. A postmortem study. *Arterioscler Thromb Vasc Biol.* 1997;17(11):3057–3063.
141. Pasterkamp G et al. Relation of arterial geometry to luminal narrowing and histologic markers for plaque vulnerability: the remodeling paradox. *J Am Coll Cardiol.* 1998;32(3):655–662.
142. Varnava AM, Mills PG, Davies MJ. Relationship between coronary artery remodeling and plaque vulnerability. *Circulation.* 2002;105(8):939–943.
143. Burke AP, Kolodgie FD, Farb A, Weber D, Virmani R. Morphological predictors of arterial remodeling in coronary atherosclerosis. *Circulation.* 2002;105(3):297–303.
144. Schoenhagen P et al. Relation of matrix-metalloproteinase 3 found in coronary lesion samples retrieved by directional coronary atherectomy to intravascular ultrasound observations on coronary remodeling. *Am J Cardiol.* 2002;89(12):1354–1359.
145. Schoenhagen P et al. Association of arterial expansion (expansive remodeling) of bifurcation lesions determined by intravascular ultrasonography with unstable clinical presentation. *Am J Cardiol.* 2001;88(7):785–787.
146. Schoenhagen P et al. Extent and direction of arterial remodeling in stable versus unstable coronary syndromes: an intravascular ultrasound study. *Circulation.* 2000;101(6):598–603.
147. Schoenhagen P, Ziada KM, Vince DG, Nissen SE, Tuzcu EM. Arterial remodeling and coronary artery disease: the concept of "dilated" versus "obstructive" coronary atherosclerosis. *J Am Coll Cardiol.* 2001;38(2):297–306.
148. Smits PC et al. Coronary artery disease: arterial remodelling and clinical presentation. *Heart.* 1999;82(4):461–464.
149. Yamagishi M et al. Morphology of vulnerable coronary plaque: insights from follow-up of patients examined by intravascular ultrasound before an acute coronary syndrome. *J Am Coll Cardiol.* 2000;35(1):106–111.
150. Mann JM, Davies MJ. Vulnerable plaque. Relation of characteristics to degree of stenosis in human coronary arteries. *Circulation.* 1996;94(5):928–931.
151. Ambrose JA et al. Angiographic progression of coronary artery disease and the development of myocardial infarction. *J Am Coll Cardiol.* 1988;12(1):56–62.
152. Giroud D, Li JM, Urban P, Meier B, Rutishauer W. Relation of the site of acute myocardial infarction to the most severe coronary arterial stenosis at prior angiography. *Am J Cardiol.* 1992;69(8):729–732.
153. Nakamura M et al. Impact of coronary artery remodeling on clinical presentation of coronary artery disease: an intravascular ultrasound study. *J Am Coll Cardiol.* 2001;37(1):63–69.
154. Vink A et al. Plaque burden, arterial remodeling and plaque vulnerability: determined by systemic factors? *J Am Coll Cardiol.* 2001;38(3):718–723.
155. Gibbons GH, Dzau VJ. The emerging concept of vascular remodeling. *N Engl J Med.* 1994;330(20):1431–1438.
156. Chatzizisis YS et al. Role of endothelial shear stress in the natural history of coronary atherosclerosis and vascular remodeling: molecular, cellular, and vascular behavior. *J Am Coll Cardiol.* 2007;49(25):2379–2393.
157. Stone PH et al. Regions of low endothelial shear stress are the sites where coronary plaque progresses and vascular remodelling occurs in humans: an in vivo serial study. *Eur Heart J.* 2007;28(6):705–710.
158. Davies MJ. Glagovian remodelling, plaque composition, and stenosis generation. *Heart.* 2000;84(5):461–462.
159. Isner JM, Donaldson RF, Fortin AH, Tischler A, Clarke RH. Attenuation of the media of coronary arteries in advanced atherosclerosis. *Am J Cardiol.* 1986;58(10):937–939.
160. Kohchi K, Takebayashi S, Hiroki T, Nobuyoshi M. Significance of adventitial inflammation of the coronary artery in patients with unstable angina: results at autopsy. *Circulation.* 1985;71(4):709–716.
161. Laine P et al. Association between myocardial infarction and the mast cells in the adventitia of the infarct-related coronary artery. *Circulation.* 1999;99(3):361–369.
162. Wolinsky H, Glagov S. A lamellar unit of aortic medial structure and function in mammals. *Circ Res.* 1967;20(1):99–111.
163. Davies MJ. The composition of coronary-artery plaques. *N Engl J Med.* 1997;336(18):1312–1314.
164. Friedrich GJ et al. Detection of intralesional calcium by intracoronary ultrasound depends on the histologic pattern. *Am Heart J.* 1994;128(3):435–441.
165. Kondos GT et al. Electron-beam tomography coronary artery calcium and cardiac events: a 37-month follow-up of 5635 initially asymptomatic low- to intermediate-risk adults. *Circulation.* 2003;107(20):2571–2576.
166. Greenland P, LaBree L, Azen SP, Doherty TM, Detrano RC. Coronary artery calcium score combined with

Framingham score for risk prediction in asymptomatic individuals. *JAMA*. 2004;291(2):210–215.
167. Burke AP et al. Pathophysiology of calcium deposition in coronary arteries. *Herz*. 2001;26(4):239–244.
168. Kragel AH, Reddy SG, Wittes JT, Roberts WC. Morphometric analysis of the composition of coronary arterial plaques in isolated unstable angina pectoris with pain at rest. *Am J Cardiol*. 1990;66(5):562–567.
169. Kragel AH, Gertz SD, Roberts WC. Morphologic comparison of frequency and types of acute lesions in the major epicardial coronary arteries in unstable angina pectoris, sudden coronary death and acute myocardial infarction. *J Am Coll Cardiol*. 1991;18(3):801–808.
170. Mann J, Davies MJ. Mechanisms of progression in native coronary artery disease: role of healed plaque disruption. *Heart*. 1999;82(3):265–268.
171. Qiao Y, Farber A, Semaan E, Hamilton JA. Images in cardiovascular medicine. Healing of an asymptomatic carotid plaque ulceration. *Circulation*. 2008;118(10):e147–e148.
172. Burke AP et al. Healed plaque ruptures and sudden coronary death: evidence that subclinical rupture has a role in plaque progression. *Circulation*. 2001;103(7):934–940.
173. Roberts WC, Jones AA. Quantitation of coronary arterial narrowing at necropsy in sudden coronary death: analysis of 31 patients and comparison with 25 control subjects. *Am J Cardiol*. 1979;44(1):39–45.

Pathophysiology of Carotid Atherosclerosis

Heather A. Hall and Hisham S. Bassiouny

2.1 Introduction

Stroke continues to be a significant cause of morbidity and mortality throughout the world. According to the World Health Organization, 15 million people suffer stroke worldwide annually and of these, 5 million die, and another 5 million are permanently disabled. In the United States, about 795,000 people suffer from stroke, and 143,579 people die from stroke annually. In Canada, stroke accounted for 7% of all deaths in 2000, and in Europe, nearly 650,000 stroke deaths occur per year.[1–3] Approximately 85% of all strokes are ischemic, and though many are termed cryptogenic, at least 20% of ischemic strokes can be attributed to carotid bifurcation disease.[4,5]

Atherosclerosis is a systemic disease in which many factors have been implicated in its pathogenesis. These include hypertension, cigarette smoking, diabetes, hyperlipidemia, and hyperhomocysteinemia. The earliest report associating cervical carotid artery disease with stroke was by Savory in 1856, and similar case reports followed, reemphasizing the relationship between carotid artery occlusive disease and stroke.[6] The frequency of atherosclerotic plaque formation involving the extracranial carotid bifurcation at regions of flow division and low shear stress suggests that fluid dynamics and vessel geometry also play a key role in the inception of atherosclerotic plaque at such regions. Both in vitro and in vivo models have demonstrated this association between flow dynamics and localization of plaque formation.[7–10]

Current noninvasive imaging modalities allow for assessment of plaque structural morphology in addition to measuring degree of stenosis. These tools currently allow for detection of plaque formation as well as surveillance of plaque progression and composition and can identify vulnerable plaques potentially at risk for disruption and thromboembolic ischemic cerebral or retinal events.

2.2 Mechanisms of Atherogenesis

2.2.1 Anatomy of the Arterial Wall

Implicit in our understanding of carotid artery bifurcation atherosclerosis pathobiology is knowledge of the structural microanatomy of a normal artery wall. The response of an artery to injury, subsequent changes in the thickness and composition of the arterial wall, and its role in subsequent symptom causation can then be examined. The primary role of the carotid arterial system is to act as a nonthrombogenic conduit for blood flow to the brain and is inherently a highly responsive and adaptive organ.

As indicated in Chap. 1, the mural structure of the carotid artery is composed of three layers: the *tunica intima*, *tunica media*, and *tunica adventitia*. Each layer plays a specific and essential role in the overall function of the artery (Fig. 2.1).

The intima, or inner lining of the vessel directly adjacent to blood flow, is an extremely dynamic layer

H.A. Hall
Section of Vascular Surgery, University of Chicago, Chicago, IL, USA

H.S. Bassiouny (✉)
Department of Surgery, University of Chicago, Chicago, IL, USA

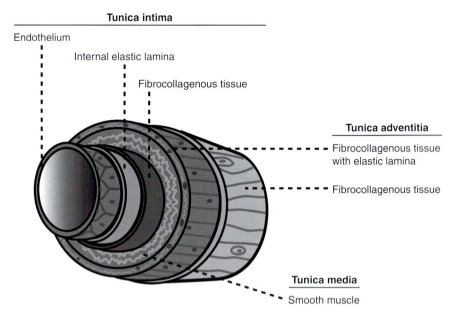

Fig. 2.1 Mural structure of the carotid artery (Illustration by Matthew Maday)

composed of a monolayer of endothelial cells. Endothelial cells have surface receptors interacting with blood proteins and molecules to regulate vascular permeability as well as playing a key role in platelet aggregation and resistance to thrombosis. The ability of the endothelial monolayer to repair itself and maintain function has a significant role in the development of atherosclerotic plaque. Beneath the intima lies a single layer of elastic fibers forming a matrix called the internal elastic lamina.

The media, or middle layer, is composed of an inner circumferential layer and an outer longitudinal layer of smooth muscle cells surrounded by a matrix of elastin, collagen, and proteoglycans.[11] The carotid artery is considered a muscular artery as it has a greater content of smooth muscle cells than central, elastic, arteries. Hemodynamic stresses applied to the wall of the artery as well as the effects of systemic inflammatory molecules impact the media in a way that alters the composition of this layer. Of note, pathologic changes seen in the composition and architecture of the media are largely secondary effects of intimal injury and repair. When the medial layer functions properly, it provides structure but is also important in maintaining vascular tone. In response to alteration in function of the intima, the media responds with proliferation of smooth muscle cells, as well as further promoting the migration of leukocytes and monocytes into this layer. Within the media layer, the derangements of cells and extracellular matrix initiate formation of the carotid plaque (Fig. 2.2).

Beneath the media lies another matrix of elastic fibers, the external elastic lamina, which underlies the adventitial, outer layer of the artery. This layer is remarkably strong, composed mostly of collagen as well as autonomic nerve fibers that extend into the media. While the intima relies on oxygen diffusion from the luminal blood supply, the media obtains oxygen necessary for its function by diffusion from the arterial lumen through the intima luminal blood supply, as well as the vasa vasorum that enter through the adventitial layer.

2.2.2 Response to Endothelial Damage and the Formation of Atherosclerotic Plaque

The term atherosclerosis comes from the Greek *athero*, meaning gruel, and *sclerosis*, meaning hardening. Atherosclerosis begins at the adluminal surface, at the interface between blood and the arterial wall. When physical or metabolic injury disrupts endothelial integrity, the endothelium transduces stress or strain into a biochemical signal. There is an alteration in expression of cellular adhesion molecules (such as VCAM-1 and ICAM) and other surface receptors and a resultant alteration in blood cell adhesion. This results in endothelial cytoskeletal rearrangement and an increase in cell permeability. A simplistic model of intimal disruption is an experimental balloon-injury model,[12] in which platelets adhere to the

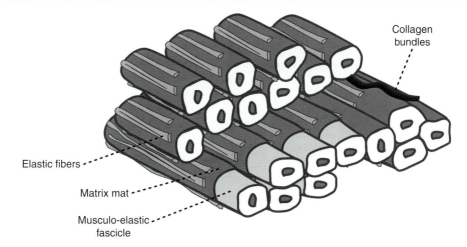

Fig. 2.2 Organization of cells and matrix fibers in the carotid artery. Each musculo-elastic fascicle contains a group of commonly oriented cells, invested by a matrix mat consisting of basal lamina and a meshwork of collagen fibrils, surrounded by a system of elastic fibers oriented in the same direction (Illustration by Matthew Maday)

disrupted intima and degranulate, releasing cytokines and growth factors which induce vascular smooth muscle cell proliferation and migration from the medial layer to the subintimal space resulting in the formation of a neointima. Factors released and contributing to smooth muscle cell proliferation include platelet-derived growth factor (PDGF), epidermal growth factor (EGF), and transforming growth factor beta (TGF-β).[13] In addition, the adhesiveness of platelets and subsequent degranulation results in the further recruitment of other inflammatory cells to the area of intimal damage.

As endothelial cell injury becomes more chronic, intimal cells become more permeable to circulating cells. The endothelial monolayer in conjunction with formerly circulating cells, now resident in the media layer, begins to secrete proinflammatory cytokines that participate in attracting various inflammatory cells (such as monocytes, T cells, and macrophages) into the subendothelial layer.[14,15] The smooth muscle cells of the underlying media respond to these local effects by proliferating, and in the milieu of the forming lesion, smooth muscle cells also begin to alter their function from a contractile to a synthetic phenotype. In addition, there is an alteration in extracellular matrix composition and organization. Macrophages, now within the media, begin to engulf surrounding lipids and become so-called lipid-laden macrophages.[16–18] While the initial intent of recruiting circulating cells and the subsequent inflammatory cascade is to heal local endothelial injury, repeated damage results in the formation of a fatty streak and the beginning of an atherosclerotic plaque.

This process begins early in life, and whether or not such early lesions progress to pathologic or even symptomatic lesions may be largely dependent on individual hemodynamic, metabolic, environmental, and genetic risk factors. Persistence of such risk factors perpetuates the inflammatory response and plaque progression. The arterial wall does not thicken after initial injury and smooth muscle cell proliferation, rather only after the smooth muscle cells migrate into the intima.[19] Propagation of the immune response within the wall of the artery, as well as altered smooth muscle cell function, leads to formation of a fibrous cap. Once the fibrous cap forms, the lesion is termed an atheroma, and may protrude into the arterial lumen causing a reduction in luminal diameter or cross-sectional area. An atheroma is an active lesion, producing cytokines and undergoing constant remodeling. Over time, smooth muscle cell proliferation continues, and the production of matrix metalloproteinases (MMPs) is altered such that increases in MMP-9 and MMP-2 remodel the artery and lead to dilation of the arterial segment.[20,21] This process initially dilates the artery enough to compensate for the luminal loss to plaque (Glagovian remodeling); however over time, this adaptive enlargement to developing plaque is self limited and fails to compensate for luminal loss once plaque occupies more than 40–50% of the cross-sectional area. Further plaque progression can lead to progressive focal arterial stenosis.

2.3 Hemodynamic Force Localization of Plaque at the Carotid Bifurcation

2.3.1 Wall Shear Stress and Other Forces on the Arterial Wall

Hemodynamic forces at the carotid bifurcation play a significant role in the localization of intimal thickening at predictable regions of the vessel wall. The magnitude and rate of change of blood flow at the luminal surface have been closely tied to the pathogenesis of atherosclerotic plaque formation. Laminar flow results in a gradient of fluid velocities as you move from the wall towards the center of a tube. Friction between fluid along the wall and the wall itself creates a tangential force exerted by flowing fluid on the wall of the tube, and this is referred to as "wall shear stress." The greater the velocity elevation, the greater the wall shear stress. Arterial segments with low and oscillatory wall shear stress appear to be atheroprone. In vivo and in vitro research has shown that disturbed flow and low shear conditions predispose to endothelial dysfunction[7–10,22] (Fig. 2.3).

Blood flow within a dynamic artery is certainly more complex than laminar flow through a rigid, strictly linear tube. Pulsatile flow due to the cardiac cycle creates what is referred to as "oscillatory shear stress." An arterial wall is also highly dynamic, and pulsatile flow alters its radius, shape, curvature, and length so that blood flow is not strictly laminar. In addition, when blood flow separates at an arterial bifurcation, there is a complex pattern of fluid velocities. The highest velocities at the center of flow come in contact with the flow divider, and flow separation occurs until some distance into the subsequent branches (Fig. 2.4).

2.3.2 Effect of Wall Shear Stress and Other Forces on Endothelial Function and Remodeling

The endothelial monolayer is highly responsive to changes in wall shear stress magnitude and direction. Physiologic variations of shear stress regulate immediate changes in vascular diameter and when sustained induce slow, adaptive, structural-wall remodeling.[21] These flow-induced forces may act independently of previous mentioned risk factors for atherosclerosis.[23] Changes occur in local concentrations of growth factors, biochemical pathways, gene expression, and cytoskeleton arrangements, and continued remodeling of the vessel wall takes place. Further changes in vessel geometry occur as a result of atheroma

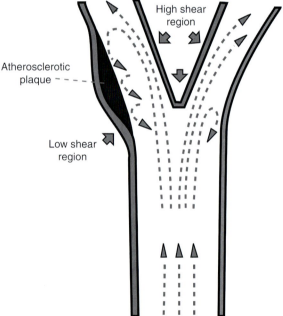

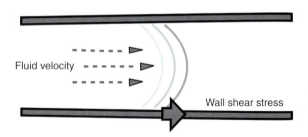

Fig. 2.3 Wall shear stress. Friction between fluid along the wall and the wall itself creates a tangential force exerted on the wall, and this is referred to as "wall shear stress" (Illustration by Matthew Maday)

Fig. 2.4 Wall shear stress with boundary layer separation. Blood flow near the center of the artery is laminar. Blood flow near the intima, referred to as the boundary layer, is slower and has more disturbed currents. This is referred to as boundary layer separation. The areas of lower shear force ($< 4\,\text{dyn/cm}^2$) have been found to induce endothelial injury and are, as demonstrated at the carotid bifurcation, typically found on the outer walls at arterial branch points (Illustration by Matthew Maday)

formation, and further modify local near wall shear stress direction, oscillation, and magnitude.

It has long been hypothesized that functional alterations in the endothelial monolayer occur as a result of low wall shear stress and increased residence time of atherogenic blood particles.[24] Wall shear stress induces changes in endothelial cell morphology and spatial orientation. Increased wall shear stress causes endothelial cells to elongate and align in the direction of flow, whereas endothelial cells exposed to low wall shear stress remain more rounded and have no preferred orientation.[25,26] Low wall shear stress may also increase intercellular permeability and consequently increase the vulnerability of these regions of the vessel to atherosclerosis.[27]

Shear stress not only affects the shape and orientation of the cell, but alters the cell's production and release of vasoactive substances (i.e., prostacyclin, nitric oxide, and endothelin-1). An acute increase in wall shear stress in vitro elicits rapid cytoskeletal remodeling and activates a signaling cascade in endothelial cells, with the consequent acute release of endothelial-derived relaxing factor (EDRF), i.e., nitric oxide and prostacyclin.[28] Nitric oxide in particular appears to be a key mediator in the atheroprotective effect of high wall shear stress.[29] High laminar shear stress sharply reduces endothelial cell levels of precursor preproendothelin mRNA. This decreases the level of endothelin-1 peptide, which exerts a constricting and mitogenic effect on vascular smooth muscle cells.[30] Finally, prolonged oscillatory shear stress induces expression of endothelial leukocyte adhesion molecules, which are important in mediating leukocyte localization in the arterial wall.[31]

In summary, high wall shear stress influences the orientation of endothelial cells and the subsequent production and release of factors that inhibit coagulation, permit migration of leukocytes, and induce smooth muscle proliferation, while simultaneously promoting endothelial cell survival. Conversely, low wall shear stress shifts the profile of secreted factors and expressed surface molecules to one that favors the opposite effects, thereby contributing to the development of atherosclerosis.[27] This complex endothelial cell response to shear stress may also provide a mechanism by which known risk factors act to promote atherosclerosis.[30] In regions of moderate to high shear stress, where flow remains unidirectional and axially aligned, intimal thickening is limited. Intimal thickening and atherosclerosis develop largely in regions of relatively low wall shear stress, flow separation, and departure from axially aligned, unidirectional flow. Wall shear stress mapping has the potential to become part of the multifactorial, multidisciplinary approach to early atherosclerosis detection, and following plaque progression.

2.4 Progression of Carotid Bifurcation Atherosclerosis

Focal endothelial dysfunction and the formation of fatty streaks within human arterial walls begin at a young age. Many factors influence whether a plaque will continue to grow and develop, become quiescent, rupture, or thrombose. The composition of a plaque and the ongoing presence of physical and biochemical stress influence plaque vulnerability to disruption. The interaction of the flow forces with plaque structural components, such as hard or soft regions, will determine the degree in biomechanical stress on the fibrous cap and likelihood of its structural failure, notwithstanding the role of MMP's in influencing the structural integrity of the fibrous cap extracellular matrix.

The composition and heterogeneity of atherosclerotic plaque influences progression by virtue of ongoing remodeling of the arterial wall.[32] Modeling has shown that stress distribution and magnitude are influenced by the shape and the composition of the fibrous plaque.[33] In addition, vulnerable plaques become more susceptible to rupture as the fibrous cap thins with remodeling of the extracellular matrix by metalloproteinases (MMPs) secreted by leukocytes within the intima.[34,35] The inflammatory response in the juxtaluminal fibrous cap and necrotic core is a key mechanism in human atherosclerotic plaque vulnerability.[36] In vulnerable atherosclerotic plaques, the fibrous cap thins out and is more likely to disrupt, resulting in thromboembolic events and cerebrovascular ischemia.[37]

Inflammation is a key element of atherosclerotic plaque vulnerability and disruption, and fibrous cap inflammation is more likely to occur in noncalcified plaques as compared to calcified plaques, indicating that plaque calcification is a marker of stability.[38] Symptomatic plaques are less calcified and more inflamed than asymptomatic plaques.[39]

2.4.1 How to Assess Carotid Stenosis

2.4.1.1 Arteriography

Arteriography is still considered the "gold standard" for diagnosing carotid artery luminal stenosis against which all other imaging modalities are compared. With defined risks inherent in angiography, there is a perpetual move toward noninvasive evaluation. This shift culminated in investigations by Strandness at the University of Washington, with criteria for estimating carotid stenosis using velocity measurements obtained by duplex ultrasound.[40] Criteria for carotid stenosis, intervention, and outcomes have been validated in several large trials including the North American Symptomatic Carotid Endarterectomy Trial (NASCET),[41] European Carotid Surgery Trial (ECST),[42] and the Asymptomatic Carotid Atherosclerosis Trial (ACAS).[43] These trials are the basis of current indications for surgical intervention in patients with carotid stenosis. However, it must be mentioned that the data remain marginal for surgical intervention on patients with asymptomatic plaques, given that the number needed to treat is at least 20 patients to prevent one stroke in 5 years.[43] It has become clear that stenosis alone is not sufficient to predict which asymptomatic plaques will progress to become symptomatic. Plaque morphology and histobiochemical analysis have emerged as additional factors in assessing plaque at risk. Imaging modalities that remain central to the evaluation of carotid artery disease include angiography, duplex ultrasound, computed tomography angiography (CTA), and magnetic resonance angiography (MRA). Further refinements in these imaging modalities have further altered the data obtainable from each exam. Newer ways of evaluating carotid plaque structural characteristics continue to evolve and allow for identification of features such as extensive necrosis, fibrous cap thinning, and intraplaque hemorrhage. These plaque characteristics connote vulnerability and propensity to embolization, transient ischemic attack (TIA), and stroke.

2.4.1.2 Duplex Ultrasound

Duplex ultrasound has become the screening and diagnostic imaging modality of choice in carotid occlusive disease largely because of its low cost, accuracy, and noninvasiveness. Early studies have arrived at velocity criteria for the diagnosis and classification of carotid disease, and the most widely used in the 1980s and 1990s have been those developed by Strandness and Zweibel[40,44,45] (Table 2.1). It should be pointed out that the early velocity criteria were developed for stenosis expressed as a percentage of the bulb diameter based on microcalcification on the arterial wall as seen on angiograms and using mechanically rotating transducers. It should also be noted that with modern linear array transducers spectral broadening cannot be used as a criterion. A recent meta-analysis showed that ultrasound was best for more critical lesions, those at least 70% or greater, with a sensitivity of 89% and specificity of 84%. Examination of lesions between 50% and 69% using velocity criteria yielded a sensitivity of only 36% and a specificity of 91%.[46] Using arteriography as the gold standard, the Strandness criteria are less reliable in patients with contralateral occlusion, high-grade contralateral stenosis, or less than 70% ipsilateral stenosis.[47] However, for plaques producing moderate or mild stenosis B-mode combined with color flow in cross-sectional views provide accurate measurements of lumen and vessel diameters from which the percentage diameter stenosis can be calculated (see Chap. 28).

An analysis of the Strandness criteria for ICA stenosis (European Carotid Surgery Trial [ECST] method, i.e., in relation to bulb diameter) conducted at the University of Chicago correlated ultrasonographic velocity measurements with CT angiogram measurements. The rationale for the study was to better outline the boundary of the ICA plaque by CT rather than using an estimated line as was done with angiography in developing the Strandness criteria when microcalcification in the arterial wall was not present. The optimal threshold velocity to identify at least a 50% stenosis of the ICA were a PSV of 155 cm/s and an internal carotid artery/common carotid artery (ICA/CCA) ratio of at least two.[38] Velocity criteria for a stenosis of at least 80% were found to be peak systolic velocity (PSV) >370 cm/s, end diastolic velocity (EDV) >140 cm/s, and an ICA/CCA ratio of at least 6.0.[38]

A full description of currently used techniques for grading internal carotid stenosis will be found in Chap. 28.

2.4.1.3 Computed Tomography (CT)

The advancement of high-resolution multidetector CT (MDCT) has allowed CT angiography to be performed to evaluate the carotid bifurcation in a noninvasive

Table 2.1 Summary of the Strandness and Zweibel duplex criteria for ICA stenosis

Strandness Stenosis (%) in relation to bulb diameter	Duplex findings	Zweibel Stenosis (%) in relation to distal ICA diameter	Duplex findings
0	PSV < 125 cm/s No spectral broadening Bulb flow reversal	0	PSV < 110 cm/s EDV < 40 cm/s PSV ICA/CCA <1.8 EDV ICA/CCA <2.4 Spectral broadening < 30 cm/s
1–15	PSV < 125 cm/s No or minimal spectral broadening Bulb flow reversal absent	1–39	PSV < 110 cm/s EDV < 40 cm/s PSV ICA/CCA <1.8 EDV ICA/CCA <2.4 Spectral broadening < 40 cm/s
16–49	PSV > 125 cm/s Marked spectral broadening	40–59	PSV < 130 cm/s EDV < 40 cm/s PSV ICA/CCA <1.8 EDV ICA/CCA <2.4 Spectral broadening < 40 cm/s
50–79	PSV > 125 cm/s EDV < 140 cm/s	60–79	PSV > 130 cm/s EDV > 40 cm/s PSV ICA/CCA >1.8 EDV ICA/CCA >2.4 Spectral broadening > 40 cm/s
80–99	PSV > 125 cm/s EDV > 140 cm/s	80–99	PSV > 250 cm/s EDV > 100 cm/s PSV ICA/CCA >3.7 EDV ICA/CCA >5.5 Spectral broadening > 80 cm/s
100	No flow	100	No flow

fashion. Early studies evaluating this technology were performed with single-slice scanners at a time when resolution was inferior. Currently, however, high-resolution CT scanners can not only evaluate the presence and degree of stenosis but also offer further information regarding plaque morphology and composition. Cinat published a study of eight patients and found a 72.6% agreement between CT assessment of plaque composition and histological examination, and a higher degree of calcification within the plaque improved sensitivity to near 100%.[48] Conversely, noncalcified components such as necrotic core, lipid volume, intraplaque hemorrhage, and connective tissue confound the ability of CT to accurately determine plaque histopathology. Further studies with larger sample sizes looking at MDCT evaluation of plaque composition may contribute to our understanding of assessing overall plaque risk.

2.4.1.4 Magnetic Resonance Imaging (MRI)

It has been shown that MRI is useful to accurately evaluate plaque size and composition and can thus aid in identifying vulnerable plaques. A study by Takaya et al. prospectively followed 154 patients with initially asymptomatic carotid stenosis by ultrasound for a mean of 38.2 months. MRI was also performed at baseline. Among this group of asymptomatic patients, MRI plaque characteristics including a thin or ruptured fibrous cap, intraplaque hemorrhage, larger lipid-rich necrotic core, and larger maximum wall thickness were all associated with subsequent cerebrovascular events.[49] This was a small study but does lay the groundwork for larger prospective studies to examine the role of MRI in identifying atherosclerotic plaques at higher risk of causing ischemic events. Although MRI avoids the use of ionizing radiation, the disadvantages associated with this imaging

Table 2.2 Different types of human atherosclerotic lesions in pathology

Type	Terms for atherosclerotic lesions in histological classifications	Appearance of lesions often based on the unaided eye	
I	Initial lesion		Early lesions
IIa	Progression-prone type II lesion	Fatty dot or streak	
IIb	Progression-resistant type II		
III	Intermediate lesion (preatheroma)		
IV	Atheroma	Atheromatous plaque	
Va	Fibroatheroma (type V lesion)	Fibrolipid plaque, Fibrous plaque, plaque	
Vb	Calcific lesion (type VII lesion)	Calcified plaque	Advanced lesions
Vc	Fibrotic lesion (type VIII lesion)	Fibrous plaque	Raised lesions
VI	Lesion with surface defect, and/or hematoma-hemorrhage, and/or thrombotic deposit	Complicated lesion, complicated plaque	

Source: Adapted from Stary et al.[51]
Note: Type I to type Va are early, type Vb advanced, and type Vc and VI are raised lesions

modality make its usefulness in imaging the carotid bifurcation limited in some patients. Long scanning times increase overall motion artifact, and the risk of gadolinium-induced nephrogenic systemic fibrosis can occur in up to 3% of patients with renal insufficiency.[50]

2.4.1.5 Histopathology

Advancements in current imaging modalities are allowing more detailed assessment of carotid plaque characteristics in vivo. Numerous studies are attempting to standardize in vivo appearance on imaging to ex vivo histology evaluation. The American Heart Association has published various reports including one by the Committee on Vascular Lesions of the Council on Arteriosclerosis that defines and classifies advanced types of atherosclerotic lesions based on histology[51] [Chap. 1]. The Committee on Vascular Lesions also attempted to correlate the appearance of lesions on clinical imaging studies with histological lesion types (Table 2.2). Correlation of images to ex vivo plaque is helping advance our understanding of plaque morphology and vulnerability.

2.5 Stroke and Carotid Bifurcation Atherosclerosis

2.5.1 Historical Perspective

One of the earliest reports linking stroke and carotid artery disease was made by Savory in 1856 who reported a case of a young woman with left monocular symptoms and right hemiplegia attributed to occlusion of the left cervical internal carotid artery and bilateral subclavian arteries found at autopsy.[6] Gowers in 1875 also described left carotid artery occlusion in a patient with a right hemiplegia and loss of sight in the left eye.[52] Subsequent case reports increasingly linked carotid artery occlusive disease to the development of neurological symptoms, namely, stroke and transient ischemic attacks.[53] In a major leap forward, Edgar Moniz developed cerebral angiography in 1927, and in 1937, he described internal carotid occlusion as documented by angiography.[54,55] Even today, arteriography of the carotid artery and its branches remains the gold standard to which newer imaging modalities are compared.

In 1951, Dr. Fisher published a landmark paper in the history of carotid artery disease in which he described occlusion of the extracranial carotid artery and its relation to cerebrovascular disease.[56] This included the first description of transient hemispheric attack and monocular vision loss (now termed amaurosis fugax) as attributable to carotid disease and as potential precursors of stroke. Prior to this, some 55% of strokes were attributed to vasospasm. The idea of a carotid bruit as an indicator of underlying carotid disease, and its use as a screening tool for diagnosis was also described by Fisher in 1957.[57] Dr. Fisher commented in his 1951 paper… "Some day vascular surgery will find a way to by-pass the occluded portion of the internal carotid artery during the period of ominous fleeting symptoms."[56] Today, it is well accepted that carotid artery occlusive disease is a risk factor for transient ischemic attack (TIA) and stroke, and medical disease modification as well as surgical intervention, carotid endarterectomy, for carotid disease have been shown to provide benefit in reducing the risk of stroke and stroke-related death.

The first successful carotid reconstruction was completed by Carrea in Argentina in 1951, on a 51-year-old man who presented with right hemiplegia and left eye blindness. The patient was diagnosed with severe left internal carotid artery stenosis on a percutaneous carotid angiogram. The stenotic segment of the internal carotid artery was resected, and an end-to-end anastomosis was performed between the external carotid and the distal internal carotid artery. Patency was confirmed by angiogram and the patient regained strength in his right side over time.[58] Reports of similar operations were reported by others in the coming decade including Eastcott in 1954.[59] Based on the idea of endarterectomy introduced by Cid dos Santos in 1947 for aortoiliac atherosclerosis,[60] the first carotid endarterectomy was performed in 1953 by Strully, Hurwitt, and Blankenberg on a patient 2 weeks after the patient had a stroke. There was no back-bleeding from the distal ICA however, and the vessel was ligated.[61] The first successful carotid endarterectomy was performed by DeBakey in 1952, though that particular case was not published until 1975.[62] Carotid endarterectomy was performed by Cooley, Al-Naaman, and Carton in 1956 and was the first to be published in the literature.[63] During this time, other studies showed improvement in patients given anticoagulants for cerebral thrombosis.[64–66] The story continues with improvement in medical prevention and treatment of atherosclerotic disease and the current debate over the use of carotid endarterectomy versus carotid artery stenting in the interventional treatment of both symptomatic and asymptomatic carotid artery disease.

2.6 Role of Imaging in Identifying the Vulnerable Asymptomatic Plaque

Stenosis of the carotid artery is noninvasively assessed with duplex ultrasound, as well as by CT-angiography or MR-angiography. However, despite large trials and refinement of criteria, stenosis alone is inadequate in predicting which asymptomatic plaques are at risk for causing cerebrovascular symptoms. Recently, additional data garnered from standard imaging modalities has been investigated to help identify those plaques at risk for causing cerebrovascular symptoms. The development of high-resolution B-mode ultrasound has improved the ability of duplex scanning to evaluate not only severity of stenosis but also morphology of the plaque. Candidate descriptors of carotid plaque morphology include echolucency, calcification, and intraplaque hemorrhage, as well as other characteristics such as plaque volume, surface irregularity, fibrous cap thickness, and the size and location of the necrotic core. Assessing additional plaque features via ultrasound is important for the stratification of high-risk patients.[67,68]

2.6.1 Echolucency/Gray Scale Median

Carotid atherosclerosis with echolucent plaque is closely related to the occurrence of cerebrovascular events.[69,70] The more echolucent a plaque on ultrasound, the more likely it is to cause TIA or stroke in the future. Initially, plaque echolucency was subjective and qualitative, thus making it difficult to correlate and attribute risk.[71–74] Echolucency has been further defined and quantified using the method of image normalization and measurement of the gray scale median (GSM). GSM is a computer-quantified measurement of plaque echolucency,[75–77] and several studies have shown a correlation between low GSM and plaque instability [78–80]; (Chaps. 12, 15, 24, 29, 33, 36, 37).

2.6.2 Calcification

Calcification is a relatively common structural feature of the atherosclerotic plaque and is enhanced with advanced age, chronic renal failure, diabetes, and inflammation[81] (Chap. 1). Calcified atherosclerotic plaques are less prone to disrupt and result in symptoms than noncalcified plaques.[82] This implies that calcification imparts structural stability to the fibrous cap.[38] A study of patients undergoing carotid endarterectomy (CEA) found that those patients with calcified carotid plaques had fewer cerebrovascular events than those with noncalcified plaques.[83] Grogan et al. showed that using B-mode ultrasound, symptomatic plaques are more echolucent and less calcified than asymptomatic plaques and are associated with a greater degree of histopathologic plaque necrosis.[84] Calcification, however, is not a normal feature of the aging process, but a dynamic process in the progression of atherosclerosis.[85,86] It is a result of a complex interplay between inflammatory cytokines and the activation of bone building cells.[87]

The presence and degree of carotid plaque calcification can be accurately quantified with ex vivo CT and is inversely related to plaque macrophage infiltration and symptomatic outcome.[39] In vivo quantitative assessment of carotid plaque calcification may help in the future to identify patients with asymptomatic but vulnerable carotid plaques who are at risk for development of cerebrovascular events and benefit from carotid interventions.

2.6.3 Intraplaque Hemorrhage

Intraplaque hemorrhage is a plaque characteristic thought to correlate with symptomatology. The American Heart Association Type VI plaque is characterized by surface irregularity, intraplaque hemorrhage, or thrombus, and is designated as a complicated plaque. Although there is some controversy over whether intraplaque hemorrhage alone is a predictor of future ischemic events, it is a marker of plaque inflammation and instability. A study by Hatsukami et al. looked at 43 plaques from both symptomatic and asymptomatic patients undergoing carotid endarterectomy for highly stenotic lesions and compared histologic findings to preoperative images.[73] In this study, they found no difference between symptomatic and asymptomatic patients with regard to the presence or volume of intraplaque hemorrhage, nor did they see a difference in calcification, fibrous intimal tissue, lipid core, or necrotic core. These findings show a limited use for intraplaque hemorrhage alone as a surrogate for plaque vulnerability. On the contrary, other studies utilizing either ultrasonography or MRI to detect intraplaque hemorrhage have indeed shown intraplaque hemorrhage to be a plaque characteristic that is predictive of cerebrovascular events.[88,89]

References

1. Centers of Disease Control and Prevention [homepage on the Internet]. Atlanta: Centers of Disease Control and Prevention; [cited 2010 Mar 17]. Available from: http://www.cdc.gov/
2. Roger VL et al. Heart disease and stroke statistics – 2010 update: a report from the American Heart Association. *Circulation*. 2010;121(7):e46–e215.
3. Heart and Stroke Foundation of Canada. *The Growing Burden of Heart Disease and Stroke in Canada 2003*. Ottawa: Heart and Stroke Foundation of Canada; 2003.
4. Donnan GA, Fisher M, Macleod M, Davis SM. Stroke. *Lancet*. 2008;371(9624):12–23.
5. Chaturvedi S et al. Carotid endarterectomy – an evidence-based review: report of the Therapeutics and Technology Assessment Subcommittee of the American Academy of Neurology. *Neurology*. 2005;65:794–801.
6. Savory WS. Case of a young woman in whom the main arteries of both upper extremities and of the left side of the neck were throughout completely obliterated. *Med Chir Trans Lond*. 1856;39:205–219.
7. Caro CG, Fitz-Gerald JM, Schroter RC. Arterial wall shear stress and distribution of early atheroma in man. *Nature*. 1969;223:1159–1161.
8. Friedman MH, Hutchins GM, Bargeron CB, Deters OJ, Mark FF. Correlation between intimal thickness and fluid shear in human arteries. *Atherosclerosis*. 1981;39:425–436.
9. Ku DN, Giddens DP, Zarins CK, Glagov S. Pulsatile flow and atherosclerosis in the human carotid bifurcation: positive correlation between plaque location and low and oscillating shear stress. *Arteriosclerosis*. 1985;5:293–302.
10. Zarins CK et al. Carotid bifurcation atherosclerosis: quantitative correlation of plaque localization with flow velocity profiles and wall shear stress. *Circ Res*. 1983;53:502–514.
11. Clark J, Glagov S. Transmural organization of the arterial wall. The lamellar unit revisted. *Arteriosclerosis*. 1985;5:19–34.
12. Baumgartner HR, Studer A. Consequences of vessel catheterization in normal and hypercholesterolemic rabbits. *Pathol Microbiol*. 1966;29:393–405.
13. Bowen-Pope DF, Ross R, Seifert RA. Locally acting growth factors for vascular smooth muscle cells: endogenous synthesis and release from platelets. *Circulation*. 1985;72:735–740.

14. Faggiotto A, Ross R, Harker L. Studies of hypercholesterolemia in the nonhuman primate. *Arteriosclerosis*. 1984;4:323–340.
15. Gerrity RG, Naito HK, Richardson M, Schwartz CJ. Dietary induced atherogenesis in swine. *Am J Pathol*. 1979;95:775–792.
16. Fowler S, Shio H, Haley WJ. Characterization of lipid-laden aortic cells from cholesterol-fed rabbits. IV. Investigation of macrophage-like properties of aortic cell populations. *Lab Invest*. 1979;41:372–378.
17. Schaffner T et al. Arterial foam cells with distinctive immunomorphologic and histochemical features of macrophages. *Am J Pathol*. 1980;100:57–80.
18. Haberland ME, Fong D, Cheng L. Malondialdehyde-altered protein occurs in atheroma of Watanabe heritable hyperlipidemic rabbits. *Science*. 1988;241:215–218.
19. Clowes AW, Ryan GB, Breslow JL, Karnovsky MJ. Absence of enhanced intimal thickening in the response of the carotid arterial wall to endothelial injury in hypercholesterolemic rats. *Lab Invest*. 1976;35(1):6–17.
20. Godin D, Ivan E, Johnson C, Magid R, Galis Z. Remodeling of carotid artery is associated with increased expression of matrix metalloproteinases in mouse blood flow cessation model. *Circulation*. 2000;102:2861–2866.
21. Glagov S. Intimal hyperplasia, vascular remodeling, and the restenosis problem. *Circulation*. 1994;89:2888–2891.
22. Lind L, Andersson J, Larsson A, Sandhagen B. Shear stress in the common carotid artery is related to both intima-media thickness and echogenecity. The Prospective Investigation of the Vasculature in Uppsala Seniors study. *Clin Hemorheol Microcirc*. 2009;43(4):299–308.
23. Gibson CM et al. Relationship of vessel wall shear stress to atherosclerosis progression in human coronary arteries. *Arterioscler Thromb*. 1993;13:310–315.
24. Glagov S, Zarins C, Giddens DP, Ku DN. Hemodynamics and atherosclerosis: insights and perspectives gained from studies of human arteries. *Arch Pathol Lab Med*. 1988;112:1018–1031.
25. Levesque MJ, Nerem RM. The elongation and orientation of cultured endothelial cells in response to shear stress. *J Biomech Eng*. 1985;107:341–347.
26. Levesque MJ, Liepsch D, Moravec S, Nerem RM. Correlation of endothelial cell shape and wall shear stress in a stenosed dog aorta. *Arteriosclerosis*. 1986;6:220–229.
27. Okano M, Yoshida Y. Junction complexes of endothelial cells in atherosclerosis-prone and atherosclerosis-resistant regions on flow dividers of brachiocephalic bifurcations in the rabbit aorta. *Biorheology*. 1994;31:155–161.
28. Ballermann BJ, Dardik A, Eng E, Liu A. Shear stress and the endothelium. *Kidney Int Suppl*. 1998;67:S100-S108.
29. Traub O, Berk BC. Laminar shear stress: mechanisms by which endothelial cells transduce an atheroprotective force. *Arterioscler Thromb Vasc Biol*. 1988;18:677–685.
30. Sharefkin JB, Diamond SL, Eskin SG, McIntire LV, Dieffenbach CW. Fluid flow decreases preproendothelin mRNA and suppresses endothelin-1 peptide release in cultured human endothelial cells. *J Vasc Surg*. 1991;14:1–9.
31. Chappell DC, Varner SE, Nerem RM, Medford RM, Alexander RW. Oscillatory shear stress stimulates adhesion molecule expression in cultured human endothelium. *Circ Res*. 1998;82:532–539.
32. Glagov S, Bassiouny HS, Giddens DR, Zarins CK. Intimal thickening: morphogenesis, functional significance and detection. *J Vasc Invest*. 1995;1:1–14.
33. Beattie D, Xu C, Vito R, Glagov S, Whang MC. Mechanical analysis of heterogeneous, atherosclerotic human aorta. *Trans ASME*. 1998;120:602–607.
34. Welgus HG et al. Neutral metalloproteinases produced by human mononuclear phagocytes. Enzyme profile, regulation, and expression during cellular development. *J Clin Invest*. 1990;86(5):1496–1502.
35. Galis ZS, Sukhova GK, Lark MW, Libby P. Increased expression of matrix metalloproteinases and matrix degrading activity in vulnerable regions of human atherosclerotic plaques. *J Clin Invest*. 1994;94(6):2493–2503.
36. Ross R. Atherosclerosis – an inflammatory disease. *N Engl J Med*. 1999;340:115–126.
37. Naghavi M et al. From vulnerable plaque to vulnerable patient: a call for new definitions and risk assessment strategies – part I. *Circulation*. 2003;108:1664–1672.
38. Wahlgren CM, Zheng W, Shaalan W, Tang J, Bassiouny HS. Human carotid plaque calcification and vulnerability. Relationship between degree of plaque calcification, fibrous cap inflammatory gene expression and symptomatology. *Cerebrovasc Dis*. 2009;27:193–200.
39. Shaalan WE et al. Degree of carotid plaque calcification in relation to symptomatic outcome and plaque inflammation. *J Vasc Surg*. 2004;40:262–269.
40. Strandness D Jr. Extracranial arterial disease. In: Duplex Scanning in Vascular Disorders. 2nd ed. New York: Raven; 1993.
41. North American Symptomatic Carotid Endarterectomy Trial Collaborators. Beneficial effect of carotid endarterectomy in symptomatic patients with high-grade carotid stenosis. *N Engl J Med*. 1991;325(7):445–453.
42. European Carotid Surgery Trialists' Collaborative Group. MRC European Carotid Surgery Trial: interim results for symptomatic patients with severe (70-99%) or with mild (0-29%) carotid stenosis. *Lancet*. 1991;337(8752):1235–1243.
43. The Asymptomatic Carotid Atherosclerosis Study Group. Study design for randomized prospective trial of carotid endarterectomy for asymptomatic atherosclerosis. *Stroke*. 1989;20(7):844–849.
44. Zwiebel WJ. Spectrum analysis in carotid sonography. *Ultrasound Med Biol*. 1987;13(10):625–636.
45. Zwiebel WJ. *Introduction to Vascular Ultrasonography*. Philadelphia: W.B. Saunders; 1992.
46. Wardlaw JM, Chappell FM, Best JJ, Wartolowska K, Berry E. Non-invasive imaging compared with intra-arterial angiography in the diagnosis of symptomatic carotid stenosis: a meta-analysis. *Lancet*. 2006;367(9521):1503–1512.
47. AbuRahma AF et al. Effect of contralateral severe stenosis or carotid occlusion on duplex criteria of ipsilateral stenoses: comparative study of various duplex parameters. *J Vasc Surg*. 1995;22(6):751–761.
48. Cinat M et al. Helical CT angiography in the preoperative evaluation of carotid artery stenosis. *J Vasc Surg*. 1998;28:290–300.

49. Takaya N et al. Association between carotid plaque characteristics and subsequent ischemic cerebrovascular events. A prospective assessment with MRI – initial results. *Stroke*. 2006;37:818–823.
50. Issa N et al. Nephrogenic systemic fibrosis and its association with gadolinium exposure during MRI. *Cleve Clin J Med*. 2008;75:95-97. 103-4, 106 passim.
51. Stary HC et al. A definition of advanced types of atherosclerotic lesions and a histologic classification of atherosclerosis, a report from the committee on vascular lesions of the Council on Arteriosclerosis, American Heart Association. *Circulation*. 1995;92:1355–1374.
52. Gowers W. On a case of simultaneous embolism of central retinal and middle cerebral arteries. *Lancet*. 1875;2:794.
53. Hunt JR. The role of the carotid arteries, in the causation of vascular lesions of the brain, with remarks on certain special features of the sympomatology. *Am J Med Sci*. 1914;147(5):704–712.
54. Moniz E. L'encephalographie arterielle, son importance dans la localisation des tumeurs cerebrales. *Rev Neurol (Paris)*. 1927;2:72-90. [Translated from the French by Espinosa RE and reprinted in: Bruwer AJ. Classic descriptions in diagnostic roentgenology. Springfield: Charles C. Thomas; 1964.]
55. Moniz E, Lima A, de Lacerda R. Par thrombose de la carotide interne. *Presse Med*. 1937;45:977–980.
56. Fisher CM. Occlusion of the internal carotid artery. *Arch Neurol Psychiatry*. 1951;65:346–377.
57. Fisher CM. Cranial bruit associated with occlusion of the internal carotid artery. *Neurology*. 1957;7:299–306.
58. Carrea R, Molins M, Murphy G. Surgical treatment of spontaneous thrombosis of the internal carotid artery in the neck: carotid carotideal anastamosis. *Acta Neurol Latinoam*. 1955;1:71–78.
59. Eastcott HHG, Pickering GW, Robb CG. Reconstruction of internal carotid artery in a patient with intermittent attacks of heiplegia. *Lancet*. 1954;2:994–996.
60. dos Santos JC. Sur la deobstruction des thromboses arterielles anciennes. *Mem Acad Chir*. 1947;73:409–411.
61. Strully KJ, Hurwitt ES, Blankenberg HW. Thromboendarterectomy for thrombosis of the internal carotid artery in the neck. *J Neurosurg*. 1953;10:474–482.
62. DeBakey ME. Successful carotid endarterectomy for cerebrovascular insufficiency; nineteen year follow-up. *JAMA*. 1975;233:1083–1085.
63. Cooley DA, Al-Naaman YD, Carton CA. Surgical treatment of arteriosclerotic occlusion of common carotid artery. *J Neurosurg*. 1956;13:500–506.
64. Hedenius P. The use of heparin in internal diseases. *Acta Med Scand*. 1941;107:170–182.
65. Millikan CH, Siekert RG, Shick RM. Studies in cerebrovascular disease, III: the use of anticoagulant drugs in the treatment of insufficiency or thrombosis within the basilar arterial system. *Proc Staff Meet Mayo Clin*. 1955;30:116–126.
66. Fisher CM. The use of anticoagulants in cerebral thrombosis. *Neurology*. 1958;8:311–332.
67. Grønholdt ML, Nordestgaard BG, Schroeder TV, Vorstrup S, Sillesen H. Ultrasonic echolucent carotid plaques predict future strokes. *Circulation*. 2001;104:68–73.
68. Hennerici M, Baezner H, Daffertshofer M. Ultrasound and arterial disease. *Cerebrovasc Dis*. 2004;17(suppl 1):19–33.
69. Polak JF et al. Hypoechoic plaque at US of the carotid artery: an independent risk factor for incident stroke in adults aged 65 years or older. *Radiology*. 1998;208:649–654.
70. Mathiesen EB, Bønaa KH, Joakimsen O. Echolucent plaques are associated with high risk of ischemic cerebrovascular events in carotid stenosis: the Tromsø study. *Circulation*. 2001;103:2171–2175.
71. Bassiouny HS et al. Juxtalumenal location of plaque necrosis and neoformation in symptomatic carotid stenosis. *J Vasc Surg*. 1997;26:585–594.
72. Gray-Weale AC, Graham JC, Burnett JR, Byrne K, Lusby RJ. Carotid artery atheroma: comparison of preoperative B-mode ultrasound appearance with carotid endarterectomy specimen pathology. *J Cardiovasc Surg (Torino)*. 1988;29:676–681.
73. Hatsukami TS et al. Carotid plaque morphology and clinical events. *Stroke*. 1997;28:95–100.
74. Carr S, Farb A, Pearce WH, Virmani R, Yao JS. Atherosclerotic plaque rupture in symptomatic carotid artery stenosis. *J Vasc Surg*. 1996;23:755–765.
75. el Barghouty N, Nicolaides A, Bahal V, Geroulakos G, Androulakis A. The identification of the high risk carotid plaque. *Eur J Vasc Endovasc Surg*. 1996;11:470–478.
76. Sabetai MM et al. Reproducibility of computer-quantified carotid plaque echogenicity. Can we overcome the subjectivity? *Stroke*. 2000;31:2189–2196.
77. Lal BK et al. Pixel distribution analysis of B-mode ultrasound scan images predicts histologic features of atherosclerotic carotid plaques. *J Vasc Surg*. 2002;35:1210–1217.
78. Tegos TJ et al. Echomorphologic and histopathologic characteristics of unstable carotid plaques. *Am J Neuroradiol*. 2000;21:1937–1944.
79. Grønholdt MLM, Nordestgaard BG, Wiebe BM, Wilhjelm JE, Sillesen H. Echo-lucency of computerized ultrasound images of carotid atherosclerotic plaques are associated with increased levels of triglyceride-rich lipoproteins as well as increased plaque lipid content. *Circulation*. 1998;97:34–40.
80. Sabetai MM et al. Hemispheric symptoms and carotid plaque echomorphology. *J Vasc Surg*. 2000;31:39S-49S.
81. Pecovnik-Balon B. Cardiovascular calcification in patients with end-stage renal disease. *Ther Apher Dial*. 2005;9:208–210.
82. Nandalur KR et al. Calcified carotid atherosclerotic plaque is associated less with ischemic symptoms than is noncalcified plaque on MDCT. *AJR Am J Roentgenol*. 2005;184:295–298.
83. Hunt JL et al. Bone formation in carotid plaques: a clinicopathalogiccal study. *Stroke*. 2002;33:1214–1219.
84. Grogan JK et al. B-mode ultrasonographic characterization of carotid atherosclerotic plaques in symptomatic and asymptomatic patients. *J Vasc Surg*. 2005;42:435–441.
85. Doherty TM, Detrano RC. Coronary arterial calcification as an active process: a new perspective on an old problem. *Calcif Tissue Int*. 1994;54:224–230.
86. Wexler L et al. Coronary artery calcification: pathophysiology, epidemiology, imaging methods, and clinical implications – a statement for health professionals from the

American Heart Association Writing Group. *Circulation.* 1996;94:1175–1192.
87. Doherty TM et al. Calcification in atherosclerosis: bone biology and chronic inflammation at the arterial crossroads. *Proc Natl Acad Sci USA.* 2003;100:11201–11206.
88. Moody AR et al. Characterization of complicated carotid plaque with magnetic resonance direct thrombus imaging in patients with cerebral ischemia. *Circulation.* 2003;107(24): 3047–3052.
89. AbuRahma AF, Kyer PD 3rd, Robinson PA, Hannay RS. The correlation of ultrasonic carotid plaque morphology and carotid plaque hemorrhage; clinical implications. *Surgery.* 1998;124(4):721–726.

Vascular Hemodynamics of the Carotid Bifurcation and Its Relation to Arterial Disease

Andreas Anayiotos and Yannis Papaharilaou

3.1 Introduction

The hemodynamic hypothesis of atherosclerosis postulates that blood flow characteristics are a synergistic factor in the development of the disease in large arteries. This was first reported in 1968 by Fry[1] who postulated that acute vascular endothelial damage is associated with increased blood velocity gradients and wall shear stress (WSS). However, Caro et al. reported in 1971[2] that atherosclerotic plaques usually develop in the outer walls of bifurcations and branches which are areas of low WSS. Numerous studies followed, based on the observation that atherosclerotic disease occurs at branches, arterial bifurcations, and regions of high curvature. Friedman et al.[3] used laser Doppler anemometry to make velocity measurements very near the walls of human arterial casts; these measurements were then correlated with the histology of the artery from which the cast was made. They observed that the shapes of the velocity profiles along the outer walls of aortic bifurcations were qualitatively different for each cast and determined by the longitudinal variation of cross-sectional area. Ku et al.[4] performed laser Doppler studies on an idealized cast of a carotid bifurcation and reported that low and oscillating WSS characterized the flow effects on the outer wall of the model and that these areas correlated with areas of plaque development in cadaver specimens of the carotid bifurcation. Numerous other studies have been performed for the carotid bifurcation and other branches. The focus of these studies had been to investigate the flow field and associate hemodynamic parameters with regions of disease development.[5–12] Flow parameters such as oscillatory shear index (OSI), particle residence times (PRT), and WSS spatial and temporal gradients (WSSSG and WSSTG) have also been suggested as measures of disease susceptibility. More recent studies have looked into the actual effect WSS has on the local arterial endothelium. Levesque and Nerem performed flow studies on cultured bovine aortic endothelial cells in parallel plate chambers.[13] They found that (a) endothelial cells orient with the flow direction under the influence of shear stress, (b) there is a strong correlation between the degree of alignment and endothelial cell shape, and (c) endothelial cells become more elongated when exposed to higher shear stresses. They also reported that endothelial cells have a shape which is more ellipsoidal in regions of high shear stress and more polygonal in regions of low shear stress. Studies on cultured bovine aortic endothelial cells exposed to physiologic WSS showed that flow-induced platelet-derived growth factor-β (PDGF-β) chain expression in endothelial cells appeared to be mediated, in part, by a protein kinase-C (PKC) independent pathway.[14] In contrast, low WSS leads to the expression of VCAM-1 monocyte adhesion molecule[15] and to a reduction in nitric oxide (NO) release.[16] NO inhibits inflammation of the endothelium and monocyte adhesion.[17] Thus, low WSS promotes monocyte adhesion which is considered to be an important early step in atherogenesis (see Chap. 1).

A. Anayiotos (✉)
Department of Mechanical and Materials Engineering, Cyprus University of Technology, Limassol, Cyprus

Y. Papaharilaou
Institute of Applied and Computational Mathematics, Foundation for Research and Technology Hellas, Heraklion, Crete, Greece

The carotid bifurcation of the common carotid artery (CCA) to the internal carotid artery (ICA) and the external carotid artery (ECA) is a vascular site frequently afflicted by atherosclerotic plaque. The plaque usually localizes at the outer walls of the branches and the common carotid near the bifurcation. The carotid bifurcation is one of the most frequently studied sites evaluating the hemodynamic hypothesis of atherosclerosis. Earlier experimental model studies[4,6,18] investigated the carotid bifurcation flow field in rigid and compliant models for idealized geometries. They have provided limited velocity and WSS measurements and correlated plaque location with regions of low and oscillating WSS. A complementary approach to this is the reconstruction of the complex three-dimensional (3D) flow field of the carotid bifurcation using computational fluid dynamic techniques. In 1991, Perktold et al.[19] were the first to provide detailed numerical results of the 3D carotid bifurcation flow field in an idealized rigid wall model. In their subsequent studies, they investigated the variation of the flow field under (a) different bifurcation angles,[20] (b) a non-Newtonian blood flow model,[21] and (c) a compliant artery wall model.[22] These studies confirmed the existence of a complicated flow field at the bifurcation, with a high WSS region at the flow divider, and regions of low and oscillating WSS at the outer walls of the bifurcation. The effects of compliance and non-Newtonian rheology were minor to the main features of the carotid flow field. Similar results were reported by others,[23,24] and the effect of carotid artery geometry on the magnitude and distribution of WSS gradients was demonstrated.[24]

3.2 Clinical Measurement of the Carotid Artery Hemodynamics in Health and Disease

3.2.1 Ultrasound Measurements

The carotid bifurcation lies superficially and thus can easily be accessed by duplex ultrasound scanning techniques used to examine the carotid arteries for the detection and assessment of possible underlying arterial disease. By using gray-scale B-mode (2D Echo), color Doppler, and spectral Doppler imaging (pulsed Doppler), an evaluation of the vessel morphology and vessel hemodynamics can be made non-invasively. B-mode provides anatomical information; color Doppler provides a visual image of flow and its direction so that the sample volume of the pulsed Doppler can be positioned precisely at any selected position within the vessel. Thus, increased velocities produced by pressure gradients at different grades of stenosis can easily be recorded. From these velocities and velocity ratios (e.g., peak systolic velocity at the stenosis divided by peak systolic velocity proximal to the stenosis), the degree of stenosis can be graded. Also, by sampling across the diameter of the lumen, information on the velocity profile can be obtained. The available techniques and their clinical applications are described in detail in subsequent chapters.

3.2.2 Magnetic Resonance Imaging (MRI) Flow Measurement Techniques

There are two basic physical principles that govern the modulation of the nuclear magnetic resonance (NMR) signal from spins in motion. One is the inflow or time-of-flight (TOF) effect, and the other is the phase shift effect. An excellent review of the basic flow imaging techniques based on the effects of blood flow on the magnetic resonance imaging (MRI) signal is given by Axel and Morton.[25]

The magnetic resonance angiography (MRA) techniques most often used for evaluating the anatomy of the carotid bifurcation consist of two-dimensional time-of-flight (2D TOF) and three-dimensional time-of-flight (3D TOF).[26] A 3D TOF maximum intensity projection (MIP) image is shown in Fig. 3.1, and a cross-sectional image of the carotid arteries is shown in Fig. 3.2.

The second category of MR angiography techniques is that relying on the flow-induced phase shifts. Phase-contrast phenomena are analogues to Doppler shift effects in ultrasound studies. Magnetic spins undergo a frequency shift when moving along a magnetic field gradient; this frequency shift is proportional to their velocity component parallel to the applied gradient direction. The product of this frequency shift and the magnetic field gradient pulse duration gives rise to the overall phase shift relative to stationary spins.

There are essentially three types of flow quantification methods using velocity-induced phase shifts.

The first category comprises of phase-sensitive angiographic methods. One such method detects flow through a loss of phase coherence due to velocity dispersion within a volume element (voxel). Two images are acquired, one with flow compensation and one without. Image subtraction suppresses the signal from stationary tissue, leaving only that from flowing blood.[25] A second phase-sensitive angiographic method uses small flow encoding gradient pulses to produce discrete velocity-induced phase shifts. Subtraction of echoes acquired from inverted and non-inverted flow encoding gradient pulses removes stationary tissue signal from the image.[27]

The second category of flow quantification methods is the direct phase velocity mapping methods that use the flow-induced phase shifts to measure velocity directly from the phase of the image voxel. Phase velocity mapping was first demonstrated by Bryant et al. in 1984 and has been extensively validated for flow measurement both in vivo and in vitro.[28]

The Fourier velocity encoding methods are the third category of methods for flow quantification using velocity-induced phase shifts to measure the intravoxel velocity distribution.[29]

The effects of various imaging parameters and flow conditions on the accuracy of MR flow quantification have been reported by Firmin et al.[30] and Buonocore and Bogren.[31]

Recent advances in phase-contrast-based MR techniques allow the time-resolved measurement of the 3D velocity field. A recent study has applied the flow-sensitive four-dimensional (4D) MRI technique to assess hemodynamic parameters such as WSS and OSI in the entire thoracic aorta based on the measured velocity field.[32]

MRA produces a good quality three-dimensional image of the carotid bifurcation with good sensitivity for detecting high-grade carotid stenosis. Slow, turbulent, and stagnant flow is poorly visualized by MRA; therefore, the degree of stenosis is hard to evaluate.

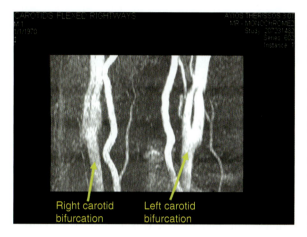

Fig. 3.1 Maximum intensity projection (MIP) image of the left and right carotid artery bifurcation

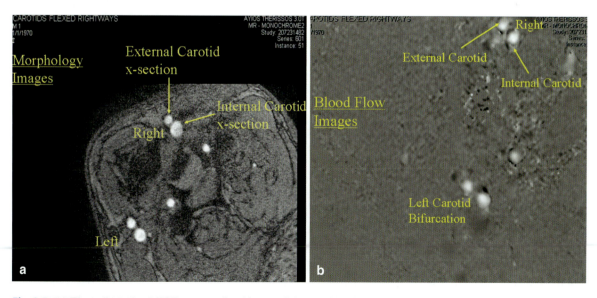

Fig. 3.2 (a) Three-dimensional TOF cross-sectional image of the carotid and vertebral arteries. (b) Two-dimensional echo phase-contrast angiography cross-sectional image of the blood flow of the carotid arteries

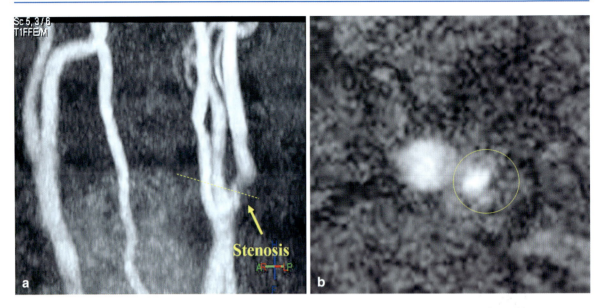

Fig. 3.3 (**a**) Maximum intensity projection MR image of a carotid bifurcation ICA stenosis. (**b**) Cross-sectional image of the ICA and ECA

One of the inherent problems with the carotid bifurcation image is the loss of flow signal and low signal to noise ratio regions at the outer wall of the CCA near the bifurcation. This may be due to saturation of inflowing spins, fluctuating flow phenomena (pulsatile flow), flow recirculation, susceptibility effects, and/or highly disturbed or transiently turbulent flow at stenotic or kinking vessels.[33] An example of a maximum intensity projection MR image of a moderately stenotic artery is shown in Fig. 3.3.

Even normal or very mildly stenotic arteries may appear diseased on MRA as disturbed flow in the carotid bulb contributes to loss of signal intensity. Irregular stenoses which disturb flow are particularly susceptible to overestimation.[34,35]

Techniques combining 3D and 2D TOF may improve the performance of MRA but are not routine clinical tests and may increase test cost if used.[34]

3.2.3 Image-Based Computational Fluid Dynamics Modeling

Recently, numerical simulation methods have been combined with imaging techniques such as MRI, computed tomography (CT), and ultrasound to provide arterial models from anatomical images with more accurate wall characteristics as well as boundary conditions.[36–41] In 1991, Taylor et al. were among the first to propose using clinical imaging data for the reconstruction of realistic models of arterial segments.[36] They had proposed that this could be used as a clinical decision support tool. Subsequent studies of the numerical flow field in the carotid bifurcation of patients with MRI provided validation.[37] Cebral et al.[39] used sequential MRI to obtain patient-specific anatomic information of the carotid arteries and then reconstructed the geometry to obtain 3D models. Flow computations were performed, and detailed information about the 3D velocity flow field and WSS distribution were provided. The comparison between the MRI velocity field and the computational fluid dynamic (CFD) velocity fields at selected locations was satisfactory. Steinman et al.[40] used MRI to reconstruct the geometry of the carotid bifurcation from patients and to successfully measure the wall thickness of the artery. Using similar imaging techniques, Zhao et al.[41] studied the carotid bifurcation in patients' arteries and compared CFD simulations with MRI phase-contrast images. The comparison showed good agreement for the main velocity component in both the CCA and the disturbed flow region in the carotid sinus. Comparison of in-plane velocity vectors showed less satisfactory consistency and revealed that the MR measurements obtained were inadequate to depict the secondary flow pattern.

Glor et al.[42] studied the carotid bifurcation by MRI and CFD and reported that, qualitatively, all WSS parameters are highly reproducible. Quantitatively, the reproducibility was over 90% for OSI and WSS, but only 60% for WSSTG since these parameters are very sensitive to subtle variations in local geometry and mesh design, especially near the bifurcation. Thomas et al.[33] assessed the carotid bifurcation geometry in young versus adult subjects and the risk of atherosclerosis development. The authors found modest interindividual variations in young adults and major interindividual variations in older vessels, with a complex interrelationship between vascular geometry, local hemodynamics, vascular aging, and atherosclerosis. They conclude that if there is a geometric risk for atherosclerosis, its early detection is challenging.

3.3 Atherosclerosis and Vascular Hemodynamics

The mechanical force applied on the endothelial layer of the arterial wall due to the flow of blood can be divided into two components. One component acts normal to the wall and represents pressure, and the other acts tangential to the wall and represents shear stress. Although pressure affects all parts of the arterial wall, shear stress principally affects the endothelium. In large arteries and in uniform sections of the vessel away from bifurcations, the mean WSS typically ranges between 20 and 40 dyn/cm^2. However, in regions of disturbed and separated flow, the shear stress will be negative or zero within the separation region and up to 40 and 50 dyn/cm^2 in its vicinity. These values vary both in magnitude and sign throughout the cardiac cycle. The morphology and orientation of endothelial cells often reflect the hemodynamic conditions they have been exposed to. The alignment of the endothelial cells reflects the mean direction of the shear stress. In regions of axial laminar flow, shear stress is unidirectional, and endothelial cells tend to align to the flow direction. However, in regions of disturbed flow where there is no prevailing mean shear stress direction, the endothelial cells show no preferred orientation.[13]

Hemodynamic interactions between the endothelial cell and shear stress are mediated through the cell surface. In vitro studies[43,44] have demonstrated that it is not only shear stress magnitude but also spatial and temporal gradients of shear that affect endothelial behavior. In order to understand these complex interactions, it is necessary to study the hemodynamic forces at a subcellular scale. It has been shown that endothelial cells are able to differentiate their response to flow environment conditions such as the frequency of the blood oscillatory motion.

One of the primary functions of the endothelium is vasoregulation. A number of vasoregulatory factors associated with the endothelium have been identified. Nitric oxide is the principal endothelium-derived relaxing factor with its release modulated by shear stress. Additional control of the vasoregulatory process is provided by prostacyclin, a vasodilator which is synthesized and released by the endothelial cells in the presence of high shear stress. Endothelin, a vasoconstrictor, is also synthesized and released by endothelial cells in response to changes in the shear stress exposure of the endothelium.

Atherosclerosis alters the mechanical properties of arteries. The initial response of the vessel to the development of an atherosclerotic lesion is dilatation. This response allows the vessel to maintain a normal-size lumen and continues until the lesion occupies approximately 40% of the vessel cross-sectional area. Further growth of the lesion cannot be accommodated by dilatation and inevitably leads to stenosis.

At an early stage, atherosclerotic lesions are soft and have minimal impact on the wall stiffness. As the lesions enlarge, they cause a degradation of the load-bearing components of the wall that may lead to a reduction in wall stiffness. Eventually, calcification of the atherosclerotic plaque leads to a significant stiffening of the artery.

Certain sites in the human circulation are more prone to the development of atherosclerotic lesions. Such sites are associated with disturbed and separated flow typically found in the vicinity of bifurcations and branches or regions of significant curvature or stenosis. Certain arteries are more susceptible to disease than others partly due to the differences in the structural properties of the wall but primarily due to the differences in the hemodynamic conditions. It has been demonstrated that atherosclerotic lesions are predominantly found in sites exposed to low time-averaged WSS[45] usually associated with flow separation and flow reversal. The exposure of the endothelium to low mean and oscillatory shear stress and separated flow triggers the secretion from endothelial cells of shear-stress-regulated factors that promote coagulation, leukocyte migration, and smooth muscle proliferation, hence promoting the development of atherosclerosis. These conditions also affect the survival of endothelial cells.[46]

It has also been established that the flow environment can affect the mass transport characteristics of the arterial wall.[47–49] In the early studies by Caro and Nerem[47] and Caro,[48] blood serum was mixed with 14C-4-labeled cholesterol, and the uptake of the label by an excised serum-perfused canine common carotid artery was measured ex vivo. Two perfusion rigs were run simultaneously. Segments of the excised left and right carotid arteries were mounted to the flow rigs and perfused with different rates of shear. The investigators found that a substantial increase in the uptake of the label from the wall occurred with increase of WSS. A later study by Deng et al.[49] showed that there is a higher accumulation of low-density lipoproteins in areas of the canine carotid wall surface exposed to low WSS and where the permeability of the endothelium is enhanced. They also found that luminal lipid concentration affects the rate of infiltration of lipids into the wall.

A study of time-varying flow in a realistic physical model of the aortic bifurcation of a subject with mild atherosclerosis indicated a negative correlation between intimal thickness and shear stress.[5] The same study showed a positive correlation between oscillatory shear and intimal thickness. The authors concluded that the presence of low and oscillatory WSS generates hemodynamic conditions that favor the development of atherosclerotic disease.

Atherosclerotic lesions may trigger a wall remodeling and adaptation process similar to that initiated by changes in flow rate.[50] It has also been postulated that atherosclerotic lesions may develop as a reaction to endothelial cell injury associated with greater wear and tear induced by high spatial gradients of WSS. This has been supported by in vitro experiments which have shown a strong influence of spatial gradients of shear stress in the migration–proliferation behavior of endothelial cells.[43] However, in the in vitro model study by White et al.[44] it was shown that temporal gradients of shear caused human endothelial cell proliferation whereas spatial gradients of shear had the same effect on cell proliferation as steady uniform shear stress. Although both studies used the sudden-expansion flow chamber to generate high spatial shear gradients, White et al.[44] introduced sudden onsets of flow to generate temporal gradients of shear.

He and Ku[51] used numerical methods to study the flow in a left coronary artery bifurcation model based on mean geometric parameters under pulsatile flow. A coronary waveform with a mean Reynolds number of 240 and a Womersley number of 2.8 was prescribed at the inlet. Skewed velocity profiles were found in both the left anterior descending (LAD) and circumflex arteries toward the inner walls of the bifurcation. Time-averaged shear stress was significantly lower on the outer walls as compared to the inner walls of both daughter vessels in the vicinity of the bifurcation. It was also found that oscillatory shear was higher on the outer walls as compared to the inner walls. According to He and Ku,[51] the localization of sites exposed to low and oscillatory shear correlates well with the distribution of atherosclerotic lesions reported in the literature.

3.3.1 Hemodynamic Parameters Used as Indices of Susceptibility to Arterial Disease

Beyond WSS, which is a well-established hemodynamic parameter and widely used as a surrogate marker for disturbed flow, other shear-stress-related parameters have been proposed as indices of susceptibility to vascular dysfunction. These include the temporal and spatial gradients of WSS magnitude and the temporal gradient of WSS angle. The latter is a measure of the WSS vector direction variation in the cardiac cycle. A more complex WSS-derived index is the OSI which involves the calculation of the instantaneous and cycle-averaged of WSS angle introduced by Ku et al.[4]

To obtain a measure of the continuous oscillatory motion of the WSS vector, a modified oscillatory shear index was introduced by Papaharilaou et al.[52] based on the definition of Ku et al.[4] and the formulation introduced by Moore et al.[53] As both shear vector magnitude and direction change with time in a continuous fashion, the OSI is defined as follows:

$$mOSI = \frac{\int_0^T w|\tau \cdot n_{mean}|dt}{\int_0^T |\tau \cdot n_{mean}|dt},$$

where τ is the instantaneous WSS; n_{mean} is the mean shear direction defined as:

$$n_{\text{mean}} = \int_0^T (\tau/\|\tau\|) \mathrm{d}t,$$

where T is the period of the flow waveform; and w is a weighting factor defined as:

$$w = 0.5(1 - \cos a),$$

where a is the angle between τ and n_{mean}. This modified definition of the oscillatory shear index allows for the inclusion in the calculation of a continuous range of instantaneous shear vector angles with respect to the mean shear direction, in contrast to the earlier definition by Ku et al.[4] which only allows for inclusion in the calculation of instances where the instantaneous WSS vector is directed opposite of the cycle-averaged WSS vector. The range of values for the modified index is $0 < \text{OSI} < 0.5$, where 0 corresponds to unidirectional shear flow and 0.5 to the purely oscillatory shear case.

In an effort to better quantify the influence of hemodynamics on the development of vascular wall disease, a new approach has been introduced whereby the total arterial wall surface area exposed to unfavorable hemodynamic conditions is used as a measure of the potential effect of flow-induced forces on the vascular wall. For this, thresholds of well-established hemodynamic indices such as cycle-averaged WSS and oscillatory shear stress are utilized to characterize the flow conditions as unfavorable. Along this line of thought, Himburg et al.[54] introduced the relative residence time (RRT) index which combines the cycle-averaged WSS and OSI indices. Low cycle-averaged WSS and high OSI can be associated with increased near-wall residence times and a high RRT value.

The dominant harmonic frequency introduced by Himburg et al.[54] is defined as the strongest harmonic of the Fourier power spectra of the time-varying WSS waveform. In a later study, Himburg and Friedman[55] found a strong inverse correlation between high harmonic content and low cycle-averaged WSS in the porcine iliac artery.

The helicity angle difference (HAD) introduced by Hyun et al.[56] provides a measure of the presence of secondary flow and as such is primarily an indicator of flow rotation or vorticity.

The harmonic index (HI) introduced by Gelfand et al.[57] is defined as follows:

$$\text{HI} = \frac{\sum_{n=1}^{\infty} T[n\omega_o]}{\sum_{n=0}^{\infty} T[n\omega_o]},$$

where $T[n\omega_o]$ is the magnitude of the Fourier series decomposed shear stress signal. HI could be thought of as a measure of the relative contribution of the time-varying intensity to the total signal intensity. This parameter ranges from zero (steady nonzero WSS signal) to one (purely oscillatory WSS signal with a cycle average of zero). HI allows the parameterization of the frequency content of the shear stress signal relative to cycle-averaged shear stress and thus allows detection of frequency spectrum intensity relative to predicted atherogenic regions.

In a recent study by Lee et al.,[58] the correlation between the various hemodynamic parameters at the carotid bifurcation was investigated within a sample of 50 carotid bifurcation geometries obtained from 25 healthy volunteers. Their findings indicate that beyond cycle-averaged WSS which is a well-established surrogate marker for disturbed flow, RRT and dominant harmonic frequency (DH) are among the other hemodynamic indices studied as the most suitable candidates for a single, independent surrogate marker for carotid arterial wall disease. In the same study, helicity angle difference (HAD) was found to be an independent predictor of flow disturbances.

3.3.2 Geometric Parameters as Predictors of Disturbed Flow

Until recently, there was no basic method to identify the anatomic geometric features of specific arteries on the arterial tree. However, recent advances in clinical imaging techniques have allowed more precise segmentation of arteries by CT or MRI and the production of 3D solid bodies or 3D virtual models of the arterial geometry.[36]

The method consists of an anatomical data acquisition procedure of multiple sequentially obtained high-resolution transverse slices of the cross section of the artery. The slices are usually more than 100 and cover the whole spatial domain of interest. Each image is then processed to extract the lumen and arterial wall boundaries. Three-dimensional surface reconstruction of the images is usually performed by a purpose-developed software such as Vascular Modeling Toolkit (VMTK),[59] and this essentially provides the solid body of the whole artery. Abnormal, small-scale surface irregularities introduced during the imaging and reconstruction processes are smoothed out using a special feature of the above or any similar software package.

Using such models, Antiga and Steinman[59] have identified and proposed a method to identify specific anatomic geometric features of virtual models of patient-specific arteries such as vessel centerlines, bifurcation angles, planarity angles, curvatures, tortuosities, etc. The importance of this method is that it allows the researcher to compare these parameters from patient to patient and quantify geometric differences.

The effect of specific geometric parameters on disturbed flow features has been studied by Lee et al.[60] on 50 healthy volunteers. In their study, they identified 14 intercorrelated geometric parameters of the CB from MR images and used multivariate regression based on an a priori selection of a subset of four of these parameters to identify two: proximal area ratio (CCA area/ICA area at the initial axis) and tortuosity that were predictors of disturbed hemodynamics.

Zhang et al.,[61] using the same 50-volunteer sample, extended the previous work to simultaneously analyze the combined role of all geometric variables using factor analysis based on principal component analysis (PCA). The purpose of their study was to investigate the relationship between geometric features and hemodynamic quantities that can be considered to typify "disturbed flow." Their results have demonstrated that bifurcation expansion (CCA area/ICA area at the initial axis) and ICA planarity angle (non-collinearity of the CCA and ICA initial axes) are strong predictors of disturbance in all parameter combinations.

Despite the fact that CCA planarity angle and bifurcation expansion cannot be evaluated with great accuracy from the MR images, these geometric factors can be used as predictors of atherogenic flow conditions and should be carefully evaluated in future studies of atherosusceptibility.

3.4 Influence of Posture Change on the Geometry and Hemodynamics of the Carotid Bifurcation

Recent reports highlight the importance of motion and posture on peripheral arteries such as the carotid, femoral, popliteal, and brachial since they may alter morphology and hemodynamic characteristics. Two overviews[62,63] assessed the progress that has been achieved with image-based CFD studies in understanding the relationship between hemodynamics and disease development. They specifically mention that it is important to better understand how local hemodynamic fields respond to normal physiological and postural variations. Cheng et al.[64] studied the in vivo deformations of the superficial femoral artery during maximum knee and hip flexion using magnetic resonance angiography. They reported significant morphological changes such as shortening, lengthening, and twisting clockwise and counterclockwise. These changes varied from patient to patient. Glor et al.[65] performed an ultrasound imaging study of the carotid bifurcation and looked at the effects of head rotation in nine patients. They reported that head rotation changed the distribution of WSS and OSI due to flow rate change in the rotated position. They also reported "planarification" of the common carotid artery and changes in centerline location of the vessel with rotation.

Such changes may alter the hemodynamic variables that are generally associated with the development of atherosclerosis, such as low and oscillating WSS, OSI, WSSTG, and PRT.

The authors' studies[66] have focused on geometric differences in the carotid bifurcation with posture change on 10 healthy volunteers. Each subject was imaged in the supine position at a normal position of the head, and at the prone position with the head rotated to the right about 80–90°. This was done in two different scanning sessions on the same day corresponding to the two head postures examined. The solid surface models were constructed with slice-by-slice manual segmentation, and the 3D geometry of the carotid bifurcation was processed using the VMTK.[59] Using various features of the VMTK package, specific important geometric parameters were identified such as bifurcation angle, internal carotid artery (ICA) angle, ICA planarity angle, in-plane

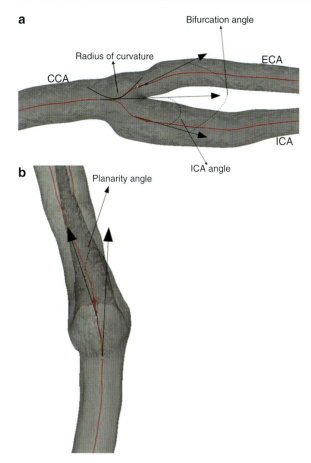

Fig. 3.4 Graphical representation of (a) the internal carotid artery (ICA) angle and the bifurcation angle, and (b) the ICA planarity angle

asymmetry angle, curvature, and tortuosity. Some of these parameters are illustrated in Fig. 3.4.

The results have shown that there are significant changes between the two postures in all 10 volunteers for both left and right carotid bifurcations in all geometric parameters. An example of the changes in both the left and right bifurcation for both neutral and rotated head position is illustrated in Fig. 3.5a and b.

The differences, however, were random in every geometric parameter, and while in some volunteers there was an increase of one geometric parameter, in other volunteers there was a decrease. Therefore, there was no preferred change in any of the geometric variables with head rotation. Hemodynamic simulations[67] have shown that the distribution of critical hemodynamic parameters such as high OSI/cycle-averaged WSS ratio, or high WSS temporal gradients, were different in the two postures.

These morphologic and hemodynamic changes in the carotid artery for different head and neck postures may be physiologically relevant and warrant further investigation. Specifically, changes in head posture may influence the morphology and degree of stenotic lesions with unknown consequences in moderate stenosis cases while the morphology of the lesion may result in a severe stenotic case with head rotation at the prone sleeping position where the exposure is several hours. With the same argument, sleeping in the prone position/rotation of the head in the case of unstable carotid plaque lesions with an embedded lipid core under a fibrous cap may result in alteration of the

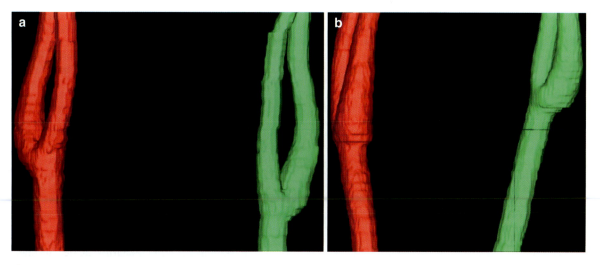

Fig. 3.5 Three-dimensional surface reconstruction images of the left and right carotid arteries of a healthy volunteer at (a) the supine (neutral) position and (b) the prone position (with rightward head rotation)

local geometry and the mechanical stress distribution around the fibrous cap. This may result in more favorable conditions for the rupture of the fibrous cap.[68] Similarly, the same argument is important in the optimization of the design and implantation of carotid stents to avoid stent fractures with head rotation.[69]

References

1. Fry DL. Acute vascular endothelial changes associated with increased blood velocity gradients. *Circ Res*. 1968;22: 165–197.
2. Caro CG, Fitz-Gerald JM, Schroter RC. Atheroma and arterial wall shear: observation, correlation and proposal of a shear dependent mass transfer mechanism for atherogenesis. *Proc R Soc Lond*. 1971;177:109–159.
3. Friedman MH, Bargeron CB, Hutchins GM, Mark FF, Deters OJ. Hemodynamic measurements in human arterial casts, and their correlation with histology and luminal area. *J Biomech Eng*. 1980;102:247.
4. Ku DN, Giddens DP, Zarins CK, Glagov S. Pulsatile flow and atherosclerosis in the human carotid bifurcation. Positive correlation between plaque location and low oscillating shear stress. *Arteriosclerosis*. 1985;5:293–302.
5. Friedman MH, Hutchins GM, Bargeron CB, Deters OJ, Mark FF. Correlation between intimal thickness and fluid shear in human arteries. *Atherosclerosis*. 1981;39:425–436.
6. LoGerfo FW, Nowak MD, Quist WC, Crawshaw HM, Bharadvaj BK. Flow studies in a model carotid bifurcation. *Arteriosclerosis*. 1981;1:235–241.
7. Motomiya M, Karino T. Flow patterns in the human carotid artery bifurcation. *Stroke*. 1984;15:50–56.
8. Liepsch D, Moravec S. Pulsatile flow of non-Newtonian fluid in distensible models of human arteries. *Biorheology*. 1984;21:571–586.
9. Cho YI, Back LH, Crawford DW. Experimental investigation of branch, flow ratio, angle, and Reynolds number effects on the pressure and flow fields in arterial branch models. *J Biomech Eng*. 1985;107:257–267.
10. Back LH, Kwack EY, Crawford DW. Flow measurements in an atherosclerotic curved tapered femoral artery model of man. *J Biomech Eng*. 1988;110:310–319.
11. Mark FF, Bargeron CB, Deters OJ, Friedman MH. Variations in geometry and shear rate distribution in casts of human aortic bifurcations. *J Biomech*. 1989;22:577–582.
12. Duncan DD et al. The effect of compliance on wall shear in casts of a human aortic bifurcation. *J Biomech Eng*. 1990; 112:183–188.
13. Levesque MJ, Nerem RM. The elongation and orientation of cultured endothelial cells in response to shear stress. *J Biomech Eng*. 1985;107:341–347.
14. Mitsumata M, Fishel RS, Nerem RM, Alexander RW, Berk BC. Fluid shear stress stimulates platelet-derived growth factor expression in endothelial cells. *Am J Physiol*. 1993; 265:H3–H8.
15. Gonzales RS, Wick TM. Hemodynamic modulation of monocytic cell adherence to vascular endothelium. *Ann Biomed Eng*. 1996;24:382–393.
16. Tsao PS, Lewis NP, Alpert S, Cooke JP. Exposure to shear stress alters endothelial adhesiveness: role of nitric oxide. *Circulation*. 1995;92:3513–3519.
17. Barbato JE, Tseng E. Nitric oxide and arterial disease. *J Vasc Surg*. 2004;40:187–193.
18. Anayiotos AS, Jones SA, Giddens DP, Glagov S, Zarins CK. Shear stress at a compliant model of the human carotid bifurcation. *J Biomech Eng*. 1994;116:98–106.
19. Perktold K, Resch M, Peter RO. Three-dimensional numerical analysis of pulsatile flow and WSS in the carotid artery bifurcation. *J Biomech*. 1991;24:409–420.
20. Perktold K, Peter RO, Resch M, Langs G. Pulsatile non-Newtonian blood flow in three-dimensional carotid bifurcation models: a numerical study of flow phenomena under different bifurcation angles. *J Biomed Eng*. 1991;13: 507–515.
21. Perktold K, Resch M, Florian H. Pulsatile non-Newtonian flow characteristics in a three-dimensional human carotid bifurcation model. *J Biomech Eng*. 1991;113:464–475.
22. Perktold K, Rappitsch G. Computer simulation of local blood flow and vessel mechanics in a compliant carotid artery bifurcation model. *J Biomech*. 1995;28:845–856.
23. Delfino A. *Analysis of Stress Field in a Model of the Human Carotid Bifurcation* [Ph.D. thesis]. Lausanne: Ecole Polytechnique Federale de Lausanne; 1996.
24. Wells DR, Archie JP Jr, Kleinstreuer C. Effect of carotid artery geometry on the magnitude and distribution of WSS gradients. *J Vasc Surg*. 1996;23:667–678.
25. Axel L, Morton D. MR flow imaging by velocity compensated/uncompensated difference images. *J Comput Assist Tomogr*. 1987;11:31–34.
26. Scarabino T et al. MR angiography in carotid stenosis: a comparison of three techniques. *Eur J Radiol*. 1998; 28(2):117–125.
27. Dumoulin CL, Hart HR. Magnetic resonance angiography. *Radiology*. 1986;161:717–720.
28. Bryant DJ, Payne JA, Firmin DN, Longmore DB. Measurement of flow with NMR imaging using a gradient pulse and phase difference technique. *J Comput Assist Tomogr*. 1984;8:588–593.
29. Dumoulin CL, Doorly DJ, Caro CG. Quantitative measurement of velocity at multiple positions using comb excitation and Fourier velocity encoding. *Magn Reson Med*. 1993;29:44–52.
30. Firmin DN, Nayler GL, Kilner PJ, Longmore DB. The application of phase shifts in NMR for flow measurement. *Magn Reson Med*. 1990;14(2):230–241.
31. Buonocore MH, Bogren H. Factors influencing the accuracy and precision of velocity-encoded phase imaging. *Magn Reson Med*. 1992;26:141–154.
32. Frydrychowicz A et al. Three-dimensional analysis of segmental wall shear stress in the aorta by flow-sensitive four-dimensional-MRI. *J Magn Reson Imaging*. 2009;30(1):77–84.
33. Thomas JB et al. Variation in the carotid bifurcation geometry of young versus older adults implications for geometric risk of atherosclerosis. *Stroke*. 2005;36:2450–2456.
34. Fisher M, Sotak CH, Minematsu K, Li L. New magnetic resonance techniques for evaluating cerebrovascular disease. *Ann Neurol*. 1992;32:115–122.
35. Riles T et al. Comparison of magnetic resonance angiography, conventional angiography, and duplex scanning. *Stroke*. 1992;23:341–346.

36. Taylor CA et al. Predictive medicine: computational techniques in therapeutic decision-making. *Comput Aided Surg*. 1999;4(5):231–247.
37. Botnar R et al. Hemodynamics in the carotid artery bifurcation: a comparison between numerical simulations and in vitro MRI measurements. *J Biomech*. 2000;33:137–144.
38. Papaharilaou Y, Doorly DJ, Sherwin SJ. The influence of out-of-plane geometry on pulsatile flow within a distal end-to-side anastomosis. *J Biomech*. 2002;35:1225–1239.
39. Cebral JR, Yim PJ, Lohner R, Soto O, Choyke PL. Blood flow modeling in carotid arteries with computational fluid dynamics and MR imaging. *Acad Radiol*. 2002;9:1286–1299.
40. Steinman DA et al. Reconstruction of carotid bifurcation hemodynamics and wall thickness using computational fluid dynamics and MRI. *Magn Reson Med*. 2002;47:149–159.
41. Zhao SZ, Papathanasopoulou P, Long Q, Marshall I, Xu XY. Comparative study of magnetic resonance imaging and image-based computational fluid dynamics for quantification of pulsatile flow in a carotid bifurcation phantom. *Ann Biomed Eng*. 2003;31(8):962–971.
42. Glor FP et al. Reproducibility study of magnetic resonance image-based computational fluid dynamics prediction of carotid bifurcation flow. *Ann Biomed Eng*. 2003;2:142–151.
43. Tardy Y, Resnick N, Nagel T, Gimbrone MA Jr, Dewey CF Jr. Shear stress gradients remodel endothelial monolayers in vitro via a cell proliferation-migration-loss cycle. *Arterioscler Thromb Vasc Biol*. 1997;17:3102–3106.
44. White CR, Haidekker M, Bao X, Frangos JA. Temporal gradients in shear, but not spatial gradients, stimulate endothelial cell proliferation. *Circulation*. 2001;103:2508–2513.
45. Caro CG, Fitz-Gerald JM, Schroeter RC. Arterial wall shear stress and distribution of early atheroma in man. *Nature*. 1969;223:1159–1161.
46. Traub O, Berk BC. Laminar shear stress: mechanisms by which endothelial cells transduce an atheroprotective force. *Arterioscler Thromb Vasc Biol*. 1998;18:677–685.
47. Caro CG, Nerem RM. Transport of 14C-cholesterol between serum and wall in perfused dog common carotid artery. *Circ Res*. 1973;32:187–194.
48. Caro CG. Transport of 14C-4-cholesterol between perfusing serum and dog common carotid artery: a shear dependent process. *Cardiovasc Res*. 1974;8:194–203.
49. Deng X et al. Luminal surface concentration of lipoprotein (LDL) and its effect on the wall uptake of cholesterol by canine carotid arteries. *J Vasc Surg*. 1995;21:135–145.
50. Zarins CK, Zatina MA, Giddens DP, Ku DN, Glagov S. Shear stress regulation of artery lumen diameter in experimental atherogenesis. *J Vasc Surg*. 1987;5:413–420.
51. He X, Ku DN. Unsteady entrance flow development in a straight tube. *J Biomech Eng*. 1994;116:355–360.
52. Papaharilaou Y et al. Combined MR imaging and numerical simulation of flow in realistic arterial bypass graft models. *Biorheology*. 2002;39(3-4):525–532.
53. Moore JA, Steinman DA, Prakash S, Johnston KW, Ethier CR. A numerical study of blood flow patterns in anatomically realistic and simplified end-to-side anastomoses. *J Biomech Eng*. 1999;121:265–272.
54. Himburg HA et al. Spatial comparison between wall shear stress measures and porcine arterial endothelial permeability. *Am J Physiol Heart Circ Physiol*. 2004;286(5):H1916–H1922.
55. Himburg HA, Friedman MH. Correspondence of low mean shear and high harmonic content in the porcine iliac arteries. *J Biomech Eng*. 2006;128(6):852–856.
56. Hyun S, Kleinstreuer C, Longest PW, Chen C. Particle-hemodynamics simulations and design options for surgical reconstruction of diseased carotid artery bifurcations. *J Biomech Eng*. 2004;126(2):188–195.
57. Gelfand BD, Epstein FH, Blackman BR. Spatial and spectral heterogeneity of time-varying shear stress profiles in the carotid bifurcation by phase-contrast MRI. *J Magn Reson Imaging*. 2006;24(6):1386–1392.
58. Lee SW, Antiga L, Steinman DA. Correlations among indicators of disturbed flow at the normal carotid bifurcation. *J Biomech Eng*. 2009;131(6):061013.
59. Antiga L, Steinman D. Robust and objective decomposition and mapping of bifurcating vessels. *IEEE Trans Med Imaging*. 2004;23(6):704–713.
60. Lee SW, Antiga L, Spence JD, Steinman DA. Geometry of the carotid bifurcation predicts its exposure to disturbed flow. *Stroke*. 2008;39(8):2341–2347.
61. Zhang Q, Steinman DA, Friedman MH. Prediction of disturbed flow by factor analysis of carotid bifurcation geometry. In: Proceedings of the ASME 2009 Summer Bioengineering Conference; June 17–21, 2009; Lake Tahoe. Abstract no. 204798.
62. Taylor CA, Draney MT. Experimental and computational methods in cardiovascular fluid mechanics. *Annu Rev Fluid Mech*. 2004;36:197–231.
63. Steinman DA, Taylor CA. Flow imaging and computing: large artery hemodynamics. *Ann Biomed Eng*. 2005;33:1704–1709.
64. Cheng CP, Wilson NM, Hallett RL, Herfkens RJ, Taylor CA. In vivo MR angiographic quantification of axial and twisting deformations of the superficial femoral artery resulting from maximum hip and knee flexion. *J Vasc Interv Radiol*. 2006;17:979–987.
65. Glor FP et al. Influence of head position on carotid hemodynamics in young adults. *Am J Physiol Heart Circ Physiol*. 2004;287:H1670-H1681.
66. Aristokleous N, et al. Effect of posture change on the geometric features of the healthy carotid bifurcation. IEEE Transactions of Information Technology in Biomedicine. 2011;15:148–154.
67. Papaharilaou Y, et al. Effect of head posture changes in the geometry and hemodynamics of a healthy human carotid bifurcation. In: Summer Bioengineering Conference; June 2007; Keystone.
68. Mitsumori LM et al. In vivo accuracy of multisequence MR imaging for identifying unstable fibrous caps in advanced human carotid plaques. *J Magn Reson Imaging*. 2003;17:410–420.
69. Valibhoy AR, Mwipatayi BP, Sieunarine K. Fracture of a carotid stent: an unexpected complication. *J Vasc Surg*. 2007;45:603–606.

The Problem with Asymptomatic Carotid Stenosis

A. Ross Naylor

Truth passes through three stages. First it is ridiculed, second it is violently oppressed and then it is accepted as being self-evident

Arthur Schopenhauer (1788–1860)

4.1 Introduction

In 1978, Jessie Thompson published a retrospective review of outcomes in 270 patients with an asymptomatic carotid stenosis.[1] Within a non-randomized cohort of 132 undergoing prophylactic carotid endarterectomy (CEA), 132 (91%) remained asymptomatic over a mean follow-up period of 50 months, 6 (5%) suffered a transient ischaemic attack (TIA), while 5 (4%) suffered a stroke. By contrast, only 77/138 patients (56%) who did not undergo CEA remained asymptomatic, 37 (27%) developed a TIA, while 24 (17%) suffered a stroke. To him, and many other surgeons, these data strongly supported a policy of prophylactic CEA in patients with asymptomatic carotid disease.

By the early 1980s, however, there were growing concerns amongst neurologists about the performance of CEA around the world. The Rand Corporation thereafter performed a retrospective analysis of the "appropriateness" of CEA in 1,302 Medicare patients undergoing surgery in 1981 and concluded that 64% of indications were either "equivocal" or "inappropriate."[2]

As a consequence, there emerged a clamor for practice to be driven by evidence, rather than the style of intuitive reasoning espoused by leading contemporary surgeons. Two large randomized trials evaluated the roles of CEA and best medical therapy (BMT) in recently symptomatic patients, and their findings changed practice immediately.[3,4] More importantly, the symptomatic trials established a consensus of practice among surgeons, neurologists, and stroke physicians that endures to this day, largely because the trials were statistically robust and consistent in their findings. Unfortunately, despite the performance of two similarly large randomized trials in asymptomatic patients,[5,6] no similar consensus has been forthcoming.

4.2 The Randomized Trials in Asymptomatic Patients

The Asymptomatic Carotid Atherosclerosis Study (ACAS) and the Asymptomatic Carotid Surgery Trial (ACST) were published in 1995 and 2004, respectively (Table 4.1). Both concluded that CEA conferred a "50%" relative risk reduction in the 5-year risk of stroke, from approximately "12%" down to "6%."[5,6] Based upon these data, the American Heart Association (AHA) concluded that "prophylactic CEA was recommended in highly selected patients with high grade asymptomatic stenoses provided it was performed by surgeons with less than 3% morbidity & mortality."[7]

A.R. Naylor
Vascular Surgery Group, Division of Cardiovascular Sciences, Leicester Royal Infirmary, Leicester, Leicestershire, UK

Table 4.1 Traditionally reported 5-year outcomes from the ACAS[5] and ACST[6] trials

Trial	n =	5-year stroke CEA (%)	BMT (%)	ARR (%)	RRR (%)	NNT	Strokes prevented/1,000 CEAs at 5 years
ACAS	1,662	5.1	11.0	5.9	54	17	59
ACST	3,120	6.4	11.8	5.4	46	19	53

CEA carotid endarterectomy, *BMT* best medical therapy, *ARR* absolute risk reduction in stroke at 5 years, *RRR* relative risk reduction in stroke at 5 years, *NNT* number needed to treat to prevent one stroke at 5 years

This recommendation has been now adopted by virtually every country performing carotid surgery.

4.3 What Is the Problem?

As was alluded to earlier, the symptomatic trials changed practice largely because interdisciplinary consensus was achieved and maintained. However, despite level I (Grade A) evidence supporting intervention by CEA, the management of asymptomatic carotid disease continues to polarize opinion around the world. It is inevitable that different health systems will embrace CEA in asymptomatic patients with varying degrees of enthusiasm, but the magnitude of variation does seem remarkable given that management decisions and fiscal priorities are based upon interpretation of the same data. Accordingly, the literature is full of contradictions in terms of what should now be considered optimal practice. As will be seen, these differences in opinion follow common themes including a lower overall benefit conferred by CEA in asymptomatic patients, inappropriate interpretation of the published data, perceived conflicts of interest by those offering CEA and CAS to asymptomatic patients, poor utilization of health resources, an inability to identify "high risk for stroke" patient cohorts, and (most importantly) a growing belief that improvements in BMT may have rendered the findings of ACAS and ACST obsolete.

For example, the Iberian Medical Tourism Network has concluded that the evidence supporting intervention is already compelling. Not only does their website provide patients with quotations for CEA or carotid artery stenting (CAS), but it also informs the reader that the indications for CAS in asymptomatic patients are "essentially the same as for standard open CEA."[8] Clearly, there is no need for any level I evidence in this organization. There is also a much greater enthusiasm for intervention in asymptomatic patients in the USA (compared with the UK). In 2005, 135,701 revascularizations (CEA/CAS) were performed in the US, of which 122,986 (92%) were in asymptomatic patients.[9] By contrast, only 20% of all carotid reconstructions in the UK were undertaken in asymptomatic individuals in 2006–2008.[10]

There are even polarized opinions within the same country about whether the available evidence supports screening for asymptomatic carotid disease. For example, the Society for Vascular Surgery (the professional body for US vascular surgeons) actively campaigns for carotid screening,[11] a cause now taken up by several commercial organizations.[12] Yet, based upon the same published data, the US Preventive Services Task Force[13] actively campaigns against screening, concluding that any benefit would be "limited by a low overall prevalence of treatable disease in the general asymptomatic population and harms from treatment."

There are also considerable interdisciplinary variations in practice, possibly because the treatment of asymptomatic disease represents a considerable source of income to surgeons and interventionists. The Society for Vascular Surgery has concluded that while there is Grade 1 evidence for performing CEA in asymptomatic patients with 60–99% stenoses, they have proposed that there is no evidence supporting the routine use of CAS in "standard risk" patients.[14] Not surprisingly, several interventionists disagree with this surgeon-led initiative.[15–17] For some interventionists,[16] developing the role for CAS in asymptomatic patients is now a race at "breakneck speed," while for others, a failure to offer treatment to patients with 80–99% asymptomatic stenoses verges on the indefensible.[15] More worrying and perhaps reflecting a wider body of opinion than just the German Pro-CAS Registry, Theiss et al. observed that "although it has been claimed that patients should only be treated within trials, the promising results reported by the majority of authors involved in CAS are leading to its everyday use in many parts of the world."[17] In short, there is a growing body of opinion that there is no need for CAS to prove either equivalence or superiority in randomized trials for it to be adopted into routine clinical practice.

Now, contrast these pro-interventional opinions with those of a growing body of neurologists and stroke physicians. Within a year of publication of the ACAS alert, Barnett et al. questioned whether the published evidence justified the huge increase in CEA numbers.[18] Two years later, a consortium of Canadian stroke neurologists actively campaigned against both screening and intervention with CEA in asymptomatic patients.[19] By 2003, neurologists were calling for the randomized trials to be repeated;[20] by 2008, editorials began to suggest that many patients should probably be treated conservatively;[21] while by 2009, a comprehensive systematic review of the published literature was interpreted to show that medical therapy was now the most clinical and cost-effective treatment for patients with asymptomatic carotid disease.[22]

Advocates of intervention may find the last recommendation incomprehensible (especially as the 2006 AHA guidelines again reaffirmed the beneficial role of CEA,[7]) but they should take careful note of the widespread uncertainty exposed in a 2008 New England Journal of Medicine audit of practice.[23] In this study, a case scenario was presented to the reader (67-year-old non-smoking male with hypertension, hyperlipidemia, and a 70–80% asymptomatic carotid stenosis), and three experts then gave their opinion as to how he should be treated. Following this, almost 5,000 readers voted their recommendation for treatment. Interestingly, almost half (49%) said they would treat him medically, 32% recommended CEA, while 19% said they would perform CAS. This pattern of response was consistently reproduced across every continent, including North America. Of particular interest was the observation that in addition to the NEJM worldwide audit observing that the single most common recommendation was BMT, up to a quarter of respondents recommended CAS, despite there being no level I evidence supporting CAS in "standard risk" asymptomatic patients.

Notwithstanding criticisms that the NEJM readership may be unrepresentative of who normally makes management decisions in this type of patient, the most interesting observation was the fact that the majority viewpoint was actually contrary to published evidence. Secondary analyses from the ACST suggest that the very patient who probably has most to gain from prophylactic CEA is the young male with asymptomatic carotid disease.[6,24] If the patient had been female, or older than 75 years (see later), then a trend towards adopting a more conservative management strategy would have been more understandable.

4.4 Why Are There Such Polarized Opinions?

It should now be clear that there are a number of discordant interdisciplinary opinions ranging from whether we should even intervene at all, to the other extreme where the only debate is whether treatment should be by CEA or CAS. This section will detail why there is such a surprising lack of consensus despite the performance of high quality randomized trials.

4.5 Interpretation of the AHA Guidelines

The first comment relates to the vox populi interpretation of the AHA guidelines. What exactly does "highly selected" or "high grade stenosis" mean (does anyone pay any attention?) and is there any evidence that the 3% risk threshold is either audited or respected? Unfortunately, there is a perception amongst many neurologists that surgeons (interventionists) simply view the AHA guidelines as being supportive of *any* intervention in *any* asymptomatic patient with a 60–99% stenosis, i.e., few will pay any attention to the "highly selected" or "high grade stenosis" caveats.

4.6 Clinical Governance

Second, there is little evidence that clinical governance is working, leading to widespread concerns amongst stroke physicians that many procedures are probably being performed with risks that are higher than was observed in ACAS and ACST. The AHA guidelines recommend that the procedural risk should be less than 3%.[7] If it exceeds 4%, no benefit accrues to the patient. If it exceeds 6%, actual harm is being conferred. But does anyone really pay that much attention? ACAS and ACST used selected surgeons (based on their track record), and 40% of surgeon applicants in ACAS were rejected.[25] Accordingly, there have been long standing concerns regarding generalizability of the trial results into routine clinical practice.

Systematic reviews suggest that vascular units must perform more than 79 CEAs per year in order to ensure optimal outcomes,[26] but community-based studies suggest that in many countries a large number of surgeons perform very few CEAs. One representative example is a 10-year audit of practice from Maryland in the United States (22,772 CEAs) which found that 48% of surgeons performed only one CEA per year and with poorer outcomes than their higher volume colleagues.[27] Accordingly, it is impossible to ensure that these low volume surgeons provide a safe service to their patients. For example, Irvine et al. have highlighted just how difficult it is to identify the surgeon (or interventionist) whose performance is substandard relative to the number of CEAs (CAS procedures) performed each year.[28] He observed that in order to reliably determine whether a surgeon had a death/stroke rate that was twice the 3% threshold for operating upon asymptomatic patients, he/she would need to operate upon at least 280 patients. Simple maths reveals that for a surgeon performing only 10 CEAs per year, it would take 28 years to determine whether he/she was performing in a substandard manner. For a surgeon performing only one CEA per year, that goal is impossible.

This might, therefore, explain why community-based audits regularly find procedural risks after CEA in asymptomatic patients that are well in excess of 4%.[29,30] It is a sobering fact that NASCET and ACAS trial hospitals currently comprise only 3% of all institutions performing CEA in the United States, performing only 6% of all endarterectomies. However, they still consistently report a lower operative risk compared with non-trial hospitals.[31] In a review of two multistate audits of practice in the US, Bunch and Kresowik observed that seven of ten states reported 30-day death/stroke rates that were in excess of 3% in 2001. More important, if patients with remote symptoms (i.e., > 6 months prior) and those with "non-hemispheric" or vertebrobasilar symptoms were excluded (i.e., they now fulfilled ACST entry criteria), the procedural risk increased to a very worrying 5.9%. When the same audit was repeated in 2004, the 30-day risk had only declined slightly to 5.4%.[29] In neither of these audits, however, did the authors comment that at these levels of risk, no benefit was being conferred to the patient. It should also be noted that similar criticisms also apply to CAS practitioners (see later) as a number of CAS Registries publish risks that are well in excess of the 3% AHA threshold.[30]

4.7 Surgeon's Beliefs

Third is the widespread held belief that by performing CEA or CAS on vast numbers of asymptomatic patients, the surgeon (or interventionist) will somehow confer significant reductions in the overall burden of stroke in his/her community. Even if it were possible to identify and then operate upon every single patient with an asymptomatic 60–99% stenosis, it is an indisputable fact that at least 95% of all strokes destined to occur will still happen.[32,33] Moreover, it is actually a logistical impossibility to undertake this magnitude of workload. For a population of one million, approximately 1% (10,000) will have an asymptomatic 60–99% stenosis. Notwithstanding the length of time it would take to screen and find the 10,000 individuals with a significant carotid stenosis and work them up for treatment, if a hospital were then to perform one CEA (or CAS) on every working day of the week, it would take 38 years to treat the 10,000 patients. If five interventions were performed every day in the city, it would still take 8 years. Accordingly, given that it would take years to screen and find the 10,000 asymptomatic patients in the general population and then many more years to treat them (never mind the new population of patients emerging with asymptomatic carotid disease in the interim), it is highly likely that the overall reduction in stroke would be about a 1–2%. Hardly a ringing endorsement for efficiency and utilization of resources!

4.8 Failure to Prioritize Patients

Fourth is a failure by health systems to prioritize patients. Notwithstanding the uncomfortable fact that the treatment of asymptomatic patients is an important source of revenue to surgeons and interventionists worldwide, the first priority must always be the rapid treatment of symptomatic patients. Evidence suggests that this is not the case.[33] There is now compelling evidence[34,35] that patients presenting with a TIA or minor stroke gain maximum benefit if subjected to CEA within 2 weeks of onset of symptoms (185 strokes prevented per 1,000 CEAs at 5 years). The same stricture will also apply to CAS. If the delay is 2–4 weeks, the number of strokes prevented falls to 98, and if it exceeds 12 weeks, only 8 strokes are prevented at 5 years per 1,000 interventions. In practice, very rapid treatment of symptomatic patients will prevent almost four times as many strokes in the long term than performing CEA or CAS on an equivalent number of asymptomatic patients. Accordingly, practices need to change. If it is regularly taking a surgeon more than 4 weeks to treat symptomatic patients, is it still acceptable to continue to treat any asymptomatic patients at all? This is a very important issue to confront, especially as 92% of all carotid interventions in the US are now undertaken in asymptomatic individuals.[9]

4.9 Financial Burden

Fifth; The inevitable consequence of treating huge numbers of asymptomatic patients is the financial burden imposed upon health systems. This is a highly controversial subject that is rarely broached in any discussion about clinical effectiveness and optimal utilization of resources. The following section will deal with practice in the USA (largely because they have published the best data), but there are important messages for every health system. The Centres for Medicare and Medicaid Services predicts that US Health care spending will nearly double to $4.3 trillion by 2017, i.e., consuming about 20% of GDP.[35] It is quite a daunting prospect for lower paid workers and their families. By 2005, family insurance premiums for a US federal employee on the minimum wage consumed up to 75% of his/her full time earnings.[36] Similarly, General Motors (GM) previously spent $6 billion annually on health care (twice as much as it did on steel), while Health care costs added about $1,500 to the price of each car.[37] Commenting upon the unparalleled accelerating costs of US Health care, Professor Brian Rubin (himself a surgeon) observed that "evidence based studies would hopefully determine which therapies offered an adequate return on investment."[38]

Given Rubin's aspiration about the role of evidence in determining optimal (and cost-effective) practices, an alternative interpretation of the ACAS data makes for bleak reading. Returning to the US statistics,[9] 122,986 revascularizations in asymptomatic patients were performed in 2005 (91% CEA, 9% CAS). Because McPhee et al. determined the average total hospital costs for CEA and CAS, it is now possible to model cost against benefit in terms of strokes prevented for asymptomatic patients. Using the ACAS data summarized in Table 4.1, 59 ipsilateral strokes will be prevented at 5 years by performing 1,000 CEAs assuming a 2.3% procedural risk. The parallel figure for "any strokes" prevented is 51. If these values are now extrapolated into McPhee et al.'s data, it becomes apparent that in 2005, only 7,256 ipsilateral strokes would have been prevented at 5 years (i.e., 59 × 122.986). The parallel number of "any strokes" prevented would be 6,272.

If one now focuses solely upon ipsilateral strokes prevented (similar calculations for "any stroke" are actually not that different), this means that 115,730 patients (94%) underwent an ultimately unnecessary procedure. Using the total hospital costs published by McPhee et al., this equates to US$2.18 billion dollars spent in 1 year alone in patients ultimately undergoing an unnecessary intervention. No health system can either justify or maintain this level of spending on "unnecessary" interventions.

4.10 Inability to Stratify Risk

Sixth is the simple fact that despite two very large randomized clinical trials (RCTs) comparing CEA with BMT, it is still not known which asymptomatic patient is at a higher or lower risk of suffering a stroke. Even more fundamental, we have still not even determined whether women gain significant benefit from surgery. In ACAS, CEA did not confer significant benefit in women,[5] even when a secondary analysis excluded the operative risk.[39] ACST (at first) claimed that women gained significant benefit at 5 years,[6] but this was only true if the operative risk was excluded.[24] When the operative risk was included, all significant benefit ceased.[24] In the 2005 Cochrane Review,[40] Chambers and Donnan combined the ACAS and ACST data (including the operative risk) and observed that while males gained a highly significant twofold reduction in the risk of late stroke (OR 2.0, 95% CI 1.5–2.8), CEA conferred no overall benefit in women (OR 1.0, 95% CI 0.7–1.6).

The reason for the apparent lack of benefit in women is probably a combination of there being a slightly higher operative risk in women than in men (4.0% vs 2.4% in ACST, 3.6% vs 1.7% in ACAS) in conjunction with a lower 5-year risk of stroke in women randomized to medical therapy compared with men (8.7% vs 12.1% in ACAS, 7.5% vs 10.6% in ACST). That there is a gender difference in risk was also supported in Bond's recent systematic review[41] (29,345 CEAs) which showed that the 30-day risk of death/stroke after CEA was significantly higher than in men (OR 1.28, 95% CI 1.12–1.46).

Moreover, simply stating that because women live longer than men they will have a greater time to gain benefit is not sustainable. Notwithstanding the fact that ACST showed that patients older than 75 gained no benefit from CEA,[6] emerging data from the ACST show that even after 10 years of follow-up, it was still not possible for women to overcome the 4.0% procedural risk and then demonstrate significant benefit in terms of late strokes prevented. This author concedes that some women will benefit from intervention (probably the younger, fitter patient), but it would be wrong to suggest that the available evidence supports treating all women under the age of 75 as if they gained the same long term benefit as men. This is a fundamental issue to be resolved as most national guidelines (with the exception of the 2009 European Society of Vascular Surgery Guidelines[42]) do not currently discriminate in their advice regarding the relative effectiveness of treatment of males and females.

4.11 Severity of Stenosis as an Indicator of Risk

Seventh, and back to a recurring theme, is our continued inability to "pick winners." In the symptomatic trials, increasing stenosis severity conferred increasing benefit in terms of strokes prevented by CEA.[43] Not surprisingly, therefore, there is an intuitively held belief that asymptomatic patients with 80–99% stenoses will face a very much higher annual risk of stroke, to the extent that it would be almost unethical not to treat them.[15] This observation is not, however, supported by evidence. Contrary to intuitive thinking, neither ACAS nor ACST found any evidence that there was any association between stenosis severity and late stroke risk.[5,6] This observation was later corroborated in a review of 26 natural history studies,[43] which correlated the severity of stenosis at study entry with the average annual risk of stroke thereafter. Across a wide range of stenoses (including 80–99%), the annual risk of stroke rarely exceeded 3% and none exceeded 4%. One exception refers to a subgroup analysis in the ACSRS study which showed that patients with a 90–99% stenosis *plus* a history of contralateral TIA *plus* renal impairment faced a 6.5% annual risk of stroke.[44] All other patients in the 90–99% stenosis category, however, faced a 1% annual ipsilateral stroke risk. In practice, the number of patients likely to fulfill all three of these three caveats is inconsequential.

The lack of any clear association between stenosis severity and stroke risk suggests that asymptomatic carotid plaques are, for the most part, "stable." Further evidence to support this statement comes from a secondary analysis in the ECST which showed that while ipsilateral stroke risk increased in proportion to stenosis severity in symptomatic patients, this only held true for the first 2 years after randomization.[3] Thereafter, there was *no* association between stenosis severity and stroke risk, suggesting that by 2 years after the index event, most previously symptomatic plaques had "stabilized."

4.12 Data from Registries

Eighth is a plea for caution regarding a growing tendency to over-interpret findings from the "high risk for CEA" CAS Registries, championed by some as being an alternative to RCTs.[45] There are now a large number of these studies in the literature, though very few have been published in peer-reviewed journals. Each was developed to prove efficacy for proprietary stents and protection devices from rival manufacturers. The vast majority of patients entering these Registries were asymptomatic and between 25% and 40% had restenosis after endarterectomy (i.e., non-atherosclerotic disease). A recent review of the data from these studies suggests that many have published 30-day risks that were well in excess of the 3% threshold recommended by the AHA and quite a proportion published risks in excess of 5%.[39] Because none of the factors deemed to render the asymptomatic patient "higher risk for CEA" are associated with an increase in the natural history risk of stroke, the 3% AHA threshold of procedural risk must continue to apply.[46]

There has, however, been a more recent trend toward improved outcomes following CAS in "high risk for CEA" asymptomatic patients (i.e., approaching 3% in patients younger than 80 years).[47] This has led to the suggestion that this might constitute evidence for offering CAS to "standard risk" asymptomatic patients. However, readers must ensure that "apples are not being compared with oranges." Only one published Registry (Acculink for Revascularization of Carotids in High-Risk Patients or ARCHeR) has stratified outcomes relative to the nature of the underlying disease.[48] Within ARCHeR, the overall 30-day risk of death/stroke was 6.9% after CAS. However, the procedural risk in patients with non-atherosclerotic disease (i.e., predominantly restenosis) was reported as being 0.7%. This means that the 30-day risk in patients with atherosclerotic disease must have been about 9.6% (i.e., 14 times higher).[49] As a consequence, it would not be appropriate to uncritically extrapolate data from non-randomized CAS Registries in order to advise on the optimal management of patients with asymptomatic atherosclerotic disease if the real procedural risks in patients with atherosclerotic disease were being diluted by the inclusion of a significant minority of low risk patients with non-atherosclerotic disease.[50]

4.13 Declining Risk and Modern "Best Medical Therapy"

Ninth and perhaps the most important of all is a growing awareness that the natural history risk of stroke in patients with asymptomatic carotid stenosis being treated medically is declining, probably as a consequence of improvements in the modern concept of best medical therapy. This is a very important issue to be resolved as every current guideline of practice assumes that the risk of stroke (on medical therapy) is similar to that observed when ACAS published 14 years ago and when ACST published 5 years ago. If, however, the annual rate of fatal/major stroke falls below 1.1%, no benefit will ever accrue to any patient from either CEA or CAS.[51]

The first real evidence that the stroke risk might be declining became apparent following a reanalysis of the ACAS and ACST data. Table 4.1 provides the "traditional" way in which the data are presented. Many uncritical observers have then concluded that both trials reported similar outcomes, but what is often not recognized, however, is that the two trials were not using the same definition of "stroke."

In its original paper, ACAS published 5-year risks for both "ipsilateral" stroke and "any" stroke. The 11.0% in Table 4.1 refers to the 5-year risk of "ipsilateral" stroke in the BMT arm. The 5-year risk of "any" stroke was 17.5%. By contrast, ACST initially only published 5-year outcomes for "any" stroke. In 2009, ACST began to report their 10-year data at International Meetings and, for the first time, included data on the 5 and 10-year risks of ipsilateral stroke. Table 4.2 now presents the ACAS and ACST data of the BMT arms of these trials in a slightly different format so that changing trends in the 5-year risk of "any" stroke and "ipsilateral" stroke can be analyzed separately. Note that between 1995 and 2004, the 5-year risks of "any" stroke in the non-operated patients fell by 33% from 17.5% to 11.8%. There was also a 52% decline in the 5-year risk of "ipsilateral" stroke from 11.0% to 5.3%. When ACST released its second 5-year period of data in 2009 (i.e., years 6–10), the risk of "any" stroke had fallen by a further 39% from 11.8% to 7.2%, while the 5-year risk of "ipsilateral" stroke fell by 32% from 5.3% to 3.6%. If one now looks at the 14-year period between ACAS publishing its first 5-year stroke risks in 1995 with comparable data released by ACST in 2009, the 5-year risk of "any" stroke has fallen by 59% from 17.5% to 7.2%, while the 5-year risk of "ipsilateral" stroke has fallen by 67% from 11.0% to 3.6%.

Further evidence suggesting that there has been a sustained reduction in the annual risk of stroke in patients with asymptomatic carotid disease has also emerged. Figure 4.1 details the temporal changes in the average annual risks of "any" stroke and "ipsilateral" stroke in a series of randomized and non-randomized cohorts of asymptomatic patients with 50–99% stenoses published between 1985 and 2008. Even though this figure does not include the latest data from ACST, there is clear evidence of a sustained decline in the average annual risk of stroke over the last 25 years.[52]

More recently, a systematic review and meta-analysis of all of the natural history data in patients with

Table 4.2 Temporal changes in the 5-year risk of "any" stroke and "ipsilateral" stroke in the best medical treatment arm of the ACAS and ACST (*)

Trial	Years	Year published	"Any" stroke (%)	"Ipsilateral" stroke (%)
ACAS	1–5	1995	17.5	11.0
ACST	1–5	2004	11.8	5.3 [a]
ACST	6–10	2009	7.2 [a]	3.6 [a]

Source: Reprinted from the Naylor et al.,[52] Copyright 2009, with permission from Elsevier
[a] Derived from oral presentations of the 10-year ACST data

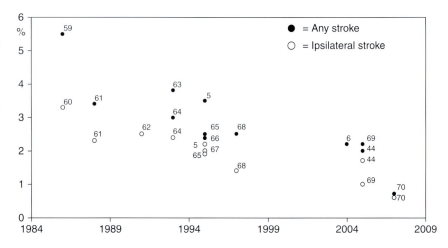

Fig. 4.1 Annual rates of ipsilateral and "any" stroke in patients with an asymptomatic 50–99% stenosis stratified by date of publication (Adapted from the Naylor et al.,[52] Copyright 2009, with permission from Elsevier. The author acknowledges that many of these studies were sourced from Abbott et al.[53])

an asymptomatic 50–99% stenosis have been performed by Abbott.[22] She observed that the average annual rate of ipsilateral stroke had fallen by an absolute value of 1.4% from 1985 through to 2007, while the average annual rate of "any territory" stroke had declined by an absolute value of 2.3%. She concluded that BMT was now three to eight times more cost-effective than CEA/CAS (in terms of stroke prevention) and that until there was a reliable way of targeting CEA or CAS towards "high risk for stroke" individuals, most asymptomatic patients should not now be treated by either intervention.[22] Since Abbott published this meta-analysis, another natural history series lends further support to evidence suggesting that there has been a decline in the annual risk of stroke. Marquardt et al. analyzed annual rates of stroke in a cohort of patients who were recruited in the last 10 years (i.e., they would be more likely to have received the modern concept of best medical therapy[54]). This group observed that 101 asymptomatic patients with a 50–99% stenosis were followed up for a mean of 3 years. During this time, the average annual rate of ipsilateral stroke was only 0.34% (95% CI 0.01–1.87). The average annual rate of ipsilateral disabling stroke in this series was 0% (95% CI 0.0–0.99).

What might have accounted for these sustained reductions in the annual risk of stroke? The most likely explanation is the continued improvement in what constitutes the modern concept of "best medical therapy." In the early 1990s, when ACAS was recruiting, most patients randomized to medical therapy were started on aspirin and advised to stop smoking. Thereafter, the quality of medical therapy improved throughout the period of time that ACST recruited, however, even that bears little comparison with what would now be considered really optimal practice (i.e., low-dose ACE inhibition, multi-agent hypertensive therapy, more aggressive hypertension therapy in diabetics, more aggressive lifestyle modification, dual antiplatelet therapy (aspirin and dipyridamole), higher dose statin therapy, discontinuation of HRT in post-menopausal women, and better glycemic control in diabetics).

Given the conclusions from Abbott's systematic review and the data from Table 4.2 and Fig. 4.1, it is hard not to speculate that if the planned/ongoing asymptomatic trials comparing CEA and CAS also included an adequately powered medical limb using the therapeutic strategy outlined above, it is possible that most patients would probably no longer need to undergo any intervention at all.

4.14 Conclusions

The use of stenosis severity as the sole arbiter of who might benefit from CEA (or CAS) has failed. Despite the performance of two high-quality, level I randomized trials, we still cannot identify which patients are "high risk for stroke" in order that resources can be targeted at a smaller cohort of "high risk" patients. As a consequence, vast amounts of resources are wasted in treating huge numbers of patients, while contributing little to reducing the overall burden of stroke.

Abbott has argued that in the absence of reliable methods for identifying which patients are truly "high risk," no patient should now undergo CEA or CAS.[22] If this approach is to be countered, future resources must be directed at developing clinical biomarker and imaging modalities capable of identifying a smaller cohort of patients who would specifically benefit from CEA or CAS.

Although never evaluated (as yet) in randomized trials, a number of imaging modalities have shown promise. For example, Spence et al. observed that the annual risk of stroke was only 1% in patients with an asymptomatic 60–99% stenosis if there was no evidence of embolization on transcranial Doppler (TCD)[55] compared with a 15% annual risk in patients with TCD evidence of embolization. Other predictive options include identifying intraplaque hemorrhage on MR[56] or using image normalized grey scale median measurement,[57] the use of CT to identify a preexisting infarction or methods for evaluating the patency of the circle of Willis. In a recent subgroup analysis from the ACSRS, patients with a 60–99% stenosis and an ipsilateral infarct on CT scan faced a 3.6% annual rate of stroke over the next 8 years, as compared with only 1.0% in patients with similar stenoses but no infarction.[58]

The management of patients with asymptomatic carotid disease remains enduringly controversial.

References

1. Thompson JE, Patman RD, Talkington CM. Asymptomatic carotid bruit: long term outcome of patients having endarterectomy compared with unoperated controls. *Ann Surg*. 1978;188(3):308–316.
2. Winslow CM et al. The appropriateness of carotid endarterectomy. *NEJM*. 1988;318:721–727.
3. European Carotid Surgery Trialists' Collaborative Group. Randomised trial of endarterectomy for recently symptomatic carotid stenosis: final results of the MRC European Carotid Surgery Trial (ECST). *Lancet*. 1998;351: 1379–1387.
4. Barnett HJM et al. Benefit of carotid endarterectomy in patients with symptomatic moderate or severe stenosis. *N Engl J Med*. 1998;339:1415–1425.
5. Executive Committee for the Asymptomatic Carotid Atherosclerosis Study. Endarterectomy for asymptomatic carotid artery stenosis. *JAMA*. 1995;273:1421–1428.
6. Asymptomatic Carotid Surgery Trial Collaborators. The MRC Asymptomatic Carotid Surgery Trial (ACST): carotid endarterectomy prevents disabling and fatal carotid territory strokes. *Lancet*. 2004;363:1491–1502.
7. Goldstein LB et al. Primary prevention of ischemic stroke. A guideline from the American Heart Association/American Stroke Association Stroke Council: Cosponsored by the Atherosclerotic Peripheral Vascular Disease Interdisciplinary Working Group; Cardiovascular Nursing Council; Clinical Cardiology Council; Nutrition, Physical Activity, and Metabolism Council; and the Quality of Care and Outcomes Research Interdisciplinary Working Group. *Stroke*. 2006;37:1583–1663.
8. Iberian Medical Tourism Network. Carotid Angioplasty with Stenting (CAS) [Internet]. 2011. Available at: http://www.fly2doc.com/public/Text.php?text_id=88. Cited January 27, 2011.
9. McPhee JT, Schanzer A, Messina LM, Eslami MH. Carotid artery stenting has increased rates of post-procedure stroke, death and resource utilization than does carotid endarterectomy in the United States, 2005. *J Vasc Surg*. 2008;48:1442–1450.
10. Halliday AW et al. Long waiting times for carotid endarterectomy in the UK. *BMJ*. 2009;338:1847–1851.
11. Society for Vascular Surgery (SVS). SVS position statement on vascular screening [Internet]. 2011. Available at: http://www.vascularweb.org/about/positionstatements/Pages/svs-position-statement-on-vascular-screening.aspx. Updated January 2011, cited January 27, 2011.
12. Life Line Screening. Preventive health screening [Internet]. 2011. Available at: http://www.lifelinescreening.co.uk/faqs/preventive-health-screening.aspx. Cited January 27, 2011).
13. US Preventive Services Task Force. Screening for carotid artery stenosis: US Preventive Services Task Force Recommendation Statement. *Ann Intern Med*. 2007;147:854–859.
14. Hobson RW et al. Management of atherosclerotic carotid artery disease: clinical practice guidelines of the Society for Vascular Surgery. *J Vasc Surg*. 2008;48:480–486.
15. Wholey MH, Barbato JE, Al-Khoury GE. Treatment of asymptomatic carotid disease with stenting. *Semin Vasc Surg*. 2008;21:95–99.

16. Fayad P. Endarterectomy and stenting for asymptomatic carotid stenosis: a race at breakneck speed. *Stroke.* 2007;38(part 2):707–714.
17. Theiss W et al. Pro-CAS: a prospective registry of carotid angioplasty and stenting. *Stroke.* 2004;35:2134–2139.
18. Barnett HJM, Eliasziw M, Meldrum HE, Taylor DW. Do the facts and figures warrant a tenfold increase in the performance of carotid endarterectomy on asymptomatic patients? *Neurology.* 1996;46:603–608.
19. Perry JR, Szalai JP, Norris JW. Consensus against both endarterectomy and routine screening for asymptomatic carotid artery stenosis: the Canadian Stroke Consortium. *Arch Neurol.* 1997;54:25–28.
20. Chaturvedi S. Should the multicenter carotid endarterectomy trials be repeated? *Arch Neurol.* 2003;60:774–775.
21. Abbott A. Asymptomatic carotid artery stenosis: it's time to stop operating. *Nat Clin Pract Neurol.* 2008;4:4–5.
22. Abbott AL. Medical (non-surgical) intervention alone is now the best for prevention of stroke associated with asymptomatic severe carotid stenosis: results of a systematic review and analysis. *Stroke.* 2009;40:e573-e583.
23. Klein A, Solomon CG, Hamel MB. Management of carotid stenosis – polling results. *N Engl J Med.* 2008;358:e23.
24. Rothwell PM. ACST: which subgroups will benefit most from carotid endarterectomy. *Lancet.* 2004;364:1122–1123.
25. Moore WS et al. Selection process for surgeons in the Asymptomatic Carotid Atherosclerosis Study. *Stroke.* 1991;22:1353–1357.
26. Holt PJE, Poloniecki JD, Loftus IM, Thompson MM. Meta-analysis and systematic review of the relationship between hospital volume and outcome following carotid endarterectomy. *Eur J Vasc Endovasc Surg.* 2007;33:645–651.
27. Nazarian SM et al. Statistical modeling of the volume-outcome effect for carotid endarterectomy for 10 years of a statewide database. *J Vasc Surg.* 2008;48(2):343–350.
28. Irvine CD, Grayson D, Lusby RJ. Clinical governance and the surgeon. *Br J Surg.* 2000;87:766–770.
29. Bunch CT, Kresowik TF. Can randomized trial outcomes for carotid endarterectomy be achieved in community wide practice? *Semin Vasc Surg.* 2004;17:209–213.
30. Naylor AR. When and how to treat asymptomatic carotid disease. In: Jacobs M, Branchereau A, eds. *Innovations in Cardiovascular Surgery.* Turin: Edizioni Minerva Medica; 2009:119–132.
31. Wennberg DE, Lucas FL, Birkmeyer JD, Bredenberg CE, Fisher ES. Variation in carotid endarterectomy mortality in the Medicare population. *JAMA.* 1998;279:1278–1281.
32. Hankey GJ. Asymptomatic carotid stenosis: how should it be managed? *Med J Aust.* 1995;163:197–200.
33. Naylor AR. Time is brain! *Surgeon.* 2007;5:23–30.
34. Rothwell PM et al. Endarterectomy for symptomatic carotid stenosis in relation to clinical subgroups and timing of surgery. *Lancet.* 2004;363:915–924.
35. Naylor AR. Occam's Razor: intervene early to prevent more strokes. *J Vasc Surg.* 2008;48:1053–1059.
36. California Healthcare Foundation. Health Insurance: Can Californians Afford It? [Internet]. 2005. Available at: http://www.sullivaninservices.com/HealthInsuranceAffordability.pdf. Cited January 27, 2011.
37. Chalice R. *Improving Healthcare using Toyota Lean Production Methods.* 2nd ed. Milwaukee: Quality; 2007.
38. McKinsey Global Institute. Accounting for the cost of US health care: a new look at why Americans spend more [Internet]. 2008. Available at: http://www.mckinsey.com/mgi/reports/pdfs/healthcare/US_healthcare_Executive_summary.pdf. Updated December 8, 2008; cited March 9, 2011.
39. Young B et al. An analysis of peri-operative surgical mortality and morbidity in the asymptomatic carotid atherosclerosis study. *Stroke.* 1996;27:2216–2224.
40. Chambers BR, Donnan GA. Carotid endarterectomy for asymptomatic carotid stenosis. *Cochrane Database Syst Rev.* 2005, Issue 4. doi: 10.1002/14651858.CD001923.pub2.
41. Bond R, Rerkasem K, Cuffe R, Rothwell PM. A systematic review of the associations between age and sex and the operative risks of carotid endarterectomy. *Cerebrovasc Dis.* 2005;20:69–77.
42. Liapis C et al. ESVS guidelines: invasive treatment for carotid stenosis: indications and techniques. *Eur J Vasc Endovasc Surg.* 2009;37(suppl):1–19.
43. Naylor AR, Rothwell PM, Bell PRF. Overview of the principal results and secondary analyses from the European and the North American randomised trials of carotid endarterectomy. *Eur J Vasc Endovasc Surg.* 2003;26:115–129.
44. Nicolaides AN et al. Severity of asymptomatic carotid stenosis and risk of ipsilateral hemispheric ischaemic events: results from the ACSRS. *Eur J Vasc Endovasc Surg.* 2005;30:275–284.
45. Gray WA. The rise of the registry: of signal importance in carotid artery stenting. *Endovasc Today.* 2007;6:47–51.
46. Naylor AR. Intervention for carotid artery disease: time to confront some inconvenient truths! *Expert Rev Cardiovasc Ther.* 2007;5:1053–1063.
47. Gray WA, Chaturvedi S, Verta P. Thirty-day outcomes for carotid artery stenting in 6320 patients from two prospective, multicentre, high-surgical-risk registries. *Circ Cardiovasc Intervt.* 2009;2:159–166.
48. Gray WA et al. Protected carotid stenting in high surgical risk patients: the ARCHeR results. *J Vasc Surg.* 2006;44:258–269.
49. Katzen BT, Laird JR, Ohki T. The SAPPHIRE and ARCHeR Updates [Internet]. Available at: www.evtodayarchive.com/03_archive/0903/171.html. Cited January 27, 2011.
50. Naylor AR. One size does not fit all! *Vasc News.* 2008;40:6.
51. Arazi HC et al. Carotid endarterectomy in asymptomatic stenosis: a decision analysis. *Clin Neurol Neurosurg.* 2008;110:472–479.
52. Naylor AR, Gaines PA, Rothwell PM. Who benefits most from treating asymptomatic carotid disease: patients or professionals? *Eur J Vasc Endovasc Surg.* 2009;37: 625–632.
53. Abbott AL, Bladin CF, Levi CR, Chambers BR. What should we do with asymptomatic carotid stenosis? *Int J Stroke.* 2007;2:27–39.
54. Marquardt L, Geraghty OC, Mehta Z, Rothwell PM. Low risk of ipsilateral stroke in patients with asymptomatic carotid stenosis on best medical therapy: a prospective, population based study. *Stroke.* 2010;41:e11-e17.
55. Spence DJ, Tamayo A, Lownie SP, Ng WP, Ferguson GG. Absence of microemboli on transcranial Doppler identifies low risk patients with asymptomatic carotid stenosis. *Stroke.* 2005;36:2373–2378.

56. Altaf N, MacSweeney ST, Gladman J, Auer DP. Carotid intraplaque haemorrhage predicts recurrent symptoms in patients with high-grade carotid stenosis. *Stroke*. 2007;38:1633–1635.
57. Nicolaides AN et al. Effect of image normalisation on carotid plaque classification and the risk of ipsilateral ischemic events: results from the Asymptomatic Carotid Stenosis and Risk of Stroke Study. *Vascular*. 2005;13:211–221.
58. Kakkos S et al. Silent embolic infarcts on computed tomography brain scans and risk of ipsilateral hemispheric events in patients with asymptomatic internal carotid artery stenosis. *J Vasc Surg*. 2009;49:902–909.
59. Johnson JM, Kennelly MM, Decesare D, Morgan S, Sparrow A. Natural history of asymptomatic carotid plaque. *Arch Surg*. 1985;120:1010–1012.
60. Chambers BR, Norris JW. Outcome in patients with asymptomatic neck bruit. *NEJM*. 1986;315:860–865.
61. Satiani B, Porter RM, Biggers KM, Das BM. Natural history of non-operated significant carotid stenosis. *Ann Vasc Surg*. 1988;2:271–278.
62. Norris JW, Zhu CZ, Bornstein NM, Chambers BR. Vascular risks of asymptomatic carotid disease. *Stroke*. 1991;22:1485–1490.
63. Bock RW et al. The natural history of asymptomatic carotid artery disease. *J Vasc Surg*. 1993;17:160–169.
64. Hobson RW et al. Efficacy of carotid endarterectomy for asymptomatic carotid stenosis: the Veterans Affairs Cooperative Study Group. *NEJM*. 1993;345:209–212.
65. Mansour MA et al. The natural history of moderate 50–79% internal carotid artery stenosis in symptomatic, non-hemispheric and asymptomatic patients. *J Vasc Surg*. 1995;21:346–357.
66. Cote R, Battista RN, Abrahamowicz M, Langlois Y, Bourque F, Mackey A. Lack of effect of aspirin in asymptomatic patients with carotid bruits and substantial carotid narrowing: the Asymptomatic Cervical Bruit Study Group. *Ann Int Med*. 1995;123:649–655.
67. European Carotid Surgery Trialists Collaborative Group. Risk of stroke in the distribution of an asymptomatic carotid artery. *Lancet*. 1995;345:209–212.
68. Mackey AE et al. Outcome of asymptomatic patients with carotid disease. *Neurology*. 1997;48:896–903.
69. Abbott AL et al. Embolic signals and prediction of ipsilateral stroke or transient ischaemic attack in asymptomatic carotid stenosis: a multicentre Prospective Cohort Study. *Stroke*. 2005;36:1128–1133.
70. Goessens BMB et al. Asymptomatic carotid artery stenosis and the risk of new vascular events in patients with manifest arterial disease: the SMART study. *Stroke*. 2007;38:1470–1475.

Part II

Imaging Techniques

Principles of Ultrasonic Imaging and Instrumentation

Kirk W. Beach

5.1 Introduction

Vivid images of the carotid bifurcation and atherosclerotic plaques can be obtained using real time transcutaneous ultrasound (Fig. 5.1). Compared to other imaging methods, ultrasound has several advantages for studying the dynamic processes that characterize arterial pathology. Acquiring data at rates as high as 10,000 samples per second, while measuring motions less than 0.001 mm (1 µm) and strains in millimeter voxels less than 0.1%, ultrasound is ideally suited to obtain information about complicated turbulent blood flow in real time, as well as the associated dynamics of the arterial walls containing those flows. However, the identification of intraplaque tissue types visualized in ultrasound images has been elusive. Differentiating the types of plaque tissues is considered to be important. Although some severely stenotic carotid plaques are vulnerable to rupture-releasing emboli causing stroke, nearly 80% of severely stenotic plaques never cause clinical stroke.[1] Intraplaque tissue type is thought to be a critical factor in stratifying the risk of plaque rupture. Because of the need to identify plaque contents, other imaging methods, including MRI, are being developed to identify plaque tissues such as hemorrhage or lipid.[2] Although there is a logical connection between intraplaque tissue types and plaque rupture leading to embolic stroke, risk stratification on the basis of plaque content remains promising rather than proven. Because the theoretical relationship between plaque content and stroke risk is only a speculation, empirical correlation between plaque content and stroke is required in studies of large numbers of patients. Such studies are more easily done with a low cost method such as ultrasound if the method is effective.

In this chapter, the advantages and limitations of pulse-echo ultrasound examination are described based on physical principles. Both imaging and Doppler methods are considered. Imaging capabilities are compared to anatomic and physiologic goals. Acquisition and processing are discussed. Transmission ultrasound methods are not considered here as these methods have not, as yet, served any needs of medical imaging. Also, continuous wave methods are not considered here because these methods provide no information unavailable from pulsed-echo methods in the carotid arteries. This chapter does not provide detail about basic ultrasound physics which is well covered in numerous other text books.

5.2 Carotid Anatomy

The normal carotid artery is 8 mm in diameter with a wall comprising an intima–media complex with a thickness of 0.5 mm (IMT) contained in a 0.5-mm thick adventitia. Diffusion can supply nutrition and remove waste through a nonvascular tissue layer thickness of about 0.5 mm so the normal media does not require an embedded microvasculature, but the adventitia layer does require an embedded microcirculation. The muscular cells in the adventitia are near 0.01 mm in diameter and 0.1 mm long. They are arranged in layers perforated with an arteriolar supply and venular drainage connecting the vasa vasorum on

K.W. Beach
Department of Surgery and Bioengineering, University of Washington, Seattle, WA, USA

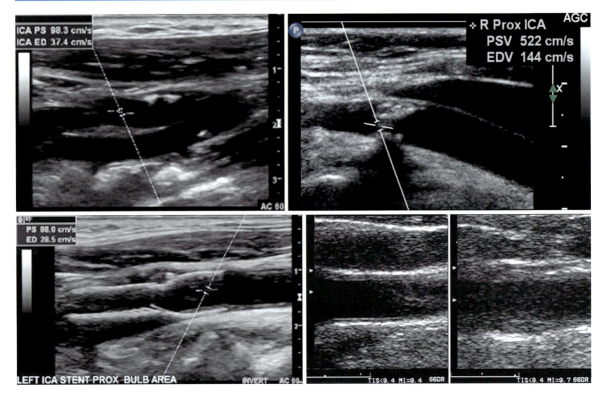

Fig. 5.1 Carotid bifurcations in longitudinal view. B-mode images showing wall features. Internal carotid artery extends to the left; common carotid artery is on the right. (*Top left*) Plaque with no stenosis; (*top right*) plaque with severe stenosis; (*bottom left*) carotid stent; (*bottom middle*) intima-Media layer on superficial and deep walls; (*bottom right*) minimal carotid plaque on deep wall

the adventitial surface to a network of 0.007-mm diameter capillaries. The capillaries are spaced at 0.1 mm intervals throughout the normal tissue. Thus, 0.5% of the tissue volume is capillary blood with an additional percentage of the volume in arteriolar and venular blood. Atherosclerotic plaques have a thickness between 1 and 8 mm with an average length of 18 mm. The microvascular blood supply to a plaque from the vasa vasorum is an extension of the supply to the normal wall. However, the neovascularization of the plaque often has microvessels with a greater size.

The normal carotid artery lies beneath 20 mm of skin, fat, and muscle, requiring an imaging depth of 40 mm to accommodate variability between patients.

5.2.1 Ultrasound Frequency, Wavelength and Resolution

Ultrasound examination of the carotid arteries is usually performed with ultrasound frequencies (F) between 5 and 15 MHz, having wavelengths (λ) between 0.3 and 0.1 mm (assuming an ultrasound speed (C) of 1.5 mm/µs).

$$F[\text{cy}/\mu s] * \lambda[\text{mm}/\text{cy}] = C[\text{mm}/\mu s]$$

$$\text{cy}/\mu s = \text{MHz}$$

$C = 1.54$ mm/µs in liver, 1.45 mm/µs in fat, 1.58 mm/µs in blood

Ultrasound instruments are capable of managing an echo amplitude range of 1,000,000–1, (120 dB); the difference in echo amplitude between blood and fibrous tissue is 1,000:1 (60 dB). Thus, an ultrasound pulse subject to 60 dB of attenuation has sufficient dynamic range above noise to return an adequate echo from blood without exceeding limits for echoes from fibrous tissue. At a typical attenuation rate of 1 dB/cm/MHz, echoes returning from a depth of 200 wavelengths are attenuated by 60 dB. 200 wavelengths of 0.2 mm ultrasound (7.5 MHz) provide a field depth of 40 mm. The depth resolution of broad band

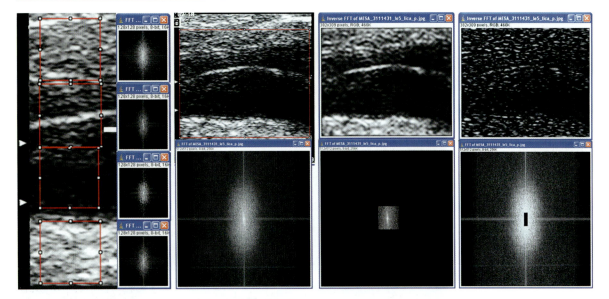

Fig. 5.2 Anisotropic resolution in ultrasound images. 2-dimensional Fourier transform of an ultrasound image shows higher spatial frequencies in the vertical direction than in the horizontal direction, verifying the better resolution in the vertical direction than in the horizontal direction. (*Left*) Four regions of interest (ROI) showing lower spatial frequencies in the lateral direction, shallow to and deep to the focal region (shown by the ≫ marks). (*Top middle left*) 2-D B-mode image; (*bottom middle left*) Fourier transform of full image. (*Bottom middle right*) 2-D Fourier transform, low pass filtered; (*top middle right*) inverse Fourier transform of low pass filtered image. (*Bottom right*) 2-D Fourier transform, high pass filtered; (*top right*) inverse Fourier transform of high pass filtered image

ultrasound can be near the central wavelength of ultrasound. The lateral resolution is much poorer (larger) than the depth resolution (Figs. 5.2 and 5.3). The lateral resolution is larger than the wavelength multiplied by the image depth divided by the transducer aperture width. In carotid ultrasound, for a depth of 20 mm and aperture of 10 mm, the lateral resolution is greater than double the depth resolution, when measured in a uniform "tissue phantom." The lateral resolution is degraded by refraction as the ultrasound passes through superficial fat, connective tissue, and muscle, so the lateral resolution observed in a phantom is never achieved in medical ultrasound imaging. Refraction, however, does not degrade depth resolution.

The cross-sectional image of a normal common carotid artery (Fig. 5.4) shows the intima–media thickness (IMT) in the depth direction if the examiner orients the ultrasound scan plane exactly perpendicular to the artery wall, which is a specular reflector. The feature is visible only on a small angle of the deep wall where the ultrasound beams are exactly perpendicular to the wall. Of course, the anatomic structure extends around the entire circumference, but because of the poor lateral resolution and requirement for a strong specular reflection, to visualize the IMT, the majority of the structure is not visualized.

The specular reflections that form the IMT image are due to a change in acoustic impedance (Z) as the ultrasound passes from one tissue to another. The power of the reflected echo is dependent on the squared fractional difference in impedance of the shallower tissue (Z_1) and the deeper tissue (Z_2), which is expressed as a reflection coefficient $(R^2 = ((Z_2 - Z_1)/(Z_2 + Z_1))^2)$. Because the impedance changes are of the same magnitude at the superficial wall as that at the deep wall, the IMT image at the superficial wall should be similar to the IMT image at the deep wall. However, the IMT is visible on the deep wall more frequently than on the superficial wall. Although the reflections of the pair of surfaces at the superficial wall are similar to the reflections of the pair of surfaces at the deep wall, the hypoechoic space between the surface reflections is obscured at the superficial wall by echoes from the adventitia, reflected by the adventitia–media interface. Similar echoes at the deep wall from the blood, reflected by

Fig. 5.3 2-Dimensional ultrasound sector scan and trapezoidal images with 2-D Fourier transforms. The higher spatial frequencies are parallel to the ultrasound scan lines. (*Top*) Phased array sector scan with the ultrasound beam patters originating from a single location. (*Bottom*) Phased-linear array *trapezoidal* showing the parallel (*vertical*) scan lines over the central field and the weaker angled scan lines near the lateral regions of the image. B-mode image ultrasound scan lines are shown as *white arrows*

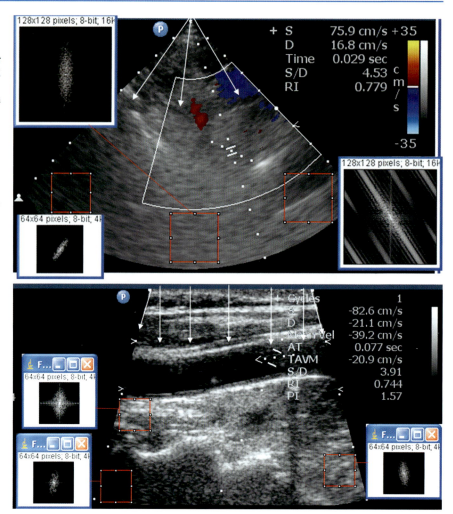

the blood–media interface, are so weak that they do not obscure the image of the anechoic medial layer.

5.2.2 Matching Resolution with Anatomy

Because arteries, veins, and obstructive carotid plaques are larger than the 0.2-mm resolution of ultrasound (at 7.5 MHz), these structures can be resolved in ultrasound images. However, cells and microvascular structures with smaller dimensions cannot be resolved. When ultrasound microbubble contrast agents are present in the microvessels, the microbubbles can be visualized, at least in groups, but they cannot be resolved as independent scatterers (see Chaps. 7–9).

5.3 Ultrasound Technology

5.3.1 Transducers

Conventional ultrasound transducers often consist of a wafer of electrically insulating ceramic crystal material (PZT, Lead Zirconate Titanate) coated with conducting metal electrodes on the opposite surfaces. This crystal is "polarized", by heating and cooling the crystal while a high voltage is applied across the crystal via the conducting electrodes. After it is polarized, the crystal will expand when a voltage of one polarity is applied, or contract if a voltage of the opposite polarity is applied. This is called the

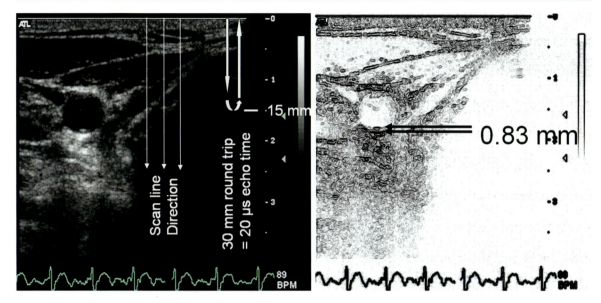

Fig. 5.4 Common carotid cross-sectional image and edge detected image. (*Left*) B-mode (brightness-mode) ultrasound image showing the common carotid artery in cross section. On the deep wall, a *spot* appears showing the intima-media thickness (IMT) only where the ultrasound scan lines are perpendicular to the arterial wall. Direction of ultrasound scan lines is shown. Round trip of an echo is depicted. (*Right*) Edge detection version of the image on the left. To improve the "image quality," a combination of edge detection and filtering is often displayed on ultrasound images

piezoelectric property of a crystal. By applying a sudden voltage pulse to the transducer (1 ns long), the transducer will change suddenly in thickness, launching an ultrasound impulse. The acoustic impedance of the PZT is much higher than air, so ultrasound reaching the crystal transducer surface from within the crystal transducer is reflected back into the crystal if it is suspended in air (without backing material or ultrasound gel in contact with tissue). The ultrasound is "trapped" in the piezoelectric crystal material. The result is a long duration oscillation as the ultrasound travels back and forth from surface to surface at a specific frequency determined by the thickness of the PZT wafer. The speed of ultrasound in the crystal C (PZT) combined with the thickness (T) determine the ultrasound frequency (F). Thus, the wavelength is $((\lambda(\text{PZT}) = C(\text{PZT})/F = 2T))$. Such crystals are used for timing of the transmit frequency of a radio station and as timers for the microprocessor in computers.

If instead, the surface of the crystal is acoustically coupled to another material, which absorbs ultrasound (backing material) and/or coupled to tissue with an acoustic matching layer and ultrasound gel, then the ultrasound energy will leave the transducer and become attenuated causing the specific frequency (narrow band) oscillation to stop after a short time.

The majority of carotid images are created using a linear array of ultrasound transducers. The array may consist of a row of 128 rectangular elements of piezoelectric material such as PZT. Each element is about 10 mm long and 0.25 mm wide, arranged in a row to form a rectangular footprint 10 mm wide and 40 mm long (Fig. 5.5).

The backing layer absorbs much of the vibration energy, damping the natural oscillation of the PZT crystal on both transmit and receive to shorten both the transmitted pulse and the received response to returning echoes. This damping serves to improve depth resolution, but degrades transmit efficiency and receive sensitivity, and therefore degrades depth penetration into the tissue. In modern "composite" transducers, damping is provided within the piezoelectric layer by absorbing material interspersed between PZT rods. Between the transducer array and the patient's skin is an acoustic matching layer, a focal lens for fixed focus in the "elevation" (cross image) direction, and ultrasound "gel." The electrodes on the back and front face of the piezoelectric transducer array (Fig. 5.6) are used to apply the transmit voltage

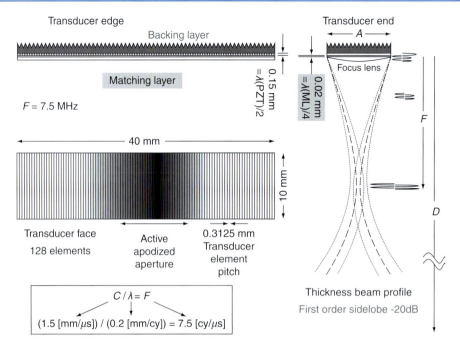

Fig. 5.5 Ultrasound scanhead construction with apodized active aperture and cross-sectional (thickness) beam profile. (*Top left*) Edge view of transducer array with backing layer to "damp" transducer oscillations, the array of 128 transducer elements with thickness equal to half the wavelength and face with matching layer and focal lens. (*Bottom left*) Face view of the ultrasound transducer array showing a region shaded to indicate apodization. *Shading* is *darker* where the transmit voltage is highest and the receive amplification is greatest. Apodization "softens" the edges of the aperture, by reducing both the transmit intensity and the receive sensitivity at the edges to suppress side lobes in that direction. (*Right*) End view of transducer array showing backing, transducer, matching and focal lens layers. The low ultrasound speed in the focal lens material retards the ultrasound phase in the center to draw the focus (F) nearer to the transducer than the natural focus (D). There is a "natural focus" at the "transition zone" which is at a depth of 50 mm ($D = A^2/(4\lambda)$, if $A \gg \lambda/4$)

and later collect the received voltages generated by the echoes from tissue. The electrodes also serve to shield the transducer from stray electrical signals in the air and to protect the patient from the high transmit voltages applied to the ultrasound transducer.

Both coupling and damping of the transducer can be achieved within the transducer without a backing layer or matching layer. Two methods are used: (1) break the ceramic piezoelectric material into small rods and form the wafer transducer by embedding the rods, oriented across the wafer, into another material such as epoxy, and (2) use a different piezoelectric wafer material such as polyvinylidene fluoride (PVDF) which has an acoustic impedance very close to tissue. The first method, forming a composite wafer of PZT embedded in epoxy serves to both decrease the acoustic impedance of the wafer and to damp oscillations in the wafer by converting the ultrasound into heat. By matching the acoustic impedance of the transducer to the tissue, more of the generated acoustic energy is delivered from the transducer to the tissue, and more of the reflected acoustic energy in the echo is transferred into the transducer (rather than being reflected) during receiving. The improved acoustic energy transfer during receiving means that less acoustic energy is needed for good imaging, thus the exposure of the patient to ultrasound can be reduced. The improved acoustic energy transfer during transmit means that less electrical power is needed to generate the pulses sent into the tissue, so that a portable ultrasound system can use smaller batteries.

In the composite transducer, the spacing and diameter of the rods must be very small compared to the wavelength of ultrasound. The acoustic impedance of the composite transducer wafer is determined by a weighted average of the impedance of the matrix ($Z(epoxy) = 3$ MRayl) and of the piezoelectric ceramic ($Z(PZT) = 30$ MRayl). Thus, by adjusting the size and spacing of the ceramic (PZT), the acoustic impedance of the composite layer can be reduced to a value closer to the acoustic

5 Principles of Ultrasonic Imaging and Instrumentation

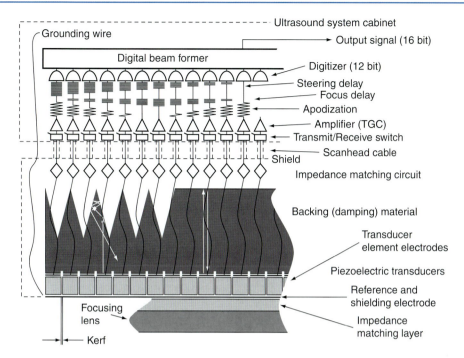

Fig. 5.6 Detail of an ultrasound transducer array and receiver signal path. Transmit signal, after transmit beam forming (not shown), the transmit signal connects to the scanhead cable at the input of the Amplifiers, via a Transmit/Receive switch to protect the amplifiers. The transmit signal passes through the cable, electrical impedance matching circuit and to the transducers. The ultrasound formed in the piezoelectric transducers passes both into the backing material and also toward the patient through the shield electrode, acoustic impedance matching layer, focusing lens, coupling gel, and skin. Applied transmit voltage may vary from 4 to 400 V, lasting 1 μs or less. Returning echoes from tissues in the patient pass through the lens, acoustic impedance matching layer and shield electrode into the transducer where the compression/decompression waves generate +/− voltages near 1 μV. The duration of the echo series lasts 60 μs for a depth of 45 mm. These received voltage fluctuations pass through the matching circuit, cable, T/R switch, amplifiers, apodization attenuators, focus delays, steering delays, and digitizers to be combined becoming the signal for demodulation. The beam former includes the apodization and delays to each channel to focus the ultrasound and suppress diffraction sidelobes. At the same time, an ultrasound pulse traveling into the backing material is absorbed, but could be reflected from the posterior face. If the face is perpendicular to the path, then the ultrasound pulse will be reflected back to the transducer, causing a "backing ghost" line in the image. By tilting the back surface of the backing material, the ultrasound can be redirected to increase absorption and to cause the returning ultrasound to form an unfavorable intersection with the transducers to suppress the "backing ghost." The damping material suppresses the natural (ringing) oscillations of the transducer, shortening the response time, increasing bandwidth, and improving resolution. Modern composite transducers have the damping material within the piezoelectric transducer layer, interspersed between columns of piezoelectric material. With composite transducers, the backing material can be eliminated. The composite structure also serves to lower the impedance of the piezoelectric layer to reduce the need for a matching layer to couple to tissue. Transducer elements are separated by a "kerf" usually formed by a saw cut through the transducer blank and back electrodes into the backing material. In this diagram, 12 channels are included within the aperture. If 16 channels are used in the receive aperture, the digital combination of these 16 (2^4) digital channels increases the dynamic range by 4 bits from 12 bits per channel to 16 bits for the combined output

impedance of tissue (Z(tissue) = 1.5 MRayl). Units of impedance (MegaRayl = MRayl = $10^6 kg/(m^2 s)$ = $10^5 g/(cm^2 s)$) are named after John William Strutt (Lord Rayleigh), Chancellor of Cambridge University and winner of the 1904 Nobel Prize in Physics for investigations of the properties of gasses.

Figure 5.6 shows the detail of an ultrasound transducer array and receiver signal path. The transmit signal, after beam forming (not shown in figure), connects to the scanhead cable at the input of the amplifiers, via a transmit/receive switch to protect the amplifiers. The transmit signal passes through the cable, electrical impedance matching circuit, and to the transducers. The ultrasound formed in the piezoelectric transducers passes both into the backing material and toward the patient through the shield electrode, acoustic impedance matching layer, focusing lens, coupling gel, and skin. Applied transmit voltage may vary from 4 to 400 V, lasting 1 μs or less.

Returning echoes pass through the lens, acoustic impedance matching layer, and shield electrode into the transducer where the compression/decompression waves generate voltages near ±1 μV. The duration of the echo series lasts 60 μs for a depth of 45 mm. These received voltages pass through the matching circuit, cable, transmit/receive switch, and into the "beam former," comprised of amplifiers, apodization attenuators, focus and steering phase delays, and digitizers and adder, to form the single channel signal for demodulation.

Beam forming includes applying a delay to each channel to focus the ultrasound, and amplification to each channel to apodize the beam. Any transducer aperture with sudden edges forms a diffraction pattern which consists of a central lobe and possibly side lobes. Whether side lobes are present and the angle of each side lobe (φ) from the central lobe is determined by the ultrasound wavelength (λ) and the aperture width (A).

$$\sin \varphi = ((2n+1)/2)(\lambda/A)$$

where the order of the side lobe ($n = 1, 2, 3$, and 4) is a positive or negative integer. The display of ultrasound images is based on the assumption that the echoes return from the central lobe. However, strong reflectors in the side lobes will generate echoes that also appear in the image. Side-lobe echoes can be suppressed by spreading the side lobes: by using multiple ultrasound wavelengths (a broad band transducer) and/or by attenuating the edges of the aperture so that the width (A) is not well defined. Apodization is achieved in the scanplane direction by electronically reducing the transmit voltage at the aperture edge and reducing the amplification of the echoes at the aperture edge (Fig. 5.5). The improvements in the appearance of ultrasound images made possible by new electronic scan heads replacing "mechanical" scan heads is the ability to implement electronic beam forming, consisting of apodization, dynamic-receive focusing, and dynamic aperture. Echoes from a 7.5 mm depth arrive at 10 μs after transmission, echoes from 30 mm depth arrive at 40 μs after transmission; during that interval between 10 and 40 μs, the beam-forming electronics can readjust the receiving focus and can increase the aperture, to optimum values for that depth. As yet, no ultrasound scan heads apodize the aperture in the cross-image direction, although this could be done either by shaping the transducer elements or by adding attenuation to the ends of the transducer elements.

An ultrasound pulse traveling into the backing material is absorbed, but will reflect from the posterior face. If the face is perpendicular to the path, then the ultrasound pulse will be reflected back to the transducer, causing a "backing ghost" line in the image. By tilting the back, the ultrasound can be redirected to increase absorption and cause the returning ultrasound to form an unfavorable intersection with the transducers to suppress the "backing ghost."

The damping material also suppresses the natural (ringing) oscillations of the transducer, shortening the response time, increasing bandwidth, and improving resolution. Modern composite transducers have the damping material within the piezoelectric transducer layer, interspersed between columns of piezoelectric material. With composite transducers, the backing material can be eliminated.

Transducer elements are separated by a "kerf" usually formed by a saw cut through the transducer blank and back electrodes into the backing material.

If 16 channels are used in the receive aperture, the digital combination of these 16 digital channels increases the dynamic range by 4 bits from 12 bits per channel to 16 bits for the combined output.

Several properties contribute to the merit of the ultrasound transducer. Transducer alignment is important to optimize focusing in the lateral direction of the image. During manufacture, the backing layer, back electrode layer, transducer layer and front electrode layer may be assembled by a combination of casting, gluing and cutting. Then the kerf saw will make 127 cuts to form the separate elements. Electrode connections can then be made to each element. During these steps, the transducer elements might move. Because the ultrasound wavelength (for 7.5 MHz ultrasound) is 0.2 mm, and phase differences near 0.01 rad can be important, the alignment of each transducer is checked for 0.002 mm displacement error before proceeding to apply additional electrode, matching, and focusing layers. Transducer damping is important to optimize depth (range) resolution to near the 0.2-mm limit (the ultrasound wavelength). Backing material can be made of epoxy mixed with grains of sand or metal to absorb the ultrasound. It is important to shape the backside of the damping layer with serrations to prevent reflections back to the transducer because reflections from within the backing material or from the back surface will appear as stationary objects in the ultrasound image. Each transducer forms a signal "channel" to the ultrasound "beam former" for both transmitting and receiving the ultrasound. The kerf space between the transducer elements is often filled with epoxy or a similar material, but mechanical coupling between the elements must be suppressed to avoid signal interaction between the signal channels. Because groups of elements comprise an aperture in the lateral image direction, to form the ultrasound beam transmitted into tissue, each element must be uniform in transmit efficiency and receive sensitivity so that the electronic amplification and delay applied to each transducer have the expected relationship to the adjacent ultrasound.

Each transducer element is coupled to the scanhead cable through an electronic matching circuit so that the transmitted voltage is efficiently coupled to the transducer element. Fortunately the same circuit serves during receiving to efficiently couple the voltage generated by the transducer into the scanhead cable. Although the transmit voltage might be 100 V (0 to peak), the received voltage is often only a few microvolts, so these circuits must be able to handle a wide dynamic range of voltages.

In the thickness direction (Fig. 5.5, right), the ultrasound transducer is uniform, forming a sharp edge aperture. Diffraction of the ultrasound wave causes the formation of sidelobes in the thickness direction. The geometric sine of the angular distance of the first sidelobe is equal to 1.5 times the wavelength divided by the aperture. Thus, for the 10 mm wide transducer array with a 0.2 mm wavelength, the first order sidelobe is angled about 2° from the main lobe. The transmit intensity of the sidelobe is about 0.1 (-10 dB) compared to the main lobe, and the receive sidelobe is also 0.1 (-10 dB) compared to the main lobe, so the net effect is 0.01 (-20 dB) below the main lobe. Such a large difference is sufficient for differentiating some solid tissues. Unfortunately, this 20-dB interference becomes a problem when viewing blood or other fluid-filled spaces which generate echoes of -60 dB compared to solid tissue. Highly echogenic structures outside the plane of the image, if at the depth of the vessel, can form echo images that appear to be within the vessel.

5.3.2 Beam Patterns

Each transducer element has a natural beam pattern (Fig. 5.7) determined by the aperture size and shape. With a rectangular transducer, a simple approximation of the beam pattern can be deduced by considering the smaller dimension of the aperture, and assuming that the aperture extends an infinite distance "perpendicular to the page." From an end view of an array, 10 mm wide and 40 mm in the direction perpendicular to the page, this is a satisfactory approximation. By considering the transducer response when receiving and adding the effects of the ultrasound compressions and decompressions on various portions of the transducer, the sensitivity pattern of the transducer can be determined. Using the principle of reciprocity (the transmit beam pattern is the same as the receive beam pattern), the transmit beam pattern can be determined. By this method, the width of the central lobe from $+\lambda/W$ to $-\lambda/W$ can be derived and the locations of higher order side lobes as well (Fig. 5.7).

The same derivation applies to each transducer element (Fig. 5.8, left). The location of diffraction lobes can also be derived from a similar analysis (Fig. 5.8, right). If the Kerf between the transducers is small, then the + and − first-order grating lobe, fortunately fall at the same angle as the null between the zero order and first-order element sidelobe. Thus, the grating lobe is absent. However, when steering the central lobe, the sidelobe is also steered toward the same direction, and now appears as it is angled within the transducer element central lobe.

In B-mode (brightness mode) imaging with a short broad band transmit burst, this is not a severe problem, because each ultrasound frequency within the broad band pulse has a different diffraction angle. Thus, the lobes are smeared. However, in Doppler, the narrow band burst has well-defined sidelobes. In addition, phased steering is common in Doppler to achieve a favorable Doppler examination angle to the vessel axis. Of course, during demodulation, Doppler processing is sensitive to echoes from blood, 60 dB below the strongest echoes. Thus, signals from sidelobes will often affect Doppler signals, even though they are not observed on a B-mode image. Dual waveforms (Fig. 5.9) are present in about 1% of carotid examinations, but only with beam steering from a linear array scanhead. Although it is possible that the dual

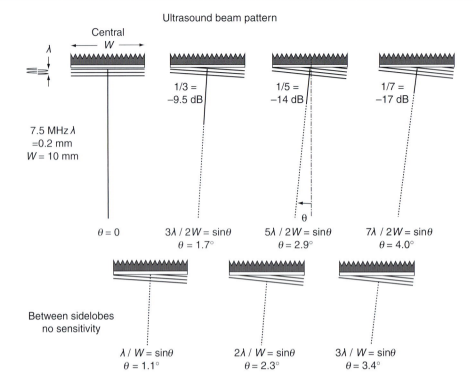

Fig. 5.7 Sidelobes in the image thickness direction. (*Top left*) Each compression phase of the echoes from the intended beam axis arrives at the transducer at the same time, compressing the entire transducer. (*Bottom left*) A compression from an off-axis echo source will impinge on only a portion of the transducer generating a positive voltage. A following decompression will simultaneously impinge on another portion of the transducer, producing a counteracting negative voltage. At the angle where the compression and decompression areas have equal transducer areas, the combined result will be zero. (*Top middle and right*) For some beam angles, areas of compression and decompression cannot be equal, so the transducer has a sensitivity that is reduced to the fraction of unequal areas. These angles are sidelobes. (*Bottom middle and right*) For some beam angles, the areas of compression always equal the areas of decompression. For these angles, the sensitivity of the transducer is zero. By the rule of reciprocity, the beam patterns for ultrasound transmitting are the same as the beam patterns for receiving

waveforms shown in Fig. 5.9 come from a single sample volume, all of these have come from linear array systems with steered ultrasound beams. It is possible that each of these waveforms comes from different lobes of the beam pattern. Dual sample volumes can be created in two other ways: "high pulse repetition frequency (PRF)" and ultrasound reflection.

5.3.2.1 High Pulse Repetition Frequency (PRF)

In pulsed Doppler, the depth of the sample gate is determined by a delay time (τ) between the transmit burst and the received sample gate. The time interval between bursts is 1/PRF. So, additional deeper sample gates exist for times $\tau + n/\text{PRF}$, where n is a positive integer. We assume that the ultrasound from the deeper sample gates is attenuated below noise, but in some cases, this assumption is not true. Doppler velocity measurements from deep vessels require the use of a low PRF. Unfortunately, the low PRF limits the range of velocities that can be measured without the ambiguity of aliasing. When measuring high velocities in deep vessels, some instruments allow the introduction of a "high PRF-Doppler" function that shows the location of the deeper sample gates, so that one of the deeper gates can be directed into the region of high velocity in the vessel. In that case, the examiner must ensure that the shallow gate is located in solid tissue rather than in another blood vessel.

5.3.2.2 Ultrasound Reflection

Any flat interface with an impedance change can reflect a portion of the ultrasound beam, splitting the sample volume into two locations in tissue.

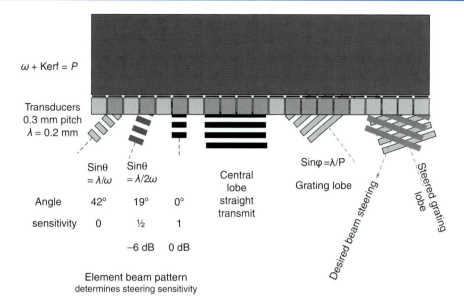

Fig. 5.8 Single element beam patterns and grating lobes. (*Far left*) Zero sensitivity angle of single transducer element beam pattern where the area of compression and decompression are equal. (*Next left*) Half amplitude, which is also quarter power (= 6 dB) angle of single transducer element beam pattern. (*Third left*) Center of single transducer element beam pattern with full intensity and sensitivity (0 dB). (*Center*) Four element aperture phased to transmit straight down. (*Middle right*) The divisions in the transducer array act like a diffraction grating. The first grating lobe is at the same angle as the single transducer zero sensitivity/power angle, if the Kerf is zero so $\omega = P$. For a wide Kerf, $\omega < P$ and $\varphi < \theta$. (*Far right*) If phase steering is applied to tilt the desired beam to the left, the right grating sidelobe also becomes angled slightly toward the left from the original right position. As it moves into the single element aperture angle, it becomes more prominent

5.3.3 Electronic Beam Former

Two kinds of transmit bursts are used for ultrasound examinations (Fig. 5.10): (1) for high-depth resolution in B-mode imaging, a short duration, broad frequency band, high voltage pulse is transmitted. This generates an ultrasound impulse with high mechanical index (MI) resulting in nonlinear propagation of ultrasound and harmonic echoes. (2) For Doppler, a long duration, narrow frequency band, low voltage beep is transmitted. This generates a low MI oscillation with a well-defined frequency and phase. In either case, the transmit burst has a duration less than 1 μs (microsecond). Either burst passes into the transmit beam former, which is connected via transmit/receive switch, multi-pin plug, multichannel coaxial cable, and matching circuits to the transducer array. For an examination depth of 37.5 mm, the ultrasound traveling at 1.5 mm/μs can complete the 75 mm round trip to the farthest depth in 50 μs. This 50 μs period allows new transmit bursts 20,000 times/s or a PRF of 20 kHz.

The transmit burst is routed to the electronic beam former which separates the signal into 128 channels and then modifies the transmit burst for each transducer element. Because the examination data are acquired one line at a time, only a portion of the elements are used during each pulse-echo cycle (Fig. 5.11). For transmit, typically 32 elements surrounding the central ray of the beam pattern will be used. For transmit, a single focal depth is selected, indicated by a carrot in Fig. 5.11. During the 45 μs available for receive, echoes return to the transducer from successively deeper depths, at a rate of 0.75 mm/μs. Because later echoes returning from deeper depths are weakened by absorption of the ultrasound in tissue, increasing amplification is applied, in concert with electronically increasing the focal length of the beam former to follow the echo depth and increasing the width of the aperture to retain uniform lateral resolution. Although these methods are effective in the lateral direction of the image, they do not apply to the thickness direction of the image.

A 2-dimensional B-mode image can be formed using 100 imaging lines. Each line is formed by an aperture around a central location. If 100 lines are generated from a transducer with 128 channels, then each line will be centered on a transducer beginning with transducer element 15 and ending with element 114.

Fig. 5.9 Dual Doppler signals

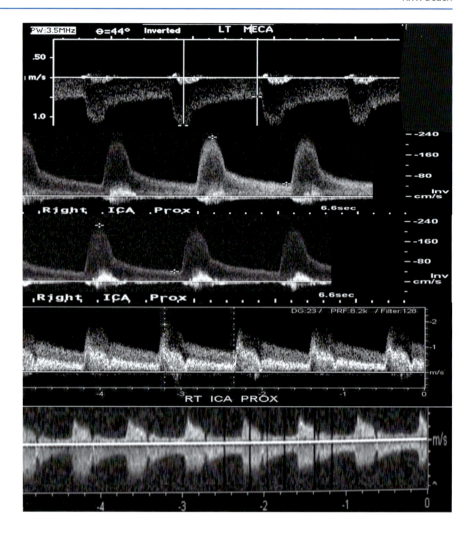

This allows an aperture 31 elements wide from element 1 to 31, centered on 15. If the PRF is 20 kHz (Pulse Repetition Interval (PRI) = 0.05 ms), and one burst is used for each line, then the image is formed in 5 ms allowing a frame rate of 200 frames per second (fps). Often the image frame rate will be synchronized with standard video-display frame rates of 30 fps (USA), or 25 fps (Europe). This allows the acquisition of several images of ultrasound to be combined to form a single display image.

A single-line Doppler examination can be performed at a PRF of 20 kHz coupled with FFT spectral analysis using 128 pulse-echo cycles (PEC) per line providing 156 lines of spectral display per second. For a 2-dimensional color Doppler examination, an ensemble of 8 PEC is used for each line. This requires 40 ms, 8 times as long to form a 2-dimensional color Doppler image compared to a B-mode image, which matches a frame rate of 25 fps.

5.3.4 Safety

Diagnostic ultrasound is considered to be safe, as no ill effects have been found in patients. Traditionally, ultrasound intensities as high as 100 mW/cm^2 have been used in diagnostic instruments. This is near the intensity of sunlight (25 mW/cm^2). However, sunlight (which heats skin) is absorbed in the first mm of skin thickness, but only a small percentage of the ultrasound is absorbed and converted to heat in the skin. In M-mode (motion mode) imaging and pulsed Doppler, the intensity is delivered along a single line; every pulse is transmitted along the one line. In 2-dimensional (2-D) imaging, each line in the image follows a different path, so the ultrasound is distributed across the image field. In order to achieve higher echo signal levels in 2-D imaging, higher energy ultrasound–transmit bursts can be used. To document the safety or potential hazard of these higher

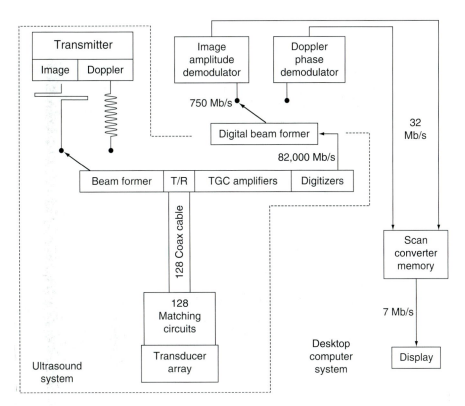

Fig. 5.10 Ultrasound system architecture. Ultrasound system includes transmitter, transmit beam former, switching, cable, scanhead, analog amplifiers and digitizers. Computer system includes demodulators and display. Digital beam former for receiving may be either outside or inside the computer. Note the required data capacity of the communication channels decreases along the received signal path from the transducer interface to the display. The major limitation in ultrasound system design is moving data along the path and into temporary storage along the way

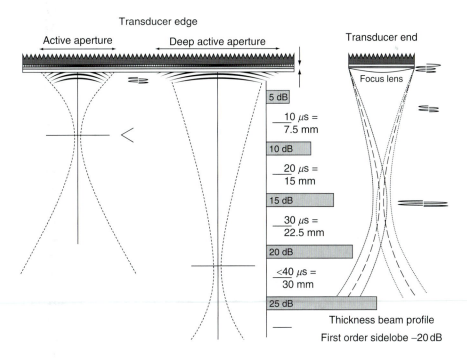

Fig. 5.11 Ultrasound beam patterns with sidelobes in the thickness direction and apodization in the lateral direction. During transmit on each line, one depth of focus is selected for use across the entire image. During receive of each line, a series of adjustments are synchronized with the time (microseconds) after the transmit burst to correspond to the depth of the reflector generating that portion of the echo: the amplification is increased ("Time-Gain Compensation" = TGC [dB]), focus is extended and aperture width is increased to achieve uniform lateral resolution and brightness in the image from all depths

Fig. 5.12 RF line showing voltage vs. "fast time." The Echoes from various depths along the line of the *arrow* are shown. "Fast Time" is the time for echoes to return from each depth in the image along a single line from a single transmit burst. "Slow Time" is the time that it takes for a series of scan lines to be acquired and form a portion of the image from a series of transmit bursts

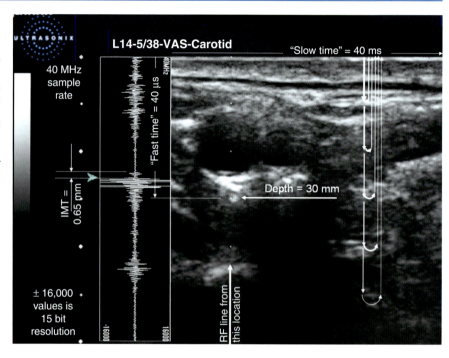

levels, two new measurement parameters "thermal index" (TI) and "mechanical index" (MI) have been introduced to replace intensity (mW/cm^2). Thermal index is the temperature rise expected in tissue during an examination. TI includes the attenuation of ultrasound in tissue. A temperature rise of 1°C is considered acceptable. TI is based on a theoretical computation including: (1) heat delivery based on intensity and attenuation (absorption rate), (2) heat capacity and examination time, and (3) heat loss by conduction and convection (blood flow). With ultrasound examination, the temperature rise occurs only in the small region of the image plane. By comparison, a similar temperature rise occurs in MR imaging, but involves a much larger volume. MI is the chance, that during the decompression half cycle of the ultrasound wave, a small air bubble will expand to cause tissue damage. MI is based on an empirical analysis of peak "negative" pressure computed from instantaneous intensity and tissue impedance (a linear assumption) and duration of the negative pressure computed from the ultrasound frequency. The actual effects of MI are non-linear and dependent on oscillation duration, the presence and nature of gas bubbles in the ultrasound field and the properties of gasses dissolved in the tissue. Although modern instruments display TI and MI, these parameters are rarely considered in clinical ultrasound examination.

5.3.5 Demodulation

Each 2-D ultrasound image is formed from a parallel array of data lines acquired sequentially from left to right. The voltage oscillations in the echo from one pulse-echo cycle are displayed in Fig. 5.12 along a vertical "fast time" axis representing depth. The oscillations are at the ultrasound frequency of near 8 MHz. The system is designed to acquire and process echo frequencies between 5 and 14 MHz over a field width of 38 mm (Model L14-5/38 scanhead). Older ultrasound systems process the echoes using analog electronics. In this instrument, after amplification, the echo voltages are converted to a series of digital measurements at a sample rate of 40 MHz. Each microsecond in "fast time" is equivalent to 0.75 mm in depth, representing a round trip distance of 1.5 mm because the speed of ultrasound in tissue is 1.5 mm/μs. Thus, for the 40 mm of depth represented here, the time to acquire the echoes from one line is 53 μs; the number of samples is 2,120. Each digital sample can be recorded by a 14-bit number plus a sign (the highest number that can be represented in 14 bits is 16,383). With the sign (an additional bit) each digitized point can be processed by a desktop computer using 16-bit numbers.

The information in the echo can be "demodulated" into two characteristic parameters: amplitude and phase

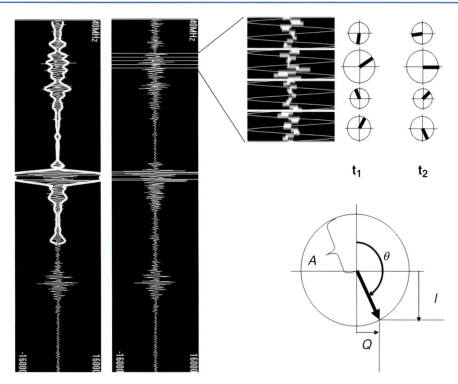

Fig. 5.13 RF line showing voltage vs. "fast time" representing echoes as a function of depth. (*Left*) Conventional amplitude demodulation (analog or digital). (*Middle left*) A portion of the echo is divided into 4 pixels, each spanning 0.25 mm in depth. (*Middle right*) The RF voltage oscillations are compared with a sample of the transmit Doppler frequency to measure amplitude and phase. (*Top right*) The amplitude from each pixel can be represented as the diameter of the phase diagram circle, the phase angle can be represented as the angle of a vector in "complex algebra." Data from the second column were gathered from the same location, but at a later time. The change in phase during the interval indicates motion. The motion can be converted to Doppler velocity by dividing the distance moved by the time between samples. The "Doppler frequency shift" (f'') is equal to the change in phase ($\Delta\theta$) divided by the time between the samples $f = ((\Delta\theta \text{ [radians]})/(t_2 - t_1))/2\pi$. The Doppler velocity ($V$) is equal to the change in phase ($\Delta\theta$) times half the wavelength (for round trip = $\lambda/2$) divided by time. $V = (\Delta\theta/4\pi)\lambda/(t_2 - t_1)$ (*Bottom right*) Pixel phase diagram represented as either Amplitude and Phase (a, θ) or complex algebra ($I + Qj$)

(Fig. 5.13). Amplitude can be determined in several ways, but each method requires a distance (depth) interval for determining the amplitude. Distance is usually equal to the length of the transmit burst, so the interval includes several cycles of ultrasound oscillation. Once that depth interval is established, the amplitude is determined by a method such as: peak detection, integrated backscatter, or average amplitude. If digital demodulation is used for both amplitude and phase, the echo is divided into uniform segments and the amplitude and phase are measured in each segment, as a pair of values (Fig. 5.13, right). The amplitude information is used for B-mode imaging displays such as the common 2-dimensional "real time" B-mode and also for the M-mode imaging used in cardiology. The phase information has not been found to be useful alone, but when the phase is compared to a phase gathered along the same line at a different time, phase change is used to measure tissue motion for applications such as Doppler velocimetry in blood and tissue Doppler in muscle.

The limits of digital technology are reached by the task of moving the echo data from one stage in the ultrasound instrument to another (Fig. 5.10) The "Radio Frequency" (RF) echo information is often sampled at 40 MHz through a 16-bit digitizer on each of the 128 channels. Thus, the data rate out of the digitizers is 128 times 16 times 40 MHz = 82 G bits per second (82 Gb/s). The handling of such data rates is at the limit of current technology. Thus, the data are combined into fewer bits/second by a series of steps, some performed in dedicated hardware and some in computer software. The first step is the beam former where the echo data received on each channel is amplified to compensate for attenuation, phase shifted to adjust the focus, attenuated to apodize the aperture, and combined into a single-beam-formed data path. The beam-forming process can reduce the number of data bits by a factor of 100. To demodulate the beam-formed data, the depth can be divided into intervals 0.4 μs (16 RF samples) long representing 0.3 mm (0.75 mm/μs) and the amplitude and phase measured resulting in a 2.5 MHz (1/(0.4 μs)) digitized amplitude signal. At each depth interval, the phase can be represented as a second number at 2.5 MHz. The amplitude and phase are often represented with a complex algebraic expression by two numbers called I and Q (Fig. 5.13). The amplitude, represented as a 16-bit number, can have over 64,000 values, represented in gray scale. This number is usually converted to a 64-level gray scale by taking the logarithm of the amplitude. The phase, represented as a circle, is often divided into 100 angular divisions. A change in phase angle at a particular depth between one pulse-echo line and another indicates that the tissue at that depth has moved toward or away from the transducer. A phase change of 0.01 of a full circle (3.6° or 0.06 rad) indicates that the tissue has moved 0.005 wavelengths of ultrasound. At 7.5 MHz with a 0.2 mm wavelength, this motion is 1 μm. In Doppler velocimetry, with a PRF of 10 kHz, the velocity is 1 μm/0.1 ms = 0.01 m/s = 1 cm/s. This is a slow speed for blood, but a common speed for arterial walls. Such signals generated by wall motion, are very strong. Because these signals interfere with the Doppler signal from blood, these strong wall motion signals are called "clutter." To measure blood velocity, a wall filter is used to reject these slow clutter velocities. This filtered band, often rejecting Doppler shifts below 100 Hz, can be seen as a dark band near zero velocity on a spectral waveform. Doppler examination of stenotic cardiac valves often requires a "high pass" clutter filter at 400 Hz to reject strong Doppler signals from fast-moving valve leaflets. In arteries, bruits may be wall vibrations above 100 Hz and interfere with the blood Doppler signal. In a reverse vein bypass graft, it is possible that valve-leaflet motion can cause clutter at a frequency above the wall filter.

5.4 B-Mode Imaging

5.4.1 Image Processing

In modern ultrasound systems, the 2-dimensional B-mode image is formed in several steps. A matrix of lines is arranged on the display plane with each line positioned to represent the origin of each ultrasound line at the scanhead, and the angle and length of the beam directed into tissue. A 2-dimensional image typically includes between 50 and 200 adjacent, equally spaced lines. A 2-D B-mode image can be created using a sequence of steps. First, a noise image is generated setting the transmit power to zero (Fig. 5.14). This allows the system to determine the baseline noise. Because the noise is primarily generated in the transducer and is affected by the damping applied, including the damping provided by the tissue which is imaged, the noise level varies with lateral position along the scanhead and with time. The noise image shown includes the effect of the time gain control (TGC), designed to compensate for weak signals coming from deep tissues due to attenuation. The amplitude of each region in this baseline image is subtracted from the amplitude in the next image, which is formed with the transmitter set at normal output voltage. Echoes from the most echoic tissues have amplitudes 1,000 times as strong as the echoes from the least echoic tissues, and intermediate echoes are 100 or 10 times as bright as the least echoic. To represent that range of echoes in the image, with 64 levels of brightness, the least echoic tissues with the lowest amplitude echoes can be displayed as brightness level 3, those echoes ten times as strong as the lowest amplitude are displayed as brightness level 23, those 100 times as the lowest amplitude are displayed as brightness level 43 and those 1,000 times as strong are displayed as brightness 63. This is a logarithmic conversation of echo amplitude to gray scale.

Coherent speckle in an ultrasound image is sometimes called noise and sometimes called tissue texture. However, speckle is not noise in the conventional sense, because the speckle pattern is identical if acquired from a stationary object in a series of images. Noise would be random in time, and averaging the RF signals between frames before demodulation, would suppress the noise. But speckle survives frame-to-frame averaging. It is dependent on angle of view and on ultrasound frequency/wavelength. If a lower ultrasound frequency (longer wavelength) is used to image the tissue, then the speckle pattern becomes more widely spaced. So speckle spacing does not show a property of the tissue, but rather a property of the ultrasound. Most broadband-ultrasound image systems now filter the echo into several ultrasound frequency bands before demodulation, amplitude

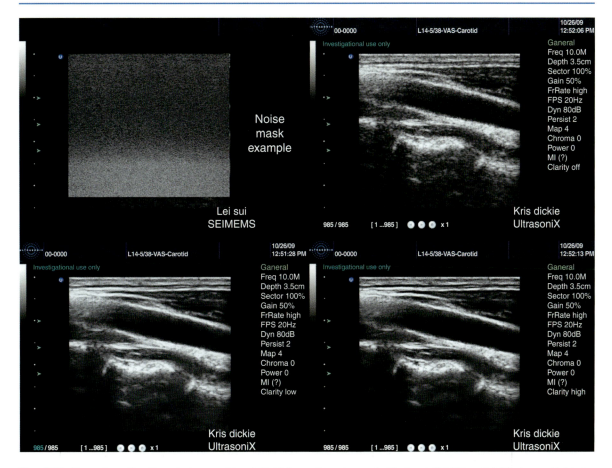

Fig. 5.14 Formation of a B-mode image. (*Top left*) Noise mask acquired with transmit power set to zero. (*Top right*) 2-Dimensional B-mode ultrasound image after subtraction of the noise mask. (*Bottom left*) Mild spatial filtering applied to the 2-D B-mode image. (*Bottom right*) Moderate spatial filtering applied to the 2-D B-mode image

demodulate in each band, and then combine the amplitude results to form an image with speckle suppressed. Another method used to suppress coherent speckle and make the image more attractive is spatial smoothing.

More complicated 2-D B-mode imaging methods can be applied including combining images taken with different transmit focal depths. Another method is to form several images, each with a different angle of view. By using 3 or 5 angles of view, speckle is suppressed and specular reflectors are enhanced (Fig. 5.15). Acquiring data for 5 images at different angles takes 5 times as long as acquiring data for one image, so in 5-angle compound imaging, the frame rate is reduced by a factor of 5.

5.4.2 Measuring Plaque Echodensity

Because the brightness of some plaque images appears high and of others appears low, the quantitative measurement of B-mode image brightness (Fig. 5.16) offers the promise of determining the echogenicity of the tissue components of the plaque and from that determining the content of the tissue.[4–8] A series of efforts to measure the RF echo frequency and echo brightness have demonstrated the merit of this approach for characterizing tissue in general and for identifying plaque contents. Unfortunately, in standard ultrasound examinations of young normal people, bright echoes often appear within the lumen of arteries without obstruction to flow (Fig. 5.17). Such artifacts

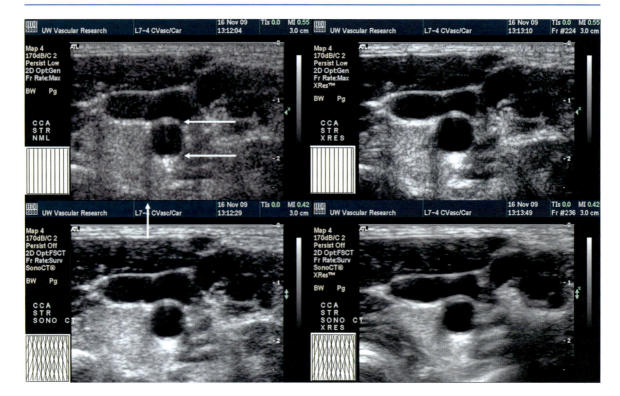

Fig. 5.15 Methods of 2-Dimensional B-mode imaging, cross section the neck. (*Top left*) 2-Dimensional B-mode ultrasound image. *Vertical arrow* marking edge shadowing below the cross section of a phase inversion reflector (Lloyds Mirror). *Horizontal arrows* mark superficial and deep IMT lines indicating that these double interface (impedance difference) specular reflectors are viewed with perpendicular ultrasound scan lines. (*Top right*) Spatial filtering applied to the 2-D B-mode image. (*Bottom left*) Multi-view, combined compound 2-dimensional B-mode ultrasound image. Note that the compound imaging fills in the edge shadowing by adding echoes from the other angle views. Note also that additional time is required to form the compound image, lowering the frame rate. (*Bottom right*) Spatial filtering applied to the multi-view, combined compound 2-dimensional B-mode ultrasound image

can be identified by expert examiners and avoided by adjusting the gain and appropriate use of color flow which in the absence of plaques will fill the lumen (Chap. 12). If the bright echoes in the lumen represent a plaque then the plaque will appear as a flow void in the color flow (Fig. 5.18).

5.4.3 Identifying Stents and Sutures

Although atherosclerotic plaques vary greatly in composition, surgical implants such as stents and sutures have uniform acoustic properties differing greatly from tissue and should therefore be uniformly visualized and conspicuous (Fig. 5.19). Because these are specular reflectors, oblique insonation sometimes renders these structures non-visible.

5.5 Phase Methods

5.5.1 Phase Image Processing

If an ultrasound image is formed from echoes reflected by uniform planar structures, adjacent RF echoes should be similar. This similarity can be appreciated in adjacent ultrasound lines taken from a layered structure such as the arterial wall, when it is oriented parallel to the ultrasound scanhead. By measuring the cross correlation between adjacent ultrasound lines, the lateral uniformity of tissue can be evaluated (Fig. 5.20). An image formed from a single 2-dimensional RF acquisition demonstrated that near the vascular walls, lateral coherence is often high. This parameter is

5 Principles of Ultrasonic Imaging and Instrumentation

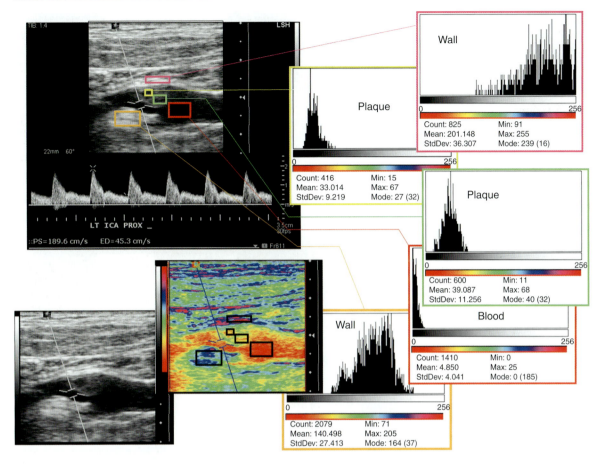

Fig. 5.16 Echogenicity of carotid plaque and surrounding tissues. Peak systolic velocity 1.89 m/s exceeding 1.25 m/s indicates a moderate carotid stenosis. *Histograms* show the image brightness for different tissues. (*Bottom left*) Original B-mode image, and B-color image. *Color scales* on histograms show the distribution of B-color[3]

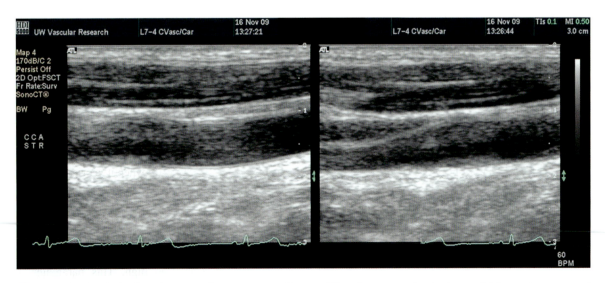

Fig. 5.17 Intraluminal echoes in a normal common carotid artery. The echoes appearing in the arterial lumen image are not anatomical structures. The blood velocities through this young normal artery are normal

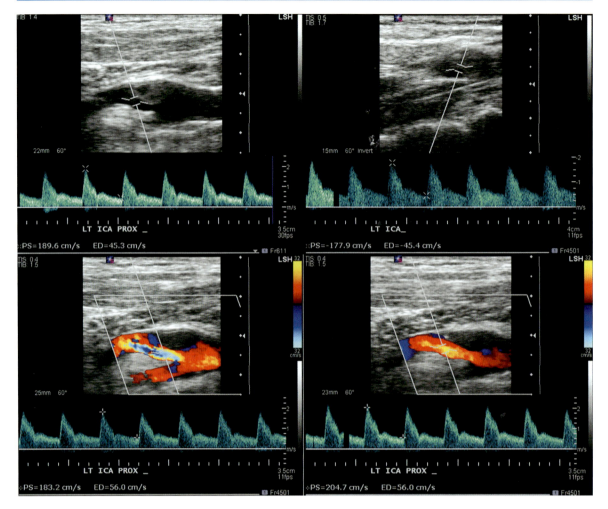

Fig. 5.18 2-dimensional brightness mode and color Doppler images of a carotid plaque and stenosis. (*Top left*) Longitudinal image of carotid plaque. (*Bottom left*) Systolic color Doppler image of carotid plaque with aliasing and reversal. (*Top right*) Longitudinal image of carotid plaque from a different sectional plane. (*Bottom right*) Diastolic color Doppler image of carotid plaque with aliasing and reversal. The systolic velocity greater than 1.25 m/s indicates a moderate stenosis. The diastolic velocity less than 1.4 m/s indicates that the stenosis is not severe

independent of echo strength and therefore might offer a method of differentiating different materials in atherosclerotic plaque. Of course, if the wall is tilted down to the right, then the phase of the echoes from the next line to the right will be shifted slightly deeper; phase processing (as it is used in Doppler) on adjacent line echoes (rather than on later echoes from the same line) divided by the spacing between the lines (rather than the time interval) can be used to measure the slope of the wall layers (rather than the velocity).

5.6 Doppler

5.6.1 Superimposed Doppler Data

There is a variety of methods for acquiring 2-dimensional ultrasound images which can be combined by superimposing the images. In Fig. 5.14, the noise image was subtracted from the B-mode. In Fig. 5.15, compounding, the brightest echo for each pixel (a particular location in the image) is used to

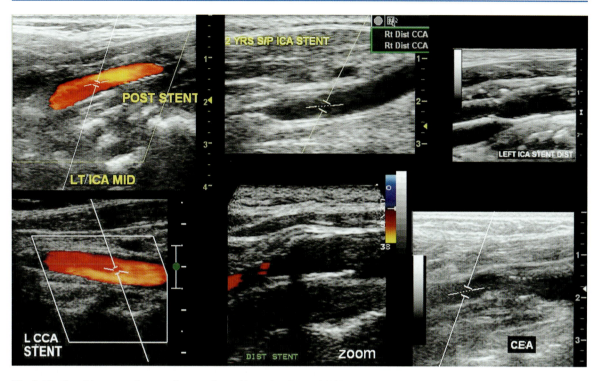

Fig. 5.19 Carotid stents and sutures in treated carotid arteries. Stent visibility varies due to several factors including the intersection between the ultrasound beams and the specular reflecting stent. (*Lower right*) CEA Carotid Endarterectomy

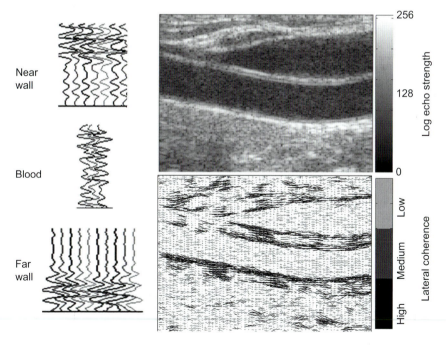

Fig. 5.20 2-dimensional ultrasonic lateral coherence imaging of a normal carotid artery. (*Left*) Array of adjacent RF lines spanning 80 RF samples (2 µs = 1.5 mm) in depth from different regions of interest in the tissue. (*Top right*) Conventional 2-dimensional brightness-mode Image. (*Bottom right*) 2-dimensional lateral coherence image. High coherence = 9 adjacent ultrasound scan lines have high cross correlation. Medium coherence = 6 adjacent ultrasound scan lines have high cross correlation. Low coherence = 3 adjacent ultrasound scan lines have high cross correlation. The lateral coherence image contains no information about echo brightness, the cross correlation between lines is normalized by signal strength

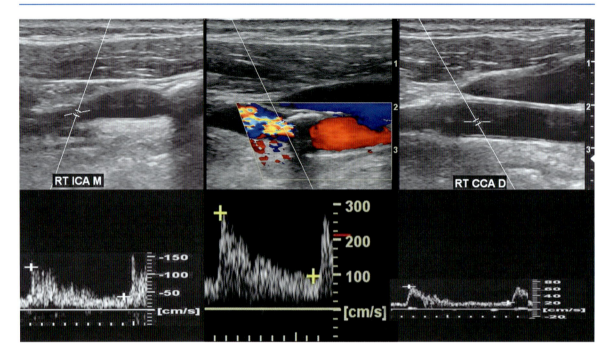

Fig. 5.21 Calcified carotid plaque in overlapping images causing a stenosis classified with spectral Doppler examination. Blood flow is toward the head from right to left in the image. (*Right*) Normal carotid blood flow in the common carotid artery with no visualized atherosclerosis but shadowing on the left. (*Middle*) Elevated velocities in the region just distal to a stenosis which exhibits a region of shadowing due to calcification. (*Left*) Post-stenotic turbulence in the internal carotid artery. Shadowing can be seen on the right edge of the image

emphasize bright specular (perpendicular) reflectors. In other image formats, the echoes can be filtered for the presence of harmonic echoes to display the presence of a microbubble ultrasound contrast (Chaps. 7–9). Doppler demodulation can also be used to generate 2-dimensional images. Although the acquisition of a 2-D color Doppler image requires more time, than a 2-D B-mode image, a full set of B-mode and color Doppler images can be acquired within 50 ms, allowing a "real time" frame rate of 20 fps. By combining 2-D B-mode and color Doppler (Fig. 5.18) into a single superimposed image, new insight into carotid pathology is revealed. On the left, the color Doppler overlay of the AP longitudinal plane of a carotid artery clearly reveals a flow void. This is also revealed on a longitudinal view on the right. The severity of the stenosis is quantified from the velocity measurement in the spectral waveform (Chap. 30).

5.6.2 Identifying Stenosis

Although some carotid stenoses can be seen on ultrasound B-mode images, the presence of shadowing due to the absorption of ultrasound by calcifications in plaque might mask the visualization of the plaque (Fig. 5.21). As an alternative, blood velocity measurements with ultrasonic Doppler have been accepted as the standard method of examination for carotid stenosis. A moderate stenosis is characterized by relatively normal flow velocity proximal to the stenosis, a high velocity greater than 1.25 m/s in the stenosis and the post-stenotic jet, and spectral broadening indicating turbulence in the region extending for 1 or 2 cm distal to the stenosis (Fig. 5.21). A severe stenosis has higher systolic velocities and diastolic velocity exceeding 1.4 m/s (Chap. 30).

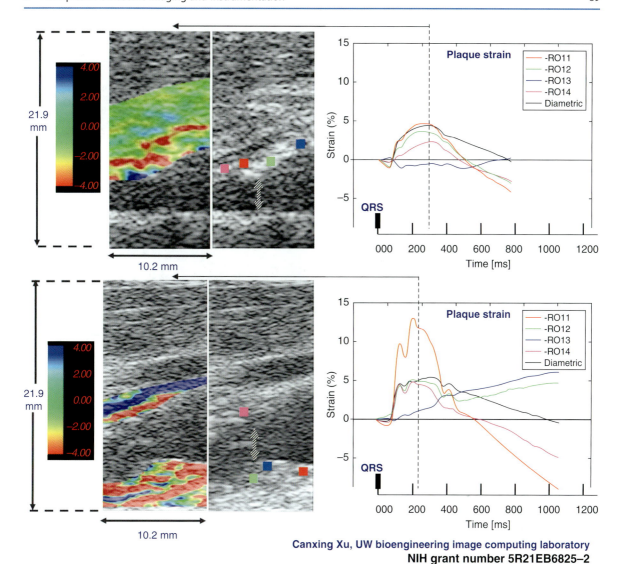

Fig. 5.22 Unidirectional plaque strain during systole in two patients with carotid stenosis. (*Top*) Patient **NEO006R**; (*bottom*) Patient **NEO008L**. (*Left*) Strain image comparing the tissue at the ECG QRS to the maximum tissue strain at about 230 ms after ECG QRS. SCALE range + 4% to −4%. (*Middle*) 2-Dimensional B-mode image of stenosis with artery diameter and strain waveform sample locations. *Vertical arrow* shows the location of the diameter waveform. *Colored boxes* show location of the tissue strain. (*Right*) 1-dimensional diametric (*black*) and NEGATIVE strain waveforms from four locations in the atherosclerotic plaque and wall. Most wall thickness strain waveforms include the wave shape features such as dicrotic and anacrotic waves, familiar in arterial plethysmography

5.6.3 Motion of Arterial Wall Tissue

Because of the cardiac cycle driving pressure pulsations and pulsatile blood flow in arteries, some information might be revealed by measuring the resulting waveforms of diameter and of strain in the arterial wall tissues (Fig. 5.22) (see Chaps. 19 and 20). As the diameter increases in systole, the thickness of the normal artery wall thins by the same percentage. In the strain waveform of the wall thickness, features such as the dicrotic wave can be seen. These waveforms differ along the length of an artery if an atherosclerotic plaque is present (Fig. 5.23). Surprisingly, sometimes the diametric waveform is inverted, and the strain waveforms can be either upright or inverted.

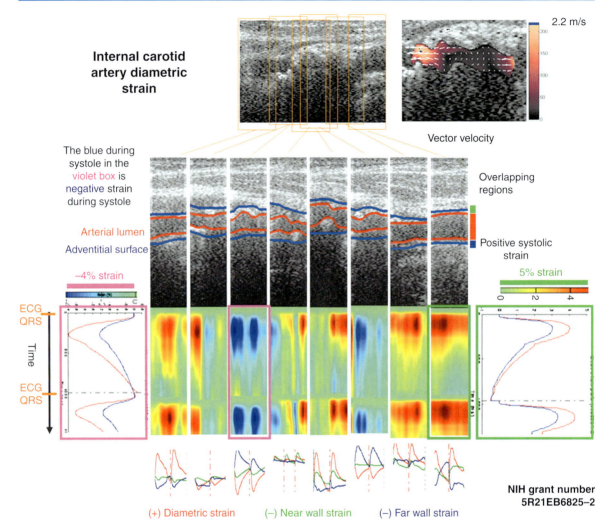

Fig. 5.23 Diametric strain and wall strain of a carotid artery with an atherosclerotic plaque. (*Top middle*) 2-D B-mode image showing frames for analysis below. (*Top right*) 2-D B-mode image with superimposed vector velocity. (*Middle*) Location images with luminal wall (*red*) and adventitial boundary (*blue*) marked by the sonographer on the superficial wall and deep wall. (*Middle*) Diametric change (*color*) as a function of position (lateral) and time (vertical) at different locations. (*Middle left and right*) Waveforms for the diameter at two of the eight locations (left with paradoxical pulsation is location 3, right is location 8). (*Bottom*) Waveforms for diameter (*red*) and inverse wall strain (superficial wall = *green*, deep wall = *blue*). Atherosclerotic Plaque Neovascular Inflation, NIH Grant Number 5R21EB6825-2

The assumption that the wall thickness strain waveform is the same shape and percentage magnitude as the inverted diametric strain waveform is based on the simple assumption that the wall volume is constant, so if the artery circumference increases, the wall thickness must decrease. However, because of the microcirculation in the wall, blood flow into and out of the wall can change the volume. This method might therefore provide insight into the volume changes of arterioles and venules in the arterial wall and plaque.

Unexpected tissue motions such as rotation might be interpreted incorrectly by the integrated tissue velocity method used to find displacement, and thus strain measurements should be interpreted with caution.

5.6.4 Tissue Vibrometry

Turbulence distal to a stenosis is a common feature of severe carotid atherosclerosis. Auscultation for carotid

Fig. 5.24 Vibration signature in spectral waveforms. Vibrations have a characteristic double sideband "Bessel Function" distribution, with the fundamental frequency equal to the lowest harmonic. The amplitude of the vibration can be determined by the number of harmonics that can be seen. (*Top*) Vibration harmonics dominate the appearance of the waveform. (*Bottom*) Vibration harmonics are nearly hidden by the blood velocity signal. This signal appears when the vibration frequency is lower than the pulse repetition frequency (PRF ~ 10 kHz) but higher than the inverse FFT period (~100 Hz)

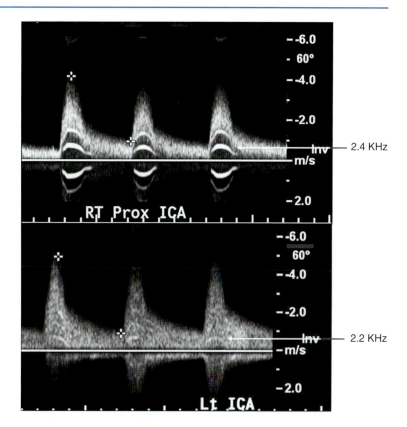

bruits is a standard method during a physical examination. Quantitative methods for measuring bruit characteristics, although of proven merit,[9–11] have been abandoned in favor of Duplex velocimetry. However, the vibrations can be imaged and the acoustic power can be directly measured in tissue, supplementing the conventional duplex examination. A characteristic vibration signal is often displayed in a Doppler spectral waveform (Fig. 5.24). Information about vibrations can be displayed in a variety of ways (Fig. 5.25), showing the spatial extent in tissue, amplitude, duration frequency and relation to the Doppler velocimetry measurements. These methods offer the promise of providing information on the stress imposed on the plaque.

5.6.5 Measuring Doppler Frequency

Although FFT spectral waveform processing of single-gate-pulse Doppler signals with a time resolution of 10 ms has become the workhorse of carotid artery examination and stenosis classification, increased data processing speeds in software rather than application-specific hardware, offers the possibility of exploring alternative methods of signal analysis. By exploring subregions in the post-stenotic "turbulence," new information about flow characteristics can be observed (Fig. 5.26). In this examination, oscillations in a portion of the post-stenotic zone are not propagated laterally into other post-stenotic regions. Such details about hemodynamics might provide new understanding about tissue remodeling. Comparing the results of alternative Doppler signal processing methods allow the examiner to avoid pitfalls. The green waveforms on the left are done with conventional autocorrelation mean processing. Velocity measurements taken from the autocorrelation waveform (green) have much lower values than those taken from the upper edge of the FFT spectral waveforms (gray). However, if short-time autocorrelation is used (Fig. 5.26, lower right), and the distribution of the results is displayed, the upper envelope is similar to the envelope for the FFT process.

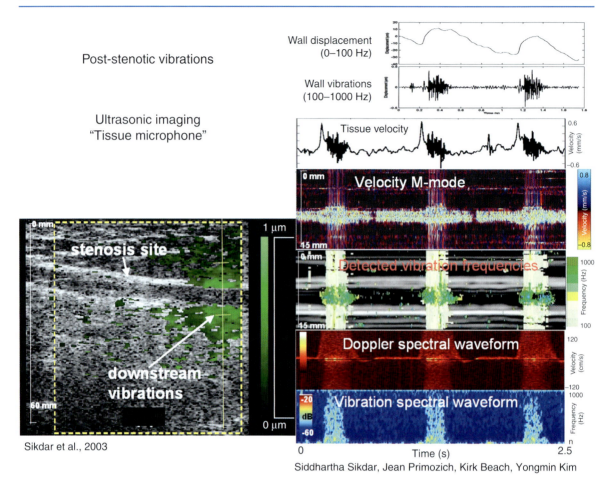

Fig. 5.25 Cross-axis Doppler measurements of both blood and tissue velocity showing post-stenotic tissue vibrations induced by deceleration turbulence. (*Left*) 2-dimensional B-mode image with green overlay of vibrations, selected for large echo amplitude and oscillation frequency between 100 and 1,000 Hz. Integration of tissue velocity provides displacement amplitude. (*Right, 1*) Integrated tissue velocity bandpass between 0.1 and 100 Hz to give displacement of the superficial wall. (*Right, 2*) Integrated tissue velocity bandpass between 100 and 1,000 Hz to give vibration displacement of the superficial wall. (*Right, 3*) Tissue velocity of the superficial wall. (*Right, 4*) Velocity M = mode showing both wall and blood velocity. (*Right, 5*) Blood vibration and wall vibration superimposed on amplitude demodulated 1-dimensional brightness-mode motion-mode. (*Right, 6*) Cross-axis Doppler spectral waveform. (*Right, 7*) Cross-axis vibration spectrum

5.6.6 Doppler Angle

A third of a century ago, the combination of ultrasonic 2-dimensional B-mode imaging with pulsed Doppler in the duplex scanner allowed the direct measurement of the Doppler examination angle.[12] The Doppler effect provides a measurement of the component of blood velocity in the direction of the Doppler ultrasound beam. Trigonometry allows the calculation of the velocity magnitude by dividing the magnitude of the component by the cosine of the ultrasound beam angle.

$$V = V(\text{component})/\cos\theta$$

However, this assumes that the heading of the blood velocity is known. Whenever the Doppler equation is tested by measuring the velocity in an artery at a series of different Doppler examination angles, measurements at smaller examination angles always produce lower results than those taken at higher angles (Fig. 5.27). This implies that Doppler data taken at a Doppler examination angle of 0°, as is done in cardiology, will provide the lowest measurement. Unfortunately, anatomic restrictions prevent the acquisition of Doppler data at an angle of zero degrees from arteries and veins except in rare cases like the middle cerebral artery. Taking Doppler data at an examination

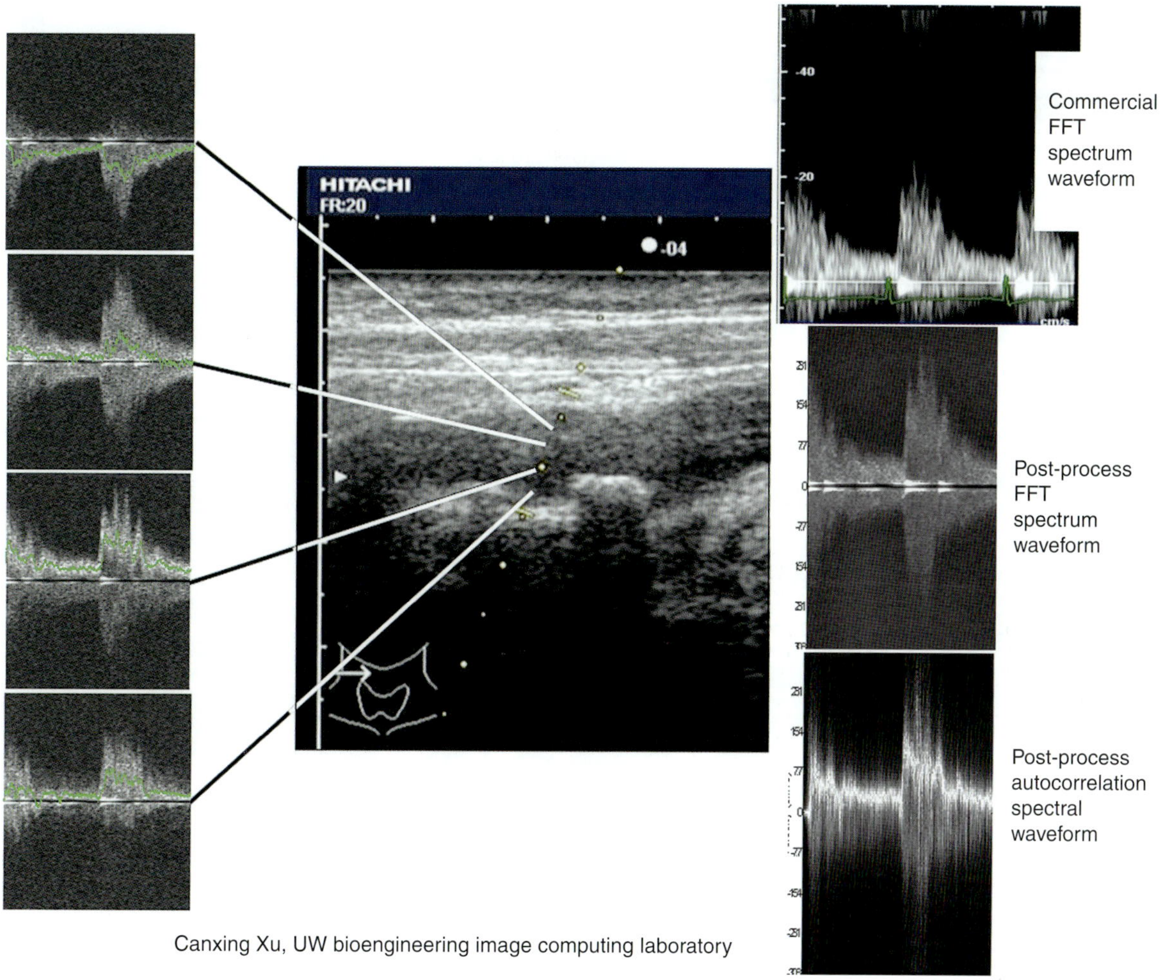

Fig. 5.26 Doppler waveform processing options in post-stenotic flow. (*Center*) Calcified Plaque on the deep wall indicated by ultrasound shadowing. (*Left*) Multigate FFT waveforms and short time autocorrelation mean velocities (*green*). Note the flow reversal in the superficial zone and the oscillations in sample volume 3. (*Top right*) FFT spectral waveform from a sample volume spanning the artery diameter generated by a commercial FFT processor. (*Middle right*) Spectral waveform from the same sample volume generated by a 256 point FFT MatLAB routine. (*Bottom right*) Autocorrelation spectral waveform generated by a six sample ensemble. Note that in regions where velocities are measured, the B-mode image shows significant echogenicity

angle of 90° (Fig. 5.28) provides a partial explanation for the limitations of the Doppler equation. At 90°, according to the Doppler equation, the Doppler shift is expected to be zero. But, in arteries, at 90°, velocity components can be measured both toward and away from the ultrasound transducer, indicating complicated helical flow. Even by examining the cross section at several angles, the exact nature of the helical flow is not obvious (Fig. 5.29). Although this problem has been recognized for decades, commercial Vector Doppler systems[13] that allow convenient examination of the complex flow patterns have become available only recently (Fig. 5.30) and clinical results from stenoses are not yet available. Whether the Vector Doppler system will allow the correct computation of volume flow rate and Bernoulli pressure depression in peripheral arteries remains to be shown.

5.7 Reprise

The relationship between carotid artery atherosclerotic stenosis and embolic stroke has been explored for over half a century. Much of the attention has been focused

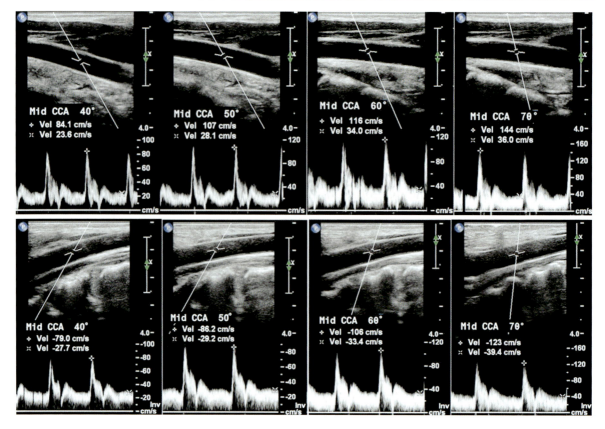

Fig. 5.27 Common carotid artery Doppler angle test. Angle adjusted velocity measurement as a function of Doppler examination angle. Head is to the left. As the Doppler examination angle is increased from 40° to 70°, the measured "angle adjusted velocity" increases

on the morphology, composition and dynamics of the carotid plaque and hemodynamics of the carotid stenosis. Cardiac factors, such as arrhythmia, and cerebral factors including collateralization and vasodilation/vasoconstriction, have also received some attention. Most studies have included laboratory investigations at convenient annual intervals. Although atherosclerosis develops over decades, the final events that lead to embolic stroke may evolve over very short times and/or irregular events. Cardiac arrhythmia, apnea leading to hypercapnic cerebral vasodilation, and episodic hypertension might be critical factors. Patient examination methods for stroke risk classification should be based on theoretical concepts about the causes of stroke validated by clinical trials. Imaging methods, including, ultrasonic methods, should be tailored to provide the information required for validation.

Ultrasound has several advantages over other examination methods. In addition to the potential for low cost, portable (wearable) applications for continuous measurement, ultrasound is capable of: (1) sub millisecond time resolution, (2) sub millimeter spatial and sub-micron displacement resolution in the depth direction, and (3) real time monitoring. Thus, it is likely that ultrasonic methods will evolve to serve the clinical and epidemiological needs of future studies of carotid atherosclerotic disease.

Acknowledgments Thanks to Ajay Anand, Kris Dickie, Siddhartha Sikdar, Edward Stutzman, Lei Sui, and Canxing Xu for providing images. Thanks to Jean Primozich for the first vibration waveforms and for studies on the effect of Doppler examination angles. Thanks to Professor Yongmin Kim for his collaboration on advanced ultrasound methods. Special thanks to David Phillips for teaching me about the physics of ultrasound and for conceiving ultrasound displacement measurements. Greatest thanks to Professor D. Eugene Strandness, Jr. for inviting me into this fascinating endeavor. Thanks also to the taxpayers of the United States and their support through the National Institute of Health.

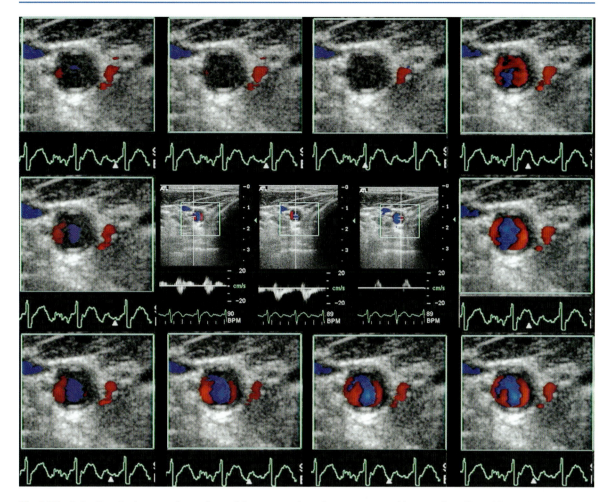

Fig. 5.28 Color Doppler image and waveform of the cross section of a common carotid artery. Complicated flow, which appears to be a dual helix

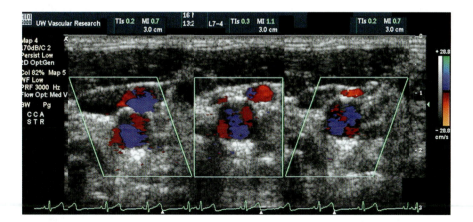

Fig. 5.29 Cross-section color Doppler in a normal common carotid artery at end systole vs. angle of view. Normal carotid flow consists of complicated helical flow patterns

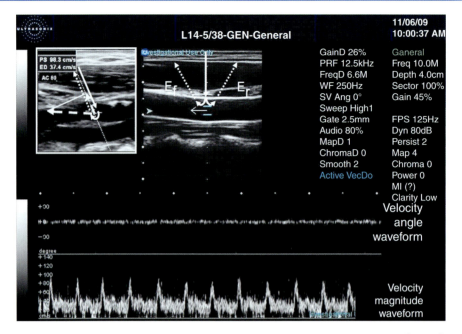

Fig. 5.30 Vector Doppler with magnitude and angle waveforms. (*Upper*) 2-D B-mode image with perpendicular Doppler ultrasound beam pattern and automatic velocity tracking vector. (*Solid arrow*) Vector Doppler transmit beam pattern. (*Dashed arrow*) Vector Doppler received beam patterns. (*Middle*) Angle waveform display. (*Lower*) Velocity magnitude waveform display. Cross-bisector velocity (*VA*) is proportional to $E_f - E_r$. Para-Bisector Velocity (*VX*) is proportional to $E_f +$ E_r. Velocity Magnitude = SQRT($VA^2 + VX^2$). Velocity Angle = ATAN (*VA/VX*). (*Left inset*) Conventional Doppler measures the velocity component along the co-linear transmit beam profile and receive beam profile. The examiner can manually mark the axis of the artery to indicate the assumed heading of the blood velocity. By dividing the velocity component by the cosine of the angle, a value for the para-axial velocity is computed Ultrasonix, Richmond, BC

References

1. Barnett HJ et al. Benefit of carotid endarterectomy in patients with symptomatic moderate or severe stenosis. *N Engl J Med*. 1998;339:1415–1425.
2. Sadat U et al. Utility of high resolution MR imaging to assess carotid plaque morphology: a comparison of acute symptomatic, recently symptomatic and asymptomatic patients with carotid artery disease. *Atherosclerosis*. 2009;207(2):434–449.
3. Comess KA, Beach KW, Hatsukami T, Strandness DE Jr, Daniel W. Pseudocolor displays in B-mode imaging applied to echocardiography and vascular imaging: an update. *J Am Soc Echocardiogr*. 1992;5:13–32.
4. Griffin M, Nicolaides A, Kyriacou E. Normalisation of ultrasonic images of atherosclerotic plaques and reproducibility of grey scale median using dedicated software. *Int Angiol*. 2007;26:372–377.
5. Kakkos SK et al. Texture analysis of ultrasonic images of symptomatic carotid plaques can identify those plaques associated with ipsilateral embolic brain infarction. *Eur J Vasc Endovasc Surg*. 2007;33:422-429.
6. Biasi GM et al. Carotid plaque echolucency increases the risk of stroke in carotid stenting: the Imaging in Carotid Angioplasty and Risk of Stroke (ICAROS) study. *Circulation*. 2004;110:756–762.
7. Tegos TJ, Kalomiris KJ, Sabetai MM, Kalodiki E, Nicolaides AN. Significance of sonographic tissue and surface characteristics of carotid plaques. *AJNR Am J Neuroradiol*. 2001;22:1605–1612.
8. Tegos TJ et al. Determinants of carotid plaque instability: echoicity versus heterogeneity. *Eur J Vasc Endovasc Surg*. 2001;22:22–30.
9. Duncan GW, Gruber JO, Dewey CF Jr, Myers GS, Lees RS. Evaluation of carotid stenosis by phonoangiography. *N Engl J Med*. 1975;293:1124–1128.
10. Knox R, Breslau P, Strandness DE Jr. Quantitative carotid phonoangiography. *Stroke*. 1981;12:798-803.
11. Plett MI et al. In vivo ultrasonic measurement of tissue vibration at a stenosis: a case study. *Ultrasound Med Biol*. 2001;27:1049–1058.
12. Barber FE, Baker DW, Nation AW, Strandness DE Jr, Reid JM. Ultrasonic duplex echo-Doppler scanner. *IEEE Trans Biomed Eng*. 1974;2:109–113.
13. Dunmire B, Beach KW, Labs K, Plett M, Strandness DE Jr. Cross-beam vector Doppler ultrasound for angle-independent velocity measurements. *Ultrasound Med Biol*. 2000;26:1213–1235.

Despeckling 6

Christos P. Loizou and Constantinos S. Pattichis

6.1 Introduction

The wide use of ultrasound imaging equipment, including mobile and portable telemedicine ultrasound scanning instruments and computer-aided systems, necessitates the need for better image processing techniques, in order to offer a clearer image to the medical practitioner. This makes the use of efficient despeckle filtering an important task.

The use of ultrasound in the diagnosis and assessment of arterial disease is well established because of its noninvasive nature, its low cost, and the continuing improvements in image quality.[1] Speckle, a form of locally correlated multiplicative noise, corrupts medical ultrasound imaging, making visual observation difficult.[2,3] The presence of speckle noise in ultrasound images has been documented since the early 1970s when researchers, such as Burckhardt,[2] Wagner et al.,[3] and Goodman,[4] described the fundamentals and the statistical properties of the speckle noise. Speckle is not truly a noise in the typical engineering sense (see Chap. 5), since its texture often carries useful information about the image being viewed. It is the primary factor, which limits the resolution in diagnostic ultrasound imaging, thereby limiting the detectability of small, low-contrast lesions and making the ultrasound images generally difficult for the non-specialist to interpret.[2,3,5,6] Due to the speckle presence, even ultrasound experts with sufficient experience may not often draw useful conclusions from the images.[6] Speckle noise also limits the effective application of image processing and analysis algorithms (i.e., edge detection, segmentation) and display in 2D and volume rendering in 3D. Therefore, speckle is most often considered a dominant source of "noise" in ultrasound imaging and should be filtered out[2,5,6] without affecting important features of the image. In this chapter, the authors present a comparative evaluation of selected despeckle filtering techniques based on texture analysis, image quality evaluation metrics, as well as visual assessment by experts on 440 ultrasound images of the carotid artery bifurcation as previously published by the authors' team[7-9] and a review of the relevant literature and discuss applications.

Early attempts to suppress speckle noise were implemented by averaging uncorrelated images of the same tissue recorded under different spatial positions.[5,8,10,11] While these methods are effective for speckle reduction, they require the capture of multiple images of the same object.[12] Speckle reducing filters originated from the synthetic aperture radar (SAR) community.[8] These filters were applied to ultrasound imaging since the early 1980s.[13] Filters that are used widely in both SAR and ultrasound imaging include the Frost,[14] Lee,[8,15,16] and Kuan[12,17] (Table 6.1).

Table 6.1 summarizes the despeckle filtering techniques that are presented in this chapter, grouped under the following categories: linear filtering (local statistics filtering, homogeneity filtering), nonlinear filtering (median filtering, linear scaling filtering, geometric filtering, logarithmic filtering, homomorphic

C.P. Loizou (✉)
Department of Computer Science, School of Sciences, Intercollege, Limassol, Cyprus

C.S. Pattichis
Department of Computer Science, University of Cyprus, Nicosia, Cyprus

Table 6.1 An overview of despeckle filtering techniques

Speckle reduction technique	Method	Investigator	Filter name
Linear filtering	Moving window utilizing local statistics		
	(a) mean (m), variance (σ^2)	[7]-[15], [14]-[19], [7]	DsFlsmv
	(b) mean, variance, 3rd and 4th moments (higher statistical moments), and entropy	[8]-[15], [9]	DsFlsmvsk1d DsFlsmvsk2d
	(c) Homogeneous mask area filters	[7], [9], [34]	DsFlsminsc
	(d) DsFwiener filtering	[7], [2]-[15], [16], [9]	DsFwiener
Nonlinear filtering	Median filtering	[2]-[35]	DsFmedian
	Linear scaling of the gray level values	[7]-[9], [48]	DsFls
			DsFca
			DsFlecasort
	Based on the most homogeneous neighborhood around each pixel	[7], [9], [19]	DsFhomog
	Nonlinear iterative algorithm (Geometric Filtering)	[7], [9], [10]	DsFgf4d
	The image is logarithmically transformed, the Fast Fourier transform (FFT) is computed, de-noised, the inverse FFT is computed and finally exponentially transformed back	[2], [7], [19], [20]	DsFhomo
Diffusion filtering	Nonlinear filtering technique for simultaneously performing contrast enhancement and noise reduction	[2], [5], [7], [9], [13], [14], [21], [22]-[25]	DsFad
	Exponential damp kernel filters utilizing diffusion	[5], [7], [9]	
	Speckle reducing anisotropic diffusion based on the coefficient of variation	[7], [9], [26]	DsFsrad
	Coherence enhancing diffusion	[7], [9], [26]	DsFnldif
Wavelet filtering	Only the useful wavelet coefficients are utilized	[9], [16], [27]-[30], [31], [37]	DsFwaveltc

Source: Loizou et al.[7]

filtering), anisotropic diffusion filtering (anisotropic diffusion, speckle reducing anisotropic diffusion, coherent nonlinear anisotropic diffusion), and wavelet filtering. Furthermore, in Table 6.1, the methodology used, the main investigators, and the corresponding filter names are given.

The Lee and Kuan filters have the same structure, although the Kuan is a generalization of the Lee filter. Both filters form the output image by computing the central pixel intensity inside a filter-moving window, which is calculated from the average intensity values of the pixels and a coefficient of variation inside the moving window. Kuan considered a multiplicative speckle model and designed a linear filter, based on the minimum-mean-square error (MMSE) criterion that has optimal performance when the histogram of the image intensity is Gaussian in distribution. The Lee[8] filter is a particular case of the Kuan filter based on a linear approximation made for the multiplicative noise model. The Frost[14] strikes a balance between the averaging and the all-pass filters. It was designed as an adaptive Wiener filter that assumed an autoregressive exponential model for the image.

In the nonlinear filtering group, the gray level values are linearly scaled to despeckle the image.[9,18] Some of the nonlinear filters are based on the most homogeneous neighborhood around each image pixel.[7] Geometric filters[10] are based on nonlinear iterative algorithms, which increment or decrement the pixel values in a neighborhood based upon their relative values. The method of homomorphic filtering[19,20] is similar to the logarithmic point operations used in histogram improvement, where dominant bright pixels are de-emphasized. In the homomorphic filtering, the fast Fourier transform (FFT) of the image is calculated, then de-noised, and then the inverse FFT is calculated.

Figure 6.1 illustrates the image of a normal carotid arterial wall (see Fig. 6.1a) and the image of a carotid arterial wall with an atherosclerotic plaque (see Fig. 6.1e) and their respective despeckled images (see Fig. 6.1b and f). Figure 6.1c–h show an enlarged

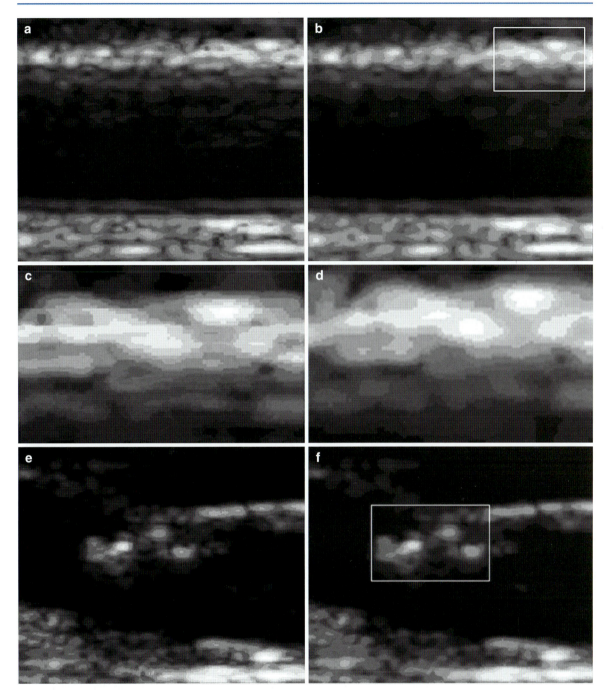

Fig. 6.1 Results of despeckle filtering based on linear filtering (first order local statistics, *DsFlsmv*). Normal arterial wall: (**a**) original, (**b**) despeckled, (**c**) enlarged region marked in (**b**) of the original, (**d**) enlarged region marked in (**b**) of the despeckled image. Symptomatic plaque: (**e**) original, (**f**) despeckled, (**g**) enlarged region marked in (**f**) of the original, (**h**) enlarged region marked in (**f**) of the despeckled image. Regions were enlarged by a factor of three. (Reprinted from Loizou and Pattichis[9]. (Spanias A, ed. Synthesis lectures on algorithms and software for engineering; #1))

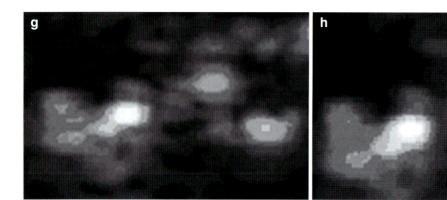

Fig. 6.1 (continued)

window from the original and despeckled images (shown in a rectangle in Fig. 6.1b and f).

The diffusion filtering category includes filters based on anisotropic diffusion,[2,21,22–25] speckle reducing anisotropic diffusion,[5] and coherence anisotropic diffusion.[26] These nonlinear filtering techniques have recently appeared in the literature. They perform contrast enhancement and noise reduction simultaneously by utilizing the coefficient of variation.[5] In the wavelet category, filters for suppressing the speckle noise have also been documented. These filters are making use of a realistic distribution of the wavelet coefficients,[2,16,27–32] where only the useful wavelet coefficients are utilized. Different wavelet shrinkage approaches have been investigated, usually based on Donoho's work.[31]

6.1.1 Limitations of Despeckle Filtering Techniques

Despeckling is always a trade-off between noise suppression and loss of information, something that experts are very concerned about. It is therefore desirable to keep as much of important information as possible. The majority of speckle reduction techniques have certain limitations that can be briefly summarized as follows:

1. They are sensitive to the size and shape of the sliding moving pixel window (usually 7×7 pixels wide). The use of different window sizes greatly affects the quality of the processed images. If the window is too large, over smoothing will occur, subtle details of the image will be lost in the filtering process and edges will be blurred. On the other hand, a small window will decrease the smoothing capability of the filter and will not reduce speckle noise, thus making the filter not effective. Our experiments showed that a 7×7 window size is a fairly good choice.

2. Some of the despeckle methods based on window approaches require thresholds to be used in the filtering process, which have to be empirically estimated. The inappropriate choice of a threshold may lead to average filtering and noisy boundaries, thus leaving the sharp features unfiltered.[7,10,15]

3. Most of the existing despeckle filters do not enhance the edges, but they only inhibit smoothing near the edges. When an edge is contained in the filtering window, the coefficient of variation will be high and smoothing will be inhibited. Therefore, speckle in the neighborhood of an edge will remain after filtering. Despeckle filters are not directional in the sense that in the presence of an edge, all smoothing is precluded. Instead of inhibiting smoothing in directions perpendicular to the edge, smoothing in directions parallel to the edge is allowed.

4. Different criteria for evaluating the performance of despeckle filtering are used by different studies. Although most of the studies use quantitative criteria such as the mean-square error (MSE) and speckle index (C), there are additional quantitative criteria, such as texture analysis and classification, image quality evaluation metrics, and visual assessment by experts that could be investigated.

To the best of the authors' knowledge, there is only one study which investigated despeckle filtering on ultrasound images of the carotid artery and proposed speckle reducing anisotropic diffusion as the most appropriate method.[5] This technique was compared with the Frost,[14] Lee,[15] and the homomorphic filtering[20] and documented that anisotropic diffusion performed better.

In the authors' study, they compared the performance of ten despeckle filters on 440 ultrasound images of the carotid artery bifurcation. The performance of these filters was evaluated using texture analysis, the kNN classifier (see the Sect. 6.3), image quality evaluation metrics, and visual evaluation by two experts. The results of the authors' study demonstrated that despeckle filtering improved the class separation between ultrasound images of asymptomatic and symptomatic carotid plaques.

In the following section, a brief overview of despeckle filtering techniques is presented followed by the methodology, which includes the material, recording of ultrasound images, texture and statistical analysis, the kNN classifier, image quality evaluation metrics, and the experiment carried out for visual evaluation. The results and discussions follow. The final section presents a summary, future directions, and a proposal for a despeckling filtering and evaluation protocol. The despeckle filtering toolbox proposed,[9] which includes the MATLAB (MathWorks, Natick, Massachusetts, USA) code for despeckling, image quality evaluation, and texture analysis, is also available for download at http://www.ehealthlab.cs.ucy.ac.cy/.

6.2 Despeckle Filtering Algorithms

To be able to derive an efficient despeckle filter, a speckle noise model is needed. The speckle noise model for ultrasound images may be approximated as multiplicative.[2–4] The signal at the output of the receiver demodulation module of the ultrasound imaging system may be defined as:

$$y_{i,j} = x_{i,j} n_{i,j} + a_{i,j} \quad (6.1)$$

where $y_{i,j}$ represents the noisy pixel in the middle of the moving window, $x_{i,j}$ represents the noise-free pixel, $n_{i,j}$ and $a_{i,j}$ represent the multiplicative and additive noise, respectively, and i,j are the indices of the spatial locations that belong in the 2D space of real numbers, $i,j \in \Re^2$. Logarithmic compression is applied to the envelope detected echo signal in order to fit it in the display range.[26,33] It has been shown that logarithmic compression affects the speckle noise statistics in such a way that the local mean becomes proportional to the local variance rather than the standard deviation.[9,26,28,30,33] More specifically, logarithmic compression affects the high-intensity tail of the Rayleigh and Rician probability density function (PDF) more than the low intensity part. As a result, the speckle noise becomes very close to white Gaussian noise corresponding to the uncompressed Rayleigh signal.[33] Referring to Eq. 6.1, since the effect of additive noise is considerably smaller compared with that of multiplicative noise, it may be written as:

$$y_{i,j} \approx x_{i,j} n_{i,j}. \quad (6.2)$$

Thus the logarithmic compression transforms the model in Eq. 6.2 into the classical signal in additive noise form as:

$$\log(y_{i,j}) = \log(x_{i,j}) + \log(n_{i,j}), \quad (6.3a)$$

$$g_{i,j} = f_{i,j} + nl_{i,j}. \quad (6.3b)$$

For the rest of the chapter, the term $\log(y_{i,j})$, which is the observed pixel on the ultrasound image display after logarithmic compression, is denoted as $g_{i,j}$, and the terms $\log(x_{i,j})$ and $\log(n_{i,j})$, which are the noise-free pixel and noise component after logarithmic compression, as $f_{i,j}$ and $nl_{i,j}$, respectively (see Eq. 6.3b).

6.2.1 Local Statistical Filtering

Most of the techniques for speckle reduction filtering in the literature use local statistics. Their working principle may be described by a weighted average calculation using subregion statistics to estimate statistical measures over different pixel windows varying from [3 × 3] up to [15 × 15]. All these techniques assume that the speckle noise model has a multiplicative form as given in Eq. 6.2.[7–16,26,28]

6.2.1.1 First Order Statistics Filtering (DsFlsmv, DsFwiener)

The filters utilizing the first order statistics such as the variance and the mean of the neighborhood may be described with the model as in (Eq. 6.2). Hence the algorithms in this class may be traced back to the following equation[5,7–17]:

$$f_{i,j} = \bar{g} + k_{i,j}(g_{i,j} - \bar{g}) \quad (6.4)$$

where $f_{i,j}$, is the estimated noise-free pixel value, $g_{i,j}$, is the noisy pixel value in the moving window, $\bar{g}$, is the local mean value of an $N_1 \times N_2$, region surrounding and including pixel $g_{i,j}$, $k_{i,j}$ is a weighting factor, with $k \in [0 \ldots 1]$, and i, j, are the pixel coordinates. The factor $k_{i,j}$ is a function of the local statistics in a moving window. It can be found in the literature[8,9,12,15] and may be derived in different forms that:

$$k_{i,j} = (1 - \bar{g}^2 \sigma^2)/(\sigma^2(1 + \sigma_n^2)) \quad (6.5)$$

$$k_{i,j} = \sigma^2/(\bar{g}^2 \sigma_n^2 + \sigma^2) \quad (6.6)$$

$$k_{i,j} = (\sigma^2 - \sigma_n^2)/\sigma^2. \quad (6.7)$$

The values σ^2, and σ_n^2, represent the variance in the moving window and the variance of noise in the whole image respectively. The noise variance may be calculated for the logarithmically compressed image as explained in Loizou et al. (2008).[9] If the value of $k_{i,j}$ is one (in edge areas), this will result in an unchanged pixel, whereas a value of zero (in uniform areas) replaces the actual pixel by the local average, $\bar{g}$, over a small region of interest (see Eq. 6.4). In this study, the filter DsFlsmv uses equation (Eq. 6.5). The filter DsFwiener uses a pixel-wise adaptive Wiener method[2–6,14] implemented as given in (Eq. 6.4), with the weighting factor $k_{i,j}$, as given in (Eq. 6.7). For both despeckle filters DsFlsmv and Wiener, the moving window size was 5×5.

6.2.1.2 Homogenous Mask Area Filtering (DsFlsminsc)

The DsFlsminsc is a 2D filter operating in a 5×5 pixel neighborhood by searching for the most homogenous neighborhood area around each pixel, using a 3×3 subset window.[9,34] The middle pixel of the 5×5 neighborhood is substituted with the average gray level of the 3×3 mask with the smallest speckle index, C, where C for log-compressed is calculated as in Loizou et al. (2008)[9] The window with the smallest C is the most homogenous semi-window, which presumably does not contain any edge. The filter is applied iteratively until the gray levels of almost all pixels in the image do not change.

6.2.2 Median Filtering (DsFmedian)

The filter DsFmedian[35] is a simple nonlinear operator that replaces the middle pixel in the window with the median-value of its neighbors. The moving window for the DsFmedian filter used for the experiments presented in this chapter was [7×7].

6.2.3 Maximum Homogeneity over a Pixel Neighborhood Filtering (DsFhomog)

The DsFhomog filter is based on an estimation of the most homogeneous neighborhood around each image pixel.[36] The filter takes into consideration only pixels that belong in the processed neighborhood (7×7 pixels), under the assumption that the observed area is homogeneous. For a complete mathematical derivation of the filter, see Loizou et al. (2008).[9] The DsFhomog filter does not require any parameters or thresholds to be tuned, thus making the filter suitable for automatic interpretation.

6.2.4 Geometric Filtering (DsFgf4d)

The concept of the geometric filtering is that speckle appears in the image as narrow walls and valleys. The geometric filter, through iterative repetition, gradually tears down the narrow walls (bright edges) and fills up the narrow valleys (dark edges), thus smearing the weak edges that need to be preserved.

The DsFgf4d filter[10] investigated in this chapter uses a nonlinear noise reduction technique. It compares the intensity of the central pixel in a 3×3 neighborhood with those of its eight neighbors and, based upon the neighborhood pixel intensities, increments or decrements the intensity of the central pixel such that it becomes more representative of its surroundings. The operation of the geometric filter DsFgf4d has been described in Loizou et al.[7,9]

6.2.5 Homomorphic Filtering (DsFhomo)

The *DsFhomo* filter performs homomorphic filtering for image enhancement, by calculating the Fast Fourier Transform (FFT) of the logarithmic compressed image, applying a de-noising homomorphic filter function $H(.)$ $H(.)$ is a homomorphic function), and then performing the inverse FFT of the image.[19,20] The homomorphic filter function, $H(.)$, may be constructed either using a band-pass Butterworth or a high-boost Butterworth filter. In this study, a high-boost Butterworth filter was used with the homomorphic function.[18] The functions and the filter realization can be found in an article by Loizou et al. (2008).[9] This form of filtering sharpens features and flattens speckle variations in an image.

6.2.6 Diffusion Filtering

Diffusion filters remove noise from an image by modifying the image via solving a partial differential equation (PDE). The smoothing is carried out depending on the image edges and their directions. Anisotropic diffusion is an efficient nonlinear technique for simultaneously performing contrast enhancement and noise reduction. It smoothes homogeneous image regions but retains image edges[5,24,25] without requiring any information from the image power spectrum. It may thus directly be applied to logarithmic compressed images. Consider applying the isotropic diffusion equation given by $dg_{i,j,t}/dt = \text{div}(d\nabla g)$ using the original noisy image, $g_{i,j,t=0}$, as the initial condition, where $g_{i,j,t=0}$ is an image in the continuous domain, i,j specifies spatial position, t is an artificial time parameter, d is the diffusion constant, and ∇g is the image gradient. Modifying the image according to this linear isotropic diffusion equation is equivalent to filtering the image with a Gaussian filter. In this work, the authors have used conventional anisotropic diffusion (*DsFad*) and coherent nonlinear anisotropic diffusion (*DsFnldif*). The theoretical background and the mathematical derivation of the filters can be found in Loizou et al. (2008).[9]

6.2.7 Wavelet Filtering (DsFwaveltc)

Speckle reduction filtering in the wavelet domain, used in this study, is based on the idea of the Daubenchies Symlet wavelet and on soft-thresholding de-noising. It was first proposed by Donoho[31] and also investigated by others.[27,28,37] The Symmlets family of wavelets, although not perfectly symmetrical, was designed to have the least asymmetry and highest number of vanishing moments for a given compact support.[31] The *DsFwaveltc* filter, implemented in this study, is well described in Loizou et al. (2008).[9]

6.3 Evaluation Methodology

In this section, the authors present the material, the ultrasound imaging scanners used for the image acquisition as well as texture analysis, distance measures, univariate statistical analysis, and the kNN classifier, which are used to evaluate despeckle filtering. Also a number of image quality metrics are presented for evaluating the quality between the original and the despeckled images. Finally the procedure of visual evaluation carried out by the experts is introduced.

6.3.1 Material and Recording of Ultrasound Images

A total of 440 ultrasound images of the carotid artery bifurcation, 220 with asymptomatic and 220 with symptomatic plaques producing greater than 70% stenosis in relation to the bulb, were used in this study. Carotid plaques were labeled as symptomatic in the presence of ischemic ipsilateral hemispheric symptoms: stroke with good recovery, transient ischemic attack (TIA), or amaurosis fugax. These images are part of a database of images obtained as part of a diagnostic service. They were acquired using the ATL HDI-3,000 ultrasound scanner (Phillips Ultrasound Inc., Bothell, WA, USA). The ultrasonographers were aware of the plan to create a database. Thus, equipment settings and image capture was as described in Chap. 12. The ATL HDI-3,000 ultrasound scanner is equipped with 64 elements fine pitch high-resolution, 38 mm broadband array, a multielement ultrasound scan head with an operating frequency range of 4–7 MHz, an acoustic aperture of 10×8 mm and a transmission focal range of 0.8–11 cm.[38] In this work all images were recorded as displayed in the ultrasound monitor, after logarithmic compression. The images were recorded digitally on a magneto-optical drive, with a resolution of 768 × 756 pixels with 256 gray levels. The image resolution was 16.66 pixels/mm.

6.3.2 Image Normalization and Plaque Segmentation

The need for image standardization or post-processing has been suggested in the past, and normalization using only blood echogenicity as a reference point has been applied in ultrasound images of carotid artery.[8,10] Brightness adjustments of the ultrasound images have been shown to improve image compatibility, by reducing the variability introduced by different gain settings and facilitate ultrasound tissue comparability.[9]

The images were normalized manually by linearly adjusting the image so that the median gray level value of the blood was 0–5, and the median gray level of the adventitia (artery wall) was 180–190 (see Chap. 12). The scale of the gray level of the images ranged from 0 to 255.[39]

This normalization using blood and adventitia as reference points was necessary in order to extract comparable measurements in case of processing images obtained by different operators or different equipment.[9,39]

Plaque segmentation was performed by an experienced ultrasonographer as described in Chap. 12.

6.3.3 Despeckle Filtering

Ten despeckle filters were applied on the 440 logarithmically compressed ultrasound images. These filters are (see Table 6.1) the *DsFlsmv*, *DsFlsminsc*, *DsFmedian*, *DsFwiener*, from the linear filtering group, *DsFhomog*, *DsFgf4d*, *DsFhomo*, from the non-linear filtering group, *DsFad*, *DsFnldif*, from the diffusion filtering group, and the *DsFwaveltc* wavelet despeckle filter.

6.3.4 Texture Analysis

Following the despeckling, texture features may be extracted from the original and the despeckled images.

Texture analysis is one of the most important features used in image processing and pattern recognition. It can provide information about the arrangement and spatial properties of fundamental image elements. Texture provides useful information for the characterization of atherosclerotic plaque. More details about texture feature extraction and algorithms used can be found in Chap. 14. In this study a total of 56 different texture features were extracted both from the original and the despeckled ultrasound images as follows:

1. Statistical Features (SF): (a) Mean, (b) Median, (c) Variance (σ^2), (d) Skewness (σ^3), (e) Kurtosis (σ^4), and (f) Speckle index (σ/m).
2. Spatial Gray Level Dependence Matrices (SGLDM) as proposed by Haralick et al.[40]: (a) Angular second moment, (b) Contrast, (c) Correlation, (d) Sum of squares: variance, (e) Inverse difference moment, (f) Sum average, (g) Sum variance, (h) Sum entropy, (i) Entropy, (j) Difference variance, (k) Difference entropy, and (l) and (m) Information measures of correlation. Each feature was computed using a distance of one pixel. Also for each feature, the mean values and the range of values were computed, and were used as two different feature sets.
3. Gray Level Difference Statistics (GLDS): (a) Contrast, (b) Angular second moment, (c) Entropy, and (d) Mean.
4. Neighborhood Gray Tone Difference Matrix (NGTDM): (a) Coarseness, (b) Contrast, (c) Business, (d) Complexity, and (e) Strength.
5. Statistical Feature Matrix (SFM): (a) Coarseness, (b) Contrast, (c) Periodicity, and (d) Roughness.
6. Laws Texture Energy Measures (TEM): For the laws TEM extraction, vectors of length $l = 7$ $L = (1, 6, 1, 5, 20, 15, 6, 1)$ $E = (-1, -4, -5, 0, 5, 4, 1)$ and $S = (-1, -2, 1, 4, 1 - 2, -1)$ were used, where L performs local averaging, E acts as an edge detector, and S acts as a spot detector. The following TEM features were extracted: (a) LL – texture energy (TE) from LL kernel, (b) EE – TE from EE kernel, (c) SS – TE from SS kernel, (d) LE – average TE from LE and EL kernels, (e) ES – average TE from ES and SE kernels, and (f) LS – average TE from LS and SL kernels.
7. Fractal Dimension Texture Analysis (FDTA) : Hurst coefficient, $H^{(k)}$, for resolutions $k = 1, 2, 3, 4$.
8. Fourier Power Spectrum (FPS): (a) Radial sum, and (b) Angular sum.

6.3.5 Distance Measures

In order to identify the most discriminant features separating the two classes under investigation, i.e., asymptomatic and symptomatic ultrasound images (identifying features that have the highest discriminatory power), before and after despeckle filtering, the distance between asymptomatic and symptomatic images was calculated for the set of all ultrasound images, before and after despeckle filtering for each feature as follows[41]:

$$\text{dis}_{zc} = |m_{za} - m_{zs}|/\sqrt{\sigma_{za}^2 + \sigma_{zs}^2} \quad (6.8)$$

where z is the feature index, c if o indicates the original image set and if f indicates the despeckled image set, m_{za} and m_{zs} are the mean values and σ_{za} and σ_{zs} are the standard deviations of the asymptomatic and symptomatic classes respectively. The most discriminant features are the ones with the highest distance values.[8,9,41] If the distance after despeckle filtering is increased, i.e.:

$$\text{dis}_{zf} > \text{dis}_{zo} \quad (6.9)$$

then it can be derived that the classes may be better separated.

For each feature, a percentage distance was computed as

$$\text{feat\_dis}_z = (\text{dis}_{zf} - \text{dis}_{zo})100. \quad (6.10)$$

For each feature set, a score distance was computed as

$$\text{Score\_Dis} = (1/N)\sum_{z=1}^{N}(\text{dis}_{zf} - \text{dis}_{zo})100 \quad (6.11)$$

where N is the number of features in the feature set. It should be noted that for all features, a larger feature distance shows improvement.

6.3.6 Univariate Statistical Analysis

The Wilcoxon rank sum test for paired samples is a non-parametric alternative for the paired samples t-test, when the distribution of the samples is not normal. The Wilcoxon test for paired samples ranks the absolute values of the differences between the paired observations in sample one and sample two and calculates a statistic on the number of negative and positive differences. If the resulting p-value is small ($p < 0.05$), then it can be accepted that the median of the differences between the paired observations is statistically significantly different from zero. The Wilcoxon matched-pairs signed rank sum test was used in order to detect if for each texture feature, a significant (S) or not significant (NS) difference exists between the original and the despeckled images at $p < 0.05$. The test was applied on all the 220 asymptomatic and 220 symptomatic, original and despeckled images of the carotid artery.

6.3.7 kNN Classifier

The k-nearest-neighbor (kNN) classification is one of the most fundamental and simple classification methods and should be one of the first choices for a classification study when there is little or no prior knowledge about the distribution of the data. K-nearest-neighbor classification was developed because of the need to perform discriminant analysis when reliable parametric estimates of probability densities are unknown or difficult to determine.

The statistical k-nearest-neighbor (kNN) classifier using the Euclidean distance with $k = 7$ was also used in this study to classify a plaque image as asymptomatic or symptomatic.[41] The leave-one-out method was used for evaluating the performance of the classifier, where each case is evaluated in relation to the rest of the cases. This procedure is characterized by no bias concerning the possible training and evaluation bootstrap sets. The kNN classifier was chosen because it is simple to implement and computationally very efficient. This is highly desired due to the many feature sets and filters tested.

6.3.8 Image Quality Evaluation Metrics

For medical images, quality can be objectively defined in terms of performance in clinically relevant tasks such as lesion detection and classification, where typical tasks are the detection of an abnormality, the estimation of some parameters of interest, or the combination of the above.[42,43] Most studies today have assessed the equipment performance by testing diagnostic performance of multiple experts, which also suffer from intra- and inter-observer variability. Although this is the most important method of assessing the results of image degradation, few studies have attempted to perform physical measurements of degradation.[44,45] Image quality is important when evaluating or segmenting atherosclerotic carotid plaques[46] or the intima-media-complex (IMC) in the carotid artery,[47] where speckle obscures subtle details[7,9] in the image. In a recent study,[9] the authors have shown that speckle reduction improves the visual perception of the expert in the assessment of ultrasound imaging of the carotid artery.

When speckle noise is apparent in the image, the expert's differing experiences with noise are bound to lead to different weightings of the artifact.[42] Researchers showed that experts and non-experts examine different critical image characteristics to form their final opinion with respect to image quality.[9,43] Thus image quality evaluation metrics can be used for the evaluation of despeckle filtering.

Differences between the original, $g_{i,j}$, and the despeckled, $f_{i,j}$, images were evaluated using image quality evaluation metrics. The following measures, which are easy to compute and have clear physical meaning, were computed[8,9]:

(a) The MSE.[9,48]
(b) The root MSE (RMSE), which is the square root of the squared error averaged over an $M \times N$ window.[9,49]
(c) The error summation in the form of the Minkowski metric (Err1, Err2), which is the norm of the dissimilarity between the original and the despeckled images.[9,44]
(d) The Geometric Average Error (GAE).[9,42]
(e) The signal to noise ratio (SNR) which is given in Loizou et al. (2008) and Sakrison.[9,45]
(f) The peak SNR (PSNR) is computed as in Loizou et al. (2008) and Sakrison.[9,45]
(g) The mathematically defined universal quality index (Q)[50] models any distortion as a combination of three different factors, which are loss of correlation, luminance distortion, and contrast distortion and is derived by Wang.[50]
(h) The structural similarity index (SSIN) between two images,[44] which is a generalization of the Q.
(i) The speckle index C, which is an average measure of the amount of speckle presented in the image area with size $M \times N$, as a whole (over the whole image).[7–9]

It is noted that a new image quality metric based on natural scene statistics, and mutual information between the original and the filtered images has recently been proposed by Sheikh et al.[51]

6.3.9 Visual Evaluation by Experts

Visual evaluation can be broadly categorized as the ability of an expert to extract useful anatomical information from an ultrasound image. The visual evaluation varies of course from expert to expert and is subject to the observer's variability.[43] The visual evaluation, in this study, was carried out according to the ITU-R recommendations with the Double Stimulus Continuous Quality Scale (DSCQS) procedure.[42] A total of 100 ultrasound images of the carotid artery bifurcation (50 asymptomatic and 50 symptomatic) were evaluated visually by two vascular experts, a cardiovascular surgeon, and a neurovascular specialist before and after despeckle filtering. For each case, the original and the despeckled images (despeckled with filters *DsFlsmv*, *DsFlsminsc*, *DsFmedian*, *DsFwiener*, *DsFhomog*, *DsFgf4d*, *DsFhomo*, *DsFad*, *DsFnldif*, and *DsFwaveltc*) were presented without labeling at random to the two experts. The experts were asked to assign a score in the one to five scale corresponding to low and high subjective visual perception criteria. Five was given to an image with the best visual perception. Therefore the maximum score for a filter is 500, if the expert assigned the score of five for all the 100 images. For each filter, the score was divided by five to be expressed in percentage format. The experts were allowed to give equal scores to more than one image in each case. For each class and for each filter, the average score was computed.

The two vascular experts evaluated the area around the distal common carotid, 2–3 cm proximal to the bifurcation and the bifurcation itself. It is known that measurements taken from the far wall of the carotid artery are more accurate than those taken from the near wall.[39] Furthermore, the experts were examining the image in the lumen area, in order to identify the existence of a plaque or not.

6.4 Results

In this section, the authors will present the evaluation of the ten despeckle filters described in the previous section that were applied on the images of the carotid artery bifurcation from 220 asymptomatic and 220 symptomatic patient. A total of 56 texture features were computed and the most discriminant ones are presented. Furthermore the performance of these filters is investigated for discriminating between asymptomatic and symptomatic images of plaques using the statistical kNN classifier. Moreover, nine different image quality evaluation metrics were computed, as well as visual evaluation scores carried out by two experts.

6.4.1 Real Carotid Ultrasound Image

Figure 6.2 shows an ultrasound image of the carotid together with the despeckled images. The best visual

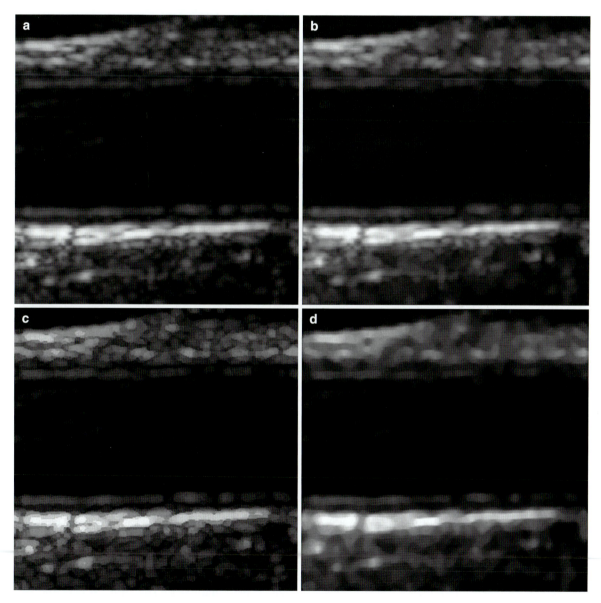

Fig. 6.2 Original ultrasound image of the carotid artery (2–3 cm proximal to bifurcation) given in (**a**), and the despeckled filtered images given in (**b–k**) (Reprinted from Loizou et al.[7] © IEEE 2005)

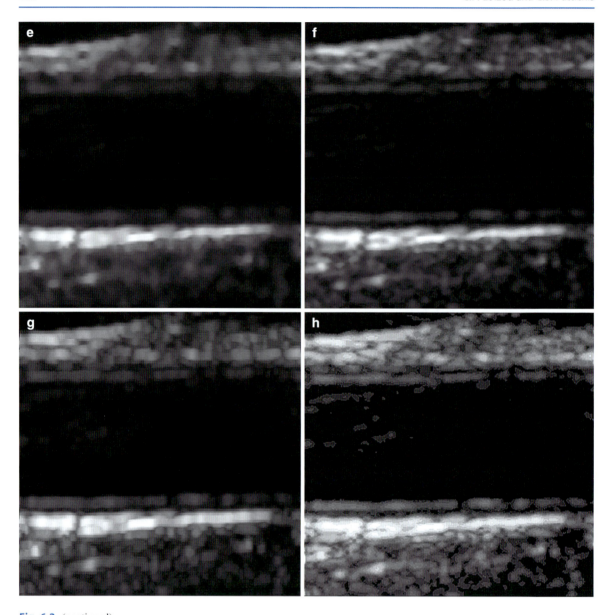

Fig. 6.2 (continued)

results as assessed by the two experts were obtained by the filters *DsFlsmv* and *DsFlsminsc*, whereas the filters *DsFgf4d*, *DsFad*, and *DsFnldif* also showed good visual results but smoothed the image considerably and thus edges and subtle details may have been lost. Filters that showed a blurring effect were the *DsFmedian*, *DsFwiener*, *DsFhomog*, and *DsFwaveltc*. Filters *DsFwiener*, *DsFhomog*, and *DsFwaveltc* showed poorer visual results.

6.4.2 Texture Analysis: Distance Measures

Despeckle filtering and texture analysis were carried out on 440 ultrasound images of the carotid bifurcation. Table 6.2 tabulates the results of $feat\_dis_z$ (Eq. 6.10), and $Score\_Dis$ (Eq. 6.11), for SF, SGLDM range of values, and NGTDM feature sets for the ten despeckle filters. Only the results of these

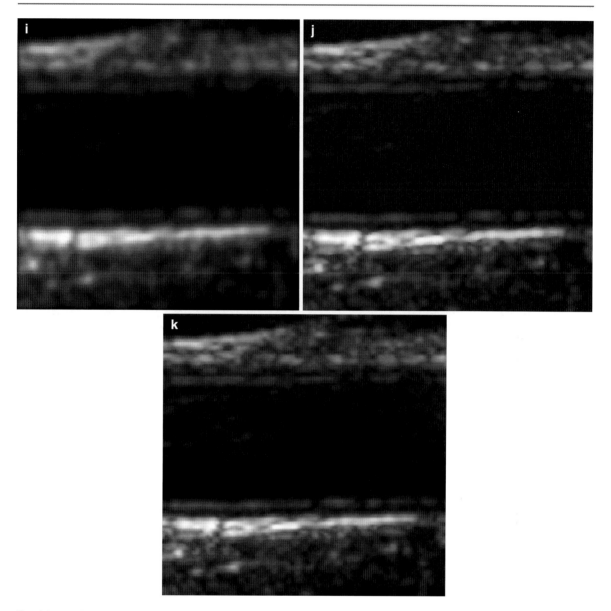

Fig. 6.2 (continued)

feature sets are presented, since the latter were the ones with the best performance. The filters are categorized as linear filtering, nonlinear filtering, diffusion filtering, and wavelet filtering. Also the number of iterations (Nr. of It.) for each filter is given, which was selected based on C and on the visual evaluation of the two experts. When C was minimally changing, the filtering process was stopped. The bold values represent the values that showed an improvement after despeckle filtering compared to the original.

The last row in each sub-table shows the $Score\_Dis$ for all features, where the highest value indicates the best filter in the sub-table. Additionally, a total score distance $Score\_Dis\_T$ was computed for all feature sets shown in the last row of Table 6.2. Some of the despeckle filters shown in Table 6.2 are changing a number of texture features, by increasing the distance between the two classes, (positive values in Table 6.2), and therefore making the identification and separation between asymptomatic and symptomatic plaques

Table 6.2 Feature distance (Eq. 6.10) and Score_Dis (Eq. 6.11) for SF, SGLDM range of values, and NGTDM texture feature sets between asymptomatic and symptomatic carotid plaque ultrasound images

Feature	Linear filtering				Nonlinear filtering			Diffusion		Wavelet
	DsFlsmv	DsFlsminsc	DsFwiener	DsFmedian	DsFhomog	DsFgf4d	DsFhomo	DsFad	DsFnldif	DsFwaveltc
Nr. of It.	4	1	2	2	1	3	2	20	5	5
SF-statistical features										
Mean	**14**	**22**	**19**	**4**	**11**	**3**	**164**	**18**	**5**	**15**
Median	−5	−17	−26	−5	−5	−15	110	−29	−6	−15
σ^2	**18**	**38**	**18**	**7**	**13**	−2	**140**	**9**	**7**	**18**
σ^3	**12**	**16**	**5**	**9**	**7**	−0.1	**149**	**17**	**7**	**8**
σ^4	−12	−14	−7	−6	−4	−3	117	−21	**6**	−9
C	**0.4**	**0.3**	**0.3**	**0.4**	**0.3**	**0.4**	0.08	**0.3**	**0.4**	**0.3**
Score_dis	27	45	9	9	22	−17	680	−6	19	17
SGLDM range of values – spatial gray level dependence matrix										
ASM	−21	−0.5	−29	**2**	−4	−8	−47	−25	−17	−20
Contrast	**47**	**107**	**14**	**64**	**32**	−3	**165**	**104**	**13**	**22**
Correlation	**12**	**59**	**15**	**24**	−5	**2**	10	**54**	−4	−4
SOSV	**9**	**40**	**18**	**10**	**16**	−2	**101**	**9**	**8**	**20**
IDM	−50	−11	−48	**2**	−29	−8	94	−54	−34	−43
SAV	**17**	**24**	**23**	**7**	**15**	**3**	**169**	**22**	**6**	**18**
$\sum var$	**19**	**38**	**18**	**9**	**15**	−2	**90**	**9**	**8**	**20**
$\sum Entr$	−34	−14	−49	3	−19	−4	−11	−47	−30	−36
Score_dis	−1	243	−38	121	21	−22	571	72	−50	−23
NGTDM – Neighborhood gray tone difference matrix										
Coarseness	**30**	**87**	**4**	**9**	−16	−7	**72**	−36	−37	−33
Contrast	**7**	−0.3	−9	**8**	**0.4**	−4	**105**	**5**	−27	−15
Busyness	**17**	**26**	−30	**8**	**1**	−4	**48**	−14	−39	**8**
Completion	**64**	**151**	**21**	**53**	**80**	**2**	**150**	**63**	**18**	**27**
Score_dis	118	264	−14	78	66	−13	375	18	−85	−13
gatheredScore_dis_Tgathered	144	551	−43	208	108	−52	1,626	84	−116	−19

Source: Loizou et al.[7]
ASM angular 2nd moment, *SOSV* sum of squares variance, *IDM* inverse difference moment, *SAV* sum average, $\sum var$ sum variance, *HF* homogeneity, *GF* geometric, *HM* homomorphic
Bolded values show improvement after despeckle filtering

more feasible. A positive feature distance shows improvement after despeckle filtering, whereas a negative shows deterioration.

In the first part of Table 6.2, the results of the SF features are presented, where the best *Score_Dis* is given for the filter *DsFhomo* followed by the *DsFlsminsc*, *DsFlsmv*, *DsFhomog*, *DsFnldif*, *DsFwaveltc*, *DsFmedian*, and *DsFwiener*, with the worst *Score_Dis* given by *gf4d*. All filters reduced the speckle index, C. Almost all filters reduced significantly the variance, σ^2, and the kurtosis, σ^3, of the histogram, as it may be seen from the bolded values in the first part of Table 6.2.

In the second part of the Table 6.2, the results of the SGLDM range of values features set are tabulated. The filters with the highest *Score_Dis* in the SGLDM range of values features set are *DsFhomo*, *DsFlsminsc*, *DsFmedian*, *DsFad*, and *DsFhomog*, whereas all other the filters (*DsFnldif*, *DsFwiener*, *DsFwaveltc*, *DsFgf4d*, *DsFlsmv*) are presenting a negative *Score_Dis*. Texture features, which improved in most of the filters, are the contrast, correlation, sum of squares variance, sum average, and sum variance.

In the third part of Table 6.2, for the NGTDM feature set, almost all filters showed an improvement in *Score_Dis*. Best filters in the NGTDM feature set were the *DsFhomo*, *DsFlsminsc*, *DsFhomog*, and *DsFlsmv*. Texture features improved at most were the completion, coarseness, and contrast. The completion of the image was increased by all filters.

Finally, in the last row of Table 6.2, the total score distance, *Score_Dis_T*, for all feature sets is shown, where best values were obtained by the filters *DsFhomo*, *DsFlsminsc*, *DsFmedian*, *DsFlsmv*, *DsFhomog*, and *DsFad*.

6.4.3 Texture Analysis: kNN Classifier (Table 6.3)

Table 6.3 shows the percentage of correct classifications score for the kNN classifier with $k = 7$ for classifying a subject as asymptomatic or symptomatic. The classifier was evaluated using the leave-one-out method (see Chaps. 14 and 15), on 220 asymptomatic, and 220 symptomatic images of carotid plaques on the original and despeckled images. The percentage of correct classifications score is given for the following feature sets: Statistical Features, SF, Spatial Gray Level Dependence Matrix Mean Values, SGLDMm, Spatial Gray Level Dependence Matrix Range of Values, SGLDMr, Gray Level Difference Statistics, GLDS, Neighborhood Gray Tone Difference Matrix, NGTDM, Statistical Feature Matrix, SFM, Laws Texture Energy Measures, TEM, Fractal Dimension Texture Analysis, FDTA, and Fourier Power Spectrum, FPS. Filters that showed an improvement in classifications success score compared to that of the original image set were in average (last row of Table 6.3) the filter *DsFhomo* (3%), *gf4d* (1%), and *DsFlsminsc* (1%).

Feature sets, which benefited mostly by the despeckle filtering were the SF, GLDS, NGTDM, and TEM when counting the number of cases that the correct classifications score was improved. Less improvement was observed for the feature sets FDTA, SFM, SGLDMm, FPS, and SGLDMr. For the feature set SGLDMr, better results are given for the *DsFlsminsc* filter with an improvement of 2%. This is the only filter that showed an improvement for this class of features. For the feature set TEM, the filter *DsFlsmv* shows the best improvement with 9%, whereas for the FPS feature set, the filter *DsFlsminsc* gave the best improvement with 5%. The filter *DsFlsminsc* showed improvement in the GLDS and NGTDM feature sets, whereas the filter *DsFlsmv* showed improvement for the feature sets SF and TEM.

6.4.4 Image Quality Evaluation Metrics (Table 6.4)

Table 6.4 tabulates the image quality evaluation metrics for the 220 asymptomatic and 220 symptomatic ultrasound images between the original and the despeckled images respectively. Best values were obtained for the *DsFnldif*, *DsFlsmv*, and *DsFwaveltc* with lower MSE, RMSE, Err3, and Err4, and higher SNR and PSNR. The GAE was 0.00 for all cases, and this can be attributed to the fact that the information between the original and the despeckled images remains unchanged. Best values for the universal quality index, Q, and the structural similarity index, SSIN, were obtained for the filters *DsFlsmv* and *DsFnldif*.

Table 6.3 Percentage of correct classifications for the kNN classifier with $K = 7$ for the original and the filtered image sets

Feature set	No. of Feat.	Original	Linear filtering			Nonlinear filtering			Diffusion		Wavelet
			DsFlsmv	DsFlsminsc	DsFwiener	DsFhomog	DsFgf4d	DsFhomo	DsFmedian	DsFad	DsFnldif	DsFwaveltc
SF	5	59	**62**	**61**	**61**	63	59	65	57	**60**	52	**61**
SGLDMm	13	65	63	64	62	**69**	67	68	63	61	**66**	63
SGLDMr	13	70	66	**72**	64	65	70	69	66	64	65	65
GLDS	4	64	63	**66**	61	64	**66**	**72**	**69**	59	58	62
NGTDM	5	64	63	**68**	60	63	**65**	57	**69**	**60**	61	62
SFM	4	62	62	60	62	55	**65**	**68**	58	59	56	55
TEM	6	59	**68**	52	**60**	**66**	**60**	**65**	59	53	**60**	**60**
FDTA	4	64	63	**66**	53	53	62	**73**	**68**	55	54	62
FPS	2	59	54	**64**	59	59	59	59	58	52	48	55
Average		63	63	**64**	60	62	**64**	**66**	63	58	58	61

Source: Loizou et al.[7]

SF statistical features, *SGLDMm* spatial gray level dependence matrix mean values, *SGLDMr* spatial gray level dependence matrix range of values, *GLDS* gray level difference statistics, *NGTDM* neighborhood gray tone difference matrix, *SFM* statistical feature matrix, *TEM* laws texture energy measures, *FDTA* fractal dimension texture analysis, *FPS* Fourier power spectrum, *HF* homogeneity, *GF* geometric, *HM* homomorphic

Bolded values indicate improvement after despeckling

Table 6.4 Image quality evaluation metrics computed for the 220 asymptomatic and 220 symptomatic images

	Linear filtering				Nonlinear filtering			Diffusion		Wavelet
Feature set	DsFlsmv	DsFlsminsc	DsFwiener	DsFmedian	DsFhomog	DsFgf4d	DsFhomo	DsFad	DsFnldif	DsFwaveltc
Asymptomatic images										
MSE	13	86	19	131	42	182	758	132	8	11
RMSE	3	9	4	10	6	13	27	11	2	3
Err3	7	17	5	25	14	25	38	21	5	4
Err4	11	26	7	41	24	40	49	32	10	5
GAE	0	0	0	0	0	0	0	0	0	0
SNR	25	17	23	16	21	14	5	14	28	25
PSNR	39	29	36	29	34	27	20	28	41	39
Q	0.83	0.78	0.74	0.84	0.92	0.77	0.28	0.68	0.93	0.65
SSIN	0.97	0.88	0.92	0.94	0.97	0.88	0.43	0.87	0.97	0.9
Symptomatic images										
MSE	33	374	44	169	110	557	1,452	374	8	23
RMSE	5	19	6	13	10	23	37	19	3	5
Err3	10	33	9	25	20	43	51	31	5	6
Err4	16	47	11	38	30	63	64	43	7	8
GAE	0	0	0	0	0	0	0	0	0	0
SNR	24	13	22	16	17	12	5	12	29	25
PSNR	34	23	33	26	28	21	17	23	39	36
Q	0.82	0.77	0.7	0.79	0.87	0.75	0.24	0.63	0.87	0.49
SSIN	0.97	0.85	0.89	0.81	0.94	0.85	0.28	0.81	0.97	0.87

Source: Loizou et al.[7]

MSE Mean-square error, *RMSE* Randomized mean-square error, Err3, Err4: Minowski metrics, *GAE* Geometric average error, *SNR* Signal to noise radio, *PSNR* Peak signal to noise radio, *Q* universal quality index, *SSIN* structural similarity index

6.4.5 Visual Evaluation by Experts
(Table 6.5)

Table 6.5 shows the results of the visual evaluation of the original and despeckled images made by two experts, a cardiovascular surgeon and a neurovascular specialist. The last row of Table 6.5 presents the overall average percentage (%) score assigned by both experts for each filter.

For the cardiovascular surgeon, the average score showed that the best despeckle filter is the *DsFlsmv* with a score of 62%, followed by *DsFgf4d*, *DsFmedian*, *DsFhomog*, and original with scores of 52%, 50%, 45%, and 41% respectively. For the neurovascular specialist, the average score showed that the best filter is the *DsFgf4d* with a score of 72%, followed by *DsFlsmv*, original, *DsFlsminsc*, and *DsFmedian* with scores of 71%, 68%, 68%, and 66% respectively. The overall average % score shows that the highest score was given to the filter *DsFlsmv* (67%), followed by *DsFgf4d* (62%), *DsFmedian* (58%), and original (54%). It should be emphasized that the despeckle filter *DsFlsmv* is the only filter that was graded with a higher score than the original by both experts for the asymptomatic and symptomatic image sets.

The difference in the scorings between the two vascular specialists may be explained by the fact that the cardiovascular surgeon was primarily interested in the plaque composition and texture evaluation whereas the neurovascular specialist was interested to evaluate the degree of stenosis and the lumen diameter in order to identify the plaque contour. Filters *DsFlsmv* and *DsFgf4d* were identified as the best despeckle filters, by both specialists as they improved visual perception with overall average scores of 67% and 62% respectively. The filters *DsFwaveltc* and *DsFhomo* were scored by both specialists with the lowest overall average scores of 28% and 29% respectively.

By examining the visual results of Fig. 6.1, the statistical results of Tables 6.2–6.5, and the visual evaluation of Table 6.5, the authors conclude that the best filters are *DsFlsmv* and *DsFgf4d*, which may be used for both plaque composition enhancement and plaque texture analysis, whereas the filters *DsFlsmv*, *DsFgf4d*, and *DsFlsminsc* are more appropriate for identification of the severity of stenosis and therefore may be used when the primary interest is to outline the plaque borders.

6.5 General Discussion

Despeckle filtering is an important operation in the enhancement of ultrasound images of the carotid artery, both in the case of texture analysis, and in the case of image quality evaluation and visual evaluation by the experts. In this study, a total of ten despeckle filters were comparatively evaluated on 440 ultrasound images of the carotid artery bifurcation and the validation results are summarized in Table 6.6.

As summarized in Table 6.6, filters *DsFlsmv*, *sFlsminsc*, and *DsFhomo* gave the best overall results in separating asymptomatic and symptomatic classes. As mentioned above and also can be seen from Tables 6.3 and 6.5, filters that improved statistical classification are not the same as those that improved visual classification by experts (filters *DsFlsminsc*, *DsFgf4d*, and *DsFhomo* improved statistical classification by an average of 1.3%, see Table 6.3, while

Table 6.5 Percentage scoring of visual evaluation of the original and despeckled images [50 asymptomatic (A) and 50 symptomatic (S)] by the experts

| Experts | A/S | Original | Linear filtering | | | Nonlinear filtering | | | Diffusion | Wavelet |
			DsFlsmv	DsFlsminsc	DsFmedian	DsFhomog	DsFgf4d	DsFhomo	DsFnldif	DsFwaveltc
Cardiovascular surgeon	A	33	75	33	43	47	61	19	43	32
	S	48	49	18	57	43	42	20	33	22
Average %		41	62	26	50	45	52	19	38	27
Neurovascular specialist	A	70	76	73	74	63	79	23	52	29
	S	66	67	63	58	45	65	55	41	28
Average %		68	71	68	66	54	72	39	47	28
Overall average %		54	**67**	47	**58**	50	**62**	29	43	28

Source: Loizou et al.[7]
HF homogeneity, *GF* geometric, *HM* homomorphic

Table 6.6 Summary findings of despeckle filtering in ultrasound imaging of the carotid artery

Despeckle filter	Statistical and texture features Table 6.2	Statistical analysis Table 6.3	kNN classifier Table 6.4	Image quality evaluation Table 6.5	Optical perception evaluation Tables 6.5, 6.6
Linear filtering					
DsFlsmv	✓	✓		✓	✓
DsFlsminsc	✓	✓	✓		
Nonlinear filtering					
DsFgf4d		✓	✓		✓
DsFhomo	✓		✓		
Diffusion filtering					
DsFnldif				✓	
Wavelet filtering					
DsFwaveltc				✓	

filters *DsFlsmv*, *DsFmedian*, *DsFgf4d* improved visual classification by an average of 8.3%, see Table 6.5).

Overall, filters *DsFlsminsc*, *DsFgf4d*, and DsFhomo gave only a marginal improvement in the percentage of correct classifications success rate (see Table 6.3). Moreover, filters *DsFlsmv*, *DsFnldif*, and *DsFwaveltc* gave better image quality evaluation results (see Table 6.4). Filters *DsFlsmv* and *DsFgf4d* improved the visual assessment carried out by the experts (see Table 6.5). It is clearly shown that filter *DsFlsmv* gave the best performance, followed by filters *DsFlsminsc* and *DsFgf4d* (see Table 6.6). Filter *DsFlsmv* or *DsFgf4d* can be used for despeckling asymptomatic images where the expert is interested mainly in the plaque composition and texture analysis. Filters *DsFlsmv* or *DsFgf4d* or *DsFlsminsc* can be used for despeckling of symptomatic images where the expert is interested in identifying the degree of stenosis and the plaque borders. Filters *DsFhomo*, *DsFnldif*, and *DsFwaveltc* gave poorer performance.

Filter *DsFlsmv* gave very good performance, with respect to: (1) preserving the mean and the median of the gray scale as well as decreasing the variance and the speckle index of the image, (2) increasing the distance of the texture features between the asymptomatic and symptomatic classes, (3) marginally improving the classification success rate of the kNN classifier for the classification of asymptomatic and symptomatic images in the cases of SF, SMF, and TEM feature sets, and (4) improving the image quality of the image. The *DsFlsmv* filter, which is a simple filter, is based on local image statistics. It was first introduced in Loizou et al. (2006), Lee (1980), and Lee (1981)[8,15,16] and it was tested on a few SAR images with satisfactory results. It was also used for SAR imaging as per an article by Frost et al.[14] and image restoration as per an article by Kuan et al.[17] again with satisfactory results.

Filter *DsFlsminsc* gave the best performance with respect to: (1) preserving the mean gray scale, as well as decreasing its variance and the speckle index and increasing the contrast of the image, (2) increasing the distance of the texture features between the asymptomatic and the symptomatic classes, and (3) improving the classification success rate of the kNN classifier for the classification of asymptomatic and symptomatic images in the cases of SF, SGLDMr, GLDS, NGTDM, FDTA, and FPS feature sets. Filter *DsFlsminsc* was originally introduced by Nagao et al.[34] and was tested on an artificial and a SAR image with satisfactory performance. In this study, the filter was modified, by using the speckle index instead of the variance value for each sub window as described in a previous paper.[9]

Filter *DsFgf4d* gave very good performance with respect to: (1) decreasing the speckle index, (2) marginally increasing the distance of the texture features between the asymptomatic and the symptomatic classes, and (3) improving the classification success rate of the kNN classifier for the classification of asymptomatic and symptomatic images in the cases of SGLDMm, GLDS, NGTDM, SFM, and TEM feature sets. The geometric filter *DsFgf4d* was introduced by

Crimmins,[10] and was tested visually on a few SAR images with satisfactory results.

Filters used for speckle reduction in ultrasound imaging by other investigators include: *DsFmedian*,[35] *DsFwiener*,[14] *DsFhomog*,[9,18] *DsFhomo*,[19,20] *DsFad*,[5] and *DsFwaveltc*.[31] However, these filters were evaluated on a small number of images, and their performance was tested based only on the mean, median, standard deviation of the images, and speckle index of the image before and after filtering.

The *DsFmedian* and the *DsFwiener* filters were originally used by many researchers for suppressing the additive and later for suppressing the multiplicative noise in different types of images.[2–8,14,35] The results of this study showed that the *DsFwiener* and *DsFmedian* filters were not able to remove the speckle noise and produced blurred edges in the filtered image (Fig. 6.1). In this study, the *DsFmedian* filter performed poorer as shown in Tables 6.2, 6.3, and 6.4.

6.5.1 Comparison and Discussion of Despeckle Filtering Techniques

The *DsFhomog*[9,18] and *DsFhomo*[2,19,20] filters were recently used by some researchers for speckle reduction but the authors' results in Tables 6.2 and 6.3, and the visual evaluation of the experts in Table 6.5 showed poor performance especially for the *DsFhomo* filter.

Anisotropic diffusion is an efficient nonlinear technique for simultaneously performing contrast enhancement and noise reduction. It smoothes homogeneous image regions but retains image edges.[25] Anisotropic diffusion filters usually require many iteration steps compared with the local statistic filters. In a recent study,[5] speckle reducing anisotropic diffusion filtering was proposed as the most appropriate filter for ultrasound images of the carotid artery. However, in this study, *DsFad*, as shown in Tables 6.2–6.6, performed poorer compared to *DsFlsmv*, *DsFgf4d*, and *DsFlsminsc*.

Furthermore, wavelet filtering proposed by Donoho[31] was investigated for suppressing the speckle noise in SAR images,[16,37] real world images,[27] and ultrasound images[28] with favorable results. In this study, it is shown that the *DsFwaveltc* filter gave poorer performance for removing the speckle noise from the ultrasound images of the carotid artery (Tables 6.2 and 6.3).

In conclusion, despeckle filtering is an important operation in the enhancement of ultrasonic imaging of the carotid artery. In this study, it was shown that simple filters based on local statistics (*DsFlsmv* and *DsFlsminsc*) and geometric filtering (*DsFgf4d*) could be used successfully for the processing of these images. In this context, despeckle filtering can be used as a pre-processing step for the automated segmentation of the IMT[52] and the carotid plaque, followed by the carotid plaque texture analysis, and classification. This field has also been investigated by the authors' group.[9,53] The authors' findings show promising results. However, further work is required to evaluate the performance of the suggested despeckle filters on a larger scale as well as their impact in clinical practice. In addition, the usefulness of the proposed despeckle filters, in portable ultrasound systems and in wireless telemedicine systems, still has to be investigated.

6.6 Summary and Future Directions

6.6.1 Summary

Despeckle filtering has been a rapidly emerging research area in recent years. The basic principles, the theoretical background, and the algorithmic steps of a representative set of despeckle filters have been covered in this chapter. Moreover, selected representative applications of image despeckling covering a variety of ultrasound image processing tasks have been presented. Most importantly a despeckle filtering and evaluation protocol is documented in Table 6.7. The source code of the algorithms discussed in this book has been made available on the web, thus enabling researchers to more easily exploit the application of despeckle filtering in relation to their problems under investigation.

In this chapter, a total of ten different despeckle filters have been documented based on linear filtering, nonlinear filtering, diffusion filtering, and wavelet filtering. The authors have evaluated despeckle filtering on 440 (220 asymptomatic and 220 symptomatic) ultrasound images of the carotid artery bifurcation, based on visual evaluation by two medical experts, texture analysis measures, and image quality

Table 6.7 Despeckle filtering and evaluation protocol

1. Recording of ultrasound images: Ultrasound images are acquired by ultrasound equipment and stored for further image processing. Regions of interest (ROI's) could be selected for further processing.
2. Normalize the image: The stored images may be retrieved and a normalized procedure may be applied (as described for example in the evaluation section, i.e., Methodology).
3. Apply despeckle filtering: Select the set of filters to apply despeckling together with their corresponding parameters (like moving window size, iterations, and other).
4. Texture features analysis: After despeckle filtering, the user may select ROI's (i.e., the plaque or the area around the IMT) and extract texture features. Distance metrics between the original and the despeckled images may be computed (as well as between different classes of images if applicable).
5. Compute image quality evaluation metrics: On the selected ROI's, compute image quality evaluation metrics between the original noisy and the despeckled images.
6. Visual quality evaluation by experts: The original and/or despeckled images may be visually evaluated by experts.
7. Select the most appropriate despeckle filter/filters: Based on steps 3–6, construct a performance evaluation table and select the most appropriate filter(s) for the problem under investigation.

Source: Loizou and Pattichis[9]

evaluation metrics. A linear despeckle filter based on local statistics (*DsFlsmv*) improved the class separation between the asymptomatic and the symptomatic classes, gave only a marginal improvement in the percentage of correct classifications success rate based on texture analysis and the kNN classifier, and improved the visual assessment by the experts. It was also found that the *DsFlsmv* despeckle filter can be used for despeckling asymptomatic images where the expert is interested mainly in the plaque composition and texture analysis, whereas a geometric despeckle filter (*DsFgf4d*) can be used for despeckling of symptomatic images where the expert is interested in identifying the degree of stenosis and the plaque borders. The results of this study suggest that the first order statistics despeckle filter, *DsFlsmv*, may be applied on ultrasound images to improve the visual perception and automatic image analysis. Furthermore, despeckle filtering was investigated as a preprocessing step for the automated segmentation of the IMT,[52] media and intima layers,[47] the carotid plaque,[46] followed by the carotid plaque texture analysis, and classification (as documented in the above paragraph). In a recent study,[54] where the texture characteristics of the media and intima layer of the CCA were investigated, the authors found significant differences among texture features extracted from the IL, ML, and IMC from different age groups. Furthermore, for some texture features, the authors found that they follow trends that correlate with a patient's age. For example, the gray-scale median GSM of the ML decreases linearly with increasing MLT and with increasing age. The authors' findings suggest that ultrasound image texture analysis of the media layer has potential as a biomarker for the risk of stroke.

Despeckle filters *DsFlsmv*, *DsFlsminsc*, and *DsFgf4d* gave the best performance for the segmentation tasks. It was shown in Loizou et al. (2006 and 2009)[8,54] that when normalization and speckle reduction filtering is applied on ultrasound images of the carotid artery prior to IMT segmentation, the automated segmentation measurements are closer to the manual measurements. This field has also been investigated by the authors' group.[9,53] The authors' findings showed promising results. However, further work is required to evaluate the performance of the suggested despeckle filters on a larger scale as well as their impact in clinical practice. In addition, the usefulness of the proposed despeckle filters, in portable ultrasound systems and in wireless telemedicine systems, still has to be investigated.

For those readers whose principal need is to use existing image despeckle filtering technologies and apply them on different type of images, there is no simple answer regarding which specific filtering algorithm should be selected without a significant understanding of both the filtering fundamentals and the application environment under investigation. A number of issues would need to be addressed. These include availability of the images to be processed/analyzed, the required level of filtering, the application scope (general-purpose or application-specific), the application goal (for extracting features from the image or for visual enhancement), the allowable computational complexity, the allowable implementation complexity, and the computational requirements (e.g., real-time or offline). The authors believe that a good understanding of the contents of this chapter can help the readers make the right choice of selecting the most appropriate filter for the application under development. Furthermore, the despeckle filtering evaluation protocol documented in Table 6.6 could also be exploited.

6.6.2 Future Directions

The despeckle filtering algorithms, and the measures for image quality evaluation introduced in this chapter, can also be generalized and applied to other image and video processing applications. Only a small number of filtering algorithms and image quality evaluation metrics were investigated in this chapter, and numerous extensions and improvements can be envisaged.

In general, the development of despeckle filtering algorithms for image despeckling is a well investigated field and many researchers have been involved in this subject, but there is still not an appropriate method proposed, which will satisfy both the visual and the automated interpretation of image processing and analysis tasks. Most importantly, more comparative studies of despeckle filtering are necessary, where different filters could be evaluated by multiple experts as well as based on image quality and evaluation metrics as also proposed in this chapter.

The issue of video despeckling is still in its infancy, although it is noted that the proposed methodology and filtering algorithms documented in this chapter may be also investigated in video sequences (by frame filtering). There are many issues related to video despeckle filtering that remain to be solved. In general, the development of a multiplicative model based on video sequences is required, since most of the models developed for video filtering were for additive noise.[55,56] Furthermore, the utilization of the motion-details by using motion estimation, in order to estimate pixels that need to be filtered in the neighboring frames should also be utilized as already proposed in Zlokoliza.[57]

Despeckle filtering may be also applied in the pre-processing of ultrasound images for other organs, including the detection of hyperechoic or hypoechoic lesions in the kidney, liver, spleen, thyroid, kidney, echocardiographic images, mammography, and others. It may be particularly effective when combined with harmonic imaging, since both can increase tissue contrast. Speckle reduction can also be extremely valuable when attempting to fuse ultrasound with Computed Tomography (CT), MRI, Positron Emission Tomography (PET), or Optical Coherence Tomography (OCT) images. For example, when a lesion is suspected on a CT scan but is not clearly visible, despeckle filtering can be applied in order to accentuate subtle borders that may be masked by speckle.

Ultrasound imaging instrumentation, linked with imaging hardware and software technology, has been rapidly advancing in the last two decades. Although these advanced imaging devices produce higher quality images and video, the need still exists for better image and video processing techniques including despeckle filtering. Toward this direction, it is anticipated that the effective use of despeckle filtering (by exploiting the filters and algorithms documented in this chapter) will greatly help in producing images with higher quality. These images would be not only easier to visualize and to extract useful information, but would also enable the development of more robust image pre-processing and segmentation algorithms, minimizing routine manual image analysis and facilitating more accurate automated measurements of both industrially and clinically relevant parameters.

References

1. Lamont D et al. Risk of cardiovascular disease measured by carotid intima-media thickness at age 49–51: life course study. *BMJ*. 2000;320:273–278.
2. Burckhardt CB. Speckle in ultrasound B-mode scans. *IEEE Trans Sonics Ultrason*. 1978;25(1):1–6.
3. Wagner RF, Smith SW, Sandrik JM, Lopez H. Statistics of speckle in ultrasound B-scans. *IEEE Trans Sonics Ultrason*. 1983;30:156–163.
4. Goodman JW. Some fundamental properties of speckle. *J Opt Soc Am*. 1976;66(11):1145–1149.
5. Yongjian Y, Acton ST. Speckle reducing anisotropic diffusion. *IEEE Trans Image Process*. 2002;11(11):1260–1270.
6. Prager RW, Gee AH, Treece GM, Berman L. *Speckle Detection in Ultrasound Images Using First Order Statistics*. Cambridge: University of Cambridge; 2002:1–17.
7. Loizou CP et al. Despeckle filtering in ultrasound imaging of the carotid artery. *IEEE Trans Ultrason Ferroelectr Freq Control*. 2005;52(10):1653–1669.
8. Loizou CP, Pattichis CS, Pantziaris MS, Tyllis T, Nicolaides AN. Quantitative quality evaluation of ultrasound imaging

in the carotid artery. *Med Biol Eng Comput.* 2006;44 (5):414–426.
9. Loizou CP, Pattichis CS. *Despeckle filtering algorithms and software for ultrasound imaging.* San Rafael: Morgan & Claypool; 2008 (Spanias A, ed. Synthesis lectures on algorithms and software for engineering; #1).
10. Busse L, Crimmins TR, Fienup JR. A model based approach to improve the performance of the geometric filtering speckle reduction algorithm. *IEEE Ultrason Symp.* 1995;2:1353–1356.
11. Lee JS. Speckle analysis and smoothing of synthetic aperture radar images. *Comput Graphics Image Process.* 1981;17:24–32.
12. Kuan DT, Sawchuk AA, Strand TC, Chavel P. Adaptive restoration of images with speckle. *IEEE Trans Acoust Speech Signal Process.* 1989;35(3):373–383.
13. Insana M, Hall TJ, Gledndon GC, Posental SJ. Progress in quantitative ultrasonic imaging. *SPIE Proceedings on Medical Imaging III: Image Formation* 1989:1092–1099.
14. Frost VS, Stiles JA, Shanmungan KS, Holtzman JC. A model for radar images and its application for adaptive digital filtering of multiplicative noise. *IEEE Trans Pattern Anal Mach Intell.* 1982;4(2):157–165.
15. Lee JS. Digital image enhancement and noise filtering by using local statistics. *IEEE Trans Pattern Anal Mach Intell.* 1980;2(2):165–168.
16. Lee JS. Refined filtering of image noise using local statistics. *Comput Graphics Image Process.* 1981;15:380–389.
17. Kuan DT, Sawchuk AA, Strand TC, Pierre C. Adaptive noise smoothing filter for images with signal dependent noise. *IEEE Trans Pattern Anal Mach Intell.* 1985;7 (2):165–177.
18. Christodoulou CI, et al. Despeckle filtering in ultrasound imaging of the carotid artery. In: Conference Proceedings of the 2nd Joint EMBS-BMES Conference; 2002; Houston; vol. 2:1027–1028.
19. Solbo S, Eltoft T. Homomorphic wavelet based-statistical despeckling of SAR images. *IEEE Trans Geosci Remote Sensing.* 2004;42(4):711–721.
20. Saniie J, Wang T, Bilgutay N. Analysis of homomorphic processing for ultrasonic grain signal characterization. *IEEE Trans Ultrason Ferroelectr Freq Control.* 1989;3:365–375.
21. Jin S, Wang Y, Hiller J. An adaptive non-linear diffusion algorithm for filtering medical images. *IEEE Trans Inf Technol Biomed.* 2000;4(4):298–305.
22. Weickert J, Romery B, Viergever M. Efficient and reliable schemes for nonlinear diffusion filtering. *IEEE Trans Image Process.* 1998;7:398–410.
23. Rougon N, Preteux F. Controlled anisotropic diffusion. In: Conference on Nonlinear Image Processing VI, IS&T/SPIE Symposium on Electron Imaging, Science and Technology; San Jose; 1995:1–12.
24. Black M, Sapiro G, Marimont D, Heeger D. Robust anisotropic diffusion. *IEEE Trans Image Process.* 1998;7 (3):421–432.
25. Perona P, Malik J. Scale-space and edge detection using anisotropic diffusion. *IEEE Trans Pattern Anal Mach Intell.* 1990;12(7):629–639.
26. Abd-Elmoniem K, Youssef A-B, Kadah Y. Real-time speckle reduction and coherence Enhancement in ultrasound imaging via nonlinear anisotropic diffusion. *IEEE Trans Biomed Eng.* 2002;49(9):997–1014.
27. Zhong S, Cherkassky V. Image denoising using wavelet thresholding and model selection. In: Proceedings of the IEEE International Conference on Image Processing; 2000; Vancouver:1–4.
28. Achim A, Bezerianos A, Tsakalides P. Novel Bayesian multiscale method for speckle removal in medical ultrasound images. *IEEE Trans Med Imaging.* 2001;20 (8):772–783.
29. Zong X, Laine A, Geiser E. Speckle reduction and contrast enhancement of echocardiograms via multiscale nonlinear processing. *IEEE Trans Med Imaging.* 1998;17(4):532–540.
30. Hao X, Gao S, Gao X. A novel multiscale nonlinear thresholding method for ultrasonic speckle suppressing. *IEEE Trans Med Imaging.* 1999;18(9):787–794.
31. Donoho DL. Denoising by soft thresholding. *IEEE Trans Inf Theory.* 1995;41:613–627.
32. Wink AM, Roerdink JBTM. Denoising functional MR images: a comparison of wavelet denoising and Gaussian smoothing. *IEEE Trans Med Imaging.* 2004;23(3):374–387.
33. Dutt V. *Statistical analysis of ultrasound echo envelope* [Ph. D. dissertation]. Rochester: Mayo Graduate School; 1995.
34. Nagao M, Matsuyama T. Edge preserving smoothing. *Comput Graphics Image Process.* 1979;9:394–407.
35. Huang T, Yang G, Tang G. A fast two-dimensional median filtering algorithm. *IEEE Trans Acoust Speech Signal Process.* 1979;27(1):13–18.
36. Ali SM, Burge RE. New automatic techniques for smoothing and segmenting SAR images. *Signal Process.* 1988;14:335–346.
37. Gupta S, Chauhan RC, Sexana SC. Wavelet-based statistical approach for speckle reduction in medical ultrasound images. *Med Biol Eng Comput J.* 2004;42:189–192.
38. A Philips Medical System Company. Comparison of image clarity, SonoCT real-time compound imaging versus conventional 2D ultrasound imaging. ATL Ultrasound, Report; 2001.
39. Elatrozy T et al. The effect of B-mode ultrasonic image standardization of the echodensity of symptomatic and asymptomatic carotid bifurcation plaque. *Int Angiol.* 1998;17(3):179–186.
40. Haralick RM, Shanmugam K, Dinstein I. Texture features for image classification. *IEEE Trans Syst Man Cybern.* 1973;SMC-3:610–621.
41. Christodoulou CI, Pattichis CS, Pantziaris M, Nicolaides AN. Texture-based classification of atherosclerotic carotid plaques. *IEEE Trans Med Imaging.* 2003;22(7):902–912.
42. Winkler S. *Vision Models and Quality Metrics for Image Processing Applications* [Ph.D.]. Lausanne: University of Lausanne-Switzerland; 2000.
43. Krupinski E, Kundel H, Judy P, Nodine C. The medical image perception society, key issues for image perception research. *Radiology.* 1998;209:611–612.
44. Wang Z, Bovik A, Sheikh H, Simoncelli E. Image quality assessment: from error measurement to structural similarity. *IEEE Trans Image Process.* 2004;13(4):600–612.
45. Sakrison D. On the role of observer and a distortion measure in image transmission. *IEEE Trans Commun.* 1977;25: 1251–1267.

46. Loizou CP, Pattichis CS, Pantziaris M, Nicolaides AN. An integrated system for the segmentation of atherosclerotic carotid plaque. *IEEE Trans Inf Technol Biomed*. 2007;11(5):661–667.
47. Loizou CP, Pattichis CS, Nicolaides AN, Pantziaris M. Manual and automated media and intima thickness measurements of the common carotid artery. *IEEE Trans Ultrason Ferroelectr Freq Control*. 2009;56(5):983–994.
48. Chen TJ et al. A novel image quality index using Moran I statistics. *Phys Med Biol*. 2003;48:131–137.
49. Gonzalez R, Woods R. *Digital Image Processing*. 2nd ed. Upper Saddle River: Prentice-Hall Inc.; 2002:419–420.
50. Wang Z, Bovik A. A universal quality index. *IEEE Signal Process Lett*. 2002;9(3):81–84.
51. Sheikh HR, Bovik AC, de Veciana G. An information fidelity criterion for image quality assessment using natural scene statistics. *IEEE Trans Image Process*. 2005;14(12):2117–2128.
52. Loizou CP, Pattichis CS, Pantziaris MS, Tyllis T, Nicolaides AN. Snakes based segmentation of the common carotid artery intima media. *Med Biol Eng Comput*. 2007;45:35–49.
53. Pattichis CS et al. Cardiovascular: ultrasound imaging in vascular cases. In: Akay M, ed. *Wiley Encyclopaedia of Biomedical Engineering*. Hoboken: Wiley; 2006:1–12.
54. Loizou CP, Pantziaris M, Pattichis MS, Kyriakou E, Pattichis CS. Ultrasound image texture analysis of the intima and media layers of the common carotid artery and its correlation with age and gender. *Comput Med Imaging Graphics*. 2009;33(4):317–324.
55. Jung J-H, Hong K, Yang S. Noise reduction using variance characteristics in noisy image sequence. In: International Conference on Consumer Electronics; 2005; Las Vegas:213–214.
56. Bertalmio M, Caselles V, Pardo A. Movie Denoising by average of warped lines. *IEEE Trans Image Process*. 2007;16(9):233–247.
57. Zlokoliza V. *Advanced Nonlinear Methods for Video Denoising* [Ph.D. dissertation]. Belgium: Ghent University; 2006.

Vascular Ultrasound Imaging with Contrast Agents: Carotid Plaque Neovascularization and the Hyperplastic Vasa Vasorum Network

Michalakis A. Averkiou, Christophoros Mannaris, and Andrew Nicolaides

7.1 Introduction

Despite continuing advances in the sensitivity of diagnostic ultrasound systems, Doppler-based imaging techniques are unable to detect low velocity blood flow in the microcirculation. The main difficulty these techniques share is that blood is a weak reflector of ultrasound with received amplitude 40–60 dB smaller than that of tissue. As a result, Doppler-based techniques rely solely on the movement of red blood cells to differentiate blood flow from tissue. The removal of this tissue signal places a lower limit on the ability to detect low velocity blood flow (<1 cm/s). A method to overcome these difficulties is to inject brighter reflectors than blood into the vascular system. Gas-filled microbubbles are one such reflector.

Computed tomography (CT) and magnetic resonance (MR) imaging modalities have long used intravenously injected contrast material to visualize blood flow in the microcirculation and larger vessels. The use of microbubbles enables ultrasound to complement CT and MR in a number of clinical areas where perfusion is an important clinical differentiator. Ultrasound contrast agents have recently been transitioning from research to clinical use. The portability and real-time nature of ultrasound combined with contrast is finding new clinical utility in vascular imaging. The spatial and temporal resolution obtainable with ultrasound contrast is providing new physiologic and pathophysiologic information not available before.

Ultrasound contrast agents have been utilized in liver oncology (tumor detection) and echocardiography (myocardial perfusion and left ventricle opacification) as a new tool with the proven ability to image flow at the level of the microcirculation, both noninvasively and in real-time. The same imaging and quantification techniques and lessons learned from oncology need to be extended to vascular imaging.

Ultrasound microbubble contrast agents given intravenously were used in the early 1990s to enhance the echogenicity of blood and improve the ultrasound visualization of the residual lumen in patients with severe internal carotid stenosis.[1] It was soon found that they could detect the presence of "trickle flow" and identify falsely diagnosed carotid occlusions.[2,3] More recently they have been used to improve the diagnosis of intracranial stenosis.[4,5]

Cardiovascular disease is the number one killer in the world and stroke is the most common cause of disability.[6] Ischemic stroke is often the result of atherosclerotic plaque rapture (Chaps. 1 and 2). The lack of the proper tools that accurately identify vulnerable carotid plaques (the degree of internal carotid stenosis is the sole criterion for intervention) results in many asymptomatic patients having an unnecessary operation. Histologic studies have recognized that plaque inflammation and the presence of plaque neovascularization are strong predictors of instability in atheromatous lesions and symptomatic carotid disease.[7,8] The ability to measure the hyperplastic network of vasa vasorum and the angiogenesis (new vessel growth) of the plaques may help the identification of

---

M.A. Averkiou (✉) • C. Mannaris
Department of Mechanical and Manufacturing Engineering, University of Cyprus, Nicosia, Cyprus

A. Nicolaides
Imperial College and Vascular Screening and Diagnostic Centre, London, UK

asymptomatic patients with vulnerable plaques. Recent developments in diagnostic ultrasound and specifically the introduction of contrast agents and nonlinear imaging techniques have led to the ability not only to image but also quantify blood perfusion in the vasa vasorum and plaque neovascularization.[9,10]

Recent perfusion studies in asymptomatic patients using SonoVue (Bracco S.P.A., Milan, Italy) have demonstrated that plaque perfusion originates in the adventitia and is present in the isoechoic or hyperechoic fibrous and fibrofatty tissue, but not in calcific tissue with acoustic shadow or hypoechoic areas.[11,12] In another study, the vascularity seen on ultrasound was visually graded and correlated to immunohistochemistry of the excised carotid plaques (symptomatic and asymptomatic) using markers such as CD31 and CD34. There was a strong linear relationship between perfusion seen on ultrasound and neovascularization seen on histology ($r = 0.68$; $P = 0.002$).[13] These findings were confirmed by subsequent studies.[14]

Quantification of plaque perfusion using contrast quantification analysis software was performed in a series of 81 plaques.[9] Time to peak was shorter and enhanced intensity was greater in soft plaques than in mixed plaques. In this study, soft plaques were defined as those with echogenicity less than that of the surrounding adventitia for more than 80% of the plaque area without acoustic shadowing; mixed plaques were those containing <90% of circumferential calcification, or associated echodense and anechoic regions occupying <80% of the plaque area.

A similar approach was used in another study of 104 plaques of which 35 were symptomatic and 69 asymptomatic.[15] In this study, a real-time contrast-enhanced carotid cine loop was obtained. Baseline intensity before injection of contrast agent and peak intensity after injection were obtained from the signal intensity versus time curve. The ratio of the enhanced intensity in the plaque to that in the carotid lumen was also calculated. It was found that the enhanced intensity in the plaque and the ratio of enhanced intensity in the plaque to that in the lumen were higher in the symptomatic than in the asymptomatic plaques.

A different approach was used in a study of 37 patients with 16 symptomatic and 21 asymptomatic plaques.[16] Late-phase contrast-enhanced ultrasound was performed 6 min after the bolus of contrast was injected. Normalized late-phase plaque echogenicity was greater in the symptomatic than in the asymptomatic group. Sensitivity and specificity were 75% and 86% respectively. There was a negative linear relationship between late-phase plaque echogenicity and gray scale median ($r = -0.44$). The authors have suggested that microbubbles are likely to be retained in the symptomatic plaques.

The published studies have already indicated the potential clinical applications of contrast agents. It is expected that in asymptomatic patients considered for surgery, contrast carotid examinations could provide a more reliable assessment of cerebrovascular risk.[11,17] In addition, contrast-enhanced carotid ultrasound imaging may provide valuable information for assessing the response to antiatherosclerotic therapies by monitoring the effectiveness of the treatment.[6,14] However, currently, there is no agreement on how best to quantify and standardize the methods of image acquisition and analysis of the microbubble signal. Once this is achieved, prospective studies will be needed in patients with asymptomatic carotid stenosis having best medical therapy in order to determine the predictive value of different plaque perfusion measurements.

The aim of this chapter is to present the principles of microbubble imaging and its application to vascular ultrasound with quantification techniques for the study of carotid plaque neovascularization and the hyperplastic vasa vasorum network.

7.2 Principles of Microbubble Imaging

7.2.1 Microbubble Nonlinearity

Ultrasound contrast agents are gas-filled microbubbles with typical diameters of 2.5 μm. The gas is typically air or a perfluorocarbon that is stabilized with a lipid or polymeric shell. The nonlinear properties of microbubbles have been discussed in detail by Leighton.[18] An acoustic wave generated by an ultrasound system consists of alternating high and low pressures at frequencies of 1.2–15 MHz. When an acoustic wave encounters a microbubble, it alternately compresses the microbubble on the positive pressure, and expands it on the negative pressure. On the positive portion of the wave, the microbubbles are compressed in a different fashion than the way they expand

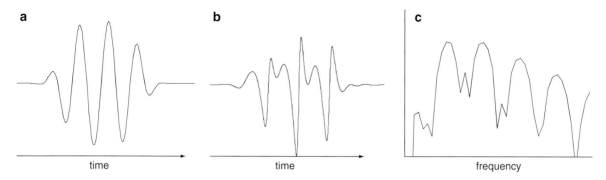

Fig. 7.1 (**a**) Incident ultrasonic wave; (**b**) nonlinear scattered signal from bubbles; (**c**) frequency spectrum of bubble echoes showing harmonic components

in the negative portion. During the expansion phase of oscillation, a gas bubble's radius can increase by as much as several 100%. During the contraction phase of oscillation, a gas bubble's radius is limited, due to the gas inside the bubble rapidly stiffening as the molecules are forced closer together, making it less compressible. This results in an asymmetric-nonlinear bubble oscillation. Instead of producing a sinusoidal echo with a clean frequency spectrum like the transmitted signal in Fig. 7.1a, it produces an odd looking echo with asymmetric top and bottom as shown in Fig. 7.1b. This asymmetry produces harmonics which can be utilized to enhance the signals from the bubbles and effectively distinguish them from the surrounding tissue. Figure 7.1c shows the frequency spectrum of the bubble echoes seen in Fig. 7.1b. The first major hump is the fundamental, and the subsequent ones are the second, third, and fourth harmonics.

7.2.2 Microbubble Disruption

Bubbles in a liquid tend to diffuse and disappear unless they are stabilized by a shell. Once the shell is disrupted, the gas inside will diffuse into the surrounding fluid. The Mechanical Index (MI), originally formulated to predict the onset of cavitation in fluids, also gives an indication of the likelihood of bubble disruption. The MI is defined as:

$$\mathrm{MI} = P_-/\sqrt{f}$$

where P_- is the peak negative pressure in MPa and f is the ultrasound wave frequency in MHz. Equivalently,

$$\mathrm{MI} = P_- * \sqrt{T}$$

where T is the ultrasound wave period in μs. From the above equations, the authors deduce that the harder one tries to expand the bubble (peak negative pressure) and the longer it is expanded (period of ultrasound wavelength), the more likely it is to break. This is also affected by the properties of the particular microbubble shell. More elastic shells are harder to break, as they stretch in the negative pressure without rupturing. It has been well established that the acoustic power level used during routine examinations destroys most contrast microbubbles.[19,20]

The blood flow in a normal capillary bed is on the order of 1 mm/s, and a typical capillary is about 1 mm long.[21] Thus, if the contrast within a capillary is destroyed, it will take about a second or more to refill the capillary. Given the branching structure of the microvasculature and the thickness of a typical scan plane, it can take several seconds to replenish the contrast in the scan plane, depending on the flow rate to the organ.

During real-time scanning at normal ultrasound output power levels, the contrast is never given a chance to fill the microvasculature. This was first observed by Porter and colleagues when they found that triggered imaging allows much better visualization of contrast within the myocardium.[22,23] This led to the widespread use of electrocardiogram (ECG) triggering during myocardial contrast echo, users often triggering only once every 4 or more cardiac cycles. Similar techniques have been used to image flow in the parenchyma of abdominal organs.[24–26] In recent years, new nonlinear imaging techniques have been developed that are far more sensitive to very small echoes from microbubbles, making it possible to image them relatively non-destructively in real-time at very low acoustic pressures. Low MI real-time scanning is currently the operating mode of choice for cardiac, abdominal, and vascular contrast imaging.

7.2.3 Low Mechanical Index Imaging

Low MI scanning is important for two reasons. First, at low MI, bubble destruction is avoided. Although microbubbles differ in their shell composition, the authors' work to date indicates that at an MI of about 0.1 or below, the microbubbles available today for clinical use are not significantly destroyed, yet give a good harmonic (nonlinear) contrast signal. The second reason for low MI scanning is the reduction of the harmonic component in the tissue echoes relative to bubble echoes. While tissue harmonics have benefited routine diagnostic scanning, it is the background "noise" signal that the contrast signal must rise above. Because tissue is less nonlinear than bubbles, it requires a higher MI than the contrast microbubbles for a certain harmonic response. Therefore, at low MI, the contrast to tissue ratio is higher than at high MI, helping to remove the tissue signal and leave only the contrast.

7.2.4 Nonlinear Imaging Methods

The nonlinear behavior of microbubbles in an acoustic field can be utilized to enhance the contrast relative to tissue. A number of techniques have been developed to help distinguish bubbles from tissue, all of which rely on the higher nonlinearity of bubbles when compared to tissue. Nonlinear pulsing schemes consist of transmitting a series of pulses and then combining the scattered signals in a way that all linear components cancel and nonlinear components enhance.[27] All of these techniques have their advantages and disadvantages for any particular clinical application, but also depend on the specific hardware of the diagnostic ultrasound system.

7.2.4.1 Harmonic Imaging

Before the various pulsing schemes are described, harmonic imaging that was the first form of nonlinear imaging used in the early 1990s will be briefly described. "Conventional" harmonic imaging relies on transmitting at a fundamental frequency f_0 and forming an image from the second harmonic component $2f_0$ of the backscattered echoes by the use of filters to remove the fundamental component.[28] While effective, this restricts the bandwidth available for imaging to ensure that the received harmonic signal can be separated from the fundamental signal. If the bandwidth of the fundamental signal overlaps with that of the second harmonic, they cannot be completely separated in the receive process. Thus, in conventional harmonic imaging, even though a narrower transmit bandwidth is used, there is still some loss of nonlinear signals.

7.2.4.2 Pulse Inversion

The bandwidth and sensitivity limitations of "conventional" harmonic imaging are overcome with multipulse pulsing schemes as they isolate (separate) the nonlinear signals instead of filtering them, even when fundamental and harmonic components of the bubble echoes overlap. This allows the use of broader transmit and receive bandwidths for improved resolution, and increased sensitivity to contrast agents.

In pulse inversion (PI), two pulses are transmitted down each ray line, instead of only a single pulse, as is done with conventional harmonic or fundamental imaging. The first is a normal pulse and the second is an inverted replica of the first so that wherever there was a positive pressure on the first pulse, there is an equal negative pressure on the second. The scattered sound from microbubbles from the two inverted pulses is shown in Fig. 7.2a and c and their addition to form the PI signal in Fig. 7.2e. In Fig. 7.2b and d, the spectra of the individual scattered response are depicted with the fundamental being the first hump and the higher harmonics the subsequent humps. In the spectrum of the added response, (f) the fundamental is removed whereas the second (and rest of even harmonic components) are retained. Pulse inversion effectively detects harmonic response and eliminates linear response. This means that scattered sound from linear targets such as tissue at low MI would be eliminated with this process, and thus the formed image would show only the microbubbles.

7.2.4.3 Power Modulation

Another pulsing scheme is power modulation (PM) where the amplitude of the second pulse is half of

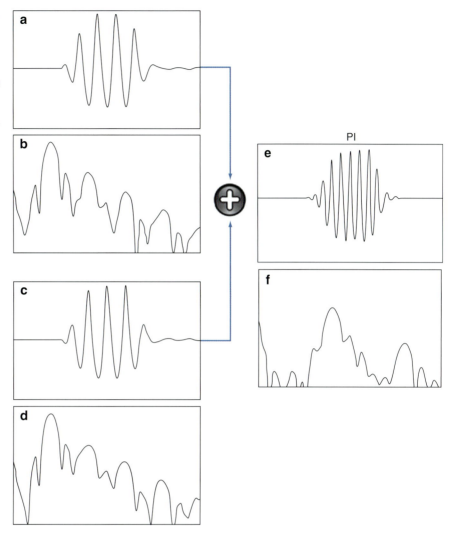

Fig. 7.2 The pulse inversion technique for nonlinear detection of bubble echoes. (**a**) Scattered sound from bubbles with a normal pulse; (**b**) frequency spectrum of (**a**); (**c**) scattered sound from bubbles with an inverted pulse; (**d**) frequency spectrum of (**c**); (**e**) pulse inversion result – the addition of scattered pulses (**a**) and (**c**); (**f**) frequency spectrum of (**e**)

that of the first, while the phase is the same (the second pulse is not inverted). The scattered sound from the half pulse (Fig. 7.3c) is scaled by a factor of 2 and then subtracted from the first (Fig. 7.3a). This also results in cancellation of all linear scattered energy and enhancement of the nonlinear. The spectrum of the resulting pulse (Fig. 7.3f) shows that the nonlinear scattered response has all harmonic components, including a nonlinear fundamental component. In essence, PM detects the differential nonlinear response generated from two different excitations. The lower frequency nonlinear signal has the luxury of lower attenuation upon return to the transducer relative to second harmonic which is detected with PI. The increased sensitivity of PM over PI makes it ideal for penetration-limited scenarios and in cases where sensitivity is important. However, the resolution and overall esthetics of PM is inferior to that of PI.

7.2.4.4 Power-Modulated Pulse Inversion

A third pulsing scheme considered here is power-modulated pulse inversion (PMPI) (referred to as Contrast Pulse Sequence or CPS by certain ultrasound manufacturers). In this case, the second pulse is half the amplitude of the first and also inverted. The scattered sound from the half-inverted pulse (Fig. 7.4c) is scaled by a factor of 2 and then added to the scattered sound from the first pulse (Fig. 7.4a). This also results in cancellation of all linear scattered energy and enhancement of the nonlinear. The spectrum of the resulting pulse (Fig. 7.4f) shows that the nonlinear scattered response has all harmonic

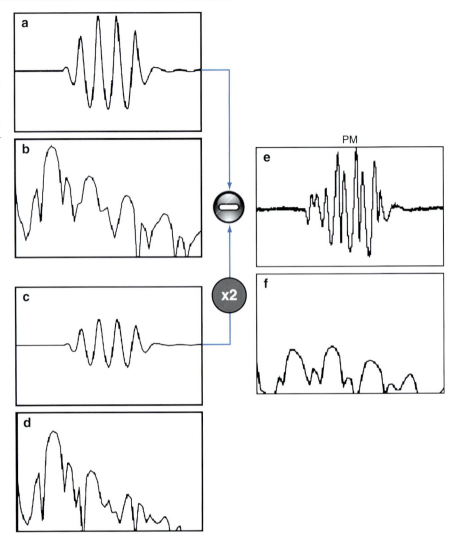

Fig. 7.3 The power modulation technique for nonlinear detection of bubble echoes. (**a**) Scattered sound from bubbles with a normal pulse; (**b**) frequency spectrum of (**a**); (**c**) scattered sound from bubbles with a half pulse; (**d**) frequency spectrum of (**c**); (**e**) power modulation – the scaling and addition of scattered pulses (**a**) and (**c**); (**f**) frequency spectrum of (**e**)

components, including a nonlinear fundamental component as is the case for PM, but now the level of the second harmonic component is considerably higher but still slightly lower than PI (compare Fig. 7.4f with Fig. 7.3f and 7.2f). Ideally, PMPI offers a good compromise between PM and PI, by having the nonlinear fundamental for sensitivity and by also having a good second harmonic for resolution.

Often much of the difference seen between the various pulsing sequences is not only due to the method itself but also due to the choice of other parameters during the optimization process, such as where the receiver filters are placed with respect to the fundamental or harmonic and how accurately the ultrasound transmitters can generate the various pulses (full, half, inverted). Most commercial systems have difficulties to perfectly invert a pulse whereas they are able to apply scaling and reduce it by half. The inability to perfectly invert pulses results in incomplete cancellation of the tissue in PI and to a lesser degree in PMPI. As mentioned earlier, the nonlinear fundamental is more sensitive but has worse esthetics (resolution) due to it its lower frequency. For vascular contrast imaging, PM and PMPI are the schemes of choice for good penetration and bubble sensitivity, while maintaining adequate resolution.

7.2.5 Contrast Side-by-Side Display

As imaging techniques have improved in their ability to detect microbubbles and reject tissue, it has become

Fig. 7.4 The power-modulated pulse inversion technique for nonlinear detection of bubble echoes. (**a**) Scattered sound from bubbles with a normal pulse; (**b**) frequency spectrum of (**a**); (**c**) scattered sound from bubbles with a half-inverted pulse; (**d**) frequency spectrum of (**c**); (**e**) power modulation – the scaling and addition of scattered pulses (**a**) and (**c**); (**f**) frequency spectrum of (**e**)

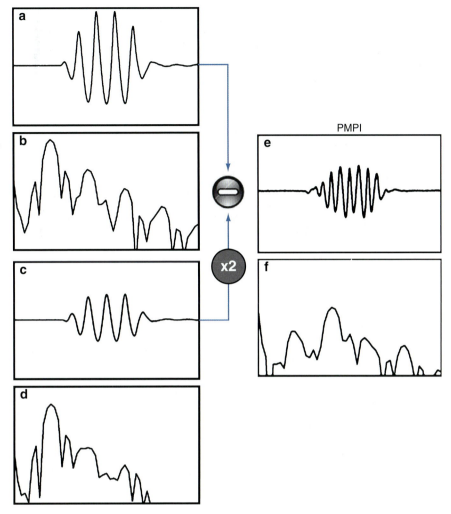

difficult to visualize the scan plane (find the plaque for example) in a contrast imaging mode prior to the arrival of contrast at the site. For this reason, a dual imaging mode (referred to as Contrast Side-by-Side by some manufacturers) display has been developed with contrast imaging mode on the left (Fig. 7.5a), and conventional (tissue) imaging on the right (Fig. 7.5b). The tissue image gives the user landmark information for guidance before and during a contrast injection. Both the contrast and the tissue images are acquired at low MI (less than 0.1) so as to not destroy additional microbubbles. For carotid and plaque neovascularization imaging, a good scanning range is $0.05 < MI < 0.08$.

7.3 Vascular Ultrasound Imaging with Contrast Agents

7.3.1 Ultrasound Examination

Vascular contrast ultrasound imaging is performed after a baseline vascular study (without contrast agents) is completed. For carotid scanning, linear array transducers in the frequency range of 7–15 MHz are used. An example of baseline images is shown in Fig. 7.6, where in the left square a B-mode image of the carotid plaque taken with the L12-5 probe of the Philips iU22 (Philips, Seattle, Washington, USA)

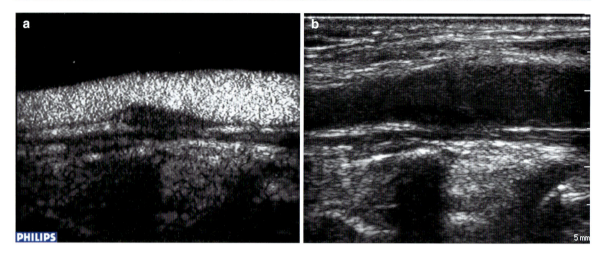

Fig. 7.5 Image of a carotid plaque in contrast side-by-side imaging. (**a**) Contrast image with PM technique at MI = 0.06; (**b**) conventional fundamental image also at MI = 0.06

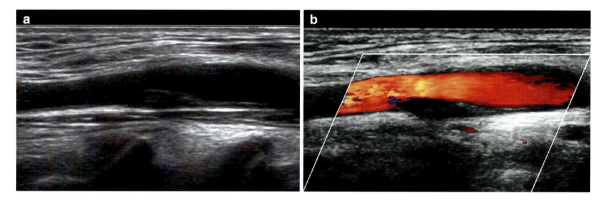

Fig. 7.6 B-mode image of a carotid plaque (**a**) taken with the L12-5 linear array of the Philips iU22 and the corresponding Doppler color flow image (**b**)

ultrasound scanner is shown, and in the right the equivalent Doppler color flow image is shown. The same linear array used for baseline study is used for the contrast study as well. Nonlinear pulsing schemes are implemented for this application (see discussion in sections above) and are optimized for good bubble sensitivity and resolution for this frequency range. In most ultrasound systems today, PM or PMPI techniques are used for vascular contrast studies. Where available, the use of the dual contrast display is preferred because it allows for the display of the fundamental/tissue carotid image on one image and the contrast image on the other, both formed with low MI to avoid bubble destruction as shown in Fig. 7.5.

Additionally, effort is placed to ensure that no tissue is seen at all in the contrast image before contrast injection by limiting the time gain compensation (TGC) gain in the area where the tissue cancellation is incomplete.

The contrast agent that is approved for clinical use in Europe by the European Medicines Evaluation Agency (EMEA) is SonoVue which consists of sulfur hexafluoride–filled microbubbles in the range 1–10 μm diameter and mean diameter 2.5 μm.[29] The agent comes in vials of 5 mL after reconstitution with saline. Bolus injections of 1.2–2.4 mL may be used. In other clinical applications such as liver, kidney, and breast, injections of 2.4 mL are most common (and

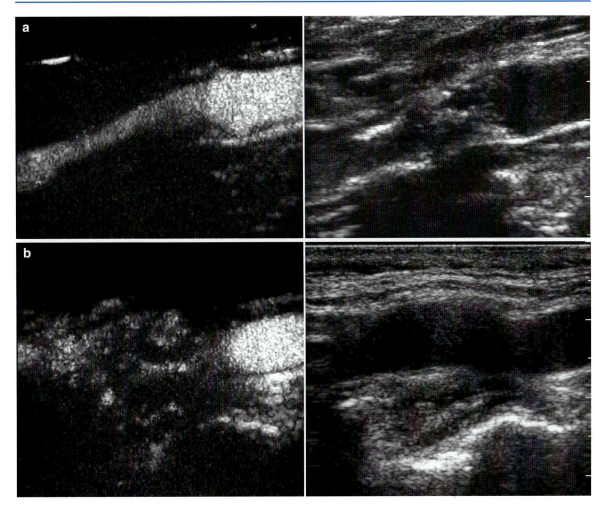

Fig. 7.7 Clinical examples of vascular contrast imaging. (**a**) A carotid with a large plaque and high degree of stenosis; (**b**) a completely occluded carotid; (**c**) trickle flow due to severe stenosis; and (**d**) hyperplastic vasa vasorum

also recommended by the manufacturer) and in some cases even the whole vial (5 mL) is used. However, for carotid scanning, 1.2 mL is preferred in order to avoid high concentrations of microbubbles in the carotid which, as it will be demonstrated in the next section, leads to the generation of artifacts at the far wall.

In order to quantify the plaque neovascularization and the hyperplastic vasa vasorum, loops of 60 s are collected by holding the transducer still over a fixed plane. Plaque neovascularization consists of very small microvessels/capillaries with very slow flow rates. Often, the individual microvessels are clearly depicted but sometimes are also seen as a very small enhancement of the image signal in the plaque area (see for example the white dots in Fig. 7.5a). Some other times, this enhancement is not possible to appreciate by just examining the images. Similarly, the hyperplastic vasa vasorum is often seen as a slight enhancement of the vessel wall after contrast injection and it may vary from clear observable enhancement to a minute increase in brightness. Quantification approaches are used to clearly observe and quantify the amount of blood present in these tiny vessels. In addition to loops, parts of the carotid may be surveyed during the contrast injection in order to visualize the flow in the carotid in the area of the plaque, and to better identify the intima-media thickness.

In Fig. 7.7, various clinical examples of carotid plaques, plaque neovascularization, and vasa vasorum enhancement are shown. In Fig. 7.7a, a carotid with a large plaque and high degree of stenosis is shown. By examining the B-mode image, one

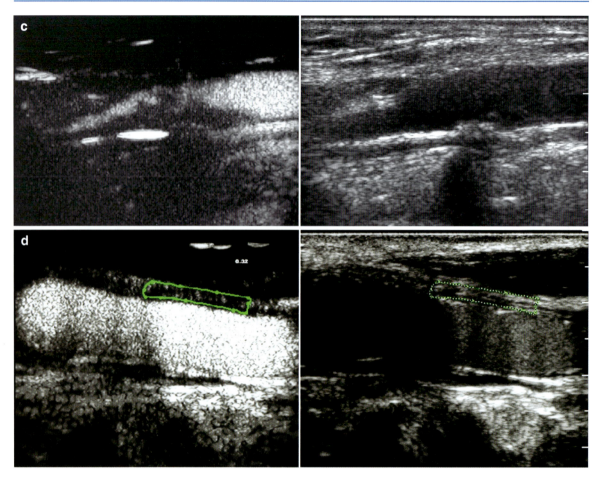

Fig. 7.7 (continued)

would possibly evaluate this as a fully occluded carotid; however, clear flow is seen in the contrast image. It is also noted that no plaque perfusion is observed as the plaque in the contrast image is seen as completely black. An example of a fully occluded plaque is shown in Fig. 7.7b, where in the B-mode image, the plaque is not seen at all (it is a black plaque) and yet in the contrast image, a complete occlusion is observed. An example of trickle flow is shown in Fig. 7.7c. With conventional ultrasound (without contrast agents), this carotid was diagnosed as fully occluded as no Doppler signals were detected. However, with a small bolus injection of 1.2 mL SonoVue, a narrow open path was confirmed. Hyperplastic vasa vasorum is shown in Fig. 7.7d. In the area outlined in green, definite microvessels with slow flow were detected.

7.3.2 Quantification of Microcirculation

Indicator dilution techniques allow for measurements of flow parameters such as flow rate, volume, and mean transit time. The basis of this method is that by injecting an indicator and making measurements during its transit, the flow of the medium in which the indicator is diluted can be evaluated. The indicator can be a dye, an isotope, a gas or even heat or cooling. In the case of contrast ultrasound, the indicator is the microbubble contrast agent. If the amount of the indicator m in a bolus injection is known, and the indicator concentration as a function of time is measured in a region of interest (ROI), then both the volumetric blood flow rate (F) and the blood volume (V) can be calculated in terms of area under the curve (AUC) and mean transit time (MTT):

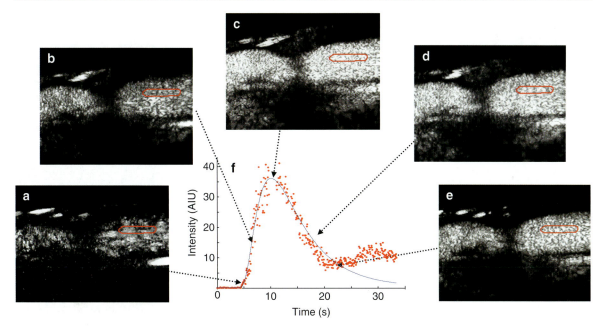

Fig. 7.8 Demonstration of how a time–intensity curve is created. The *red points* in the curve are the average intensity of the ROI in every individual frame of the loop. The *blue line* is the lognormal curve fitted for these data. (**a**–**e**) The images at specific times in the loop

$$F = m \cdot (\text{AUC})^{-1}$$

$$V = F \cdot \text{MTT}$$

These relations are known as the Stewart-Hamilton relations[30–32] and their derivation makes no assumptions about the shape of the indicator dilution curves. In contrast imaging, the backscattered intensity $I(t)$ is measured instead of the microbubble concentration, therefore F and V cannot be measured directly. However, at low microbubble concentrations, the backscattered intensity is proportional to the concentration,[33] implying that one can measure quantities that are proportional to F and V.

Different indicator dilution models have been suggested for contrast ultrasound. In the present work, the lognormal function is used. The lognormal distribution function with a delay t_0 is given by:

$$I(t) = \frac{\text{AUC}}{\sqrt{2\pi}\sigma(t-t_0)} e^{\frac{[\ln(t-t_0)-\mu]^2}{2\sigma^2}} + I_0 \quad \text{with} \quad t > t_0,$$

where $I(t)$ is the backscattered signal intensity (which is proportional to indicator concentration) as a function of time. The variables μ and σ are the mean and standard deviation of the normal distribution of the logarithm of the independent variable t. I_0 is the baseline intensity offset due to the noise level present in the image and the background backscatter from tissue (without bubbles). MTT, defined as the first moment of the probability density function $(I(t) - I_0)$ minus the bolus arrival time t_0, and t_p, is given by:

$$\text{MTT} = e^{\mu + \frac{\sigma^2}{2}}, \quad t_p = e^{\mu - \sigma^2}$$

Indicator dilution methods are applied to quantification of vascular contrast imaging and more specifically to quantification of the perfusion of plaques and the vasa vasorum. A ROI may be placed either in the lumen or the plaque and the average intensity as a function of time is plotted to form a time–intensity curve (TIC), as shown in Fig. 7.8. The intensity from every image in a loop is shown as red dots and typical images that produced this type of TIC are shown in Fig. 7.8a–e. A lognormal function is then fitted to the

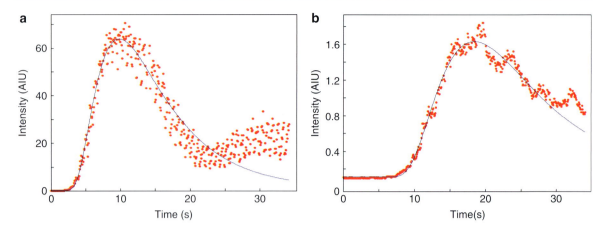

Fig. 7.9 Quantification results. A time–intensity curve from a ROI in the lumen of the carotid in (**a**) and from a ROI in a vascularized plaque in (**b**). *Red dots* are the image data and the *blue line* is the best fit to the data with the lognormal function

points of the TIC (shown as a blue line in the curve). From the lognormal function, we can extract the following hemodynamic-related parameters: area under the curve (AUC), mean transit time (MTT), wash-in time (WIT), peak intensity (I_p).

In Fig. 7.9, quantification results from analysis of the blood flow in the carotid and in the plaques are shown. In Fig. 7.9a, a TIC of the carotid is shown. The lognormal model is fitted through the data. It is also interesting to note that the recirculation of the contrast agent (second pass through the ROI in the carotid) is clearly seen around 20s as a hump in the TIC. By comparing the I_p of the two curves, one can observe that it is much larger for the carotid than the plaque (a value of 70 versus 2, measured in arbitrary (linear) intensity units). This is expected as the amount of bubbles (and consequently blood) in the carotid is much higher than that of the plaque microvessels. In addition, both WIT and MTT are larger for the plaque neovessels indicating slower flow rates and smaller blood volumes. Another important observation is that the arrival time of blood in the plaque (Fig. 7.9b) is around 10 s versus 4 s for the carotid. Since the plaque neovascularization is fed from outside smaller vessels, this delayed arrival is expected and could also be used as a differentiator of plaque neovascularization from possible artifacts. It is hypothesized that progression or regression of plaque neovascularization caused by therapy (such as statins) would cause observable changes in the hemodynamic-related parameters (WIT, MTT, etc.) extracted from indicator dilution models, e.g., the lognormal function.

7.3.2.1 Propagation in a Nonlinear Bubbly Fluid: An Artifact for Plaques in the Far Wall

One issue often encountered in the quantification of the plaque neovascularization or vasa vasorum perfusion is an artifact where signal in the image is falsely registered in cases where the ROI (plaque or vasa vasorum) is at the far wall. Pixels in the plaque are seen to increase their intensity as if microvessel blood flow is present (see for example the gray pixels in the plaque of Fig. 7.10a in the blue ROI). This is caused by the propagation of the ultrasound pulse in a very nonlinear (bubbly) medium[34] such as is the case of the blood in the carotid. The pulses used for nonlinear pulsing schemes are highly distorted during their passage in the carotid above the plaque or vasa vasorum of interest at the distal wall. This results in incomplete cancellation of the linear targets (the tissue) and their depiction as nonlinear, which is in turn interpreted as microbubbles or blood. In Fig. 7.10b, the TICs from those two ROIs where the y-axis is the intensity normalized with respect to its maximum value are shown. It is seen that the arrival in the two ROIs is almost simultaneous and this would not be physiologically possible since the plaque neovascularization is fed from smaller vessels on the vessel wall and the near vicinity. In addition, one can also observe in Fig. 7.10a that enhancement is also seen in the tissue below the carotid wall where normal tissue is present and it is known that it is an artifact also as it is not blood. In fact, this image was taken with side-by-side

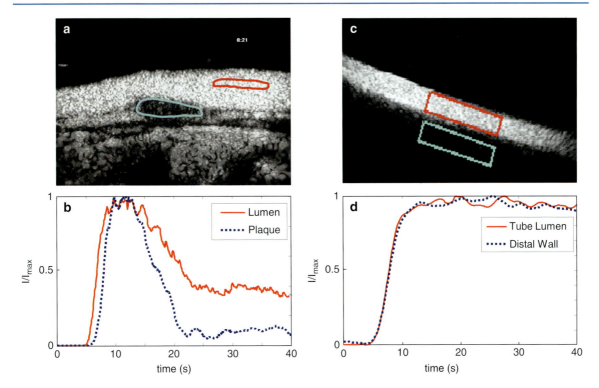

Fig. 7.10 Image artifact from propagation in a bubbly liquid. (**a**) Image of a carotid plaque at the distal wall with falsely registered signal; (**b**) time–intensity curves for the ROIs shown in (**a**); (**c**) image of SonoVue flow in a flow phantom; and (**d**) time–intensity curves for the ROIs in (**c**)

imaging and the tissue image (not shown here) had a great resemblance with the contrast image in the artifacted area below the carotid.

In order to further demonstrate this artifact, the authors also collected images from a flow phantom with similar SonoVue concentrations to that used clinically, as shown in Fig. 7.10c. In Fig. 7.10d, the TICs from the two ROIs are shown, again with the y-axis being the normalized intensity. Again, similar signal is observed in the blue ROI (even though it is not observable with naked eye) where clearly no bubbles are present since the tube terminates above the blue ROI.

The problem is reduced when lower bubble concentrations are used for the clinical exam. Instead of 2.4 mL of Sonovue, 1.2 mL may be used. Even at this lower concentration, the artifact is not eliminated totally. Another option is to always study plaques and sections of the vasa vasorum that are at the proximal wall. Until a final solution for eliminating this artifact is found (possible improvements on the pulsing scheme), it is advised that quantification of plaques and the vasa vasorum at the distal wall is avoided.

7.3.3 Quantification Results and Clinical Importance

Data from 22 carotids with 50% or greater stenosis (some of them were completely occluded) were collected and a total of 31 plaques were analyzed. Thirteen of those had some level of perfusion and neovascularization and 9 had active (thickened) vasa vasorum. The quantification analysis consisted of forming TICs and then fitting the data to the lognormal function discussed above and extracting hemodynamic-related parameters (WIT, MTT, AUC, I_p, etc.). The authors' findings are briefly summarized here.

The degree of stenosis was calculated with the ECST criteria (Chaps. 2, 30 and 36) with both vascular contrast ultrasound and conventional ultrasound. In all cases studied, the degree of stenosis found with contrast was lower. It is not apparently clear why there is a discrepancy between the stenosis calculation found from contrast images and from velocity information. One possible explanation is the sensitivity of color flow Doppler. Often, obstacles in the path to the vessel can attenuate the ultrasound wave considerably to the point that no flow information is registered. The use of a nonlinear pulsing scheme and by looking into the nonlinear component of the scattered signal only eliminates some of the path-induced noise. In addition, the sensitivity to detect blood flow (even with extremely low velocities) is much higher for CEUS than it is for Doppler, hence the ability of CEUS to measure blood flow in the microcirculation (established in liver oncology[35]). Another explanation is the variable collateral circulation which determines the pressure gradient across a stenosis and the resulting velocity detected by Doppler (Chap. 30).

From TICs in the carotid, the recirculation time, the time it takes for a tracer to have a second pass in a ROI, was observed and measured (it is seen as a hump in the TIC, see for example Fig. 7.9a). For the patients studied, the average recirculation time was 18.4 s with standard deviation of 3.5, standard error of 1.17, and standard error average of 6.34.

The vessels feeding the plaque and the vasa vasorum are much smaller vessels than the carotid and there is a definite arrival delay between the two. The delay of arrival Δt_a is measured from the time–intensity curves. The authors have found that Δt_a for plaques is 1.93 s (taken from 14 plaques) and 3.35 s for the vasa vasorum (taken from 7 enhancing vasa vasorum sections). These indicative times may also be used in deciding whether circulation in a region in the plaque or the vasa vasorum is real or caused by the nonlinear propagation artifact. It would be of interest to monitor this parameter in therapies aimed at plaque remodeling and reducing the cardiovascular risk.

From quantification studies in oncology,[35,36] it is suggested that the WIT and the MTT are possibly the most important parameters to evaluate in order to deduce blood flow rate both in the carotid and also in the plaque. From the authors' studies, the average WIT and MTT for the carotid is lower than those for the plaque microcirculation and the vasa vasorum. The increase of the WIT from the carotid to the microcirculation is almost twofold whereas the increase of MTT is about 10%. The WIT for plaques and vasa vasorum is about the same, whereas the MTT of the vasa vasorum is found to be about 20% greater than that of plaque microcirculation. The authors propose as possible imaging biomarkers both the WIT and the MTT and place more emphasis on the WIT as it is already known that this parameter is closely related to flow rate and was found to be a good imaging biomarker in liver oncology patients as well.[35]

The intensity of the pixels in a ROI is proportional to the total blood volume in the area. Thus it may be used as an indicator of the degree of neovascularization. However, the nature of diagnostic ultrasound is such that user machine settings may influence this value. By taking the ratio of the plaque (or the vasa vasorum) intensity over the carotid (lumen), the user influence on the settings is suppressed. It is hypothesized that plaques with more perfusion activity (higher signals in the ROI) may be more dangerous. The plaque/lumen intensity ratio shows that type 1 plaques that are pure cholesterol or necrotic material do not have any perfusion, as expected. Type 4 plaques have variable perfusion, but they are clinically safe, and are not associated with events. What is exciting is that in type 2 and 3 plaques, some show high and some low perfusion. High perfusion is associated with neovascularization and macrophages, and our hypothesis is that this finding may differentiate between subtypes of high-risk and low-risk plaques type 2 and 3. More research is needed in this area in the future.

7.4 Concluding Remarks

Vascular contrast ultrasound is an emerging technique that adds clinical value and research information toward the identification of vulnerable plaques. It is quick to perform, inexpensive, and less invasive compared with CT, MRI, or PET imaging. The imaging of the plaque microcirculation is performed with nonlinear imaging techniques, with power modulation and power-modulated pulse inversion being the most suitable for this application. The quantification of the blood flow in the microcirculation of the plaques and the vasa vasorum is performed on contrast image loops and with the aid of indicator dilution techniques. In asymptomatic patients with carotid plaques, vascular contrast ultrasound is an adjunct tool to plaque morphology studies by providing valuable information on the degree of neovascularization and the extent of vasa vasorum activity. Large prospective studies are needed to clarify the prognostic value of plaque vascularization in asymptomatic patients. Finally, vascular contrast ultrasound with the quantification of plaque neovascularization and vasa vasorum perfusion may in the future be applied in therapy monitoring for treatments aimed at plaque remodeling and reducing cardiovascular risk.

Acknowledgments The authors acknowledge the help of Marios Lampaskis and Christina Keravnou with patient data analysis. This work is supported by the Cyprus Research Promotion Foundation through the grant Vasorum (Grant number: Ygeia/0506/06).

References

1. Sitzer M, Fürst G, Siebler M, Steinmetz H. Usefulness of an intravenous contrast medium in the characterization of high-grade internal carotid stenosis with color Doppler-assisted duplex imaging. *Stroke*. 1994;25(2):385–389.
2. Ferrer JM et al. Use of ultrasound contrast in the diagnosis of carotid artery occlusion. *J Vasc Surg*. 2000;31(4):736–741.
3. Holden A, Hope JK, Osborne M, Moriarty M, Lee K. Value of a contrast agent in equivocal carotid ultrasound studies: pictorial essay. *Australas Radiol*. 2000;44(3):253–260.
4. Hansberg T, Wong KS, Droste DW, Ringelstein EB, Kay R. Effects of the ultrasound contrast-enhancing agent Levovist on the detection of intracranial arteries and stenoses in Chinese by transcranial Doppler ultrasound. *Cerebrovasc Dis*. 2002;14(2):105–108.
5. Tateishi Y et al. Contrast-enhanced transcranial color-coded duplex sonography criteria for basilar artery stenosis. *J Neuroimaging*. 2008;18(4):407–410.
6. Rajaram V et al. Role of surrogate markers in assessing patients with diabetes mellitus and the metabolic syndrome and in evaluation lipid-lowering therapy. *Am J Cardiol*. 2004;93(11A):32C-48C.
7. McCarthy MJ et al. Angiogenesis and the atherosclerotic carotid plaque: an association between symptomatology and plaque morphology. *J Vasc Surg*. 1999;30(2):261–268.
8. Mofidi R et al. Association between plaque instability, angiogenesis and symptomatic carotid occlusive disease. *Br J Surg*. 2001;88(7):945–950.
9. Huang PT et al. Contrast-enhanced sonographic characteristics of neovascularization in carotid atherosclerotic plaques. *J Clin Ultrasound*. 2008;36(6):346–351.
10. Feinstein SB. Contrast ultrasound imaging of the carotid artery vasa vasorum and atherosclerotic plaque neovascularization. *J Am Coll Cardiol*. 2006;48(2):236–243.
11. Vicenzini E et al. Detection of carotid adventitial vasa vasorum and plaque vascularization with ultrasound cadence contrast pulse sequencing technique and echo-contrast agent. *Stroke*. 2007;38:2841–2843.
12. Giannoni MF, Vicenzini E. Focus on the "unstable" carotid plaque: detection of intraplaque angiogenesis with contrast ultrasound. Present state and future perspectives. *Curr Vasc Pharmacol*. 2009;7(2):180–184.
13. Shah F et al. Contrast-enhanced ultrasound imaging of atherosclerotic carotid plaque neovascularization: a new surrogate marker of atherosclerosis? *Vasc Med*. 2007;12(4):291–297.
14. Coli S et al. Contrast-enhanced ultrasound imaging of intraplaque neovascularization in carotid arteries: correlation with histology and plaque echogenicity. *J Am Coll Cardiol*. 2008;52(3):223–230.
15. Xiong L et al. Correlation of carotid plaque neovascularization detected by using contrast-enhanced US with clinical symptoms. *Radiology*. 2009;251(2):583–589.
16. Owen DR et al. Inflammation within carotid atherosclerotic plaque: assessment with late-phase contrast-enhanced US. *Radiology*. 2010;255(2):638–644.
17. Staub D et al. Vasa vasorum and plaque neovascularization on contrast-enhanced carotid ultrasound imaging correlates with cardiovascular disease and past cardiovascular events. *Stroke*. 2010;41(1):41–47.
18. Leighton TG. *The Acoustic Bubble*. San Diego: Academic; 1997.
19. Villarraga HR, Foley DA, Aeschbacher BC, Klarich KW, Mulvagh SL. Destruction of contrast microbubbles during ultrasound imaging at conventional power output. *J Am Soc Echocardiogr*. 1997;10(8):783–791.
20. Walker KW, Pantely GA, Sahn DJ. Ultrasound-mediated destruction of contrast agents. Effect of ultrasound intensity, exposure, and frequency. *Invest Radiol*. 1997;32(12):728–734.
21. Berne RM, Levy MN, eds. *Cardiovascular Physiology*. 2nd ed. St. Louis: C.V. Mosby Co; 1972:265.
22. Porter T, Xie F. Transient myocardial contrast following initial exposure to diagnostic ultrasound pressures with minute doses of intravenously injected microbubbles: demonstration and potential mechanisms. *Circulation*. 1995;92:2391–2395.
23. Porter TR, Xie F, Kricsfeld D, Armbruster R. Improved myocardial contrast with second harmonic transient ultrasound response imaging in humans using intravenous perfluorocarbon-exposed sonicated dextrose albumin. *J Am Coll Cardiol*. 1996;27(6):1497–1501.
24. Heckemann RA et al. Liver lesions: intermittent second-harmonic gray-scale US can increase conspicuity with microbubble contrast material-early experience. *Radiology*. 2000;216(2):592–596.
25. Kim TK, Choi BI, Hong HS, Choi BY, Han JK. Improved imaging of hepatic metastases with delayed pulse inversion harmonic imaging using a contrast agent SH U 508A: preliminary study. *Ultrasound Med Biol*. 2000;26(9):1439–1444.
26. Wilson SR, Burns PN, Muradali D, Wilson JA, Lai X. Harmonic hepatic US with microbubble contrast agent: initial experience showing improved characterization of hemangioma, hepatocellular carcinoma, and metastasis. *Radiology*. 2000;215(1):153–161.
27. Averkiou MA, Mannaris C, Bruce M, Powers J. Nonlinear pulsing schemes for the detection of ultrasound contrast agents. In: Proceedings of the 155th Meeting of the ASA, Acoustics 2008; 2008; Paris:915–920.
28. Averkiou MA, Roundhill DN, Powers JE. New imaging technique based on the nonlinear properties of tissues. *Proc IEEE Ultrason Symp*. 1997;2:1561–1566.

29. Greis C. Technology overview: SonoVue (Bracco, Milan). *Eur Radiol*. 2004;14(suppl 8):11–15.
30. Stewart GN. Researches on the circulation time and on the influences which affect it. IV. The output of the heart. *J Physiol*. 1897;22:159–183.
31. Henriques V. Über die Verteilung des Blutes vom linken Herzen zwischen dem Herzen und dem übrigen Organismus. *Biochem Ztschr*. 1913;56:230–248.
32. Hamilton WF, Moore JW, Kinsman JM, Spurling RG. Simultaneous determination of the pulmonary and systemic circulation times in man and of a figure related to cardiac output. *Am J Physiol*. 1928;84:338–344.
33. Lampaskis M, Averkiou MA. Investigation of the relationship of non-linear backscattered ultrasound intensity with microbubble concentration at low MI. *Ultrasound Med Biol*. 2010;36(2):306–312.
34. Tang MX, Elson DS, Li R, Dunsby C, Eckersley RJ. Effects of nonlinear propagation in ultrasound contrast agent imaging. *Ultrasound Med Biol*. 2010;36(3):459–466.
35. Averkiou MA et al. Quantification of tumor microvascularity with respiratory gated contrast enhanced ultrasound for monitoring therapy. *Ultrasound Med Biol*. 2010;36(1):68–77.
36. Lassau N et al. Metastatic renal cell carcinoma treated with sunitinib: early evaluation of treatment response using dynamic contrast-enhanced ultrasonography. *Clin Cancer Res*. 2010;16(4):1216–1225.

Nonlinear Contrast Intravascular Ultrasound

David E. Goertz, Martijn E. Frijlink, Nico de Jong, and Antonius F.W. van der Steen

8.1 Introduction

8.1.1 Background

Intravascular ultrasound (IVUS) is an established clinical tool for assessing coronary artery atherosclerosis. Its use has contributed to an improved understanding of the natural history of atherosclerosis[1] and, increasingly, IVUS data are used as an endpoint in therapeutic trials.[2] For diagnostic purposes, it is employed as an adjunct to angiography, in order to provide additional insight into the extent and severity of atherosclerosis. It frequently reveals the presence of angiographically occult (i.e., non-stenotic) lesions.[3] Such "non-culprit" lesions are now recognized to be responsible for a high proportion of ensuing cardiac events resulting in either fatalities or requiring further interventional treatment.[4] A significant issue in cardiology is therefore to develop imaging methods to identify specific atherosclerotic lesions that are vulnerable to rupture.[5,6] Candidate markers of lesion vulnerability currently under investigation include plaque morphology, volume, mechanical integrity, and composition.[7,8] IVUS is well suited to indicate morphology and plaque burden, which has been the primary form of data analysis.[3] Mechanical properties relevant to plaque vulnerability can be derived using IVUS elastography techniques,[9] and efforts are being made to perform radiofrequency (RF) IVUS signal analysis to gain insight into plaque composition.[10] More recently, there is a growing recognition of the significance of *vasa vasorum* in plaque development and stability.

The vasa vasorum are the microvascular bed responsible for nourishing the portion of the walls of arteries and veins that lie beyond the diffusion limit of the lumen.[11] It is now well recognized that pathologic neovascularization occurs during plaque development, and that the resulting microvessels have abnormal spatial distributions and branching patterns.[12,13] Further, there is evidence suggesting that the spatial location of vasa vasorum may provide an indication of lesion vulnerability.[14] Neovascular vasa vasorum are part of an apparent positive feedback loop of inflammation and angiogenesis,[15–17] and are associated with macrophages and often intraplaque hemorrhage, and thereby an increased risk of rupture.[18,19] There is therefore considerable interest in targeting the neovascular vasa vasorum as a therapeutic strategy as well as to understand the potentially deleterious effects other angiogenically active therapies may have on the plaque vasa vasorum.[20] While imaging has been successful in detecting carotid artery vasa vasorum,[21,22] at present there are no established methods of in vivo imaging of vasa vasorum in coronary arteries.

D.E. Goertz (✉)
Department of Imaging Research, Sunnybrook Health Sciences Centre, Toronto, ON, Canada

M.E. Frijlink
Department of Probe Research & Development, Esaote Europe BV, Maastricht, The Netherlands

N. de Jong
Department of Biomedical Engineering, Erasmus MC and University of Twente, Rotterdam, The Netherlands

A.F.W. van der Steen
Department of Biomedical Engineering, Erasmus MC, Rotterdam, The Netherlands

8.1.2 Contrast IVUS Background

IVUS is one candidate imaging modality for accomplishing this. Due to high levels of relative tissue/catheter motion, it is unlikely that conventional high-frequency microvascular flow imaging methods[23,24] will be effective in detecting vasa vasorum. IVUS in combination with microbubbles may be one approach for overcoming these issues. There have been a number of recent reports of extraluminal image enhancement following the bolus injection of contrast agent, which has been attributed to the presence of adventitial vasa vasorum.[25–27] The basis of the approach employed in these reports is to compare post-contrast injection images with a baseline image derived from a single point in the cardiac cycle.[28] The sensitivity and robustness of this technique ultimately relies upon the assumption of similarity between images acquired at the same point in the cardiac cycle, and as such, it is susceptible to noncyclical catheter-vessel motion or nonuniform rotation velocity of the transducer element. These general issues were also encountered when such approaches were implemented in the context of lower frequency diagnostic ultrasound. This has motivated the development of contrast IVUS detection techniques based on bubble-specific signatures (e.g., nonlinear), which are now dominant at lower diagnostic frequencies (<10 MHz).

In this chapter, recent work relating to the development and investigation of nonlinear IVUS contrast agent imaging is discussed. The chapter begins with a discussion of contrast agent behavior at high frequencies, provides an overview of instrumentation for nonlinear IVUS imaging, and presents initial results obtained with this approach.

8.2 Contrast Behavior at High Frequencies

8.2.1 Frequency and Microbubble Sizes

The stimulation of nonlinear microbubble behavior, which gives rise to acoustic signatures that are significantly different from those of tissue, has enabled the detection of microvascular flow with ultrasound, even in the presence of substantial tissue motion. Initial implementations used second harmonic signals (twice the transmit frequency) which were isolated through the use of filtering. Detection techniques have evolved to include nonlinearities that are manifested within other bandwidths (e.g., subharmonic, superharmonic), and within the transmit bandwidth itself. These approaches involve the use of specialized pulse-sequences (e.g., pulse-inversion) that typically vary the phase and/or amplitude of successive pulses to isolate nonlinear energy (Chap. 7).

As indicated in Chap. 7, a pre-condition of most detection approaches is that bubbles are induced to behave in a nonlinear manner at the frequencies being employed. As substantial bubble vibrations are most readily achieved when they are stimulated near their resonant frequency (or twice in the case of superharmonics), current contrast agents have been fabricated to be comprised primarily of bubbles that are resonant in the lower diagnostic frequency range. As the resonance size of bubble scales varies inversely with frequency, it is reasonable to hypothesize that higher frequencies will perform more effectively with smaller bubbles. A good indicator of the frequency range an agent will be most active is to examine its frequency-dependent attenuation properties: Attenuation will be higher in the vicinity of where bubbles are resonant. The majority of clinically available agents have attenuation peaks in the lower frequency range: for example, for Optison™ (GE Healthcare, Princeton, New Jersey, USA) it is 3 MHz[29], for Sonovue® (Bracco Diagnostics Inc., Geneva, Switzerland) it is 2 MHz[30], and for Sonazoid™ (Amersham Health, Buckinghamshire, United Kingdom) it is 4–5 MHz[31]. The exception to this is Definity™ (Lantheus Medical Imaging, Billerica, Massachusetts, USA), which in its native form has an attenuation peak near 10 MHz (Fig. 8.1a), with considerable activity up to at least 50 MHz which is associated with a substantial subpopulation of bubbles 1–2 μm and below (Fig. 8.1b).[32] It is also notable that it has been shown that Definity™ can be manipulated with simple in-vial "decantation" procedures, compatible with clinical use, to improve its relative activity at higher frequencies through the preferential elimination of larger bubbles (Figs. 8.1c and d).[32] This procedure produces similar attenuation patterns to experimental agents manufactured to be comprised of such populations.[33]

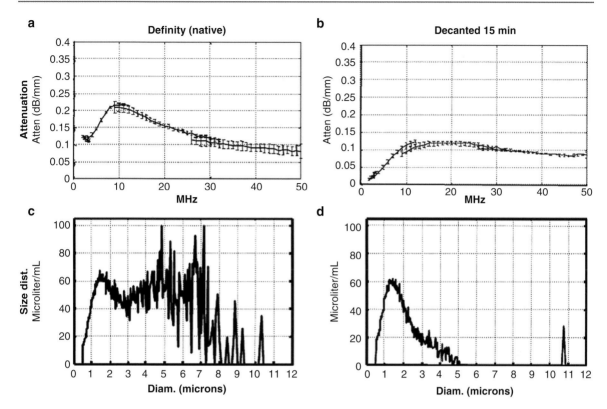

Fig. 8.1 (**a**) Attenuation as a function of frequency for "native" Definity shows a significant degree of activity at IVUS frequencies. (**b**) Size distribution of Definity shows a bimodal population of bubbles active at lower frequencies (>3 μm) as well as a significant number of bubbles below 2 μm. With in vial decantation, the relative activity at high frequencies is increased (**c**), reflecting the preferential elimination of large bubbles from the suspension (**d**) (Reprinted from Goertz et al.,[32] copyright 2007, with permission from Elsevier)

8.2.2 Nonlinear Microbubble Behavior at IVUS Frequencies

Lipid-encapsulated agents (Definity™ and experimental agents) containing populations of microbubbles below 2 μm have been shown to exhibit substantial nonlinear behavior at frequencies above 15 MHz.[34–36] In addition to their size, it also appears that an additional factor enabling the nonlinear behavior of small bubbles at high frequencies is that the lipid shell properties (i.e., viscosity) also fortuitously scale with frequency in a manner that enables substantial bubble oscillations.[32] The feasibility of exploiting this energy for imaging purposes at high frequencies was initially demonstrated with ultrasound biomicroscopy imaging systems in the context of small animal imaging applications using Definity™ and experimental small bubble agents.[34,35] The nonlinear behavior observed with Definity™ and manipulated Definity™ populations is of particular significance for clinical applications of IVUS contrast as it is an approved agent. In a preclinical context, it is possible to employ a wider range of agents, specifically optimized for use at high frequencies, with nonlinear IVUS due to lack of regulatory considerations.

It is also of interest that other microbubble detection approaches are also under investigation that, for example, combine low and high frequencies to facilitate the detection of larger (off-resonance) bubbles at higher frequencies.[37–39] While these are promising for a range of applications, it must also be considered that as the sample volume scales down with frequency so does the volume of blood and therefore the concentration of contrast agent. Since smaller bubbles can be present in higher number densities than larger bubbles,[32] the potential to have a smaller bubble present within a given sample volume will also be higher. This is particularly relevant in the context of microvascular imaging, where the blood compartment occupies only a fraction of the sample volume. The use of small bubble agents (and detection techniques such as sub- and second harmonic which detect smaller bubbles) may therefore be favorable from this perspective.

8.3 Instrumentation for Nonlinear IVUS Imaging

8.3.1 System Overview

Nonlinear contrast IVUS has to date been implemented using single element rotating transducers, which are the most commonly employed IVUS catheters. In B-scan imaging mode, short (high-resolution) pulses are sent at regular intervals during continuous rotation. The primary difference between conventional B-scan imaging and contrast imaging instrumentation requirements is that nonlinear contrast imaging requires careful control of the transmit pulse and receive processing in order to isolate the nonlinear signals of interest and separate them from tissue signals.

The prototype system employed to conduct initial nonlinear contrast work has been described in detail previously.[40] Briefly, the system has a rotational unit, and employs either off-the-shelf catheters directly, or modified versions using specialized transducers. Transmit pulses are sent into the catheter and receive pulses are recorded after appropriate signal conditioning to permit the effective extraction of nonlinear signals. A pulse-inversion sequence approach[41] has been employed and experiments have been constructed at a catheter rotation rate of 5–7 Hz. The use of pulse-inversion as opposed to direct filtering of nonlinear signals permits the use of broader bandwidth pulses (thereby improving depth resolution), though more basic implementations are also possible using narrowband pulses in combination with filtering alone (e.g., Granada et al.[42]). In the context of mechanically scanned transducers, it must be also be considered that transducer translation causes a decorrelation of the signal that can lead to an incomplete cancellation of the tissue signal when applying pulse-inversion approaches, particularly within the transmit bandwidth.[43,44] For harmonic and subharmonic (one half the transmit frequency) signals, the suppression of the transmit signal has been found to be sufficient in the presence of this decorrelation.

However, the use of amplitude modulation approaches, which exploit nonlinear signals in the transmit bandwidth will be more impacted by this decorrelation, which will act to decrease the contrast-to-tissue ratio.

In addition to forming contrast images, the same data sets can also be used to form B-scan images. Either second harmonic (transmit 20 MHz, receive 40 MHz) or subharmonic (transmit 30 MHz, receive 15 MHz) imaging is possible with the appropriate selection of transmit pulses and electronics.

8.3.2 Transducers

The transducer is a key element in any nonlinear contrast imaging system, with its efficiency and bandwidth being of central importance in determining microbubble detection sensitivity and spatial resolution. To date, both off-the shelf catheters (30 MHz center frequency) and custom dual-frequency (20–40 MHz and 15–30 MHz) transducer elements situated on conventional catheters[45,46] have been evaluated. While both approaches have been shown to be feasible, it is clear that the continuing development of improved sensitivity and bandwidth transducers,[47,48] also beneficial for conventional B-scan IVUS imaging, can be expected to result in the enhanced performance of contrast IVUS techniques.

8.4 Harmonic IVUS Contrast Imaging

8.4.1 Phantom Experiments

The feasibility and performance of harmonic IVUS contrast imaging was initially investigated using tissue mimicking phantoms and an experimental small bubble agent. For these experiments, the IVUS transducer was situated in a semicircular 1.4 mm diameter notch in the boundary between a suspension of agent and a block of tissue mimicking material.[40] Figure 8.2 shows example images from these experiments using an experimental small bubble agent. In B-scan imaging mode, the agent can be seen to have a lower signal strength than from the tissue mimicking material. In harmonic imaging mode, the tissue signals are suppressed to below the noise floor, while the agent

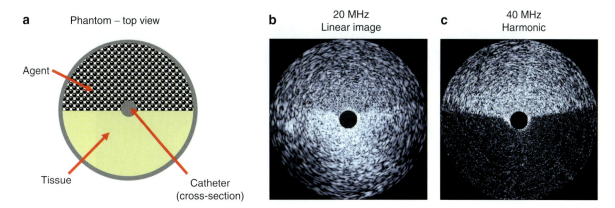

Fig. 8.2 (**a**) Experiment for imaging agent adjacent to a tissue mimicking phantom (*bottom half* – "T") and agent (*upper half* – "A") for a 20 MHz transmit frequency. (**b**) Image constructed in F20 mode (0.3 MPa) indicates contrast signals are lower than tissue signals. (**c**) H40 with filtering and PI, the tissue signal has been suppressed to below the noise floor. Images are 12 mm in diameter. The dynamic range of F40 image is 40 dB, the harmonic images are 25 dB (Reprinted from Goertz et al.,[40] copyright 2006, with permission from Elsevier)

signal is retained, thereby providing a means by which to segment the agent and tissue compartments.

A more realistic phantom experiment is shown in Fig. 8.3, where a catheter was placed within a 4 mm diameter flow phantom, and two smaller 0.75 mm vessels (situated at 4 o'clock and 12 o'clock) were located outside the main lumen. In B-scan imaging mode, these vessels are not readily distinguished (Fig. 8.3a), and would be even less evident if they were of a microvascular size of the order of or smaller than the system resolution. In harmonic mode (Fig. 8.3b), agent is detected within the main lumen as well as in the smaller vessels, while tissue signals are suppressed. Signals in the more distant vessel (12 o'clock) approach the noise floor however, which warrants discussion. Improving the signal strength can be accomplished in several ways. From a technical perspective, the signal to noise ratio will increase proportional to the transducer sensitivity, which has the potential to improve significantly. Another option in principle is to increase the transmit amplitude. However, a fundamental limitation of second harmonic imaging is that nonlinear propagation in tissue gives rise to a pressure-dependant tissue second harmonic signal that eventually begins to degrade the "contrast-to-tissue" signal ratio. An example of this is shown in Figs. 8.3c and d. This motivates the exploration of other detection strategies, such as subharmonic imaging, examined in a subsequent section.

8.4.2 In Vivo Harmonic Contrast Imaging

The general approach employed for contrast IVUS to date is to locate the transducer in a region of interest and then locally release a bolus of agent upstream of the transducer. The majority of the agent then washes through the main lumen while a portion of the agent is taken up by the vasa vasorum through vascular paths connected to the main lumen. In clinical experiments reported by Carlier et al.[25] this has been accomplished by the IVUS catheter that is situated within a delivery catheter through which agent is injected. For the nonlinear IVUS contrast work to date, in vivo validation has been conducted in atherosclerotic rabbit abdominal aortas, with atherosclerosis being initiated through the technique of local vessel injury followed by a cholesterol diet.[49] Due to limitations in the vessel size of this model, a smaller delivery catheter must be employed (5 French) which cannot accommodate an IVUS catheter within its lumen. The IVUS catheter was therefore introduced through the femoral artery, and the delivery catheter was passed through the carotid artery and its tip located 2–3 cm upstream of the IVUS catheter tip.

Examples of in vivo results obtained with this approach are shown in Fig. 8.4 for fundamental and harmonic imaging modes using 15 min decanted Definity™.[50] In fundamental mode prior to injection (Fig. 8.4a), the vena cava can be seen at 10 o'clock, while the main aortic lumen boundary and plaque are

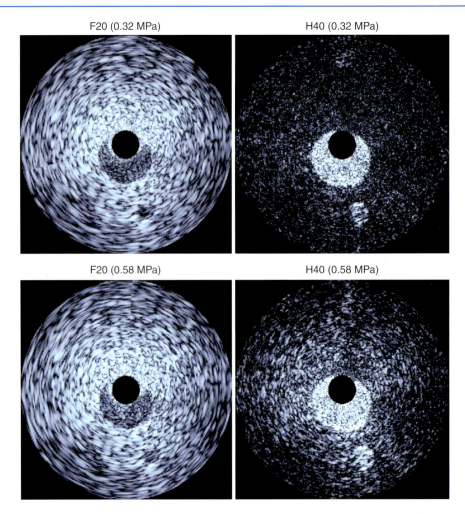

Fig. 8.3 Coronary phantom images for a 20 MHz transmit frequency. F20 images at two pressure levels (**a**, **b**) show agent within the main lumen and the "v1" vessel (5 o'clock) outside the main lumen. In H40 mode at 0.32 MPa (**c**), the CTR improves substantially for the main lumen, the "v1" vessel, while the "v2" vessel (12 o'clock) is at the edge of detection. As at a 0.58 MPa transmit level (**d**), the H40 tissue signal becomes prominent, though the CTR is still better relative to F20. Images are 12 mm in diameter. Display dynamic ranges are 40 dB for F20 and 25 dB for H40 (Reprinted from Goertz et al.,[40] copyright 2006, with permission from Elsevier)

difficult to visualize. Following contrast injection, the passage of the bolus transiently obscured imaging through attenuation effects, and by 5 s post injection, the intensity of the image had recovered. Echogenicity enhancement was then evident in the vena cava, but was not apparent in the adventitia, except in a small region at 4 o'clock (Fig. 8.4b). The harmonic imaging results are substantially different. Prior to injection, it can be seen that the tissue signals have been largely suppressed, with only a small amount of tissue signal artifact remaining (Fig. 8.4c). Post-injection, the agent was first briefly visualized in the main lumen and before imaging was obscured by the attenuation effects. At approximately 5 s post injection, a ring at the boundary of the main lumen could be seen (Fig. 8.4d). This can be attributed to the presence of a small amount of more slowly moving agent adjacent to the aortic wall, which was also observed in dynamic phantom experiments. This effect enabled the lumen boundary to be easily distinguished. There was then an eccentric circumferential region devoid of enhancement, with a thickness larger in the 2 o'clock direction than in the 8 o'clock direction. Outside this hypoechoic region, numerous locations of enhancement were observed that were associated with the presence of agent. While toward 10 o'clock, the

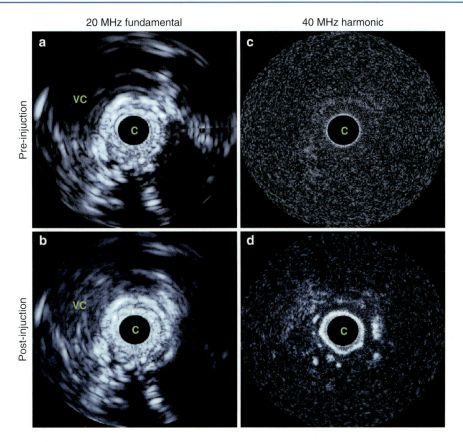

Fig. 8.4 In vivo results in an atherosclerotic rabbit aorta using decanted Definity™. (**a**) Fundamental mode prior to agent injection, where "c" is the catheter, the vena cava is "vc." (**b**) Fundamental mode 10 s post injection where changes in adventitial enhancement are not evident, except for in a region at 4 o'clock and within the vena cava. (**c**) Harmonic mode prior to injection shows the tissue signals to be largely suppressed. (**d**) A 10 s post-injection harmonic mode shows significant adventitial enhancement, consistent with the detection of adventitial microvessels. Scale of images is 12 mm across. The dynamic ranges of the fundamental and harmonic images are 40 and 25 dB, respectively (Reprinted with permission from Goertz et al.[50])

enhancement is associated with vena cava, the other locations are consistent with the detection of microvessels outside the main vessel lumen. The delayed arrival of enhancement in this region, relative to the main lumen, is also expected due to the longer traveling distance and slower blood velocities within the vasa vasorum.

Following the imaging experiments, tissue was harvested and serial histologic sections were made around the imaged region. Hematoxylin and eosin stained sections from this region show the presence of a large, eccentric plaque within the aorta (Fig. 8.5a). The plaque thins toward the 7 o'clock position and the vena cava is situated to the left of the aorta. Accounting for the different orientation of the histology sections, these features are generally consistent with the IVUS images. CD31 staining for endothelial cells revealed the plaque to be avascular. The media also had very little evidence of the presence of blood vessels (Fig. 8.5b). Contrast enhancement of harmonic IVUS images between the lumen and adventitial regions would therefore not be expected, and was not in fact observed. Within the adventitia, there is extensive evidence of microvessels, particularly toward the bottom and right. The histology therefore indicates the general presence of microvessels in regions where harmonic IVUS has detected contrast enhancement. Aside from the vena cava, there was an absence of larger vessels in the sections examined. While a specific comparison between histology microvessels and IVUS images cannot be made, these results do support the conclusion that harmonic IVUS has detected adventitial microvessels. Following the convention detailed in Kwon et al.[12] and Edelman et al.[51] these

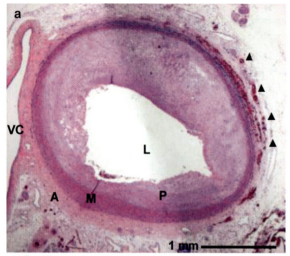

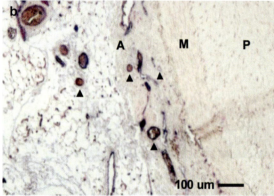

Fig. 8.5 (**a**) Overview hematoxylin/eosin stained section from the aorta examined with IVUS in Fig. 8.4. *VC* vena cava, *L* aortic lumen, *M* media, *P* atherosclerotic plaque, *A* adventitia. A large eccentric plaque is evident, which thins toward the vena cava. (**b**) CD31 stained section highlights endothelial cells (*purple*) and reveals the presence of numerous adventitial microvessels (many containing erythrocytes), some examples of which are denoted with ▲ (Reprinted with permission from Goertz et al.[50])

results indicate the presence of vasa vasorum. Despite the inherent limitations of second harmonic contrast imaging, this is a viable approach for bubble-specific imaging of the vasa vasorum.

8.4.3 IVUS Tissue Harmonic Imaging

As indicated above under "Phantom Experiments," the use of higher transmit pressure levels improves the contrast signals, but also increases second harmonic energy associated with nonlinear propagation. In the context of contrast imaging, this is an undesirable effect which limits system performance. As at lower frequencies however, the tissue propagation harmonic can also be exploited for the purposes of tissue imaging and thereby overcome many imaging artifacts and thereby improve image quality. Tissue harmonic imaging has also been investigated with the nonlinear IVUS instrumentation reported here,[45] which may be advantageous for the reduction of artifacts associated with stents and calcifications, and catheter sheaths.

8.5 Subharmonic IVUS Contrast Imaging

8.5.1 Phantom Experiments

Subharmonic IVUS contrast imaging has been investigated at transmit frequencies of 30 and 40 MHz, using both off-the-shelf and custom transducers. An example vessel phantom experiment illustrating the feasibility of subharmonic imaging with an experimental small bubble agent at 40 MHz transmit frequency is shown in Fig. 8.6.[40] In linear imaging mode (Fig. 8.6a), it is difficult to distinguish the two smaller vessels (4 o'clock and 12 o'clock). In subharmonic mode (Fig. 8.6b), the main lumen and two smaller vessels can be readily observed, with the tissue signals suppressed below the noise floor. As transmit pressure is increased, the contrast signal strength in subharmonic imaging mode (Fig. 8.6d) is also increased without the appearance of tissue propagation harmonic.

Figure 8.7 shows an example phantom experiment using Definity™, conducted with a specialized 30–15 MHz dual-frequency transducer.[52] In this case, the signal of the contrast agent in linear imaging mode (Fig. 8.7a) is similar to that of tissue, reflecting the increased echogenicity of Definity™ relative to the small bubble agent, due to the presence of larger bubbles. In subharmonic mode (Fig. 8.7b), a high signal to noise ratio is observed, demonstrating the feasibility of performing subharmonic imaging with subharmonic IVUS and a clinically available agent.

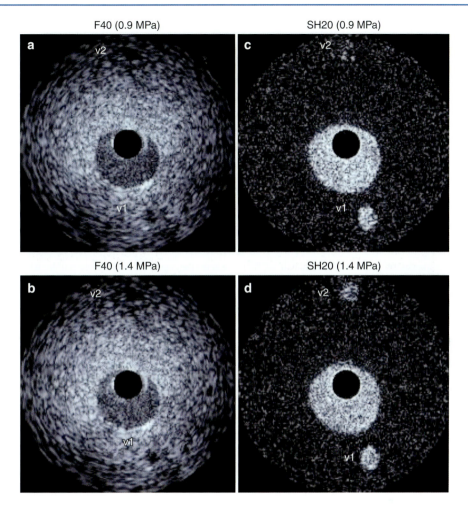

Fig. 8.6 Vessel phantom images using a small bubble agent for a 40 MHz transmit frequency. F40 images at two pressure levels (**a**, **b**) show agent within the main lumen and the "v1" vessel (5 o'clock) outside the main lumen. (**c**) In SH20 mode at 0.9 MPa, the CTR improves substantially for the main lumen, the "v1" vessel, while the "v2" vessel (12 o'clock) is at the edge of detection. (**d**) At a 1.4 MPa transmit level, the tissue signal does not increase, as in the H40 case, and the CTR for the "v2" vessel undergoes further improvements. Images are 12 mm in diameter. Display dynamic ranges are 40 dB for F40 and 25 dB for SH20 (Reprinted from Goertz et al.,[40] copyright 2006, with permission from Elsevier)

8.5.2 In Vivo Experiments

In vivo validation experiments were performed in atherosclerotic rabbit abdominal aortas at a transmit frequency of 30 MHz (subharmonic 15 MHz) using Definity™.[52] These experiments began with 3D IVUS imaging of the abdominal aorta using a pullback of a 40 MHz catheter with a Galaxy system (Boston Scientific Inc., Freemont CA, USA). This was done to ascertain the presence and extent of the atherosclerotic plaque and the resulting images, referred to as "BSci40" images, were used to compare with subsequently acquired data from the prototype IVUS system.

Following this, a 5 French agent delivery catheter with a helical release hole pattern was introduced through the carotid and its tip was situated approximately 1 cm below the lower renal artery branch point. The subharmonic IVUS catheter was then advanced through the femoral artery into the abdominal aorta and its transducer was located within 2–8 mm of a lumbar artery branch point. This procedure was guided by angiography, with radiopaque contrast released proximally through the delivery catheter. The location adjacent to a limbic branch point facilitated the co-registration of the images with histology derived from tissue harvested from these locations.

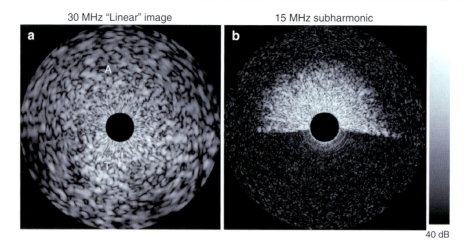

Fig. 8.7 Example images of phantom (bottom half – "T") and Definity agent (upper half – "A") for (**a**) conventional linear imaging at 30 MHz, where little difference is observed between agent and tissue and (**b**) for subharmonic imaging, where the agent is readily detectable while tissue signals are suppressed. Images are 12 mm in diameter (Reprinted from Goertz et al.,[52] copyright 2007, with permission from Elsevier)

An example longitudinal view of the BSci40 pullback data is shown in Fig. 8.8a, where the limbic artery branches and atherosclerotic plaque are evident. A cross-sectional image, taken in the vicinity of where the subharmonic imaging plane was located, is shown in Fig. 8.8b. The atherosclerotic plaque can be clearly demarcated as a slightly elliptical ring about the main lumen with a thickness ranging from 0.3 to 0.7 mm. The vena cava is also evident ("vc") along with several other vessels. "s" is a shunt vessel that, from an examination of the 3D data set, connects the immediately distal lumbar artery to the vena cava, joining it at a point approximately 1–2 mm proximal to (i.e., upstream of) the imaging plane. A small (~300 μm) microvessel "m" can also be seen 1 mm outside the aortic lumen at 7 o' clock. Two larger hypoechoic "vessels" can be seen also, one of which ("u" at 5 o'clock) is thought to be the ureter and the outer ("v" at 6 o'clock) a blood vessel. The F30 image from the prototype IVUS for this region is shown in Fig. 8.8c. While the image quality of the fundamental image has not been optimized, a number of common features can be observed, supporting that this is a similar location to that depicted with the BSci40 images, and is consistent with the angiogram guidance. Note also that there is a slight underrotation of the catheter due to nonuniform rotation of this older model catheter.

An example series of F30 and SH15 images acquired following a contrast injection is shown in Figs. 8.9a–e. Figure 8.9a shows the F30 and SH15 images immediately prior to the release of contrast agent, where in the SH15 image, the tissue signals are suppressed to near the noise floor. Shortly after the injection begins (~1–3 s), imaging was transiently obscured (not shown) due to the high attenuation levels associated with the passage of the bolus through the main lumen. By 3 s post injection, F30 imaging has recovered in amplitude and a ring of enhancement is evident in the SH15 image arising from agent at the boundary of the aortic lumen. This feature was previously observed with harmonic imaging in phantoms and harmonic experiment[50] and is consistent with the effects of more slowly moving flow near the vessel boundary. A smaller vessel is also observed at 6 o'clock, consistent with the "m" vessel in the BSci40 images. Moreover, several faint and discrete enhancements begin to appear within the adventitial region. At 5 s, the SH15 image (Fig. 8.9c) shows a fading ring and agent within the shunt vessel "s." Immediately outside the ring, there is no enhancement, consistent with an avascular plaque. Of particular interest is that there are also a number of small discrete enhancements within the adventitial region just outside the hypoechoic plaque region (e.g., 8–11 o'clock). Histology revealed that microvessels were present in the adventitia, as also found in other similar experiments.[50] Following the convention employed in Edelman et al. and Herrmann et al.,[51,53] these data support the detection of vasa vasorum. By 7 s (Fig. 8.9d), the ring has faded indicating the clearance

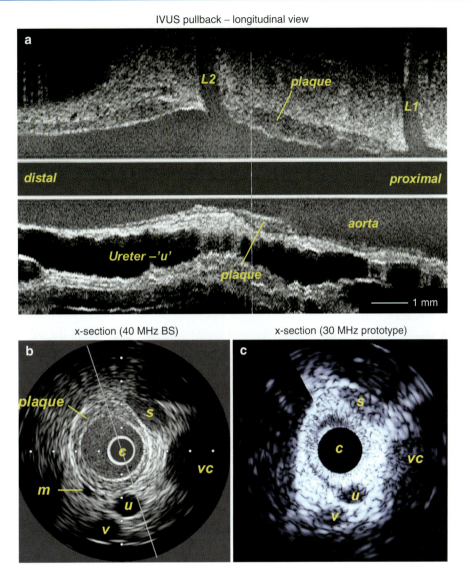

Fig. 8.8 (**a**) An example longitudinal section through a 3D BSci40 IVUS image of an atherosclerotic rabbit abdominal aorta. The plaque is evident, as well as two lumbar artery branches (L1 and L2). (**b**) A cross-sectional BSci image from the plane indicated in longitudinal section (1 mm between scale dots) clearly indicates an eccentric plaque, the vena cava (*vc*), a shunt vessel (*s*), a small vessel (*m*), a ureter (*u*), and another vessel (*v*). (**c**) A F30 prototype image (12 mm across) taken in this region shows several of these features (*s*, *vc*, *u*, and *v*), albeit with degraded image quality (Reprinted from Goertz et al.,[52] copyright 2007, with permission from Elsevier)

of the bolus from within the aortic lumen. The vessels "s" and "m" clearly have agent within then and, additionally, there is now agent return evident in the vena cava. A number of small adventitial enhancements also persist. At 10 s (Fig. 8.9e), the main lumen is more homogeneously enhanced, consistent with the effects of agent recirculation. The rabbits employed in this study were approximately 2 kg. This corresponds to an expected average blood recirculation time (defined as total volume/cardiac output[54]) of 20s. The observed arrival of recirculated agent is earlier than this, as would be expected when it is released and imaged within a large vessel with high blood velocities. The recirculation time will be longer for

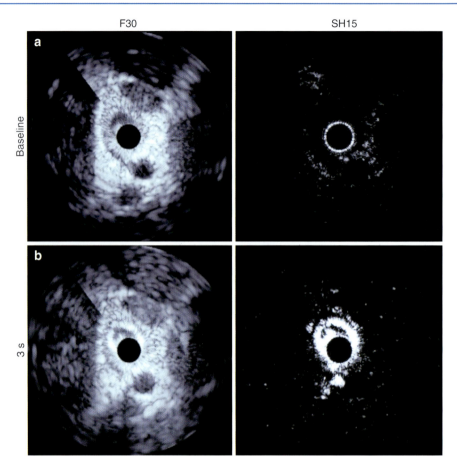

Fig. 8.9 Example of in vivo results in an atherosclerotic rabbit aorta for F30 (*left*) and SH15 imaging (*right*). (**a**) Baseline image immediately prior to contrast release shows the tissue signals suppressed to near the noise floor in SH15 images. (**b**) By 3 s post injection, after the passage of the main bolus, a ring is present at the aortic lumen boundary, and adventitial enhancement is evident in the SH15 images. (**c**) At 5 s, adventitial enhancement has increased, in a small vessel ("m" in Fig. 8.6b), the shunt ("s" in Fig. 8.6b) as well as in areas outside the lumen that are consistent with the location of vasa vasorum (e.g., 8–11 o'clock). (**d**) Ring has faded, and vena cava return is now apparent (3 o'clock). (**e**) Recirculation of agent is now evident as more homogenous enhancement within the aortic lumen. Images are 12 mm across (Reprinted from Goertz et al.,[52] copyright 2007, with permission from Elsevier)

larger animals (e.g., ~50s for 70 kg human) and the dilution ratio will be higher, both factors that will act to reduce this effect considerably.

8.6 Molecular Imaging

The use of targeted microbubble contrast agents in conjunction with IVUS holds considerable potential for gaining insight into the molecular status of atherosclerotic plaques, which may in turn impact plaque staging. These include markers for neovascular endothelial cells, inflammation, and thrombus. A number of reports have indicated the feasibility of imaging microbubbles targeted to endothelial cell adhesion molecules and fibrin at both lower frequencies and with conventional IVUS.[55,56] These studies relied upon simple enhancement of echogenicity to determine the presence of microbubbles and as such require the accumulation of considerable amounts of agent at the target sites. The authors, therefore, investigated the feasibility of performing bubble-specific imaging of targeted agent using the prototype nonlinear IVUS system.[57,58]

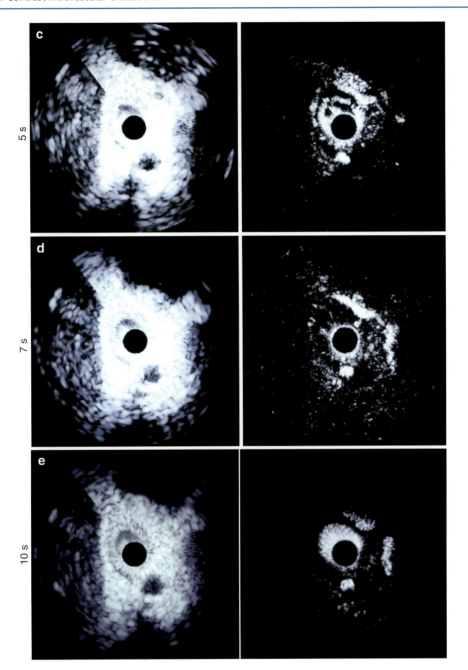

Fig. 8.9 (continued)

The agent examined was an experimental biotinated, lipid-encapsulated formulation comprised substantially of micron- and submicron-sized bubbles, which were targeted to an avidin-coated agar substrate (Fig. 8.10a). In fundamental (i.e., conventional "linear" imaging) mode (Fig. 8.10b), the agent is difficult to distinguish from background tissue signals. However, in second harmonic (not shown) and subharmonic (Fig. 8.10c) modes, the agent is clearly detected, with tissue signals being suppressed to below the noise floor. These results demonstrate the feasibility of harmonic imaging as a strategy for improving the sensitivity and specificity of targeted contrast agent detection at high ultrasound frequencies.

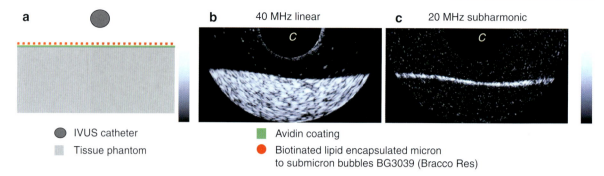

Fig. 8.10 Example of nonlinear IVUS imaging of targeted microbubbles in vitro. (**a**) Microbubbles are targeted to the surface of a tissue mimicking phantom, with the IVUS transducer axis oriented perpendicular to the surface. (**b**) An example 40 MHz "conventional" linear image of the bubbles and tissue phantom, where it is difficult to distinguish the bubbles form the tissue. (**c**) Subharmonic image derived from the same data clearly shows the microbubble layer while suppressing the tissue signal

8.7 Summary and Future Perspectives

Nonlinear IVUS contrast imaging has been shown to be feasible as an approach for imaging vasa vasorum associated with atherosclerosis in a preclinical context. It has been shown to be viable with a clinically available agent as well as with experimental agents comprised primarily of smaller bubbles. The approaches investigated are compatible with implementation on commercial platforms and early results in animal experiments are now being reported with these systems.[42] At the time of writing, these approaches were not available for clinical use, though it is anticipated that they will be in the near future. This technology is in its early stages of development and there is considerable room for improving its performance.

Despite recent advances, a great deal remains unknown about the specific mechanisms of vasa vasorum involvement in the progression and instability of plaques. Within this context, IVUS contrast imaging is suitable for longitudinal studies of the role of vasa vasorum in the pathogenesis of atherosclerosis as well as for preclinical therapeutic studies. Such experiments may be particularly relevant due to the lack of other techniques capable of in vivo high-resolution monitoring of vasa vasorum, and should also provide a foundation for understanding the potential role and limitations of contrast IVUS in future clinical applications. It is anticipated that they will conceivably have application to gain further insight into the natural history of atherosclerosis, the effects of novel therapeutic strategies, and possibly as a marker of plaque vulnerability.

References

1. Schoenhagen P, Ziada KM, Vince DG, Nissen SE, Tuzcu EM. Arterial remodeling and coronary artery disease: the concept of "dilated" versus "obstructive" coronary atherosclerosis. *J Am Coll Cardiol*. 2001;38:297–306.
2. Nicholls SJ et al. Application of intravascular ultrasound in anti-atherosclerotic drug development. *Nat Rev Drug Discov*. 2006;5(6):485–492.
3. Nissen SE, Yock P. Intravascular ultrasound: novel pathophysiological insights and current clinical applications. *Circulation*. 2001;103(4):604–616.
4. Glaser R et al. Clinical progression of incidental, asymptomatic lesions discovered during culprit vessel coronary intervention. *Circulation*. 2005;111(2):143–149.
5. Schaar JA et al. Terminology for high-risk and vulnerable coronary artery plaques. Report of a meeting on the vulnerable plaque, June 17 and 18, 2003, Santorini, Greece. *Eur Heart J*. 2004;25(12):1077–1082.
6. Waxman S, Ishibashi F, Muller JE. Detection and treatment of vulnerable plaques and vulnerable patients: novel approaches to prevention of coronary events. *Circulation*. 2006;114(22):2390–2411.
7. Virmani R, Kolodgie FD, Burke AP, Farb A, Schwartz SM. Lessons from sudden coronary death: a comprehensive morphological classification scheme for atherosclerotic lesions. *Arterioscler Thromb Vasc Biol*. 2000;20(5):1262–1275.
8. Virmani R, Burke AP, Farb A, Kolodgie FD. Pathology of the vulnerable plaque. *J Am Coll Cardiol*. 2006;47(8 suppl):C13-C18.
9. Schaar JA et al. Characterizing vulnerable plaque features with intravascular elastography. *Circulation*. 2003;108(21):2636–2641.
10. Nair A et al. Coronary plaque classification with intravascular ultrasound radiofrequency data analysis. *Circulation*. 2002;106(17):2200–2206.
11. Williams JK, Heistad DD. Structure and function of vasa vasorum. *Trends Cardiovasc Med*. 1996;6(2):53–57.
12. Kwon HM et al. Enhanced coronary vasa vasorum neovascularization in experimental hypercholesterolemia. *J Clin Invest*. 1998;101(8):1551–1556.

13. Zhang Y, Cliff WJ, Schoefl GI, Higgins G. Immunohistochemical study of intimal microvessels in coronary atherosclerosis. *Am J Pathol.* 1993;143(1):164–172.
14. Moreno PR, Purushothaman KR, Fuster V, et al. Plaque neovascularization is increased in ruptured atherosclerotic lesions of human aorta: implications for plaque vulnerability. *Circulation.* 2004;110(14):2032–2038.
15. Kumamoto M, Nakashima Y, Sueishi K. Intimal neovascularization in human coronary atherosclerosis: its origin and pathophysiological significance. *Hum Pathol.* 1995;26(4):450–456.
16. de Boer OJ, van der Wal AC, Teeling P, Becker AE. Leucocyte recruitment in rupture prone regions of lipid-rich plaques: a prominent role for neovascularization? *Cardiovasc Res.* 1999;41(2):443–449.
17. Moulton KS et al. Inhibition of plaque neovascularization reduces macrophage accumulation and progression of advanced atherosclerosis. *Proc Natl Acad Sci USA.* 2001;100(8):4736–4741.
18. Kolodgie FD et al. Intraplaque hemorrhage and progression of coronary atheroma. *N Engl J Med.* 2003;349(24):2316–2325.
19. Milei J et al. Carotid rupture and intraplaque hemorrhage: immunophenotype and role of cells involved. *Am Heart J.* 1998;136(6):1096–1105.
20. Moulton KS. Angiogenesis in atherosclerosis: gathering evidence beyond speculation. *Curr Opin Lipidol.* 2006;17(5):548–555.
21. Kerwin W et al. Quantitative magnetic resonance imaging analysis of neovasculature volume in carotid atherosclerotic plaque. *Circulation.* 2003;107(6):851–856.
22. Feinstein SB. The powerful microbubble: from bench to bedside, from intravascular indicator to therapeutic delivery system, and beyond. *Am J Physiol Heart Circ Physiol.* 2004;287(2):H450-H457.
23. Kruse DE, Ferrara KW. A new high resolution color flow system using an eigendecomposition-based adaptive filter for clutter rejection. *IEEE Trans Ultrason Ferroelectr Freq Control.* 2002;49(10):1384–1399.
24. Goertz DE, Yu JL, Kerbel RS, Burns PN, Foster FS. High-frequency 3-D color-flow imaging of the microcirculation. *Ultrasound Med Biol.* 2003;29(1):39–51.
25. Carlier S et al. Vasa vasorum imaging: a new window to the clinical detection of vulnerable atherosclerotic plaques. *Curr Atheroscler Rep.* 2005;7(2):164–169.
26. Kakadiaris I et al. Intravascular ultrasound-based imaging of vasa vasorum for the detection of vulnerable atherosclerotic plaque. *J Am Coll Cardiol.* 2006;47(4 suppl A):264A.
27. Vavuranakis M et al. A new method for assessment of plaque vulnerability based on vasa vasorum imaging, by using contrast-enhanced intravascular ultrasound and differential image analysis. *Int J Cardiol.* 2008;130(1):23–29.
28. O'Malley SM, Vavuranakis M, Naghavi M, Kakadiaris IA. Intravascular ultrasound-based imaging of vasa vasorum for the detection of vulnerable atherosclerotic plaque. *Med Image Comput Comput Assist Interv.* 2005;8(Pt 1):343–351.
29. Shi WT, Forsberg F. Ultrasonic characterization of the nonlinear properties of contrast microbubbles. *Ultrasound Med Biol.* 2000;26(1):93–104.
30. Gorce JM, Arditi M, Schneider M. Influence of bubble size distribution on the echogenicity of ultrasound contrast agents: a study of Sonovue. *Invest Radiol.* 2000;35(11):661–671.
31. Sarkar K, Shi WT, Chatterjee D, Forsberg F. Characterization of ultrasound contrast microbubbles using in vitro experiments and viscous and viscoelastic interface models for encapsulation. *J Acoust Soc Am.* 2005;118(1):539–550.
32. Goertz DE, de Jong N, van der Steen AF. Attenuation and size distribution measurements of Definity and manipulated Definity populations. *Ultrasound Med Biol.* 2007;33(9):1376–1388.
33. Goertz DE, Frijlink ME, Voormolen MM, de Jong N, van der Steen AF. High frequency attenuation measurements of lipid encapsulated contrast agents. *Ultrasonics.* 2006;44(suppl 1):e131–e134.
34. Goertz DE et al. High frequency nonlinear B-scan imaging of microbubble contrast agents. *IEEE Trans Ultrason Ferroelectr Freq Control.* 2005;52(1):65–79.
35. Goertz DE, Frijlink ME, de Jong N, van der Steen AF. High frequency nonlinear scattering from a micrometer to submicrometer sized lipid encapsulated contrast agent. *Ultrasound Med Biol.* 2006;32(4):569–577.
36. Cheung K et al. In vitro characterization of the subharmonic ultrasound signal from Definity microbubbles at high frequencies. *Phys Med Biol.* 2008;53(5):1209–1223.
37. Bouakaz A, Versluis M, Borsboom J, de Jong N. Radial modulation of microbubbles for ultrasound contrast imaging. *IEEE Trans Ultrason Ferroelectr Freq Control.* 2007;54(11):2283–2290.
38. Masoy SE, Standal O, Nasholm P, Johansen TF, Angelsen B. SURF imaging: in vivo demonstration of an ultrasound contrast agent detection technique. *IEEE Trans Ultrason Ferroelectr Freq Control.* 2008;55(5):1112–1121.
39. Vos HJ, Goertz DE, de Jong N. Pulse repetition rate excitation of contrast agents. In: IEEE Ultrasonics Symposium; October 2–6, 2006; Vancouver:216–219.
40. Goertz DE, Frijlink ME, de Jong N, van der Steen AF. Nonlinear intravascular ultrasound contrast imaging. *Ultrasound Med Biol.* 2006;32(4):491–502.
41. Simpson DH, Chin CT, Burns PN. Pulse inversion Doppler: a new method for detecting nonlinear echoes from microbubble contrast agents. *IEEE Trans Ultrason Ferroelectr Freq Control.* 1999;46(2):372–382.
42. Granada JF, Feinstein SB. Imaging of the vasa vasorum. *Nat Clin Pract Cardiovasc Med.* 2008;5(suppl 2):S18-S25.
43. Frijlink ME, Goertz DE, Bouakaz A, van der Steen AF. A simulation study on tissue harmonic imaging with a single-element intravascular ultrasound catheter. *J Acoust Soc Am.* 2006;120(3):1723–1731.
44. Frijlink ME, Goertz DE, de Jong N, van der Steen AF. Pulse inversion sequences for mechanically scanned transducers. *IEEE Trans Ultrason Ferroelectr Freq Control.* 2008;55(10):2154–2163.
45. Frijlink ME et al. Harmonic intravascular ultrasound imaging with a dual-frequency catheter. *Ultrasound Med Biol.* 2006;32(11):1649–1654.
46. Vos HJ et al. Transducer for harmonic intravascular ultrasound imaging. *IEEE Trans Ultrason Ferroelectr Freq Control.* 2005;52(12):2418–2422.
47. Yuan Y, Rhee S, Jiang XN. 60 MHz PMN-PT based 1–3 composite transducer for IVUS imaging. In: IEEE Ultrasonics Symposium; November 2–5, 2008; Beijing:682–685.

48. Degertekin FL, Guldiken RO, Karaman M. Annular-ring CMUT arrays for forward-looking IVUS: transducer characterization and imaging. *IEEE Trans Ultrason Ferroelectr Freq Control*. 2006;53(3):474–482.
49. Schaar JA et al. Three-dimensional palpography of human coronary arteries. Ex vivo validation and in-patient evaluation. *Herz*. 2005;30(2):125–133.
50. Goertz DE et al. Contrast harmonic intravascular ultrasound: a feasibility study for vasa vasorum imaging. *Invest Radiol*. 2006;41(8):631–638.
51. Edelman ER, Nugent MA, Smith LT, Karnovsky MJ. Basic fibroblast growth factor enhances the coupling of intimal hyperplasia and proliferation of vasa vasorum in injured rat arteries. *J Clin Invest*. 1992;89(2):465–473.
52. Goertz DE et al. Subharmonic contrast intravascular ultrasound for vasa vasorum imaging. *Ultrasound Med Biol*. 2007;33(12):1859–1872.
53. Herrmann J et al. Coronary vasa vasorum neovascularization precedes epicardial endothelial dysfunction in experimental hypercholesterolemia. *Cardiovasc Res*. 2001;51(4):762–766.
54. Schmidt-Nielsen K. *Scaling: Why Is Animal Size So Important?* Cambridge: Cambridge University Press; 1984.
55. Ellegala DB et al. Imaging tumor angiogenesis with contrast ultrasound and microbubbles targeted to alpha(v)beta3. *Circulation*. 2003;108(3):336–341.
56. Demos SM et al. In vivo targeting of acoustically reflective liposomes for intravascular and transvascular ultrasonic enhancement. *J Am Coll Cardiol*. 1999;33(3):867–875.
57. Goertz DE, van Wamel A, Frijlink ME, de Jong N, van der Steen AFW. Nonlinear imaging of targeted microbubbles with intravascular ultrasound. In: IEEE International Ultrasonics Symposium; September 18–21, 2005; Rotterdam: 2003–2006.
58. Goertz DE, Frijlink ME, Krams R, de Jong N, van der Steen AF. Vasa vasorum and molecular imaging of atherosclerotic plaques using nonlinear contrast intravascular ultrasound. *Neth Heart J*. 2007;15(2):77–80.

Molecular Imaging of Carotid Plaque with Targeted Ultrasound Contrast

Joshua J. Rychak and Alexander L. Klibanov

9.1 Introduction

Just about a decade ago, targeted or molecular[1] imaging with ultrasound contrast agents was deemed impossible. However, with the advances of ultrasound imaging equipment and improved design of ultrasound contrast agents, the old point of view could be reconsidered. Currently, ultrasound contrast agents are widely investigated as the imaging tools for molecular imaging of the specific markers, mostly for the targets located within the vascular bed.[2] Most of the studies are performed in vivo in the animal model setting and clinical trials are expected to follow in the near future. Unique advantages of ultrasound imaging are the ease of use, real-time (>20 frames per second) imaging in 2D and 3D, low equipment cost, and high mobility and portability (full-scale D2 and 3D ultrasound imaging systems are already implemented as laptops). Modern ultrasound contrast agents (microbubbles, typically several micrometers in diameter) provide superb detection sensitivity (i.e., the ability to image individual microbubbles in the vasculature in real time) and therefore are associated with a low required dose of injected contrast, especially as compared with computer tomography (CT) and magnetic resonance imaging (MRI) contrast agents.

J.J. Rychak
Department of Research, Targeson Inc., San Diego, CA, USA

A.L. Klibanov (✉)
Department of Medicine, Cardiovascular Division, University of Virginia, Charlottesville, VA, USA

This unique combination of ultrasound imaging capabilities makes ultrasound a useful choice for the investigation of vascular plaques, either with transcutaneous imaging devices, or with the use of intravascular ultrasound (Chap. 8). Molecular markers on the vascular endothelium in the areas of plaque vulnerability are well known: P- and E-selectins, ICAM-1, VCAM-1, etc.[3] Such markers can be selectively imaged by targeted microbubbles. The purpose of this chapter is to evaluate the targeted ultrasound imaging strategies that are currently available in the field and discuss their application for imaging of atherosclerotic plaques in the carotid vasculature setting.

9.2 Molecular Imaging with Microbubble Contrast: General Considerations

The general strategy of molecular imaging with microbubble contrast agents is exactly the same as in case of other ligand–receptor imaging modalities: the ligand is attached to the label, injected in the body (usually intravenously), and following a dwell time period, imaging is performed. Dwell time is needed for two reasons. First, one is to allow the labeled ligand to circulate within the body and have a chance to accumulate in the target regions, such as areas of high concentration of the target receptor, where the targeting ligand could attach. The second reason is to allow the removal of excess of the labeled ligand from the bloodstream to reduce the nonspecific tissue background response. Both of these steps are accomplished in the case of targeted ultrasound contrast agents. However, unlike the case of other labels (such as radioactive probes used in nuclear medicine, or optical dyes used in optical imaging, which mostly clear through the kidney excretion), the gas contained inside the microbubble contrast agent is mostly removed from the body by exhalation.[4]

Traditionally, microbubbles used for molecular imaging need to be stabilized to be able to circulate in the bloodstream for at least several minutes. Early generation of agents with thin-shelled microbubbles such as Albunex (Molecular Biosystems Inc., San Diego, California, USA; Mallinckrodt Inc., Hazelwood, Missouri, USA; Nycomed, Oslo, Norway) or Levovist (Schering AG, Berlin, Germany) lose gas quite rapidly after intravenous administration. Two main strategies to extend circulation time of microbubbles exist. The most popular strategy is to use a poorly soluble gas core for the microbubble construction, such as (progressively lesser solubility): sulfur hexafluoride (Sonovue microbubble, Bracco S. P.A., Milan, Italy); perfluoropropane (Optison [GE Healthcare, Milwaukee, Wisconsin, USA] and Definity [Lantheus Medical Imaging, North Billerica, Massachusetts, USA]/Luminity [Lantheus Medical Imaging, United Kingdom Ltd.]); perfluorobutane (BR14 [Bracco, Milan, Italy], Sonazoid [GE Healthcare, Milwaukee, Wisconsin, USA], MicroMarker [Visualsonics Inc., Toronto, Ontario, Canada; Bracco, Geneva, Switzerland], Targestar [Targeson, Inc., San Diego, California, USA]). These low solubility gases allow microbubbles with thin flexible shells (such as a lipid monolayer) that do not provide good barrier properties for gas exchange to circulate in the bloodstream for many minutes, instead of just seconds as it happens with air- or nitrogen-filled bubbles. Many of the microbubble preparations described above have achieved clinical approval or are at preclinical application stage (or have been in widespread clinical trials).

An alternative approach, that so far has reached only the widespread clinical trials stage, is to use a thicker polymer shell (tens or even hundreds of nm thick); the polymer needs to be biocompatible and biodegradable, such as poly-butyl-cyanoacrylate, Sonovist (Schering AG, Berlin, Germany)[5] or polylactide/PLGA (PB-127 [Point Biomedical, San Carlos, California, USA],[6] Imagify [Acusphere Inc., Lexington, Massachusetts, USA][7]). The latter agent combines both approaches: It uses a polymer foam shell doped with phospholipids, and decafluorobutane gas core, to improve stability and circulation time. Thick-shell microbubbles based on the telechelic cross-linked polyvinyl alcohol gel shell have been proposed also.[8] Unfortunately, detection of thick-shelled microbubbles by ultrasound imaging requires high-mechanical index (MI) destructive pulses, and this is not efficient with low-MI real-time imaging.[9]

9.3 Targeted Microbubble Imaging Techniques: Attaining High Signal-to-Background Ratio

Active microbubble targeting requires decorating the microbubble shell with a specific ligand, which has to be firmly anchored to the shell and should not be pulled out easily if firm binding to the target is to be achieved. In some instances, the targeting ligand, e.g., lipid, such as phosphatidylserine,[10] or protein, such as avidin,[11] is not tethered to the shell, but it is actually part of the shell. However, more often the targeting ligand is attached to the microbubble shell via a flexible tether/spacer arm, e.g., polyethylene glycol (PEG) polymer with a molecular mass of several thousands and degree of polymerization of up to ~100. Use of the long tether improves targeting efficacy[12,13].

Detection of microbubbles by ultrasound imaging is quite sensitive: Individual microbubble particles, with picogram mass and size of several micrometers, can be detected by ultrasound.[14] Figure 9.1 provides an image of the dilute microbubble dispersion in saline; each speckle on the screen of the imaging system corresponds to an individual microbubble in the imaging plane of the ultrasound transducer. The size and shape of the speckles is defined by the point-spread function determined by the imaging equipment.

The ability to detect targeted microbubbles in their target location is greatly enhanced by the recent advances in ultrasound imaging equipment, using multipulse techniques, such as Cadence Contrast Pulse Sequences[15] or Pulse-Inversion Amplitude Modulation.[16] These techniques take advantage of nonlinear properties of microbubble scattering behavior and allow complete suppression of the background tissue ultrasound signal, while providing efficient detection of microbubbles. One technique of microbubble detection in the tissue is by subtraction[17]: If a higher-intensity ultrasound pulse is applied, microbubbles deposited in the target are destroyed,

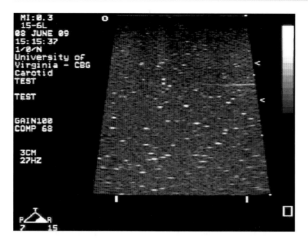

Fig. 9.1 Ultrasound imaging of a very dilute dispersion of decafluorobutane microbubbles, coated with a monolayer of phosphatidylcholine and PEG stearate in normal saline. Individual contrast speckles represent images of individual microbubbles suspended in the aqueous medium (mean bubble size ~2 um, microbubble mass ~ 1 pg). Imaging performed with L15-6 transducer and Philips Sonos 7500 imaging system (Philips, Andover, Massachusetts, USA)

and the level of residual circulating microbubbles can be evaluated. This technique can be not only applied for the modern linear array or phase array devices, capable of multipulse sequences, but also in the single-element mechanically steered transducer systems, such as a high-frequency small-animal imaging system, Visualsonics vevo770 (Visualsonics, Toronto, Ontario, Canada).[18]

The time between microbubble bolus administration and imaging is relatively short, as compared with other contrast imaging modalities, such as positron emission tomography (PET), single photon emission-computed tomography (SPECT), or MRI. Ultrasound imaging of targeted microbubbles in murine models is typically performed 5–10 min after bolus injection of contrast agent (may be somewhat longer for larger animals[19] and humans). During this period, microbubble concentration in the bloodstream is decreased greatly, and, thus nonspecific background signal from circulating ultrasound contrast is reduced. The mechanism of this rapid blood contrast reduction is mostly due to gas loss from the microbubble core due to gas exchange through the thin (several nm) bubble shell and exhalation.[4] This may be useful, because it implies rapid reduction of nonspecific background signal in the bulk of blood. Hypothetically, gas loss from microbubbles that are already attached to the target, especially at the areas of slower blood flow, might be slower, which would potentially help boost signal-to-noise ratio. However, this also means that the flux of circulating bubbles through the potential target areas will be reduced quite rapidly with the reduction of the level of circulating microbubbles, and may need some improvement for effective target delineation.

Improvement of targeting efficacy is possible by using the radiation force of the ultrasound field: a pressure wave that can displace microbubbles without destroying them. This technique was first shown to deflect microbubbles from the center of the 0.2 mm diameter tube in a flow-through setting so that they would be forced to touch the wall of the tube and be retained there despite the flow.[20] This approach may be quite useful for targeting, because normally, in larger vessels, such as arterioles and postcapillary venules, most of the circulating particles are distributed in the bulk of the blood and do not come in close contact with the vessel wall. These microbubbles normally pass through the lumen of the vessel without a chance to touch the target endothelium surface so that specific vessel wall disease markers are not probed efficiently.

Following the initial ultrasound-induced deflection and retention studies with non-targeted microbubbles, it was shown that improvement of targeting of microbubbles with the specific ligand–receptor interaction could be achieved in model systems in vitro[21,22], and later in vivo[23] in a murine vascular inflammation model: Anti-P-selectin antibody targeting of microbubbles in the inflamed femoral vasculature was greatly enhanced by radiation force application, especially in the arterial fast-flow conditions with high wall shear stress.

In addition to the increase of the concentration of microbubbles close to the target surface, radiation force application may decelerate and even transiently stop the bubble motion along the axis of the vessel, which increases the time of contact between the ligand-carrying microbubble and the target, especially in wide vessels.[24] This is also helpful for the success of the targeting event, because in many of ligand-targeted microbubble situations, adhesion in the fast (physiological) flow conditions is inefficient,[25] and time for the contact between the ligand-carrying bubble and receptor-expressing endothelial target is critical for the success of the targeting event. This improvement of targeting efficacy may be of special importance for the success of clinical applications, because higher targeting efficacy, e.g., by nearly two orders of magnitude,[22] implies respectively a much lower injected dose of contrast agent.

9.4 Ultrasound Molecular Imaging of General Inflammatory Conditions: Phosphatidylserine Microbubbles

Based on the existing data,[3] one may expect that an inflammatory condition exists in the area of plaque development. One of the important steps of this event is the accumulation of leukocytes (e.g., neutrophils), which are brought into the tissue via the vascular route. Activated endothelium in the inflamed vasculature expresses P- and E-selectins, as well as other adhesion molecules on the cell surface. Leukocytes in the bloodstream, when exposed to these markers, become involved in a cascade of events that starts with slow rolling, leading to firm adhesion, diapedesis, and entry into the tissue of interest.[26] Leukocytes that adhere to the vessel wall in the region of interest can be detected by molecular imaging techniques, including targeted contrast ultrasound. Leukocyte detection by phosphatidylserine-targeted microbubble contrast has been in the preclinical study stage for nearly a decade.[10]

Phosphatidylserine is a known natural enhancer of particle binding and uptake by any phagocytic cell, including neutrophils. Therefore, if there are neutrophils present on the vessel wall, and phosphatidylserine-carrying microbubbles are injected in the bloodstream, they selectively bind to these cells and mark the area of inflammation (Fig. 9.2). This approach has been successfully tested in the models of inflammation, including tumor necrosis factor (TNF)-alpha-induced response,[10] or ischemia-reperfusion injury,[19] including myocardial ischemia. Actual clinical application of this targeted imaging approach may be the closest to practical use, because there are phosphatidylserine-shelled microbubbles authorized for clinical application already: Sonazoid is an approved microbubble contrast agent in use for liver radiology indications in Japan. The mechanism of Sonazoid microbubble accumulation in normal liver tissue is by Kupffer cell uptake.[27] However, one can

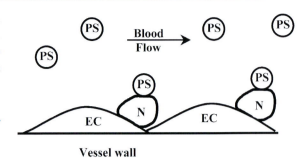

Fig. 9.2 Targeting active inflammatory event with phosphatidylserine microbubbles. In the inflamed vasculature, activated endothelial cells (*EC*) are overexpressing ICAM-1, VCAM-1, and P- and E-selectin. Circulating neutrophils (*N*) attach to these receptors on endothelial lining via their specific ligands, such as PSGL-1 and VLA-4, first by slow rolling, followed by firm adhesion. Before these activated neutrophils transfer out of the vessel into the interstitial space, phosphatidylserine-containing microbubbles (*PS*) can bind to them, and be retained on the target after circulating bubbles disappear from the circulation

expect that these microbubbles would bind to any actively phagocytic leukocyte. Therefore, clinical testing of these microbubbles for inflammation imaging could be achievable without the need for the development of a novel contrast agent.

9.5 Molecular Imaging of the Atherosclerotic Plaque Markers

Despite the potential applicability of simple phosphatidylserine microbubbles for imaging general inflammatory conditions as described above, this approach does not provide information on the exact molecular pattern of the compounds expressed on the vascular endothelium in the regions of interest. True molecular imaging of these markers requires the use of more specific targeting ligands that will specifically attach to the molecules that are upregulated in the active plaque regions. Receptors of interest are numerous, such as P- and E-selectin, ICAM-1, VCAM-1, vascular endothelial growth factor (VEGF) receptor 1 and 2, LOX-1, and matrix metalloproteinases. In addition to endothelial-related markers, targeting of adherent platelets (which express P-selectin and GP IIbIIIa) may also be of interest.

Microbubbles targeted to most of these markers (or their combinations) have been in the experimental testing stage for the past decade. The studies were

Fig. 9.3 Targeted ultrasound contrast molecular imaging of the atherosclerotic murine vasculature. Microbubbles decorated with anti-VCAM-1 antibody, 7,500 molecules per um² of microbubble surface (**a**) or control microbubbles (**b**) were injected in an apoE −/− mouse following a 10-week high-cholesterol diet. Imaging was performed with Siemens Sequoia 15L8 transducer (Siemens Medical Solutions, Malvern, Pennsylvania, USA) in CPS mode; image presented as CPS-grayscale mix

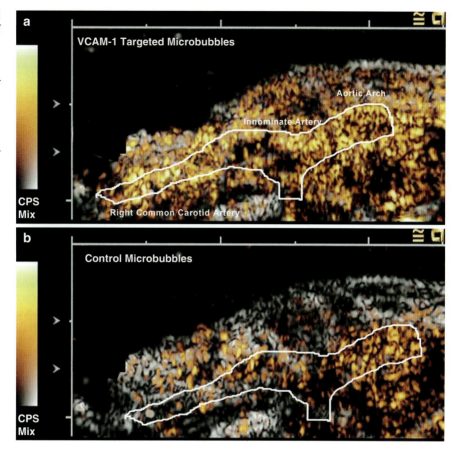

first initiated in the setting of an in vitro system (with avidin as the model target coating a Petri dish) and biotin-carrying microbubbles[28] and soon expanded into more realistic targets. First, microbubbles were decorated with antibodies against ICAM-1 to target ICAM-1-expressing activated human endothelium in vitro.[29] Next, anti-P-selectin antibody was attached to the bubble shell for targeting and ultrasound imaging of model inflammatory conditions in murine setting.[17] Later, in order to improve targeting efficacy, especially in fast-flow conditions, a combination of two ligands on the bubble surface was applied: Sialyl Lewis X (a ligand targeting P- and E-selectin) was combined with anti-ICAM-1 antibody.[30] Polymeric version of sialyl Lewis X allowed successful microbubble targeting in fast-flow conditions in vitro and in vivo[31]: This ligand adheres to selectin target much faster than the anti-P-selectin antibody does, hence it is more efficient in fast-flow microbubble targeting physiological situations. Anti-ICAM-1 and anti-VCAM-1 antibodies were attached to the polylactide microbubble surface with the intent to target these receptors; in vitro detection sensitivity of 40 particles per mm² was achieved.[32] Recently, Kaufmann et al[33] demonstrated that microbubbles targeted to P-selectin or to VCAM-1 successfully accumulated in and enhance ultrasound images of inflamed plaque in the model of atherosclerosis in mice.

A combination of a sialyl Lewis ligand and anti-VCAM-1 antibody on the same bubble further improves targeting efficacy as proven in vitro in the parallel plate chamber flow studies.[34] In vivo examples of the successful application of P-, E-selectin and VCAM-1 targeting by such microbubbles that were decorated with both polymeric sialyl Lewis X and anti-VCAM-1 antibody have been reported for apoE -/- mice on high-cholesterol diet.[35] An example of ultrasound contrast imaging (Fig. 9.3) showed significant anti-VCAM-1-targeted (a), but not control (b), microbubble accumulation in the vasculature of atherosclerotic mice. The locations of ascending aorta, innominate artery, and proximal portion of the right common carotid artery in this study (marked on Fig. 9.3a as blue contour) were determined by long axis view ultrasound imaging using B-mode and color Doppler.

Targeting adherent platelets on the vessel wall may be another viable strategy for active plaque imaging (in addition to being the essential component of blood clot, adherent platelets may be also present in the inflamed vasculature).[17] Following activation, P-selectin appears on platelet surface and can be targeted by the respective sialyl Lewis oligosaccharide ligands. Such microbubble targeting was successfully demonstrated recently in very high shear flow conditions (up to 40 dyn/cm^2 wall shear stress) in the parallel plate flow chamber of an in vitro model.[36] Another platelet surface marker, GP IIbIIIa, has been tested as a receptor for clot imaging with targeted microbubbles in vitro and in vivo.[37] Possibly, a combination of both of these ligands on microbubble surface may be useful for targeting.

An important technological consideration for the ligand-microbubble design is the technique for ligand attachment. In the numerous preclinical animal studies, biotinylated ligands, such as antibodies, are attached to the microbubble shell via a streptavidin protein linker[17,18]. Many biotinylated ligands (mostly antibodies) against numerous receptors are available commercially, or could be easily prepared by routine biotinylation. However, streptavidin is a foreign protein to humans, and a risk of anaphylactic reaction associated with its administration to patients should be avoided. Therefore, covalent attachment of ligands to the microbubble shell is preferable.[29] Still, the use of antibodies, with their bulky and potentially immunogenic FC-fragment, is questionable, so humanized or fully human FV antibody fragments should be preferred. The best strategy would be to use small (e.g., peptide or peptidomimetic) ligands, which should not be immunogenic per se, and would be easy to attach to the microbubble surface covalently and in an oriented manner.[38]

9.6 Future Applications and Specific Ultrasound/Carotid Considerations

Attention should first turn to the pioneering work of the Feinstein group,[39] who had brought into the clinic the use of non-targeted perfusion microbubbles to evaluate the functional neovasculature within the active carotid plaque. Based on their success, further characterization of the molecular pattern of plaque neovasculature could be considered. Several receptors might be used for targeted microbubble imaging of plaque and specifically for the characterization of plaque vulnerability. As indicated above, they include targets such as VEGF receptors (overexpressed on endothelial vasa vasorum neovasculature in the active plaque area) and matrix metalloproteinases,[40] as well as LOX-1.[41] Antibodies and other ligands have been available for these receptors; such compounds have been attached to the microbubble shell routinely. It is crucial to target the receptors on vascular endothelial luminal surface, because current microbubble size (several microns) restricts all the targeting efforts to the intravascular space. One such example of ultrasound molecular imaging of plaque neovasculature with microbubbles carrying an antibody against VEGF Receptor 2 is provided in Fig. 9.4, demonstrating successful targeting of microbubbles in an atherosclerosis model apoE −/− mouse on a high-cholesterol diet, but not in control mice.

Recently, a BR-55 peptide-carrying microbubble preparation targeted to VEGF Receptor 2 has been described.[38] This agent may be approaching clinical trials in the near future. It has been shown to attach selectively and enhance ultrasound signal of the solid tumor vasculature in a rat model. This contrast agent might be useful for targeted imaging of the vasa vasorum neovasculature of atherosclerotic plaque, and characterization of plaque in the carotid arteries is the obvious step to be taken.

The superficial location of the carotid bifurcation makes imaging of the plaque by ultrasound in this setting much easier compared with other vessels, e.g., coronary. Direct access (no ribcage) to the imaging area and the shallow location of the vessels allow successful use of higher frequencies for transcutaneous ultrasound imaging. Based on the frequency range of available clinical system transducers, it should be possible to achieve spatial resolution approaching 0.2 mm or even better. Intravascular ultrasound (IVUS, up to 60 MHz frequency of operation) will improve spatial resolution several-fold (Chap. 8). However, compared with coronary vasculature, in the case of carotid artery imaging, IVUS image quality improvement is not going to be as dramatic when compared with ~1–2-mm spatial resolution normally applicable for human cardiac ultrasound. The invasiveness of

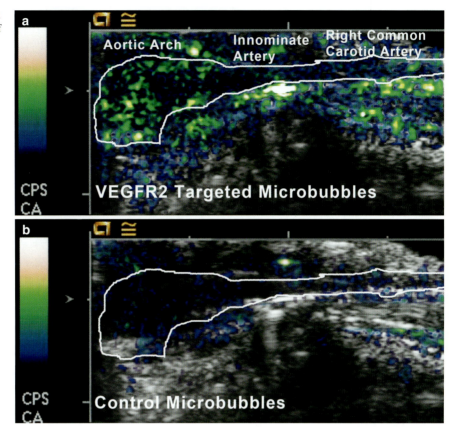

Fig. 9.4 Targeted ultrasound contrast molecular imaging of the atherosclerotic murine vasculature. Microbubbles decorated with anti-VEGFR2 antibody were injected in an apoE −/− mouse on a high-cholesterol diet (**a**) or wild-type control C57BL/6 mice (**b**). Imaging performed with Siemens Sequoia 15L8 transducer in CPS mode

IVUS may make it less attractive for purely diagnostic imaging, especially if pharmacological (e.g., statin) plaque treatment strategy is selected. IVUS ultrasound with targeted contrast could aid in the proper stent placement guidance in the region of a high-risk plaque. However, the spatial resolution of high-frequency ultrasound may actually be too high to be useful for molecular ultrasound contrast imaging. Furthermore, at higher frequencies, microbubble detection is not as efficient as it is at 1–10 MHz. Therefore, a fine detail image of plaque structure at 0.05-mm resolution might not be valuable if it is accompanied by a significant loss of the targeted microbubble imaging capability.

9.7 Conclusion

Overall, ultrasound molecular imaging with targeted microbubbles may become a powerful tool for detection and characterization of the carotid plaque. Microbubble contrast agents suitable for this application are either already available commercially, or are approaching the clinical trial stage.

9.8 Acknowledgment and Disclosures

A.L. Klibanov is supported in part via NIH R33CA102880 and R01EB002185. Valuable discussions with K. Ley, J. Lindner, M. Lawrence, and J. Hossack are gratefully acknowledged by authors. A.L. Klibanov and J.J. Rychak are shareholders of Targeson Inc; J.J. Rychak is employed by Targeson Inc.

References

1. Weissleder R, Mahmood U. Molecular imaging. *Radiology*. 2001;219(2):316–333.
2. Villanueva FS. Molecular imaging of cardiovascular disease using ultrasound. *J Nucl Cardiol*. 2008;15(4):576–586.

3. Galkina E, Ley K. Leukocyte influx in atherosclerosis. *Curr Drug Targets*. 2007;8(12):1239–1248.
4. Hutter JC, Luu HM, Mehlhaff PM, Killam AL, Dittrich HC. Physiologically based pharmacokinetic model for fluorocarbon elimination after the administration of an octafluoropropane-albumin microsphere sonographic contrast agent. *J Ultrasound Med*. 1999;18(1):1–11.
5. Harris JR, Depoix F, Urich K. The structure of gas-filled *n*-butyl-2-cyanoacrylate (BCA) polymer particles. *Micron*. 1995;26(2):103–111.
6. Patrianakos AP, Hamilos MI. Drug evaluation: PB-127, a novel contrast agent for the detection of myocardial perfusion. *Curr Opin Investig Drugs*. 2007;8(3):248–255.
7. Straub JA et al. Porous PLGA microparticles: AI-700, an intravenously administered ultrasound contrast agent for use in echocardiography. *J Control Release*. 2005;108(1):21–32.
8. Paradossi G, Cavalieri F, Chiessi E, Ponassi V, Martorana V. Tailoring of physical and chemical properties of macro- and microhydrogels based on telechelic PVA. *Biomacromolecules*. 2002;3(6):1255–1262.
9. Chlon C et al. Effect of molecular weight, crystallinity, and hydrophobicity on the acoustic activation of polymer-shelled ultrasound contrast agents. *Biomacromolecules*. 2009;10(5):1025–1031.
10. Lindner JR et al. Noninvasive ultrasound imaging of inflammation using microbubbles targeted to activated leukocytes. *Circulation*. 2000;102(22):2745–2750.
11. Korpanty G, Grayburn PA, Shohet RV, Brekken RA. Targeting vascular endothelium with avidin microbubbles. *Ultrasound Med Biol*. 2005;31(9):1279–1283.
12. Kim DH, Klibanov AL, Needham D. The influence of tiered layers of surface-grafted poly(ethylene glycol) on receptor-ligand-mediated adhesion between phospholipid monolayer-stabilized microbubbles and coated class beads. *Langmuir*. 2000;16(6):2808–2817.
13. Ham AS, Klibanov AL, Lawrence MB. Action at a distance: lengthening adhesion bonds with poly(ethylene glycol) spacers enhances mechanically stressed affinity for improved vascular targeting of microparticles. *Langmuir*. 2009;25(17):10038–10044.
14. Klibanov AL et al. Detection of individual microbubbles of ultrasound contrast agents: imaging of free-floating and targeted bubbles. *Invest Radiol*. 2004;39(3):187–195.
15. Phillips P, Gardner E. Contrast-agent detection and quantification. *Eur Radiol*. 2004;14(suppl 8):P4–P10.
16. Eckersley RJ, Chin CT, Burns PN. Optimising phase and amplitude modulation schemes for imaging microbubble contrast agents at low acoustic power. *Ultrasound Med Biol*. 2005;31(2):213–219.
17. Lindner JR et al. Ultrasound assessment of inflammation and renal tissue injury with microbubbles targeted to P-selectin. *Circulation*. 2001;104(17):2107–2112.
18. Rychak JJ et al. Microultrasound molecular imaging of vascular endothelial growth factor receptor 2 in a mouse model of tumor angiogenesis. *Mol Imaging*. 2007;6(5):289–296.
19. Christiansen JP, Leong-Poi H, Klibanov AL, Kaul S, Lindner JR. Noninvasive imaging of myocardial reperfusion injury using leukocyte-targeted contrast echocardiography. *Circulation*. 2002;105(15):1764–1767.
20. Dayton P, Klibanov A, Brandenburger G, Ferrara K. Acoustic radiation force in vivo: a mechanism to assist targeting of microbubbles. *Ultrasound Med Biol*. 1999;25(8):1195–1201.
21. Zhao S et al. Radiation-force assisted targeting facilitates ultrasonic molecular imaging. *Mol Imaging*. 2004;3(3):135–148.
22. Rychak JJ, Klibanov AL, Hossack JA. Acoustic radiation force enhances targeted delivery of ultrasound contrast microbubbles: in vitro verification. *IEEE Trans Ultrason Ferroelectr Freq Control*. 2005;52(3):421–433.
23. Rychak JJ, Klibanov AL, Ley KF, Hossack JA. Enhanced targeting of ultrasound contrast agents using acoustic radiation force. *Ultrasound Med Biol*. 2007;33(7):1132–1139.
24. Patil AV, Rychak JJ, Allen JS, Klibanov AL, Hossack JA. Dual frequency method for simultaneous translation and real-time imaging of ultrasound contrast agents within large blood vessels. *Ultrasound Med Biol*. 2009;35(12):2021–2030.
25. Takalkar AM, Klibanov AL, Rychak JJ, Lindner JR, Ley K. Binding and detachment dynamics of microbubbles targeted to P-selectin under controlled shear flow. *J Control Release*. 2004;96(3):473–482.
26. Ley K, Gaehtgens P, Spanel-Borowski K. Differential adhesion of granulocytes to five distinct phenotypes of cultured microvascular endothelial cells. *Microvasc Res*. 1992;43(2):119–133.
27. Watanabe R, Matsumura M, Munemasa T, Fujimaki M, Suematsu M. Mechanism of hepatic parenchyma-specific contrast of microbubble-based contrast agent for ultrasonography: microscopic studies in rat liver. *Invest Radiol*. 2007;42(9):643–651.
28. Klibanov AL et al. Targeting of ultrasound contrast material. An in vitro feasibility study. *Acta Radiol Suppl*. 1997;412:113–120.
29. Villanueva FS et al. Microbubbles targeted to intercellular adhesion molecule-1 bind to activated coronary artery endothelial cells. *Circulation*. 1998;98(1):1–5.
30. Weller GE, Villanueva FS, Tom EM, Wagner WR. Targeted ultrasound contrast agents: in vitro assessment of endothelial dysfunction and multi-targeting to ICAM-1 and sialyl Lewisx. *Biotechnol Bioeng*. 2005;92(6):780–788.
31. Klibanov AL et al. Targeted contrast agent for molecular imaging of inflammation in high-shear flow. *Contrast Media Mol Imaging*. 2006;1(6):259–266.
32. Ottoboni S et al. Characterization of the in vitro adherence behavior of ultrasound responsive double-shelled microspheres targeted to cellular adhesion molecules. *Contrast Media Mol Imaging*. 2006;1(6):279–290.
33. Kaufmann BA et al. Molecular imaging of the initial inflammatory response in atherosclerosis: implications for early detection of disease. *Arterioscler Thromb Vasc Biol*. 2009;30(1):54–59.
34. Ferrante EA, Pickard JE, Rychak J, Klibanov A, Ley K. Dual targeting improves microbubble contrast agent adhesion to VCAM-1 and P-selectin under flow. *J Control Release*. 2009;140(2):100–107.
35. Cho YK et al. Dual-targeted contrast enhanced ultrasound imaging of atherosclerosis in apolipoprotein e gene knockout mice. *Circulation*. 2006;114(18):759.

36. Guenther F, Klibanov AL, Ferrante E, Bode C, von zur Muhlen C. An ultrasound contrast agent targeted towards P-selectin detects activated platelets at supra-arterial shear flow ex-vivo. In: Contrast Media Research Symposium; Copenhagen; 2009:21–23.
37. Schumann PA et al. Targeted-microbubble binding selectively to GPIIb IIIa receptors of platelet thrombi. *Invest Radiol*. 2002;37(11):587–593.
38. Pochon S et al. BR55: a lipopeptide-based VEGFR2-targeted ultrasound contrast agent for molecular imaging of angiogenesis. *Invest Radiol*. 2010;45(2):89–95.
39. Staub D et al. Vasa vasorum and plaque neovascularization on contrast-enhanced carotid ultrasound imaging correlates with cardiovascular disease and past cardiovascular events. *Stroke*. 2010;41(1):41–47.
40. Fuster V, Badimon J, Chesebro JH, Fallon JT. Plaque rupture, thrombosis, and therapeutic implications. *Haemostasis*. 1996;26(suppl 4):269–284.
41. Dunn S et al. The lectin-like oxidized low-density-lipoprotein receptor: a pro-inflammatory factor in vascular disease. *Biochem J*. 2008;409(2):349–355.

Part III

Measurement and Image Analysis

Methodological Considerations of Ultrasound Measurement of Carotid Artery Intima-Media Thickness and Lumen Diameter

John C.M. Wikstrand

10.1 Introduction

Atherosclerosis and its complications, myocardial infarction, stroke, and sudden death, are the industrialized world's major health problem. Not many decades ago, there was a belief that atherosclerotic changes and their complications were a manifestation of aging – hence unavoidable and beyond human control. A much more optimistic attitude is prevailing today. However, until recently, little advance had been made in the fundamental interpretation of early atherosclerotic manifestations in man, because these manifestations had been inaccessible to direct observation and quantification. With the introduction of medical ultrasound in this field, a new era had begun. It became possible to measure and quantify atherosclerosis in carotid arteries noninvasively,[1] and study early changes long before a decrease in lumen diameter would occur.

B-mode ultrasound has been developed to a valuable noninvasive, sensitive, and reproducible technique for measurement of carotid artery intima-media thickness (IMT) and lumen diameter, and for identifying and quantifying atherosclerotic burden and cardiovascular risk. As summarized in this textbook, the application of the technique ranges from determining prevalence of atherosclerosis in large-scale epidemiological studies, research on the etiology and pathophysiology of early atherosclerotic development, and also for investigating preventive measures in randomized clinical trials. However, the method has some limitations.

As indicated in earlier chapters (Chaps. 1 and 2), the arterial wall contains three distinct separate layers: intima, media, and adventitia (Fig. 10.1). Atherosclerosis is a disease affecting the intima leading to intimal thickening, but there is no method available at present which can measure only intima thickness in vivo. However, IMT may be measured with ultrasound and an increase in IMT in atherosclerotic-prone areas is used as an indicator of intimal thickening. The first limitation is thus that a surrogate variable for intimal thickening that is IMT is measured. This may underestimate intimal thickening since media thickness may decrease in connection with intimal thickening during atherosclerosis development. In rare cases, a primary increase in media thickness may also occur, which can increase IMT. This may lead to an overestimation of intima thickness when IMT is used as a surrogate variable for intimal thickening.

This chapter will discuss some of the fundamental principles of the ultrasound method that do not allow valid measurements of near-wall intima-media thickness. Thus, another limitation of the method is that valid measurements of IMT can only be performed in the far wall. Furthermore, with the present technique, noninvasive recordings of the intima-media complex can only be performed on superficial arteries such as carotid and femoral arteries.

Figure 10.2 shows an ultrasound recording from a carotid artery illustrating the typical double-line pattern from both the near and also the far wall of a carotid artery. Figure 10.3 shows the definition of

---

J.C.M. Wikstrand
Wallenberg Laboratory for Cardiovascular Research,
Sahlgrenska Academy, Gothenburg University,
Gothenburg, Sweden

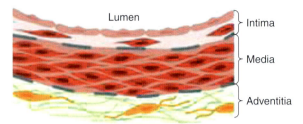

Fig. 10.1 Anatomy of the arterial wall with its three different layers (From Wikstrand.[2] Reprinted with permission)

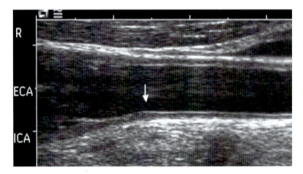

Fig. 10.2 Ultrasound recording from a carotid artery showing the typical double-line pattern from both the near and far wall of the artery. The *arrow* indicates the transition from common carotid artery to carotid artery bulb. (*ECA* external carotid artery, *ICA* internal carotid artery) (From Wikstrand.[2] Reprinted with permission)

leading and far edge of the near-wall intima/lumen interface echo in a section of the common carotid artery. The typical double-line pattern from both the near and also the far wall is clearly illustrated also in this figure.

10.2 Theoretical Considerations: Visibility of Below-Resolution Structures

Small structures, the dimensions of which are far beyond the resolution limits of the equipment, can be detected and produce a clearly visible ultrasound echo.[2,3] The explanation for this phenomenon is that each tissue interface, no matter what size, produces an echo if there is sufficient difference in structure, i.e., in acoustic impedance between two structures (i.e., the very thin interface between two fluids such as oil and water will produce a clear echo that is much thicker than the interface itself, which is infinitely thin). Thus, the thickness of an echo defining an interface is not related to the thickness of the actual structure of interest (for further comments, see below). The anatomical delineation of a biological structure is always defined by a leading edge, i.e., the upper demarcation line of an echo (Fig. 10.3).

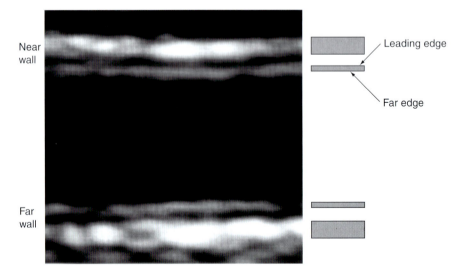

Fig. 10.3 Definition of leading edge and far edge of the near-wall intima/lumen interface in a section of the common carotid artery. The typical double-line pattern from both the near and far wall is also clearly illustrated (From Wikstrand.[2] Reprinted with permission)

10.3 In Vitro Experiments

10.3.1 Pignoli and Coworkers

Pignoli and coworkers published their important observations on ultrasound measurement of intima plus media thickness in 1986.[1] They concluded that B-mode imaging represented a useful approach for measurement of the intima-media complex of human arteries in vivo. However, their experiments were performed on far walls only because the typical double-line pattern on which measurements were made could be more consistently visualized on far walls compared with near walls with their equipment. Therefore, they concluded that the results of their experiments could only be applied to far-wall measurements.

However, with better equipment, the typical double-line pattern can easily be recorded also from the near wall of the carotid artery in the majority of cases (Figs. 10.2 and 10.3), and the question arises: Can near-wall intima-media thickness be measured in these images, i.e., can the adventitia/media interface and the intima/lumen interface be clearly defined from near-wall images?

10.3.2 Wendelhag and Coworkers 1991[3]

A B-mode two-dimensional image from the carotid artery may be described as containing seven echo zones: three from the near wall, three from the far wall, and an echo-free zone in between (Figs. 10.2 and 10.3).[3] When inspecting the three echo zones from the near and far walls, respectively, and comparing it with a picture of the anatomy of the arterial wall (Fig. 10.1), one may be deluded into believing that this similarity implies that the three echo zones anatomically correspond to intima, media, and adventitia, and that the echo-free space in the middle corresponds to the lumen of the artery. This was actually also argued to be the case when the technique was new.[4] However, keeping the fundamental principles of the ultrasound method in mind (summarized above), this cannot be the case. The author's group decided to perform a couple of in vitro experiments during 1990 to prove their case.

The in vitro experiments were designed to illustrate two things of fundamental importance when interpreting the ultrasound image of an artery[1]: *The thickness of the echo created by the interface between the liquid (blood) in the lumen and the intima of the vessel wall has no anatomical relationship to the thickness of the intima itself;* and[2] *the transition between the vessel wall and the vessel lumen in the near wall is defined by the leading edge of the echo from the lumen/intima interface, not by the far edge of this echo.* Thus, the thickness of the echo created by the interface between the intima and the liquid (blood) in the lumen in the near wall can have no anatomical relationship to the thickness of the intima (this echo is actually anatomically located outside the vessel wall and in the lumen itself).

The in vitro experiments were performed on human arteries removed at autopsy (for details, see Wendelhag[3]).

10.3.2.1 Experiment 1: Trepanation Experiment

The vessel was cut open longitudinally and mounted, slightly stretched, with pins on a rectangular rubber sheet. Now with a corneal trepanation instrument, intima and part of the media was removed at various depths (Fig. 10.4). The vessel was then placed in a bath with buffer solution. The ultrasound transducer was mounted in a fixture in the bath at a distance of about 10 mm above the vessel specimen. The intimal surface faced the transducer. The results clearly illustrate that a sharp demarcation echo still can be recorded between the buffer solution and the blood vessel even after the trepanation procedure has removed the intima. The echo was there irrespective of the depth of the trepanation into the media (the echo looked the same even if the intima was removed). The conclusion is that the thickness of the intima cannot be measured by measuring the thickness of the echo created by the difference in acoustic impedance between liquid (blood or buffer solution) and the intima.

10.3.2.2 Experiment 2: Using an Air Bubble

In the second experiment, part of an intact carotid artery was mounted in the bath with buffer solution. The transducer was mounted as before at a distance of 10 mm above the near wall of the vessel. The artery was closed at one end, while the other end was

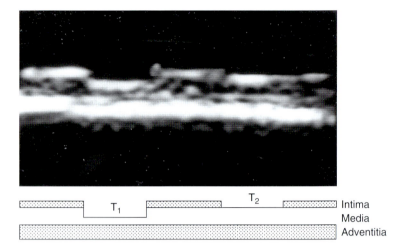

Fig. 10.4 Illustration of ultrasound image in which the intima and part of the media were removed at various depths using a corneal trepanation instrument (see text for comments) (From Wendelhag.[3] Reprinted with permission)

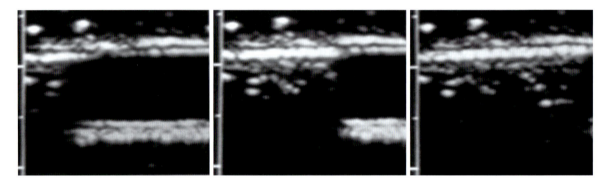

Fig. 10.5 Illustration of an ultrasound image in which an air bubble is introduced between the vessel wall and the liquid solution in the vessel wall lumen. The image shows (from *left* to *right*) how the leading edge of the near-wall intima/lumen interface echo coincides with the leading edge of the echo from the vessel wall/air bubble echo when the air bubble moves to the right. Note the increasing size of the echo shadow created by the air bubble when the bubble extends to the right. For further comments, see text (From Wendelhag.[3] Reprinted with permission)

connected to a syringe filled with buffer solution and some air. Using the syringe, an air bubble was now slowly created above the buffer solution and in direct contact with the near-wall intima.

The results showed, as expected, that a sharp, high-contrast echo was created by the intima/air interface (Fig. 10.5). The most important observation, of course, was that the leading edge of the near-wall intima/air bubble interface echo corresponded to the leading edge of the near-wall intima/buffer interface echo. When the air bubble extends along the vessel wall, the near-wall "intima" echo disappears completely, it is so to say swallowed by the echo from the air bubble. The results of this experiment clearly illustrate that the near wall/lumen transition is defined by the leading edge of this echo (line 2 in Fig. 10.6), not by the far edge (line 3 in Fig. 10.6).

10.3.3 Wong and Coworkers 1993[4]

As a reaction to the in vitro experiments performed by the author's group,[3] Gene Bond's group at Bowman Gray School of Medicine in Winston-Salem decided to re-evaluate in vitro measurements of arterial wall segment thickness obtained by histology and by ultrasound recordings. Wong et al interpreted the similarity of the echo picture with anatomy to indicate that the thicknesses of the echoes (Fig. 10.3) corresponded to the thicknesses of intima, media, and adventitia, respectively (Fig. 10.1). They therefore embarked on trying to correlate the thickness of single echoes by measuring on leading and far edges of the different echoes.[4] They concluded, however, that their experiments showed that it was not possible to accurately measure single layers in the arterial wall with

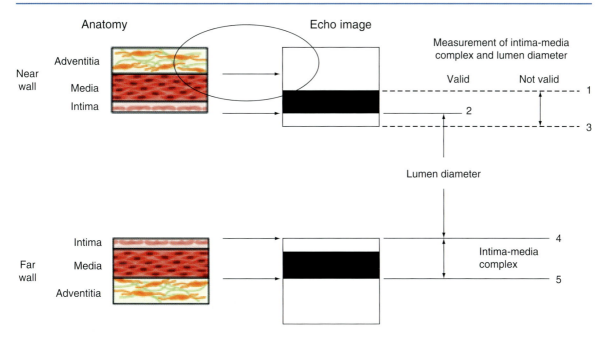

Fig. 10.6 Illustration of the anatomical correlates to echoes that may be recorded from a carotid artery. Observe that all valid measurements are performed on leading edges of the different echoes, that a thickness of an echo has no correlate to a thickness of an anatomical structure, and that the thickness of an anatomical entity is always defined by the distance between the leading edges of two different echoes. The figure also illustrates that the near-wall adventitia/media interface cannot be identified in the ultrasound image (*encircled*, see text for comments). Valid measurements may be done of the far-wall intima-media thickness, but not of the near-wall intima-media thickness. Lumen diameter may be measured in a valid way. *1* far edge of near-wall adventitia echo, *2* leading edge of echo from near-wall intima/lumen interface, *3* far edge of echo from near-wall intima/lumen interface, *4* leading edge of echo from far-wall lumen/intima interface, *5* leading edge of echo from far-wall media/adventitia interface (From Wikstrand.[2] Reprinted with permission)

ultrasound, nor was it possible to accurately measure the IMT in the near wall. Their experiments corroborated our findings that only far-wall intima-media thickness could be accurately measured.

10.4 Near-Wall Adventitia/Media Interface and Near-Wall IMT

The following important question arises: *Is it possible to identify the leading edge of an echo from the interface between adventitia and media in the near wall?* If this echo cannot be identified in the image, near-wall IMT cannot, of course, be measured.

The first prerequisite for being able to define the adventitia/media interface of the near wall is that the thickness of the echoes produced by the lower part of the adventitia is not overlapping a possible echo produced by the adventitia/media interface. The adventitia, in contrast to the media, is normally quite echogenic with bright echoes produced also by the adventitia tissue adjacent to the adventitia/media interface. Therefore, any possible echo from the adventitia/media interface is lost in the echo produced by the lower parts of the adventitia (Fig. 10.6, see encircled part). This is the reason why valid measurements of near-wall intima-media thickness cannot be done. This problem cannot be overcome by making the reading on the far edge of the adventitia echo, since by definition, the location of this echo is always clearly below the true location of the adventitia-media transition (and thus lead to an underestimation of the near-wall IMT, Fig. 10.6, see encircled part). Furthermore, the location of the far edge of the adventitia echo is dependent on several factors which are not possible to standardize or control for, such as gain-setting (the echo will be thicker the higher the gain), and individual composition of adventitia tissue, which means that the underestimation will vary from case to case.

10.5 Near-Wall Intima/Lumen Interface

The near-wall intima/lumen interface is defined by the leading edge of the second echo from the near wall (Figs. 10.3 and 10.6; marked with *2* in Fig. 10.6), which is well defined in most images from the common carotid artery. This echo is well defined since normally the media has a low echogenic structure and therefore does not produce any echoes disturbing the mostly highly echogenic intima/lumen interface. Defining and delineating the intima/lumen interface in the near wall should be done on the leading edge of this second echo. Unfortunately, groups dealing with measurement of what incorrectly is defined as near-wall "IMT" rarely measure on the leading edge of this echo (although always well defined if the echo exists at all), but on the far edge of this echo, which is against fundamental principles for ultrasound delineation of anatomical structures. One might speculate that this is a futile way of trying to compensate for not being able to define the leading edge of the adventitia-media echo of the near wall (and measure on the far edge of the adventitia echo instead) only to have the effect of increasing the measurement error. Also, in this case, the measurement error will vary from case to case because the thickness of the intima-lumen echo is also dependent on several factors which are not possible to standardize or control for, such as gain-setting and individual composition of the intima.

Ultrasound recordings of near-wall images are not redundant, however. On the contrary this segment of the wall should be clearly visualized. This will guarantee that the vessel is being imaged in an optimal way, i. e., presenting an ultrasound image with the largest (true) diameter, and thus a guarantee that the far-wall intima-media thickness will be correctly measured (90° angle between ultrasound array and arterial wall). A poorly visualized near wall may indicate a non-optimal imaging view. Furthermore, the leading edge of the near-wall intima/lumen interface is used when measuring lumen diameter (see below and Fig. 10.6).

10.6 Near-Wall Total Wall Thickness and Adventitia Thickness

Total wall thickness of the near wall may be measured as the distance from the leading edge of the near-wall adventitia echo to the near-wall intima/lumen interface. In a symmetrical vessel, adventitia thickness may then be calculated as near-wall total wall thickness minus far-wall intima-media thickness.

10.7 Measurements of Lumen Diameter

In measurement of the lumen diameter of the common carotid artery, this should be done from the leading edge of the near-wall intima-lumen echo to the leading edge of the echo from the far-wall lumen/intima interface (distance between echoes marked 2 and 4 in Fig. 10.6). The two leading edges defining lumen diameter of the common carotid artery can be easily recorded in most cases. From lumen diameter *(LD)* and far-wall common IMT, the cross-sectional common carotid intima-media *area (A)* may be calculated as $(A) = \pi (0.5\ LD + IMT)^2 - \pi (0.5\ LD)^2$.[2] This is a useful variable to calculate when interpreting changes in intima-media thickness if changes in lumen diameter have also been recorded in a prospective study. This is because changes in intima-media thickness over time could be just secondary to changes in lumen diameter and not to atherosclerotic changes per se. A change in lumen diameter will automatically lead to a secondary (functional) change in intima-media thickness (compare with inflating a balloon).

There is one good example in the literature when changes in IMT were misinterpreted because of this phenomenon.[5] In this study, an increase in IMT was recorded after institution of treatment with a diuretic (but not on a calcium antagonist), which was erroneously interpreted to indicate a progression of atherosclerosis on the diuretic. However, calculations showed that the cross-sectional intima-media area was unchanged, and that the increase in intima-media thickness was secondary to the decrease in lumen diameter probably caused by the diuretic treatment (not observed on the calcium antagonist).

10.8 Far-Wall IMT

The leading edge echo from the lumen/intima interface and from the media/adventitia interface of the far wall can be recorded for the common carotid artery and carotid artery bulb in the majority of cases, thus enabling valid measurements of far-wall intima-media thickness (distance between echoes marked 4 and 5 in Fig. 10.6).

However, present experience from several groups indicates that it is difficult to achieve reliable high-quality measurements of intima-media thickness of the internal carotid artery in prospective studies. This is probably due to anatomical reasons, it is hard getting the ultrasound transducer in a good recording position for the curved internal carotid artery located deeply high up on the neck below the mandible (especially so in overweight people). Furberg and coworkers reported that less than 50% of the internal near-wall intima-media complex could be visualized on duplicate baseline scans, and less than 70% from far-wall scans.[5] The author's recommendation is to refrain from trying to measure the intima-media complex from the internal carotid artery. It is likely that including these measurements in scientific studies will decrease precision and lead to increases in sample size, or even dilute positive results in an otherwise well-designed study, especially so if near-wall measurements are also included.

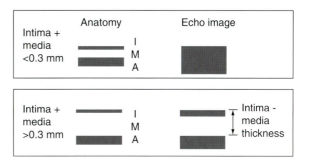

Fig. 10.7 *Upper panel*: Illustration of the axial resolution of the ultrasound system. The theoretical axial resolution of a 7-MHz transducer is approximately 0.3 mm. This means that if intima plus media is thinner than 0.3 mm, the two echo interfaces merge and cannot be separated, and measurement of the intima-media complex is not possible (*upper panel*). *Lower panel*: If intima-media thickness is thicker than 0.3 mm, two separate echoes may be recorded, and intima-media thickness measured (From Schmidt.[6] Reprinted with permission)

10.9 Axial Resolution

The theoretical axial resolution of a 7-MHz transducer is approximately 0.3 mm.[6] This means that if the intima-media complex is thinner than 0.3 mm, the leading edges of the two echo interfaces from far-wall intima and adventitia respectively cannot be separated and measurement of the intima-media complex is not possible (Fig. 10.7, upper panel). However, if the intima-media complex is thicker than 0.3 mm, two separate echoes may be recorded, and intima-media thickness measured (Fig. 10.7, lower panel).

10.10 Reading

A computerized analyzing system for measurement of IMT and lumen diameter in carotid and femoral arteries has been developed by the author's group in collaboration with Chalmers University of Technology.[2,3,6–8] The present system, used also by many other research groups in this field both in Europe and also in the USA, includes automatic detection of echo interfaces (10-mm long sections of the artery, see below), and also includes optional interactive modification of the delineated echo interfaces to be done by the technician performing the readings. The advantages of such a system are that it greatly increases the speed of measurements, and also reduces the variability between readers.[6,7] Furthermore such a system reduces the problem with drift over time in prospective studies. (Further information on the reading system may be obtained by contacting Professor Tomas Gustavsson at Chalmers University of Technology, University of Gothenburg, Gothenburg Sweden.

10.10.1 Comment on Measurement Precision of IMT

Reports from ultrasound studies often give results with 2 or 3 decimals of a mm, and the question arises whether it is possible to measure with such precision? Yes, it is possible (provided that measurements have been performed on leading edges of echoes).

One image point (pixel) in the digitized ultrasound image (7-MHz transducer) is approximately 0.08 mm (may vary somewhat from equipment to equipment). In each single measurement point, the maximal deviation from the true value will be maximum half a pixel, that is 0.04 mm. However, intima-media thickness is measured as a distance between two echo interfaces, which means that a pair of measurement points is marked. The maximal deviation from the true distance will therefore be 0.08 mm, and varies from the true value with a standard deviation of 0.03 mm (Fig. 10.8).[2,6]

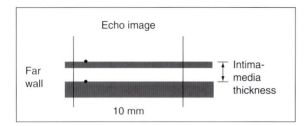

Fig. 10.8 IMT is measured as a distance between two echo interfaces, which means that a pair of measurement points is marked. The maximal deviation from the true distance will be 0.08 mm (see text for comments), and varies from the true value with a standard deviation of 0.03 mm (From Schmidt.[6] Reprinted with permission)

Measurements along a 10-mm section of the artery in the digitized image means approximately 125 measurement points (10/0.08 = 125). Assume (arbitrarily) that at least ten of these are independent. This means that in measurement of one image, the measurement error over a 10-mm section will be $0.03/\sqrt{10} \approx 0.009$ mm (10 independent pairs of measurement points), and for just one maximum value in the section $0.03/\sqrt{1} \approx 0.03$ mm (1 pair of measurement points). These calculations are applicable for one individual. The precision increases when more than one image from an arterial segment is recorded and a mean value is calculated (measurement error for left and right with two 10-mm sections images from each side gives a mean of four images and a precision of $0.03/\sqrt{40} \approx 0.005$ mm). If a composite of common carotid and carotid bulb (mean) is used based on duplicate scans from each 10-mm section from both right and left sides (eight scans in total), the precision is $0.03/\sqrt{80} \approx 0.003$ mm. When a mean value from a group of subjects is calculated, the precision increases further.

Observe that the precision is much higher from a 10-mm section (with 125 pairs of measurement points) of an artery compared to just 1 point (i.e., one single maximum value from just 1 pair of measurement points). The coefficient of variation is also lower for the former compared to the latter.[2,6] It might be advisable to present both mean values and also maximum value measurements in scientific reports.

The author's advice would be to define a composite mean of 10-mm sections from far-wall common carotid and carotid artery bulb IMT as the primary variable of interest.[2,9,10] In order to reduce variability in recordings and measurements of IMT and lumen diameter due to phase in the cardiac cycle, the author recommends recording of images in end-diastole via ECG-triggering (top of R-wave is easy to use).[2,3,6,7]

10.10.2 Measurement of Plaque Area

An atherosclerotic plaque in the ultrasound image may be defined as a focal thickening of the intima-media complex that is 50% thicker than that of the adjacent region, or as a focal thickening over 1.5 mm.

The author's analyzing system also permits measurements of plaque area to be performed by the reader by manually delineating the plaque. However, this is a time-consuming procedure, and not all patients have plaques, which may lead to missing data for plaque area for many subjects in a study. Furthermore, since this reading does not include any component of automatic edge detection, it has the inherent weaknesses of reader variability and drift in readings over time.

In a study of patients with familial hypercholesterolemia, a rather close relationship between change in carotid plaque area and change in IMT in the carotid artery bulb over a 2-year period was observed (Fig. 10.9, upper panel).[11] Therefore, changes over time in IMT in the carotid artery bulb may well mirror changes in plaque area, and be used as a surrogate variable for plaque area changes.

Carotid bulb IMT may be measured in the majority of cases with a low dropout rate. Areas with plaques should not be excluded when measuring, e.g., IMT in a 10-mm section of the carotid artery bulb, since this will of course introduce a serious selection bias. On the contrary, when performing our recordings, our protocol states that recordings should be made over a 10-mm long longitudinal section of the carotid artery bulb showing the thickest part of the intima-media complex (90° angle between ultrasound array and arterial wall, see comment above).

10.11 IMT and Extent of Coronary Atherosclerosis

As commented upon in several chapters in this book, there is a relationship between carotid IMT and coronary heart disease (Chaps. 22 and 23). Hulthe and

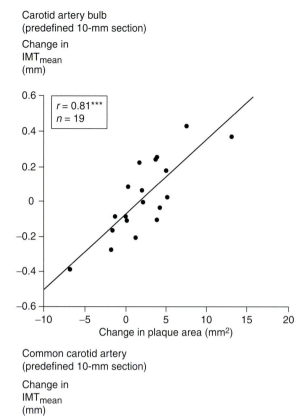

Fig. 10.9 Scatterplots showing relationships between 2-year change in atherosclerotic plaque area and change in IMT measured in a pre-specified 10-mm long section of the carotid artery bulb (*upper panel*), and common carotid artery (*bottom*). Note the close relationship between change in atherosclerotic plaque area and IMT in the carotid artery bulb (From Wendelhag.[11] Reprinted with permission)

coworkers investigated the relationship between the extent of coronary atherosclerosis as measured with quantitative angiography and peripheral atherosclerosis as measured by ultrasound in three different arterial regions: the common carotid artery, the carotid artery bulb, and the common femoral artery.[12] The results showed a significant correlation between carotid bulb IMT and diameter stenosis of the included coronary segments (Fig. 10.10, upper panel), and of carotid plaques and diameter stenosis. However, there was no significant correlation between common carotid (or femoral) artery IMT and diameter stenosis of the included coronary segments (Fig 10.10, lower panel). Although this study was small, and results should be confirmed by other similar studies, the results point to a very important aspect of ultrasound measurements of atherosclerosis: Measurements performed in the common carotid may not relate to coronary atherosclerosis in the same way as measurements performed in the carotid artery bulb. The findings from this study and also the findings from the Wendelhag study[11] underline the importance of measuring IMT not only in the common carotid artery, but also in the carotid artery bulb, and present data separately.

10.12 Precaution: Investigating High-Risk Individuals in Prospective Ultrasound Studies

Dropouts due to hard cardiovascular endpoints such as death, myocardial infarction, and stroke may create a serious selection bias when interpreting prospective randomized studies using surrogate endpoints if high-risk subjects have better (or worse) survival on one treatment compared to the other.[13,14] In such studies, data on ultrasound findings on IMT may be misleading. One example of such a study[14] is commented upon by Fagerberg in this book (Chap. 26).

10.13 International Guidelines

In spite of the tremendous increase in the number of articles published presenting data on ultrasound measurements of IMT, there are no international guidelines on how the technique should be applied as

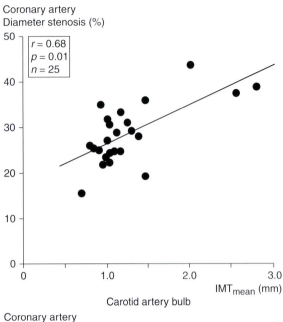

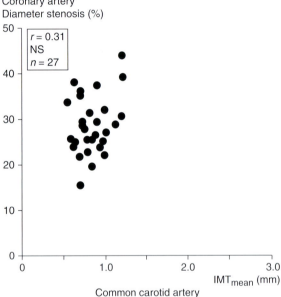

Fig. 10.10 Scatterplots showing the relationships between coronary artery disease as measured by quantitative angiography (diameter stenosis) and IMT of the carotid artery bulb (*upper panel*) and the IMT of the common carotid artery (*bottom panel*), respectively (From Hulthe.[12] Reprinted with permission)

regulatory authorities on randomized controlled outcome studies is not clear, and may vary between countries (and between Europe and the USA).

10.13.1 The Near-Wall Issue

It has been claimed that near-wall measurements are reliable because there is a relatively good correlation between far-wall IMT and "near-wall IMT" in cross-sectional studies. However, in prospective studies, it is the very small changes in IMT over time (delta values) that are in the focus. No data has yet been published from prospective ultrasound studies illustrating a good correlation between delta values (baseline minus follow-up) from measurements of near-wall "IMT" changes vs. far-wall IMT changes during follow-up.

It would be very interesting to get scientific reports on the analysis of the relationship between the changes during follow-up in far-wall IMT (composite of common and bulb) vs. change in near "IMT" (composite of common and bulb) from some of the large randomized studies including near-wall measurements in their outcome variable.[17] This would be a type of test of the validity of including measurements of near-wall "IMT" as an outcome variable in prospective studies. Results from such analyses would be very valuable when defining international guidelines in the future. Therefore, authors of studies including near-wall measurements in prospective studies should be urged to publish such data.

Furthermore it would be very interesting to see publications presenting a re-analysis of randomized clinical studies including a composite of far-wall common carotid and far-wall carotid artery bulb IMT only as the primary outcome variable of interest, and excluding near-wall and internal carotid artery components. The question in focus is: *"Is the treatment effect diluted by including near-wall and internal carotid artery measurements?"* From an ethical standpoint, each study should try to estimate the treatment effect as precisely as possible, whether positive or negative.

In the future, knowledge of how to best define a primary outcome ultrasound variable, both in epidemiological studies and of course also in randomized clinical trials, is needed. Decisions should be based on the huge experiences already gathered by all research groups in the field.

a research tool in an optimal and standardized way. Two consensus articles have touched on the problem.[15,16] Both recommend IMT to be measured preferably in the far wall, but what endpoint to use as the primary outcome measure in ultrasound studies has not been discussed. Furthermore, the view of

Whatever endpoint that is decided upon, it must include measurements from the far-wall carotid artery bulb. This is the section of the artery where atherosclerotic plaques develop and aggravate in people suffering from the disease, and where valid measurements of IMT also can be performed in the majority of people.

10.14 Conclusion

The joint experience from many research laboratories around the world shows that high-quality 2-D ultrasound images can be recorded from the common carotid artery and the carotid artery bulb. In most cases, the image from the carotid artery shows a typical double-line pattern similar in appearance from the near and far wall of the artery. In spite of the similarity of the near-wall and far-wall images, the thickness of the intima-media complex can only be measured in a valid way in the far-wall position. This is because it is only in the far wall that the intima-media complex is defined by leading edges from echoes of interest. In vitro experiments and measurements of arterial wall segment thicknesses obtained by histology and by vascular ultrasound also confirm that only far-wall IMT, in contrast to near-wall thickness, may be accurately measured. The anatomical location of a biological structure is always defined by a leading edge of an echo, and the thickness of a structure as the distance between the leading edges of two different echoes.

It has been claimed that near-wall measurements are reliable because there is a relatively good correlation between far-wall IMT and "near-wall IMT" in cross-sectional studies. However, in prospective studies, it is the very small changes in IMT over time (delta values) that are in the focus. No data has yet been published from prospective ultrasound studies illustrating a good correlation between delta values (baseline minus follow-up) from measurements of near-wall "IMT" changes vs. far-wall IMT changes during follow-up.

If analyses of the near wall are to be performed by some groups also in the future, it is the author's recommendation that near- and far-wall measurements should also be separately presented in scientific reports. The author would also strongly suggest that the near-wall intima-lumen transition is defined by (i.e., measured from) the leading edge (valid edge) of the echo from the intima/lumen interface, and not on the far edge. The far edge has no anatomical correlate and is furthermore gain dependent.

If lumen diameter is measured in the carotid artery, this measurement should be carried out according to the leading edge principle. If changes in common carotid lumen diameters are observed in prospective studies, analyses of common carotid artery cross-sectional area may help in interpreting the results.

Present experience from several groups indicates that it is difficult to achieve reliable high-quality measurements of IMT of the internal carotid artery in prospective studies. In measurements of IMT, it would seem advisable therefore to focus on far-wall common carotid artery and carotid artery bulb recordings. Better precision and probably smaller sample sizes can be achieved by measuring on 10-mm sections of the artery sections of interest than just single maximum values. The author's advice would be to define a composite mean of 10-mm sections from the far-wall common carotid and far-wall carotid artery bulb IMT as the primary outcome variable.

The author concludes that main outcome variables in ultrasound studies of atherosclerosis should be from the far wall. It would seem advisable to focus on far-wall common carotid artery and carotid artery bulb IMT. It is likely that including near-wall measurements and measurements from the internal carotid artery will decrease measurement precision and lead to increases in sample size in scientific studies or even dilute positive results in an otherwise well-designed study.

Acknowledgments I would like to thank all coworkers and colleagues who for over 20 years have taken part in developing current knowledge around the ultrasound technique of measuring IMT, and I would like to name especially Associate Professor Inger Wendelhag and Professor Tomas Gustavsson for their outstanding contributions.

References

1. Pignoli P, Tremoli E, Poli A, Oreste P, Paoletti R. Intimal plus medial thickness of the arterial wall: a direct measurement with ultrasound imaging. *Circulation*. 1986;74:1399-1406.
2. Wikstrand J. Methodological considerations of ultrasound measurement of carotid artery intima-media thickness and

lumen diameter. *Clin Physiol Funct Imaging*. 2007;27: 341-345.
3. Wendelhag I, Gustavsson T, Suurküla M, Berglund G, Wikstrand J. Ultrasound measurement of wall thickness in the carotid artery: fundamental principles, feasibility and description of a computerized analysing system. *Clin Physiol*. 1991;11:565-577.
4. Wong M, Edelstein J, Wollman J, Bond MG. Ultrasonic-pathological comparison of the human arterial wall. Verification of intima-media thickness. *Arterioscler Thromb*. 1993;13:482-486.
5. Furberg CD, Borhani NO, Byington RP, Gibbons ME, Sowers JR. Calcium antagonists and atherosclerosis. The multicenter isradipine/diuretic atherosclerosis study. *Am J Hypertens*. 1993;6:24S-29S.
6. Schmidt C, Wendelhag I. How can the variability in ultrasound measurement of intima-media thickness be reduced? Studies of interobserver variability in carotid and femoral arteries. *Clin Physiol*. 1999;19:45-55.
7. Wendelhag I, Liang Q, Gustavsson T, Wikstrand J. A new automated computerized analysing system simplifies readings and reduces the variability in ultrasound measurement of intima-media thickness. *Stroke*. 1997;28:2195-2200.
8. Liang Q, Wendelhag I, Wikstrand J, Gustavsson T. A multiscale dynamic programming procedure for boundary detection in ultrasonic artery images. *IEEE Trans Med Imaging*. 2000;19:127-142.
9. Hedblad B, Wikstrand J, Janzon L, Wedel H, Berglund G. Low dose metoprolol CR/XL and fluvastatin slow progression of carotid intima-media thickness (IMT). Main results from the Beta-blocker Cholesterol-lowering Asymptomatic Plaque Study (BCAPS). *Circulation*. 2001;103:1721.
10. Wiklund O et al. Effect of controlled release/extended release metoprolol on carotid intima-media thickness in patients with hypercholesterolemia: a 3-year randomized study. *Stroke*. 2002;33:572-577.
11. Wendelhag I, Wiklund O, Wikstrand J. On quantifying plaque size and intima-media thickness in carotid and femoral arteries. Comments on results from a prospective ultrasound study in patients with familial hypercholesterolemia. *Arterioscler Thromb Vasc Biol*. 1996;16:843-850.
12. Hulthe J et al. Atherosclerotic changes in the carotid artery bulb as measured by B-mode ultrasound are associated with the extent of coronary atherosclerosis. *Stroke*. 1997;28:1189-1194.
13. Wikstrand J, Wiklund O. Frontiers in cardiovascular science. Quantitative measurements of atherosclerotic manifestations in humans. *Arterioscler Thromb*. 1992;12:114-119.
14. Suurküla M, Agewall S, Fagerberg B, Wendelhag I, Wikstrand J on behalf of the Risk Factor Intervention Study (RIS) group. Multiple risk intervention in high-risk hypertensive patients. A 3-year ultrasound study of intima-media thickness and plaques in the carotid artery. *Arterioscler Thromb Vasc Biol*. 1996;16:462-470.
15. Touboul PJ et al. Mannheim carotid intima-media thickness consensus (2004–2006). *Cerebrovasc Dis*. 2007;23:75-80.
16. Stein JH et al. Use of carotid ultrasound to identify subclinical vascular disease and evaluate cardiovascular disease risk: a consensus statement from the American Society of Echocardiography carotid intima-media thickness task force. *J Am Soc Echocardiogr*. 2008;21:93-111.
17. Crouse JR et al. Effect of rosuvastatin on progression of carotid intima-media thickness in low-risk individuals with subclinical atherosclerosis. *JAMA*. 2007;297:1344-1353.

Automated Measurement of Carotid Artery Intima-Media Thickness

11

Filippo Molinari and Jasjit S. Suri

11.1 Introduction

Atherosclerosis is a degenerative process that, during years, leads to the accumulation of lipids and other blood-borne materials into the arterial walls.[1] The most important consequences correlated to the progression of atherosclerosis are: (1) the narrowing of the artery lumen, (2) the thickening of the wall, (3) the loss of elasticity, and (4) the reduction of the artery blood flow.[1]

The atherosclerotic process influences almost all the major arteries of the body. However, atherosclerosis affecting the carotid arteries should be considered with particular care. In fact, carotid atherosclerosis is the primary cause of stroke and the third leading cause of death in the industrialized countries.[2]

Carotid intima-media thickness (IMT) is the most widely used and accepted marker of atherosclerosis. Even though in the Mannheim consensus IMT was suggested as risk marker[3] but not as risk indicator, the Rotterdam study showed that IMT had an important diagnostic and predictive value for incident myocardial infarction.[4] Ultrasound is the most widely used technique for the in vivo measurement of carotid IMT. Ultrasound has many advantages over other radiological or imaging methods: absence of non-ionizing radiation; quick examination; geometric measurements of wall thickness, diameters, areas; and for 3-D images, volumes, are relatively simple, and cost is relatively low. In addition, ultrasound scanners are portable and freely available in hospitals and clinics making investigations with ultrasound very diffused with the coverage of a very large percentage of the population of a country.

Perhaps the major drawback of ultrasound is that it is highly operator-dependent. This means that a number of technical and methodological requirements need to be fulfilled in order to perform a correct and effective computer-based IMT measurement.[3,5] The image should be acquired by a trained sonographer using a high-frequency linear probe and insonating the common carotid artery. The optimal location of IMT measurement is within 1 cm from the carotid bulb. Both the anterolateral and the posterolateral longitudinal views should be acquired.

In clinical practice, the carotid IMT value is routinely manually measured during an ultrasound examination of the supra-aortic vessels. The sonographer acquires a longitudinal projection of the artery and then places two markers on the image: the first in correspondence of the lumen-intima (LI) interface and the second of the media-adventitia (MA) interface. Since manual measurement is operator-dependent, it is likely to be prone to errors, time consuming, and subjected to inconsistencies[6] (Chap. 10). Optimal imaging technique and performing computer algorithms enable the fast and accurate evaluation of the artery wall and IMT measurement.

It has been demonstrated that the use of computer techniques for aiding IMT measurement can reduce the inter- and intra-observer variability.[7] Minimization of the user dependence of IMT measurement is,

F. Molinari (✉)
BioLab, Department of Electronics, Politecnico di Torino, Torino, Italy

J.S. Suri
Global Biomedical Technologies Inc. (Affiliated with Idaho State University), Roseville, CA, USA

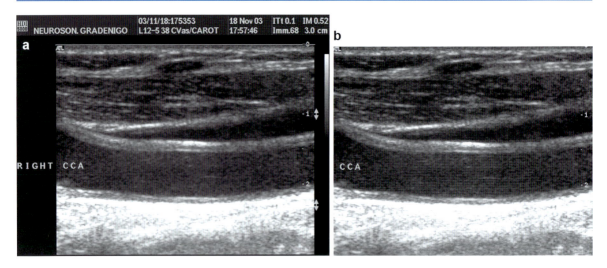

Fig. 11.1 (a) Original raw B-mode ultrasound image. It can be noticed that the region containing the ultrasound data is surrounded by a black frame which may contain other data (i.e., the TGC settings, the grayscale map, markups, and the usual indication of the patient's data, institution, and date which are located on *top*). (b) Cropped image where only the region corresponding to the ultrasound data has been preserved

therefore, becoming a major requirement, especially in large and multicentre studies.

Since the first computer approach proposed by Pignoli and Longo,[8] many techniques were proposed for IMT measurement in longitudinal B-mode carotid artery images. In a recent review,[9] Molinari et al. revisited and commented upon all the most disseminated and adopted methods for computer-based IMT measurements. It was found that the best performing techniques are characterized by an IMT measurement bias as low as 0.01 mm.[10,11] However, the detailed analysis of the available computer methods for IMT measurement revealed that, overall, the best performing techniques suffer from some of the following limitations.

- Usually, to obtain high performance (i.e., a low IMT measurement bias), a technique must be tuned on a specific set of images or, alternatively, on a specific ultrasound scanner. In many studies, there is no discussion about how the techniques have been optimized. Therefore, it becomes very difficult to obtain the same performance when working with different images or with different scanner settings.
- There is always a certain degree of user interaction, even in some techniques that are referred to as "automated". In fact, the ultrasound image has some standard features that are not very suitable to automated processing. An example is provided in Fig. 11.1. Figure 11.1a represents the raw B-mode ultrasound image as acquired by the scanner. Clearly, the ultrasound data representing the carotid artery are located into a region that is only part of the entire image frame. For a computer algorithm, the frame surrounding the ultrasound data region could constitute a problem since it is not homogeneous and black, but it can contain bars, scales, and markups. Therefore, in most techniques, the image is provided to the computer method after a cropping. The result of cropping is represented in Fig. 11.1b in which only the region containing the ultrasound data has been preserved. Most of the time this preliminary cropping is manually made.
- The carotid morphology could constitute a problem for many computer methods. In fact, it is possible to find not only longitudinal and straight vessels but also curved vessels or vessels that cannot be represented as horizontally placed in the image frame. Figure 11.2 reports an example of such different morphological representations of a carotid artery.

Even though the user should always be granted with the possibility of manually correcting the computer measurements, automation would play a fundamental role when large datasets must be processed.

In this chapter, some approaches leading to a completely automated segmentation of the carotid artery wall and IMT measurement will be shown.

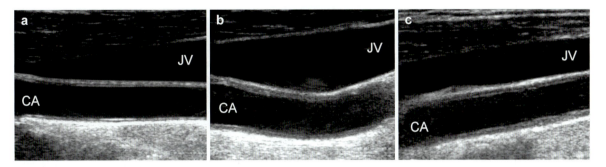

Fig. 11.2 Different carotid appearances in the B-mode ultrasound images. (**a**) Straight and horizontal carotid. (**b**) Curved carotid. (**c**) Straight but non-horizontal carotid. (*CA* carotid artery, *JV* jugular vein)

The computer methods for the automated recognition of the carotid artery in the image frame (as depicted in Fig. 11.1) will be discussed, as well as the recent studies leading to an automated segmentation. Finally, the possible metrics that can be used to characterize the system performance will be discussed. In this final section about performance, the authors will discuss both how to assess the quality of the computer-generated boundary lumen-intima (CGB_{LI}) and media-adventitia boundaries (CGB_{MA}) and how to measure the IMT estimation bias. In the rest of the chapter, attention will be placed on the distal wall of the carotid artery only, since the segmentation of the near wall is still problematic, due to poor definition of the wall layers (Chap. 10). Also, the chapter will always consider performance assessment made against manual tracings, which are considered as ground truth (GT).

11.2 Automated Carotid Artery Recognition and Creation of a Guidance Zone

Figure 11.1 depicts a raw B-mode image as acquired by a scanner. The first problem that must be considered in automated computer methods is the cropping of the image. Then, the carotid artery must be recognized in the image frame. Once recognized, the distal wall of the carotid artery can be segmented in order to extract the CGB_{LI} and CGB_{MA}.

Therefore, conceptually, the overall processing system can be considered as the logical sequence of two stages:
- Stage I: carotid artery recognition
- Stage II: carotid artery distal wall segmentation and IMT measurement

In this section, the possible strategies for Stage I will be discussed, whereas in the next section, some possibilities for Stage II will be presented.

11.2.1 Automated Cropping of the B-Mode Image

Typical B-mode ultrasound images need to be cropped to discard the surrounding black frame containing device headers and image/patient data. If the image is DICOM (digital imaging and communications in medicine) formatted, the field named SequenceOfUltrasoundRegions can be used. This field contains four subfields that mark the location of the image containing the ultrasound representation. These fields are named RegionLocation (with their specific labels being x_{min}, x_{max}, y_{min}, and y_{max}), and they mark the horizontal and vertical extension of the image. The raw B-mode image is then cropped in order to extract only the portion that contains the ultrasound scan image.

If the image is not DICOM formatted, or if the DICOM headers are incomplete, an automated cropping is still possible by relying on image gradients. When computed outside the region of the image containing the ultrasound data, the gradients, both vertical and horizontal, are zero. Hence, the beginning of the image region containing the ultrasound data can be calculated as the first row/column with gradient different from zero. Similarly, the end of the ultrasound region is computed as the last non-zero row/column of the gradient.

The output of this procedure, which we developed and tested,[12] is represented by the cropped image of Fig. 11.1b.

11.2.2 Carotid Artery Recognition Based on Integrated Approach

Molinari et al. developed a generalized architecture for vessel wall segmentation in 2009.[13] Their technique exploited the image information in order to automatically detect the near and far adventitia. The basic idea was to consider the carotid artery as a dark region (the lumen) comprised by two bright stripes (the near and far wall adventitia layers). Therefore, the carotid artery was recognized when the boundaries of the near and far wall adventitia were traced.

This procedure combined feature extraction, fitting, and classification approach. The image was considered column-wise, and the local intensity maxima of each column were processed by a linear discriminator to detect which were located on the wall of the common carotid artery. These points were called "seed points." Seed points were then linked to form line segments. An intelligent procedure removed short or false line segments and joined close and aligned segments. This step avoided over-segmentation of the artery wall. Linear discriminators were used to perform the above-mentioned operations. The parameters of the linear discriminators were derived after pilot studies were conducted on a subset of images. Once the line segments had been connected, an intelligent validation procedure selected the two that were in correspondence of the near and far adventitia layers. Figure 11.3 depicts this procedure. Starting from the identified line segments (Fig. 11.3a), the procedure finds the ones corresponding to the near (AD_N) and far (AD_F) adventitia layers (Fig. 11.3b). The AD_F profile is used to drive the segmentation of Stage II. A region of interest (ROI) is drawn starting from the AD_F boundary. The pixels within the ROI constituted the guidance zone for segmentation. Complete description of the linear discriminators and of the procedures for fitting and classification can be found in previous publications.[13,14]

This technique has the advantage of being completely user-independent. Its integrated approach exploits the morphological features of the artery wall allowing for segmentation in more than 95% of the cases. The authors have validated this method against human tracings[15] using the mean absolute distance as performance metric.

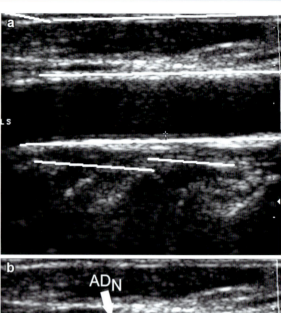

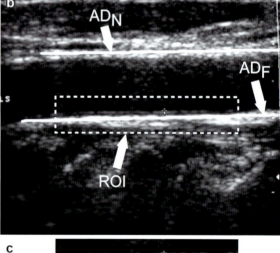

Fig. 11.3 (a) Cropped B-mode image with line segments overlaid in *white*. (b) The line segments that are identified by the discriminant procedure are in correspondence of the near (AD_N) and far (AD_F) adventitia layers. The AD_F profile is used to draw a region of interest (ROI) which will be used in Stage II for wall segmentation. (c) Guidance zone obtained by AD_F

11.2.3 Carotid Artery Recognition Based on Local Statistics and Signal Analysis

Another well-performing technique for carotid artery recognition and creation of a guidance zone was developed by Molinari et al.[15-18] Carotid characteristics can

be thought of as a mixture model with varying intensity distributions. This is because:
(a) Pixels belonging to the vessel lumen are characterized by low mean intensity and low standard deviation.
(b) Pixels belonging to the adventitia layer of the carotid wall are characterized by high mean intensity and low standard deviation.
(c) All remaining pixels should have high mean intensity and high standard deviation.

On the basis of this assumption, the technique first identified all the possible pixels belonging to the carotid artery lumen. For each pixel, the authors considered a 10 × 10 neighborhood of which they calculated the mean value and the standard deviation. The mean values and the standard deviations were normalized to 0 and 1 and were grouped into 50 classes each having an interval of 0.02. The bidimensional histogram (2DH) was then a joint representation of the mean value and standard deviation of each pixel neighborhood. In previous studies, it was shown that pixels belonging to the lumen of the artery are usually classified into the first classes of this 2DH[17,18]: an expert sonographer manually traced the boundaries of the common carotid artery (CCA) lumen and observed the distribution of the lumen pixels on the 2DH. Overall results revealed that pixels of the lumen had mean values classified in the first four classes and a standard deviation in the first seven classes. Therefore, it was possible to consider a pixel as belonging to the carotid lumen if its neighborhood intensity was lower than 0.08 and if its neighborhood standard deviation was lower than 0.14. Figure 11.4 shows an example of automated identification of lumen pixels. From the cropped image (Fig. 11.4a), the 2DH is derived (Fig. 11.4b). The gray area of the histogram represents the location of the pixels possibly belonging to the carotid artery lumen. All the pixels falling into the gray region of panel B are represented in gray in Fig. 11.4c. It is possible to observe that this procedure is very effective in recognizing all the pixels that belong to a lumen vessel.

Once the lumen had been identified, this procedure scanned the image column-wise. By relying on intensity-based criterion, the near and far adventitia layers were found. The intensity profile of every column was processed starting from the bottom of the image (i.e., from the pixel with higher row index). The first local intensity maxima with intensity falling into the 90th percentile of the intensity distribution of the column was marked as AD_F. Then, the row index was decreased, and by moving towards the top of the image, the procedure marked by L is the first local intensity minimum falling into the gray region of the 2DH. Finally, the row index was decreased again until another local intensity maximum was found. This was marked as AD_N. The picture in Fig. 11.4d shows an example of AD_F, AD_N, and L location on a column of the image in Fig. 11.4a.

This procedure proved robust and processed almost every kind of image independently of the carotid artery morphology.[12,15,17,18] If a column missed one of the three points, that column was discarded and not used for final segmentation. The sequence of all the marked AD_F points formed the AD_F profile, which was used to derive a guidance zone (with a procedure similar to that of Fig. 11.3).

11.2.4 Carotid Artery Recognition Based on Hough Transform

The Hough transform (HT) is a mathematical tool used to find specific shapes in the images. The object must be mathematically modeled, then it is searched through the image. In advanced implementations, the HT can search given shapes independently of the scale. This means that the morphology of the object must be described, but not its color or size.

Golemati et al.[19,20] developed automated methodology for recognizing the carotid artery using the HT. The peculiarity of this technique is that it can locate the carotid artery both in longitudinal and transverse projections. With reference to Fig. 11.5, a longitudinal (Fig. 11.5a) and a transverse projection (Fig. 11.5b) can be observed. When in longitudinal projection, the carotid artery consists of two bright lines (the adventitia layers). When in transverse projection, the carotid artery consists of a circular dark area (the lumen). Therefore, it is possible to describe the carotid artery morphology as a set of two parallel lines in longitudinal B-mode and as a circle in transverse.

Golemati et al. adopted this technique for carotid artery wall segmentation. This approach proved robust to the presence of small plaques.[20] Clearly, however, this approach cannot be generalized since it cannot

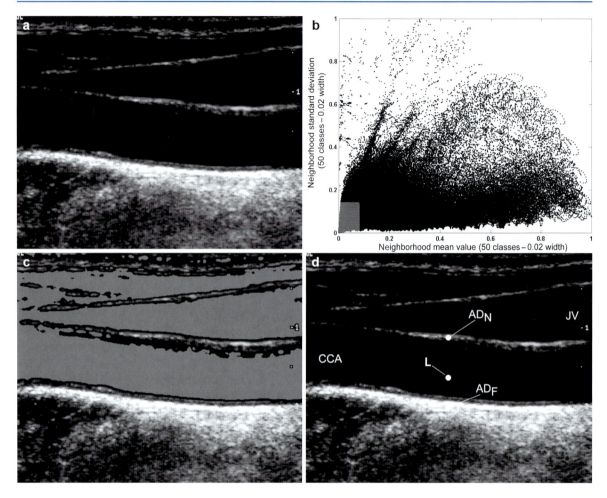

Fig. 11.4 (**a**) Cropped B-mode image. (**b**) Bidimensional histogram of the mean and standard deviation of a 10 × 10 pixels neighborhood. The classes with pixels possibly belonging to the CA lumen are depicted in gray. (**c**) Lumen pixels overlaid to the B-mode image. (**d**) Sample identification of the near (AD_N) and far (AD_F) adventitia layers and of the lumen (L) on a single column of the image

cope with different carotid artery morphologies. When the morphology of the vessel changes, then its mathematical representation must be re-defined. If the common carotid artery were straight but not horizontal, the Hough transform would not recognize the correct dominant lines. Therefore, this system could be difficult to adapt to a real clinical scenario.

Validation of this technique was done against human tracings by using the cross-table: the authors computed the number of pixels correctly segmented (true positives and true negatives) and those incorrectly traced (false positives or false negatives). Sensitivity was 96% and 82% in longitudinal and transverse projections, respectively; specificity was 96% in both the projections.

11.2.5 Carotid Artery Recognition Based on Template Matching

In 2008, Rossi et al.[21] proposed a very powerful technique that automatically locates the carotid artery in the image frame. They considered only longitudinal B-mode images. Two basic assumptions constituted the key points of their technique:

1. They argued that processing all the columns of a B-mode image is useless and prone to errors. In fact, ultrasound images are usually characterized by a low signal-to-noise ratio (SNR). Low SNR values increase the variability in the computer-generated boundaries (CGBs) and make them little accurate. However, since the carotid artery has a

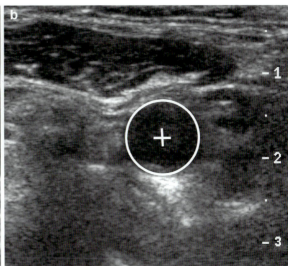

Fig. 11.5 Example of CA recognition based on the Hough transform. (**a**) Longitudinal B-mode image, where the CA appears as a *dark stripe* with *bright boundaries*. The *straight lines* delimiting the lumen are automatically detected. (**b**) Transverse B-mode image, where the CA appears as a *dark circle*. The *white circle* is automatically traced by the Hough transform

well-defined morphology and, considering the absence of plaques, regular layer profiles, it is better to process only a few columns of the image. In fact, the first step of their methodology consisted in a heavy decimation of the column number. This also ensured a lower computational burden (i.e., the expected diameter range and an a priori knowledge of the typical pattern in the echo envelope of the arterial wall–lumen complex).

2. Subsequently, they showed that template matching is very effective in detecting the carotid artery when some parameters of the artery have been a priori selected.

Based upon such consideration, they used parametrical template matching to locate the lumen position along the considered image columns. Figure 11.6 shows a sample output of this algorithm.

This technique was validated against human tracings and on a very large dataset of 6,185 frames acquired on 45 patients. The authors considered the carotid artery as correctly identified if the CGB differed from GT by less than 1.5 mm. Success rate was 98%. This technique had a very low computational cost and could be implemented in real time. The only drawback of this technique, which is common to most of the template matching algorithms, is the choice of the a priori parameters. This technique was specifically tuned for a given scanner. Therefore, when used for different scanners, redefinition of the parameters is required.

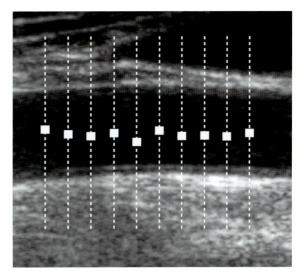

Fig. 11.6 Automated CA recognition as proposed by Rossi et al.[21] The longitudinal B-mode image is first column decimated (the considered columns are represented by *white dashed lines*). The intensity envelope of each column is processed by a parametric template matching algorithm in order to detect the position of the lumen. The sequence of the lumen points (*white squares*) determines the guidance zone

11.3 Common Segmentation Strategies

In this section, an overview of the most used methods for carotid artery wall segmentation (i.e., for performing Stage II) will be presented. These methods aim at tracing the lumen-intima (LI) and media-adventitia (MA) far wall boundaries, which will then be used to compute IMT. The discussion about how to compute IMT from the CGBs will be presented in the last section of this chapter.

11.3.1 Edge-Based Tracking and Gradient-Based Techniques

Edge-based and gradient approaches track the position of the LI/MA interfaces on the intensity profiles of the image columns. The adventitia layer is usually very bright, being formed by dense and fibrous tissue. Therefore, it is relatively easy to mark, on the intensity profile of a region of the far wall of the common carotid artery, the transition between the lumen and the artery wall (LI) and then the transition between the media and the adventitia layer (MA). Figure 11.7 illustrates an example of intensity and edge-based segmentation. Figure 11.7a shows the original cropped B-mode image. The intensity profile of the column marked by the dashed line is indicated by Figure 11.7c. The LI and MA interface points are clearly observable. However, it can be noticed that LI is usually a low intensity peak, while the MA point cannot be located with precision since often the adventitia layer is then represented by a very bright white that creates a wide peak (in correspondence of the MA arrow in Fig. 11.7c).

Gradient-based approaches were introduced in order to cope with this problem of detectability of the LI/MA points. Usually, a gradient of the image is computed, and then the LI/MA points are searched along every column of the image. This technique was adopted by Touboul et al.[7] that used an IMT measurement system based on edge detection in several multicentre clinical and epidemiological studies.[5,22]

In 2001, Liguori et al.[23] proposed a segmentation technique based on edge detection that used image gradients. They considered the artery as horizontally placed in the B-mode image. For each column of the image, they calculated the gradient of the intensity profile. They assumed that all the pixels of the artery lumen were black and that the carotid wall layers originated with gradient transitions. Experimentally, however, due to noise, the measured intensity gradient was different from what is expected. In order to facilitate edge detection, Liguori et al. adopted a statistical thresholding to reduce noise before computing the image gradient. Even though this methodology was not well characterized in terms of segmentation and IMT measurement performance, Liguori et al. provided a very exhaustive and complete metrological characterization.

A common problem of gradient-based approaches is noise. Several solutions have been proposed, but the most performing and innovative gradient-based approach is represented by the recent work of Faita et al.[10] The gradient-based segmentation, as already noted by Liguori et al.,[23] mainly suffers from the problem of superimposed noise, which precludes a proper individualization of the LI and MA transitions. In their study, Faita et al. improved the gradient performance by a first-order absolute moment edge-operator (FOAM) and a pattern recognition approach. The FOAM operator was defined as:

$$e(x,y) = \frac{1}{A_\theta} \int\int_\theta |I_1(x,y) - I_2(x-x', y-y')| \cdot G(x,y,\sigma_r) dx' dy', \quad (11.1)$$

where $I_1(x,y) = I(x,y) \, G(x,y,\sigma_1)$ and $I_2(x,y) = I \times (x,y) \, G(x,y,\sigma_2)$ were computed by low-pass filtering of the input image $I(x,y)$ by a Gaussian kernel with standard deviations equal to σ_1 and σ_2, respectively. This low-pass filtering step was required in order to cope with images having low values of signal to noise. The third Gaussian kernel $G(x,y,\sigma_r)$ is the regularization and weighting term. The "·" sign in Eq. 11.1 indicates the bidimensional convolution (i.e., filtering) by the kernel $G(x,y,\sigma_r)$. When computed in a homogeneous region, the FOAM operator $e(x,y)$ is zero valued. When computed in the presence of a gray level discontinuity, the value of $e(x,y)$ increases. In the authors' study, they used $\sigma_1 = \sigma_r = 0.3$ mm and σ_2 equal to 0.6 mm. Such values were tuned accordingly to the image resolution, as suggested in previous work.[10] Figure 11.7b shows the FOAM operator

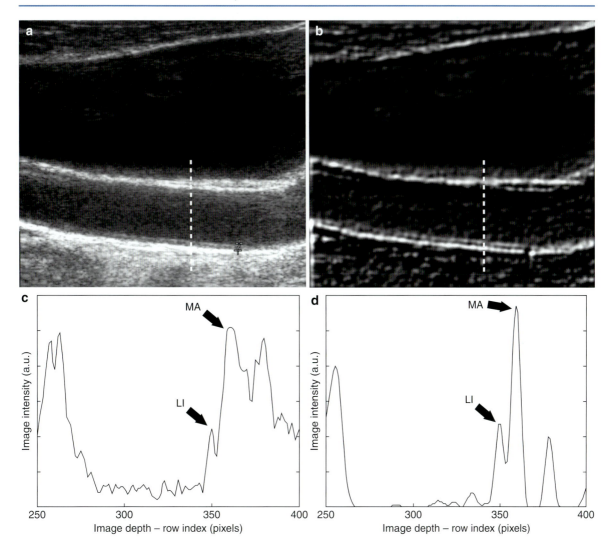

Fig. 11.7 CA far wall segmentation based on intensity criterion and on gradient approach. (**a**) Original cropped B-mode image. (**b**) FOAM edge-operator. (**c**) Intensity profile of the original image, relative to the *dashed line* in *panel A*. (**d**) Intensity profile of the FOAM operator relative to the same column of the image (*dashed white line*). It can be noticed that edge operators increase the detectability of the layers transitions. Specifically, FOAM is particularly effective in increasing the LI/MA peaks while attenuating noise

associated to the image of Fig. 11.7a. Figure 11.7d represents the intensity profile of the FOAM operator relative to the same column of Fig. 11.7c. It can be observed that the LI/MA transitions are now much more evident, and that the gradient has a very good SNR value.

Gradient-based and edge-based techniques have the advantage of being computationally very light. Therefore, they can be considered as an optimal choice for the development of online segmentation systems.

11.3.2 Snake-Based LI/MA Segmentation

A snake is a deformable parametric model that describes an evolving contour. Two forces drive the evolution of the contour: an internal force that is originated by the mathematical formulation of the model itself and that ensures a certain morphological coherence to the snake, and an external force that is given by the image. The external force drives the snake towards the image transitions.

Several authors[17,18,24–29] developed segmentation schemes based on snakes. One of the most widely used snakes is based on the Williams and Shah definition.[30] If a snake contour is represented by $v(s) = [x(s), y(s)]$, where $(x, y) \in \Re^2$ denotes the spatial coordinates of an image and $s \in [0, 1]$ represents the parametric domain, then a snake adapts itself by a dynamic process that minimizes an energy function defined as:

$$\begin{aligned}E_{\text{snake}}(v(s)) &= E_{\text{int}}(v(s)) + E_{\text{image}}(v(s)) \\ &\quad + E_{\text{external}}(v(s)) \\ &= \int_s (\alpha(s)E_{\text{cont}} + \beta(s)E_{\text{curv}} \\ &\quad + \gamma(s)E_{\text{image}} + E_{\text{external}})\mathrm{d}s.\end{aligned} \quad (11.2)$$

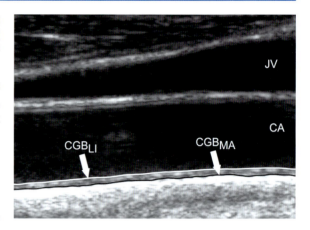

Fig. 11.8 Example of snake-based segmentation. The LI and MA profiles were obtained by using the Williams and Shah snake with parameters $\alpha(s) = 0.6$, $\beta_i(s) = 0.4$, and $\gamma_i(s) = 2$

At each iteration step, the energy function in Eq. 11.2 is evaluated for the current point in $v(s)$ and for the points in an $m \times n$ neighborhood along the *arc* length s of the snake contour. Subsequently, the point on $v(s)$ is moved to the new position in the neighborhood that gives the minimum energy. The term $E_{\text{int}}(v)$ in Eq. 11.2 denotes the internal energy derived from the physical characteristics of the snake and is given by the continuity $E_{\text{cont}}(v)$ and the curvature term $E_{\text{cont}}(v)$. This term controls the natural behavior of the snake. The term $\alpha(s)$ discourages stretching and makes the model behave like an elastic string by introducing tension. The second order term controlled by $\beta(s)$ prevents excessive bending and makes the model behave like a stiff rod. The weighting parameters $\alpha(s)$ and $\beta(s)$ can be used to control the strength of the model's tension and stiffness, respectively. Altering the parameters $\alpha, \beta,$ and γ affect the convergence of the snake. The term E_{image} in Eq. 11.2 represents the image energy due to some relevant features such as the gradient of edges, lines, regions, and texture.[28] It attracts the snake to low-level features such as brightness and edge data. Finally the term E_{external} is the external energy of the snake, which is defined by the user and is optional.

The calculation of the snake parameters is critical to obtain an accurate convergence. Many authors derive the parameters during pilot studies conducted on relatively large image datasets. However, it is clear that once selected, the snake parameters will strongly influence the segmentation performance. Therefore, snake-based techniques still lack in versatility. Some studies have demonstrated that when processing vessels with plaques, the redefinition of the elasticity and stiffness parameters is mandatory.[18,25]

Figure 11.8 presents a sample output of a snake-based procedure. The CGBs are overlaid on the original image. In this example, the snake parameters were chosen as: $\alpha_i(s) = 0.6$, $\beta_i(s) = 0.4$, and $\gamma_i(s) = 2$.

11.3.3 Dynamic Programming Techniques

Dynamic programming techniques were introduced starting in the early 1990s to reduce the variability in ultrasound measurements.[6,31–33] Evidence was that manual measurements were subjected to high variability introduced by the operator skills and by overt drifts over time.[34,35] In 1997, Wendelhag et al.[31] first introduced a dynamic programming procedure for the automatic detection of echo interfaces. This technique combined multiple measurements of echo intensity, intensity gradient, and boundary continuity. The system also included optional interactive modification by the human operator. An initial set of ultrasound images was manually segmented by expert operators and served as reference (ground truth). The estimated values of the three boundary features (echo intensity, intensity gradient, and boundary continuity) were linearly combined in order to create a cost function. Each image point was associated with a specific cost that in turn correlated with the likelihood of that point being located at the echo interface. Therefore, points being located at the interfaces between different artery layers were expected to be associated with a low cost, whereas points located far from the interfaces were associated with a high cost. The weights of the linear combination originating the cost function were determined by training the system and considering the ground truth as reference. Dynamic programming was used in order to reduce the computational cost given by the need of inspecting all the points of the image.

A major advantage of this methodology was complete automation: the dynamic programming approach allowed for analyzing the cost associated to every pixel in the image, thus avoiding the need for any human action. Also, this technique permitted the human correction of evident erroneously segmented points. The major limitation relied in the need for training of the system. The three boundary features (echo intensity, intensity gradient, and boundary continuity) are dependent on the ultrasound scanner used and on the scanner settings. Therefore, retraining is required when the scanner is changed.

In 2000, Liang et al.[36] proposed a dynamic programming technique based on multiscale analysis. Basically, this technique can be thought of as the evolution of the previous one by Wendelhag et al.[31] Dynamic programming was applied in an iterative fashion, starting from the image in a coarse representation and then applying step-by-step refinement iteration. Hence, the global position of the artery in the image was estimated on a coarse scale (thus reducing computational cost), while precise position of the wall layers was estimated in a fine scale (thus ensuring accurate performance). This improved technique reduced the computational burden, whereas the segmentation performance remained unchanged.

11.4 Automated Optimization of Computer-Generated Boundaries: The Greedy Approach

The greedy algorithm (GA) is an iterative technique that searches the global optimum of a problem by a series of local optimizations. Greedy algorithms have been extensively used in segmentation procedures for error correction and performance optimization.[37,38] The basic idea is to fuse two given boundaries in such a way that the fused boundary is closer to the ideal boundary or ground truth (GT) compared to the two given boundaries.

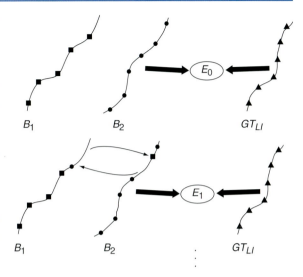

Fig. 11.9 Schematic representation of the greedy algorithm (GA). The initial boundaries B_1 and B_2 are fused together in order to decrease the overall distance E_0 from ground truth (GT_{LI}). Points are swapped between the boundaries until error decreases. The process is iteratively repeated until the error cannot be further lowered or until all the points have been swapped

A possible greedy implementation, which gave optimal performance in the IMT measurement framework,[39] is the one proposed by Suri et al.[37] that is very well described using a the "ball-basket" method. The greedy technique will be explained with reference to Fig. 11.9. Let's consider the LI interface. Start with the two boundaries, namely, B_1 and B_2 that represent the LI-automated tracings of two techniques. The ideal boundary is represented by GT_{LI}. Let's suppose that B_1 has P_1 number of points and B_2 has P_2 number of points. This starting condition is reported by the upper panel of Fig. 11.9. The first vertex of B_2 is swapped with the closest one of B_1, and the system error (i.e., the distance of this new boundary with respect to the ideal boundary, GT) is computed. This error is indicated by E_1 in Fig. 11.9 (lower panel). This cycle in Fig. 11.9 is iterated for every point of the B_2 boundary, obtaining P_2 values of system error. If the minimum of the P_2 values of system error is lower than the initial system error between B_1 and GT_{LI} (indicated by E_0 in Fig. 11.9), the corresponding vertex of B_2 is substituted to the closest vertex of B_1. At this point, the procedure iterates until there are no more vertex swaps that decrease the system error or until all the P_2 vertices of B_2 have been inserted into B_1. The final boundary is the new greedy GA_{LI}. The GA_{LI} final boundary is interpolated by a bicubic spline to smooth out any minor oscillations in the boundary profile. The same structure can be used for the MA profile.

The greedy approach can be very effective for merging together profiles obtained by different techniques. Certainly, GA is best suited for profiles obtained by completely automated techniques. In fact, considering that noise has different effects on different processing techniques, the GA could be very important to improve the overall system performance in automated methods, where the effect of noise cannot be fully controlled. In a pilot study conducted by the authors,[39] using two automated techniques they developed,[15] they obtained an improvement in the system performance of about 3.6% in the IMT measurement error.

11.5 Performance Metrics and Quality Tests for Boundary Tracings and IMT Estimates

Presently, it is very difficult to compare the system performance one obtains with other published works. This is because the validation procedure and the performance metrics used are very different. Molinari et al. recently reviewed some of the most performing techniques for carotid artery segmentation and IMT measurement and provided, for every discussed technique, a detailed description of the validation method and of the performance metric.[9]

In this section, the issue of validation and of performance assessment in a framework of carotid artery computer segmentation and IMT estimation will be briefly covered.

11.5.1 Assessing the Quality of the Computer-Generated Boundaries

The first performance evaluation is about the quality of the computer-generated boundaries. Specifically, the question could be: "How much do my CGBs differ from manual segmentations (i.e., from ground truth)?".

In the rest of this section, it is assumed that validation will be made against manual tracings, as it is commonly accepted in this kind of problem. Usually, many trained operators manually segment the same image set, drawing the boundaries of the LI and MA interfaces, which will be called GT_{LI} and GT_{MA}. Therefore, the question is to compute how much CGB_{LI} differs from GT_{LI} and how much CGB_{MA} differs from GT_{MA}.

To provide an answer to this question, one has to establish a performance metric.

11.5.1.1 Mean Absolute Point-By-Point Distance (MAD)

This is probably the most widely used and yet simple performance metric. Given the CGB and GT boundaries, the mean absolute distance (MAD) metric computes the distance between a point of CBG and the corresponding point of GT. The MAD can be expressed as:

$$\text{MAD} = \frac{1}{N} \sum_{y=1}^{N} |\text{CGB}(y) - \text{GT}(y)|, \quad (11.3)$$

where y is an index spanning the columns of the image (i.e., the points of the CGB and GT profiles). Clearly, this performance metric makes sense when CGB and GT have the same number of points. Figure 11.10 sketches a condition in which MAD is suitable to measure the distance between CGB and GT. In this case, (1) CGB and GT are constituted by the same number of points, (2) the points are aligned along the same columns, and (3) the profiles are almost perpendicular to the columns (represented by the dashed lines in Fig. 11.10). Clearly, if one of the above-mentioned conditions is not true, MAD becomes a biased metric.

This metric is not particularly suited to compare CGB and GT in a real scenario. In fact, usually CGBs consist of 100–200 points, whereas GT boundaries are usually made of 10–20 points. The different number of points makes MAD unreliable.

11.5.1.2 Hausdorff Distance Metric (HDM)

The Hausdorff distance metric (HDM) has a specific rationale in this field. In fact, the HDM between two boundaries is a measure of the longest distance that one has to travel if moving from a given point on a boundary and going to the other boundary. In other words, given the boundaries CGB and GT, one has to calculate the Euclidean distances of each vertex of CGB from the vertices of GT. Let's indicate with d_{12} the minimum distance of the most distant vertex of B_1

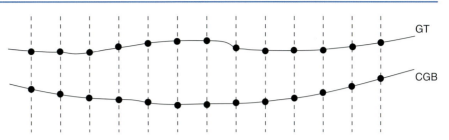

Fig. 11.10 Schematic representation of a condition in which the mean absolute distance (MAD) metric is suitable. The two boundaries GT and CGB are constituted of the same number of points, and the points are aligned on the same columns. Also, the boundaries are almost perpendicular to the column edges (*dashed lines*)

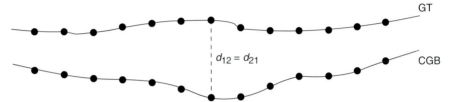

Fig. 11.11 Representation of the Hausdorff distance metric (HDM) computation in a condition where $d_{12} = d_{21}$

from the vertices of B_2. Similarly, let's define d_{21} the minimum distance of the most distant vertex of B_2 from the vertices of B_1. The HDM can then be mathematically defined as:

$$\mathrm{HDM} = \max\{d_{12}, d_{21}\}. \tag{11.4}$$

In a real case, since linear or quasi-linear profiles are being considered, often $d_{12} = d_{21}$. Figure 11.11 provides an example of HDM computation. The major limitation of HDM is that only distances between vertices are measured. Therefore, this measure is significant when the two boundaries have almost the same number of vertices. Also, if the spatial sampling of the vertices of the two boundaries is very different, the HDM may lead to unreliable results.

However, the HDM can be used to measure the distance between different sets of CGBs, for instance when comparing the performance of different segmentation techniques. Its dependence on the number of vertices and on their sampling makes this metric little usable for IMT measurement.

11.5.1.3 Polyline Distance Metric (PDM)

The polyline distance measure (PDM) as performance metric was introduced by Suri et al. in 2000.[37] Given the two boundaries CGB and GT, first, the distance of the vertices of CGB from the segments of the boundary GT is computed. This distance is indicated as $d(CGB,GT)$. Then, the distance of the vertices of GT to the vertices of CGB is computed and indicated as $d(GT,CGB)$. Figure 11.12 shows, as example, a simple visual explanation of the distance of a vertex of CGB from the closer segments of GT (indicated by $d_\perp$ in the figure). The final PDM measure is the average distance of the two distances normalized to the overall number of points (i.e., the sum of the points of CGB and GT) and can be written as:

$$\mathrm{PDM} = \frac{d(\mathrm{CGB},\mathrm{GT}) + d(\mathrm{GT},\mathrm{CBG})}{(\text{\# of vertices of CGB} + \text{\# of vertices of GT})} \tag{11.5}$$

It was shown that PDM is almost independent of the number of points of the boundaries.[37] Hence, PDM was proposed as a good metric when in presence of boundaries with a different number of points: in real condition, this is the best performance metric to estimate the IMT value. In fact, it is possible to compute the IMT as:

$$\begin{aligned}\mathrm{IMT}_{\mathrm{CGB}} &= \mathrm{PDM}(\mathrm{CGB}_{\mathrm{LI}}, \mathrm{CGB}_{\mathrm{MA}}) \\ \mathrm{IMT}_{\mathrm{GT}} &= \mathrm{PDM}(\mathrm{GT}_{\mathrm{LI}}, \mathrm{GT}_{\mathrm{MA}}),\end{aligned} \tag{11.6}$$

where $\mathrm{IMT}_{\mathrm{CGB}}$ is the IMT estimated by the computer tracings, whereas $\mathrm{IMT}_{\mathrm{GT}}$ is the IMT manually measured by the operators.

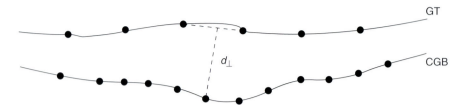

Fig. 11.12 Representation of the polyline distance metric (PDM) computation. In this example, the distance of one vertex of CGB from the line segment of GT is indicated by $d_\perp$

11.5.2 Percent Statistic Test (PST)

The percent statistic test was firstly introduced by Chalana and Kim[40] and then modified by Alberola-Lòpez et al.[41] Basically, it is used to test if the computer-generated boundaries differ from manual tracings as much as the manual tracings differ from one another. This test is very important since many authors pointed out the variability between human tracings made by different experts.[8,10,16–18,27,28,34] The basic idea is that if the computer-generated boundary behaves like a human-generated boundary, then it must have the same probability of falling within the interobserver range as the manual segmentation. Let D_m be the maximum distance between any two tracings (i.e., $D_m = \max_{i,j} \{D_{ij}\}$ for $i \neq j$). A tracing falls in the interobserver range if the distances separating it from the other tracings are all lower than D_m. Assuming the human tracings as independent and identically distributed, the probability p of the computer-generated boundary falling into the interobserver range is equal to $p = \frac{n-1}{n+1}$, being $n + 1$ the total number of tracings (i.e., n human tracing and 1 computer-generated boundary) and $n - 1$ the number of contours minus the two contours with distance D_m. Defining X_j as the event of "the computer-generated tracing lies within the interobserver range for the j-th image," then X_j is a random variable with Bernoulli distribution of parameters p and $q = 1 - p$. Having a database consisting of N images, the variable $Z = \sum_{j=1}^{N} \frac{X_j}{N}$ can be considered as normally distributed with mean value equal to p and standard deviation equal to pq/N. As whether the computer-generated tracing falls outside the interobserver range more often than the human tracings is being determined, the one sided confidence interval for the variable Z, i. e., the θ value for which $P(p - Z > \theta) = \alpha$, where $1 - \alpha$ is the significance level, is being sought. It was shown that $\theta = \sqrt{pq/N} z_{1-\alpha}$,[41] where $z_{1-\alpha}$ is the value of a normal standard variable leaving an area equal to $1 - \alpha$ to its right. Therefore, the acceptance region for this test is where the critical value Z_0 is greater than $p - \theta$.

The PST is a very good indication of reliability of the CGBs in its complex. This test is particularly important since it also takes into consideration the variability in manual tracings (i.e., in GT boundaries). Therefore, this test can also be used to provide a reliable insight into the quality of the operator traced profiles.

11.5.3 A Metrological Note on IMT Measurement and Uncertainty

The analysis of the uncertainty related to computer measurement of the IMT is not straightforward. However, if a simplified condition is considered, an order of magnitude can be given that can be used as further reference to assess the IMT computation quality.

If the segmentation error is calculated column-wise on the image, it can be expressed as $e = |y_{CGB} - y_{GT}|$, where the two measures can be considered statistically independent since they derive from different measurement methodologies. The application of the ISO uncertainty propagation law to the previous equation leads to the uncertainty expression of the error:

$$U_e = \sqrt{U_{yCGB}^2 + U_{yGT}^2} \qquad (11.7)$$

Liguori et al.[23] demonstrated that the uncertainty affecting the algorithm's measurements can be modeled essentially as the uncertainty of $\pm 1/2$ pixel introduced by spatial quantization. Having this quantization error in a triangular probability density function, it can be said that $U_{yCGB} = \frac{1}{2\sqrt{12}}$. This uncertainty essentially models the uncertainty in the y-coordinate positioning of a point of the CGB.

The uncertainty related to the operators depends on the fact that different operators trace different profiles. Form a large and multi-institutional dataset of 300 images, the authors measured a standard deviation value equal to 0.125 pixels and assigned this value to U_{yGT}. Hence, they found an uncertainty value U_e error equal to 0.19 pixels.

For the IMT calculation, having an ultrasound equipment with spatial resolution extremely close to that of Liguori et al.,[23] the authors can say that, as Liguori et al. has already pointed out, $U_{IMT} = 0.2$. This means that for an IMT of 1 mm and an axial resolution better than 100 μm, U_{IMT} is better than 0.02 mm.

From a clinical point of view, the IMT values are used to assess cardiovascular risk and to decide if a patient needs to undergo prophylactic therapy. Usually, if IMT is lower than 0.9 mm, the adult subject is considered normal. If IMT is greater than 0.9 mm, then prophylactic therapy will be considered. Thus, the uncertainty affecting the CGB measures can be considered compatible with the clinical needs provided that its U_{IMT} is of the order of magnitude indicated herein.

11.6 Conclusions and Future Perspectives

In this chapter, the most widely used techniques that are leading to a completely automated carotid IMT measurement in ultrasound imaging were summarized. Currently, the overall system performance of automated methods is lower than that of semi-automated and user-driven methods. The best performing semi-automated methods may have an IMT measurement bias lower than 10 μm, whereas automated techniques, on the average, have a bias of about 35–50 μm.

Nevertheless, automated methods are rapidly growing, and it is expected that performance will be comparable to semi-automated techniques in the near future. The performance gap between semi-automated and fully automated techniques will be filled only by using superior optimization techniques, such as the greedy approach, or by combining different methodologies.

There is still the need for a wider validation, made on multi-institutional databases, possibly acquired by different sonographers and using different scanners. Further, a need is necessary to build common databases where research groups and commercial entities can test their algorithms on this database. Lastly, a need for commercial entities to partner with University hospitals that face the real time challenges, and whose solutions need to be established. We anticipate releasing a commercial system called AtheroEdge® from Global Biomedical Technologies, Roseville, CA, USA, which is aimed at supporting different fields of medicine for Atherosclerosis Disease Management. Taking these health care challenges and getting them regulatory clearance so that these solid commercial systems can then be run at different hospital-based and clinical-based settings are the final stages.

References

1. Badimon JJ, Ibanez B, Cimmino G. Genesis and dynamics of atherosclerotic lesions: implications for early detection. *Cerebrovasc Dis*. 2009;27(suppl 1):38–47.
2. World Health Organization. Cardiovascular diseases [Internet]. 2011. Available at: http://www.who.int/cardiovascular_diseases/en/. Cited April 5, 2011.
3. Touboul PJ et al. Mannheim intima-media thickness consensus. *Cerebrovasc Dis*. 2004;18:346–349.
4. van der Meer IM et al. Predictive value of noninvasive measures of atherosclerosis for incident myocardial infarction: the Rotterdam Study. *Circulation*. 2004;109: 1089–1094.
5. Touboul PJ et al. Mannheim carotid intima-media thickness consensus (2004-2006). An update on behalf of the Advisory Board of the 3rd and 4th watching the risk symposium, 13th and 15th European stroke conferences, Mannheim, Germany, 2004, and Brussels, Belgium, 2006. *Cerebrovasc Dis*. 2007;23:75–80.
6. Schmidt C, Wendelhag I. How can the variability in ultrasound measurement of intima-media thickness be reduced? Studies of interobserver variability in carotid and femoral arteries. *Clin Physiol*. 1999;19:45–55.
7. Touboul PJ et al. Use of monitoring software to improve the measurement of carotid wall thickness by B-mode imaging. *J Hypertens Suppl*. 1992;10:S37–S41.
8. Pignoli P, Longo T. Evaluation of atherosclerosis with B-mode ultrasound imaging. *J Nucl Med Allied Sci*. 1988;32:166–173.
9. Molinari F, Zeng G, Suri JS. A state of the art review on intima-media thickness (IMT) measurement and wall segmentation techniques for carotid ultrasound. *Comput Methods Programs Biomed*. 2010;100(3):201–221.
10. Faita F et al. Real-time measurement system for evaluation of the carotid intima-media thickness with a robust edge operator. *J Ultrasound Med*. 2008;27:1353–1361.
11. Stein JH et al. A semiautomated ultrasound border detection program that facilitates clinical measurement of ultrasound carotid intima-media thickness. *J Am Soc Echocardiogr*. 2005;18:244–251.

12. Molinari F, Liboni W, Giustetto P, Badalamenti S, Suri JS. Automatic computer-based tracings (ACT) in longitudinal 2-D ultrasound images using different scanners. *J Mech Med Biol*. 2009;9:481–505.
13. Molinari F, Zeng G, Suri JS. An integrated approach to computer- based automated tracing and its validation for 200 common carotid arterial wall ultrasound images: a new technique. *J Ultrasound Med*. 2010;29:399–418.
14. Molinari F, Zeng G, Suri J. Automatic Recognition and Validation of the Common Carotid Artery Wall Segmentation in 100 Longitudinal Ultrasound Images: An Integrated Approach Using Feature Selection, Fitting & Classification. SPIE Medical Imaging 2009: Image Processing; San Diego, SPIE, 2009: 1–10.
15. Molinari F, Zeng G, Suri JS. Intima-media thickness: setting a standard for completely automated method for ultrasound. *IEEE Trans Ultrason Ferroelectr Freq Control*. 2010;57:1112–1124.
16. Delsanto S, Molinari F, Giustetto P, Liboni W, Badalamenti S. CULEX-completely user-independent layers extraction: ultrasonic carotid artery images segmentation. *Conf Proc IEEE Eng Med Biol Soc*. 2005;6:6468–6471.
17. Delsanto S et al. Characterization of a completely user-independent algorithm for carotid artery segmentation in 2-D ultrasound images. *IEEE Trans Instrum Meas*. 2007;56:1265–1274.
18. Molinari F et al. User-independent plaque segmentation and accurate intima-media thickness measurement of carotid artery wall using ultrasound. In: Suri JS, Kathuria C, Chang R-F, Molinari F, Fenster A, eds. *Advances in Diagnostic and Therapeutic Ultrasound Imaging*. Norwood: Artech House; 2008:111–140.
19. Golemati S, Stoitsis J, Balkizas T, Nikita K. Comparison of B-mode, M-mode and Hough transform methods for measurement of arterial diastolic and systolic diameters. *Conf Proc IEEE Eng Med Biol Soc*. 2005;2:1758–1761.
20. Golemati S, Stoitsis J, Sifakis EG, Balkizas T, Nikita KS. Using the Hough transform to segment ultrasound images of longitudinal and transverse sections of the carotid artery. *Ultrasound Med Biol*. 2007;33:1918–1932.
21. Rossi AC, Brands PJ, Hoeks AP. Automatic recognition of the common carotid artery in longitudinal ultrasound B-mode scans. *Med Image Anal*. 2008;12:653–665.
22. Touboul PJ et al. Carotid artery intima media thickness, plaque and Framingham cardiovascular score in Asia, Africa/Middle East and Latin America: the PARC-AALA study. *Int J Cardiovasc Imaging*. 2007;23:557–567.
23. Liguori C, Paolillo A, Pietrosanto A. An automatic measurement system for the evaluation of carotid intima-media thickness. *IEEE Trans Instrum Meas*. 2001;50:1684–1691.
24. Cheng DC, Schmidt-Trucksass A, Cheng KS, Burkhardt H. Using snakes to detect the intimal and adventitial layers of the common carotid artery wall in sonographic images. *Comput Methods Programs Biomed*. 2002;67:27–37.
25. Delsanto S et al. User-independent plaque characterization and accurate IMT measurement of carotid artery wall using ultrasound. *Conf Proc IEEE Eng Med Biol Soc*. 2006;1:2404–2407.
26. Loizou CP, Pantziaris M, Pattichis MS, Kyriacou E, Pattichis CS. Ultrasound image texture analysis of the intima and media layers of the common carotid artery and its correlation with age and gender. *Comput Med Imaging Graph*. 2009;33:317–324.
27. Loizou CP, Pattichis CS, Nicolaides AN, Pantziaris M. Manual and automated media and intima thickness measurements of the common carotid artery. *IEEE Trans Ultrason Ferroelectr Freq Control*. 2009;56:983–994.
28. Loizou CP, Pattichis CS, Pantziaris M, Tyllis T, Nicolaides A. Snakes based segmentation of the common carotid artery intima media. *Med Biol Eng Comput*. 2007;45:35–49.
29. Mao F, Gill J, Downey D, Fenster A. Segmentation of carotid artery in ultrasound images: method development and evaluation technique. *Med Phys*. 2000;27:1961–1970.
30. Williams DJ, Shah M. A fast algorithm for active contours and curvature estimation. *CVGIP Image Underst*. 1992;55:14–26.
31. Wendelhag I, Liang Q, Gustavsson T, Wikstrand J. A new automated computerized analyzing system simplifies readings and reduces the variability in ultrasound measurement of intima-media thickness. *Stroke*. 1997;28: 2195–2200.
32. Wendelhag I, Wiklund O, Wikstrand J. Arterial wall thickness in familial hypercholesterolemia. Ultrasound measurement of intima-media thickness in the common carotid artery. *Arterioscler Thromb*. 1992;12:70–77.
33. Wendelhag I, Gustavsson T, Suurkula M, Berglund G, Wikstrand J. Ultrasound measurement of wall thickness in the carotid artery: fundamental principles and description of a computerized analysing system. *Clin Physiol*. 1991;11:565–577.
34. Wendelhag I, Wiklund O, Wikstrand J. On quantifying plaque size and intima-media thickness in carotid and femoral arteries. Comments on results from a prospective ultrasound study in patients with familial hypercholesterolemia. *Arterioscler Thromb Vasc Biol*. 1996;16:843–850.
35. Furberg CD, Byington RP, Craven TE. Lessons learned from clinical trials with ultrasound end-points. *J Intern Med*. 1994;236:575–580.
36. Liang Q, Wendelhag I, Wikstrand J, Gustavsson T. A multiscale dynamic programming procedure for boundary detection in ultrasonic artery images. *IEEE Trans Med Imaging*. 2000;19:127–142.
37. Suri JS, Haralick RM, Sheehan FH. Greedy algorithm for error correction in automatically produced boundaries from low contrast ventriculograms. *Pattern Anal Appl*. 2000;3:39–60.
38. Verbeek JJ, Vlassis N, Krose B. Efficient greedy learning of Gaussian mixture models. *Neural Comput*. 2003;15: 469–485.
39. Molinari F, Zeng G, Suri J. Greedy technique and its validation for fusion of two segmentation paradigms leads to an accurate intima-media thickness measure in plaque carotid arterial ultrasound. *J Vasc Ultrasound*. 2010;34(2):63–73.
40. Chalana V, Kim Y. A methodology for evaluation of boundary detection algorithms on medical images. *IEEE Trans Med Imaging*. 1997;16:642–652.
41. Alberola-Lopez C, Martin-Fernandez M, Ruiz-Alzola J. Comments on: a methodology for evaluation of boundary detection algorithms on medical images. *IEEE Trans Med Imaging*. 2004;23:658–660.

12. Image Normalization, Plaque Typing, and Texture Feature Extraction

Maura Griffin, Efthyvoulos Kyriacou, Stavros K. Kakkos, Kirk W. Beach, and Andrew Nicolaides

12.1 Introduction

In the 1980s and early 1990s, ultrasonic plaque characterization was highly subjective. When the examination was performed in a dimly lit room, the gain was usually reduced by the operator; when it was performed in a brightly lit room, the gain was increased. Although the human eye could adjust to the image brightness to a certain extent, reproducible measurements of echodensity when the same patient was scanned in another room and on different equipment were not possible. Ultrasonic image normalization which has been introduced in the late 1990s has enabled us to overcome this problem.

Computer-assisted plaque measurements of echodensity were initially made from digitized B-mode images of plaques taken from a duplex scanner with fixed instrument settings including gain and time control.[1] Because the frequency distribution of gray values of the pixels within the plaque was skewed, it was suggested that the gray scale median (GSM) value rather than the mean should be used as the measurement of echodensity (gray scale on a computer is usually in the range of 0–255; 0 = absolute black, 255 = absolute white). The authors' initial study performed without image normalization had demonstrated that plaques with a GSM of less than 32, i.e., echolucent plaques, had a fivefold increase in the prevalence of silent ipsilateral brain infarcts on CT-brain scans.[1] Biasi's team found similar results, but their cutoff point was higher than 32 because they had used a higher gain setting.[2] Soon it became apparent that ultrasonic image normalization was necessary so that images captured under different instrument settings, from different scanners, by different operators, and through different peripherals such as video or magneto-optical disk could be comparable. As a result, a method was developed to normalize images by means of digital image processing using blood and adventitia as two reference points.[3]

The aim of this chapter is to present the technique of image acquisition, image normalization, and their value in obtaining reproducible measurements of gray scale, texture features, and plaque classification; also, to indicate their potential in identifying unstable (high risk) atherosclerotic plaques.

12.2 Development of Image Normalization

With the use of commercially available software (Adobe Photoshop™ version 3.0 or later, Adobe Systems Inc., San Jose, CA, USA) and the "histogram"

M. Griffin
Vascular Screening and Diagnostic Centre, London, UK

E. Kyriacou
Department of Computer Science and Engineering, Frederick University Cyprus, Lemesos, Cyprus

S.K. Kakkos
Department of Vascular Surgery, University of Patras Medical School, Patras, Achaia, Greece

K.W. Beach
Department of Surgery and Bioengineering, University of Washington, Seattle, WA, USA

A. Nicolaides (✉)
Imperial College and Vascular Screening and Diagnostic Centre, London, UK

facility, the gray scale median (GSM) of the two reference points (blood and adventitia) in the original B-mode image was determined. Algebraic (linear) scaling of the image was performed with the "curves" option of the software so that in the resultant image, the GSM of blood was equal to 0 and that of the adventitia to 190. Thus, the gray scale value (brightness) of all pixels in the image including those of the plaque became adjusted on a linear scale defined by these two reference points.[3]

Selection of the two reference points was based on the argument that a black area representing blood and a relatively bright area of adventitia could always be present in a B-mode image of a vessel. Determination of the optimum gray values of the two reference points was made by first selecting a number of images that in the eyes of two experienced ultrasonographers appeared to be of high quality and subsequently measuring the gray scale value of blood and adventitia. The gray value of blood was found to be in the range of 0–5, and that of adventitia, 180–190. Selecting the gray value of adventitia as 190 meant that calcification would be represented with higher values often close to and including 255.[3]

Two major reproducibility studies have been performed by the authors' team in order to establish the validity of the method of image normalization and the value of GSM measurements.[4,5] These studies have demonstrated that GSM after image normalization is a highly reproducible measurement that could be used in natural history studies of asymptomatic carotid atherosclerotic disease, aiming to identify patients at higher risk of stroke. For the first time, it became possible to obtain the same GSM value for a plaque even when a patient was scanned by different ultrasonographers on different equipment on different days. A recent third reproducibility study by Seo and his team[6] in 30 patients scanned on two different scanners has confirmed the authors' findings. The correlation of the GSM of the plaques between the systems was high ($Y = 1.01X - 0.47$, $R^2 = 0.938$); in addition, the intra- and interobserver variability in 100 plaques were $5.1 \pm 2.3\%$ and $6.2 \pm 2.5\%$, respectively. As a result of these studies, guidelines for equipment settings and image normalization technique were produced (see below). Key issues for the successful reproducibility of normalized images were (a) imaging the vessel with the ultrasound beam at right angles to the vessel wall, (b) overall gain setting by minimizing but not abolishing "noise" in the vessel lumen, and (c) that only the inner two fourths of the brightest section of adventitia should be sampled for normalization. This meant that training of both the ultrasonographer and the operator performing image normalization was essential.

12.3 Guidelines for Maximization of Reproducibility of GSM

12.3.1 Image Acquisition

As mentioned above, a number of prerequisites for image acquisition and normalization are essential for achieving a high reproducibility of GSM (and other texture features).[7] These are listed below:

1. Maximum dynamic range was used which ensured the greatest possible display of gray scale values and hence texture detail.
2. Persistence was set on low and frame rate on high, ensuring good temporal resolution.
3. The time gain compensation curve (TGC) was sloping through the tissues but was positioned vertically through the lumen of the vessel because the ultrasound beam is not attenuated as it passes through blood. This ensured that the adventitia of the anterior and posterior walls had similar brightness.
4. The overall gain was adjusted to give optimum image quality. This was achieved by adjustment of the gain control to minimize but not abolish noise. In practice, the gain was turned down so that noise was abolished, and then it was gradually turned up until some noise appeared in the lumen. This ensured that the gain was not reduced too much to lose low-intensity features in the plaque and that there was a black area without noise in the lumen to be used for normalization.
5. A linear post-processing curve was used. In the absence of a linear curve, the one closest to linear was used.
6. The ultrasound beam was at 90° to the arterial wall.
7. The minimum depth was used so that the plaque occupied a large part of the image.
8. The position of the probe was adjusted so that adventitia adjacent to the plaque was clearly visible as a hyperechoic band that could be used for normalization.

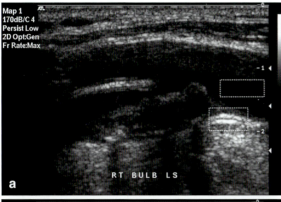
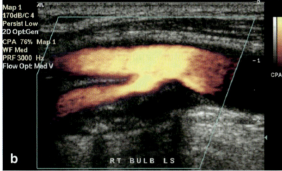
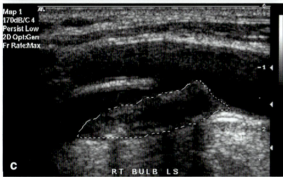

Fig. 12.1 Atherosclerotic plaque at origin of right internal carotid artery producing a severe stenosis. (**a**) Black and white image. *Rectangular box* in vessel lumen shows an area of blood free from noise used for image normalization. *Rectangular box* over arterial wall is an outline of magnified area shown in Fig. 12.2. (**b**) Power Doppler highlighting the outline of plaque. (**c**) Plaque outlined by ultrasonographer at the time of image capture using the on-screen calipers of the ultrasound equipment

In images that contained hypoechoic plaques or plaques whose edge was not clearly visible, a second image was saved using the color or power Doppler facility to indicate the outline of the plaque, taking care to avoid color overspill (Fig. 12.1a, b). If the outline of the plaque could not be clearly defined with color, a third black and white image was saved

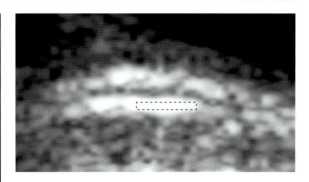

Fig. 12.2 Magnified area of arterial wall from Fig. 12.1a showing the most echogenic segment of arterial wall adjacent to the plaque. The *rectangle* demonstrates the correct sampling of adventitia (central two-fourths of the adventitia)

with the plaque outlined using the on-screen calipers of the ultrasonic equipment (Fig. 12.1c).

12.3.2 Technique of Image Normalization and Measurement of GSM Using Adobe Photoshop

The details and reproducibility of this method have been described in several publications.[3–5] Briefly, the GSM of blood (B) and adventitia (A) were obtained using the "histogram" facility of the program. This was achieved by selecting an area of noiseless blood from the vessel lumen and the inner two fourths of the brightest area of adventitia adjacent to the plaque (Fig. 12.2). Zooming so that the area of adventitia was enlarged made this procedure easier to perform. Also, selecting the inner two fourths of the brightest area of adventitia was essential for ensuring reproducibility. Normalization was subsequently performed using the "curves" facility and adjusting the straight line of the "curves" diagram so that the value of B would become zero and the value A would become 190 in the final image. Thus, all the pixels in the image would adjust automatically according to the new linear scale defined by these two reference points. Subsequently, the plaque in the final image was outlined with the mouse, and the GSM was obtained from the "histogram" facility.

The use of Adobe Photoshop™ was adequate for image normalization and measurements of GSM as a measure of plaque overall echodensity, although time consuming. However, this software could not provide any measurements of texture, i.e., the spatial distribution of pixels with different gray scale values within the plaque area. This has now been overcome by dedicated software.[7]

12.3.3 Dedicated Software

The Plaque Texture Analysis software (Iconsoft International Ltd, PO Box 172, Greenford, London UB6 9ZN, UK) which is a dedicated research software package for image normalization and extraction of plaque texture features including GSM became available in 2004. This software has five modules[7]:

1. *Image Histogram Normalization*: It provides a user-friendly way to normalize images with blood and adventitia as reference points (Fig. 12.3).
2. *Measurements*: It provides a means of scale calibration and of making measurements of distance or area in mm and mm^2, respectively (distances such as intima media thickness or IMT, plaque thickness, and plaque area).
3. *Pixel Density Standardization*: It provides a method of normalizing images to a standard pixel density (20 pixels per mm). This is because a number of texture features are pixel density dependent.[8] In images from different duplex scanning equipment, pixel density has been found to vary from 10 to 30 pixels per mm. Also, various degrees of image magnification applied by the operator do

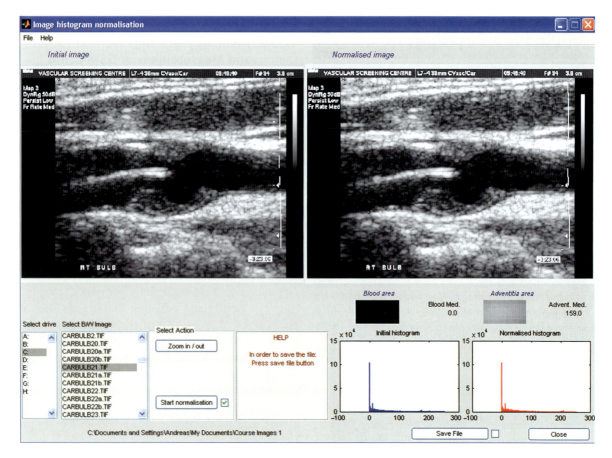

Fig. 12.3 Image normalization module. Image before normalization is on the *left* and normalized image on the *right*. In the original image, the gray value of blood was 0 and of adventitia 159. The normalized image can be saved using the "Save File" button at the bottom of the screen

12 Image Normalization, Plaque Typing, and Texture Feature Extraction

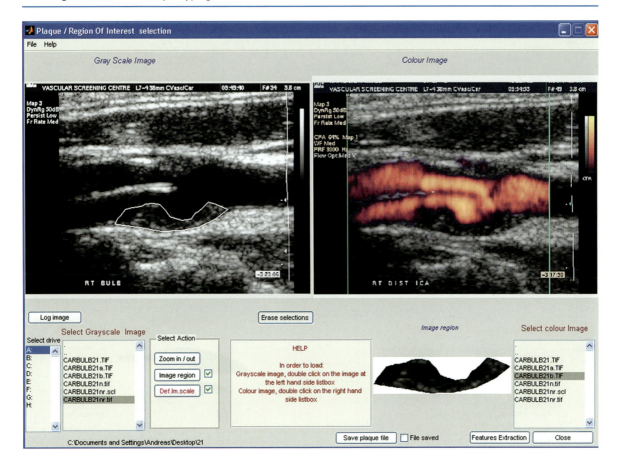

Fig. 12.4 Image crop module. The black and white normalized and standardized image is on the *left*, and the image with color flow (in this case power Doppler) is on the *right*. The outlined plaque is automatically extracted as a separate image that can be saved as a new file

alter the pixel density. Thus, the value of 20 pixels per mm has been suggested for a standard image.

4. *Image Crop*: This module has two windows, one for the normalized black and white image and the other for the color flow image or image with the plaque outlined by the ultrasonographer (Fig. 12.4). The plaque in the normalized image is outlined with the mouse and saved as a new file with the same name and extension ".plq." Both components of a plaque (anterior and posterior wall) can be selected (Fig. 12.5). By pressing the "Features Extraction" button in this window or using the "Feature Extraction" module, a variety of texture features are automatically calculated (Fig. 12.6) including GSM and can be saved in a database that can be opened by "Windows Excel." Data can then be transferred to statistical package for social sciences (SPSS) or any other statistical package.

5. *Texture Feature Extraction*: It extracts a number of plaque texture features including GSM (Fig. 12.6) and saves them on a file for subsequent statistical analysis (see section under "Texture features" below). It classifies plaques according to the Geroulakos classification[9] (Chap. 37). In addition, images of plaques are color contoured: pixels with a gray scale value in the range of 0–25 are colored black. Pixels with values 26–50, 51–75, 76–100, 101–125, and values greater than 125 are colored blue, green, yellow, orange, and red, respectively. In addition, this module allows printing of the plaque images and selected features in the form of a report or saving the latter in a folder (Fig. 12.7). For asymptomatic plaques, this report also provides the calculated annual stroke risk based on the Cox proportional hazard model of the ACSRS study[10] (Chap. 36).

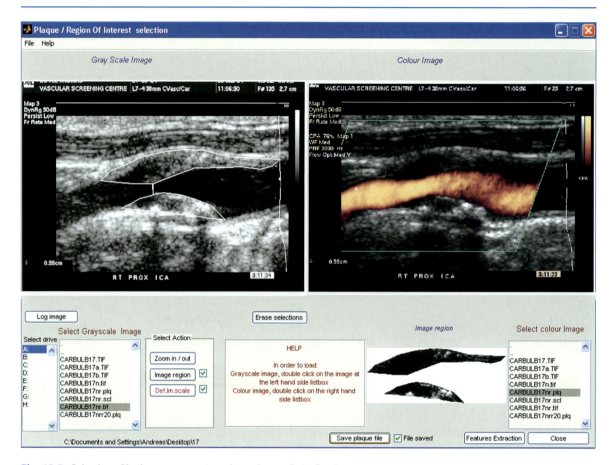

Fig. 12.5 Selection of both components (anterior and posterior) of a plaque

For the purpose of automatic classification by computer, the Geroulakos classification has been redefined in terms of pixels and gray levels as shown below:

Type 1. Uniformly echolucent (black): (Less than 15% of the plaque area is occupied by colored areas, i.e., with pixels having a gray scale value greater than 25). If the fibrous cap is not visible, the plaque can be detected as a black filling defect only by using color flow or power Doppler.

Type 2. Mainly echolucent: (Colored areas occupy 15–50% of the plaque area).

Type 3. Mainly echogenic: (Colored areas occupy 50–85% of the plaque area).

Type 4 and 5. Uniformly echogenic: (Colored areas occupy more than 85% of the plaque area).

Examples of plaque types 1–4/5 are shown in Fig. 12.8a–e. For plaques type 5, only the calcified or visible bright areas of the plaque are selected, ignoring the areas of acoustic shadows where information on plaque texture is lacking (Fig. 12.9).

12.4 Comparison of GSM Obtained Using Adobe Photoshop™ with GSM Obtained Using the Plaque Texture Analysis Software

In a comparison and reproducibility study, two operators normalized and measured the GSM of the 33 plaques using both methods.[7] Each image and plaque was initially processed using Adobe Photoshop and subsequently using the "Plaque Texture Analysis" software before proceeding to the next image. This ensured that the same area of adventitia and plaque were outlined when using each type of software. The two observers did not know the results of each other. For each observer, the GSM values obtained with each software package were compared. The GSM values obtained by each operator using the "Plaque Texture Analysis" software were also compared.

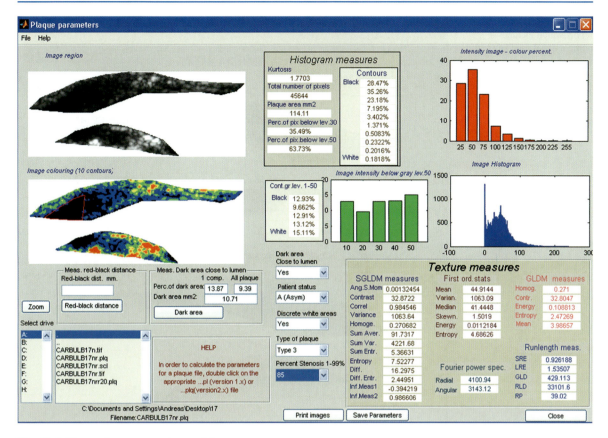

Fig. 12.6 Texture feature extraction module

There was a linear relationship between the GSM obtained using the Adobe Photoshop program and the Plaque Texture Analysis program with a correlation coefficient (r) of 0.990 (95% CI 0.984–0.996) for the first observer and 0.987 (95% CI 0.973–0.994) for the second observer (Fig. 12.10). The corresponding Bland–Altman plots are shown in Fig. 12.11. The interobserver GSM reproducibility using the Plaque Texture analysis by the two operators and corresponding Bland–Altman plot are shown in Fig. 12.12. The correlation coefficient (r) was 0.933 (95% CI 0.864–0.967) ($p < 0.0001$). There was a large discrepancy in one observation. This was the result of a different selection of plaque area by each observer in a heterogenous plaque in which the outline of the plaque close to the lumen was not outlined by color and an additional image with an outline of the plaque using the on-screen calipers was not available. As a result, one observer included a large black area in the plaque selection that resulted in an erroneous low GSM.

The results indicated a high intraobserver reproducibility of GSM when the same plaque images were analyzed using both Adobe Photoshop and the dedicated software. In addition, there was a high interobserver reproducibility when the dedicated software was used by each observer.[7]

Reproducibility studies of visual classification of plaque echogenicity and of classification by computer-assisted plaque echogenicity (GSM) were performed in a longitudinal population-based ultrasound survey (Tromsø study).[11] A total of 198 and 222 paired images were selected from the baseline and the follow-up study, respectively. Despite good agreement in the on-line visual classification (Kappa 0.52–0.57), there was substantial drift on plaque echogenicity during the survey period. However, inter- and intraobserver agreement on computer-assisted GSM classification of the same plaques was higher with kappa values (95% CI) of 0.77 (0.73–0.80) and 0.79 (0.75–0.84), respectively. Thus, computer-assisted off-line classification had better reproducibility.

Fig. 12.7 Print preview of report which includes a number of selected key texture features

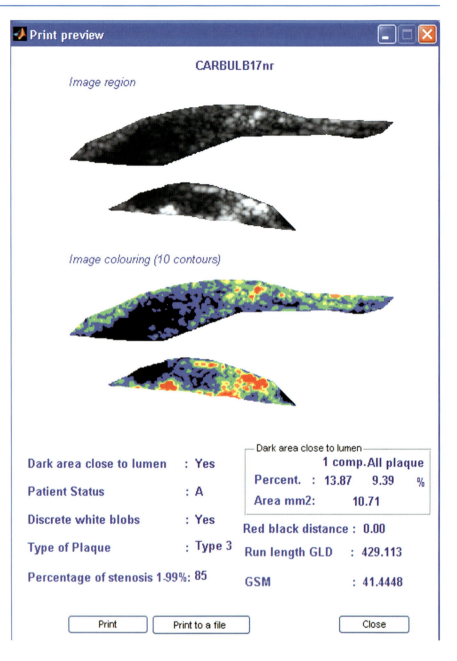

12.5 Effect of Image Normalization on Plaque Classification

The effect of image normalization on plaque classification and risk of ipsilateral ischemic neurological events in patients with asymptomatic carotid stenosis was tested in the first 1,115 patients recruited to the ACSRS study with a follow-up of 6–84 months (mean 42).[9] Duplex scanning was used for grading the degree of internal carotid stenosis according to Doppler velocity measurements at an angle of 60° and for plaque characterization visually (Types 1–5) that was performed before and after image normalization and by the "Plaque Texture Analysis" software.

Images that were recorded on video tapes (S-VHS) were digitized off-line on a PC using a video grabber card (Videologic, TV Snap version 1.0.3 c 1990–1994) at a resolution of 640 × 480 pixels at the coordinating center by two members of the team who

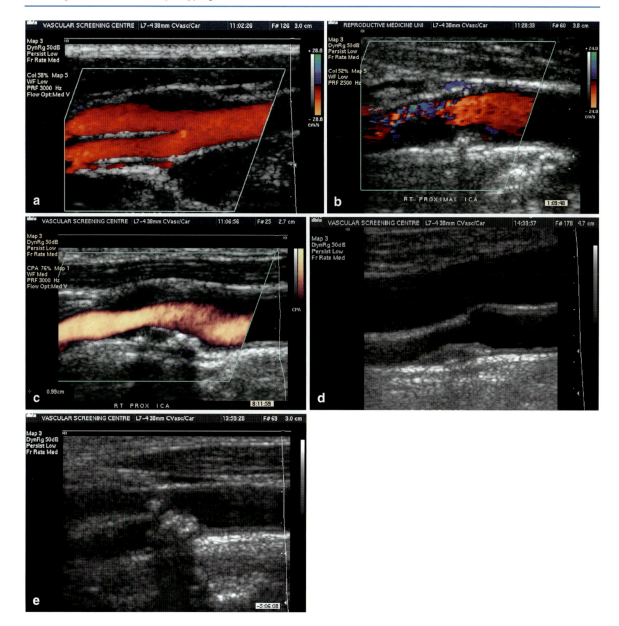

Fig. 12.8 (**a**) Type 1, (**b**) type 2, (**c**) type 3, (**d**) type 4, and (**e**) type 5 plaques

were experienced in carotid scanning. These two members performed plaque classification. Image normalization was performed by the same members of the team several months later using linear scaling with blood (gray scale value assigned: 0) and adventitia (gray scale value assigned: 190) as reference points using Adobe Photoshop™, and the plaques were reclassified without access to the results of the initial classification. As indicated above, before image normalization, plaques with a calcified cap that had more than 15% of the plaque obscured by an acoustic shadow were classified as type 5. After image normalization, only the calcified area and the area of the plaque adjacent to the calcification that was outside the acoustic shadow were considered.

The relationship between plaque classification before image normalization and after image normalization is shown in Table 12.1. Before image

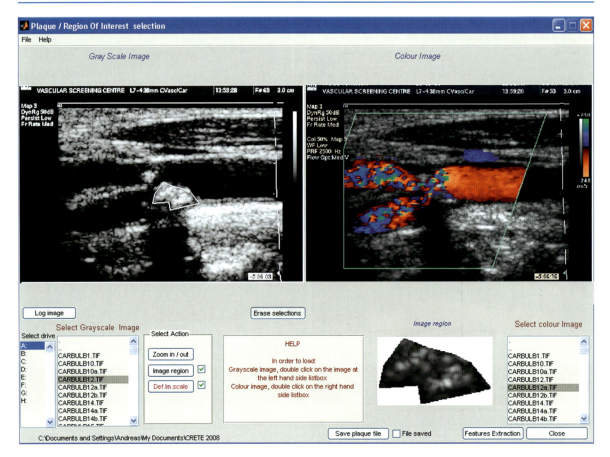

Fig. 12.9 Selection of the calcified or visible bright areas of the plaque are selected, ignoring the area of acoustic shadow where information on plaque texture is lacking

normalization, 131 plaques were classified as type 1, 288 as type 2, 319 as type 3, 166 as type 4, and 188 as type 5. It can be seen that after image normalization, 66% of type 1, 49% of type 2, 46% of type 3, 66% of type 4, and 82% of type 5 were reclassified as a different plaque type (kappa statistic 0.22).

The ipsilateral neurological events (AF, TIAs, and stroke) that occurred during follow-up in patients with different types of plaque before and after image normalization are shown in Tables 12.2 and 12.3, respectively. It can be seen that after image normalization, the incidence of events in relation to different plaque types has changed. After image normalization, there was a decreased incidence in patients with plaques type 4 and 5, with the vast majority of events occurring in plaque types 1, 2, and 3. Before image normalization, only 82 (71%) of the 116 neurological events occurred in plaque types 1–3, but after image normalization, the number increased to 109 (94%).

When plaque types 1–3 were compared with plaque types 4 and 5 before image normalization, the relative risk of having an event was 1.12 (95% CI 0.76–1.66) (Chi Sq. $p = 0.45$). Also, only 37 (73%) of the 51 ischemic strokes occurred in patients with plaque types 1–3 (Table 12.2). When plaque types 1–3 were compared with plaque types 4 and 5 after image normalization, the relative risk of having an event was 4.8 (95% CI 2.27–10.28) (Chi Sq. $p = 0.0001$). Also, 49 (96%) of the 51 ischemic strokes occurred in patients with plaque types 1–3 (Table 12.3).

When echolucent plaques (type 1 and 2) were compared with echogenic (type 3 and 4), the incidence of ipsilateral neurological events was 61 (14.9%) out of 409 in the former and 53 (8.3%) out of 635 in the latter (Table 12.3) (RR 1.6 95% CI 1.16–2.32) (Chi Sq. $p = 0.003$).

When heterogenous plaques (type 2 and 3) were compared with homogenous plaques (type 1 and 4),

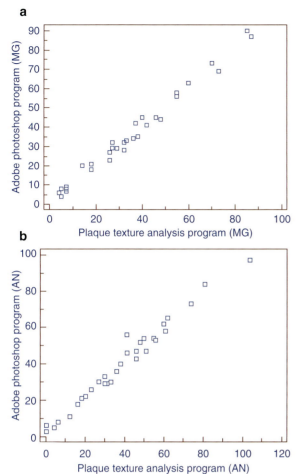

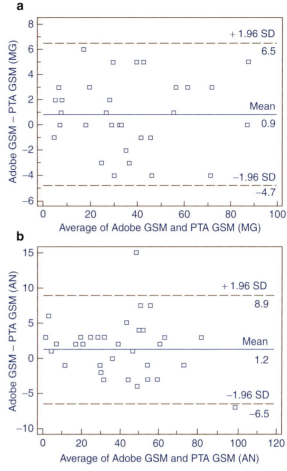

Fig. 12.10 (**a**) Scattergram of GSM obtained with both Adobe Photoshop and Plaque Texture Analysis program by first operator (MG) with a high correlation coefficient ($r = 0.990$). (**b**) Scattergram of GSM obtained with both Adobe Photoshop and Plaque Texture Analysis program by second operator (AN) with a high correlation coefficient ($r = 0.987$)

Fig. 12.11 (**a**) Bland–Altman plot obtained with both Adobe Photoshop and Plaque Texture Analysis program by first operator (MG) and (**b**) Bland–Altman plot obtained with both Adobe Photoshop and Plaque Texture Analysis program by second operator (AN)

the incidence of ipsilateral neurological events was 102 (13%) out of 782 in the former and 12 (4.6%) out of 262 in the latter (Table 12.3) (RR 2.8 95% CI 1.59–5.10) (Chi Sq. $p = 0.0001$).

In summary, image normalization resulted in 60% of plaques being reclassified. Before image normalization, a high event rate was associated with all types of plaque. After image normalization, 109 (94%) of the events occurred in patients with plaques type 1–3. Thus, asymptomatic patients with plaque types 4 and 5 classified as such after image normalization are at low risk irrespective of the degree of stenosis.

12.6 GSM Versus Integrated Backscatter (IBS)

In carotid ultrasound images, the echo amplitude from the adventitia is 1,000 times greater than from intraluminal flowing blood (Chap. 5). Echo intensity is proportional to amplitude squared, so adventitial echo intensity is 1,000,000 times greater than blood echo intensity ($1,000,000 = 10^6 = >6$ Bels = 60 deciBels). The echogenicities of the media and of the atherosclerotic plaque are between the echogenicities of adventitia and blood. Both GSM and IBS have been used for the measurement of plaque echogenicity. With both methods, a region of interest (ROI) is defined in the image by drawing an outline around the pixels representing each tissue type: adventitia, plaque, and blood. With both methods, the ultrasound system will typically digitize the Radio Frequency echo (RF, typically 7.5 MHz) from each image line at 40 million values per second (40 MHz). The digitized values within the ROI are combined to determine an echogenicity score. Then the echogenicity scores assigned to the tissue regions are compared. GSM and IBS methods differ only in the way that the echogenicity score is determined from the digitized values.

In GSM, the sampled values are segmented into groups of four digitized RF values representing an image pixel with a tissue depth of 0.075 mm (4 samples at 40 MHz = 0.1 μs ~ 0.075 mm assuming an ultrasound speed of 1.5 mm/μs). The logarithm of the squared sum of the four digitized values is displayed as brightness level on the ultrasound image screen. All of the brightness levels within the ROI are combined into a statistical distribution, and the median value is selected as the echogenicity score for the ROI. The median value has been chosen, rather than the mean or the mode, because of the skewed distribution of the brightness levels.

In IBS, the sample values are segmented by selecting all digitized RF values within the ROI from all of the image lines passing through the ROI. The mean of the logarithm of the square of all digitized values within the ROI is computed as the echogenicity score for the ROI.

With both GSM and IBS, the echogenicity score for adventitia is greater than the echogenicity score for intraluminal flowing blood; the echogenicity score for media and for atherosclerotic plaque are both between the adventitial and blood values. GSM and IBS scores are statistically correlated with a monotonic functional relationship. The classification of the scores is relative to a threshold, hyperechoic plaque scores are above a threshold, hypoechoic plaque scores are below the threshold. The threshold must be referenced to either the adventitial score or the flowing blood score, preferably both. There is no theoretical reason to choose either GSM or IBS over the other. The IBS method requires access to the echo signal path in the

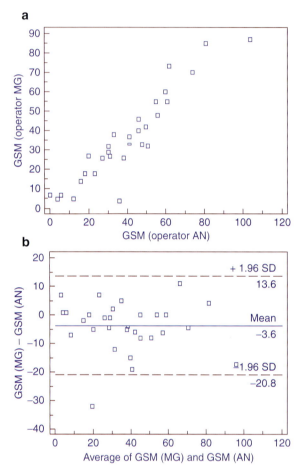

Fig. 12.12 (a) Scattergram of GSM obtained by two operators (MG and AN) using the Plaque Texture Analysis program with a high correlation coefficient ($r = 0.933$). (b) The corresponding Bland–Altman plot shows a large discrepancy in one observation between the two operators

Table 12.1 Lack of agreement between plaque classification before and after image normalization (kappa = 0.22)

Plaque type before image normalization	Plaque type after image normalization					
	1	2	3	4	5	Total
1	44 (34%)	54 (41%)	22 (17%)	11 (7%)	0	131 (100%)
2	23 (8%)	148 (51%)	97 (34%)	16 (6%)	4 (1.4%)	288 (100%)
3	10 (3%)	68 (21%)	173 (54%)	54 (17%)	4 (4%)	319 (100%)
4	0	35 (21%)	62 (37%)	57 (34%)	2 (7%)	166 (100%)
5	0	27 (19%)	96 (51%)	47 (25%)	18 (10%)	188 (100%)
Total	77 (7%)	332 (31%)	450 (41%)	185 (17%)	48 (6%)	1092 (100%)

Table 12.2 The ipsilateral AF, TIAs, and strokes that occurred during follow-up in patients with different types of plaque before image normalization

Plaque type	Events absent	AF	TIAs	Stroke	All events	Total
1	125 (95.4%)	1 (0.8%)	4 (3.1%)	1 (0.8%)	6 (4.6%)	131 (100%)
2	243 (84.4%)	3 (1.0%)	19 (6.6%)	23 (8.0%)	45 (15.6%)	288 (100%)
3	288 (90.3%)	5 (1.6%)	13 (4.0%)	13 (4.0%)	31 (9.7%)	319 (100%)
4	146 (88.0%)	6 (3.6%)	4 (2.4%)	10 (6.0%)	20 (12%)	166 (100%)
5	174 (92.5%)	4 (2.1%)	6 (3.2%)	4 (2.6%)	14 (7.5%)	188 (100%)
Total	976 (89.4%)	19 (1.7%)	46 (4.2%)	51 (4.7%)	116 (10.6%)	1092 (100%)

Table 12.3 The ipsilateral AF, TIAs, and strokes that occurred during follow-up in patients with different types of plaque after image normalization

Plaque type	Events absent	AF	TIAs	Stroke	All events	Total
1	70 (91.0%)	2 (2.6%)	1 (1.3%)	4 (5.2%)	7 (9.1%)	77 (100%)
2	278 (84.1%)	7 (2.1%)	23 (6.7%)	24 (7.1%)	54 (15.9%)	332 (100%)
3	419 (93.1%)	10 (2.2%)	17 (3.8%)	21 (4.7%)	48 (10.7%)	450 (100%)
4	180 (97.3%)	0	3 (1.6%)	2 (1.1%)	5 (2.7%)	185 (100%)
5	46 (95.8%)	0	2 (4.2%)	0	2 (4.2%)	48 (100%)
Total	976 (89.4%)	19 (1.7%)	46 (4.2%)	51 (4.7%)	116 (10.6%)	1092 (100%)

ultrasound system; the GSM method can be applied to post-processed ultrasound images which include a linear gray scale stripe in the image field, even if the image has been subjected to several compression steps.

12.7 Acoustic Densitometry

Acoustic densitometry which is available on some ultrasound scanning equipment was initially developed for quantitative cardiac tissue characterization. It could delineate cardiac cycle dependent changes in normal myocardium and differentiate between normal and myopathic myocardium.[12] More recently, it has been applied to the study of carotid bifurcation plaques.[13] Acoustic densitometry provides two-dimentional integrated backscatter (IBS) images in which the gray level is displayed proportionally to the IBS power. The IBS value is internally calibrated in decibels, having a dynamic range of 0–64 dB in the SONOS 5500 system. For all patients, IBS images are acquired with the same time gain compensation setting and gain control values. IBS values are obtained from plaque area (pl), vessel lumen (lm), and adventitia (ad) at the same depth of the plaque. Two reference values are used: vessel lumen and adventitia. The IBS index has been defined as $((pl - lm)/(ad - lm)) \times 100$. Thus, a lower IBS index corresponds to lower echogenicity. In cases of echolucent plaques, color Doppler images are used to help identify the plaque outline. In the study by Yamagami et al.,[13] the intraobserver and interobserver coefficients of variation for IBS index measurements were 8.9% and 9.2%, respectively.

Acoustic densitometry has demonstrated that higher IL-6 and hsCRP blood levels are associated with lower echogenicity of carotid plaques, suggesting a link between inflammation and plaque instability.[13] Correlation with histology has demonstrated that IBS measurements can differentiate between the various components of plaque (hemorrhage/lipid, fibrous component, and calcification).[14–16] More recently, prospective randomized controlled studies have demonstrated that statin therapy increases plaque echogenicity within 6 months[17,18] (see Chap. 35).

12.8 Pixel Distribution Analysis (PDA)

This is a refinement of the GSM analysis of carotid plaque proposed by Lal and his colleagues.[19,20] Plaques scanned with ultrasound were subjected to histological examination after carotid endarterectomy. After image normalization, pixel distribution within the images was analyzed. The grayscale ranges of known tissues obtained from control subjects was used to define the amount of intraplaque hemorrhage, lipid, fibromuscular tissue, and calcium within the plaque images. This analysis was correlated with tissue composition on the corresponding histologic sections. It was found that in control subjects, the median gray scale value (and range) was 2 (0–4) for blood, 12 [8–26] for lipid, 53 (41–76) for muscle, 172 (112–196) for fibrous tissue, and 221 (211–255) for calcium. PDA-derived predictions for blood, lipid, fibromuscular tissue, and calcium within the plaques correlated with the histologic estimates of each tissue. A higher amount of blood and lipid was seen within symptomatic plaques compared with asymptomatic plaques, and a larger amount of calcification was noted within asymptomatic plaques. In addition, lipid cores were larger, and their distance from the lumen was lower in symptomatic plaques.

A similar approach was used by Madycki and his team in a study of 76 patients scheduled for carotid endarterectomy.[21] They chose five partitions of gray scale values corresponding to the echogenicity of blood (0–9), lipid, [10–31] muscle (32–74), fibrous tissue (75–111), and for calcified tissues (112–255). These reference points were normalized for every tissue in every subject: blood – lumen of the artery, lipid – subcutaneous tissue, muscle – sternomastoid muscle, fibrous – anterior rectus abdominis sheath, and calcium – the transverse process of a cervical vertebra. These gray scale partitions were given five different colors depending on the gray scale range. MRI brain scans were performed routinely 2 days prior to and 2 days after the operation. Transcranial Doppler (TCD) (Chap. 34) was used perioperatively to monitor microembolic (ME) signals in the middle cerebral artery. Excised carotid plaques were classified into three types according to histological criteria: (1) combined plaque (presence of thrombus, ulceration, disintegration, or intraplaque hemorrhage), (2) Fibrous plaque, and (3) solid plaque according to previously published criteria.[22] In this series, Madycki and his team found that 17 (22%) of the 76 patients had new ischemic lesions on the postoperative MRI. ME signals were a potent predictor of new lesions. Also, GSM had a median of 16 (0–29) for the group with and of 38 (12–49) for the group without new perioperative brain infarcts. Patients with a percentile content of partitions 1, 2, and 3 (hypoechoic) exceeding 72% of the plaque area were associated with a higher rate of perioperative complications including brain infarcts and a higher rate of ME.

A slightly different approach (fully described in Chap. 33) was used by Sztajzel and his colleagues in 28 patients (31 plaques) scheduled for carotid endarterectomy.[23] Thirteen patients were symptomatic and 15 asymptomatic. After image normalization, a profile of the regional GSM as a function of distance from the plaque surface was generated, realizing a stratified determination of the GSM. Plaque pixels were further mapped into three different colors depending on their GSM value (<50 red, 50–80 yellow, and >80 green). Histological examination was performed on the excised plaques. It was found that predominance of the red color on the plaque surface was associated with symptomatic patients and a necrotic core located near the surface or a thin fibrous cap.

In a subsequent study, the authors' team investigated the diagnostic value of a juxtaluminal black (hypoechoic) area without a visible echogenic cap (JBA) in ultrasonic images of internal carotid artery plaques.[24] Ultrasonic images of plaques from 324 patients with asymptomatic ($n = 139$) and symptomatic ($n = 185$) internal carotid 50–99% stenosis in relation to the bulb referred for duplex scanning were studied. The JBA in mm^2 as outlined with color or power Doppler and the GSM were obtained after image normalization of the gray scale image. Cutoff points for GSM and JBA (combined highest sensitivity with highest specificity) were determined from ROC curves. It was found that the presence of a JBA equal or greater than 8 mm^2 was associated with a high prevalence of symptomatic plaques in all grades of stenosis. In a multiple logistic regression model, increasing stenosis (mild, moderate, severe), GSM ≤ 15, and JBA ≥ 8 mm^2 were associated with hemispheric symptoms. This model could identify a high risk group of 188 plaques which contained 142 (77%) of the 185 symptomatic plaques (OR 6.7; 95% CI 4.08–10.91), ($p < 0.001$), (Sensitivity: 77%; specificity 66%; PPV 75%; NPV 68%). The results of this study indicate the potential diagnostic value of the presence of a JBA, and for the first time suggest a cutoff point of 8 mm^2 for JBA. It can be argued that a juxtaluminal black area without a visible fibrous cap may represent a necrotic lipid core or a hemorrhage in the presence of a fibrous cup which is too thin to be visualized by ultrasound; also, an intraluminal thrombus on the plaque surface. Whatever the case, the risk of emboli and development of carotid territory symptoms would be high.

A prospective study investigated whether the distribution of pixel intensities could predict the instability of asymptomatic plaque.[25] GSM values were assigned for blood, lipid, muscle/fibrous tissue, and calcification by comparison to endarterectomy specimens. The percent area of each tissue component was subsequently estimated for 297 asymptomatic plaques, causing 40–99% stenosis in 250 patients. Eight infarcts occurred during a follow-up period of 22 ± 15 months. Plaques in the top tertile for the percent area of lipid-like echogenicity showed an association with future infarction according to Kaplan–Meier analysis. This remained significant after adjustment for the severity of carotid stenosis (hazard ratio 4.4) according to Cox proportional hazards analysis.

A similar approach to carotid plaque image analysis which is presented in detail in Chap. 32 has been used with intravascular ultrasound (IVUS) and has been called "virtual histology."[26,27] An advantage of IVUS is that the transducer is in the vessel lumen and thus very close to the plaque. As a consequence, higher frequencies producing higher resolution than that from external probes can be used. The reflected signals from the artery wall provide a color-coded map of the atherosclerotic plaque. Different constituents of the plaque produce different reflected signals, and these are assigned different colors: dark green for fibrous, yellow/green for fibrofatty, white for calcified, and red for necrotic lipid core. This color-coded map assists the interventionalist in understanding how the lesion will behave at the moment of treatment, whether it will resist stent deployment or be liable to produce emboli.[26–28] A high correlation was found with true histology when performed in 15 patients having carotid endarterectomy.[29] It has been suggested that IVUS-virtual histology has the potential to improve the results of carotid artery stenting by optimizing the criteria of patient and lesion selection.[30]

Based on the above studies, it has become obvious that the spatial distribution of pixels has the potential to provide more information on plaque stability or instability than GSM alone.

12.9 Texture Features

In addition to GSM measurements, plaque typing, and PDA described above, another approach has been to perform texture analysis using established statistical texture analysis computer programs. A number of such texture features have been found to be associated with symptomatic carotid plaques in ultrasonic images.[8,31–34] More recently, they have been shown to be useful in automatic tumor detection in MRI and CT liver[35,36] and mammographic images.[37] Examples of such texture features are listed below:

1. *First order statistics (FOS)*: FOS-mean, FOS-variance, FOS-median (GSM), FOS-mode, FOS-skewness, FOS-kurtosis, FOS-energy, FOS-entropy, and total number of pixels which can be used to calculate plaque area in mm^2. The FOS analyzes the distribution of the gray levels of the pixels in the image without considering the neighborhood relationship between the pixels. This system is based on a histogram of the frequency distribution of gray levels. FOS-mean is the average gray level; FOS-variance is a measure of the intensity changes with respect to the mean intensity value; FOS-median is the middle gray level, above and below which 50% of the overall number of pixels are spread; FOS-mode is the most frequent gray level appearing in the image; FOS-skewness is a measure of the symmetry of the gray level histogram; FOS-kurtosis is a measure of the flatness of the histogram; FOS-energy is a measure of the homogeneity (uniformity in the distribution of the gray levels); and FOS-entropy addresses the issue of whether and to what extent the gray level values are evenly distributed.[35]

   The FOS provide some descriptive information about the texture but do not take into account the spatial neighborhood distribution of the gray levels of the pixels. This aspect is addressed by the second-order statistics. The latter considers both the distribution of the gray levels and the relative position of the pixels with respect to each other. These statistics are used by the co-occurrence based approach to textural analysis, which includes the spatial gray level dependence matrix (SGLDM) method and the gray level difference statistics (GLDS) methods.

2. *Spatial gray level dependence matrix (SGLDM)*: SGLDM-homogeneity, SGLDM-contrast, SGLDM-energy, SGLDM-entropy, and SGLDM-correlation.[38] SGLDM-homogeneity is a measure of the dominant neighboring gray level transitions (images without any transitions are associated with a value of 1); SGLDM-contrast is a measure of local variations in the gray level values (images with large neighboring gray level differences or large spatial

frequencies of changes in the intensity are associated with high contrast); SGLDM-energy is a measure of dominant neighboring gray level transitions (as homogeneity); SGLDM-entropy is a measure of the uniformity of the probability distribution of the gray level values in the matrix, with larger values of entropy applying to more uniform probability distributions and thus more heterogenous and complex images; and SGLDM-correlation is a measure of the gray level linear dependence in the image ("noisy" images are associated with low correlation).

3. *Gray level difference statistics (GLDS)*: GLDS-homogeneity, GLDS-contrast, GLDS-energy, GLDS-entropy, and GLDS-mean. The first four perform measurements similar to those of their counterparts in the SGLDM, whereas GLDS-mean is the average value of the gray level differences between the pairs of pixels (it is low when the gray level differences present in the image are low).[35,39]

4. *Gray level run length statistics (RUNL)*: RUNL-short run emphasis, RUNL-gray level distribution (GLD), RUNL-run length distribution, RUNL-long run emphasis, RUNL-run percentage. These measurements depend on the length of runs of consecutive pixels with the same gray value before they change to a higher or lower value.[40]

5. *Other techniques*: These include textural analysis based on fractal geometry method (SFM),[35,41] Law's texture energy method (LTE),[42] or frequency-based texture analysis[37].

A detailed explanation of the above and many other techniques is beyond the scope of this chapter. However, a mathematical definition of the above measures with an application example will be found in Chap. 14.

It should be noted that many of the above texture features are highly correlated (Fig. 12.13), while others are not (Fig. 12.14). Also, most second-order statistics are pixel density dependent and will be affected by zooming.[8] Thus, image interpolation to a standard pixel density prior to image analysis as provided by the "Plaque Texture Analysis" software is essential.

In a cross-sectional study in patients with 50–99% carotid stenosis in relation to the bulb, computerized texture analysis of ultrasonic images of symptomatic carotid plaques could identify those that were associated with brain infarction, improving the results

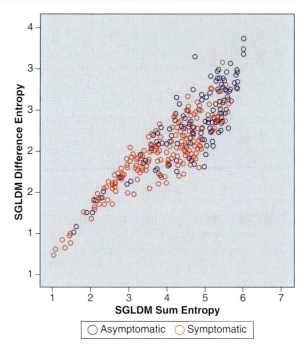

Fig. 12.13 Correlation between SGLDM-difference entropy and SGLDM-sum entropy ($r = 0.88$). Their combined ability to discriminate between symptomatic and asymptomatic plaques is not better than that achieved by each measurement on its own

achieved by GSM alone.[32] In this study, carotid plaque ultrasonic images ($n = 54$, 26 with TIAs and 28 with stroke) obtained during carotid ultrasound were normalized and standardized for pixel density and subsequently assessed visually for the presence of discrete echogenic or juxtaluminal echolucent components and overall echogenicity (plaque type). Using computer software, 51 histogram/textural features of the plaque outlines were calculated. Factor analysis was subsequently applied to eliminate redundant variables. Small cortical, large cortical, and discrete subcortical infarcts on CT-brain scan were considered as being embolic. Twenty-five cases (46%) had embolic infarcts. On logistic regression, GSM, SGLDM-correlation, and SGLDM-correlation-1 were significant ($p < 0.05$), but not RUNL-percentage, stenosis severity, type of symptoms, or echolucent juxtaluminal components. Using ROC curve methodology, SGLDM-correlation-1 improved the value of GSM in distinguishing embolic from non-embolic CT-brain infarction. This methodology can be developed into an automated computerized method of analyzing carotid plaque images.

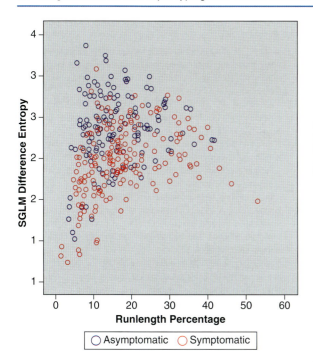
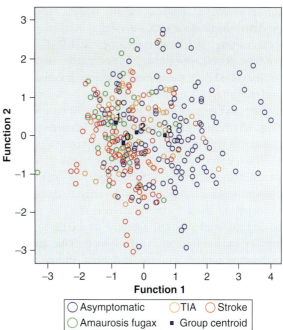

Fig. 12.14 Correlation between SGLDM-difference density and RUNL-percentage ($r = 0.22$). Their combined ability to discriminate between symptomatic and asymptomatic plaques is better than that achieved by each measurement on its own

Fig. 12.15 Canonical discriminant analysis based on SGLD-sum entropy, SGLD-difference entropy, RUNL-percentage, FOS-entropy, and FOS median

The value of texture features in identifying plaques associated with symptoms has been tested by applying these techniques to a database of carotid plaque images established for the initial testing of diagnostic algorithms.[24] The images of the database were collected prospectively from patients referred to the vascular laboratory for diagnostic carotid ultrasound in order to detect the presence and severity of internal carotid stenosis. Asymptomatic patients were referred because of hyperlipidemia, the presence of a cervical bruit, or for screening prior to cardiac surgery. Symptomatic patients presented with amaurosis fugax, ipsilateral hemispheric TIAs, or stroke, as diagnosed by referring physicians or surgeons and subsequently confirmed by a neurologist. Duplex scanning was performed on an ATL HDI 3000 ultrasound unit and a high frequency linear array transducer (4–7 MHz) (Philips/Advanced Technologies Laboratories, Bothel, WA, USA). Images were stored on magneto-optical disks. At the end of the routine clinical examination for the grading of internal carotid stenosis, plaques with ESCT stenosis (European Carotid Surgery Trial method of measuring stenosis) greater than 50% were imaged and recorded with the view to creating a database for future studies on the diagnostic value plaque texture features. The equipment presets and method described under "image acquisition of carotid plaques" above was used. The plaque images were collected consecutively with elimination of plaques that produced less than 50% (ECST) stenosis and emergency cases scanned after normal working hours. As a result, a database was created consisting of images of symptomatic and asymptomatic plaques. The ultrasonographers that performed the examinations and obtained the plaque images knew the reason for referral since they were performing routine diagnostic testing for the presence and grading of stenosis. However, for the purpose of testing new diagnostic algorithms, the images of the database were anonymized and the persons who subsequently did the image normalization and image analysis did not know whether the plaques were symptomatic or asymptomatic.

This database of images is now being used as a testing ground for the potential clinical value of different texture features and appropriate cutoff points prior to testing the latter in prospective studies. Thus, for prospective studies, cutoff points would be predetermined and not data derived.

By using SGLD-sum entropy, SGLD-difference entropy, RUNL-percentage, FOS-entropy, and FOS-median (GSM) in a canonical discriminant analysis, a potential clinically useful discrimination between symptomatic and asymptomatic plaques could be produced (Fig. 12.15). However, discrimination between plaques associated with different types of symptoms was poor.

The clinical value of all these methods in risk stratification of patients with moderate and severe asymptomatic carotid stenosis can only be determined by applying them to prospective studies of patients having optimal medical therapy or in the medical arm of randomized trials of asymptomatic patients, comparing surgery with medical therapy alone.

References

1. El-Barghouty NM, Nicolaides A, Bahal V, Geroulakos G, Androulakis A. The identification of high risk carotid plaque. *Eur J Vasc Surg*. 1996;11:470–478.
2. Biasi GM et al. Computer analysis of ultrasonic plaque echolucency in identifying high risk carotid bifurcation lesions. *Eur J Vasc Endovasc Surg*. 1999;17:476–479.
3. El-Atrozy T et al. The effect of B-mode image standardisation on the echodensity of symptomatic and asymptomatic carotid bifurcation plaques. *Int Angiol*. 1998;17:179–186.
4. Tegos TJ et al. Comparability of the ultrasonic tissue characteristics of carotid plaques. *J Ultrasound Med*. 2000;19:399–407.
5. Sabetai MM et al. Reproducibility of computer-quantified carotid plaque echogenicity. *Stroke*. 2000;31:2189–2196.
6. Seo Y et al. Echolucent carotid plaques as a feature in patients with acute coronary syndrome. *Circ J*. 2006;70:1629–1634.
7. Griffin M, Nicolaides AN, Kyriacou E. Normalisation of ultrasonic images of atherosclerotic plaques and reproducibility of grey scale median using dedicated software. *Int Angiol*. 2007;26:372–377.
8. Kakkos SK, Nicolaides AN, Kyriacou E, Pattichis CS, Geroulakos G. Effect of zooming on texture features of ultrasonic images. *Cardiovasc Ultrasound*. 2006;4:8.
9. Nicolaides AN et al. Effect of image normalization on carotid plaque classification and risk of ipsilateral hemispheric events: results from the ACSRS study. *Vascular*. 2005;13:211–221.
10. Nicolaides AN et al. Asymptomatic internal carotid stenosis and cerebrovascular risk stratification. *J Vasc Surg*. 2010;52(6):1486–1496.
11. Fosse E et al. Repeated visual and computer-assisted carotid plaque characterization in a longitudinal population-based ultrasound study: the Tromsø study. *Ultrasound Med Biol*. 2006;32:3–11.
12. Vered Z et al. Quantitative ultrasonic tissue characterization with real-time integrated backscatter imaging in normal human subjects and in patients with dilated cardiomyopathy. *Circulation*. 1987;5:1067–1073.
13. Yamagami H et al. Higher levels of interlukin-6 are associated with lower echogenicity of carotid plaques. *Stroke*. 2004;35:677–681.
14. Kawasaki M et al. Noninvasive quantitative tissue characterization and 2-dimentional color- coded map of human atherosclerotic lesions using ultrasound integrated backscatter: comparison between histology and integrated backscatter images. *J Am Coll Cardiol*. 2001;38: 486–492.
15. Baroncini LA et al. Ultrasonic tissue characterization of vulnerable carotid plaque: correlation between videodensitometric method and histological examination. *Cardiovasc Ultrasound*. 2006;4:32.
16. Nagano K et al. Quantitative evaluation of carotid plaque echogenicity by integrated backscatter analysis: correlation with symptomatic history and histologic findings. *Cerebrovasc Dis*. 2008;26:578–583.
17. Watanabe K et al. Stabilization of carotid atheroma assessed by quantitative ultrasound analysis in nonhypercholesterolemic patients with coronary artery disease. *J Am Coll Cardiol*. 2005;46:2022–2030.
18. Yamada K et al. Effects of atorvastatin on carotid atherosclerotic plaques: a randomized trial for quantitative tissue characterization of carotid atherosclerotic plaques with integrated backscatter ultrasound. *Cerebrovasc Dis*. 2009;28:417–424.
19. Lal BK et al. Pixel distribution analysis of B-mode ultrasound scan images predicts histologic features of atherosclerotic carotid plaques. *J Vasc Surg*. 2002;35:1210–1217.
20. Lal BK et al. Noninvasive identification of the unstable carotid plaque. *Ann Vasc Surg*. 2006;20:167–174.
21. Madycki G, Staszkiewicz W, Gabrusiewicz A. Carotid plaque texture analysis can predict the incidence of silent brain infarcts among patients undergoing carotid endarterectomy. *Eur J Vasc Endovasc Surg*. 2006;31:373–380.
22. Sitzer M et al. Plaque ulceration and lumen thrombus are the main sources of cerebral microemboli in high-grade internal carotid artery stenosis. *Stroke*. 1995;26:1231–1233.
23. Sztajzel R et al. Stratified gray-scale median analysis and color mapping of the carotid plaque. *Stroke*. 2005;36: 741–745.
24. Griffin M et al. Juxtaluminal hypoechoic area in ultrasonic images of carotid plaques and hemispheric symptoms. *J Vasc Surg*. 2010;52:69–76.
25. Hashimoto H, Takaya M, Niki H, Etani H. Computer-assisted analysis of heterogeneity on B-mode imaging predicts instability of asymptomatic carotid plaque. *Cerebrovasc Dis*. 2009;28:357–364.
26. Diethrich EB, Irshad K, Reid DB. Virtual histology and color flow intravascular ultrasound in peripheral interventions. *Semin Vasc Surg*. 2006;19:155–162.
27. Irshad K et al. Virtual histology intravascular ultrasound in carotid interventions. *J Endovasc Ther*. 2007;14:198–207.
28. Schiro BJ, Wholey MH. The expanding indications for virtual histology intravascular ultrasound for plaque analysis

28. prior to carotid stenting. *J Cardiovasc Surg*. 2008;49:729–736.
29. Diethrich EB et al. Virtual histology intravascular ultrasound assessment of carotid artery disease: the Carotid Artery Plaque Virtual Histology Evaluation (CAPITAL) study. *J Endovasc Ther*. 2007;14:676–686.
30. Inglese L, Fantoni C, Sardana V. Can IVUS-virtual histology improve outcomes of percutaneous carotid treatment? *J Cardiovasc Surg (Torino)*. 2009;50:735–744.
31. Tegos TJ et al. Types of neurovascular symptoms and carotid plaque textural characteristics. *J Ultrasound Med*. 2001;20:113–121.
32. Kakkos SK et al. Texture analysis of ultrasonic images of symptomatic carotid plaques can identify those plaques associated with ipsilateral embolic brain infarction. *Eur J Vasc Endovasc Surg*. 2007;33:422–429.
33. Christodoulou CI, Pattichis CS, Pantziaris M, Nicolaides A. Texture based classification of atherosclerotic carotid plaques. *IEEE Trans Med Imaging*. 2003;22:902–912.
34. Stoitsis J, Tsiaparas N, Golemati S, Nikita KS. Characterization of carotid atherosclerotic plaques using frequency-based texture analysis and bootstrap. *Conf Proc IEEE Eng Med Biol Soc*. 2006;1:2392–2395.
35. Wu Q. *Automatic Tumor Detection for MRI Liver Images* [Ph.D. thesis]. London: Imperial College; 1996:49–59.
36. Ganeshan B, Miles KA, Young RC, Chatwin CR. Texture analysis in non-contrast enhanced CT: impact of malignancy on texture in apparently disease-free areas of the liver. *Eur J Radiol*. 2009;70:101–110.
37. Manduca A et al. Texture features from mammographic images and risk of breast cancer. *Cancer Epidemiol Biomarkers Prev*. 2009;18:837–845.
38. Haralick RM, Shanmugam K, Diristein I. Textural features for image classification. *IEEE Trans Syst Man Cybern SMC-3*. 1973;6:610–623.
39. Weszka JS, Dyer CR, Rosenfeld A. A comparative study of texture measures for terrain classification. *IEEE Trans Syst Man Cybern SMC-6*. 1976;4:269–285.
40. Galloway MM. Texture classification using gray level run lengths. *Comput Graph image Process*. 1975;4:172–179.
41. Lopes R, Betrouni N. Fractal and multifractal analysis: a review. *Med Image Anal*. 2009;13:634–649.
42. Wu CM, Chen YC. Texture features for classification of ultrasonic liver images. *IEEE Trans Med Imaging*. 1992;11:141–152.

Automated Classification of Plaques

Göran ML. Bergström, Ulrica Prahl, and Peter Holdfeldt

13.1 Introduction

Atherosclerotic plaques appear in the carotid artery with normal aging, and 60–90% of the population at 60 years of age has identifiable plaques.[1,2] However, only a fraction of these plaques will eventually be complicated by rupture or thrombosis and possibly cause an ischemic stroke (Chaps. 1, 2, and 4). Thus, one major challenge for vascular medicine is to develop techniques that allow us to identify these vulnerable carotid plaques and separate them from more stable plaques. Ultrasound examinations are instrumental in this work because they provide us with detailed image information and functional estimates of degree of stenosis with the additional benefits of low cost, high throughput, and accessibility.

Carotid plaques also provide information about cardiovascular risk in other vascular territories. The mere occurrence of plaques in the carotid artery is associated with an elevated risk of all forms of cardiovascular disease,[3–5] and this risk increases with increased plaque area.[6] Moreover, the ultrasound appearance of plaque tissue (plaque morphology) appears to be related to overall cardiovascular risk.[7] A number of publications have described different aspects of plaque morphology that predict future clinical events, including ipsilateral strokes as well as events in other vascular territories.[8–10] However, because of lack of conformity in the description of these morphological techniques, it is difficult to reproduce many of these results and even more difficult to use these data in clinical practice for cardiovascular risk prediction. The reason for the lack of conformity is, in many cases, that plaque appearance is visually judged by an examiner. The result is a subjective and highly user-dependent description of different aspects of plaque morphology that is difficult to reproduce. If the image analysis could be performed automatically, it is conceivable that more objective and user-independent information would be extracted. Hence, it is important, both for research and clinical use, to establish tools to objectively characterize and stratify the cardiovascular risk of carotid plaques from a population perspective.

There are basically three aspects of carotid plaque ultrasound appearance that need to be dealt with to stratify atherosclerotic carotid disease in different subtypes: (1) plaque presence (yes/no), (2) plaque size, and (3) the properties of the reflected ultrasound from plaque tissue.

There is a reasonably broad consensus on the definition of what constitutes a plaque and how it differs from a mere intima-media thickening.[11,12] However, an automatic procedure to identify plaques within the carotid artery ultrasound image is a methodological challenge. If successful, it would reduce the time needed for evaluation of images as well as reduce the subjectivity in plaque delinearization. Automatic procedures can also allow less well-experienced readers to evaluate images with good results. However, at present, only promising, mainly semiautomatic solutions are available. In contrast, an automatic solution to analyze the properties of the

G.ML. Bergström (✉) • U. Prahl • P. Holdfeldt
Wallenberg Laboratory for Cardiovascular Research, and Center for Cardiovascular and Metabolic Research, Sahlgrenska Academy, Institute of Medicine, University of Gothenburg, Gothenburg, Sweden

reflected ultrasound from plaque tissue has been more successful and is subject to intense research interest. This is further evidenced by the number of suggestions for semi- or fully automated feature extractions and automated procedures that have been published.[13-21] This chapter describes the advantages and disadvantages as well as the technical possibilities and limitations of using semi- or fully automated procedures to accomplish plaque classification.

13.2 Technical Aspects on Classification

A procedure that is used to automatically assign objects into different classes is called a classifier. There are a number of technical aspects that need to be considered when embarking on a project to develop an automated procedure for image classification. Figure 13.1 depicts an overview of the process, which has been described in detail in an excellent review by Jain et al.[22] Briefly, the development can be described in three major steps: training, validation, and classification.

Before the classifier can be used to classify a new object, it must be trained with the help of a training data-set using pre-classified samples. The purpose of the training is to find patterns in the test data that separate the different classes from each other. Carotid plaque images from patients with and without acute embolic stroke are a common training data-set. Sometimes the images are preprocessed to enhance the important information in the images (e.g., noise removal and normalization) and thereby making the work of the classifier easier and more accurate.

In image analysis, it is possible to consider all the individual pixel values and their information. However, it is usually better to aggregate this detailed information into one or more groups so-called *features*. Examples of image features are the gray scale mean and variance, features based on gray level co-occurrence matrices (also called "gray-tone spatial-dependence matrices")[23] and features based on frequencies in the image, i.e., its Fourier spectrum. It is quite common to start with a number of features that might or might not help the classification. The training process is then run several times to test which feature or combination of features leads to the best result to separate the two classes of images from each other.

When the training process results in a satisfactory result, the classifier needs to be *validated* using a validation data-set with images that have not yet been tested. Importantly, the same preprocessing must be applied to the new images, and the features should be extracted from the new images in exactly the same way as for the training data-set. The classifier then compares the extracted feature values with information from the training process and assigns the image to a certain class.

The validation process is important because the classifier might have a good performance on the training samples but generalizes badly, i.e., it has a problem with classifying new data. This phenomenon is called *over-fitting* and occurs because the classifier learns to detect irrelevant, random patterns in the training data. The risk of over-fitting increases if the number of features is high and the amount of training data is small.

Besides selecting the feature set, one must also decide which classification technique to use. A number of classifier techniques exist, some of the most common are: *Bayesian classifiers*, which try to find the most probable class for an object by using feature statistics (mean vectors and covariance matrices); *k-nearest-neighbors (k-NN) classifiers*, which classify

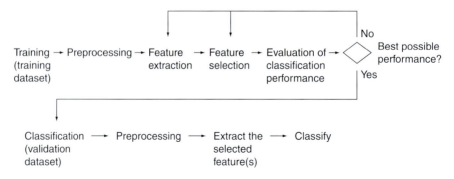

Fig. 13.1 Model for development of an automatic support system for plaque classification

objects by looking at the *k* nearest samples in the training set (most similar feature values); and *neural networks*, which are classifiers that are inspired by modern brain research. The computations are done by units called "neurons" that are organized in a network. More information about classification methodology can be found in the book by Duda et al.[24]

13.3 Preprocessing of Images to Facilitate Extraction of Image Information

As mentioned above, images are often preprocessed to facilitate the work of the classifier. One usually performed preprocessing task is to rescale the images which will normalize the image gray scale appearance in relation to different ultrasound equipment, different user settings, and differences in patient ultrasound characteristics. These factors result in differences between images that are not directly related to the actual plaque tissue, and it is an obvious concern when comparing plaques from different images. A way of reducing this problem is to *normalize* the images by linear rescaling of their intensity (gray scale) values.[25]

Structures that are small compared to the ultrasound wavelength cause diffuse echoes. The interferences between those echoes produce the characteristic granular "ultrasound look", called *speckle* in the image. Preprocessing the images with a *despeckle filter* usually improves the image quality and facilitates classification[26] (Chap. 6). Different forms of despeckle filters are usually integrated into modern ultrasound machines. A more in-depth discussion of despeckle filtering and normalization can be found in Chaps. 6 and 12.

13.4 Automatic Plaque Boundary Detection

Once preprocessing of the image has been performed, the boundaries of the plaque need to be delineated. Using computer software to partition an image into multiple sets of pixels is usually referred to as segmentation. At present, in both research and clinical work, segmentation of plaque tissue from the 2D ultrasound image of the carotid artery is mainly done manually by experienced ultrasonographers with reasonably high inter- and intra-observer reproducibility.[2,27,28]

However, if automated techniques are developed, this could speed up the analysis process and perhaps also make it possible for less-experienced staff to work with plaque segmentation. Automatic segmentation of the different layers of the vascular wall for intima-media thickness (IMT) measurements has proven very successful[29,30] (Chap. 11). The success of these techniques very much depends on the possibility to standardize the orientation of the image as well as the standardized position of the vascular wall from where the image is acquired. However, because of the irregular shape of a plaque, automatic plaque segmentation is much more difficult than detecting the almost horizontal boundaries of a "normal" vessel wall seen in the longitudinal axis. There is also a large variability of plaque shapes, making it hard for the automatic segmentation algorithm to be trained to know what a "correct" plaque should look like. Another challenge is that the plaque often develops in areas of the carotid artery where it is difficult to obtain high-quality standardized images (bulb and proximal internal carotid artery). Furthermore, when detecting the plaque-lumen border, another problem is the very weak echoes of the most echolucent plaques, making them difficult to distinguish from the low echogenicity of the blood-filled lumen.

Despite these challenges, attempts have been made to automatically segment images of carotid arteries for automatic calculation of plaque areas. In a small number of plaques, successful segmentation with an error as low as around 10% has been reported.[31] However, all plaques are different and the algorithm has to perform well in a large series of representative images. In a series of 80 plaques from longitudinal images, a good performance to detect the presence of plaque has been reported with an impressive true positive performance at around 80% and a true negative performance of similar magnitude.[32] However, the performance of the automatic procedure to calculate plaque area was less optimal with an overlap between the expert and the software of only 65–70%. A common problem of the published techniques is that they only have been tested in longitudinal sections of carotid arteries with good plaque visibility. It thus appears likely that these procedures can mainly be used for research purposes in selected populations. Development of a successful technique for clinical work is still awaited, and published data on the feasibility of plaque detection in less easily imaged sections of the carotid artery are urgently required.

A possible way to improve the performance of automatic plaque segmentation is to use image sequences instead of still images. By having multiple similar images of the same object, the detection quality might increase. Graph cuts is an interesting technique that can handle sequences of images for segmentation as well as interaction from the user.[33]

In summary, today there is no available software solution to automatically segment plaque tissue with performance comparable to that of the experienced human eye in combination with manual segmentation. Nevertheless, the present techniques could facilitate and speed up the manual segmentation work if semi-automated systems were constructed with the possibility to manually correct the automatic segmentation in a fast and efficient way.

The 2D representation of a plaque is an oversimplification that does not necessarily reflect the true 3D appearance. Attempts have been made to reconstruct 3D volumes of plaques that could possibly have higher predictive value for future clinical events than 2D areas[2,34] (Chaps. 16 and 18). Automatic segmentation of these 3D volumes offers other as yet unresolved challenges.

13.5 Automatic Analysis of the Backscattered Ultrasound from Plaque Tissue

Once the segmentation process is accomplished, the next challenge is to analyze the properties of the backscattered ultrasound from the plaque in a biologically meaningful way. Ever since ultrasound was first used to image carotid artery disease, different methods and systems have been suggested that can translate the different features of the ultrasound image and relate them to the histology of the plaque tissue.[35] The ultimate goal is to find features that can predict if the imaged plaque will eventually cause clinical problems or if it is one of many plaques that are just a coincidental finding and therefore mainly related to normal aging.

The ultrasound image features that have been tested for their predictive value can basically be divided into two groups: features related to the overall echogenicity of the plaque, which are dominating,[18,36–38] and features related to the texture of the plaque.[19,20,39] The texture of the plaque is often referred to as either homogenous (uniform distribution of echogenicity) or heterogenous (nonuniform distribution of echogenicity). The overall echogenicity of two plaques can thus be similar but their texture may differ.

A number of publications show that both overall plaque echogenicity and texture carry information on future risk of stroke as well as risk of all forms of cardiovascular events[40–46] (Chaps. 12, 15, and 36). However, many of these publications are based on classifications subjectively extracted by experienced ultrasonographers. The user dependency of these features makes them difficult to reproduce outside the specific laboratory. If automatic image analysis tools were applied, these features would be standardized and could be used by other laboratories in clinical trials and possibly implemented in clinical work flow.

Several reasonably successful automatic feature extraction processes have been described and will be covered briefly. A new feature that the authors have developed in their laboratory that makes use of several important aspects of carotid plaque ultrasound image information to extract one image feature will also be described.

During the past decade, gray scale median (GSM) has successfully been introduced as an important feature describing the overall echogenicity of the plaque ultrasound image.[14,47] The applicability of GSM measurements after image normalization (25, 36) is strengthened by the fact that it is based on the standard processed image extracted from the ultrasound scanner in combination with a commercially available software solution (Adobe Photoshop® [Adobe Systems Inc., San Jose, CA, USA] or other purposely designed software described in Chap. 12). GSM has been related to clinical events in several studies.[36,48–51] It has been demonstrated that this method has excellent reproducibility and that image standardization further reduces some of the inter-scanner and gain-level variability.[52] However, there is still a substantial measurement error related to the choice of standardization reference points.[52] Importantly, GSM has shown a predictive value in development of ipsilateral stroke in symptomatic patients[9] as well as in a recent prospective study on asymptomatic individuals with carotid artery stenosis[53] (Chap. 36).

Modern ultrasound systems use extensive post-processing such as log-compression of the backscattered signals to improve image quality. The integrated backscatter (IBS), which is based on analysis of the unprocessed radiofrequency signals, has been suggested to provide more undistorted and correct information on plaque characteristics[18,54] (Chap. 12). IBS produces a gray scale image proportional to the integrated backscatter power in dB.[13] The signal is sometimes normalized against the adventitial backscatter, producing a so-called calibrated integrated backscatter,[55] although other normalization methods are also used.[56] Histological studies suggest that this feature has some validity for in vivo characterization of plaque tissue.[54] Interestingly, published studies suggest that IBS can be used to monitor changes in plaque composition during treatment with statins.[57] However, prospective studies have not been published on the predictive value of IBS for ipsilateral stroke.

There are also a number of reports of techniques automatically extracting features related to the texture of plaque tissue[10,20,58,59] (Chaps. 12 and 14). These tools have so far been tested on relatively small series of images from asymptomatic and symptomatic carotid atherosclerosis. Results show that some of these texture features can identify atherosclerotic tissue associated with brain infarction, improving the results achieved by GSM alone.[10] However, the first study showing the predictive value of automated texture analysis for ipsilateral stroke has yet to be published.

13.6 Semi-Automated Method to Evaluate Echogenicity

On the bases of the success of GSM for image classifications, the authors were encouraged to further develop this concept by incorporating some other aspects of image information. The authors' aim was to develop an automatic software solution to classify plaques into high-echogenicity and low-echogenicity plaques according to the visual and subjective Gray-Weale classification,[60] and the novel aspect being that the software should mimic the human eye ability to incorporate information on general image noise and overall image echogenicity in the automatic procedure. The software was thus trained to correctly classify and separate a set of high-echogenicity plaques from a set of low-echogenicity plaques obtained from one of the authors' population-based studies.[61] The authors used the visual Gray-Weale[60] classification as their gold standard. The scale was slightly modified because they grouped dominantly echolucent and substantially echolucent plaques into one group called "echolucent" (hypoechoic) and dominantly echogenic and uniformly echogenic plaques into another group called "echogenic" (hyperechoic). The authors' intention was to develop a classifier that, in a similar way to that of an expert, classifies the overall echogenicity of a plaque, i.e., it estimates the relative occurrences of echolucent versus echogenic regions inside the plaque.

The authors chose to use a manual segmentation process for plaque delineation because their own and others' previous experience in this area was successful.[2,27,28] The program was thus semi-automatic and was therefore named SAMEE (Semi-Automated Method to Evaluate Echogenicity).[21]

To avoid problems with over-fitting (see above), the authors decided to base SAMEE on one single feature, percentage white (PW). PW describes the percentage of bright (echogenic) structures inside a plaque in relation to less bright (echolucent) structures. Before computing PW for a plaque, its image was normalized so that the most echolucent pixel in the image was referred to as black and the most echogenic pixel in the image was referred to as white (the image was rescaled to 0–255).

The algorithm to decide which pixels were to be considered echogenic was based on an intensity threshold (I_T), which was calculated as the sum of a constant (w_0) and two weighted intensity terms: echogenicity (I_E) and image noise (I_N). The sum of the weighted terms provides a threshold value as shown by the equation

$$I_T = w_E I_E + w_N I_N + w_0 \qquad (13.1)$$

The PW feature describes the percentage of plaque pixels with intensities above the intensity threshold. To compute the different components of the PW feature, four image regions were segmented as shown in Fig. 13.2: (1) *Image region* is segmented manually and is defined as the part of the image that contains pure ultrasound information from the tissue, (2) *plaque region* is also manually segmented, (3) *noise reference region* is automatically positioned in the vessel lumen just above (or below) the plaque region, and (4) *extended plaque region* is automatically positioned around the plaque region. I_N was calculated as the average image intensity in the noise reference region.

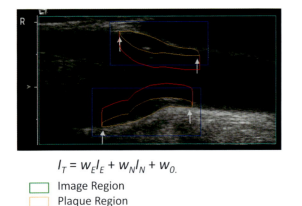

$I_T = w_E I_E + w_N I_N + w_0.$

☐ Image Region
☐ Plaque Region
☐ Extended Plaque Region (I_E, tissue echogenicity)
☐ Noise Reference Region (I_N)

Fig. 13.2 The SAMEE algorithm is based on image analysis of the following regions of the carotid ultrasound image: image region (*turquoise*), plaque region (*yellow*), extended plaque region (*blue*), and noise reference region (*red*) (Reprinted from Prahl[21], copyright 2010, with permission from Elsevier)

I_E was calculated from the image intensity in the extended plaque region. Because I_E is an assessment of the strength of the echoes inside this region, the authors first define which pixels belong to actual echoes. By using "trial and error", the authors decided to consider pixels with intensities above a cutoff value of 50 as being "real echoes" (i.e., not background noise). A histogram was formed with the intensities of these pixels, and the 85th percentile of that histogram was computed. Finally, I_E was obtained by subtracting the same cutoff value (50) from the computed percentile.

The value of the intensity threshold can be considered as an adaptive threshold that takes into account image echogenicity and noise in a similar way to the human eye. The rationale for our feature is the correlation of echo strength between the plaque and the surrounding tissue, i.e., if the echoes in the surrounding tissue are weak, the medium intensity pixels inside the plaque region are more likely to belong to actual echoes. Consequently, a low I_E results in a low I_T. If there is considerable noise inside the noise reference region (vessel lumen), the probability of noise inside the plaque region is also high. In this case, the medium intensity pixels are more likely to be artificial echoes (noise), i.e., a high I_N results in a high I_T.

To find the values of the constants for the weighted terms in the equation (Eq. 13.1), the software was then trained on a data-set consisting of 92 far-wall plaques and 47 near-wall plaques.[21,61] Based on data collected from the training set, the optimal values of the constants were $w_E = 0.5$, $w_N = 0.4$, and $w_0 = 15$ for far-wall plaques, and $w_E = 0.2$, $w_N = 0.3$, and $w_0 = 40$ for near-wall plaques. A plaque with a PW value >50.4 was classified as echogenic. This threshold was computed from the prior probabilities and the sample means and variances of the two classes, i.e., a Bayesian classifier (see above) was used. Using these criteria on the training set, the sensitivity (proportion of correctly classified echolucent plaques) and specificity (proportion of correctly classified echogenic plaques) were 96% and 81%, respectively for far-wall plaques, and 70% and 100% for near-wall plaques.

The SAMEE method was then validated with a new data-set consisting of 273 ultrasound images obtained from the same study.[61] The sensitivity for the validation data-set was 96%, and the specificity, 80%. Thus, it can be concluded that the authors' program generalizes well since it is capable of classifying new data (i.e., images not in the training set).

The authors also made a biological validation of the SAMEE algorithm, testing if the percentage white feature correlated with biomarkers of cardiovascular risk in the population. For this purpose, a data set consisting of both the plaques in the training set and the validation set as well as several new images was used (426 images from 264 subjects, with 41% of the subjects having more than one plaque). The authors used three different approaches to evaluate carotid plaque echogenicity in subjects with multiple plaques: (1) average PW (average of PW values from all plaques in each subject), (2) biggest plaque PW (PW value corresponding to the plaque with the biggest area in each subject), and (3) worst-case PW (lowest PW value identified of all plaques in each subject). The approach that showed the highest correlation with various risk factors was average PW, which was associated with several predictors of cardiovascular risk such as: lipoprotein(a), HbA1c, blood glucose, apolipoproteinB/apolipoproteinA-I ratio, adiponectin, and apolipoprotein A-I.

The SAMEE can serve as an example on how to develop automatic procedures for extraction of features from plaque ultrasound images in cardiovascular risk prediction. It combines manual segmentation procedures with automatic feature extraction. The SAMEE program and its main feature, percentage white, are constructed to handle different technical and artifact-related sources of variability and are thus intended to resemble the human ability to recognize patterns. SAMEE also correlates with GSM and is associated with a number of cardiovascular risk factors. The authors are currently testing the potential of SAMEE to predict cardiovascular events in both healthy populations as well as in clinical cohorts.

13.7 Summary

Automated classification of ultrasound images of plaque tissue is an important area for future research. Segmentation processes need to be improved as well as features that automatically handle data on plaque texture. More prospective observational studies with hard end-points are also encouraged to find out the true relevance of the different techniques to extract echogenicity and texture data. Finally, it is important to note that solid evidence showing that a feature is mechanistically linked to cardiovascular events is missing for all current features. No treatment study has yet been presented, showing that changes in plaque morphology extracted from ultrasound images result in improvement of CVD risk independent of other changes.

References

1. Joakimsen O, Bonaa KH, Stensland-Bugge E, Jacobsen BK. Age and sex differences in the distribution and ultrasound morphology of carotid atherosclerosis: the Tromso Study. *Arterioscler Thromb Vasc Biol.* 1999;19(12): 3007–3013.
2. Spence JD. Technology insight: ultrasound measurement of carotid plaque – patient management, genetic research, and therapy evaluation. *Nat Clin Pract Neurol.* 2006;2(11): 611–619.
3. Ebrahim S et al. Carotid plaque, intima media thickness, cardiovascular risk factors, and prevalent cardiovascular disease in men and women: the British Regional Heart Study. *Stroke.* 1999;30(4):841–850.
4. van der Meer IM et al. Predictive value of noninvasive measures of atherosclerosis for incident myocardial infarction: the Rotterdam Study. *Circulation.* 2004;109(9):1089–1094.
5. Wyman RA, Mays ME, McBride PE, Stein JH. Ultrasound-detected carotid plaque as a predictor of cardiovascular events. *Vasc Med.* 2006;11(2):123–130.
6. Spence JD. Ultrasound measurement of carotid plaque as a surrogate outcome for coronary artery disease. *Am J Cardiol.* 2002;89(4A):10B-15B; discussion 15B-16B.
7. Sztajzel R, Momjian-Mayor I, Comelli M, Momjian S. Correlation of cerebrovascular symptoms and microembolic signals with the stratified gray-scale median analysis and color mapping of the carotid plaque. *Stroke.* 2006;37(3): 824–829.
8. Belcaro G et al. Carotid and femoral ultrasound morphology screening and cardiovascular events in low risk subjects: a 10-year follow-up study (the CAFES-CAVE study(1)). *Atherosclerosis.* 2001;156(2):379–387.
9. Gronholdt ML, Nordestgaard BG, Schroeder TV, Vorstrup S, Sillesen H. Ultrasonic echolucent carotid plaques predict future strokes. *Circulation.* 2001;104(1):68–73.
10. Kakkos SK et al. Texture analysis of ultrasonic images of symptomatic carotid plaques can identify those plaques associated with ipsilateral embolic brain infarction. *Eur J Vasc Endovasc Surg.* 2007;33(4):422–429.
11. Touboul PJ et al. Mannheim intima-media thickness consensus. *Cerebrovasc Dis.* 2004;18(4):346–349.
12. de Bray JM, Baud JM, Daudzat M. Consensus concerning the morphology and the risk of carotid plaques. *Cerebrovasc Dis.* 1997;7:289–296.
13. Urbani MP et al. In vivo radiofrequency-based ultrasonic tissue characterization of the atherosclerotic plaque. *Stroke.* 1993;24(10):1507–1512.
14. el-Barghouty N, Geroulakos G, Nicolaides A, Androulakis A, Bahal V. Computer-assisted carotid plaque characterisation. *Eur J Vasc Endovasc Surg.* 1995;9(4): 389–393.
15. Wilhjelm JE et al. Quantitative analysis of ultrasound B-mode images of carotid atherosclerotic plaque: correlation with visual classification and histological examination. *IEEE Trans Med Imaging.* 1998;17(6):910–922.
16. Aly S, Bishop CC. An objective characterization of atherosclerotic lesion: an alternative method to identify unstable plaque. *Stroke.* 2000;31(8):1921–1924.
17. Pedro LM et al. Computer-assisted carotid plaque analysis: characteristics of plaques associated with cerebrovascular symptoms and cerebral infarction. *Eur J Vasc Endovasc Surg.* 2000;19(2):118–123.
18. Takiuchi S et al. Quantitative ultrasonic tissue characterization can identify high-risk atherosclerotic alteration in human carotid arteries. *Circulation.* 2000;102(7):766–770.
19. Christodoulou CI, Pattichis CS, Pantziaris M, Nicolaides A. Texture-based classification of atherosclerotic carotid plaques. *IEEE Trans Med Imaging.* 2003;22(7):902–912.
20. Stoitsis J, Tsiaparas N, Golemati S, Nikita KS. Characterization of carotid atherosclerotic plaques using frequency-based texture analysis and bootstrap. *Conf Proc IEEE Eng Med Biol Soc.* 2006;1:2392–2395.
21. Prahl U et al. Percentage white: a new feature for ultrasound classification of plaque echogenicity in carotid artery atherosclerosis. *Ultrasound Med Biol.* 2010;36(2) 218–226.
22. Jain AK, Duin RPW, Mao J. Statistical pattern recognition: a review. *IEEE Trans Pattern Anal Mach Intell.* 2000;2(1):4–37.
23. Haralick RM, Shanmugam K, Dinstein I. Textural features for image classification. *IEEE Trans Syst Man Cybern.* 1973;3(6):610–621.
24. Duda RO, Hart PE, Stork DG. *Pattern Classification.* New York: Wiley; 2001.

25. Griffin M, Nicolaides A, Kyriacou E. Normalisation of ultrasonic images of atherosclerotic plaques and reproducibility of grey scale median using dedicated software. *Int Angiol*. 2007;26(4):372–377.
26. Loizou CP et al. Comparative evaluation of despeckle filtering in ultrasound imaging of the carotid artery. *IEEE Trans Ultrason Ferroelectr Freq Control*. 2005;52(10): 1653–1669.
27. Persson J et al. Noninvasive quantification of atherosclerotic lesions. Reproducibility of ultrasonographic measurement of arterial wall thickness and plaque size. *Arterioscler Thromb*. 1992;12(2):261–266.
28. Kofoed SC, Gronholdt ML, Wilhjelm JE, Bismuth J, Sillesen H. Real-time spatial compound imaging improves reproducibility in the evaluation of atherosclerotic carotid plaques. *Ultrasound Med Biol*. 2001;27(10):1311–1317.
29. Wendelhag I, Liang Q, Gustavsson T, Wikstrand J. A new automated computerized analyzing system simplifies readings and reduces the variability in ultrasound measurement of intima-media thickness. *Stroke*. 1997;28(11):2195–2200.
30. Liang Q, Wendelhag I, Wikstrand J, Gustavsson T. A multiscale dynamic programming procedure for boundary detection in ultrasonic artery images. *IEEE Trans Med Imaging*. 2000;19(2):127–142.
31. Delsanto S et al. User-independent plaque characterization and accurate IMT measurement of carotid artery wall using ultrasound. *Conf Proc IEEE Eng Med Biol Soc*. 2006;1:2404–2407.
32. Loizou C, Pattichis C, Pantziaris M, Nicolaides A. An integrated system for the segmentation of atherosclerotic carotid plaque. *IEEE Trans Inf Technol Biomed*. 2007; 11(6):661–667.
33. Boykov Y, Funka-Lea G. Graph cuts and efficient n-d image segmentation. *Int J Comput Vis*. 2006;70(2):109–131.
34. Egger M, Spence JD, Fenster A, Parraga G. Validation of 3D ultrasound vessel wall volume: an imaging phenotype of carotid atherosclerosis. *Ultrasound Med Biol*. 2007;33 (6):905–914.
35. Wolverson MK, Bashiti HM, Peterson GJ. Ultrasonic tissue characterization of atheromatous plaques using a high resolution real time scanner. *Ultrasound Med Biol*. 1983;9 (6):599–609.
36. Elatrozy T, Nicolaides A, Tegos T, Griffin M. The objective characterisation of ultrasonic carotid plaque features. *Eur J Vasc Endovasc Surg*. 1998;16(3):223–230.
37. el-Barghouty N, Nicolaides A, Bahal V, Geroulakos G, Androulakis A. The identification of the high risk carotid plaque. *Eur J Vasc Endovasc Surg*. 1996;11(4):470–478.
38. Wijeyaratne SM et al. A new method for characterizing carotid plaque: multiple cross-sectional view echomorphology. *J Vasc Surg*. 2003;37(4):778–784.
39. Asvestas P, Golemati S, Matsopoulos GK, Nikita KS, Nicolaides AN. Fractal dimension estimation of carotid atherosclerotic plaques from B-mode ultrasound: a pilot study. *Ultrasound Med Biol*. 2002;28(9):1129–1136.
40. Johnson JM, Kennelly MM, Decesare D, Morgan S, Sparrow A. Natural history of asymptomatic carotid plaque. *Arch Surg*. 1985;120(9):1010–1012.
41. Sterpetti AV et al. Ultrasonographic features of carotid plaque and the risk of subsequent neurologic deficits. *Surgery*. 1988;104(4):652–660.
42. Langsfeld M, Gray-Weale AC, Lusby RJ. The role of plaque morphology and diameter reduction in the development of new symptoms in asymptomatic carotid arteries. *J Vasc Surg*. 1989;9(4):548–557.
43. Bock RW et al. The natural history of asymptomatic carotid artery disease. *J Vasc Surg*. 1993;17(1):160–169.
44. Belcaro G et al. Ultrasonic classification of carotid plaques causing less than 60% stenosis according to ultrasound morphology and events. *J Cardiovasc Surg (Torino)*. 1993;34 (4):287–294.
45. Liapis CD, Kakisis JD, Kostakis AG. Carotid stenosis: factors affecting symptomatology. *Stroke*. 2001;32 (12):2782–2786.
46. Mathiesen EB, Bonaa KH, Joakimsen O. Echolucent plaques are associated with high risk of ischemic cerebrovascular events in carotid stenosis: the Tromso study. *Circulation*. 2001;103(17):2171–2175.
47. Sztajzel R. Ultrasonographic assessment of the morphological characteristics of the carotid plaque. *Swiss Med Wkly*. 2005;135(43–44):635–643.
48. Biasi GM et al. Computer analysis of ultrasonic plaque echolucency in identifying high risk carotid bifurcation lesions. *Eur J Vasc Endovasc Surg*. 1999;17(6):476–479.
49. Matsagas MI et al. Computer-assisted ultrasonographic analysis of carotid plaques in relation to cerebrovascular symptoms, cerebral infarction, and histology. *Ann Vasc Surg*. 2000;14(2):130–137.
50. Hashimoto H, Tagaya M, Niki H, Etani H. Computer-assisted analysis of heterogeneity on B-mode imaging predicts instability of asymptomatic carotid plaque. *Cerebrovasc Dis*. 2009;28(4):357–364.
51. Reiter M et al. Increasing carotid plaque echolucency is predictive of cardiovascular events in high-risk patients. *Radiology*. 2008;248(3):1050–1055.
52. Fosse E et al. Repeated visual and computer-assisted carotid plaque characterization in a longitudinal population-based ultrasound study: the Tromso study. *Ultrasound Med Biol*. 2006;32(1):3–11.
53. Nicolaides A et al. Asymptomatic internal carotid artery stenosis and cerebrovascular risk stratification. *J Vasc Surg*. 2010;52(6):1486–1496.
54. Waki H et al. Ultrasonic tissue characterization of the atherosclerotic carotid artery: histological correlates or carotid integrated backscatter. *Circ J*. 2003;67(12):1013–1016.
55. Hirano M et al. Rapid improvement of carotid plaque echogenicity within 1 month of pioglitazone treatment in patients with acute coronary syndrome. *Atherosclerosis*. 2009;203(2):483–488.
56. Nagano K et al. Quantitative evaluation of carotid plaque echogenicity by integrated backscatter analysis: correlation with symptomatic history and histologic findings. *Cerebrovasc Dis*. 2008;26(6):578–583.
57. Yamada K et al. Effects of atorvastatin on carotid atherosclerotic plaques: a randomized trial for quantitative tissue characterization of carotid atherosclerotic plaques with integrated backscatter ultrasound. *Cerebrovasc Dis*. 2009;28(4):417–424.
58. Stoitsis J, Golemati S, Nikita KS, Nicolaides AN. Characterization of carotid atherosclerosis based on motion and texture features and clustering using fuzzy C-means. *Conf Proc IEEE Eng Med Biol Soc*. 2004;2:1407–1410.

59. Stoitsis J, Golemati S, Tsiaparas N, Nikita KS. Texture characterization of carotid atherosclerotic plaque from B-mode ultrasound using gabor filters. *Conf Proc IEEE Eng Med Biol Soc*. 2009;2009:455–458.
60. Gray-Weale AC, Graham JC, Burnett JR, Byrne K, Lusby RJ. Carotid artery atheroma: comparison of preoperative B-mode ultrasound appearance with carotid endarterectomy specimen pathology. *J Cardiovasc Surg (Torino)*. 1988;29(6):676–681.
61. Brohall G, Behre CJ, Hulthe J, Wikstrand J, Fagerberg B. Prevalence of diabetes and impaired glucose tolerance in 64-year-old Swedish women: experiences of using repeated oral glucose tolerance tests. *Diabetes Care*. 2006;29(2):363–367.

Plaque Feature Extraction

14

Christodoulos I. Christodoulou, Efthyvoulos Kyriacou, Marios S. Pattichis, and Constantinos S. Pattichis

14.1 Introduction

Feature extraction is a critical step in any pattern classification system. In order for the pattern recognition process to be tractable, it is necessary to convert patterns into features, which are condensed representations of the patterns, containing only salient information. Features contain the characteristics of a pattern in a comparable form making the pattern classification possible. The extraction of "good" features from the signal patterns and the selection from them of the ones with the most discriminatory power is very crucial for the success of the classification process. The feature extraction and selection is a dimensionality reduction process that is necessary in order to meet software and hardware constraints.

For carotid plaque characterization, texture and other features were extracted from the normalized and manually segmented ultrasound plaque images (Chap. 12) (see examples for asymptomatic and symptomatic plaques in Fig. 14.1). Texture contains important information, which is used by humans for the interpretation and the analysis of many types of images. It is especially useful for the analysis of natural scenes since they mostly consist of textured surfaces. Texture refers to the spatial interrelationships and arrangement of the basic elements of an image.[2] Visually, these spatial interrelationships and arrangements of the image pixels are seen as variations in the intensity patterns or gray tones. Therefore, texture features have to be derived from the gray tones of the image. Although texture can be easily recognized, it is quite a difficult task to define it, and subsequently interpret it, by digital computers. In this study, features containing information about plaque textural characteristics like first order statistics, gray level dependence matrices, coarseness, contrast, roughness, periodicity, and the complexity of the image are presented.

For the extraction of texture and other features, the authors selected from the literature the most popular ones and grouped them under the following four categories:

A. Single point based statistical plaque feature extraction studies (see Table 14.1)
   A.1 Single region of interest, or ROI (whole plaque)
   A.2 Multi ROIs (multiple plaque regions)
   A.3 Histogram based features
B. Spatial based plaque feature extraction studies (see Table 14.2)
   B.1 Geometrical
   B.2 Early texture features
   B.3 Morphological
   B.4 Multi-scale
C. Spatiotemporal plaque feature extraction studies (see Table 14.3)
D. 3D plaque feature extraction studies (see Table 14.4)

C.I. Christodoulou
Department of Computer Science, University of Cyprus, Nicosia, Cyprus

E. Kyriacou (✉)
Department of Computer Science and Engineering, Frederick University Cyprus, Lemesos, Cyprus

M.S. Pattichis
Department of Electrical and Computer Engineering, The University of New Mexico, Albuquerque, NM, USA

C.S. Pattichis
Department of Computer Science, University of Cyprus, Nicosia, Cyprus

Symptomatic plaques

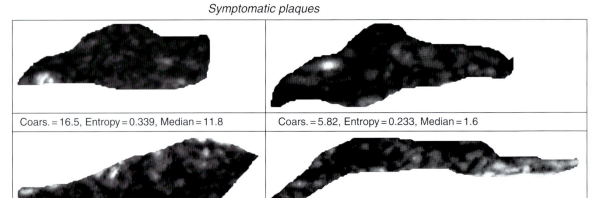

Asymptomatic plaques

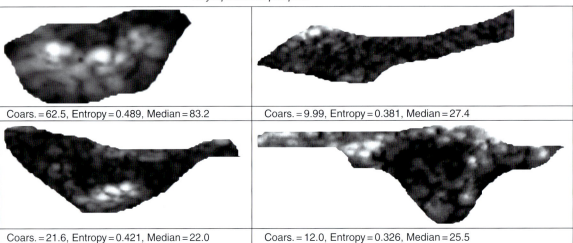

Fig. 14.1 Examples of symptomatic and asymptomatic plaques as these were segmented by the expert physician. Selected texture values are given for the features Coarseness, Entropy, and Median (Reprinted from Christodoulou et al.[1] © IEEE 2003)

In the following section, a brief overview of selected studies falling under the aforementioned four categories is given. In the subsequent section, feature selection methodologies are described. In the fourth section, results of feature extraction studies are given based on two case studies on early texture features, and morphology features, carried out by the authors' group. In the last section, the significance of these feature sets in differentiating between asymptomatic and symptomatic carotid plaque ultrasound images is described. Moreover, Chap. 15 describes computer-aided plaque classification studies based on selected feature sets presented in this chapter.

14.2 Plaque Feature Extraction Studies

14.2.1 Single Point Based Statistical Plaque Feature Extraction Studies

Single point based statistical plaque feature extraction studies, as listed in Table 14.1, are further subdivided into single ROI (whole plaque) studies, multi-ROIs (multiple plaque regions) studies, and histogram based features studies. Single ROI studies refer to the whole plaque, and these studies in general compute features such as the gray scale median (GSM) for the whole plaque region.

Table 14.1 Summary of selected single point based statistical plaque feature extraction studies

Author	Year	Ref.	N	Short description of study
A. Single point based statistical features				
A.1 Single ROI (whole plaque)				
El-Barghouty et al.	1995	3	94	*FE*: GSM
				FI: Echolucent plaques are characterized with GSM $\leq$ 32, whereas echogenic plaques with GSM $>$ 32. An association between carotid plaque echolucency and the incidence of cerebral computed tomography (CT) brain infractions was reported.
Biasi et al.	1998	4	96	*FE*: GSM
				FI: Symptoms correlated well with CT evidence of brain infarction: 32% of symptomatic patients had a positive CT scan versus 16% for asymptomatic plaques. The mean GSM value was 56 $\pm$ 14 for plaques associated with negative CT scans and 38 $\pm$ 13 for plaques from patients with positive scans.
Elatrozy et al.	1998	5	80	*FE*: GSM
				FI: GSM $<$ 40 related to ipsilateral hemispheric symptoms
Tegos et al.	2000	6	67	*FE*: GSM (measured on normalized images)
				FI: Retinal symptomatology was associated with a hypoechoic plaque appearance (GSM: 0), asymptomatic status with a hyperechoic plaque appearance (GSM: 34), and cerebrovascular symptomatology with an intermediate plaque appearance (GSM: 16). The histopathologic characteristics did not disclose differences between the three clinical groups.
Biasi et al.	2004	7	418	*FE*: GSM
				FI: Carotid plaque echolucency, as measured preprocedurally by GSM $\leq$ 25, increases the risk of stroke in Carotid artery stenting (CAS). The inclusion of echolucency measured as GSM in the planning of any endovascular procedure of carotid lesions allows stratification of patients at different risks of complications in CAS.
A.2 Multi ROIs (multiple plaque regions)				
Lal et al.	2002 2006	8,9	29	*FE*: GSM
				FI: GSM (range) in control subjects was 2 (0–4) for blood, 12 (8–26) for lipid, 53 (41–76) for muscle, 172 (112–196) for fibrous tissue, and 221 (211–255) for calcium. These features correlated significantly with the histologic estimates of each tissue respectively.
Sztajzel et al.	2005	10	28	*FE*: Stratified GSM determination as a distance from the plaque
				FI: Plaque pixels were further mapped into three different colors depending on their GSM value ($<$ 50 red; 50–80 yellow and $>$ 80 green). Histological findings demonstrated the predominance of the red color on the plaque surface was associated with symptomatic patients and a necrotic core located near the surface or a thin fibrous cap.
Madycki et al.	2006	11	76	*FE*: Gray scale values
				FI: Normalized colored gray scale values computed for patients scheduled for carotid endarterectomy (and then investigated for histology) corresponding to the echogenicity of blood (0–9), lipid (10–31), muscle (32–74), fibrous tissue (75–111), and for calcified tissue (112–255).
Hashimoto et al.	2009	12	250	*FE*: GSM
				FI: GSM values were assigned for blood, lipid, muscle/fibrous tissue, and calcification by comparison to endarterectomy specimens. Plaques in the top tertile for the percent area of lipid-like echogenicity showed an association with future infarction according to Kaplan–Meier analysis.
Prahl et al.	2010	13	97	*FE*: PW = percentage white, represents the fraction of bright structures inside a plaque
				FI: PW shows excellent reproducibility and agreement with visual assessment. Average PW values were associated with several predictors of cardiovascular risk: lipoprotein (a), HbA1c, blood glucose, apolipoprotein B/apolipoprotein A-I.

(continued)

Table 14.1 (continued)

Author	Year	Ref.	N	Short description of study
A.3 Histogram based features				
Kakkos et al.	2007 2010	14,15	137 188	*FE*: Percentage of pixels below gray level 30 (PP < 30), 50 (PP <50), of each of the 10 contours of the 0–255 gray level spectrum (PPC1-PPC10), and the first 2 contours (gray level 0–51) analyzed further into 5 sub-contours (PPCS1-PPCS5); SF, SGLDM, GLDS, RUNL, FPS.
				FI: PPCS10 (percentage of pixels 0–10), and SGLDM features were associated with unstable carotid plaques.[14]
				Texture analysis can identify carotid plaques associated with a neurological event, improving the diagnostic value of echolucency measures.[15]
Christodoulou et al.	2010	16	274	*FE*: Histogram computation in 32 equal width bins for the whole plaque, and for 3 equidistant plaque ROIs, and correlogram features.
				FI: Equidistant plaque histograms of the 3 ROIs could differentiate better between asymptomatic vs symptomatic plaques.

FE features extracted, *FI* findings, see bottom of Table 14.2 for abbreviations

Table 14.2 Summary of selected spatial-based plaque feature extraction studies

Author	Year	Ref.	N	Short description of study
B. Spatial-based features				
B.1 Geometrical				
Johnsen et al.	2005	17	1,952	*FE*: Plaque area and GSM)
				FI: This study shows that a high level of HDL cholesterol reduces plaque growth in subjects with preexisting carotid atherosclerosis.
Johnsen et al.	2007	18	6,226	*FE*: Carotid intima media thickness (IMT), total plaque area, and GSM as predictors for first-ever myocardial infarction (MI)
				FI: In a general population, carotid plaque area was a stronger predictor of first-ever MI than was IMT. Carotid atherosclerosis was a stronger risk factor for MI in women than in men. In women, the risk of MI increased with plaque echolucency.
Griffin et al.	2010	19	324	*FE*: Juxtaluminal Black (hypoechoic) Area (JBA) in mm2 and (GSM)
				FI: In a multiple logistic regression model, stenosis (mild, moderate, severe), GSM < 20 and JBA > 8 mm^2 were all strongly associated with hemispheric symptoms.
B.2 Early texture features				
Wilhjelm et al.	1998	20	52	*FE*: SF, SGLDM, and histology features
				FI: Some correlation was found between subjective, ultrasound texture features, and histological features where the best performing feature was found to be the contrast.
Christodoulou et al.	2003	1	230	*FE*: GSM, SF, SGLDM, NGTDM, SFM, FDTA, FPS
				FI: Plaques were classified into symptomatic or asymptomatic using the SOM and KNN classifiers and combining techniques with the best %CCs = 73%
Mougiakakou et al.	2007	21	108	*FE*: SF, Laws' texture energy measures
				FI: Plaques were classified into symptomatic or asymptomatic using a back propagation neural network with an overall %CCs = 99%.
B.3 Morphological				
Kyriacou et al.	2009	22	274	*FE*: Multilevel binary and gray scale morphological analysis
				FI: In this work, an integrated system for the assessment of the risk of stroke based on clinical risk factors and noninvasive investigations and carotid plaque texture analysis, and multilevel binary and gray scale morphological analysis in the assessment of atherosclerotic carotid plaques.
B.4 Multi-scale				
Asvestas et al.	2002	23	19	*FE*: Fractal Dimension (FD)
				FI: FD indicated a significant difference between the asymptomatic and symptomatic groups.

(continued)

Table 14.2 (continued)

Author	Year	Ref.	N	Short description of study
Christodoulou et al.	2008	24	274	FE: Amplitude Modulation–Frequency Modulation (AM-FM) features
				FI: AM-FM features performed slightly better than the traditional texture features in differentiating between asymptomatic and symptomatic plaques.
Tsiaparas et al.	2011	25	20	FE: multiresolution texture analysis based on the discrete wavelet transform (DWT), the stationary wavelet transform (SWT), wavelet packets (WP), and Gabor filters (GT)
				FI: WP analysis and the coiflet 1 features gave the highest classification accuracy in differentiating between asymptomatic and symptomatic plaques.

FE features extracted, FI findings, GSM Gray Scale Median, SF Statistical Features, SGLDM Spatial Gray Level Dependence Matrices, GLDS Gray Level Difference Statistics, NGTDM Neighborhood Gray Tone Difference Matrix, SFM Statistical Feature Matrix, TEM Laws Texture Energy Measures, FDTA Fractal Dimension Texture Analysis, FPS Fourier Power Spectrum, AM-FM Amplitude Modulation–Frequency Modulation

Table 14.3 Summary of selected spatiotemporal plaque feature extraction studies

Author	Year	Ref.	N	Short description of study
C. Spatiotemporal based features				
Meairs and Hennerici	1999	26	45	FE: 3D plaque surface velocities and internal carotid artery motions.
				FI: In asymptomatic patients, 3D plaque surface velocities were approximately equal to internal carotid artery velocities. In symptomatic cases, plaque surface velocities were both larger and independent than internal carotid artery motion.
Murillo et al.	2006	27	2	FE: 2D pixel motion trajectories from plaque region and internal carotid artery.
				FI: Significant motion differences between plaque and arterial motions.
Murray et al.	2007	28	2	FE: Motion velocity estimates based on new AM-FM and phase-based method.
				FI: AM-FM method provided significantly better motion estimates.
Gastounioti et al.	2010	29		FE: Block motion vector tracking using Kalman filtering.
				FI: Kalman filtering led to improved results over block-based methods.

FE features extracted, FI findings

Table 14.4 Summary of selected 3D plaque feature extraction studies

Author	Year	Ref.	N	Short description of study
3D plaque feature extraction studies				
Landry et al.	2004	30	40	FE: plaque volume change in plaques with volumes from 37.43 mm^3 to 604.1 mm^3.
				FI: 20–35% change can be detected with 95% confidence for plaques that are smaller than 100 mm^3. For larger plaques, we can detect volume changes of 10–20%.
Chiu et al.	2008	31		FE: 3D volumes of the plaque, intima, and media manually segmented 5 times in two imaging sessions.
				FI: 3D volume and volume change maps suggested for tracking plaque progression in relation to oscillatory shear and plaque regression.
Chiu et al.	2008	32		FE: Segmentation of 3D vessel wall plus plaque thickness and thickness changes.
				FI: Method showed promise for plaque volume and plaque volume changes.
Mallet et al.	2009	33	106	FE: intima media thickness, total plaque area, and vessel wall volume from a longitudinal study of carotid atherosclerosis for patients with diabetic nephropathy. 77 scanned at baseline and 2.3 ± 1 year (0.5–4.5 years). Both treated and untreated groups considered separately.
				FI: Vessel wall volume changes strongly correlated with changes in intima media thickness.
Awad et al.	2010	34		FE: 270 texture features from 3D ultrasound of carotid arteries based on the intima media boundary.
				FI: Fourier power spectrum and Laws texture energy measures gave the best results.

FE features extracted, FI findings

In one of the first studies, investigating the usefulness of GSM, El-Barghouty et al.,[3] documented that echolucent plaques are characterized with GSM ≤ 32, whereas echogenic plaques with GSM > 32 (Chap. 12). An association between carotid plaque echolucency and the incidence of cerebral computed tomography (CT) brain infractions was reported. Furthermore, Biasi et al.[4] found that symptoms correlated well with CT evidence of brain infarction: 32% of symptomatic patients had a positive CT scan versus 16% for asymptomatic plaques. The mean GSM value was 56 ± 14 for plaques associated with negative CT scans and 38 ± 13 for plaques from patients with positive scans. Elatrozy et al.[5] found that GSM < 40 was related to ipsilateral hemispheric symptoms.

The importance of image normalization is covered extensively in Chap. 12. One of the first studies that computed GSM on normalized images was by Tegos et al.[6] In this study, retinal symptomatology was associated with a hypoechoic plaque appearance (GSM: 0), asymptomatic status with a hyperechoic plaque appearance (GSM: 34), and cerebrovascular symptomatology with an intermediate plaque appearance (GSM: 16).

Biasi et al.[7] worked also on normalized images, and documented that carotid plaque echolucency, as measured preprocedurally by GSM ≤ 25, increases the risk of stroke in carotid artery stenting (CAS). Thus, the inclusion of echolucency measured as GSM in the planning of any endovascular procedure of carotid lesions allowed risk stratification of patients for complications in CAS.

The GSM can easily be computed in other plaque regions, given that these regions are manually, or automatically, or semiautomatically defined or segmented. Lal and his group[8,9] proposed that GSM (range) in control subjects was 2 (0–4) for blood, 12 (8–26) for lipid, 53 (41–76) for muscle, 172 (112–196) for fibrous tissue, and 221 (211–255) for calcium. These features correlated significantly with the histologic estimates of each tissue respectively.

Stratified GSM determination as a distance from the lumen was proposed by Sztajzel et al.[10] (Chap. 33). Plaque pixels were further mapped into three different colors depending on their GSM value (<50 red; 50–80 yellow; and >80 green). Histological findings demonstrated the predominance of the red color near the plaque surface was associated with symptomatic patients with a necrotic core located near the surface or a thin fibrous cap.

Similarly, Madycki et al.[11] proposed the following normalized colored gray scale values computed for patients scheduled for carotid endarterectomy (and then studied by histology) corresponding to the echogenicity of blood (0–9), lipid (10–31), muscle (32–74), fibrous tissue (75–111), and for calcified tissue (112–255). Moreover, Hashimoto et al.[12] assigned GSM values for blood, lipid, muscle/fibrous tissue, and calcification by comparison to endarterectomy specimens. Plaques in the top tertile for the percent area of lipid-like echogenicity showed an association with future infarction according to Kaplan–Meier analysis.

A different measure was proposed by Prahl et al.[13] He introduced percentage white (PW), that represents the fraction of bright structures inside a plaque. It was found that PW shows excellent reproducibility and agreement with visual assessment. Average PW values were associated with several markers of atherosclerotic disease: lipoprotein (a), HbA1c, blood glucose, apolipoproteinB/apolipoproteinA-I.

Several histogram based features were also proposed by Kakkos and co-workers,[14,15] and Christodoulou et al.[16] Kakkos et al. proposed the following histogram based features: percentage of pixels below gray level 30 (PP < 30), 50 (PP < 50), of each of the 10 contours of the 0–255 gray level spectrum (PPC1-PPC10), and the first 2 contours (gray level 0–51) analyzed further into 5 sub-contours (PPCS1-PPCS5). In addition, several early texture features were computed as documented in the following subsection: statistical features (SF), spatial gray level dependence matrix (SGLDM), gray level difference statistics (GLDS), gray level run length statistics (RUNL), Fourier power transform (FPS). It was found that PPCS10 (percentage of pixels 0–10) and SGLDM features were associated with unstable carotid plaques.[14] Moreover, texture analysis could identify carotid plaques associated with a neurological event, improving the diagnostic value of echolucency measures.[15]

Furthermore, Christodoulou et al.[16] proposed histogram computation in 32 equal width bins for the whole plaque, and for three equidistant plaque ROIs, and correlogram features. It was found that equidistant plaque histograms of the 3 ROIs could differentiate better between asymptomatic versus symptomatic plaques.

14.2.2 Spatial Based Plaque Feature Extraction Studies

Spatial based plaque feature extraction studies listed in Table 14.2 are further subdivided into geometrical, early texture features, and multi-scale.

In plaque geometrical studies, Johnsen and his group[17] measured plaque area and GSM, and showed that a high level of HDL cholesterol reduces plaque growth in subjects with preexisting carotid atherosclerosis and is associated with hyperechoic plaques. In another extensive study by the same group,[18] carotid intima media thickness (IMT), total plaque area, and GSM were significant predictors for first-ever myocardial infarction (MI). It was found that in a general population, carotid plaque area was a stronger predictor of first-ever MI than IMT. Also, carotid atherosclerosis was a stronger risk factor for MI in women than in men. In women, the risk of MI increased with plaque echolucency. Furthermore, Griffin et al.[19] measured juxtaluminal black (hypoechoic) area (JBA) in mm^2 and GSM, and found that in a multiple logistic regression model, stenosis (mild, moderate, severe), GSM < 20, and JBA > 8 mm^2 were all strongly associated with hemispheric symptoms.

Early texture features were investigated by a number of studies. In general, these studies extracted the following feature sets that are documented in detail at the appendix at the end of this chapter:
1. Statistical Features (SF)[35]
2. Spatial Gray Level Dependence Matrices (SGLDM) algorithm[36]
3. Gray Level Difference Statistics (GLDS) algorithm[37]
4. Neighborhood Gray Tone Difference Matrix (NGTDM)[2]
5. Statistical Feature Matrix (SFM) method[38]
6. Laws Texture Energy Measures (TEM)[39,40]
7. Fractal Dimension Texture Analysis (FDTA)[41]
8. Fourier Power Spectrum (FPS)[37,40]

The ultrasound carotid plaque feature sets SF and SGLDM, as well as histology features were investigated by Wilhjelm et al.[20] They found that some correlation existed between subjective, ultrasound texture features, and histological features where the best performing feature was found to be the contrast. Christodoulou and co-workers[1] carried out an extensive study on early texture feature analysis, where the following feature sets were investigated: SF (including GSM), SGLDM, NGTDM, SFM, TEM, FDTA, and FPS. Plaques were classified into symptomatic or asymptomatic using the self-organizing feature maps (SOM) and the K nearest neighbors (KNN) classifiers and combining techniques having as input the aforementioned texture feature sets. The best correct classifications score achieved was 73%. More details about this study are given in the following section. Furthermore, the SF and TEM texture feature sets were investigated by Mougiakagou et al.[21] Plaques were classified into symptomatic or asymptomatic using a back propagation neural network with an overall percentage of correct classifications score equal to 99%.

Morphology feature sets were also investigated by Kyriacou et al.[22] based on the works of Dougherty,[42] Dougherty and Astola,[43] and Marangos,[44] and are documented in the last sub-section of the appendix. The study by Kyriacou et al.[22] used an integrated system for the association of plaques with stroke (multilevel binary and gray scale morphological). More details on plaque morphological analysis feature sets are given also in the following section.

Multi-scale plaque feature analysis studies were carried out by Asvestas et al.,[23] Christodoulou et al.,[24] and Tsiaparas et al.[25] Asvestas et al.[23] investigated the use of fractal dimension (FD) and found that a significant difference existed between the asymptomatic and symptomatic groups. Christodoulou et al.[24] investigated the use of Amplitude Modulation–Frequency Modulation (AM-FM) features in differentiating between asymptomatic and symptomatic plaques. It was found that early AM-FM features performed slightly better than the traditional early texture features. Furthermore, Tsiaparas et al.[25] in a recent study, investigated the use of multiresolution texture analysis based on the discrete wavelet transform (DWT), the stationary wavelet transform (SWT), wavelet packets (WP), and Gabor filters (GT). They found that WP analysis and the coiflet 1 features gave the highest classification accuracy in differentiating between asymptomatic and symptomatic plaques.

14.2.3 Spatiotemporal Plaque Feature Extraction Studies

Spatiotemporal features range from block motion estimates, 2D and 3D velocity estimates, and 2D pixel trajectories (Table 14.3). An important early study by Meairs and Hennerici[26] used 4D ultrasound for motion estimation. Using 45 patients, Meairs and Hennerici showed that in asymptomatic plaques, plaque surface motion vectors were approximately equal to motion vectors of the internal carotid artery. In contrast, plaques from symptomatic patients exhibited independent motion with larger surface motion.

For B-mode ultrasound, Murillo et al.[27] computed motion trajectories over the plaques and used the results to develop realistic, synthetic models of plaque motion. Murray et al.[28] developed a new, AM-FM motion estimation model and demonstrated that it can provide dense estimates over the entire cardiac cycle. Gastounioti et al.[29] developed a Kalman filter extension to basic block matching to obtain better block motion estimates.

14.2.4 3D Plaque Feature Extraction Studies

The development of 3D techniques (Table 14.4) has been dominated by the use of geometric features. The important exceptions include the 3D motion study[26] covered earlier and a more recent texture feature study.[34]

Landry et al.[30] demonstrated that significant volume changes can be detected using 3D ultrasound. Chiu et al.[31,32] suggested the use of 3D volume maps of the plaque, intima, and the media for visualizing localized 3D changes. Here, Chiu et al. recommend the use of 3D volume and 3D volume change maps for monitoring disease progression and its relation to oscillatory shear and plaque regression. A more extensive, longitudinal study of 106 patients found strong correlations between the intima media thickness and the vessel wall volume changes.[33] Awad et al.[34] investigated the use of 270 texture features extracted from 3D ultrasound. Results indicated that Fourier power spectrum features and Laws texture energy measures gave the most promising results.

14.3 Feature Selection

Several algorithms are available for the extraction of texture features. The most popular algorithms were implemented and a great number of texture features as listed in the previous section and the appendix have been extracted from the plaque images. The selection of the ones with the most discriminatory power can reduce the dimensionality of the input data and improve the classification performance. In the authors' work, the best features were selected using univariate selection, multivariate selection, and principal component analysis (PCA).

14.3.1 Univariate Selection

From the features extracted as described above, the best performing features were identified in order to be used later for the classification of the carotid plaques. A simple way to identify potentially good features is to compute the distance between the two classes for each feature as

$$\text{dis} = \frac{|m_1 - m_2|}{\sqrt{\sigma_1^2 + \sigma_2^2}} \quad (14.1)$$

where m_1 and m_2 are the mean values, and σ_1 and σ_2 are the standard deviations of the two classes.[1] Best features are considered to be the ones with the greatest distance. The mean and standard deviation of the features extracted from all the plaques, as well as for the symptomatic and asymptomatic groups were computed, and the distance between the two classes for each feature was calculated as described in Eq. 14.1. The features were ordered according to their interclass distance, and the features with the greatest distance were selected.

14.3.2 Multivariate Selection

Beyond the above described univariate selection method where each feature is considered in isolation ignoring its relationship to other features, features are considered in groups using multivariate selection. Because of the huge number of possible feature combinations and the computational effort, search strategies have to be used[45]: (14.1) the forward selection method which starts with the selection of the best individual feature as the first feature, and subsequently a feature is added at each iteration which in combination with the already selected feature(s) improves the class separability mostly and (2) the backwards elimination method where at each iteration, the feature which contributes to the class separability less is discarded.

14.3.3 Principal Component Analysis

Another way for feature selection and dimensionality reduction is the use of principal component analysis (PCA).[46] In PCA, the data set is represented by a reduced number of uncorrelated features while retaining most of its information content. This is carried out by eliminating correlated components, which contribute only to a small amount to the total variance in the data set.

14.4 Feature Extraction Case Studies

In a number of studies[1,20,21] carried out on carotid plaque characterization by the authors' team, the above texture features were extracted and evaluated. Some of the results from these studies are summarized below. Before processing, the images were normalized by adjusting the image linearly so that the gray level value of blood to be about 0, and the gray level of adventitia to be about 190. The scale of the gray level of the images ranged from 0 to 255. In addition, images were standardized to a pixel density of 20 pixels/mm (Chap. 12). This normalization was necessary in order to extract comparable measurements in case of processing images obtained by different operators or different equipment. Plaque identification and segmentation were carried out manually by expert physicians and/or vascular ultrasonographers as described in Chap. 12.

In a dataset of 230 (115 symptomatic and 115 asymptomatic) ultrasound images of carotid atherosclerotic plaques, nine different texture feature sets as listed above with a total of 56 features were extracted from the segmented carotid plaque images (see examples in Fig. 14.1). The results obtained through the feature selection techniques and part of the selected features with the highest discriminatory power are given in Table 14.5.[1] The mean and standard deviation for the symptomatic and asymptomatic groups were computed for each individual feature. Furthermore, the distance between the two classes was computed as described above using Eq. 14.1 and the features were ordered according to their interclass distance. The best features were the ones with the greatest distance.

Best texture features as tabulated in Table 14.5 were found to be the coarseness of NGTDM with average and standard deviation values for the symptomatic plaques 9.3 ± 8.2 and for the asymptomatic plaques 21.4 ± 14.9, the range of values of angular second moment of SGLDM with 0.0095 ± 0.0055 and 0.0050 ± 0.0050, and the range of values of entropy also of SGLDM with 0.28 ± 0.11 and 0.36 ± 0.11 for the symptomatic and the asymptomatic plaques respectively. Features from other feature sets which also performed well were the median gray level value (SF) with average values for the symptomatic plaques 15.7 ± 16.6 and for the asymptomatic plaques 29.4 ± 22.9, the fractal value H1 with 0.37 ± 0.08 and 0.42 ± 0.07 respectively, the roughness of SFM with 2.39 ± 0.13 and 2.30 ± 0.10, and the periodicity also of SFM with 0.58 ± 0.08 and 0.62 ± 0.06 for the symptomatic and the asymptomatic plaques respectively. Two-dimensional scatter plots illustrating the difficulty of the problem in differentiating between asymptomatic and symptomatic plaques for the most discriminatory features are given in Fig. 14.2.

In general, texture in symptomatic plaques tends to be more dark, more heterogeneous, more rough, and less periodical, whereas in asymptomatic plaques, texture tends to be brighter, with less contrast, more homogeneous, more smooth, with large areas of small gray tone variations, and more periodical. These results tabulated in Table 14.6 are in agreement with the original assumption that smooth surface, echogenicity, and a homogenous texture are characteristics of stable plaques, whereas irregular surface, echolucency, and a heterogeneous texture are characteristics of potentially unstable plaques.

In a second dataset where the usefulness of the morphological features was investigated, a total of 274 ultrasound images of carotid atherosclerotic plaques were analyzed.[22] The morphological algorithms extracted features from the plaque images. Structural elements of several sizes are defined in the appendix at the end of the chapter. The classification for some cases was slightly improved compared to the one from the texture analysis (see Chap. 15). Using an algorithm based on decision trees[22] and

Table 14.5 Statistical analysis of 16 out of 56 texture and shape features computed from the 230 (115 symptomatic and 115 asymptomatic) ultrasound images of carotid atherosclerotic plaques of dataset 1. For each feature, the mean and standard deviation were computed (1) for the symptomatic group, and (2) for the asymptomatic group. The distance between the symptomatic and asymptomatic groups was computed as described in Eq. 14.1 and their rank order according to their interclass distance is given

		Symptomatic		Asymptomatic		Distance	
Nr	Texture feature	Mean m_1	Std σ_1	Mean m_2	Std σ_2	$dis = \frac{|m_1 - m_2|}{\sqrt{\sigma_1^2 + \sigma_2^2}}$	Rank order
Statistical Features (SF)							
2	Median	15.71	16.62	29.40	22.87	0.484	10
Spatial Gray Level Dependence Matrices (SGLDM) – Mean values							
6	Angular second moment	0.1658	0.1866	0.0646	0.1201	0.456	11
10	Inverse difference moment	0.4856	0.1827	0.3545	0.1613	0.538	6
11	Sum average	57.091	33.671	82.675	44.953	0.456	13
13	Sum entropy	3.759	1.163	4.619	1.000	0.561	5
14	Entropy	4.730	1.619	5.972	1.456	0.570	4
15	Difference variance	280.5	119.8	219.7	65.8	0.445	12
Spatial Gray Level Dependence Matrices (SGLDM) – Range of values							
19	Angular second moment	0.0095	0.0055	0.0050	0.0050	0.611	2
27	Entropy	0.277	0.109	0.365	0.106	0.571	3
31	Information measures of correlation	0.0314	0.0189	0.0214	0.0120	0.448	14
Gray Level Difference Statistics (GLDS)							
33	Angular second moment (Energy)	0.259	0.181	0.161	0.125	0.446	16
Neighborhood Gray Tone Difference Matrix (NGTDM)							
36	Coarseness	9.265	8.236	21.354	14.909	0.710	1
Statistical Feature Matrix (SFM)							
43	Periodicity	0.578	0.081	0.625	0.064	0.452	15
44	Roughness	2.386	0.127	2.301	0.100	0.527	8
Fractal Dimension Texture Analysis (FDTA)							
51	H1	0.367	0.081	0.423	0.068	0.531	7
52	H2	0.291	0.063	0.336	0.059	0.521	9

Source: Adapted from Christodoulou et al.[1]

principal component analysis, a total number of five features were selected and used in the classification scheme. Figure 14.3 is showing an example of binary morphology applied on one plaque from the asymptomatic group and one from the symptomatic group. As can be seen in Fig. 14.3 the different levels can emphasize different structures in each plaque.

14.5 Interpretation and Significance of Results

The statistics for the texture features extracted and shown in Table 14.1 indicate a high degree of overlap between the symptomatic and asymptomatic groups. Best texture features on an individual basis using their statistics as tabulated in Table 14.1 were found to be the coarseness of NGTDM, the entropy, the mean values of angular second moment and inverse difference moment of SGLDM, the median gray level value, the fractal values H1 and H2, and the roughness and periodicity of SFM. Morphological features exhibited poorer discriminatory capability between symptomatic and asymptomatic plaques, compared to texture features. As it is shown in Tables 14.5 and 14.7, the highest distance for morphological features was 0.393 whereas for texture it was 0.710.

In previous work, a relationship between plaque morphology and risk of stroke was reported.[3,5,47] In a prospective study, Polak et al.[47] found that hypoechoic

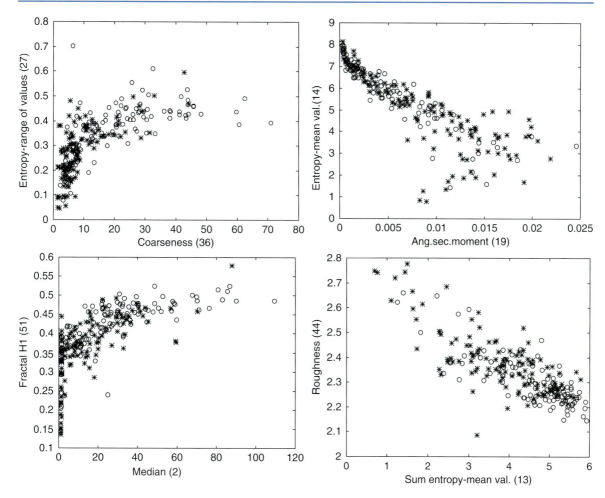

Fig. 14.2 Two-dimensional plots for the 230 carotid plaques, of several combinations of some of the best features as these are tabulated in table I (* = symptomatic, o = asymptomatic). All plots show the high degree of overlap between the symptomatic and asymptomatic plaque classes (Reprinted from Christodoulou et al.[1] © IEEE 2003)

Table 14.6 Verbal interpretation of the arithmetical values of some of the features from Table 14.5, for the symptomatic versus the asymptomatic plaques

Feature	Symptomatic	Asymptomatic
Median gray level	More dark	Brighter
Entropy	Less local uniformity in image density	Image intensity in neighboring pixels is more equal
Roughness	More rough	More smooth
Periodicity	Less periodical	More periodical
Coarseness	Less local uniformity in intensity	Large areas with small gray tone variations
Fractals H1, H2	Rough texture surface	Smooth texture surface

Source: Adapted from Christodoulou et al.[1]

carotid plaques, as seen on ultrasound images of the carotid arteries, were associated with increased risk of stroke. In their study, plaques were visually categorized as hypoechoic, isoechoic, or hyperechoic by independent readers. El-Barghouty et al.[3] reported an association between carotid plaque echolucency and the prevalence of cerebral infarction on CT-brain scans. They used the gray scale median (GSM) of the ultrasound plaque image for classifying the plaques as echolucent (GSM $\leq$ 32) or echogenic (GSM $>$ 32). Elatrozy et al.[5] also reported that carotid plaque GSM less than 40 had a strong association with ipsilateral hemispheric symptoms. In the authors' work, the best cutoff GSM value (highest sensitivity combined with highest specificity) was found to be 23 (GSM $\leq$ 23 for symptomatic plaques

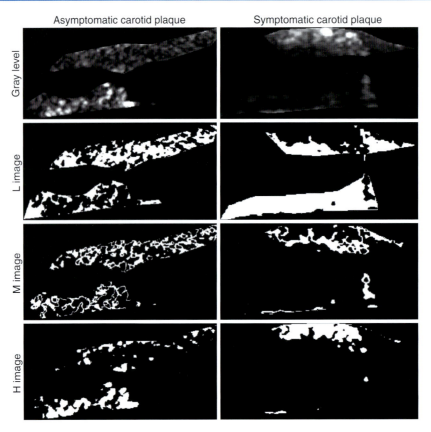

Fig. 14.3 Binary morphology example applied on one plaque from the asymptomatic and one from the symptomatic group. The three different sets are displaying three binary level images: (L, M, H) of the plaques (With kind permission from Springer Science+Business Media: Kyriacou et al.[22]. Figure 1)

Table 14.7 Statistical analysis of the four best morphological features computed from the 330 (194 asymptomatic and 136 symptomatic) ultrasound images of carotid plaques of dataset 2. For each feature, the mean and standard deviation were computed for the asymptomatic group and for the symptomatic group. The distance between the symptomatic and the asymptomatic groups was computed as described in Eq. 14.1

Feature	Symptomatic plaques		Asymptomatic plaques		Distance
	Mean m_1	Std σ_1	Mean m_2	Std σ_2	dis $= \frac{|m_1-m_2|}{\sqrt{\sigma_1^2+\sigma_2^2}}$
$P_{1,'+'}$	0.0433	0.0407	0.0249	0.0229	0.393
$P_{3,'+'}$	0.1922	0.1218	0.1355	0.0870	0.379
$P_{2,'+'}$	0.1102	0.0888	0.0713	0.0520	0.378
$P_{-4,'+'}$	0.0080	0.0061	0.0119	0.0084	0.370

Source: Adapted from Kyriacou et al.[22]

and GSM > 23 for asymptomatic plaques). The difference in the computed GSM value from the previous studies can be attributed for the El-Barghouty et al. work[1] to the fact that the gray level of the plaque images was not normalized using blood and adventitia as reference. In the case of Elatrozy et al.[5] a normalization procedure was followed, as described in Chap. 12. Furthermore, the use of color flow in the lumen allowed the correct outline of the plaque region. This was especially useful in the case of the highly echolucent (dark) plaques where the plaque boundaries were not visible on gray scale images, and therefore dark areas of the plaque were not considered. This can explain why the GSM value of 23 reported in our work is lower than the GSM values reported in the other two studies.

The results presented indicate that it is possible to use texture features from high-resolution ultrasound images of carotid plaques to demonstrate differences between symptomatic and asymptomatic plaques. State-of-the-art ongoing work includes the investigation of multi-scale texture features, and most importantly spatiotemporal, and 3D feature extraction studies. These features are ideally suitable for computer-aided plaque classification studies which are presented in the subsequent chapter (Chap. 15).

Appendix 1   Statistical Features (SF)

The SF features are resolution independent. The following SF features were computed[35]:

1. *Mean value*

   The mean of the gray level values $I_1, \ldots, I_N$ of the pixels of the segmented plaque.

   $$\bar{I} = \frac{1}{N} \sum_{j=1}^{N} I_j \qquad (14.2)$$

2. *Median value*

   The median I_{med} of the distribution of the gray level values $I_1, \ldots, I_N$ is the value of the middle item of the distribution.

3. *Standard Deviation*

   $$\sigma = \sqrt{\frac{1}{N-1} \sum_{j=1}^{N} (I_j - \bar{I})^2} \qquad (14.3)$$

4. *Skewness*

   $$\text{Skew} = \frac{1}{N} \sum_{j=1}^{N} \left[\frac{I_j - \bar{I}}{\sigma} \right]^3 \qquad (14.4)$$

   The skewness characterizes the degree of asymmetry of a distribution around its mean.

5. *Kurtosis*

   $$\text{Kurt} = \left\{ \frac{1}{N} \sum_{j=1}^{N} \left[\frac{I_j - \bar{I}}{\sigma} \right]^4 \right\} - 3 \qquad (14.5)$$

   Kurtosis measures the peakedness or flatness of a distribution in relation to a normal distribution.

Appendix 2   Spatial Gray Level Dependence Matrices (SGLDM)

The spatial gray level dependence matrices as proposed by Haralick et al.[36] are based on the estimation of the second-order joint conditional probability density functions, $f(i, j, d, \theta)$. The $f(i, j, d, \theta)$ is the probability that two pixels (k,l) and (m,n) with distance d in direction specified by the angle θ have intensities of gray level i and gray level j.[38] The estimated values for these probability density functions will be denoted by $P(i, j, d, \theta)$. In a $N_x \times N_y$ image, let $L_x = \{1, 2, \ldots, N_x\}$ be the horizontal spatial domain, $L_y = \{1, 2, \ldots, N_y\}$ be the vertical spatial domain, and $I(x,y)$ be the image intensity at pixel (x,y). Formally, for angles quantized at 45° intervals, the unnormalized probability density functions are defined by

$$\begin{aligned} P(i,j,d,0°) = &\#\{((k,l),(m,n)) \in (L_y \times L_x) \\ &\times (L_y \times L_x) : k-m=0, |l-n|=d, \\ &I(k,l)=i, I(m,n)=j\} \end{aligned} \qquad (14.6)$$

$$\begin{aligned} P(i,j,d,45°) = &\#\{((k,l),(m,n)) \in (L_y \times L_x) \\ &\times (L_y \times L_x) : (k-m=d, |l-n|=d) \\ &\text{or } (k-m=-d, l-n=d), \\ &I(k,l)=i, I(m,n)=j\} \end{aligned} \qquad (14.7)$$

$$\begin{aligned} P(i,j,d,90°) = &\#\{((k,l),(m,n)) \in (L_y \times L_x) \\ &\times (L_y \times L_x) : |k-m|=d, l-n=0, \\ &I(k,l)=i, I(m,n)=j\} \end{aligned} \qquad (14.8)$$

$$\begin{aligned} P(i,j,d,135°) = &\#\{((k,l),(m,n)) \in (L_y \times L_x) \\ &\times (L_y \times L_x) : (k-m=d, |l-n|=d) \\ &\text{or}(k-m=-d, l-n=-d), \\ &I(k,l)=i, (m,n)=j\} \end{aligned} \qquad (14.9)$$

where # denotes the number of elements in the set.

Haralick et al.[36] proposed the following texture measures that can be extracted from the spatial gray level dependence matrices:

Notation

$p(i, j)$	(i, j)th entry in the normalized spatial gray level dependence matrix, $= P(i, j)/R$, where R is a normalizing constant.
$p_x(i)$	ith entry in the marginal probability matrix obtained by summing the rows of $p(i, j)$, $= \sum_{j=1}^{N_g} p(i, j)$.
N_g	Number of distinct gray levels in the quantized image.
	$\sum_i$ means $\sum_{i=1}^{N_g}$, and $\sum_j$ means $\sum_{j=1}^{N_g}$
$p_y(i) =$	$\sum_{i=1}^{N_g} p(i, j)$.
$p_{x+y}(k) =$	$\sum_{\substack{i=1 \\ i+j=k}}^{N_g} \sum_{j=1}^{N_g} p(i, j)$, $k = 2, 3, \ldots 2N_g$
$p_{x-y}(k) =$	$\sum_{\substack{i=1 \\ |i-j|=k}}^{N_g} \sum_{j=1}^{N_g} p(i, j)$, $k = 0, 1, \ldots N_g - 1$.

Texture Measures

1. Angular second moment

$$f_1 = \sum_i \sum_j \{p(i, j)\}^2 \quad (14.10)$$

The angular second moment is a measure for homogeneity of the image.

2. Contrast

$$f_2 = \sum_{i=1}^{N_g - 1} n^2 \left\{ \sum_{\substack{i=1 \\ |i-j|=n}}^{N_g} \sum_{j=1}^{N_g} p(i, j) \right\} \quad (14.11)$$

The contrast is a measure of the amount of local variations present in the image.

3. Correlation

$$f_3 = \frac{\sum_i \sum_j (i, j)p(i, j) - \mu_x \mu_y}{\sigma_x \sigma_y} \quad (14.12)$$

where μ_x, μ_y, and σ_x, σ_y, are the mean and standard deviation values of p_x and p_y. Correlation is a measure of gray tone linear dependencies.

4. Sum of squares: variance

$$f_4 = \sum_i \sum_j (i - \mu)^2 p(i, j) \quad (14.13)$$

5. Inverse difference moment

$$f_5 = \sum_i \sum_j \frac{1}{1 + (i-j)^2} p(i, j) \quad (14.14)$$

6. Sum average

$$f_6 = \sum_{i=2}^{2N_g} i p_{x+y}(i) \quad (14.15)$$

7. Sum variance

$$f_7 = \sum_{i=2}^{2N_g} (i - f_6)^2 p_{x+y}(i) \quad (14.16)$$

8. Sum entropy

$$f_8 = \sum_{i=2}^{2N_g} p_{x+y}(i) \log\{p_{x+y}(i)\} \quad (14.17)$$

9. Entropy

$$f_9 = \sum_i \sum_j p(i, j) \log(p(i, j)) \quad (14.18)$$

10. Difference variance

$$f_{10} = \text{variance of } p_{x-y} \quad (14.19)$$

11. Difference entropy

$$f_{11} = \sum_{i=0}^{N_g - 1} p_{x-y}(i) \log\{p_{x-y}(i)\} \quad (14.20)$$

12, 13. Information measures of correlation

$$f_{12} = \frac{\text{HXY} - \text{HXY1}}{\max\{\text{HX}, \text{HY}\}} \quad (14.21)$$

$$f_{13} = (1 - \exp[-2.0(\text{HXY2} - \text{HXY})])^{1/2} \quad (14.22)$$

$$\text{HXY} = -\sum_i \sum_j p(i, j) \log(p(i, j)) \quad (14.23)$$

where HX and HY are entropies of p_x and p_y, and

$$\text{HXY1} = -\sum_i \sum_j p(i,j) \log\{p_x(i)p_y(j)\} \quad (14.24)$$

$$\text{HXY2} = -\sum_i \sum_j p_x(i)p_y(j) \log\{p_x(i)p_y(j)\} \quad (14.25)$$

For a chosen distance d (in this work, $d = 1$ was used), there are four angular gray level dependence matrices, i.e., 4 values for each of the above 13 texture measures are obtained. The mean and the range of the 4 values of each of the 13 texture measures comprise a set of 26 texture features, which can be used for classification. Some of the 26 features are strongly correlated with each other, and a feature selection procedure may be applied in order to select a subset or linear combinations of them. In this work, the mean values and the range of values were computed for each feature for $d = 1$ and they were used as two different feature sets.

Appendix 3 Gray Level Difference Statistics (GLDS)

The Gray Level Difference Statistics algorithm[37] use first order statistics of local property values based on absolute differences between pairs of gray levels or of average gray levels in order to extract texture measures. Let $I(x,y)$ be the image intensity function and for any given displacement $\delta \equiv (\Delta x, \Delta y)$, let $I_\delta(x, y) = -I(x, y) - I(x + \Delta x, y + \Delta y)|$. Let p_δ be the probability density of $I_\delta(x, y)$. If there are m gray levels, this has the form of an m-dimensional vector whose ith component is the probability that $I_\delta(x, y)$ will have value i. The probability density p_δ can be easily computed by counting the number of times each value of $I_\delta(x, y)$ occurs, where Δx and Δy are integers. In a coarse texture, if the δ is small, $I_\delta(x, y)$ will be small, i.e., the values of p_δ should be concentrated near $i = 0$. Conversely, in a fine texture, the values of p_δ should be more spread out. Thus, a good way to analyze texture coarseness would be to compute, for various magnitudes of δ, some measure of the spread of values in p_δ away from the origin. Four such measures are the following:

1. *Contrast*

$$\text{CON} = \sum_i i^2 p_\delta(i) \quad (14.26)$$

This is the second moment of p_δ, i.e., its moment of inertia about the origin.

2. *Angular second moment*

$$\text{ASM} = \sum_i p_\delta(i)^2 \quad (14.27)$$

ASM is small when the $p_\delta(i)$ values are very close and large when some values are high and others low.

3. *Entropy*

$$\text{ENT} = -\sum_i p_\delta(i) \log(p_\delta(i)) \quad (14.28)$$

This is largest for equal $p_\delta(i)$ values and small when they are very unequal.

4. *Mean*

$$\text{MEAN} = (1/m) \sum_i i p_\delta(i) \quad (14.29)$$

This is small when the $p_\delta(i)$ are concentrated near the origin and large when they are far from the origin. The above features were calculated for $\delta = (0, 1), (1, 1), (1,0), (1,-1)$ and their mean values were taken.

Appendix 4 Neighborhood Gray Tone Difference Matrix (NGTDM)

Amadasun and King[2] proposed the Neighborhood Gray Tone Difference Matrix in order to extract textural features which correspond to visual properties of texture. Let $f(k, l)$ be the gray tone of a pixel at (k, l) having gray tone value i. Then the average gray tone over a neighborhood centered at, but excluding (k, l), can be found

$$\bar{A}_i = \bar{A}(k,l)$$
$$= \frac{1}{W-1} \left[\sum_{m=-d}^{d} \sum_{n=-d}^{d} f(k+m, l+n) \right] \quad (14.30)$$

where $(m,n) \neq (0,0)$, d specifies the neighborhood size and $W = (2d+1)^2$. The neighborhood size $d = 1$ was used in this work.

Then the ith entry in the NGTDM is

$$\begin{aligned} s(i) &= \sum |i - \bar{A}_i| & \text{for } i \in N_i \text{ if } N_i \neq 0, \\ &= 0, & \text{otherwise} \end{aligned} \quad (14.31)$$

where $\{N_i\}$ is the set of all pixels having gray tone i.

The following textural features are defined as:

1. *Coarseness*

$$f_{\cos} = \left[\varepsilon + \sum_{i=0}^{G_h} p_i s(i)\right]^{-1} \quad (14.32)$$

where G_h is the highest gray tone value present in the image and ε is a small number to prevent $f_{\cos}$ to get infinite. For an $N \times N$ image, p_i is the probability of occurrence of Gray tone value i, and is given by

$$p_i = N_i/n^2, \quad \text{where } n = N - 2d. \quad (14.33)$$

Amadasun and King[2] define an image as coarse when the primitives composing the texture are large and texture tends to possess a high degree of local uniformity in intensity for fairly large areas. Large values of $f_{\cos}$ represent areas where gray tone differences are small. The definition of coarseness given here is different than the definition given in Eq. 14.41.

2. *Contrast*

$$f_{\text{con}} = \left[\frac{1}{N_g(N_g-1)} \sum_{i=0}^{G_h} \sum_{j=0}^{G_h} p_i p_j (i-j)^2\right]\left[\frac{1}{n^2} \sum_{i=0}^{G_h} s(i)\right] \quad (14.34)$$

where N_g is the total number of different gray levels present in the image. High contrast means that the intensity difference between neighboring regions is large.

3. *Busyness*

$$f_{\text{bus}} = \left[\sum_{i=0}^{G_h} p_i s(i)\right] \Big/ \left[\sum_{i=0}^{G_h} \sum_{j=0}^{G_h} i p_i - j p_j\right],$$
$$p_i \neq 0, p_j \neq 0. \quad (14.35)$$

A busy texture is one in which there are rapid changes of intensity from one pixel to its neighbor.

4. *Complexity*

$$f_{\text{com}} = \sum_{i=0}^{G_h} \sum_{j=0}^{G_h} \{(|i-j|)/(n^2(p_i + p_j))\}$$
$$\{p_i s(i) + p_j s(j)\}, p_i \neq 0, p_j \neq 0. \quad (14.36)$$

A texture is considered complex when the information content is high, i.e., when there are many primitives in the texture, and more so when the primitives have different average intensities.

5. *Strength*

$$f_{\text{str}} = \left[\sum_{i=0}^{G_h} \sum_{j=0}^{G_h} (p_i + p_j)(i-j)^2\right]\left[\varepsilon + \sum_{i=0}^{G_h} s(i)\right], \quad (14.37)$$
$$p_i \neq 0, \ p_j \neq 0.$$

A texture is generally referred to as strong when the primitives that comprise it are easily definable and clearly visible.

Appendix 5 Statistical Feature Matrix (SFM)

The statistical feature matrix[38] measures the statistical properties of pixel pairs at several distances within an image which are used for statistical analysis. Let $I(x, y)$ be the intensity at point (x, y), and let $\delta = (\Delta x, \Delta y)$ represent the intersample spacing distance vector, where Δx and Δy are integers. The δ contrast, δ covariance, and δ dissimilarity are defined as

$$\text{CON}(\delta) \equiv E\{[I(x, y) - I(x + \Delta x, y + \Delta y)]^2\} \quad (14.38)$$

$$\text{COV}(\delta) \equiv E\{[I(x, y) - \eta][I(x + \Delta x, y + \Delta y) - \eta]\} \quad (14.39)$$

$$\text{DSS}(\delta) \equiv E\{[I(x, y) - I(x + \Delta x, y + \Delta y)]\} \quad (14.40)$$

where $E\{\ \}$ denotes the expectation operation and η is the average gray level of the image.

A statistical feature matrix, (SFM) M_{sf}, is an $(L_r + 1) \times (2L_c + 1)$ matrix whose (i, j) element is the d statistical feature of the image, where $d = (j-L_c, i)$ is an intersample spacing distance vector for $i = 0, 1, \ldots, L_r, j = 0, 1, \ldots, L_c$, and L_r, L_c are the constants which determine the maximum intersample spacing distance. In a similar way, the contrast matrix (M_{con}), covariance matrix (M_{cov}), and dissimilarity matrix (M_{dss}) can be defined as the matrices whose (i, j) elements are the d contrast, d covariance, and d dissimilarity, respectively. Based on the SFM, the following texture features can be computed:

1. *Coarseness*

$$F_{\text{CRS}} = c \Bigg/ \sum_{(i,j)\in N_r} \text{DSS}(i,j)/n \qquad (14.41)$$

where c is a normalizing factor, N_r is the set of displacement vectors defined as $N_r = \{(i,j): |i|, |j| \leq r\}$, and n is the number of elements in the set. A pattern is coarser than another when they differ only in scale with the magnified one to be the coarser and having a larger F_{CRS} value. The definition of coarseness given here is different than the definition given by NGTDM in Eq. 14.32.

2. *Contrast*

$$F_{\text{CON}} = \left[\sum_{(i,j)\in N_r} \text{CON}(i,j)/4\right]^{1/2} \qquad (14.42)$$

Contrast measures the degree of sharpness of the edges in an image.

3. *Periodicity*

$$F_{\text{PER}} = \frac{\overline{M}_{\text{dss}} - M_{\text{dss}}(\text{valley})}{\overline{M}_{\text{dss}}} \qquad (14.43)$$

where $\overline{M}_{\text{dss}}$ is the mean of all elements in M_{dss} and $M_{\text{dss}}(\text{valley})$ is the deepest valley in the matrix. Periodicity measures the appearance of periodically repeated patterns in the image.

4. *Roughness*

$$F_{\text{RGH}} = (D_f^{(h)} + D_f^{(v)})/2 \qquad (14.44)$$

where D_f is the fractal dimension (see Sect. A.7) in horizontal and vertical directions. $D_f = 3 - H$ and $E\{-\Delta I\} = k(\delta)^H$ where H can be estimated from the dissimilarity matrix since the $(i, j + L_c)$ element of the matrix is $E\{-\Delta I\}$ with $\delta = (j, i)$. The larger the D_f the rougher is the image. In this study, an inter-sample spacing distance vector $\delta = (4,4)$ was used.

Appendix 6 Laws Texture Energy Measures (TEM)

Laws texture energy measures[39,40] are derived from three simple vectors of length 3, $L3 = (1, 2, 1)$, $E3 = (-1, 0, 1)$, and $S3 = (-1, 2, -1)$, which represent the one-dimensional operations of center-weighted local averaging, symmetric first differencing for edge detection, and second differencing for spot detection. If these vectors are convolved with themselves, new vectors of length 5, $L5 = (1, 4, 6, 4, 1)$, $E5 = (-1, -2, 0, 2, 1)$, and $S5 = (-1, 0, 2, 0, -1)$, are obtained. By further self-convolution, new vectors of length 7, $L7 = (1, 6, 15, 20, 15, 6, 1)$, $E7 = (-1\ -4, -5, 0, 5, 4, 1)$, $S7 = (-1\ -2, 1, 4, 1-2\ -1)$ are obtained, where $L7$ again performs local averaging, $E7$ acts as edge detector, and $S7$ acts as spot detector. If the column vectors of length l are multiplied by row vectors of the same length, Laws $l \times l$ masks are obtained. In this work, the following combinations were used to obtain 7×7 masks:

$$\text{LL} = L7^t\,L7,\ \text{LE} = L7^t\,E7,\ \text{LS} = L7^t\,S7,\ \text{EL}$$
$$= E7^t\,L7,\ \text{EE} = E7^t\,E7,\ \text{ES} = E7^t\,S7,\ \text{SL}$$
$$= S7^t\,L7,\ \text{SE} = S7^t\,E7,\ \text{SS} = S7^t\,S7$$

In order to extract texture features from an image, these masks are convoluted with the image, and the statistics (e.g., energy) of the resulting image are used to describe texture. The following texture features were extracted:

1. *LL – texture energy from LL kernel*
2. *EE – texture energy from EE kernel*
3. *SS – texture energy from SS kernel*
4. *LE – average texture energy from LE and EL kernels*

$$\text{LE} = (\text{LE} + \text{EL})/2$$

5. *ES – average texture energy from ES and SE kernels*

$$\text{ES} = (\text{ES} + \text{SE})/2$$

6. *LS – average texture energy from LS and SL kernels*

$$\text{LS} = (\text{LS} + \text{SL})/2$$

The averaging of matched pairs of energy measures gives rotational invariance.

Appendix 7 Fractal Dimension Texture Analysis (FDTA)

Mandelbrot[41] developed the fractional Brownian motion model in order to describe the roughness of nature surfaces. It considers naturally occurring surfaces as the end result of random walks. Such random walks are basic physical processes in our universe.[38] An important parameter to represent a fractal dimension is the fractal dimension D_f estimated theoretically by the equation[38]

$$E(\Delta I^2) = c(\Delta r)^{(6-2D_f)} \quad (14.45)$$

where $E(\ )$ denotes the expectation operator, ΔI is the intensity difference between two pixels, c is a constant, and Δr is the distance between two pixels.

A simpler method is to estimate the H parameter (Hurst coefficient) from

$$E(|\Delta I|) = k(\Delta r)^H \quad (14.46)$$

where $k = E(|\Delta I|)_{\Delta r = 1}$.

By applying the log function the following is obtained

$$\log E(|\Delta I|) = \log k + H \log(\Delta r). \quad (14.47)$$

From the above equation, the H parameter can be estimated and the fractal dimension D_f can be computed from the relationship

$$D_f = 3 - H. \quad (14.48)$$

A smooth surface is described by a small value of the fractal dimension D_f (large value of the parameter H) where the reverse applies for a rough surface.

Given an $M \times M$ image, the intensity difference vector is defined as

$$\text{IDV} \equiv [id(1), id(2), \ldots id(s)] \quad (14.49)$$

where s is the maximum possible scale, $id(k)$ is the average of the absolute intensity difference of all pixel pairs with vertical or horizontal distance k. The value of the parameter H can be obtained by using least squares linear regression to estimate the slope of the curve of $id(k)$ versus k in log–log scales.

If the image is seen under different resolutions, then the multiresolution fractal (MF) feature vector is defined as

$$\text{MF} \equiv (H^{(m)}, H^{(m-1)}, \ldots, H^{(m-n+1)}) \quad (14.50)$$

where $M = 2^m$ is the size of the original image, $H^{(k)}$ is the H parameter estimated from image $I^{(k)}$, and n is the number of resolutions chosen.

The multiresolution fractal (MF) feature vector describes also the lacunarity of the image. It can be used for the separation of textures with the same fractal dimension D_f by considering all but the first components of the MF vectors. In this work, H was computed for four different resolutions.

Appendix 8 Fourier Power Spectrum (FPS)

The discrete Fourier transform[37,40] of a $N \times N$ picture is defined by

$$F(u,v) = \frac{1}{N^2} \sum_{i,j=0}^{n-1} f(i,j) e^{-2\pi\sqrt{-1}(iu+jv)} \quad (14.51)$$

where $0 \leq u$ and $v \leq N - 1$.

The sample Fourier power spectrum is defined by

$$\Phi(u,v) \equiv F(u,v) F^*(u,v) = |F(u,v)|^2 \quad (14.52)$$

where Φ is the sample power spectrum, and * denotes the complex conjugate. Coarse texture will have high values of $|F|^2$ concentrated near the origin, whereas in fine texture, the values will be more spread out. The standard set of texture features used are ring and wedge shaped samples of the discrete FPS:

1. *Radial sum*

$$\Phi_{r_1,r_2} \equiv \sum_{r_1^2 \leq u^2 + v^2 \langle r_2^2} |F(u,v)|^2 \quad (14.53)$$

for various values of the inner and outer radii r_1 and r_2.

2. *Angular sum*

$$\Phi_{\theta_1,\theta_2} \equiv \sum_{\theta_1 \leq \tan^{-1}(v/u) \leq \theta_2} |F(u,v)|^2 \quad (14.54)$$

for various angles θ_1 and θ_2.

Appendix 9 Morphology Features

Morphological features are motivated from the need to study the basic structure of the plaque. In order to achieve this task, two morphological analysis methods are being described in order to quantify morphological features of the plaques. The first one is based on a multilevel approach where the image intensity was thresholded at three different levels, while the second one is based on gray scale morphological analysis. The presentation is closely related to previously published works Marangos (1989) and Kyriacou (2009).[22,44]

Morphological analysis of an image is based on the pattern spectrum used. Pattern spectra are defined in terms of translations and dilations of a single structural element. For the morphological analysis carried out in this description, the cross "+" structural element is considered. The cross structural element exhibits limited directional selectivity. This is desirable since there is no clearly preferred direction for the analysis. The set B represents the "+" structural element, and it is defined by its five pixel coordinates

$$B = \{(-1,0), (0,0), (1,0), (0,-1), (0,1)\}. \quad (14.55)$$

Discrete-set translation by points are defined using

$$B + P = \{(m+i, n+j) : (m,n) \in B\}, \text{ where } p = (i,j). \quad (14.56)$$

In $B + p$, the structural element is centered over the point $p = (i, j)$. Binary dilation is defined using

$$X \oplus B = \bigcup_{p \in B} X + p = \{a + b : a \in X \text{ and } b \in B\} \quad (14.57)$$

The definition leads to the definition of kB that denotes the k-fold expansion of B, and is given by

$$kB = \begin{cases} \{(0,0)\}, & k = 0, \\ \underbrace{B \oplus B \oplus \cdots \oplus B}_{k-1 \text{ dilations}}, & \text{for integer } k > 1. \end{cases} \quad (14.58)$$

Pattern spectra are defined in terms of openings and closings with kB. The authors do not have any clear clinical interpretation for the pattern spectra generated by closings with kB. Thus, they will only focus on the pattern spectra generated by openings with kB.[22] In what follows, detailed descriptions of the two morphological methods are provided in Sects. A.9.1 and A.9.2. In Sect. A.9.3, a summary of how the two methods can be applied will be provided.

Appendix 9.1 Multilevel Binary Morphological Analysis

In multilevel binary morphological analysis, the authors are interested in extracting different plaque components and investigating their geometric properties. They begin by generating three binary images by thresholding:

$$L = (i,j) : \text{such that } f(i,j) < 25\},$$
$$M = \{(i,j) : \text{such that } 25 \leq f(i,j) \leq 50\},$$
$$H = \{(i,j) : \text{such that } f(i,j) > 50\}.$$
$$(14.59)$$

Here, binary image outputs are represented as sets of image coordinates where image intensity meets the threshold criteria. Overall, this multilevel decomposition is closely related to a three-level quantization of the original image intensity. To see this, note that the authors can simply assign quantization levels to each of the pixels in L, M, H and then use them to provide an approximate reconstruction of the original image.

In L, the authors want to extract dark image regions representing blood, thrombus, lipid, or hemorrhage. Similarly, in H, the authors want to extract the collagen and calcified components of the plaque, while in M, the authors want to extract image components that fall between the two. Thus, to decide the threshold levels of (5), the authors varied the threshold levels so as to extract the desired components from the plaques.

In what follows, the use of morphological pattern spectra for analyzing the extracted binary images is introduced. The authors' motivation lies in analyzing the structural components of each binary image.

Normalized pattern spectra is computed for each one of the three binary images L, M, H. Thus, in the following discussion, the symbol X will be used to denote any one of the three binary images L, M, H. Binary image erosion is defined using

$$X \odot B = \bigcap_{p \in B} X - p = \{\alpha : B + a \subseteq X\} \quad (14.60)$$

An opening is then defined in terms of an erosion followed by a dilation:

$$X \circ B = (X \ominus B) \oplus B. \tag{14.61}$$

In general, an opening reduces the input image $X \circ B \subseteq X$. However, when the input image can be expressed in terms of translations of the structural element B, the opening operation will preserve the input image. The authors thus write

$$X \circ B = X \tag{14.62}$$

when

$$X = \bigcup_{p \in S} B + p = B \oplus S = S \oplus B \tag{14.63}$$

In general, for any given binary image, an opening outputs an approximation to the input image. This approximation is expressed as a union of translations of the structural element[14]:

$$X \circ B = \bigcup_{B+z \subseteq X} B + z. \tag{14.64}$$

The approximation error image is defined in terms of the set difference $X - X \circ B$. The approximation error is quantified by counting the number of pixels in the difference image. $A(S)$ is written to denote the cardinality of the set S. For measuring the binary components at different scales, a sequence of openings with the dilated structural element is considered (see Eq. 14.58):

$$X, X \circ B, X \circ 2B, \ldots, X \circ nB. \tag{14.65}$$

For our plaque images, it is noted that the plaques are segmented, and image intensity outside the plaque is assigned to zero. Thus, for a sufficiently large value of k, kB will outgrow the support of the plaque. When this happens, the opening operation will return the empty-set image. Thus, n is picked to be the smallest integer for which $X \circ (n+1)B = \emptyset$.

For computing (Eq. 14.65), it is noted that a single opening is needed each time, since the openings can be computed recursively using $X \circ (n+1)B = (X \circ nB) \circ B$. It is also clear from this recursive relationship that the openings generate decreasing images

$$X \circ nB \subseteq \ldots \subseteq X \circ 2B \subseteq X \circ B \subseteq X \tag{14.66}$$

with decreasing areas

$$A(X \circ nB) \leq \cdots \leq A(X \circ 2B) \\ \leq A(X \circ B) \leq A(X). \tag{14.67}$$

The set difference images are formed using

$$\begin{aligned} d_0(X;B) &= X - X \circ B \\ d_1(X;B) &= X \circ B - X \circ 2B \\ &\vdots \\ d_{n-1}(X;B) &= X \circ (n-1)B - X \circ nB. \end{aligned} \tag{14.68}$$

The difference images are orthogonal with respect to set intersection

$$d_i(X;B) \cap d_j(X;B) = \emptyset \quad \text{when} \quad i \neq j. \tag{14.69}$$

The image can be reconstructed using the difference images

$$\begin{aligned} X &= (X \circ nB) \cup \left(\bigcup_{i=0}^{n-1} d_i(X;B) \right) \\ &= \bigcup_{i=0}^{n} d_i(X;B). \end{aligned} \tag{14.70}$$

The authors think of the image decomposition given by Eq. 14.16 as a multi-scale decomposition where the difference images $d_i(f;B)$ represent information captured at the ith scale.

The pattern spectrum is also defined in terms of the number of elements in the difference images

$$PS_X(n, B) = A(d_n(X;B)). \tag{14.71}$$

In (Eq. 14.71), it is noted that the pattern spectra vary with the size of the plaque.

To remove this dependency, a probability density function (pdf) measure is considered defined as

$$pdf_X(k, B) = A(d_k(X;B))/A(X) \quad \text{for} \quad k \geq 0. \tag{14.72}$$

In Eq. 14.72, it is noted that the normalization is motivated by the reconstruction formula (see Eq. 14.70). Given the pdf-measure, the cumulative distribution function (cdf) can also be constructed using

$$cdf_f(k, B) = \begin{cases} 0, & k = 0, \\ \sum_{r=0}^{k-1} pdf_f(r, B), & n+1 \geq k > 0. \end{cases}$$
$$\tag{14.73}$$

Appendix 9.2 Gray Scale Morphological Analysis

For gray scale morphological analysis, it is assumed that the input image $f(i, j)$ denotes the (positive) gray scale image intensity at pixel (i, j). At every pixel, for structural element B, gray scale dilation is defined by

$$(f \oplus B)(i, j) = \max_{(m, n) \in B+(i, j)} f(m, n) \quad (14.74)$$

which represents the maximum intensity value over the support of the translated structural element. Similarly, for symmetric structural elements (as is the case for "+"), gray scale erosion is defined using the minimum value:

$$(f \odot B)(i, j) = \min_{(m, n) \in B+(i, j)} f(m, n) \quad (14.75)$$

Openings are then defined using the new definitions for gray scale erosions and dilations. Instead of the subset relation, we now have that an opening reduces image intensity in the sense that $f \circ B \leq f$ for every pixel.

Due to the bounds of the extend of the plaque, the maximum number of openings that make sense is again limited. Here, instead of the empty set, the limit is the zero-image. The difference images are formed in the same way. For the reconstruction, a finite sum is used instead of a union:

$$f = (f \circ nB) + \left(\sum_{i=0}^{n-1} d_i(f; B) \right)$$

$$= \sum_{i=0}^{n} d_i(f; B). \quad (14.76)$$

For the gray scale definition of the pattern spectrum

$$PS_f(k, B) = \| d_k(f; B) \|, \quad (14.77)$$

is used where

$$\| f \| = \sum_{(i, j)} f(i, j). \quad (14.78)$$

The original image intensity is now normalized by

$$pdf_f(k, B) = \| d_k(f; B) \| / \| f \|, \quad \text{for } k \geq 0. \quad (14.79)$$

Appendix 9.3 Morphological Analysis Application to Atherosclerotic Carotid Plaques

To summarize: For each plaque, the three binary images L, M, H are computed as outlined in Eq. 14.59. For each binary image, the *pdf* and *cdf* distributions are computed as outlined in Eqs. 14.72 and 14.73, for $k = 0, \ldots, 70$. Similarly, for gray scale morphological image analysis, the *pdf* and *cdf* distributions are computed based on gray scale erosions and dilations (see Eq. 14.77). Thus, *pdf* and *cdf* measures are computed on the original gray scale image and the three binary images that are derived from it.

For each one of the four images, the positively indexed *pdf* and *cdf* measures provide normalized size distributions of the white (or brighter) blob-components. These measures are based on binary and gray scale openings. An application of these features and their results is presented in Chap. 15.

References

1. Christodoulou CI, Pattichis CS, Pantziaris M, Nicolaides A. Texture based classification of atherosclerotic carotid plaques. *IEEE Trans Med Imaging*. 2003;22(7):902–912.
2. Amadasun M, King R. Textural features corresponding to textural properties. *IEEE Trans Syst Man Cybern*. 1989;19(5):1264–1274.
3. El-Barghouty N, Geroulakos G, Nicolaides A, Androulakis A, Bahal V. Computer assisted carotid plaque characterisation. *Eur J Vasc Endovasc Surg*. 1995;9:548–557.
4. Biasi GM et al. Plaque characterization using digital image processing and its potential in future studies of carotid endarterectomy and angioplasty. *J Endovasc Surg*. 1998;5:240–246.
5. Elatrozy T, Nicolaides A, Tegos T, Griffin M. The objective characterization of ultrasonic carotid plaque features. *Eur J Vasc Endovasc Surg*. 1998;26:223–230.
6. Tegos TJ et al. Echomorphologic and histopathologic characteristics of unstable carotid plaques. *Am J Neuroradiol*. 2000;21:1937–1944.
7. Biasi GM et al. Carotid plaque echolucency increases the risk of stroke in carotid stenting The Imaging in Carotid Angioplasty and Risk of Stroke (ICAROS) Study. *Circulation*. 2004;110:756–762.
8. Lal BK et al. Pixel distribution analysis of B-mode ultrasound scan images predicts histologic features of atherosclerotic carotid plaques. *J Vasc Surg*. 2002;35:1210–1217.
9. Lal BK et al. Noninvasive identification of the unstable carotid plaque. *Ann Vasc Surg*. 2006;20:167–174.

10. Sztajzel R et al. Stratified gray-scale median analysis and color mapping of the carotid plaque. *Stroke*. 2005;36:741–745.
11. Madycki G, Staszkiewicz W, Gabrusiewicz A. Carotid plaque texture analysis can predict the incidence of silent brain infarcts among patients undergoing carotid endarterectomy. *Eur J Vasc Endovasc Surg*. 2006;31:373–380.
12. Hashimoto H, Takaya M, Niki H, Etani H. Computer-assisted analysis of heterogeneity on B-mode imaging predicts instability of asymptomatic carotid plaque. *Cerebrovasc Dis*. 2009;28:357–364.
13. Prahl U et al. Percentage white: a new feature for ultrasound classification of plaque echogenicity in carotid artery atherosclerosis. *Ultrasound Med Biol*. 2010;36(2):218–226.
14. Kakkos SK et al. Texture analysis of ultrasonic images of symptomatic carotid plaques can identify those plaques associated with ipsilateral embolic brain infarction. *Eur J Vasc Endovasc Surg*. 2007;33(4):422–429.
15. Kakkos SK et al. Computerised texture analysis of carotid plaque ultrasonic images can identify unstable plaques associated with ipsilateral neurological symptoms. *Angiology*. 2011;62(4):317–328.
16. Christodoulou CI, Pattichis CS, Kyriacou E, Nicolaides A. Image retrieval and classification of carotid plaque ultrasound images. *Open Cardiovasc Imaging J*. 2010;2:18–28.
17. Johnsen SH et al. Elevated high-density lipoprotein cholesterol levels are protective against plaque progression: a follow-up study of 1952 persons with carotid atherosclerosis the Tromsø study. *Circulation*. 2005;112:498–504.
18. Johnsen SH et al. Carotid atherosclerosis is a stronger predictor of myocardial infarction in women than in men a 6-year follow-up study of 6226 persons: the Tromsø study. *Stroke*. 2007;38:2873–2880.
19. Griffin M et al. Juxtaluminal hypoechoic area in ultrasonic images of carotid plaques and hemispheric symptoms. *J Vasc Surg*. 2010;52(1):69–76.
20. Wilhjelm JE et al. Quantitative analysis of ultrasound Bmode images of carotid atherosclerotic plaque: correlation with visual classification and histological examination. *IEEE Trans Med Imaging*. 1998;17(6):910–922.
21. Mougiakakou S, Golemati S, Gousias I, Nicolaides A, Nikita KS. Computer-aided diagnosis of carotid atherosclerosis based on ultrasound image statistics, Laws' texture and neural networks. *Ultrasound Med Biol*. 2007;33(1):26–36.
22. Kyriacou E et al. Classification of atherosclerotic carotid plaques using morphological analysis on ultrasound images. *Appl Intell*. 2009;30:3–23.
23. Asvestas P, Golemati S, Matsopoulos GK, Nikita KS, Nikolaides AN. Fractal dimension estimation of carotid atherosclerotic plaques from B-mode ultrasound. *Ultrasound Med Biol*. 2002;28(9):1129–1136.
24. Christodoulou CI, Pattichis CS, Murray V, Pattichis MS, Nicolaides A. AM-FM representations for the characterization of carotid plaque ultrasound images. MBEC'08 4th European Conference of the International Federation for Medical and Biological Engineering; November 23–28, 2008; Antwerp.
25. Tsiaparas N, Golemati S, Andreadis I, Stoitsis J, Nikita KS. Comparison of multiresolution features for texture classification of carotid atherosclerosis from B-mode ultrasound. *IEEE Trans Inf Technol Biomed*. 2011;15(1):130–137.
26. Meairs S, Hennerici M. Four-dimensional ultrasonographic characterization of plaque surface motion in patients with symptomatic and asymptomatic carotid artery stenosis. *Stroke*. 1999;30:1807–1813.
27. Murillo SE et al. Atherosclerotic plaque motion trajectory analysis from ultrasound videos. In: CD-Rom Proceedings of the 5th IEEE EMBS Special Topic Conference on Information Technology in Biomedicine; October 26–28, 2006; Ioannina-Epirus:5p.
28. Murray V., et al. An AM-FM model for motion estimation in atherosclerotic plaque videos. In: Proceedings of the 41st Asilomar Conference on Signals, Systems and Computers; 2007; Pacific Grove:746–750.
29. Gastounioti A, Golemati S, Stoitsis J, Nikita KS. Kalman filter based block matching for arterial wall motion from B-mode ultrasound. In: IEEE International Conference on Imaging Systems and Techniques (IST); July 1–2, 2010; Thessaloniki:234–239.
30. Landry A, Spence JD, Fenster A. Measurement of carotid plaque volume by 3-dimensional ultrasound. *Stroke*. 2004;35(4):864–869.
31. Chiu B, Egger M, Spence JD, Parraga G, Fenster A. Quantification of carotid vessel wall and plaque thickness change using 3D ultrasound images. *Med Phys*. 2008;35(8):3691–3710.
32. Chiu B, Egger M, Spence JD, Parraga G, Fenster A. Development of 3D ultrasound techniques for carotid artery disease assessment and monitoring. *Int J Comput Assist Radiol Surg*. 2008;3:1–10.
33. Mallett C, House AA, Spence JD, Fenster A, Parraga G. Longitudinal ultrasound evaluation of carotid atherosclerosis in one, two and three dimensions. *Ultrasound Med Biol*. 2009;35(3):367–375.
34. Awad J, Krasinski A, Parraga G, Fenster A. Texture analysis of carotid artery atherosclerosis from three dimensional ultrasound images. *Med Phys*. 2010;37(4):1382–1391.
35. Press WH, Flannery BP, Teukolsky SA, Vetterling WT. *Numerical Recipes: The Art of Scientific Computing*. Cambridge: Cambridge University Press; 1987.
36. Haralick RM, Shanmugam K, Dinstein I. Texture features for image classification. *IEEE Trans Syst Man Cybern*. 1973;SMC-3:610–621.
37. Weszka JS, Dyer CR, Rosenfield A. A comparative study of texture measures for terrain classification. *IEEE Trans Syst Man Cybern*. 1976;SMC-6:269–285.
38. Wu CM, Chen Y-C. Statistical feature matrix for texture analysis. *CVGIP Graphical Models Image Process*. 1992;54(5):407–419.
39. Laws KI. Rapid texture identification. *SPIE*. 1980;238:376–380.
40. Wu C-M, Chen Y-C, Hsieh K-S. Texture features for classification of ultrasonic liver images. *IEEE Trans Med Imaging*. 1992;11(3):141–152.
41. Mandelbrot BB. *The Fractal Geometry of Nature*. San Francisco: Freeman; 1982.
42. Dougherty ER. *An Introduction to Morphological Image Processing*. Bellingham: SPIE Optical Engineering Press; 1992.

43. Dougherty ER, Astola J. *An Introduction to Nonlinear Image Processing*. Bellingham: SPIE Optical Engineering Press; 1994.
44. Marangos P. Pattern spectrum and multiscale shape representation. *IEEE Trans Pattern Anal Mach Intell*. 1989;11: 701–715.
45. Ripley BD. *Pattern Recognition and Neural Networks*. Cambridge: Cambridge University Press; 1996.
46. Haykin S. *Neural Networks: A Comprehensive Foundation*. New York: Macmillan College Publishing Company; 1994.
47. Polak J et al. Hypoechoic plaque at US of the carotid artery: an independent risk factor for incident stroke in adults aged 65 years or older. *Radiology*. 1998;208 (3):649–654.

Plaque Classification

15

Efthyvoulos Kyriacou, Christodoulos I. Christodoulou,
Marios S. Pattichis, Constantinos S. Pattichis,
and Stavros K. Kakkos

15.1 Introduction

This chapter presents several classification techniques that could be used in computer-aided systems for the automated characterization of carotid plaques and the identification of individuals with asymptomatic carotid stenosis at increased risk of stroke. First, recent advances in ultrasonic plaque characterization are summarized, and then the efficacy of computer-aided diagnosis based on neural and statistical classifiers is evaluated using as input the texture analysis and morphological features presented in Chap. 14. Classifiers like probabilistic neural network (PNN) and the support vector machine (SVM) are being presented with actual patient data.

E. Kyriacou (✉)
Department of Computer Science and Engineering, Frederick University Cyprus, Lemesos, Cyprus

C.I. Christodoulou
Department of Computer Science, University of Cyprus, Nicosia, Cyprus

M.S. Pattichis
Department of Electrical and Computer Engineering, The University of New Mexico, Albuquerque, NM, USA

C.S. Pattichis
Department of Computer Science, University of Cyprus, Nicosia, Cyprus

S.K. Kakkos
Department of Vascular Surgery, University of Patras Medical School, Patras, Achaia, Greece

15.2 Background

15.2.1 Visual Classification of Atherosclerotic Plaque in Ultrasound Imaging

High-resolution ultrasound provides information not only on the degree of carotid artery stenosis but also on the characteristics of the arterial wall, including the size and consistency of atherosclerotic plaques. Several studies have indicated that "complicated" carotid plaques are often associated with ipsilateral neurological symptoms and share common ultrasonic characteristics, being more echolucent (weak reflection of ultrasound and therefore containing echo-poor structures) and heterogeneous (having both echolucent and echogenic areas). In contrast, "uncomplicated" plaques which are often asymptomatic tend to be of uniform consistency (uniformly hypoechoic or uniformly hyperechoic) without evidence of ulceration.[1–5] Historically, different classifications of plaque ultrasonic appearance have been proposed in the literature. Reilly et al. in 1983[1] classified carotid plaques as homogenous and heterogeneous, defining as homogeneous plaques those with "uniformly bright echoes" that are now known as uniformly hyperechoic (type 4) (see below). Johnson et al. in 1985[6] classified plaques as dense and soft. Widder et al. in 1990[7] classified them as echolucent and echogenic based on their overall level of echo patterns. Subsequently, he recognized four types (1–4) with type 1 being the most echogenic and type 4 as the most echolucent. Gray-Weale et al. in 1988[8] suggested four types: (1) type 1, predominantly echolucent lesions; (2) type 2, echogenic lesions with substantial (>75%) components of echolucency; (3)

Table 15.1 Ultrasound carotid plaque heterogeneity and clinical implications

Author	Year	Ultrasound carotid plaque heterogeneity	Clinical implications
O'Donnell Jr et al.[2]	1985	Visual classification; distinguished fine vs rough and random vs regular texture	Histology study
Aldoori et al.[9]	1987	Visual classification	Plaque classification
Leahy et al.[3]	1988	Plaques containing echolucent components. Homogeneous plaques had uniform consistency suggestive of sclerotic plaques	Heterogeneous plaques more frequently symptomatic and associated with ipsilateral infarction on CT scan
Sterpetti et al.[10]	1988	Mixed high-, medium-, and low-level echoes. Homogenous lesions had uniformly high- to medium-level echoes	Heterogeneous plaques became symptomatic more frequently during follow-up
Langsfeld et al.[4]	1989	Predominantly echolucent plaques with a thin "egg shell" cap of echogenicity and echogenic plaques with substantial components of echolucency	Heterogeneous plaques more frequently symptomatic. Heterogeneous plaques became symptomatic more frequently during follow-up
Widder et al.[7]	1990	Visual estimation, plaques being classified into four categories (homogeneous, slightly or markedly heterogeneous and non visible)	Histology study
Giannoni et al.[11]	1991	Not provided	Heterogeneous plaques progressed and became symptomatic
ECPSG[12]	1995	Mixed composition	Heterogeneous plaques contained more calcification
Kagawa et al.[13]	1996	Plaques composed of a mixture of hyperechoic, isoechoic, and hypoechoic plaques. Normal intima-media complex used to define isoechoicity	Heterogeneous lesions consisted of a mixture of atheroma and fibrosis on histology and demonstrated calcification more frequently than the homogeneous ones
Kardoulas et al.[14]	1996	Mixed echo level pattern	Association of plaque heterogeneity with symptoms less consistent in comparison with echolucency
AbuRahma et al.[15]	1998	Plaques composed of a mixture of hyperechoic, isoechoic, and hypoechoic plaques. Normal intima-media complex used to define isoechoicity	Heterogeneous plaques more frequently symptomatic

type 3, predominately echogenic with small area(s) of echolucency occupying less than a quarter of the plaque; and (4) type 4, uniformly dense echogenic lesions. Geroulakos et al. in 1993[5] modified the Gray-Weale classification by using a 50% area cutoff point instead of 75% and by adding a fifth type, which, as a result of heavy calcification on its surface, could not be correctly classified. In recent years, the Gray-Weale and Geroulakos classifications became widely accepted.

Regarding the clinical significance of carotid plaque heterogeneity, it seems that the heterogeneous plaques described in the three studies published in the 1980s (Table 15.1) include hypoechoic plaques. Also, heterogeneous plaques in all studies listed in Table 15.1 contain hypoechoic areas (large or small). These plaques also appear to be associated with symptoms or, if found in asymptomatic individuals, they subsequently tend to become symptomatic.

15.3 Ultrasound Image Analysis: Automated Classification Using Several Features

15.3.1 Plaque Classification Studies

As described in Chap. 14, several features can be extracted from plaque images using different techniques. In the last few years, these techniques have been applied on plaques in order to achieve automatic classification. Earlier studies have been primarily focused on basic statistical features, such as the grayscale medial (GSM), the mean, the median, the standard deviation, skewness, and kurtosis.[16–21] In these earlier studies, the GSM was found to be very successful in differentiating between symptomatic and asymptomatic cases.[16,20] Depending on the image preprocessing method, threshold values for the GSM

Table 15.2 Ultrasound carotid plaque classification studies

Author	Year	Ref.	Short description of study	N	Score
Statistical analysis studies					
Geroulakos et al.	1994	19	Tested the hypothesis that the ultrasonic characteristics of carotid artery plaques were closely related to symptoms. An association was found of echolucent plaques with symptoms and cerebral infractions, which provided further evidence that echolucent plaques are unstable and tend to embolize	105	
El-Barghouty et al.	1995	20	In a study with 94 plaques, the grayscale median (GSM) of the ultrasound plaque image was used for the characterization of plaques as echolucent (GSM $\leq$ 32) and echogenic (GSM $>$ 32). An association between carotid plaque echolucency and the incidence of cerebral computed tomography (CT) brain infractions was reported	94	
Iannuzzi et al.	1995	21	Identified significant relationships between carotid artery ultrasound plaque characteristics and ischemic cerebrovascular events. The features that were more consistently associated with TIAs were low echogenicity of carotid plaques, thicker plaques, and presence of longitudinal motion	549	
Elatrozy et al.	1998	16	A study where 80 patients were examined and reported that plaques with GSM $<$ 40 are more related to ipsilateral hemispheric symptoms	80	
Wilhjelm et al.	1998	22	In a study with 52 patients scheduled for endarterectomy, a quantitative comparison between subjective classification of the ultrasound images, first- and second-order statistical features, and a histological analysis of the surgically removed plaque was presented. Some correlation was found between the three types of information where the best performing feature was found to be the contrast	52	
Rakebrandt et al.	2000	23	This study aimed to construct parametric images of B-scan texture and assess their potential for predicting plaque morphology. Sequential transverse in vitro scans of ten carotid plaques, excised during endarterectomy, were compared with macrohistology maps of plaque content	10	
Asvestas et al.	2002	24	A pilot study with 19 carotid plaques. Indicated a significant difference of the fractal dimension between the symptomatic and asymptomatic groups	19	
Kakkos et al.	2010	25	A pilot study with 188 patients with internal carotid artery $\geq$50% (ECTS). Symptomatic patients had an event within the preceding 6 months. The most recent event was considered. Logistic regression model was independently associated with severity of stenosis, percentage of pixels between gray levels 0–10, SGLDM texture features, and percentage of pixels between gray levels 11–20. Results indicated an area under the curve of the regression-derived predicted probability for amaurosis fugax, TIA, and stroke, 0.92, 0.82, and 0.85, respectively (all $P < .001$)	188	
Griffin et al.	2010	26	Ultrasonic images from 324 patients (139 asymptomatic, 185 symptomatic) with internal carotid stenosis 50–99% (ECTS). The juxtaluminal hypoechoic (black) area (JBA) and grayscale median(GSM) proved to be independent predictors of the presence of hemispheric symptoms	324	
Intelligent diagnostic systems					
Christodoulou et al.	2003, 2006	18,27	A study with 230 plaque images where ten different texture feature sets were extracted. The plaques were classified into symptomatic or asymptomatic using the SOM and KNN classifiers and combining techniques. Furthermore, a carotid plaque image retrieval system was developed based on texture, histogram, and correlogram features	230	73%
Mougiakakou et al.	2007	28	A study with 108 plaque images where first-order statistical features and Laws' texture energy measures with the neural network back propagation algorithm were used. An overall accuracy of 99.1% in the classification into symptomatic or asymptomatic plaques was reported	108	99%
Prahl et al.	2007	29	In this study, a semiautomated method for the classification of echogenic vs echolucent plaques using an adaptive threshold was developed. The plaques were labeled as echogenic or echolucent by the human expert	273	96%
Kyriacou et al.	2007, 2009	30,31	In this work, an integrated system for the assessment of the risk of stroke was developed. This was based on clinical risk factors, noninvasive investigations, carotid plaque texture analysis and multilevel binary and grayscale morphological, analysis of atherosclerotic carotid plaques.	274	73%

were provided for differentiating between symptomatic and asymptomatic plaques. Echogenic plaques tended to be asymptomatic (Table 15.2).

More extensively, *histogram features* were later used to provide plaque signature vectors.[18,27,28] Similarly, histograms of grayscale occurrences at different angles and distances (correlograms, not the same as used in spatial statistics) were reported.[18]

Standard texture features have been extensively used for the classification of carotid plaques.[18,27,28,30,31]

An early discussion of standard texture features can be found in a technical review.[32] The most commonly used texture features include: (1) spatial gray level dependence matrices (SGLDM), (2) gray level difference statistics, (3) neighborhood gray tone difference matrix, (4) statistical feature matrix, (5) Laws' texture energy measures, and (6) fractal dimension texture analysis. The basic differences between texture characteristics from symptomatic and asymptomatic cases have been discussed by Iannuzzi et al.[21] and presented in Chap. 14.

More recently, the authors have used morphological features for plaque image characterization.[18,30,31] The most successful morphological features were based on a multilevel decomposition, associated with different plaque image components. In the multilevel approach, each normalized plaque is thresholded at three different intensity ranges, low, medium, and high, creating three new images called *L*-, *M*-, and *H*-images in the rest of the document. The darkest (low) components are associated with unstable plaque components, such as lipid and hemorrhages. In contrast, more stable plaque components are captured at higher brightness levels. For each one of the three new images, the authors compute pattern spectra to provide size distributions of the plaque components.[33,34] The authors then use the pattern spectra as texture features for classification.

Additionally, features like the juxtaluminal black (hypoechoic) area (JBA) without a visible echogenic cap (Chap. 12) in ultrasonic images of internal carotid artery plaques, in combination with the grayscale median of the plaque, proved to be successful independent predictors of the presence of hemispheric symptoms.[26]

15.3.2 Classification

Several classification techniques have been used for the classification of the carotid plaques. Neural classifiers such as the self-organizing map (SOM),[18,27] back propagation (BP) neural networks,[28] and the probabilistic neural network (PNN)[30,31] are common classification examples. More recently, classification based on support vector machines (SVMs) has been used by the authors' group.[30,31] In addition, the authors have also used statistical classifiers, such as the K-nearest neighbor (KNN),[18,27] or simple statistical analysis of the plaque characteristics.[18–22] For measuring performance, the leave-one-out method has been commonly used together with receiver operating characteristic (ROC) analysis.[27,28] A brief survey of a number of classification studies and comment on the association between the extracted plaque characteristics and ipsilateral hemispheric cerebrovascular symptoms are provided. These studies are listed in Table 15.2.

Geroulakos et al.[19] tested the hypothesis that the ultrasonic characteristics of carotid artery plaques are closely related to symptoms and that the plaque structure may be an important factor in producing stroke, perhaps more than the degree of stenosis. In this work, Geroulakos et al. categorized carotid plaques into four ultrasonic types: echolucent, predominately echolucent, predominately echogenic, and echogenic. An association was found of echolucent plaques with symptoms and cerebral infractions, which provided further evidence that echolucent plaques are unstable and tend to embolize.

El-Barghouty et al.[20] in a study with 94 plaques reported an association between carotid plaque echolucency and the prevalence of ipsilateral cerebral infarcts on computed tomography (CT) brain scans. The grayscale median (GSM) of the ultrasound plaque image was used for the characterization of plaques as echolucent (GSM $\leq$ 32) and echogenic (GSM $>$ 32).

Iannuzzi et al.[21] studied 242 stroke and 336 transient ischemic attack (TIA) patients and identified significant relationships between carotid artery ultrasound plaque characteristics and ischemic cerebrovascular events. The results suggested that the features more strongly associated with stroke were either the occlusion of the ipsilateral carotid artery or wider lesions and smaller minimum residual lumen diameter. The features, which were more consistently associated with TIAs, were low echogenicity of carotid plaques, thicker plaques, and the presence of longitudinal motion.

Elatrozy et al.[16] examined 96 plaques (25 symptomatic and 71 asymptomatic) from 80 patients with more than 50% internal carotid artery stenosis. They reported that plaques with GSM less than 40 or with a percentage of echolucent pixels greater than 50% were good predictors of the presence of ipsilateral hemispheric symptoms, as echolucent pixels were defined pixels with gray level values below 40.

Wilhjelm et al.[22], in a study with 52 patients scheduled for carotid endarterectomy, made a quantitative comparison between subjective classifications of the ultrasound images, first- and second-order statistical features, and a histological analysis of the surgically removed plaque. Some correlation was found between the three types of information where the best performing feature was found to be the contrast.

Rakebrandt et al.[23] in 2000 demonstrated that texture analysis of B-mode ultrasound images of carotid plaques using histogram features (in conjunction with co-occurrence matrices, fractal models, and first-order statistics) can predict histological plaque composition.

In a pilot study with 19 carotid plaques, Asvestas et al.[24] indicated a significant difference in the fractal dimension between the symptomatic and asymptomatic groups. Moreover, the phase of the cardiac cycle (systole/diastole) during which the fractal dimension was estimated had no systematic effect on the calculations. This study suggested that the fractal dimension could be used as a single determinant for the discrimination between symptomatic and asymptomatic subjects.

Kakkos et al.[25] used histogram measures and found that a high percentage of pixels below gray level ten (i.e., the darkest parts of the plaque) was associated with symptoms (amaurosis fugax, TIA, and stroke).

In a series of 324 normalized images of carotid plaques (139 asymptomatic and 158 symptomatic), Griffin et al.[26] used the size of the juxtaluminal black (hypoechoic) area in the absence of a visible echogenic plaque (JBA) in combination with the GSM of the plaque. They demonstrated that these features were independent predictors of the presence of hemispheric symptoms.[26] This model could identify a high-risk group of 188 plaques that contained 142 (77%) of the 185 symptomatic plaques (odd ratio [OR], 6.7; 95% confidence interval [CI], 4.08–10.91), ($P < .001$), (sensitivity, 77%; specificity, 66%; positive predictive value, 75%; negative predictive value, 68%).

In most of the above studies, the characteristics of the plaques were usually subjectively defined or using simple statistical measures, and the association with symptoms was established through simple *statistical analysis*. In the following studies, *intelligent diagnostic systems* were developed for the automatic classification of plaques into symptomatic or asymptomatic.

Christodoulou et al.[27] extracted a total number of 61 texture and shape features from 230 ultrasound plaque images, and those features were analyzed using a multifeature multiclassifier methodology (Chap. 14). A correct classification rate of 73.1% was reported, indicating that it was possible to identify a group of patients at risk of stroke based on texture features and neural networks. In content-based image retrieval study, Christodoulou et al.[18] showed that correlograms gave slightly better performance than traditional texture features.

Mougiakakou et al.,[28] in a study with 108 plaque images, extracted first-order statistical features and Laws' texture energy measures that were classified with a neural network back propagation algorithm. Mougiakakou et al. claimed an overall accuracy of 99.1% in the classification of symptomatic and asymptomatic plaques.

Prahl et al.[29] developed a semiautomated method for the classification of echogenic versus echolucent plaques using heuristics and an adaptive threshold (Chap. 13). The plaques were also labeled as echogenic or echolucent by a human expert. Prahl reported that the system could correctly identify the plaques with a success rate up to 96%.

The authors recently described an integrated system for the assessment of the risk of stroke based on carotid plaque image analysis.[30,31] The system was validated on 274 images. It included semiautomatic plaque segmentation, morphological image analysis, and classification using multiple classifiers. For image features, the system compared the use of a new multilevel morphological decomposition (see below) versus standard grayscale morphological analysis. For classification, comparisons were made between a probabilistic neural network (PNN) and a support vector machine (SVM) with radial basis function (RBF) kernels. The best classification result was at 73.4% using the SVM classifier with multilevel morphological features. This study is described in the following section.

15.4 Automatic Classification Case Study

For better understanding of the steps followed during automatic classification procedure, a real case describing the procedure of classifying plaques has been selected and presented in this section.

15.4.1 Material

A total of 274 carotid plaque ultrasound images of which 137 were from asymptomatic and 137 from symptomatic patients (33 stroke, 60 TIA, and 44 AF) have been included.[31] Patients with cardioembolic symptoms or contralateral symptoms (<6 months) had been excluded from the study. Asymptomatic plaques were truly asymptomatic if they had never been associated with symptoms in the past.

15.4.2 Image Acquisition

The ultrasound images were obtained using an ATL (model HDI 3000 – Advanced Technology Laboratories, Seattle, WA, USA) duplex scanner with a 5–10-MHz multifrequency probe. Longitudinal scans were performed using duplex scanning and colour flow imaging. Images were captured according to the protocol presented in Chap. 12.[35]

15.4.3 Plaque Segmentation

Plaque identification and segmentation tasks are quite difficult and were carried out manually by individuals who were experienced in ultrasound scanning (physicians or vascular ultrasonographers). The main difficulties in plaque segmentation are due to the fact that the plaque edges cannot always be distinguished from blood based on brightness level differences or texture features. Also, calcification and acoustic shadows make the segmentation problem more complex. Thus, acoustic shadows were excluded. The identification of the outline of hypoechoic plaques was facilitated using a color Doppler or power Doppler image indicating the blood flow. Also, in addition to the blood flow image, visual inspection of a logarithmically transformed plaque image was used to help identify the correct plaque boundary. The procedure for carrying out the manual segmentation process was established by a team of experts[35] and is described in detail in Chap. 12.

15.4.4 Classification Techniques

15.4.4.1 The PNN Classifier
A probabilistic neural network (PNN) classifier was used for developing classification models for the problem under study. The PNN falls within the category of nearest-neighbor classifiers.[36] For a given vector **w** to be classified, an activation a_i is computed for each of the two classes of plaques ($i = 1, \ldots, 2$). The activation a_i is defined to be the total distance of **w** from each of the M_i prototype feature vectors $x_j^{(i)}$ that belong to the ith class:

$$a_i = \sum_{j=1}^{M_i} \exp\left[-\beta\left(w - x_j^{(i)}\right)^T \left(w - x_j^{(i)}\right)\right] \quad (15.1)$$

where β is a smoothing factor. The normalized activations

$$\tilde{a}_i = a_i / \sum_{i=1}^{N} a_i \quad (15.2)$$

provide a confidence estimate for the hypothesis that **w** belongs to class i. The authors then classify **w** into the class that yields the highest confidence. An important advantage of the PNN is that it provides confidence estimates for the classification decision. Also, to avoid dependence on the smoothing factor β, the value of β was set to the one that yielded the minimum misclassification error on the training set.

15.4.4.2 The SVM Classifier
A support vector machine (SVM) classifier was also used for the classification of plaques. SVM is based on nonlinear mapping of the initial data set using a function $\varphi(.)$, followed by the identification of a hyperplane which is able to achieve the separation of the two categories of data. The SVM is applied here using Gaussian radial basis function (RBF) kernel. Details about the implementation of the SVM algorithm used can be found in [37].

15.4.4.3 Feature Selection
A popular way to reduce the dimensionality of a feature vector is principal component analysis (PCA).[31] This method can be used in cases when the input feature vector is large, but the components of this vector are highly correlated. After applying PCA, the data set is represented by a reduced number of uncorrelated features while retaining most of the variance of the input features. In this study, dimension of feature sets was reduced by using their projections on the

components which contributed for 98% of the variance in the data set.

15.4.4.4 Classification Tests

The leave-one-out estimate was used for validating all the classification models. Here, classification performance was estimated by testing on each plaque image after the system is trained on the remaining plaques. This requires 274 classification runs, one for each plaque. The performances of the classifier systems were measured using the percentages of: (1) true positives (TP), (2) false positives (FP), (3) false negatives (FN), (4) true negatives (TN), (5) sensitivity (SE), and (6) specificity (SP). For the overall performance, the correct classification (CC) rate is provided, which gives the percentage of correctly classified plaques.[31]

15.4.5 Results

The results presented are based on the texture features extracted from the data set of 274 plaque images (137 asymptomatic and 137 symptomatic).

15.4.5.1 Results from Texture Analysis

Best texture features, as presented in Chap. 14, were found to be the inverse difference moment of SGLDM (mean) with average and standard deviation values for the symptomatic plaques 0.439 ± 0.144 and for the asymptomatic plaques 0.305 ± 0.136, the median (GSM) from the SF with 17.04 ± 14.42 and 35.16 ± 23.12, the sum average of the SGLDM (mean) with 61.45 ± 27.19 and 93.89 ± 43.42, and the entropy of the SGLDM (mean) with 6.06 ± 1.43 and 7.21 ± 1.3 for the symptomatic and asymptomatic plaques, respectively.

The probabilistic neural network (PNN), the support vector machine (SVM), and the K-nearest neighbor were tested on the same data set of the 274 manually cropped ultrasound plaque images. Principal component analysis (PCA) was used as a method for dimensionality reduction. This was applied in order to retain only those components that contributed 98% to the variance of the data set. For each one of the algorithms and for each one of the texture and morphology feature sets, the classifiers were evaluated with and without PCA analysis. Results from all classifiers and image texture sets are presented in Table 15.3.

Results using PNN and SVM classifiers were significantly high. For the PNN classifier, the highest correct classification (CC) of 71.2% was achieved using the SGLDM (mean) set without PCA, while SF gave a CC only up to 65.3%. The combination of all 54 features did not improve the best CC. For the SVM classifier, the highest CC was achieved using SF after PCA analysis with a CC 70.1%. The use of SGLDM

Table 15.3 Correct classification rate (CC) using the probabilistic neural networks (PNN) and the support vector machine (SVM) classifiers for the classification of the two classes of plaques (137 symptomatic and 137 asymptomatic) for the SF, SGLDM mean, SGLDM range, GLDS, NGTDM, TEM, and FDTA feature sets, compared to that of KNN for $k = 9$

Texture analysis algorithms – classification results					
	KNN ($k = 9$) CC %	PNN CC %		SVM (RBF kernel function) CC %	
Texture features	Original	Original	Using PCA (98%)	Original	Using PCA (98%)
SF	61.3	65.3	65.3	69.3	70.1
SGLDM (mean)	62.5	**71.2**	70.8	69.7	68.6
SGLDM (range)	64.3	61.0	62.4	64.6	64.2
GLDS	58.9	60.6	60.6	65.0	65.0
NGTDM	62.8	55.8	55.8	68.3	67.9
SFM	58.9	54.4	54.4	58.4	58.4
TEM	68.2	61.0	58.4	69.3	67.5
FDTA	56.5	59.5	59.5	61.3	62.4
All 54 features	66.1	55.5	59.9	69.7	64.2
SF & NGTDM	62.5	62.8	62.4	**71.2**	69.3
SF & SGLDM (mean)	63.7	66.8	68.6	68.6	65.7
SF & SGLDM (mean) & TEM & NGTDM	66.4	65.3	64.2	70.8	70.1

(mean) achieved results up to 69.7%. The use of all 54 features gave 69.7%. The combination of SF and NGTDM gave the same result of 71.2% as the SGLDM (mean) with the previous classifier.

15.4.5.2 Results from Multilevel Binary Morphological Analysis

The median of the estimated probability density functions (*pdfs*) and cumulative density functions (*cdfs*) (see Chap. 14) extracted from the plaques can be seen in Fig. 15.1. All figures are plotted against the radial size of the structural element. The results have been divided into the two categories of multilevel binary and grayscale morphological analysis.

From the results, it is observed that the median symptomatic *cdf* is *stochastically* smaller than the median asymptomatic *cdf* for the *L*-images. This means that the median *cdf* for the symptomatic cases assumes equal or smaller values than the asymptomatic *cdf*.

For the *M*-images, the median *cdf* of the asymptomatic cases turned out to be *stochastically* larger than

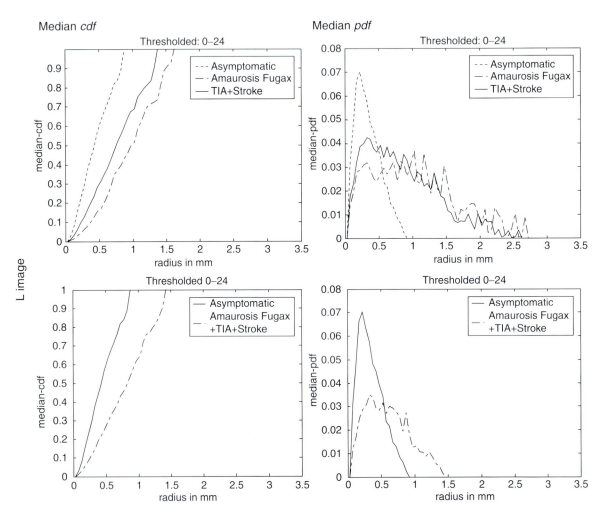

Fig. 15.1 Corresponding median values of the *pdfs* and *cdfs* of asymptomatic versus symptomatic plaques for the three different levels (*L*-, *M*-, *H*-images) of multilevel binary morphological analysis. The first line of each subplot represents the median *cdf* and *pdf* for asymptomatic vs amaurosis fugax vs (TIA & stroke) plaques, while the second line represents the median *cdf* and *pdf* for asymptomatic vs symptomatic plaques. In the plot, radius refers to radial spread of the structural element (With kind permission from Springer Science + Business Media: Kyriacou et al.[31] Fig. 3)

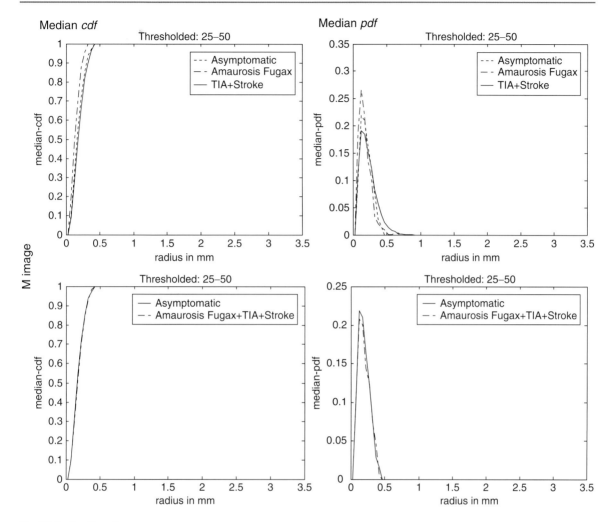

Fig. 15.1 (continued)

that of TIA and stroke but smaller to that of amaurosis fugax. Thus, the median *cdfs* of asymptomatic and symptomatic plaques are almost equal. Due to these observations, as expected, the classification results from the *M*-images were relatively lower. Finally, for the *H*-images, the median symptomatic *cdf* turned out to be *stochastically* larger than the asymptomatic *cdf*.

The authors attempted to relate their measurements to clinical expectations for a known type of dangerous plaques. Consider the case of having a plaque characterized by a dark background with isolated white blobs. This description characterizes dangerous symptomatic plaques. In this case, the uniformity in the dark regions suggests that the symptomatic *cdf* plot in the *L*-image will be slow to rise, resulting in a *cdf* that is stochastically smaller than that of the median asymptomatic case. On the other hand, the isolated white blobs will force the *cdf* of the *H*-image to be stochastically larger than that of the median asymptomatic case. Thus, in this case, both of these observations are in agreement with the authors' measurements. Naturally, how to extend these observations for different types of plaques will also need to be investigated (also see Sterpetti et al.[10])

The *cdfs* and *pdfs* of all plaques were used with the PNN and SVM classifiers. Both classifiers were tested on both the *pdf* and *cdf* feature sets. The first set included features produced for the whole range of scales (1–70), while the second set included the pattern spectra of selected scales (*L*-images: 1, 2, 3, 4, 5; *M*-images: 3, 4, 9, 11, 12; *H*-images: 2, 11, 12, 15, 18)[38]. These scales were selected because of their

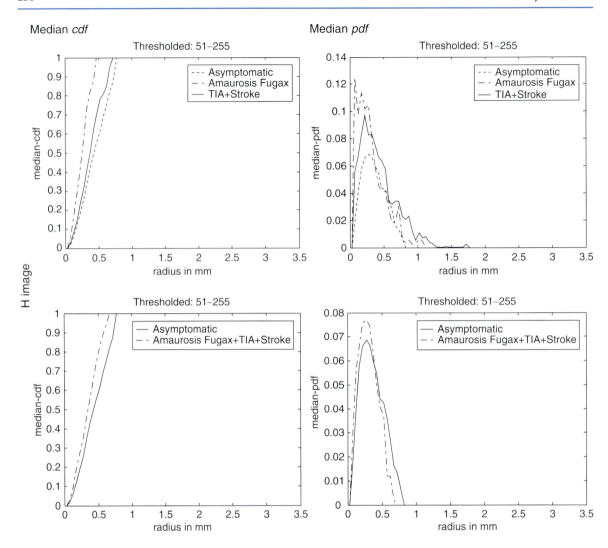

Fig. 15.1 (continued)

discriminatory power as evaluated using the C4.5 decision trees algorithm.[38,39] The C4.5 was run, and the pattern spectra scale with the highest discriminative score was computed. This best scale was then removed, and the C4.5 was run again to compute the next best scale. The procedure was repeated five times. The dimensionality of the entire *pdf*/*cdf* feature vectors from both sets was also reduced using principal components analysis (PCA). As a result of PCA, a small number of components that accounted for 98% of the total variance were selected.

Table 15.4 presents the results of the ROC analysis for the SVM and PNN classifiers for the different feature sets investigated. Classifiers were tested using features extracted from the *L*-, *M*-, and *H*-images and the combination of the three. The highest percentage of correct classifications score was 73.7% and was achieved using the SVM classifier on the features extracted from the *L*-images (*cdf* scales: 1–70 + PCA). For PNN, the highest percentage of correct classification score achieved was 70.4% for *pdf* scales 1–70 + PCA. The combination of the three feature sets gave the same highest results as those achieved with the *L*-images feature set.

15.4.5.3 Results from Grayscale Morphological Analysis

From the results, it can be observed that the median symptomatic *cdf* is *stochastically* larger than the median asymptomatic *cdf*. Recall that this means that

Table 15.4 Percentages of correct classifications (% CC), false positives (% FP), false negatives (% FN), sensitivity (% SE), and specificity (% SP) of multilevel morphological features using the SVM and PNN classifiers for the *L*-, *M*- and *H*-images in classification models developed for two groups of plaques (137 symptomatic and 137 asymptomatic) using the leave-one-out method

	SVM classifier	% CC	% FP	% FN	% SE	% SP
L-image	SVM rbf spread = 0.4 **PCA** for *pdf* scales 1, 2, 3, 4, 5, 6	70.80	42.34	16.06	83.94	57.66
	SVM rbf spread = 9.0510 *pdf* scales 1, 2, 3, 4, 5, 6	69.71	51.09	9.49	90.51	48.91
	SVM rbf spread = 0.1 **PCA** for *cdf* scales 1–70	**73.72**	**36.50**	**16.06**	**83.94**	**63.50**
	SVM rbf spread = 12.8 *cdf* scales 1–70	72.26	37.23	18.25	81.75	62.77
	SVM rbf spread = 1.6 **PCA** for *pdf* scales 1–70	70.07	43.07	16.79	83.21	56.93
	SVM rbf spread = 9.0510 *pdf* scales 1–70	70.80	41.61	16.79	83.21	58.39
	Average values	71.23	41.97	15.57	84.43	58.03
	PNN classifier					
	PNN spread = 5 **PCA** for *pdf* scales 1, 2, 3, 4, 5, 6	66.79	62.77	3.65	96.35	37.23
	PNN spread = 5 *pdf* scales 1, 2, 3, 4, 5, 6	66.79	63.50	2.92	97.08	36.50
	PNN spread = 5 **PCA** for *cdf* scales 1–70	**70.07**	**37.96**	**21.90**	**78.10**	**62.04**
	PNN spread = 5 *cdf* scales 1–70	**70.07**	**37.96**	**21.90**	**78.10**	**62.04**
	PNN spread = 5 **PCA** for *pdf* scales 1–70	70.44	40.88	18.25	81.75	59.12
	PNN spread = 5 *pdf* scales 1–70	69.71	35.77	24.82	75.18	64.23
	Average values	68.98	46.47	15.57	84.43	53.53
	SVM classifier	% CC	% FP	% FN	% SE	% SP
M-image	SVM rbf spread = 9.0510 **PCA** for *pdf* scales 2, 11, 12, 15, 18, 19	58.76	47.45	35.04	64.96	52.55
	SVM rbf spread = 12.8 *pdf* scales 2, 11, 12, 15, 18, 19	58.39	47.45	35.77	64.23	52.55
	SVM rbf spread = 6.4 **PCA** for *cdf* scales 1–70	59.12	42.34	39.42	60.58	57.66
	SVM rbf spread = 0.4 *cdf* scales 1–70	59.12	41.61	40.15	59.85	58.39
	SVM rbf spread = 9.0510 **PCA** for *pdf* scales 1–70	**62.04**	**40.88**	**35.04**	**64.96**	**59.12**
	SVM rbf spread = 0.8 *pdf* scales 1–70	60.22	45.26	34.31	65.69	54.74
	Average values	59.61	44.17	36.62	63.38	55.84
	PNN classifier					
	PNN spread = 5 **PCA** for *pdf* scales 2, 11, 12, 15, 18, 19	43.80	24.82	87.59	12.41	75.18
	PNN spread = 5 *pdf* scales 2, 11, 12, 15, 18, 19	43.80	24.82	87.59	12.41	75.18

(continued)

Table 15.4 (continued)

	SVM classifier	% CC	% FP	% FN	% SE	% SP
	PNN spread = 5 **PCA** for *cdf* scales 1–70	**59.12**	**48.18**	**33.58**	**66.42**	**51.82**
	PNN spread = 5 *cdf* scales 1–70	58.76	48.91	33.58	66.42	51.09
	PNN spread = 5 **PCA** for *pdf* scales 1–70	57.66	64.23	20.44	79.56	35.77
	PNN spread = 5 *pdf* scales 1–70	55.47	65.69	23.36	76.64	34.31
	Average values	53.1	46.11	47.69	52.31	53.89
	SVM classifier	% CC	% FP	% FN	% SE	% SP
H-image	SVM rbf spread = 0.1414 **PCA** for *pdf* scales 3, 4, 9, 11, 12	**60.58**	**45.99**	**32.85**	**67.15**	**54.01**
	SVM rbf spread = 0.1 *pdf* scales 3, 4, 9, 11, 12	59.49	47.45	33.58	66.42	52.55
	SVM rbf spread = 2.2627 **PCA** for *cdf* scales 1–70	55.47	34.31	54.74	45.26	65.69
	SVM rbf spread = 0.2 *cdf* scales 1–70	59.12	29.93	51.82	48.18	70.07
	SVM rbf spread = 0.4 **PCA** for *pdf* scales 1–70	58.39	37.96	45.26	54.74	62.04
	SVM rbf spread = 0.1 *pdf* scales 1–70	58.39	37.96	45.26	54.74	62.04
	Average values	58.57	38.93	43.92	56.08	61.07
	PNN classifier					
	PNN spread = 5 **PCA** for *pdf* scales 3, 4, 9, 11, 12	48.18	10.95	92.70	7.30	89.05
	PNN spread = 5 *pdf* scales 3, 4, 9, 11, 12	48.18	10.95	92.70	7.30	89.05
	PNN spread = 5 **PCA** for *cdf* scales 1–70	49.27	9.49	91.97	8.03	90.51
	PNN spread = 5 *cdf* scales 1–70	48.91	11.68	90.51	9.49	88.32
	PNN spread = 5 **PCA** for *pdf* scales 1–70	51.46	9.49	87.59	12.41	90.51
	PNN spread = 5 *pdf* scales 1–70	51.09	9.49	88.32	11.68	90.51
	Average values	49.52	10.34	90.63	9.37	89.66
	SVM classifier	% CC	% FP	% FN	% SE	% SP
Combination L-, M-, H-images	SVM rbf spread = 6.4 **PCA** for *pdf* scales (low: 1, 2, 3, 4, 5, 6) (med: 3, 4, 9, 11, 12) (high: 19, 12, 15, 11, 18, 2)	71.90	43.07	13.14	86.86	56.93
	SVM rbf spread = 6.4 *pdf* scales (low: 1, 2, 3, 4, 5, 6) (med: 3, 4, 9, 11, 12) (high: 19, 12, 15, 11, 18, 2)	71.90	45.26	10.95	89.05	54.74
	SVM rbf spread = 12.8 **PCA** for *cdf* scales 1–210	69.34	43.80	17.52	82.48	56.20
	SVM rbf spread = 2.2627 *cdf* scales 1–210	71.90	39.42	16.79	83.21	60.58

(continued)

Table 15.4 (continued)

SVM classifier	% CC	% FP	% FN	% SE	% SP
SVM rbf spread = 9.0510 PCA for *pdf* scales 1–210	70.80	42.34	16.06	83.94	57.66
SVM rbf spread = 6.4 *pdf* scales 1–210	**73.36**	**39.42**	**13.87**	**86.13**	**60.58**
Average values	71.53	42.22	14.72	85.28	57.78
CPNN classifier					
PNN spread = PCA for *pdf* scales (low: 1, 2, 3, 4, 5, 6) (med: 3, 4, 9, 11, 12) (high: 19, 12, 15, 11, 18, 2)	69.34	53.28	8.03	91.97	46.72
PNN spread = 5 *pdf* scales (low: 1, 2, 3, 4, 5, 6) (med: 3, 4, 9, 11, 12) (high: 19, 12, 15, 11, 18, 2)	69.71	54.01	6.57	93.43	45.99
PNN spread = 5 PCA for *cdf* scales 1–210	69.71	37.96	22.63	77.37	62.04
PNN spread = 5 *cdf* scales 1–210	68.61	40.15	22.63	77.37	59.85
PNN spread = 5 PCA for *pdf* scales 1–210	**70.44**	**42.34**	**16.79**	**83.21**	**57.66**
PNN spread = 5 *pdf* scales 1–210	**70.07**	**38.69**	**21.17**	**78.83**	**61.31**
Average values	69.65	44.41	16.3	83.7	55.6

the median *cdf* for the symptomatic cases assumes equal or larger values than the asymptomatic *cdf*. The median and box plots of *pdfs* and *cdfs* for gray-scale morphological can be seen in Fig. 15.2.

For the dangerous type of symptomatic plaque discussed above, this observation appears to be in agreement with the authors' expectations. Here, the isolated white blobs against a dark background in the symptomatic plaques lead to a larger concentration of the detected components in the lower scales of the pattern spectrum, as compared to the asymptomatic cases. In turn, as for the *H*-images, this causes a rise in the symptomatic *cdf* in contrast to the median asymptomatic *cdf* (also see[40]).

Again, the *cdfs* and *pdfs* of all plaques were used with the PNN and SVM classifiers. Both classifiers were tested on both the *pdf* and *cdf* feature sets. The first set included features produced for the whole range of scales (1–70), while the second set included the pattern spectra of selected scales (2, 3, 5, 10, 21, and 23),[38] using the C4.5 decision tree algorithm.

Table 15.5 presents the results of the ROC analysis for the SVM and PNN classifiers for the different feature sets investigated. The highest percentage of correct classifications score was 66.7% and was achieved using the SVM classifier on the second set of data (pdf scales: 2, 3, 5, 10, 21, and 23 + PCA). For PNN, the highest percentage of correct classifications score achieved was 62.04% for cdf scales 1–70.

15.5 Conclusions

This chapter demonstrates how image texture and morphology analysis algorithms are used in order to classify ultrasound images of carotid plaques. The results using different classifiers are very promising and can be used to create a system for computer-assisted identification of patients with asymptomatic carotid stenosis at increased risk of stroke.

The results using image texture analysis algorithms presented in this chapter[31] are comparable with previous work carried out with different data sets.[27]

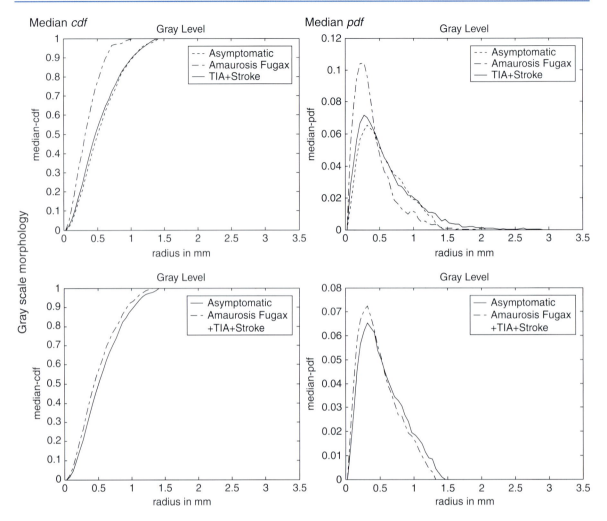

Fig. 15.2 Corresponding median values of the *pdfs* and *cdfs* of asymptomatic versus symptomatic plaques for the grayscale morphological analysis. The first row represents the median *cdf* and *pdf* for asymptomatic vs amaurosis fugax vs (TIA & stroke) plaques, while the second represents median *cdf* and *pdf* for asymptomatic vs symptomatic plaques (With kind permission from Springer Science + Business Media: Kyriacou et al.[31] Fig. 4)

The Haralick SGLDM texture features gave best results in both studies, whereas the statistical feature grayscale median (GSM) proved again a good and simple descriptor for plaque instability.

Morphological features help us understand the interrelations among different intensity regions. The authors have examined morphological results from dark, midrange, and high intensity regions. The authors have found that there was significant overlap between the pattern spectra coming from symptomatic and asymptomatic plaques. Furthermore, as the authors expected, probability density function (*pdf*) estimates were visually verified to be noisier than cumulative distribution function estimates. For larger morphological components, the *pdf* started to decrease, and the variance in the estimates increased significantly. Thus, most of the discriminating power was concentrated in the smaller components for lower scales.

The application of these techniques and their performance in a prospective study are presented in Chap. 37.

Table 15.5 Percentage of correct classifications (% CC), false positives (% FP), false negatives (% FN), sensitivity (% SE), and specificity (% SP) of grayscale morphological features using the SVM and PNN classifiers in classification models developed for two classes using the leave-one-out method in 137 symptomatic and 137 asymptomatic plaques

	SVM classifier	% CC	% FP	% FN	% SE	% SP
Gray scale	SVM rbf spread = 2.2627 PCA for *pdf* scales 2, 3, 5, 10, 21, 23	**66.79**	20.44	45.99	54.01	79.56
	SVM rbf spread = 0.5657 *pdf* scales 2, 3, 5, 10, 21, 23	65.33	28.47	40.88	59.12	71.53
	SVM rbf spread = 2.2627 PCA for *cdf* scales 1–70	63.14	42.34	31.39	68.61	57.66
	SVM rbf spread = 2.2627 *cdf* scales 1–70	62.41	32.12	43.07	56.93	67.88
	SVM rbf spread = 1.1314 PCA for *pdf* scales 1–70	60.22	43.80	35.77	64.23	56.20
	SVM rbf spread = 0.5657 *pdf* scales 1–70	**63.14**	**36.50**	**37.23**	**62.77**	**63.50**
	Average values	63.51	33.95	39.06	60.95	66.06
	PNN classifier					
	PNN spread = 5 PCA for *pdf* scales 2, 3, 5, 10, 21, 23	56.57	22.63	64.23	35.77	77.37
	PNN spread = 5 *pdf* scales 2, 3, 5, 10, 21, 23	56.57	22.63	64.23	35.77	77.37
	PNN spread = 5 PCA for *cdf* scales 1–70	60.58	36.50	42.34	57.66	63.50
	PNN spread = 5 *cdf* scales 1–70	**62.04**	**35.77**	**40.15**	**59.85**	**64.23**
	PNN spread = 5 PCA for *pdf* scales 1–70	58.76	42.34	40.15	59.85	57.66
	PNN spread = 5 *pdf* scales 1–70	60.22	48.91	30.66	69.34	51.09
	Average values	59.12	34.8	46.96	53.04	65.2

References

1. Reilly LM et al. Carotid plaque histology using real-time ultrasonography. Clinical and therapeutic implications. *Am J Surg*. 1983;146:188–193.
2. O'Donnell TF Jr et al. Correlation of B-mode ultrasound imaging and arteriography with pathologic findings at carotid endarterectomy. *Arch Surg*. 1985;120:443–449.
3. Leahy AL et al. Duplex ultrasonography and selection of patients for carotid endarterectomy: plaque morphology or luminal narrowing? *J Vasc Surg*. 1988;8:558–562.
4. Langsfeld M, Gray-Weale AC, Lusby RJ. The role of plaque morphology and diameter reduction in the development of new symptoms in asymptomatic carotid arteries. *J Vasc Surg*. 1989;9:548–557.
5. Geroulakos G et al. Characterisation of symptomatic and asymptomatic carotid plaques using high-resolution real-time ultrasonography. *Br J Surg*. 1993;80:1274–1277.
6. Johnson JM, Kennelly MM, Decesare D, Morgan S, Sparrow A. Natural history of asymptomatic carotid plaque. *Arch Surg*. 1985;120:1010–1012.
7. Widder B et al. Morphological characterization of carotid artery stenoses by ultrasound duplex scanning. *Ultrasound Med Biol*. 1990;16:349–354.
8. Gray-Weale AC, Graham JC, Burnett JR, Byrne K, Lusby RJ. Carotid artery atheroma: comparison of preoperative B-mode ultrasound appearance with carotid endarterectomy specimen pathology. *J Cardiovasc Surg (Torino)*. 1988; 29:676–681.
9. Aldoori MI et al. Duplex scanning and plaque histology in cerebral ischaemia. *Eur J Vasc Surg*. 1987;1:159–164.
10. Sterpetti AV et al. Ultrasonographic features of carotid plaque and the risk of subsequent neurologic deficits. *Surgery*. 1988;104:652–660.
11. Giannoni MF et al. Minor asymptomatic carotid stenosis contralateral to carotid endarterectomy (CEA): our experience. *Eur J Vasc Surg*. 1991;5:237–245.
12. European carotid plaque study group. Carotid artery plaque composition – relationship to clinical presentation and ultrasound B-mode imaging. *Eur J Vasc Endovasc Surg*. 1995;10:23–30.
13. Kagawa R, Moritake K, Shima T, Okada Y. Validity of B-mode ultrasonographic findings in patients undergoing

carotid endarterectomy in comparison with angiographic and clinicopathologic features. *Stroke*. 1996;27:700–705.
14. Kardoulas DG et al. Ultrasonographic and histologic characteristics of symptom-free and symptomatic carotid plaque. *Cardiovasc Surg*. 1996;4:580–590.
15. AbuRahma AF, Kyer PD 3rd, Robinson PA, Hannay RS. The correlation of ultrasonic carotid plaque morphology and carotid plaque hemorrhage: clinical implications. *Surgery*. 1998;124:721–728.
16. Elatrozy T, Nicolaides A, Tegos T, Griffin M. The objective characterisation of ultrasonic carotid plaque features. *Eur J Vasc Endovasc Surg*. 1998;16:223–230.
17. Tegos TJ et al. Comparability of the ultrasonic tissue characteristics of carotid plaques. *J Ultrasound Med*. 2000;19:399–407 (9).
18. Christodoulou CI, Kyriacou E, Pattichis CS, Nicolaides A. Multiple feature extraction for content-based image retrieval of carotid plaque ultrasound images. In: ITAB '06 Conference; October 26–28, 2006; Ioannina-Epirus.
19. Geroulakos G et al. Ultrasonic carotid artery plaque structure and the risk of cerebral infarction on computed tomography. *J Vasc Surg*. 1994;20(2):263–266.
20. El-Barghouty N, Geroulakos G, Nicolaides A, Androulakis A, Bahal V. Computer assisted carotid plaque characterisation. *Eur J Vasc Endovasc Surg*. 1995;9: 548–557 (12).
21. Iannuzzi AI et al. Ultrasonographic correlates of carotid atherosclerosis in transient ischemic attack and stroke. *Stroke*. 1995;26(4):614–619.
22. Wilhjelm JE et al. Quantitative analysis of ultrasound B-mode images of carotid atherosclerotic plaque: correlation with visual classification and histological examination. *IEEE Trans Med Imaging*. 1998;17(6):910–922.
23. Rakebrandt F, Crawford DC, Havard D, Coleman D, Woodcock JP. Relationship between ultrasound texture classification images and histology of atherosclerotic plaque. *Ultrasound Med Biol*. 2000;26(9):1393–1402.
24. Asvestas P, Golemati S, Matsopoulos GK, Nikita KS, Nicolaides A. Fractal dimension estimation of carotid atherosclerotic plaques from B-mode ultrasound: a pilot study. *Ultrasound Med Biol*. 2002;28(9):1129–1136.
25. Kakkos S et al. Computerised texture analysis of carotid plaque ultrasonic images can identify unstable plaques associated with ipsilateral neurological symptoms. *Angiology*. 2011;62:317–328.
26. Griffin M et al. Juxtaluminal hypoechoic area in ultrasonic images of carotid plaques and hemispheric symptoms. *J Vasc Surg*. 2010;52(1):69–76.
27. Christodoulou CI, Pattichis CS, Pantziaris M, Nicolaides A. Texture based classification of atherosclerotic carotid plaques. *IEEE Trans Med Imaging*. 2003;22(7):902–912.
28. Mougiakakou SG, Golemati S, Gousias I, Nicolaides AN, Nikita KS. Computer-aided diagnosis of carotid atherosclerosis based on ultrasound image statistics, Laws' texture and neural networks. *Ultrasound Med Biol*. 2007;33(1):26–36.
29. Prahl U et al. Percentage white: a new feature for ultrasound classification of plaque echogenicity in carotid artery atherosclerosis. *Ultrasound Med Biol*. 2010;36(2):218–226.
30. Kyriacou EC et al. An integrated system for assessing stroke risk. *IEEE Eng Med Biol Mag*. 2007;26(5):43–50.
31. Kyriacou E et al. Classification of atherosclerotic carotid plaques using morphological analysis on ultrasound images. *Appl Intell*. 2009;30(1):3–23.
32. Amadasun M, King R. Textural features corresponding to textural properties. *IEEE Trans Syst Man Cybern*. 1989;19 (5):1264–1274.
33. Dougherty ER. *An Introduction to Morphological Image Processing*. Bellingham: SPIE Optical Engineering Press; 1992.
34. Dougherty ER, Astola J. *An Introduction to Nonlinear Image Processing*. Bellingham: SPIE Optical Engineering Press; 1994.
35. Nicolaides A et al. The Asymptomatic, Carotid, Stenosis and Risk of Stroke (ACSRS) study. *Int Angiol*. 2003;22 (3):263–272.
36. Specht DF. Probabilistic neural networks. *INNS Neural Netw*. 1990;3(1):109–118.
37. Joachims T. Making large-scale support vector machine learning practical. In: Schölkopf B, Burges CJC, Smola AJ, eds. *Advances in Kernel Methods: Support Vector Learning*. Cambridge: MIT Press; 1999:169–184.
38. Panagiotou S. *Classification of plaques using SVM class* [M. Sc. thesis]. Nicosia, Cyprus: University of Cyprus; 2006.
39. Han J, Kamber M. *Data Mining: Concepts and Techniques*. San Francisco: Morgan Kaufmann; 2000.
40. Mavrommatis A. *Morphology of carotid US images* [M.Sc. thesis]. Nicosia, Cyprus: University of Cyprus; 2006.

16. Volumetric Evaluation of Carotid Atherosclerosis Using 3-Dimensional Ultrasonic Imaging

Grace Parraga, Andrew A. House, Adam Krasinski, J. David Spence, and Aaron Fenster

16.1 Introduction

The established measurements of carotid atherosclerosis using ultrasound include Bright or B-mode measurement of the carotid intima-media thickness (IMT)[1] and Doppler ultrasound velocity measurements.[2,3] Doppler velocity measurements are well established as a screening tool in the assessment of the severity of stenosis[2–6] (Chap. 30). The measurement of IMT from B-mode ultrasound images is a widely used phenotype and is regarded as a surrogate measurement of atherosclerosis because it has been shown to correlate with vascular outcomes.[7–9] Although the measurement of IMT has been validated in many studies, it is clear that it may reflect many distinct biological pathways and mechanisms. For example, IMT may represent hypertensive medial hypertrophy,[10,11] compensatory intimal thickening due to mechanical forces of blood flow,[12,13] or the initial "fatty streak" stage of atherosclerosis that involves accumulation of macrophage foam cells in the arterial wall.[14] IMT fluctuates over time in response to a variety of factors, which may not necessarily be related to atherosclerotic plaque formation and progression. More recently, *total plaque area* (TPA)[15] and *total plaque volume* (TPV)[16–22] have emerged as complementary ultrasonic phenotypes of carotid atherosclerosis providing specific measurements of plaque burden in two dimensions (2D) and three dimensions (3D), respectively. Total plaque area has been shown to be a stronger predictor of coronary events than IMT.[23,24] Previous work also demonstrated that TPV in particular can be used to measure changes in plaque burden[16–18,25,26] and evaluate the effects of statin therapy.[27,28] While the measurement of TPV provides valuable quantitative information about global plaque burden, it does not identify the locations in the vessel where volumetric changes are occurring. Furthermore, the measurement of TPV from 3D ultrasonic images requires trained observers who are expert in 3D image interpretation and in distinguishing vessel wall from plaque in such images. Limitations of this approach include image interpretation and measurement differences within and between observers, long training times for observers, and long duration to perform manual segmentations. In order to overcome some of these limitations and accelerate the translation of 3D measurements of carotid atherosclerosis to clinical research and clinical practice, semiautomated methods of measurement and measurements that are derived from biological components of carotid disease with readily distinguishable boundaries (enabling multiple observers to be trained in shorter time periods and with decreased interobserver variability) are required.[29]

This has driven the development and validation of a new 3D measurement of carotid atherosclerosis using ultrasound: *Vessel Wall Volume* (VWV). This is a measurement of vessel wall thickness and plaque

G. Parraga (✉) • A. Fenster
Imaging Research Laboratories, Robarts Research Institute, The University of Western Ontario, London, ON, Canada

A.A. House
Division of Nephrology, London Health Sciences Centre, London, ON, Canada

A. Krasinski • J.D. Spence
Stroke Prevention & Atherosclerosis Research Centre, Robarts Research Institute, University of Western Ontario, London, ON, Canada

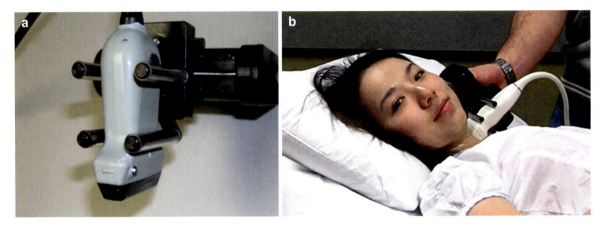

Fig. 16.1 (**a**) A mechanical linear scanning mechanism used to acquire 3D carotid ultrasound (US) images. The transducer is translated along the artery, while conventional 2D US images are acquired by a computer and reconstructed into a 3D image in real time. (**b**) Photograph of the carotid artery scanning system

within the common carotid artery and internal carotid branch. In the authors' recent experience, the measurement of 3D VWV can be more easily semiautomated, and observers can be trained to measure VWV in shorter duration and with greater intraobserver reliability.

The measurement of 3D TPV requires observers to distinguish plaque-lumen and plaque–outer vessel wall boundaries, whereas the measurement of 3D VWV requires only the segmentation of the lumen-intima/plaque and media-adventitia boundaries – which is similar to the measurement of IMT. These boundaries are more straightforward to interpret than plaque-lumen and wall boundaries in 3D images. In addition, VWV boundary measurements are more regular and circular, which simplifies the development of semiautomated segmentation techniques. In this chapter, the method used to acquire 3D images of the carotid arteries using ultrasound will be reviewed, and the use of TPV and VWV for quantifying the progression and regression of carotid atherosclerosis will be discussed.

16.1.1 3D Carotid Imaging Method Using Ultrasound

3D ultrasonic carotid imaging for visualizing and measuring TPA and VWV is reviewed here in detail. Further information about the technical and computational aspects on the subject can be found in a number of excellent recent review articles and books.[30–37] Because carotid artery imaging requires at least a scanning length of about 4 cm, real-time 3D (i.e., four-dimensional or 4D) systems have not yet been developed. Thus, all 3D systems dedicated to carotid artery imaging using ultrasound are conventional transducers that produce 2D images. Since a conventional transducer must be moved over the carotid artery to acquire all the required 2D images necessary to reconstruct the 3D image, a method to track the position and orientation of the transducer must be used. Over the past decade, two methods have been developed to image the carotid arteries: mechanical linear scanners and magnetically tracked freehand scanners. The authors have used the mechanical scanning approach, as summarized here.

16.1.2 Mechanical Linear 3D Carotid Imaging

Linear scanners use a motorized mechanism to translate the transducer linearly along the neck, as shown in Fig. 16.1. Transverse 2D images of the carotid arteries are acquired at regular spatial intervals as the transducer moves over the carotid arteries. Each image in the set of acquired 2D images is spaced equally so that all images are parallel to each other, making 3D reconstruction easy and possible in real time. The length of the scan depends on the length of the mechanical scanning mechanism, and in practice ranges from

4 to 6 cm. The resolution of the image in the 3D scanning direction (i.e., along the artery) depends on the elevational resolution of the transducer as well as the spacing between the acquired images. It can be optimized by varying the speed (of translation) and sampling interval in order to match the sampling rate to the frame rate of the ultrasound machine and to match the sampling interval to half (or smaller) the elevational resolution of the transducer.[38] Typically, the authors acquire 2D images every 0.2 mm. If the 2D images are acquired at 30 frames/s, a 4-cm length will require 200 2D images, which can be acquired in 6.7 s without cardiac gating.

The simple predefined geometry of the acquired 2D ultrasonic images allows the development of a simple algorithm to reconstruct a 3D image.[38] Thus, using this approach, a 3D image can be reconstructed as the 2D images are being acquired, and immediate viewing of the 3D carotid image after scanning is possible to determine if additional 3D scans are necessary. This specific advantage of immediate review of 3D images after a scan significantly shortens the examination time and reduces digital storage requirements because inadequate images do not require archiving.

Because the 3D carotid image is produced from a series of conventional 2D images, the resolution in the 3D image will not be isotropic. In the direction parallel to the acquired 2D image planes, the resolution of the reconstructed 3D image will be equal to the original 2D images; however, in the direction of the 3D scan along the arteries, the resolution of the reconstructed 3D image will depend on the elevational resolution of the transducer and interslice spacing.[38] Since the elevational resolution is worse than the in-plane resolution of the 2D images, the resolution of the 3D image will be the poorest in the 3D scanning direction (i.e., elevation). Therefore, to optimize resolution along the artery, a transducer with good elevational resolution should be used.

Although the 3D mechanical scanning approach requires a mechanical mover held by the operator (Fig. 16.1), it offers a number of advantages, such as short imaging times, high-quality 3D images, and fast reconstruction times. However, bulkiness and weight of the mechanism sometimes make it inconvenient or difficult to use over long periods of time. Linear scanning has been successfully implemented in many vascular imaging applications using B-mode and color Doppler images of the carotid arteries,[2,3,6,39,40] vascular test phantoms,[4,5,41] power Doppler images,[2–6,39,40] and studies of carotid atherosclerosis.[42–44] An example of a mechanical scanning mechanism and its use is shown in Fig. 16.1, and examples of linearly scanned 3D ultrasound images of carotid arteries with complex plaques are shown in Figs. 16.2 and 16.3.

16.1.3 3D Carotid Image Reconstruction

The 3D reconstruction procedure involves placing the acquired 2D ultrasonic images in their correct location within the volume, generating a 3D image. The gray-scale values of any voxel not sampled by the 2D images are then calculated by interpolating between the adjacent 2D images. As a result, all 2D image information is preserved, allowing viewing of the original 2D planes as well as any other views. The authors' methods have been developed to run on standard desktop personal computers that are more than sufficient to allow for 3D reconstructions to occur while the 2D images are being acquired (i.e., in real time). Thus, it is possible to view the complete 3D carotid image immediately after the acquisition of the 2D ultrasonic images is completed.

16.1.4 Viewing 3D Carotid Images

Many 3D viewing methods have been developed over the past decade. The method the authors use most commonly is the *cube view* approach, which is based on multiplanar rendering using texture mapping. In this technique, a 3D image is displayed as a polyhedron, and the appropriate image for each plane is "painted" on the face of the cube (texture-mapped). Users can rotate the polyhedron in order to obtain the desired orientation of the 3D image as well as move any of the surfaces (i.e., by slicing the 3D image parallelly or obliquely) to the original while the appropriate data is texture-mapped in real time onto the new face. As a result, users always have 3-dimensional image-based cues, which relate the plane being manipulated to the rest of the anatomy. These visual cues allow users to efficiently identify the desired structures.[30,31,35,36] Examples of this approach are shown in Figs. 16.2 and 16.3.

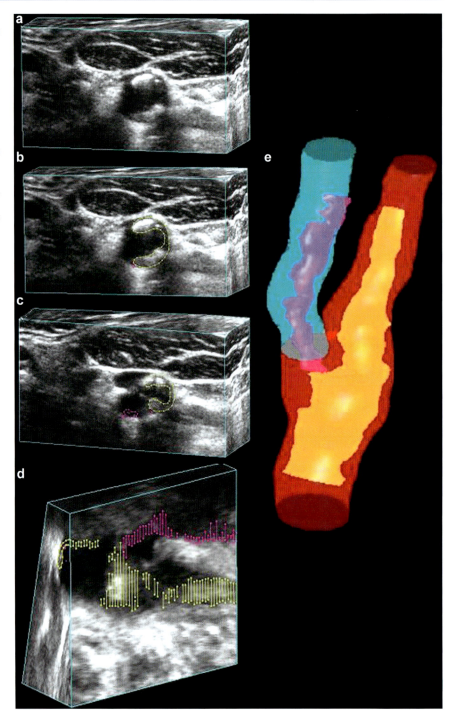

Fig. 16.2 Steps used in measurement of *TPV* from 3D images. (**a**) First, the 3D image is "sliced" to obtain a transverse view. (**b**, **c**) By using a mouse-driven crosshaired cursor, the plaque is outlined in successive image "slices" until all the plaques have been traversed. (**d**) The vessel can be sliced to reveal a longitudinal view with the outlines of the plaques. (**e**) After outlining all the plaques, the total volume can be calculated, and a mesh fitted to provides a view of the plaque surface together with the boundary of the vessel

Fig. 16.3 Steps used in measurement of *vessel wall (plus plaque)* volume from 3D images. (**a**) First, the 3D image is "sliced" to obtain a transverse view. (**b, c**) By using a mouse-driven crosshaired cursor, the vessel boundary and the lumen boundary plaque are outlined separately in successive image "slices" until all the slices have been traversed (typically 1.5 cm above and below the carotid bifurcation). (**d**) The vessel can be sliced to reveal a longitudinal view with the outlines and correct any errors. (**e**) After outlining has been completed, the *vessel wall plus plaque* volume can be calculated, and a mesh fitted to provides a view of the vessel and the lumen boundaries. Each branch of the carotid artery has been colored differently

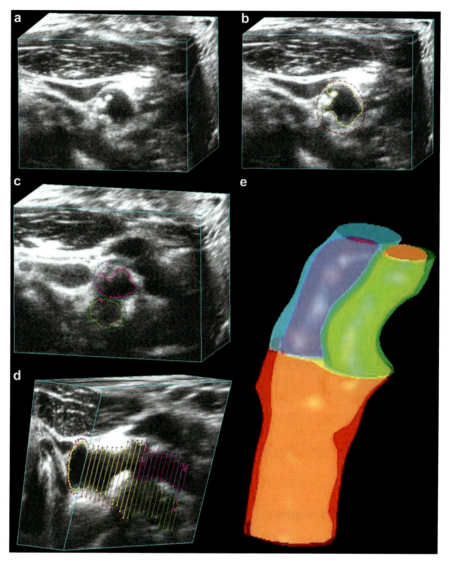

16.2 Quantification of Carotid Atherosclerosis

16.2.1 Total Plaque Volume (TPV)

The authors have quantified carotid atherosclerosis using manual planimetry to generate: *total plaque volume* (TPV) and *vessel wall volume* (VWV). To measure TPV, each 3D carotid image is "sliced" transverse to the vessel axis, starting from one end of the plaque using an interslice distance (ISD) of 1.0 mm. Using software developed in the authors' laboratory, the plaque is contoured in each cross-sectional image using a crosshaired cursor (see Fig. 16.2). As the contours are manually outlined, the visualization software calculates the area of the contours automatically. Sequential areas enclosed by the contours are averaged and multiplied by the ISD in order to calculate the incremental volume. A summation of incremental volumes provides a measure of the TPV. After measuring a complete plaque volume, the 3D image can be viewed in multiple orientations in order to verify that the entire plaque volume is outlined by the set of contours. A typical plaque volume calculation requires about 10–30 slices and approximately 15 min to complete.

16.2.2 Vessel Wall Volume (VWV)

VWV is currently derived from magnetic resonance imaging carotid magnetic resonance (MR) images, and as it represents a 3D IMT, it is an alternative method for quantifying atherosclerosis in the carotid arteries using ultrasound. Measurement of the VWV proceeds whereby each 3D carotid image is "sliced" transverse to the vessel axis, starting from one end of the 3D image using an interslice distance (ISD) of 1.0 mm. In this approach, the lumen (blood-intima boundary) and the vessel wall (media-adventitia boundary) are segmented in each slice. The area inside the lumen boundary is subtracted from the area inside the vessel wall boundary to give the vessel wall area. Sequential areas are averaged and multiplied by the ISD to give the incremental vessel wall volume. The summation of incremental volumes provides a measure of the total VWV (Figs. 16.4 and 16.5). It is also important to note that for the measurement of VWV, 3D ultrasound works well with hyperechoic plaques, but hypoechoic plaques or plaques with echolucent areas adjacent to the lumen in the absence of a visible echogenic cup represent a special challenge. In these special circumstances, it is helpful to use color flow or power Doppler to provide guidance regarding the blood/plaque boundary for VWV segmentation (Chap. 18).

16.3 3D Carotid Studies

16.3.1 Monitoring Regression of Carotid Atherosclerosis

Numerous carotid atherosclerosis measurement tools have been developed and used for monitoring of patients at risk of stroke, such as blood pressure and serum cholesterol levels. Here, the use of 3D carotid ultrasound to monitor response of carotid atherosclerosis to intensive statin treatment is summarized. To visualize changes in the carotid artery and any potential arterial remodeling that occurs during intensive statin treatment and to try to exploit the inherent advantages of 3D imaging, the authors measured[17,18,28,42,43] successive carotid artery vessel wall and lumen segmentation outlines to generate TPA, VWV, and carotid VWV thickness and thickness difference maps.

16.3.1.1 TPA Measurements of Intensive Statin Treatment of Carotid Atherosclerosis

Fifty patients with asymptomatic carotid stenosis greater than 60%, as defined by carotid Doppler flow velocities, were enrolled in this study[28] after providing written informed consent to a protocol approved by the University of Western Ontario Standing Board of Human Research Ethics, and were randomized to either placebo or atorvastatin 80 mg daily for 3 months.

The subjects were imaged using 3D carotid ultrasound while recumbent on a gurney, with their upper torso inclined approximately 15°. Both right and left carotid arteries were scanned over a scan distance of 4 cm with the bifurcation set as the center of the volume. Measurements of TPV were made using manual planimetry. From the initial cohort of 50 subjects, baseline and 3-month TPV measurements were obtained in 38 cases. Characteristics of the subjects who completed the study were analyzed at baseline and showed that there were no significant differences in risk factors between the two treatment groups. Analysis of the results (see Fig. 16.6) of the TPV measurements showed that over 3 months, plaque volume increased for those subjects administered placebo by 16.8 ± 74.1 mm^3, while for subjects treated with atorvastatin, there was significant TPV decrease of -90.3 ± 85.1 mm^3 ($p < 0.0001$).

16.3.1.2 VWV Measurements of Intensive Statin Treatment of Carotid Atherosclerosis

The same images were also used to measure VWV. A single observer blinded to subject identity, treatment, and time point performed manual segmentation of all carotid volumes. Manual planimetry was used to measure VWV as described. Briefly, to identify the media-adventitia boundary, all 3D images were viewed simultaneously in the longitudinal and axial views. This allowed the observer to identify the characteristic double line pattern in the longitudinal view, which represented the intima-lumen and media-adventitia boundaries.[45] The carotid bifurcation was used as a point of reference to reduce interscan measurement variability, and the bifurcation was first identified within both follow-up and baseline 3D images so that all measurements could be initialized with the same 2D image slice. The common carotid artery

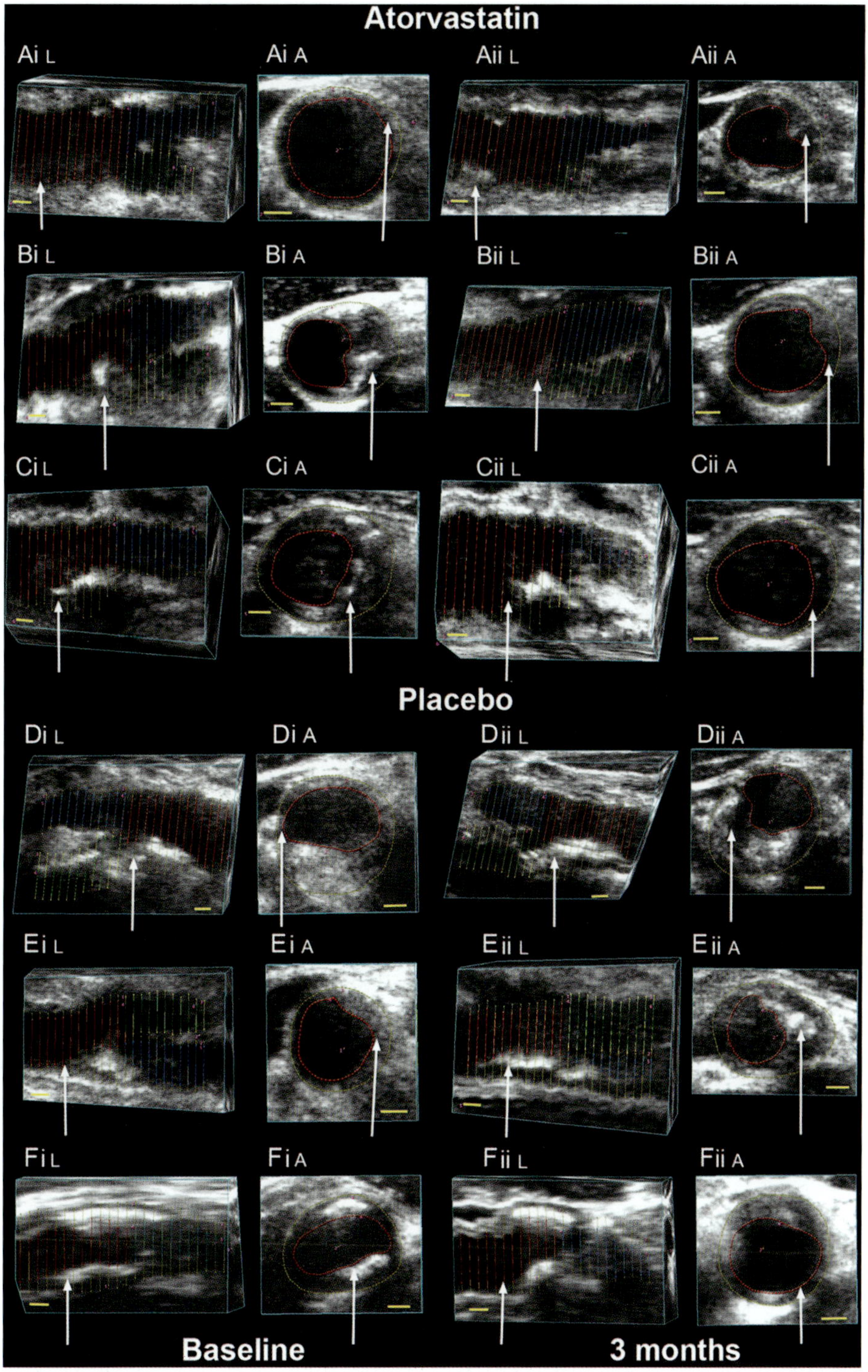

Fig. 16.4 Transverse and longitudinal 3D ultrasound of carotid atherosclerosis. Both longitudinal (*L*) and axial (*A*) views are shown. Arrows indicate regions corresponding to regions of interest in Fig. 16.6. All scale bars represent 2 mm. (**a**) A particular atorvastatin subject shown with a large positive change (increase) in VWV between baseline (**i**) and follow-up (**ii**). (**b**) An atorvastatin subject with a mean negative change (decrease) in VWV between baseline (**i**) and follow-up (**ii**). (**c**) An atorvastatin subject with a large negative change (decrease) in VWV between baseline (**i**) and follow-up (**ii**). (**d**) A particular placebo subject with a large positive change (increase) in VWV between baseline (**i**) and follow-up (**ii**). (**e**) A representative placebo subject with a mean positive change (increase) in VWV between baseline (**i**) and follow-up (**ii**). (**f**) A particular placebo subject with a large negative change (decrease) in VWV between baseline (**i**) and follow-up (**ii**)

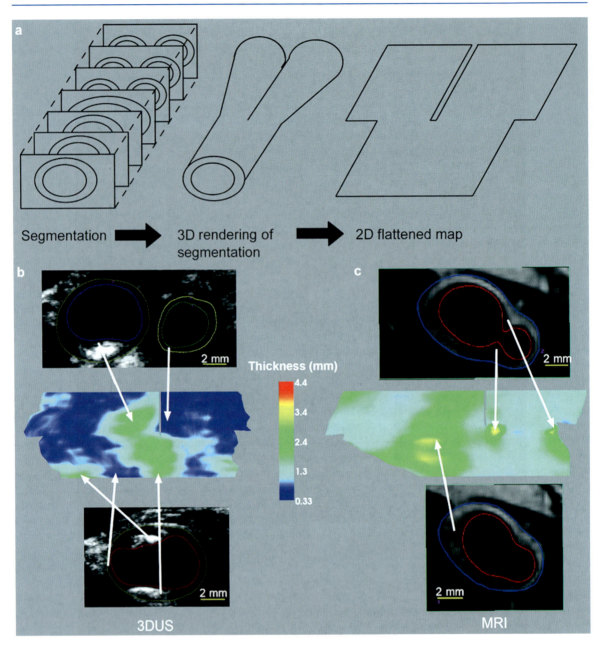

Fig. 16.5 Generation of 2D and 3D carotid thickness maps. (**a**) Schematic diagram showing the flattening process of the 3D thickness maps generated from the measurements of VWV. (**b**) Sections "sliced" from the 3D carotid images and their correspondence to the 2D flattened maps. (**c**) MRI-derived carotid image and 2D flattened map

(CCA) was segmented a maximum distance of 15 mm proximal to the bifurcation, and the internal and external carotid branches (ICA and ECA, respectively) were segmented 10 mm distal from the bifurcation. The enclosed areas were used to calculate VWV. Percent atheroma volume (PAV), a measure of atherosclerotic lesion burden previously developed for coronary intravascular ultrasound (IVUS),[46] was also derived from the manually segmented contours. PAV was calculated as the ratio of 3D VWV to the entire outer wall volume.

The results of the analysis of VWV and PAV for both treatment groups are shown in Fig. 16.4 and Table 16.1. After 3 months, subjects in the atorvastatin

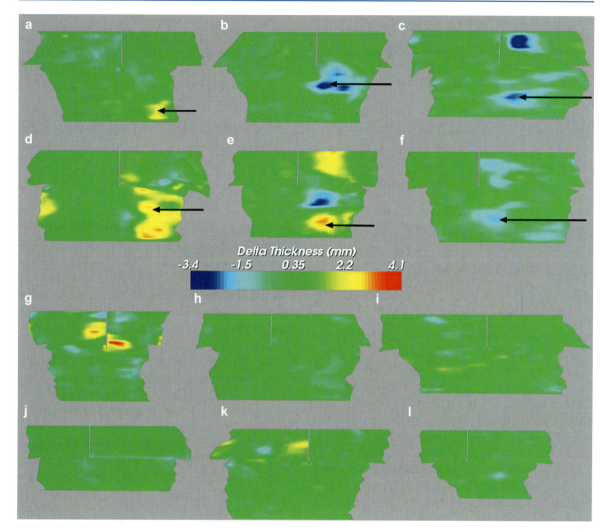

Fig. 16.6 Three-dimensional thickness difference maps. Regions of interest on maps correspond to regions of interest demonstrated in Fig. 16.5. (**a**) Carotid thickness difference map for a representative subject from the atorvastatin treatment group with largest positive change (increase) in VWV measured over a 3-month follow-up period. (**b**) Carotid thickness difference map for a representative subject from the atorvastatin treatment group with mean VWV change measured over a 3-month follow-up period. (**c**) Carotid thickness difference map for a representative subject from the atorvastatin treatment group with greatest negative change (decrease) in VWV measured over a 3-month follow-up period. (**d**) Carotid thickness difference map for a representative subject from the placebo treatment groups with the largest positive change (increase) in VWV measured over a 3-month follow-up period. (**e**) Carotid thickness difference map for a representative subject from the placebo treatment groups with mean change in VWV measured over a 3-month follow-up period. (**f**) Carotid thickness difference map for a representative subject from the placebo treatment group with greatest negative change (decrease) in VWV measured over a 3-month follow-up period. (**g–l**) Carotid thickness difference maps for six additional representative subjects from the atorvastatin (**g–i**) and placebo (**j–l**) groups

treatment group demonstrated a mean VWV change (mean ± SD) of -30 ± 110 mm^3, whereas for subjects in the placebo treatment group, a mean VWV increase of 70 ± 140 mm^3, and this difference between groups was statistically significant ($p < 0.05$). Ultrasound volumes demonstrating changes in selected subjects are seen in Fig. 16.4.

The change in PAV (mean ± SD) was $0.2 \pm 3.2\%$ for the atorvastatin treatment group and $1.9 \pm 3.8\%$ for subjects in the placebo treatment group, and this difference was not significant ($p > 0.05$) (Table 16.1). In addition, a repeated measures analysis of variance (ANOVA) demonstrated a significant interaction of time and treatment for VWV ($p < 0.05$) but not for

Table 16.1 Atherosclerosis measurements from 3D ultrasound

		Atorvastatin treatment group $n = 16$	Placebo treatment group $n = 19$	Difference between treatment groups
VWV (± SD) mm^3	Baseline	1,330 (300)	1,510 (450)	
	Follow-up	1,300 (250)	1,580 (490)	
Δ VWV (± SD) mm^3		−30 (110)	+70 (140)	$p = .03$
Δ VWV (± SD) %		−1.4 (7.7)	4.9 (10.3)	$p = .05$
PAV (± SD) %	Baseline	53.8 (8.7)	47.4 (7.5)	
	Follow-up	54.0 (8.6)	49.3 (7.7)	
Δ PAV (± SD) %		+0.2 (3.2)	+1.9 (3.8)	$p = .17$

PAV. For PAV, ANOVA also detected a significant treatment effect ($p = 0.045$).

16.3.1.3 Generation of 3D and 2D Carotid Maps

VWV segmentation has the advantage over TPV in that it allows for the generation of vessel wall and plaque thickness maps[47,48] and plaque thickness difference maps. Briefly, as shown in Fig. 16.5 and previously described,[47] for each carotid artery, a 3D carotid thickness map was generated by establishing corresponding points of the vessel wall and lumen segmentation surfaces with the resultant thickness of the vessel wall and plaque considered to be the distance between each pair of corresponding points. To map the 3D thickness map onto a 2D plane, the carotid map was bisected and flattened using arc-preserving[48] and area-preserving[49] algorithms. To generate carotid thickness difference maps,[42] carotid maps from baseline and 3-month follow-up were registered[47] and digitally subtracted.

The carotid artery thickness difference maps shown in Fig. 16.6 demonstrate localized spatial vessel wall and plaque thickness changes over 3 months for 12 representative subjects from the atorvastatin treatment (Fig. 16.6a–c, g–i) and placebo (Fig. 16.6d–f, h–i) groups.

The resultant quantification of plaque and wall thickness is represented by color maps (see color bar in Fig. 16.6), normalized for all maps according to the measured minimum and maximum thickness changes observed for all 12 subjects. Representative maps are provided for two subjects with the largest VWV increases in the atorvastatin and placebo groups (Fig.16.5a, d) as well for two subjects representing the average amount of VWV change measured (Fig. 16.5b, e) and for two subjects with the largest VWV decreases in both the atorvastatin (Fig. 16.5c) and placebo group (Fig. 16.5f). The maps show spatial changes in vessel wall and plaque thickness which, for subjects in the atorvastatin treatment group shown in Fig. 16.5a–c, can be observed as regions of decreased thickness in the common and internal carotid artery for two subjects (Fig. 16.7b, c) and a region of increased thickness in the CCA for the single subject in that treatment group that showed the corresponding greatest increase in VWV. Thickness difference maps for two representative patients in the placebo treatment group provided in Fig 16.5d and e show large increases in vessel wall thickness within the CCA and ICA. For the single subject in the placebo group that showed the greatest overall decrease in VWV, there was a corresponding small focal area of decreased vessel wall and plaque thickness in the common carotid artery.

16.3.1.4 Mapping Spatial and Temporal Changes in Carotid Atherosclerosis from 3D Images

The analysis of 3D carotid changes in carotid plaque and vessel wall has the potential to provide quantitative and dynamic measures of the volumetric and spatial changes. Thus, the authors developed a method to analyze successive carotid artery wall and lumen segmentation outlines from 3D carotid images and display these as spatial 2D maps of vessel thickness.[48,50] To demonstrate this technique, results from two studies will be shown.

(1) Three subjects with carotid plaque area greater than 0.5 cm^2 (moderate atherosclerosis subjects) were scanned twice in 2 weeks to assess the variability of the 3D measurements due to image variability, scanning parameter changes, sonographer changes, and observer variability, and (2) five subjects with carotid

Fig. 16.7 3D views of VWV measurements. The 3D image is "sliced" to obtain a transverse view (**aii** and **bii**). By using a mouse-driven cross-haired cursor, the plaque is outlined in successive image "slices" until all the plaques have been traversed. The vessel can be sliced to reveal a longitudinal view with the outlines of the plaques (**ai** and **bi**). After outlining all the plaques, the total volume can be calculated, and a mesh fitted to provides a view of the plaque surface together with the boundary of the vessel

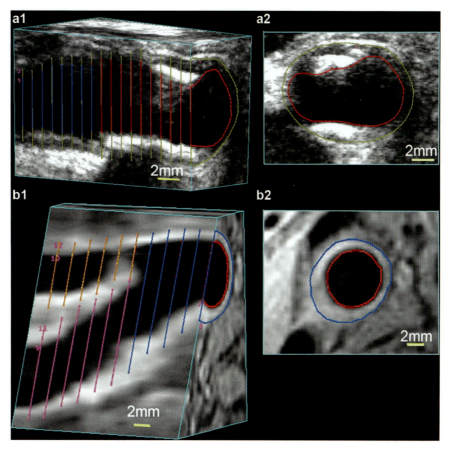

stenosis (carotid stenosis subjects) were scanned twice, once at baseline and once after 12 weeks of statin or placebo therapy, with three subjects having received 80 mg atorvastatin daily and two subjects receiving placebo treatment (discussed in section above).

The technique used to generate the 3D and 2D maps of the carotid VWV has been described in detail by Chiu et al.[48,50] and is only summarized here. Briefly, as shown in Figs. 16.5 and 16.8, mean vessel wall and lumen surfaces (shown in Fig. 16.8a) are reconstructed from the five repeated segmentations of each carotid image.[43] The 3D carotid thickness map shown in Fig. 16.8b is generated by establishing corresponding points on the vessel wall and lumen surfaces with the resultant thickness of the vessel wall and plaque calculated to be the distance between each pair of corresponding points.[50] The 3D carotid map is then "cut" (as shown in Fig. 16.8c) to generate a flattened 2D thickness map (Fig.16.8d) to map the 3D wall and plaque thickness maps shown in Fig. 16.8b onto a two-dimensional plane.[48] The flattened 2D thickness map in Fig. 16.8d shows the spatial distribution of wall and plaque thickness within the artery and provides a continuous wall and plaque surface[48,50] to facilitate the visualization and qualitative assessment of carotid artery wall and plaque thickness distribution.

In addition to generating thickness 2D maps, thickness difference 2D maps can also be generated by subtracting the 2D thickness map at baseline (scan) from the 2D thickness map obtained at a later time. The resultant thickness difference 2D map provides a continuous surface in which to examine location-specific changes in wall and plaque thickness.[48,50]

The utility of the 2D thickness change maps is shown in Figs. 16.9 and 16.10. Figure 16.9 shows "slices" of 3D carotid images of three subjects obtained at baseline and 12 weeks later. Figure 16.9a shows 3D image "slices" of a subject treated with atorvastatin at baseline and 12 weeks later, Fig. 16.9b shows 3D image "slices" of a subject

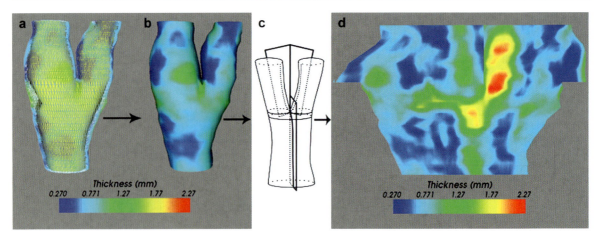

Fig. 16.8 (**a**) Five repetitions of manual image segmentation provide mean vessel wall and lumen outlines, with the distance between each pair of corresponding points on the vessel wall and lumen surfaces providing thickness of vessel wall and plaque. Once the correspondence points have been established between reconstructed vessel and lumen surfaces, a 3D image rendered thickness map is generated (**b**), with the carotid artery opened along the planes (**c**) into a flattened thickness 2D map (**d**)

treated with placebo at baseline and 12 weeks later, and Fig. 16.9c shows 3D image "slices" of a subject with moderate atherosclerosis who was scanned twice in 2 weeks.

Scan-rescan 2D thickness difference maps are shown in Fig. 16.10 for six subjects: (1) two moderate atherosclerosis subjects (Fig. 16.10a, b) scanned twice in 2 weeks, (2) three carotid atherosclerosis subjects treated with atorvastatin (Fig. 16.10d–f) and scanned at baseline and 12 weeks later, and (3) a carotid atherosclerosis subject treated with placebo (Fig. 16.10c) and scanned at baseline and 12 weeks later. These six carotid 2D thickness difference maps allow qualitative examination of plaque and wall changes in these subjects over the different scan-rescan periods. Plaque and wall thickness differences between scan and rescan are color-coded with the color scale provided for the six topology difference maps, and the color scale is normalized according to the range of thickness changes observed for statin-treated subject (shown in Fig. 16.10e with a change in VWV at rescan of 280 ± 60 mm^3 VWV in 12 weeks).

Carotid 2D thickness difference maps for a carotid stenosis subject (Fig. 16.10c) scanned after 12 weeks of treatment with placebo and for two moderate atherosclerosis subjects scanned twice within 2 weeks (Fig. 16.10a, b) indicate no change (green = 0 mm thickness difference). However, thickness difference maps for all three carotid stenosis subjects treated with atorvastatin do show plaque and wall thickness changes in the common carotid artery, with plaque and wall thickness changes ranging from −4.5 mm to +2.5 mm.

16.4 Future Perspectives

3D ultrasound has already demonstrated clear advantages in obstetrics, cardiology, and image guidance of interventional procedures. Current 3D ultrasound technology is sufficiently advanced to allow real-time 3D imaging using 2D array transducers and near real-time 3D imaging with mechanically manipulated 1D transducers. The current focus related to 3D imaging is the establishment of the utility of 3D ultrasound in clinical applications and improved image analysis techniques allowing quantitative measurements in an efficient manner. Improved software tools for image analysis are promising to make 3D ultrasound a routinely used tool.

Although the authors have shown the potential of 3D carotid imaging for monitoring carotid atherosclerosis progression and regression, this modality requires further development in order to become a routine tool for quantifying carotid disease and its changes. Chief among the required changes is the development of automated or semiautomated carotid plaque, lumen, and vessel wall segmentation. Manual

Fig. 16.9 (**a**) Carotid stenosis subject baseline scan (**i**) and 12 weeks later (**ii**) treated with atorvastatin. (**b**) Carotid stenosis subject baseline scan (**i**) and 12 weeks later (**ii**) treated with placebo. (**c**) Moderate atherosclerosis subject scan baseline scan (**i**) and 2 weeks later (**ii**).

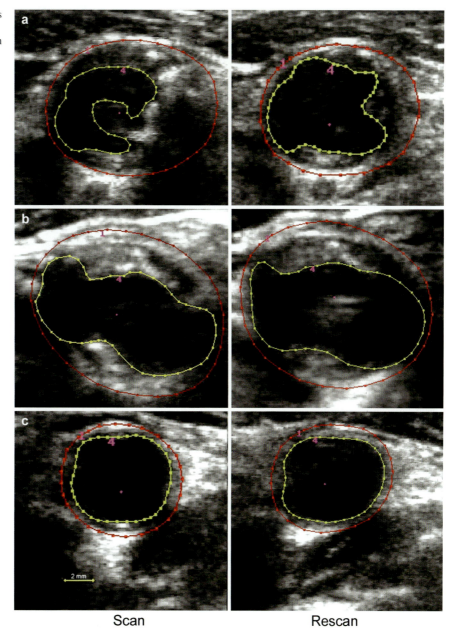

Scan   Rescan

segmentation has been demonstrated to have low intraoperator variability when used by a trained operator. However, the manual segmentation approach is slow and tedious. Thus, improved methods to segment the structures in the 3D carotid images would accelerate the use of this technology. However, before automated or semiautomated techniques are used routinely, they must be verified thoroughly. Use of manual segmentations by a trained observer can be used as the surrogate "gold" standard for analysis of accuracy, and repeated segmentations can be used for analysis of variability.

In addition to segmentation developments, analysis of changes in plaque texture may provide information on changes in plaque composition. Validation of these developments is more difficult and would require comparisons to MR plaque composition results or comparisons to histological sections of carotid vessel specimens.

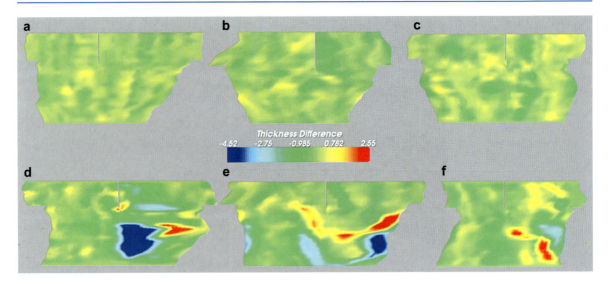

Fig. 16.10 (**a**, **b**) Moderate atherosclerosis subject difference between baseline scan and scan 2 weeks later. (**c**) Carotid stenosis subject treated with placebo – difference between baseline scan and 3-month follow-up. (**d**–**f**) Carotid stenosis subjects treated with atorvastatin, 2D difference maps between baseline scan and 3-month follow-up

Acknowledgments The authors acknowledge the financial support of the Canadian Institutes for Health Research and the Ontario Research Fund. Dr. Fenster holds a Canada Research Chair and acknowledges the support of the Canada Research Chairs Program.

References

1. Barth JD. Carotid intima media thickness and beyond. *Curr Drug Targets Cardiovasc Hematol Disord*. 2004;4(2):129–145.
2. Pretorius DH, Nelson TR, Jaffe JS. 3-dimensional sonographic analysis based on color flow Doppler and gray scale image data: a preliminary report. *J Ultrasound Med*. 1992;11(5):225–232.
3. Picot PA, Rickey DW, Mitchell R, Rankin RN, Fenster A. Three-dimensional colour Doppler imaging of the carotid artery. *SPIE Proceed Image Capture Formatting Display*. 1991;1444:206–213.
4. Guo Z, Fenster A. Three-dimensional power Doppler imaging: a phantom study to quantify vessel stenosis. *Ultrasound Med Biol*. 1996;22(8):1059–1069.
5. Dabrowski W, Dunmore-Buyze J, Cardinal HN, Fenster A. A real vessel phantom for flow imaging: 3-D Doppler ultrasound of steady flow. *Ultrasound Med Biol*. 2001;27(1):135–141.
6. Picot PA, Rickey DW, Mitchell R, Rankin RN, Fenster A. Three-dimensional colour Doppler imaging. *Ultrasound Med Biol*. 1993;19(2):95–104.
7. Barnett P, Spence J, Manuck S, Jennings S. Psychological stress and the progression of carotid artery disease. *J Hypertens*. 1997;15(1):49–55.
8. Baldassarre D, Amato M, Bondioli A, Sirtori CR, Tremoli E. Carotid artery intima-media thickness measured by ultrasonography in normal clinical practice correlates well with atherosclerosis risk factors. *Stroke*. 2000;31(10):2426–2430.
9. Baldassarre D et al. Measurement of carotid artery intima-media thickness in dyslipidemic patients increases the power of traditional risk factors to predict cardiovascular events. *Atherosclerosis*. 2007;191(2):403–408.
10. Owens GK. Control of hypertrophic versus hyperplastic growth of vascular smooth muscle cells. *Am J Physiol*. 1989;257(6 Pt 2):H1755–H1765.
11. Spence JD. Ultrasound measurement of carotid plaque as a surrogate outcome for coronary artery disease. *Am J Cardiol*. 2002;89(4A):10B–15B.
12. Stary HC et al. A definition of the intima of human arteries and of its atherosclerosis-prone regions. A report from the Committee on Vascular Lesions of the Council on Arteriosclerosis, American Heart Association. *Arterioscler Thromb*. 1992;12(1):120–134.
13. Hennerici M, Baezner H, Daffertshofer M. Ultrasound and arterial wall disease. *Cerebrovasc Dis*. 2004;17(suppl 1):19–33.
14. Stary HC et al. A definition of initial, fatty streak, and intermediate lesions of atherosclerosis. A report from the Committee on Vascular Lesions of the Council on Arteriosclerosis, American Heart Association. *Arterioscler Thromb*. 1994;14(5):840–856.
15. Spence JD, Hegele RA. Non-invasive assessment of atherosclerosis risk. *Curr Drug Targets Cardiovasc Haematol Disord*. 2004;4(2):125–128.
16. Landry A, Fenster A. Theoretical and experimental quantification of carotid plaque volume measurements made by three-dimensional ultrasound using test phantoms. *Med Phys*. 2002;29(10):2319–2327.

17. Landry A, Spence JD, Fenster A. Measurement of carotid plaque volume by 3-dimensional ultrasound. *Stroke*. 2004;35(4):864–869.
18. Landry A, Spence JD, Fenster A. Quantification of carotid plaque volume measurements using 3D ultrasound imaging. *Ultrasound Med Biol*. 2005;31(6):751–762.
19. Delcker A, Diener HC. Quantification of atherosclerotic plaques in carotid arteries by three-dimensional ultrasound. *Br J Radiol*. 1994;67(7999):672–678.
20. Delcker A, Diener HC. 3D ultrasound measurement of atherosclerotic plaque volume in carotid arteries. *Bildgebung*. 1994;61(2):116–121.
21. Delcker A, Tegeler C. Influence of ECG-triggered data acquisition on reliability for carotid plaque volume measurements with a magnetic sensor three-dimensional ultrasound system. *Ultrasound Med Biol*. 1998;24(4):601–605.
22. Palombo C et al. Ultrafast three-dimensional ultrasound: application to carotid artery imaging. *Stroke*. 1998;29(8):1631–1637.
23. Spence JD et al. Carotid plaque area: a tool for targeting and evaluating vascular preventive therapy. *Stroke*. 2002;33(12):2916–2922.
24. Johnsen SH et al. Carotid atherosclerosis is a stronger predictor of myocardial infarction in women than in men: a 6-year follow-up study of 6226 persons: the Tromso Study. *Stroke*. 2007;38(11):2873–2880.
25. Delcker A, Diener HC, Wilhelm H. Influence of vascular risk factors for atherosclerotic carotid artery plaque progression. *Stroke*. 1995;26(11):2016–2022.
26. Schminke U, Motsch L, Griewing B, Gaull M, Kessler C. Three-dimensional power-mode ultrasound for quantification of the progression of carotid artery atherosclerosis. *J Neurol*. 2000;247(2):106–111.
27. Zhao XQ et al. Effects of prolonged intensive lipid-lowering therapy on the characteristics of carotid atherosclerotic plaques in vivo by MRI: a case-control study. *Arterioscler Thromb Vasc Biol*. 2001;21(10):1623–1629.
28. Ainsworth CD et al. 3D ultrasound measurement of change in carotid plaque volume: a tool for rapid evaluation of new therapies. *Stroke*. 2005;36(9):1904–1909.
29. Zahalka A, Fenster A. An automated segmentation method for three-dimensional carotid ultrasound images. *Phys Med Biol*. 2001;46(4):1321–1342.
30. Fenster A, Downey DB, Cardinal HN. Three-dimensional ultrasound imaging. *Phys Med Biol*. 2001;46(5):R67–R99.
31. Nelson TR, Downey DB, Pretorius DH, Fenster A. *Three-Dimensional Ultrasound*. Philadelphia: Lippincott Williams & Wilkins; 1999.
32. Nelson TR, Pretorius DH. Three-dimensional ultrasound imaging. *Ultrasound Med Biol*. 1998;24(9):1243–1270.
33. Baba K, Jurkovic D. *Three-Dimensional Ultrasound in Obstetrics and Gynecology*. Pearl River: Parthenon Publishing Group; 1997.
34. Downey DB, Fenster A. Three-dimensional ultrasound: a maturing technology. *Ultrasound Q*. 1998;14(1):25–40.
35. Fenster A, Downey DB. Three-dimensional ultrasound imaging. In: Beutel J, Kundel H, Van Metter R, eds. *Handbook of Medical Imaging*, Physics and Psychophysics, vol. 1. Bellingham: SPIE Press; 2000:433–509.
36. Fenster A, Downey DB. Three-dimensional ultrasound imaging. *Annu Rev Biomed Eng*. 2000;2:457–475.
37. Fenster A, Downey DB. Basic principles and applications of 3-D ultrasound imaging. In: Stergiopoulos S, ed. *Advanced Signal Processing Handbook*. Boca Raton: CRC Press; 2001:14–34.
38. Smith W, Fenster A. Statistical analysis of decorrelation-based transducer tracking for three-dimensional ultrasound. *Med Phys*. 2003;30(7):1580–1591.
39. Downey DB, Fenster A. Vascular imaging with a three-dimensional power Doppler system. *AJR Am J Roentgenol*. 1995;165(3):665–668.
40. Fenster A, Tong S, Sherebrin S, Downey DB, Rankin RN. Three-dimensional ultrasound imaging. *Proc SPIE Phys Med Imaging*. 1995;2432:176–184.
41. Hughes SW et al. Volume estimation from multiplanar 2D ultrasound images using a remote electromagnetic position and orientation sensor. *Ultrasound Med Biol*. 1996;22(5):561–572.
42. Egger M, Chiu B, Spence JD, Fenster A, Parraga G. Mapping spatial and temporal changes in carotid atherosclerosis from three-dimensional ultrasound images. *Ultrasound Med Biol*. 2008;34(1):64–72.
43. Egger M, Spence JD, Fenster A, Parraga G. Validation of 3D ultrasound vessel wall volume: an imaging phenotype of carotid atherosclerosis. *Ultrasound Med Biol*. 2007;33(6):905–914.
44. Egger M, Krasinski A, Rutt BK, Fenster A, Parraga G. Comparison of B-mode ultrasound, 3-dimensional ultrasound, and magnetic resonance imaging measurements of carotid atherosclerosis. *J Ultrasound Med*. 2008;27(9):1321–1334.
45. Pignoli P, Tremoli E, Poli A, Oreste P, Paoletti R. Intimal plus medial thickness of the arterial wall: a direct measurement with ultrasound imaging. *Circulation*. 1986;74(6):1399–1406.
46. Nissen SE et al. Effect of recombinant ApoA-I Milano on coronary atherosclerosis in patients with acute coronary syndromes: a randomized controlled trial. *JAMA*. 2003;290(17):2292–2300.
47. Chiu B, Egger M, Spence D, Parraga G, Fenster A. Quantification of carotid vessel wall and plaque thickness change using 3D ultrasound images. *Med Phys*. 2008;35:3691–3710.
48. Chiu B, Egger M, Spence JD, Parraga G, Fenster A. Quantification of progression and regression of carotid vessel atherosclerosis using 3D ultrasound images. *Conf Proc IEEE Eng Med Biol Soc*. 2006;1:3819–3822.
49. Chiu B, Egger M, Spence DJ, Parraga G, Fenster A. Area-preserving flattening maps of 3D ultrasound carotid arteries images. *Med Image Anal*. 2008;12(6):676–688.
50. Chiu B, Egger M, Spence JD, Parraga G, Fenster A. Quantification of carotid vessel atherosclerosis. *Proc SPIE*. 2006;6143:85–94.

Carotid Plaque Surface Irregularity

Bernard Chiu, Vadim Beletsky, J. David Spence,
Grace Parraga, and Aaron Fenster

17.1 Introduction

The introduction of computer-aided analysis methods of ultrasonic images has provided new opportunities to improve the diagnosis of carotid atherosclerotic disease and to monitor treatment. Methods have been developed to assess carotid plaque heterogeneity[1,2] and echogenicity[1,3] and their improvements are continuing. The use of three-dimensional (3D) ultrasound has provided a means to quantify carotid plaque volume and has been shown to be a sensitive method to measure plaque changes[4,5] (Chap. 16). Reports have shown that the use of 3D ultrasound provides direct plaque visualization and precise measurements of plaque burden.[4-9] Thus, measurements of plaque changes using 3D ultrasound provide an aid in evaluating the effect of treatment options for patients with atherosclerosis.[10,11] While the risk of stroke has been shown to increase with the severity of carotid stenosis,[12] it is generally accepted that the risk of major vascular events is related more to plaque stability than carotid stenosis.[13-16] An ulcer or fissure in the plaque exposes the blood to thrombogenic material, resulting in possible life- or brain-threatening thrombosis and embolization.[14,17-19]

X-ray angiography has been used to detect plaque fissures and ulcers and classify them subjectively (e.g., ulcerated/irregular, no ulceration/smooth and uncertain).[13,16,17] Ultrasound imaging has also been used to detect plaque ulceration based on a measurement of depth (e.g., 2 mm[10,19]), and with a well-defined wall at the base exhibiting a region of reverse flow using Doppler ultrasound. The use of intravascular ultrasound with its higher resolution has allowed[20] the detection of smaller plaque ulcers with a depth of 0.5 mm.

3D ultrasound can also provide a means to visualize the plaque surface and detect variation in the plaque's surface morphology using various image processing and visualization techniques. However, these methods are prone to variability as setting image processing and visualization parameters are user dependent. A better method would involve quantification of the plaque surface and scoring any fissures in the surface. Typically, this would require that carotid arterial wall and lumen be segmented as a step in the quantification plaque surface.[8,9] However, manual segmentation of 3D ultrasonic images is difficult and prone to observer variability due to speckle, shadowing, and noise, which limits the broad application of these methods and measurements.

The authors have reported on the development of methods to obtain 3D ultrasonic images of the carotid arteries and image processing methods used to quantify plaque volume and thickness changes on a point-by-point basis.[21-23] These methods are particularly

B. Chiu • A. Fenster (✉)
Imaging Research Laboratories, Robarts Research Institute,
The University of Western Ontario, London, ON, Canada

V. Beletsky
Department of Clinical Neurosciences, LHSC, University of Western Ontario, London, ON, Canada

J.D. Spence
Stroke Prevention & Atherosclerosis Research Centre, Robarts Research Institute, University of Western Ontario, London, ON, Canada

G. Parraga
Imaging Research Laboratories, Robarts Research Institute,
The University of Western Ontario, London, ON, Canada

useful in monitoring plaque changes in response to therapy. This aspect is the subject of Chap. 16 in this book. The goal of this chapter is to describe the authors' methods to identify carotid plaque fissures and quantify their size using 3D images. While in this report, vessel lumen manually segmented surfaces are used, these methods would be equally applicable to segmented surfaces generated using semiautomated or automated algorithms.

17.2 Methods

17.2.1 Background on Surface Curvature Estimation

Mean and Gaussian curvatures are two local geometric descriptors of surface "roughness" in classical differential geometry. However, these two local geometric quantities are defined only for twice differentiable surfaces in differential geometric theories. Consensus is lacking on the best method for estimating surface curvatures for piecewise linear surfaces, such as triangular meshes, although the triangular mesh representation of surfaces is extensively used in the computer graphics community.[24]

Surface curvature estimation methods can be classified into two major categories. The first is based on local surface fitting (e.g., paraboloid fitting in[25]) and the second type estimates the curvatures directly from the triangular mesh.[24,26,27] However, the first class of methods often introduce overshooting and unexpected behavior between sampling points.[24] With this in mind and with the development of a method for reconstructing a triangular mesh for a stack of segmented lumen contours in the authors' previous work,[22,28] the algorithm described by Meyer et al.[24] was used to compute curvatures directly from a triangular mesh. Meyer et al.[24] designed the partition of the surface in such a way so that they could establish a tight error bound for curvature estimation. In addition, the surface partitioning scheme is nonoverlapping, which is essential for the satisfaction of Gauss–Bonnet theorem, and which was not considered by previous work.[26,27]

In this work, the authors combine mean and Gaussian curvatures in quantifying luminal surface irregularity. One main reason is that Gaussian curvature, as an intrinsic property, cannot be used to differentiate between regions curving inwards and those curving outwards, while mean curvature, as an extrinsic property, can be used for this purpose. Ulcers, as craters on the lumen surface, are characterized by regions where the luminal surface curves inwards (Fig. 17.1). Thus, there is a need to differentiate between potential regions of ulceration and outward curving regions. In the following section, the mean and Gaussian curvatures computation procedure is briefly described.

17.2.2 Computation of Surface Curvatures

17.2.2.1 Discrete Mean Curvature

The mean curvature κ_H at a point P is related to the mean curvature normal operator $\mathbf{K}$ by the equation $\mathbf{K}(P) = 2\kappa_H(P)\mathbf{n}(P)$, where $\mathbf{n}(P)$ is the normal vector of the surface. Meyer et al.[24] expressed the integral of $\mathbf{K}$ over a cell with vertex i at the center and with boundary intersecting midpoints of the edges connecting vertex i and $j \in N_1(i)$ (i.e., the gray region in Fig. 17.2a) as:

$$\iint_A \mathbf{K}(x)dA = \frac{1}{2} \sum_{j \in N_1(i)} (\cot \alpha_{ij} + \cot \beta_{ij})(\mathbf{x}_i - \mathbf{x}_j) \tag{17.1}$$

where α_{ij} and β_{ij} are the two angles opposite to the edge in the two triangles sharing the edge $(\mathbf{x}_i, \mathbf{x}_j)$, and $N_1(i)$ is the set of 1-ring neighbor vertices of vertex i.

Although Eq. 17.1 holds true for any surface partitioning as long as the edge of the cell centered at vertex i intersects the midpoints of the set of edges $\{(\mathbf{x}_i, \mathbf{x}_j) : j \in N_1(i)\}$, a surface partitioning scheme must be chosen to provide an accurate estimation of the curvature. The use of Voronoi regions minimizes the error of the curvature estimation as shown in Meyer et al.[24] Given a nonobtuse triangle, the area of the Voronoi region for P is (see Fig. 17.2b):

$$A_{\text{Voronoi}} = \frac{1}{8}|PR|^2 \cot(\angle Q) + \frac{1}{8}|PQ|^2 \cot(\angle R) \tag{17.2}$$

The Voronoi partitioning scheme, however, could not be used for triangles with an obtuse angle (Fig. 17.2c) because the circumcenter of the obtuse triangle does not lie inside the triangle. However, as long as we use a region whose edges pass through the

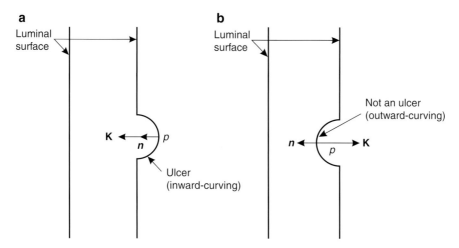

Fig. 17.1 Two shapes that have the same Gaussian curvatures, but different mean curvatures. This figure shows that (**a**) inward-curving and (**b**) outward-curving regions can have the same Gaussian curvature (κ_G). However, the outward-curving region shown in (**b**) is not an ulcer, whereas (**a**) shows an ulcer. The mean curvature normal vector $\mathbf{K}(p)$ points inward from the surface. Thus, $\kappa_H(p)$ is positive according to Eq. 17.7. In (**b**), $\mathbf{K}(p)$ points outward from the surface, and $\kappa_H(p)$ is negative. Ulcers are associated with high Gaussian and (positive) mean curvatures (Reproduced with permission from Chiu et al.[41])

midpoint of the edges of the triangles, Eq. 17.1 is still valid. To allow nonoverlapping surface partitioning, Meyer et al.[24] used a third vertex that is the midpoint of the edge opposite to the obtuse angle to define the partition. This partition is represented by the gray region in Fig. 17.2c. A new surface area for each vertex **x** can now be defined, denoted by $A_\text{mixed}(\mathbf{x})$, which is computed by the following algorithm (Fig. 17.2d):

$$A_\text{mixed}(\mathbf{x}) = \sum_{i=1}^{\#f} FA(T_i) \qquad (17.3)$$

where

$$FA(T_i) = \begin{cases} A_\text{Voronoi}, & T_i \text{ is nonobtuse.} \\ \text{Area}(T_i)/2, & T_i \text{ is obtuse and the angle of } T_i \text{ at } \mathbf{x} \text{ is } \textit{obtuse}. \\ \text{Area}(T_i)/4, & T_i \text{ is obtuse and the angle of } T_i \text{ at } \mathbf{x} \text{ is } \textit{nonobtuse}. \end{cases}$$

and $\#f$ denotes the number of triangular faces around the vertex **x**, and T_i denotes the triangle corresponding to the ith face (see Fig. 17.2a).

With A_mixed defined, the mean curvature normal operator **K** can be expressed as:

$$K(\mathbf{x}_i) = \frac{1}{2A_\text{mixed}(\mathbf{x}_i)} \sum_{j \in N_1(i)} (\cot \alpha_{ij} + \cot \beta_{ij}) \times (\mathbf{x}_i - \mathbf{x}_j) \qquad (17.4)$$

Defining **n** to be the normal vector pointing inward from the surface, the mean curvature is expressed as:

$$\kappa_H(\mathbf{x}_i) = \frac{1}{2} \mathbf{K}(\mathbf{x}_i) \cdot \mathbf{n}(\mathbf{x}_i) \qquad (17.5)$$

This equation implies that $\kappa_H > 0$ if **K** points inward from the surface. Otherwise, $\kappa_H < 0$.

17.2.2.2 Discrete Gaussian Curvature

The Gaussian curvature was computed similarly as the mean curvature. First, it is noted that from the Gauss–Bonnet theorem that the integral of the Gaussian curvature, κ_G, is:

$$\iint_A \kappa_G \, dA = 2\pi - \sum_{j=1}^{\#f} \theta_j \qquad (17.6)$$

where θ_j is the angle of the jth face around vertex $\mathbf{x}_i$ (see Fig. 17.2a), and $\#f$ denotes the number of faces around the vertex.

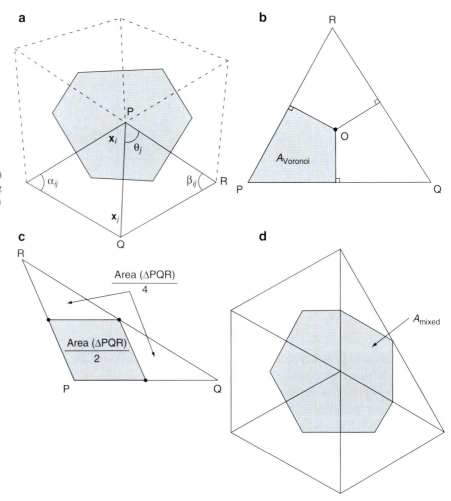

Fig. 17.2 Illustrations of the surface partitioning schemes for obtuse and nonobtuse triangles. (**a**) Voronoi region (*shaded*) in a 1-ring neighborhood that does not contain a nonobtuse triangle. (**b**) Voronoi region (*shaded*) of point P on a nonobtuse triangle. (**c**) Partitioning region (*shaded*) of point P on an obtuse triangle. (**d**) The shaded area (with area A_{mixed}) is used for surface partitioning in a 1-ring neighborhood with at least one obtuse triangle (Reproduced with permission from Chiu et al.[41])

The same partitioning scheme is used here as that used in the computation of the mean curvature normal operator, giving the following expression for the Gaussian curvature:

$$\kappa_G(\mathbf{x}_i) = (2\pi - \sum_{j=1}^{\#f} \theta_j)/A_{\text{mixed}}(\mathbf{x}_i) \qquad (17.7)$$

17.2.2.3 Smoothing of Curvatures

Since semiautomatic or manual segmentation of carotid images is prone to observer variability due to speckle, shadowing, and noise,[29,30] the authors smooth the curvature (either Gaussian or mean curvature) at each vertex using an iterative algorithm proposed in Sundaram et al.[31] to successively average the curvature at a vertex with those of its adjacent neighbors.

The smoothing algorithm is briefly summarized as follows:

1. Initialize $S_{i,0} = S_i$ and $\sigma_0 = 0.5$ mm.
2. At iteration $l + 1$, set

$$\sigma_{l+1} = 1.1\sigma_l$$

$$S_{i,l+1} = \frac{1}{2}\left(S_{i,l} + \frac{\sum_{j \in N_1(i)} w_{ij,l} S_{j,l}}{\sum_{j \in N_1(i)} w_{ij,l}}\right)$$

3. Terminate when $\sigma_l > 1$ mm
   where the following notations are used:
   $S_{i,l}$ = curvature at vertex p_i obtained at the lth iteration
   N_i = normal at vertex p_i
   $N_1(i)$ = 1-ring neighbourhood of vertex p_i
   $A_i = A_{\text{mixed}}(p_i)$.

The termination condition $\sigma_l > 1$ mm was selected because the segmentation interslice distance is 1 mm. $w_{ij,l}$, the weight of vertex p_j in the calculation of the smoothed curvature at p_i at iteration l, was obtained by the following equation:

$$w_{ij,l} = A_j(N_i \cdot N_j) \frac{\exp\left(-\frac{\|p_i - p_j\|^2}{2\sigma_l^2}\right)}{\sigma_l^2} \quad (17.8)$$

17.2.3 Area-Preserving Flattened Map

The surface curvature computed using the above method (Eq. 17.8) was superimposed on the arterial lumen to produce 3D surface curvature maps. Although 3D surface curvature maps thus constructed provide rich information on surface irregularity, the flattened representation of the 3D maps allows analysis in a single view, eliminating the need to study the 3D maps from multiple angles in an investigation, thereby allowing easy comparison between two maps obtained either in a longitudinal study for a single patient or in a cross-sectional study for different patients under different treatment arms. Thus, the area-preserving surface-flattening algorithm the authors developed in a previous publication[23] was used in displaying the surface curvature maps for the phantom and the study subjects.

17.3 Experimental Methods

17.3.1 Synthetic Surfaces

The authors validated the accuracy of the mean and Gaussian computation algorithm by using two types of synthetic surfaces: the sphere and the torus. The relationship between the number of sampling points used to represent these discrete surfaces and the numerical accuracy of the computed curvatures was also investigated. No noise was introduced in constructing these surfaces, and thus, the smoothing algorithm described above (Eq. 17.8) was not applied.

κ_G of a sphere equals $1/r^2$ everywhere, where r is the radius of the sphere, and κ_H equals $1/r$ everywhere (according to the orientation defined in Eq. 17.3). The authors use the following parameterization to construct the spheres:

$$(x, y, z) = (r \cos v \cos u, \ r \cos v \sin u, r \sin v), \quad (17.9)$$

where
$0 \leq u < 2\pi$ and $0 \leq v < \pi$. The authors generated meshes of the unit sphere (i.e., $r = 1$) by sampling u and v in 5°, 10° and 20° intervals, and then computed κ_H and κ_G for each point on the meshes using the discrete curvature operators.

The authors also generated synthetic tori using the following parameters to test the algorithm:

$$(x, y, z) = ((a + r \cos u) \cos v, (a + r \cos u) \\ \times \sin v, r \sin u). \quad (17.10)$$

The theoretical κ_H and κ_G are expressed as follows:

$$\kappa_H = \frac{a + 2r \cos u}{2r(a + r \cos u)}$$
$$\kappa_G = \frac{\cos u}{r(a + r \cos u)} \quad (17.11)$$

The authors generated three toroidal meshes (with $a = 1$, $r = 0.25$) by sampling u and v in 5°, 10° and 20° intervals, respectively, and then computed κ_H and κ_G for each point on the meshes.

17.3.2 Vascular Phantom

To test the curvature computation algorithm, a vascular mimicking phantom was constructed using a heated 85°C agar mixture consisting of the following (by % mass): 3% agar (A-7002, Sigma-Aldrich, Oakville, ON, Canada), 8% glycerol, 86% distilled water, and 3% Sigmacell® (S-5504, Sigma-Aldrich). Sigmacell® is a product consisting of 50-μm cellulose particles added as scatterers.[32] Hemispheres made of acetal with diameters 2 mm, 3 mm, and 4 mm (McMaster-Carr, Aurora, OH) were glued on a brass cylinder with 10 mm diameter. The distance between the centers of the 2 mm and 3 mm hemispheres was 11 mm, and the distance between the centers of the 3 mm and 4 mm hemispheres was 14 mm (Fig. 17.3a). The brass cylinder was composed of two longitudinal

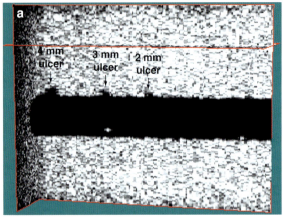
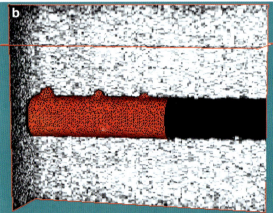
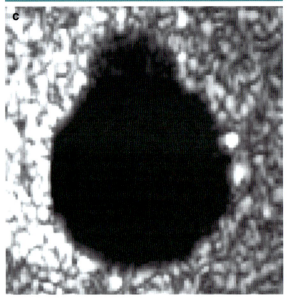

Fig. 17.3 3D ultrasound image of the phantom. (a) The longitudinal view of the phantom with the 2 mm, 3 mm, and 4 mm ulcers labeled. (b) The same longitudinal view with the segmented luminal surface superimposed on the image. (c) The transverse view of the 4-mm ulcer (Reproduced with permission from Chiu et al.[41])

halves, which were inserted into a box to create a vascular channel that was 15 mm below the surface of the phantom. The agar mixture was then poured into the vascular phantom box and allowed to cool for 30–40 min until the agar mixture solidified. Then, the brass cylinder was removed. To avoid damaging the phantom, the bottom half of the cylinder without any spheres was removed first. Then, the top half was detached from the phantom, before it was slid out.

17.3.3 3D Ultrasound Image Acquisition for Vascular Phantom

The 3D carotid imaging system was based on a mechanical linear scanning mechanism[33] as described in Chap. 16. The images of the phantom were acquired by translating an ultrasound transducer (L7-4, ATL-Philips, Bothell, Washington, USA) over the surface of the phantom along the longitudinal axis of the vessel, with the three synthetic ulcers facing the transducer. The probe was held by a mechanical assembly, and the transducer angle was fixed to be perpendicular to the phantom surface and the longitudinal axis of the vessel. Video frames from the ultrasonic equipment (HDI-5000, ATL-Philips, Bothell, Washington, USA) were digitized at 30 Hz, saved to a computer workstation, and reconstructed into a 3D image.[4,6,7,33] The acquired 2D images were parallel to each other with a pixel size of 0.13 mm × 0.13 mm. The mean spatial interval between adjacent 2D images was 0.3 mm.

17.3.4 Study Subjects

The authors used the 3D images acquired for two subjects to demonstrate the application of their algorithm. These subjects, who participated in a clinical study focusing on the effect of atorvastatin, were asymptomatic with carotid stenosis greater than 60% according to carotid Doppler flow velocities.[11] All the subjects provided written informed consent to the study protocol, which was approved by the University of Western Ontario's standing board of human research ethics. The 3D images were acquired by translating the ultrasound transducer (L12-5, ATL-Philips, Bothell, Washington, USA) along the neck of the subjects for approximately 4.0 cm, which takes approximately 8 s.

17.3.5 Carotid Segmentation and Surface Reconstruction

The vascular phantom was segmented using the semi-automatic segmentation algorithm as described by Landak et al.[34] and based on the discrete dynamic contour (DDC) model proposed by Lobregt and Viergever.[35] A transverse 2D image at approximately 8 mm away from the center of the 2 mm-hemisphere (i.e., 19 mm and 33 mm from the center of 3 mm- and 4 mm-hemisphere, respectively) was chosen as the initial 2D image, and a single observer initialized four points, from which the boundary of the phantom was determined using a cubic-spline interpolation technique.[34] The estimated boundary on the initial 2D image was then automatically deformed using the DDC model. The deformed contour was then propagated to the adjacent 2D transverse image, 1 mm away from the initial 2D image, and used as the initial contour before refining. This process was repeated until the complete vascular phantom was segmented.

From the 3D images acquired for two subjects, ulcers on the common carotid artery (CCA) lumen were identified by a physician who was experienced in analyzing carotid images. Using the knowledge of the location of the ulcers as identified by the physician, a separate observer segmented the CCA lumen using the method described in the previous paragraph, for 10 mm with 1 mm interslice distance.

Each set of 2D contours was then reconstructed into a triangulated surface mesh using a previously described method.[22,28] The reconstructed surface of the phantom is represented as a red surface superimposed on the 3D ultrasonic image of the phantom in Fig. 17.3b and the luminal surfaces for the two subjects are shown in Figs. 17.4b and 17.5b.

17.4 Results

17.4.1 Synthetic Surfaces

Table 17.1 shows the root-mean-square error (RMSE) and in the calculations of κ_H and κ_G, and the means of κ_H and κ_G. In agreement with Meyer et al.,[24] the authors observed that the computed κ_G satisfies the Gauss–Bonnet theorem regardless of the sampling interval used (i.e., the integral of κ_G over an entire sphere is equal to 4π). For example, the spherical mesh produced by sampling u and v in 20° intervals has a surface area that is 3% smaller than the continuous sphere. As a result, κ_G was overestimated by an average of 3% so that κ_G integrates to 4π over the entire discrete sphere. Similar observation applies for the spheres with sampling intervals 5° and 10°. As the spherical mesh becomes denser, the total surface area of the discrete sphere converges to the continuous sphere, resulting in a more accurate estimation of κ_G. Table 17.1 shows that both the RMSEs of κ_H and κ_G decrease as the sampling intervals decrease.

Table 17.2 shows the RMSE in the calculations of κ_H and κ_G for three tori sampled with different angular intervals. The Gauss–Bonnet theorem was also satisfied in these three tori (i.e., the integral of κ_G over whole torus is 0 as torus has 1 hole). The RMSEs of κ_H and κ_G converge to 0 as sampling intervals decrease.

17.4.2 Vascular Phantom

The surface representing the vascular phantom is shown in Fig. 17.6a with the mean curvature color-coded and superimposed on the surface. The area-preserving flattened map of the vascular phantom surface was displayed in Fig. 17.6b. The mean curvature values at all vertices were collected, and the 98th percentile of this sample was obtained. The authors used the clipping algorithm implemented in visualization toolkit (VTK)[36] to extract regions with mean curvature greater than the 98th percentile. Figure 17.6c shows the surface patches that have mean curvature greater than or equal to the 98th percentile with the boundary of a flattened map represented by the black outline. Figure 17.6c shows that the ulcers could not be detected as connected regions, and that small patches outside the ulcers were extracted erroneously.

The mean curvature was then smoothed, which is shown in Fig. 17.6d. It is important to note that the same surface is shown in Fig. 17.6a, d, only with different mean curvature values mapped onto them (i.e., the surface was not smoothed, only the curvature values were smoothed). The area-preserving flattened map of Fig. 17.6d is displayed in Fig. 17.6e. The authors computed the 98th percentile of the smoothed mean curvature and used it as the threshold to clip the surface, producing the result shown in Fig. 17.6f.

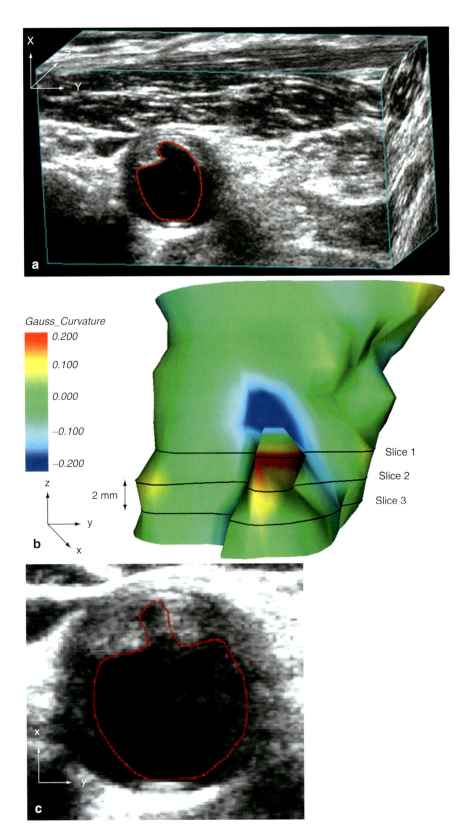

Fig. 17.4 Curvature maps for the arterial lumen of subject 1. (a) 3D image with segmented lumen. (b) 3D κ_G map for the arterial lumen of subject 1. The transverse views of (c) Slice 1, (d) Slice 2, and (e) Slice 3 as labeled in (b). (f) 2D Gaussian curvature map. κ_G of the shaded region is equal to or greater than the 98th percentile (i.e., G_{98}.) (g) 2D mean curvature map. κ_H of the shaded area is equal to or greater than the 98th percentile (i.e., M_{98}.) (f) $G_{98} \bigcap M_{98}$. (h) Result of thresholding applied to image in(f). (Reproduced with permission from Chiu et al.[41])

17 Carotid Plaque Surface Irregularity

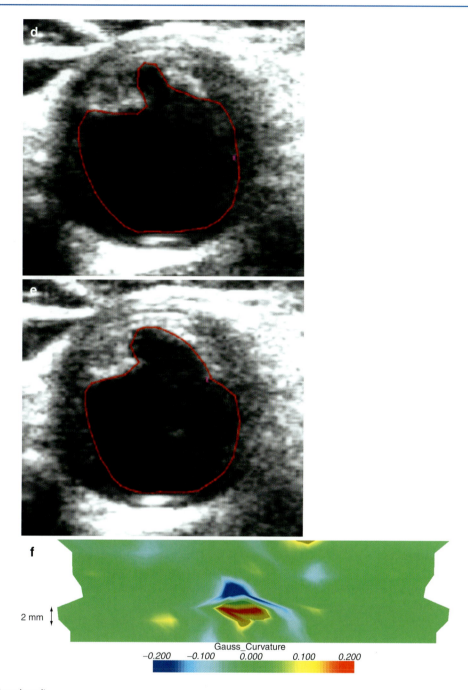

Fig. 17.4 (continued)

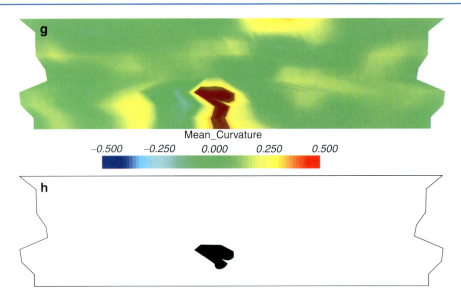

Fig 17.4 (continued)

After smoothing, only regions where ulcers were located were extracted, and the sizes of the three surface patches extracted corresponded approximately to the sizes of the ulcers.

Figure 17.7 shows the results of the experiment performed for the Gaussian curvature. The experiment performed here was the same as that described previously for the mean curvature. The results show that the regions extracted from the smoothed Gaussian curvature map identified the ulcers more accurately than that extracted from the nonsmoothed curvature map.

17.4.3 Study Subjects

Results using the phantom showed that ulcers are characterized by high Gaussian and mean curvatures. In the phantom experiment, ulcers were identified using Gaussian and mean curvatures independently and both curvatures did well in identifying ulcers. However, it was not possible to differentiate between inward- and outward-curving regions using Gaussian curvature alone. The authors had no problem in identifying ulcers in the phantom using Gaussian curvature alone because all ulcers in the phantom experiment were inward curving. However, for accurate identification of ulcers from carotid luminal surfaces of human subjects, the authors needed to combine the use of Gaussian and mean curvatures. The combined information of Gaussian and mean curvatures allowed the authors to exclude the outward-curving regions in the identification of ulcers.

Figure 17.4a shows the 3D carotid image of subject 1 with segmented lumen. Figure 17.4b shows the CCA lumen surface of subject 1, with the smoothed Gaussian curvature color-coded and superimposed on the surface. Figure 17.4c–e shows the transverse 2D images that correspond to slices 1, 2, and 3 labeled in Fig. 17.4b. Figure 17.4f shows the area-preserving flattened map with Gaussian curvature color-coded and superimposed on the map. The shaded area in this map represents regions where Gaussian curvature was greater than or equal to the 98th percentile, which was denoted by G_{98}. Figure 17.4g shows the area-preserving flattened map with mean curvature color-coded and superimposed on the map. Similarly, the shaded area in this map represents regions where mean curvature was greater than or equal to the 98th percentile, denoted by M_{98}. As a criterion, the authors identify ulcers as the intersection between G_{98} and M_{98}. Figure 17.4h shows the region identified by this method.

Figure 17.5a shows the 3D carotid image of subject 2 with segmented lumen. Figure 17.5b shows the CCA lumen surface of subject 2, with the smoothed Gaussian curvature color-coded and superimposed on the surface. Figure 17.5c, d shows transverse 2D images that correspond to slices 1 and 2 labeled in Fig. 17.5b. Unlike subject 1, there were multiple smaller ulcers in the artery of this subject. Figure 17.5e shows the area-preserving flattened map with Gaussian curvature color-coded and superimposed on the map. The shaded area represents the region G_{98}. It is noted from this figure that G_{98} covered regions with two of

Fig. 17.5 Curvature maps for the arterial lumen of subject 2. (**a**) 3D US image with segmented lumen. (**b**) 3D κ_G map for the arterial lumen of subject 2. The transverse views of (**c**) Slice 1 and (**d**) Slice 2 as labeled in (**b**). (**e**) 2D Gaussian curvature map. κ_G of the shaded area is equal to or greater than the 98th percentile (i.e., G_{98}.) (**f**) 2D mean curvature map. κ_H of the shaded area is equal to or greater than the 98th percentile (i.e., M_{98}.) (**g**) $G_{98} \cap M_{98}$ (Reproduced with permission from Chiu et al.[41])

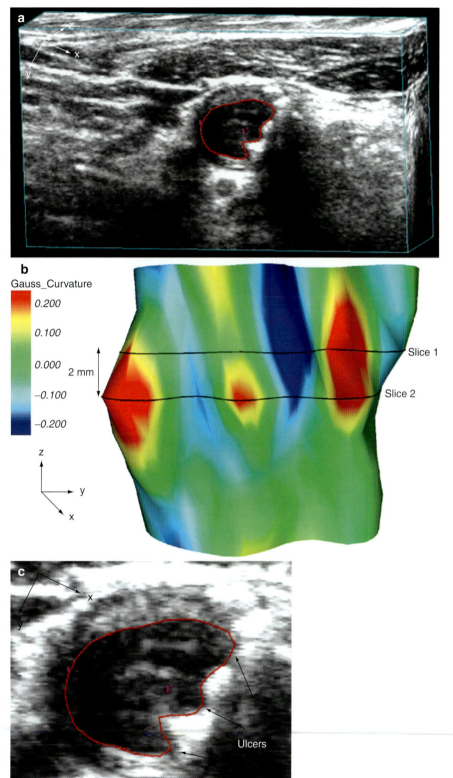

Fig. 17.5 (continued)

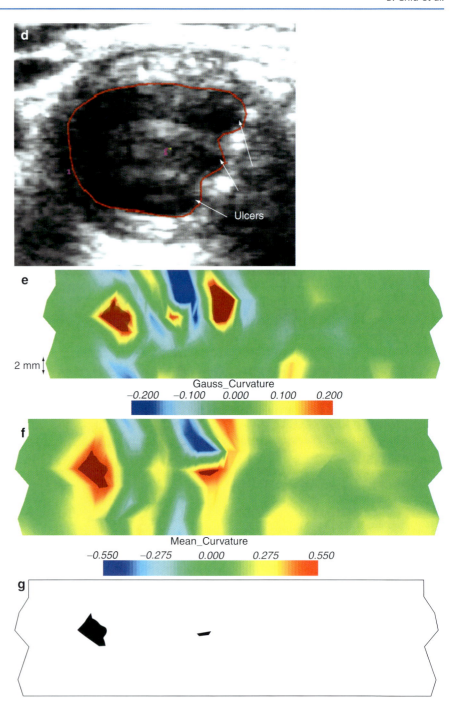

the three ulcers, but did not cover the ulcer between the two identified ulcers. In addition, the ulcer on the right of Fig. 17.5e should be much smaller than the detected region in G_{98} because the upper part of the detected region curves outward, and therefore, is not a part of the ulcer. The lower part of the detected region, however, corresponds to an ulcer shown in Fig. 17.5d.

Figure 17.5f shows the area-preserving flattened map with the mean curvature color-coded and superimposed on the map. The shaded area represents the region M_{98}. The region mentioned above, that curves outward had a negative mean curvature, and thus, was not covered by M_{98}. Figure 17.5g shows the region $G_{98} \bigcap M_{98}$, which covered two of the three ulcers.

Table 17.1 Numerical accuracy in computing mean (κ_H) and Gaussian curvature (κ_G) for three spherical meshes with different sampling intervals. For each mesh, the mean and the root-mean-square error (RMSE) of κ_H and κ_G were tabulated. Since a (continuous) sphere with unity radius has κ_H and κ_G both equalling to 1, the means of κ_H and κ_G provide a measure of the bias in the computation (Reproduced with permission from Chiu et al.[41])

Sphere, radius = 1					
Angle interval	No. of points	Mean κ_H	RMSE κ_H	Mean κ_G	RMSE κ_G
5°	2,450	1.0002	5.04×10^{-4}	1.0017	1.76×10^{-3}
10°	578	1.0007	1.89×10^{-3}	1.0070	7.01×10^{-3}
20°	128	1.0022	6.58×10^{-3}	1.0304	3.04×10^{-2}

Table 17.2 Numerical error in computing mean (κ_H) and Gaussian curvature (κ_G) for three toroidal meshes, constructed by sampling a torus with $a = 1$ and $r = 0.25$ according to Eq. 17.11. For each mesh, the root-mean-square error (RMSE) of κ_H and κ_G were tabulated (Reproduced with permission from Chiu et al.[41])

Torus, $a = 1, r = 0.25$			
Angle interval	No. of points	RMSE κ_H	RMSE κ_G
5°	5,184	0.00409	0.00727
10°	1,440	0.00862	0.0181
20°	480	0.0233	0.0517

17.5 Discussion and Conclusion

The authors have introduced an algorithm to quantify and display the irregularity of vessel wall and plaque surfaces in this chapter. First, the authors implemented the method proposed by Meyer et al.[24] for Gaussian and mean curvature computation. Since ultrasonic images are susceptible to artifacts caused by speckle, shadowing, and noise,[29,30] the authors applied a smoothing algorithm[31] to smooth the discrete curvatures computed for surfaces segmented from 3D images. The numerical accuracy of the curvature computation algorithm was validated by applying the algorithm on discrete spherical and toroidal meshes sampled at different intervals. The practicality of the method in identifying ulcers from 3D ultrasonic images was demonstrated by the application of the algorithm using 3D images of a vascular phantom and two in vivo cases.

In the authors' phantom study, the ulcers were oriented in a direction that was facing the transducer. It is known that sections of boundary perpendicular to the direction of the ultrasonic beam produce higher contrast, and sections of boundary parallel to the beam direction give lower contrast.[37] Therefore, the segmentation of the ulcers may be less accurate if the boundaries of the ulcers are parallel, instead of perpendicular, to the direction of propagation of ultrasound. The same may be true for the in vivo 3D images, causing the ulcers with boundaries parallel to the direction of ultrasound (US) transmission more difficult to be detected. Compound ultrasonic imaging is a potential solution to this problem[37,38] in which multiple ultrasonic images of the vessel are obtained from different directions, then averaged and registered to produce the final image.

To enhance the visualization and facilitate the interpretation of the 3D surface curvature maps (i.e., the luminal surface with curvatures color-coded and mapped onto it), the 3D maps were flattened to 2D using the area-preserving flattening map algorithm introduced in a previous publication.[23] 2D maps allow the study of surface curvature maps in a single view, thereby allowing easy comparison between multiple maps. For example, the improvement in ulcer identification in the phantom experiment after the introduction of curvature smoothing was clearly demonstrated by comparing the difference between Fig. 17.6c, f (or Fig. 17.7c, f).

The authors combined Gaussian and mean curvatures in detecting ulcers from luminal surfaces segmented from in vivo 3D ultrasonic images. Only regions with high Gaussian and mean curvatures were identified as ulcers. These two criteria precluded the false detection of outward-curving regions as ulcers, since outward-curving regions would have a negative mean curvature.

In demonstrating the application of the proposed algorithm for the carotid luminal surfaces of human subjects, the authors considered a physician's identification of the ulcers as the surrogate gold standard, and have segmented the arterial lumen according to this identification. As a result, the ulcer identification and the subsequent segmentation are subjective, and therefore, susceptible to observer bias and

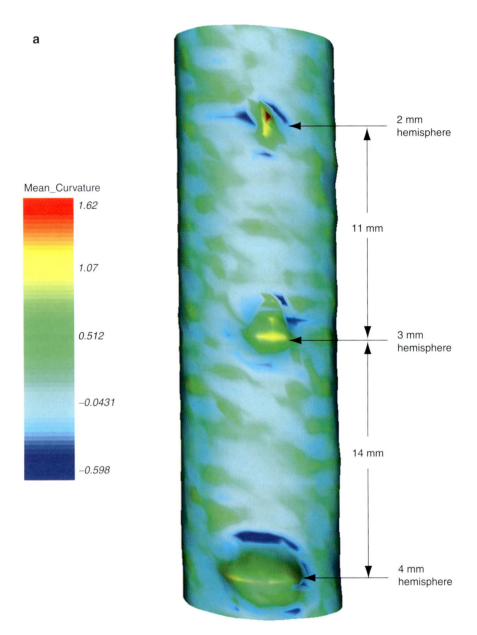

Fig. 17.6 (a) Mean curvature map of the vascular phantom and (b) its flattened map. The 98th percentile of the mean curvature at all vertices was used as a threshold to extract surface patches. (c) Shows surface patches that have mean curvature greater than or equal to this threshold. (d) Smoothed mean curvature of the phantom and (e) its flattened map. (f) Surface patches that have mean curvature greater than or equal to the 98th percentile (Reproduced with permission from Chiu et al.[41])

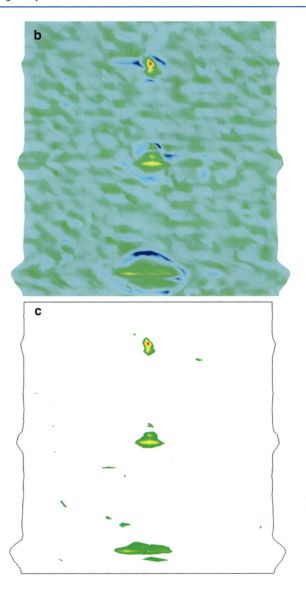

Fig. 17.6 (continued)

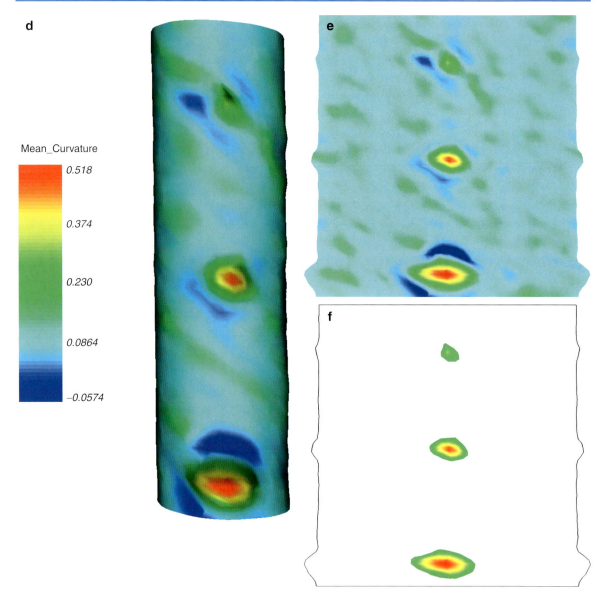

Fig. 17.6 (continued)

variability. Future studies should be performed to quantify the intra and interobserver variability in luminal segmentation. The accuracy of the segmented luminal boundaries should also be validated against corresponding histological specimens before the proposed ulcer detection algorithm is used clinically. After an ulcer has been detected using the algorithm, the location of the detected ulcer should also be verified against histological observations in future studies.

The motivation for this work stems from increasing evidence suggesting that the risk of vascular events is related to atherosclerotic plaque stability.[39,40] Plaque features related to plaque stability, such as lesion surface irregularities, ulcerations, and fissures have been shown to correlate with the risk of stroke.[13,14,16,17] An automated method described here may be used to provide a rapid and feasible method of screening a large number of images for the presence of surface irregularities. Carotid 3D ultrasonic images with irregular surface features can then be flagged for observer analysis and validation. The proposed automatic algorithm can be used in large cross-sectional studies to evaluate the correlation between the risk of vascular events and the condition of the plaque surface, and in longitudinal studies to evaluate whether there is any correlation between the change in plaque surface irregularity and symptoms of internal carotid artery occlusive diseases (e.g., transient ischemic attacks and strokes).

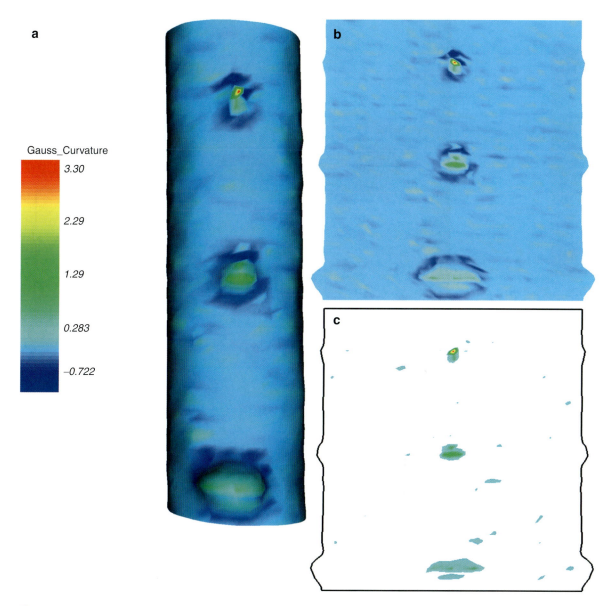

Fig. 17.7 (a) Gaussian curvature map of the vascular phantom and (b) its flattened map. (c) Shows surface patches that have Gaussian curvature greater than or equal to the 98th percentile. (d) Smoothed Gaussian curvature of the phantom and (e) its flattened map. (f) Surface patches that have Gaussian curvature greater than or equal to the 98th percentile (Reproduced with permission from Chiu et al.[41])

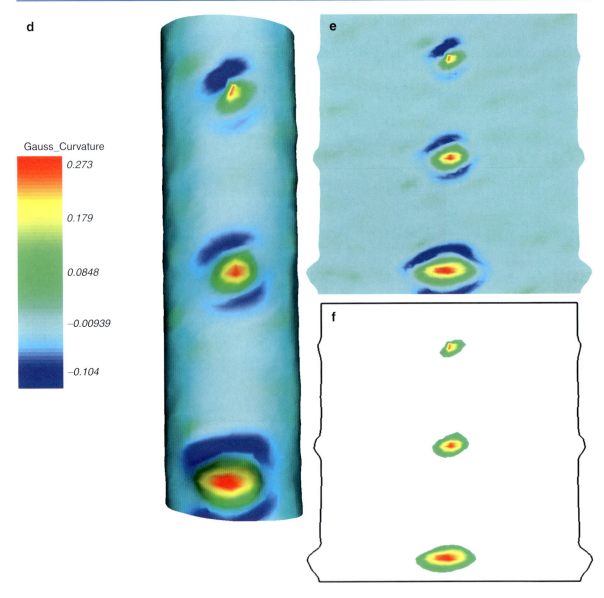

Fig. 17.7 (continued)

References

1. El-Barghouti N, Nicolaides AN, Tegos T, Geroulakos G. The relative effect of carotid plaque heterogeneity and echogenicity on ipsilateral cerebral infarction and symptoms of cerebrovascular disease. *Int Angiol.* 1996;15(4):300–306.
2. Tegos TJ et al. Determinants of carotid plaque instability: echoicity versus heterogeneity. *Eur J Vasc Endovasc Surg.* 2001;22(1):22–30.
3. Elatrozy T, Nicolaides A, Tegos T, Griffin M. The objective characterisation of ultrasonic carotid plaque features. *Eur J Vasc Endovasc Surg.* 1998;16(3):223–230.
4. Fenster A, Landry A, Downey DB, Hegele RA, Spence JD. 3D ultrasound imaging of the carotid arteries. *Curr Drug Targets Cardiovasc Haematol Disord.* 2004;4(2):161–175.
5. Fenster A, Blake C, Gyacskov I, Landry A, Spence JD. 3D ultrasound analysis of carotid plaque volume and surface morphology. *Ultrasonics.* 2006;44(Suppl 1):e153-e157.
6. Landry A, Fenster A. Theoretical and experimental quantification of carotid plaque volume measurements made by three-dimensional ultrasound using test phantoms. *Med Phys.* 2002;29(10):2319–2327.
7. Landry A, Spence JD, Fenster A. Quantification of carotid plaque volume measurements using 3D ultrasound imaging. *Ultrasound Med Biol.* 2005;31(6):751–762.

8. Egger M, Spence JD, Fenster A, Parraga G. Validation of 3d ultrasound vessel wall volume: an imaging phenotype of carotid atherosclerosis. *Ultrasound Med Biol*. 2007;33(6):905–914.
9. Egger M, Chiu B, Spence JD, Fenster A, Parraga G. Mapping spatial and temporal changes in carotid atherosclerosis from three-dimensional ultrasound images. *Ultrasound Med Biol*. 2008;34(1):64–72.
10. Schminke U, Motsch L, Hilker L, Kessler C. Three-dimensional ultrasound observation of carotid artery plaque ulceration. *Stroke*. 2000;31(7):1651–1655.
11. Ainsworth CD et al. 3D ultrasound measurement of change in carotid plaque volume: a tool for rapid evaluation of new therapies. *Stroke*. 2005;36(9):1904–1909.
12. NASCET Collaborators. Beneficial effect of carotid endarterectomy in symptomatic patients with high-grade stenosis. *N Engl J Med*. 1991;325(7):445–453.
13. Eliasziw M et al. Significance of plaque ulceration in symptomatic patients with high-grade carotid stenosis. North American Symptomatic Carotid Endarterectomy Trial. *Stroke*. 1994;25(2):304–308.
14. Fisher M et al. Carotid plaque pathology: thrombosis, ulceration, and stroke pathogenesis. *Stroke*. 2005;36(2):253–257.
15. Spence JD, Bang H, Chambless LE, Stampfer MJ. Vitamin intervention for stroke prevention trial: an efficacy analysis. *Stroke*. 2005;36(11):2404–2409.
16. Streifler JY et al. Angiographic detection of carotid plaque ulceration. Comparison with surgical observations in a multicenter study. North American Symptomatic Carotid Endarterectomy Trial. *Stroke*. 1994;25(6):1130–1132.
17. Rothwell PM, Gibson R, Warlow CP. Interrelation between plaque surface morphology and degree of stenosis on carotid angiograms and the risk of ischemic stroke in patients with symptomatic carotid stenosis. *Stroke*. 2000;31(3):615–621.
18. Sitzer M et al. Plaque ulceration and lumen thrombus are the main sources of cerebral microemboli in high-grade internal carotid artery stenosis. *Stroke*. 1995;26(7):1231–1233.
19. Sztajzel R. Ultrasonographic assessment of the morphological characteristics of the carotid plaque. *Swiss Med Wkly*. 2005;135(43–44):635–643.
20. Miskolczi L, Guterman LR, Flaherty JD, Hopkins LN. Depiction of carotid plaque ulceration and other plaque-related disorders by intravascular sonography: a flow chamber study. *AJNR Am J Neuroradiol*. 1996;17(10):1881–1890.
21. Chiu B, Egger M, Spence JD, Parraga G, Fenster A. Development of 3D ultrasound techniques for carotid artery disease assessment and monitoring. *Int J Comput Assist Radiol Surg*. 2008;3(1):1–10.
22. Chiu B, Egger M, Spence JD, Parraga G, Fenster A. Quantification of carotid vessel wall and plaque thickness change using 3D ultrasound images. *Med Phys*. 2008;35(8):3691–3710.
23. Chiu B, Egger M, Spence JD, Parraga G, Fenster A. Area-preserving flattening maps of 3D ultrasound carotid arteries images. *Med Image Anal*. 2008;12(6):676–688.
24. Meyer M, Desbrun M, Schroder P, Barr AH. Discrete differential-geometry operators for triangulated 2-manifolds. In: Hege HC, Polthier K, eds. *Visualization and Mathematics III*. 1st ed. Heidelberg: Springer; 2003:35–57.
25. Krsek P, Pajdla T, Hlavac V. Estimation of differential parameters on triangulated surface. In *Proceedings of the Czech Pattern Recognition Workshop*, February 1997, 151–155. Prague, Czech Republic: Czech Pattern Recognition Society; 1997.
26. Besl PJ, Jain RC. Invariant surface characteristics for 3D object recognition in range images. *Comp Vis Graph Image Proc*. 1986;33(1):33–80.
27. Han C, Hatsukami TS, Yuan C. Accurate lumen surface roughness measurement method in carotid atherosclerosis. *Proc SPIE*. 2001;4322:1817–1827.
28. Chiu B, Egger M, Spence JD, Parraga G, Fenster A. Quantification of carotid vessel atherosclerosis. *Proc SPIE*. 2006;6143:61430B.
29. Mao F, Gill J, Downey D, Fenster A. Segmentation of carotid artery in ultrasound images: method development and evaluation technique. *Med Phys*. 2000;27(8):1961–1970.
30. Zagzebski JA. *Essentials of Ultrasound Physics*. St. Louis: Mosby; 1996.
31. Sundaram P, Zomorodian A, Beaulieu C, Napel S. Colon polyp detection using smoothed shape operators: preliminary results. *Med Image Anal*. 2008;12(2):99–119.
32. Rickey DW, Picot PA, Christopher DA, Fenster A. A wallless vessel phantom for Doppler ultrasound studies. *Ultrasound Med Biol*. 1995;21(9):1163–1176.
33. Fenster A, Downey DB, Cardinal HN. Three-dimensional ultrasound imaging. *Phys Med Biol*. 2001;46(5):R67-R99.
34. Ladak HM et al. Prostate boundary segmentation from 2D ultrasound images. *Med Phys*. 2000;27(8):1777–1788.
35. Lobregt S, Viergever MA. A discrete dynamic contour model. *IEEE Trans Med Imaging*. 1995;14(1):12–24.
36. Schroeder WJ, Martin K, Lorensen W. *The Visualization Toolkit, an Object-Oriented Approach to 3D Graphics*. New York: Kitware Inc; 2002.
37. Rohling RN, Gee AH, Berman L. Automatic registration of 3-D ultrasound images. *Ultrasound Med Biol*. 1998;24(6):841–854.
38. Jespersen SK, Wilhjelm JE, Sillesen H. In vitro spatial compound scanning for improved visualization of atherosclerosis. *Ultrasound Med Biol*. 2000;26(8):1357–1362.
39. Barnett HJ. Stroke prevention by surgery for symptomatic disease in carotid territory. *Neurol Clin*. 1992;10(1):281–292.
40. Warlow C. MRC European Carotid Surgery Trial: interim results for symptomatic patients with severe (70–99%) or with mild (0–29%) carotid stenosis. *Lancet*. 1991;337(8752):1235–1243.
41. Chiu B, Beletsky V, Spence JD, Parraga G, Fenster A. Analysis of carotid lumen surface morphology using 3-dimensional ultrasound imaging. *Phys Med Biol*. 2009;54(5):1149–1167. doi:dx.doi.org. © IOP Publishing Ltd.

Carotid Plaque Texture Analysis Using 3-Dimensional Volume Ultrasonic Imaging

Andrew Nicolaides, Maura Griffin, Gregory C. Makris, George Geroulakos, Dawn Bond, Efthyvoulos Kyriacou, Antonios A. Polydorou, and Victoria Polydorou

18.1 Introduction

The principles of 3-dimensional (3D) image reconstruction from a series of consecutive two-dimensional (2D) ultrasound images and the measurement of plaque volume and plaque surface irregularity have been described in Chaps. 16 and 17. The application and value of 3D volume ultrasonic imaging to the measurement of plaque volume changes in response to medical therapy are presented in Chap. 25.

Relatively little has been published on carotid plaque texture analysis using 3D ultrasonic imaging (see below). So far, plaque texture analysis has been applied on conventional 2D brightness mode (B-mode) images and has been shown to have considerable success in identifying symptomatic carotid plaques (Chaps. 12, 14, 15, 24, 26, 31 and 32) including risk stratification and prediction of stroke (Chap. 36). Also, the effect of statin therapy on carotid plaque morphology has been demonstrated by several studies using conventional 2D B-mode imaging (Chap. 35). The question that has often been asked is how representative of the whole plaque are the texture features obtained from single 2D images and would texture features extracted from 3D volume reconstructions perform better. The aim of this chapter is to present the rationale and a methodology that has been developed for 3D plaque texture analysis and to demonstrate the potential for future research and clinical applications.

A. Nicolaides (✉)
Imperial College and Vascular Screening and Diagnostic Centre, London, UK

M. Griffin • D. Bond
Vascular Screening and Diagnostic Centre, London, UK

G.C. Makris
Division of Vascular Surgery, Imperial College of London, London, UK

G. Geroulakos
Department of Surgery, Charing Cross Hospital, London, UK

E. Kyriacou
Department of Computer Science and Engineering, Frederick University Cyprus, Lemesos, Cyprus

A.A. Polydorou
Interventional Cardiac and Peripheral Department, General Hospital of Athens "Evangelismos", Athens, Greece

V. Polydorou
Department of Internal Medicine, General Airforce Hospital, Athens, Greece

18.2 Lessons from Histology and Intravascular Ultrasound (IVUS) Virtual Histology

18.2.1 Lessons from Histology

The association between silent brain infarcts and carotid plaque ulceration was demonstrated by the authors' team in the early 1980s.[1] In this study, patients scheduled for carotid endarterectomy (symptomatic and asymptomatic) had a preoperative computed tomography (CT) brain scan, and carotid specimens were examined for ulceration. The prevalence of CT brain infarcts was 62% in patients with ulcerated plaques but only 8% in those without plaque ulceration.

The concept of unstable carotid plaques was subsequently supported by the work of Yao and his team.[2] They demonstrated that patients with symptomatic carotid stenosis had more frequent plaque rupture, fibrous cap thinning, and fibrous cap foam-cell infiltration than patients with asymptomatic carotid stenosis.

Subsequently, Bassiouny and his team[3] demonstrated that in a series of 99 carotid endarterectomy plaques (59 symptomatic and 40 asymptomatic), the necrotic core was twice as close to the lumen in symptomatic plaques when compared with asymptomatic plaques (0.27 ± 0.30 vs. 0.50 ± 0.50 mm; $P < 0.001$). In addition, the number of macrophages infiltrating the fibrous cap was three times greater in symptomatic than asymptomatic plaques, but the percent area occupied by the lipid necrotic core was the same in both. Their findings indicated that the proximity of plaque necrotic core to the lumen and cell infiltration of the fibrous cap were the strongest histological associations with symptoms.

Another histological study of carotid endarterectomy specimens[4] demonstrated significantly more neovessels in plaques and fibrous caps of symptomatic than asymptomatic plaques. In addition, in symptomatic plaques, neovessels were larger and more irregular and were associated with increased plaque necrosis and rupture.

More recently, a detailed histological assessment of 526 symptomatic carotid plaques from consecutive patients undergoing carotid endarterectomy[5] demonstrated that in ruptured plaques, the median representative cap thickness was 300 µ (interquartile range [IQR] 200–500 µ), and the median minimum cap thickness was 150 µ (IQR 80–210). In contrast, in nonruptured plaques, the median representative cap thickness was 500 µ (IQR 300–700 µ), and the median minimum cap thickness was 250 µ (IQR 180–400). Minimum and representative plaque thicknesses were both independently associated with cap rupture.

In terms of imaging with ultrasound, the above have a number of implications. Plaque ulceration is difficult to detect on B-mode longitudinal images but much easier on 3D volume reconstruction (Chap. 17). The necrotic core is visualized as a hypoechoic area and although it cannot be distinguished from hemorrhage, it can be argued that both are means of determining the fibrous cap thickness. A fibrous cap which is thinner than 200 µ is at the limit of most ultrasound probes, and it is unlikely to be visualized. This will result in the presence of a juxtaluminal black area (JBA) without a visible echogenic cap. This proves to be an ultrasonic characteristic of the dangerous plaque[6] (Chaps. 12 and 36). The size (volume) of this JBA can only be measured with 3D volume reconstruction (see below). Although neovascularization cannot be visualized by B-mode grayscale imaging, it can be studied and measured using plaque perfusion microbubble agents (Chap. 7). The hyperperfused plaque areas indicating neovascularization are associated with an increased number of macrophages.[7]

18.2.2 Lessons from IVUS

Some of the early work on 3D plaque characterization has been related to IVUS and coronary atherosclerosis. One of the earliest studies[8] correlated regions of calcification, fibrous tissue, and necrotic core with first order statistics, Haralick's texture features, Laws' texture energy features, neighborhood graytone difference matrix features, and texture spectrum features. Haralick's texture features yielded the most accurate results with error rates of 6.8%. Several subsequent studies have demonstrated that IVUS with virtual histology (VH-IVUS) and 3D volume reconstruction has allowed in vivo delineation of the relative contributions of necrotic core and fibrous atheroma in unstable coronary plaques.[9] The in vivo validity of VH-IVUS backscatter data from 51 ex vivo left anterior descending coronary arteries were recorded and compared with histology.[10] The overall predictive accuracies were 93.5% for fibrotic tissue, 94.1% for fibrofatty tissue, 95.8% for necrotic core, and 96.7% for dense calcium. The VH-IVUS definition of vulnerability is: a confluent necrotic core greater than 10% in direct contact with the lumen (fibrous cap <65 µ indicating a histologically unstable plaque not visualized with ultrasound) and a minor amount of calcium (<10%) present on three consecutive VH-IVUS cross-sectional frames.[9] When the same technique and criteria were applied to carotid plaques in the carotid artery plaque virtual histology evaluation (CAPITAL) study[11] (Chap. 32), the predictive accuracy for thin cap fibroatheroma plaques was 99.4%.

18.2.3 Application of Texture Analysis to 3D Reconstructed Carotid Plaques

A 3D ultrasonographic analysis of 110 symptomatic (stroke) and 104 asymptomatic atherosclerotic carotid plaques was recently performed by Heliopoulos and his colleagues.[12] They measured the mean gray value (MGV) of the 3D volume reconstruction of the plaques after image normalization using blood and adventitia as reference points (blood $= 0$–1; adventitia $= 59$–61). MGV was lower in symptomatic than asymptomatic patients for plaques producing less than 70% stenosis ($P < 0.01$) but not in those with a higher degree of stenosis.

Texture analysis tools such as the ones described in Chaps. 14 and 15 have been used to evaluate the effect of atorvastatin 80 mg daily administered to patients with carotid stenosis compared to those treated with placebo.[13] In addition to vessel wall volume measurements (VWV) (Chap. 16), 270 texture features were extracted from 3D vessel wall volume. The texture feature techniques that most differentiated between atorvastatin and placebo classes were Fourier power spectrum and Laws' texture energy measures. These texture features were more sensitive in detecting statin-related changes in carotid atherosclerosis than VWV, suggesting that texture feature classifiers can be used to detect changes in carotid plaques after therapy.

At the time of writing, the authors are not aware of any other publications on the application of texture features other than MGV to a substantial series of 3D carotid plaque volume data to differentiate symptomatic from asymptomatic carotid plaques.

18.3 3D Image Capture

18.3.1 Equipment and Settings

18.3.1.1 Equipment

The authors have used the VL13-5 probe (Fig. 18.1) with the Philips iU22 ultrasound scanner (Philips, Seattle, Washington, USA). This probe is ideally suited for carotid scans. It supports 2D and 3D image capture. It consists of a high-resolution linear array with 192 elements which is supported in a fluid

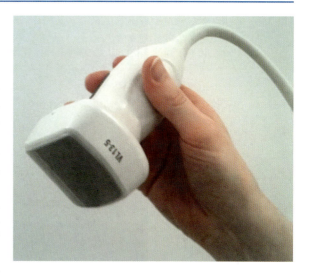

Fig. 18.1 The VL13-5 probe

chamber that mechanically acquires a series of conventional images covering the whole carotid bifurcation with one sweep in approximately 3–4 s. These images are automatically combined to create a $4 \times 2.5 \times 2.5$-cm "block" of voxels. Ultrasound images can be obtained with and without color flow or power Doppler. Because the movement of the probe is within the chamber, the probe is held still in contact with the skin. 3D image capture is activated after an optimal 2D longitudinal conventional image is visualized on the monitor and final fine adjustments have been made in terms of angle of insonation, gain, and focal zones.

The VL13-5 probe supports both SonoCT which is essential for 3D imaging and XRES. SonoCT provides real-time compound imaging. It uses transmit beam steering to obtain coplanar images from different viewing angles which are combined into a single compound image at real-time frame rates. This reduces speckle noise artifacts, but most important is the fact that it allows visualization of structures with curved or irregular borders (Fig. 18.2).

XRES is a post-processing technique which according to the manufacturer's specifications reduces "speckle, haze, and clutter artifacts and, at the same time, enhances edges by correcting discontinuity between textured regions allowing improved images close to how humans perceive tissue patterns." XRES is useful for measurements of plaque volume but should be switched off in acquiring images for texture measurements (see below).

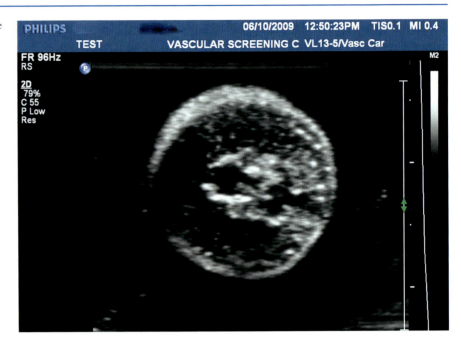

Fig. 18.2 2D B-mode image of a grape using the VL13-5 probe

18.3.1.2 Presets

2D settings were as follows: SonoCT on, XRES off, 2D PRF high and persistence low as described in Chap. 12, chroma map off, compress 55, 2D opt, wide scan off, and AGC optional. 3D settings were: tilt 0, angle 15, FR 59 Hz, and select resolution over speed for volume acquisition.

18.3.2 Image Capture

A full conventional study of the carotid bifurcation is first performed. Initially, the common carotid artery and bifurcation are inspected with transverse and longitudinal imaging in B-mode and color-mode so that the operator can fully appreciate the extent and anatomic position of the plaque or plaques. Loops are obtained where necessary in longitudinal and transverse views for subsequent reference. Grading of the stenosis is performed based on a combination of transverse color flow images, absolute velocities and/or velocity ratios obtained at 60° to the ultrasound beam as described in Chap. 30.

An important decision needs to be made prior to 3D image capture. This is whether one is dealing with a plaque that has a hypoechoic (black) area adjacent to the lumen without a visible fibrous cap. If this is the case, the appropriate use of color flow is essential in outlining this part of the plaque. The color gain is adjusted to avoid any overspill obscuring the plaque borders. Also, as indicated in Chap. 12, when in B-mode alone, the gain is adjusted so that noise in the lumen is minimized but not completely abolished. Several 3D acquisitions may have to be made to ensure complete color filling of the lumen adjacent to any hypoechoic plaque areas (Fig. 18.3). This is not necessary if the fibrous cap demarcating the plaque blood interface is visible. A similar 3D acquisition is made without the color flow (Fig. 18.4). Inspection of volume data sets can be made immediately using the QLAB software (Philips, Seattle, Washington, USA) installed on the scanner. This is particularly useful and time saving.

All 2D images, 3D acquisitions, and cine loops are automatically saved on the hard drive of the scanner and can be exported to a DVD in digital imaging and communications in medicine (DICOM), jpeg or TIF format. Loops can be exported in DICOM or audio video interleave (AVI) format. The DICOM files are then used for subsequent analysis using the Philips QLAB software either on the scanner itself which is generally inherent within the ultrasound system or on a laptop.

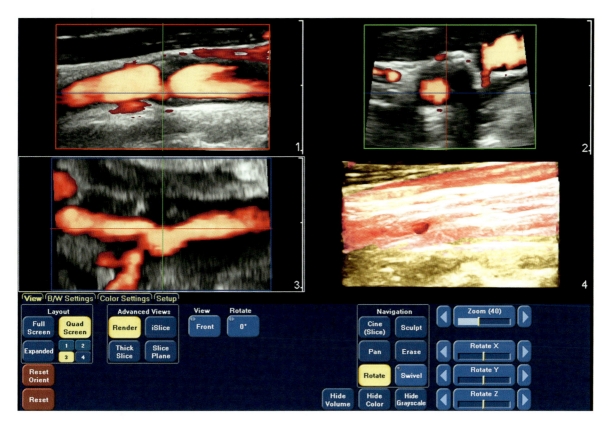

Fig. 18.3 3D image acquisition. The use of color flow to outline the interphase between lumen and hypoechoic areas of plaque

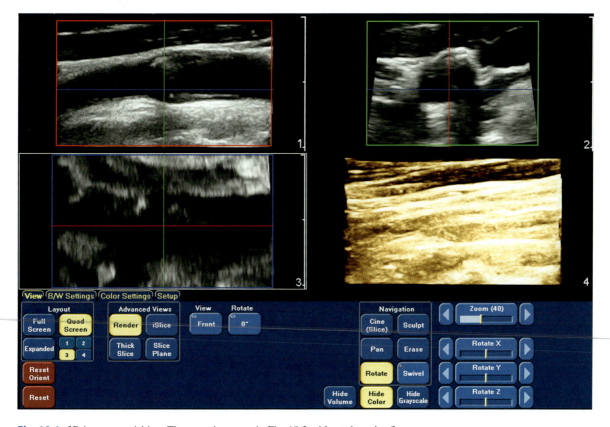

Fig. 18.4 3D image acquisition. The same image as in Fig. 18.3 without the color flow

18.4 Image Analysis

Image analysis is performed offline on a laptop using the Philips QLAB software and the Plaque Texture Analysis software version 3.3 (Iconsoft International Ltd, PO Box 172, Greenford, London UB6 9ZN, UK). The latter has been described in detail in Chap. 12.

18.4.1 3D Visualization and Image Orientation

One of the advantages of the QLAB software is that the "block" of voxels, once acquired, can be adjusted in terms of grayscale settings and rotation and, in addition, sliced in any direction required. The multiplanar display as seen in Fig. 18.3 presents four images: the plane in which the region under examination was scanned (the acquisition plane), that is, in this instance, the conventional longitudinal image as seen by the operator at the time of the 3D capture (Fig. 18.3_1), and along with this are two further planes that are generated from the original volume data set collected: Fig. 18.3_2 and 18.3_3, respectively. These three planes are orthogonal to each other resulting in transverse and coronal sections. The fourth image represents the volume-rendered image as seen Fig. 18.3_4. A measurement scale is provided on the right of each image. The level of these sections is determined by the position of the corresponding three cross wires: red, green, and blue. Moving any of the cross wires produces an automatic change in the section of the box with the corresponding color. Any of the four images can be rotated, and this produces an automatic adjustment of the other three. For example, by rotating the transverse image to approximately 90° counterclockwise and "hiding" the gray scale in the 3D reconstruction, separation of the jugular vein from the carotid bifurcation is obtained, and the latter can be seen as a red 3D image similar to an angiogram (Fig. 18.5_4). It should be emphasized that with the mechanical acquisition transducer, it is not always possible to obtain color filling of the whole lumen, especially when dealing with a long lesion, depending on the heart rate and duration of 3D capture. This is the reason why several 3D captures may be required. However, as long as there is color adjacent to the hypoechoic part of the plaque, adequate plaque segmentation can be performed.

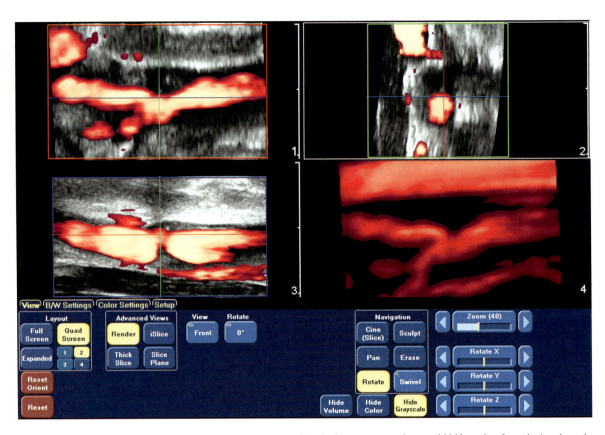

Fig. 18.5 The transverse section (*top right*) has been rotated anticlockwise to separate the carotid bifurcation from the jugular vein in the 3D reconstruction after switching off the gray scale

18.4.2 QLAB Settings

The following settings have been fixed to ensure reproducibility and image uniformity.

18.4.2.1 Set Up
Link, ruler, and MPR x-hair should be on; 3D box, rotate x-hair, and vol x-hair should be off.

18.4.2.2 Grayscale Settings Are Set at Defaults
Brightness 41, transparency 20, threshold 5, lighting 0, smoothing 10. MPR: chroma is off; gray 2. XRES is off. For texture analysis, it is essential that XRES is off because XRES changes the gray texture. So far, all texture image analysis for plaque characterization as reported by different groups and described in different chapters has been performed without XRES, and to date, there is no data on the effect of the latter on texture features.

18.4.2.3 Adjustment of Brightness
If necessary, the MPR brightness is adjusted so that there will be minimal noise in the vessel lumen. This is rarely necessary because "minimal noise in the lumen" is usually set correctly prior to capture by adjusting the gain as described above and in Chap. 12.

18.4.3 Segmentation of 3D Images

Both the 3D color flow and the 3D grayscale volume data sets are sliced at right angles to the axis of the common/internal carotid artery. Usually, this is done at 1 mm intervals, but for the sake of clarity in the demonstration below, it will be done at 2 mm intervals.

Initially, a slight rotation of the longitudinal image may be necessary to ensure that sections through the plaque are truly transverse. In the case demonstrated below, a 2° clockwise rotation was performed (Fig. 18.6). Subsequently, a landmark is identified that is easily recognizable in both the color

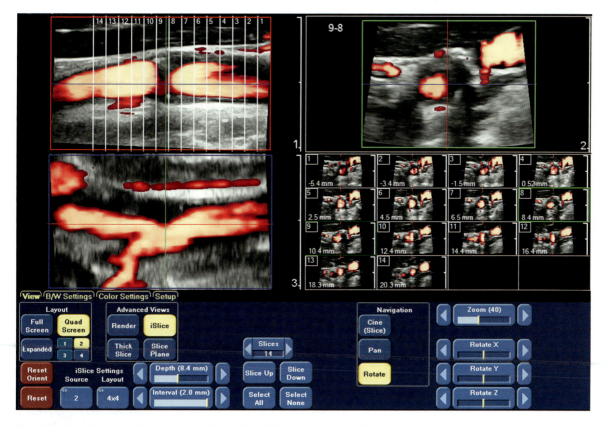

Fig. 18.6 The 2D longitudinal image (*top left*) in Fig. 18.3 has been rotated 2° clockwise and sliced at 2 mm intervals

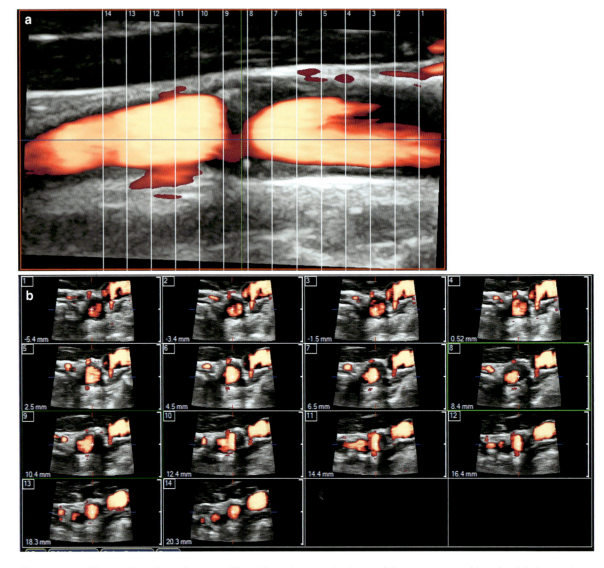

Fig. 18.7 (a) Slices 1–14 at 2 mm intervals. Slice 1 is positioned at the beginning of the plaque, slice 8 through a white landmark in the stenotic part of the plaque, and slice 14 at the most distal end of the plaque. Note: The black area in the most proximal part of the common carotid on the right is not plaque but noncolor filling. The visible IMT confirms this. (b) The 14 transverse slices obtained from Fig. 18.6

flow and grayscale images. It can be the beginning of the plaque if hyperechoic and easily defined or a landmark such as the small white area on the far wall overlapped by the white vertical line representing section 8 adjacent to the green crosshair (Figs. 18.6 and 18.7a). The sections (Figs. 18.6 and 18.7b) are produced by using the "iSlice" facility. The number of sections, distance between sections, and position of the block of sections are adjusted by using the appropriate buttons as shown in the lower part of the screen. By convention, section 1 is positioned at the more proximal end of the plaque and the last section at the distal end of the plaque. In the example shown in Figs. 18.6 and 18.7, there are 14 sections at 2 mm intervals. This process is repeated in the corresponding 3D grayscale image (Figs. 18.8 and 18.9). Section 8 is through the same position marked by the white area in both the color and grayscale image. This ensures that each section in the color image

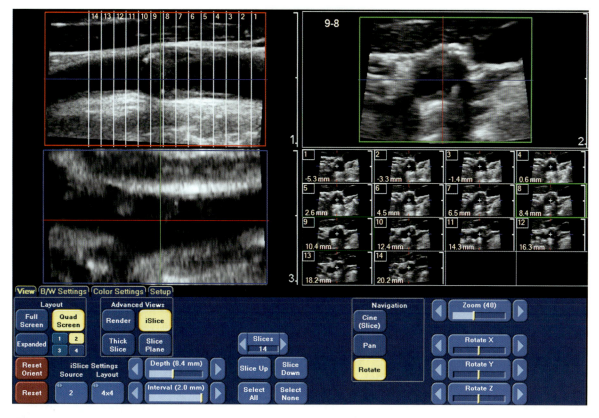

Fig. 18.8 The same 14 slices as in Fig. 18.6

corresponds as close as possible to the section with the same number in the grayscale image (Fig. 18.10).

The 14 transverse color images and the 14 transverse grayscale images are exported as TIFF images in a folder. Subsequently, corresponding color and grayscale images are placed in 14 subfolders numbered 1–14.

18.4.4 Measurement of Volume and Texture

18.4.4.1 Image Analysis

Image analysis of the 14 consecutive transverse grayscale images is performed using the Plaque Texture Analysis software version 3.3 as described in Chap. 12. For each pair of transverse images (color and grayscale), image normalization for gray scale using blood and adventitia as reference points (blood = 0 and adventitia = 190) is performed followed by image standardization to 20 pixels per mm. The color image is a useful guide to the plaque segmentation (Fig. 18.11). Finally, texture feature extraction is performed (Fig. 18.12). Processed images of each transverse section are saved on file or printed, and texture features are saved in a database (Fig. 18.13) (see Chap. 12).

18.4.4.2 Calculation of Plaque Volume and 3D Texture Features

In the above example in which the transverse sections were at 2 mm intervals, plaque volume was calculated from the areas of the 14 transverse sections shown in Fig. 18.13 using the following equation:

$$\text{Volume} = (\text{Area}_1 \times 2) + (\text{Area}_2 \times 2) \\ + \ldots\ldots\ldots + (\text{Area}_{14} \times 2) \quad (18.1)$$

Plaque volume was found to be 506 mm^3 or 0.506 mL.

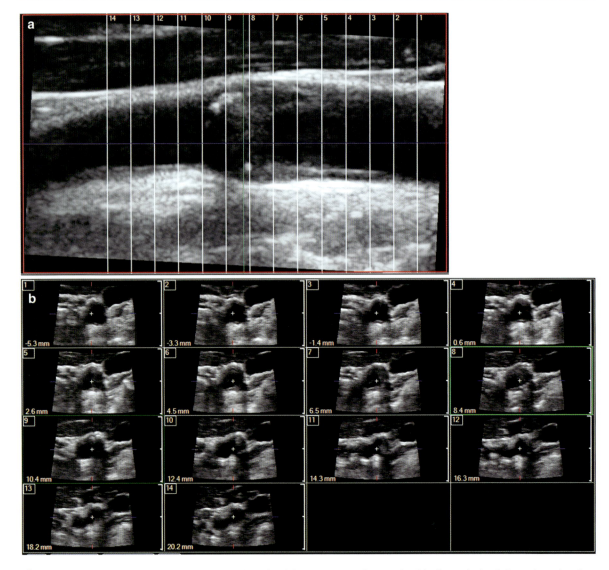

Fig. 18.9 (**a**) Slices 1–14 at 2 mm interval. Note that slice 8 is positioned through the white landmark in the stenotic part of the plaque. (**b**) The 14 transverse slices obtained from Fig. 18.8 corresponding to the 14 slices obtained from the color flow image shown in Fig. 18.7b

For any other 3D texture feature, the weighted mean value (e.g., GSM_w) is calculated as follows:

$$GSM_W = \frac{(GSM_1 * Area_1) + (GSM_2 * Area_2) + \ldots + (GSM_{14} * Area_{14})}{Area_1 + Area_2 + \ldots + Area_{14}}$$

(18.2)

In the above example, GSM_w was found to be 46.7. This is the true GSM average for the whole plaque. As can be seen in Fig. 18.13, GSM values for individual sections varied from 24.6 (lowest value in section 8) to 62 (highest value in section 7).

18.5 Application of 3D Volume and Texture Analysis in a Symptomatic and an Asymptomatic Plaque

Two examples of 3D volume and texture analysis are provided below with reference to plaque volume, juxtaluminal "black" volume (JBV) that is defined as a volume of plaque with grayscale pixel values less than 25 adjacent to the lumen in the absence of a visible fibrous cap, GSMw and spatial gray

Fig. 18.10 (a) Slice 8 from color flow image and corresponding (b) slice 8 from grayscale image

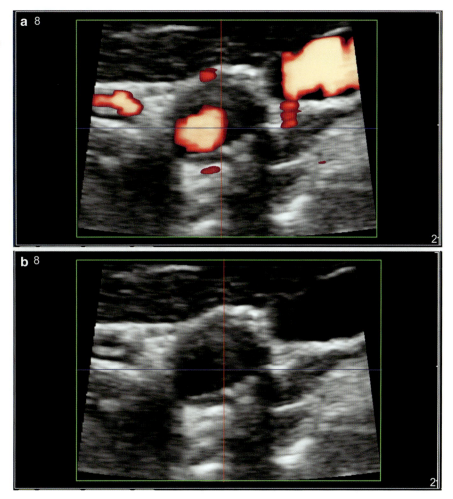

level dependence matrix (SGLDM) difference entropy as defined and shown in Chap. 12. Recent cross-sectional studies[6, 14] (Chaps. 12 and 33) have demonstrated that in conventional 2D longitudinal plaque images, the presence of a juxtaluminal hypoechoic area greater than 8 mm^2 in the absence of a visible echogenic cap is associated with symptomatic plaques. The ability to measure the volume of such hypoechoic areas adjacent to the lumen is a new challenge, and such measurement may prove a valuable predictor of future strokes. The aim of the examples below is to show the variability of texture features within the plaques and how this can be overcome by 3D indicating the potential value of the latter for both research and clinical applications.

18.5.1 First Example

This is a small volume plaque, 12 mm in length (Fig. 18.14), producing a 90–95% stenosis as shown by the high peak systolic velocity of 625 cm/s and end diastolic velocity of 336 cm/s detected (Fig. 18.15a) and the small residual lumen visualized in transverse section (Fig. 18.15b). The patient presented with a transient ischemic attack (TIA) 1 week prior to scanning. Visually, this is a predominantly echogenic plaque with an obvious hypoechoic area close to the lumen (Fig. 18.14).

18.5.1.1 Analysis of the 2D Image
Image analysis of the conventional 2D grayscale longitudinal image (Fig. 18.16a) as described in Chap. 12

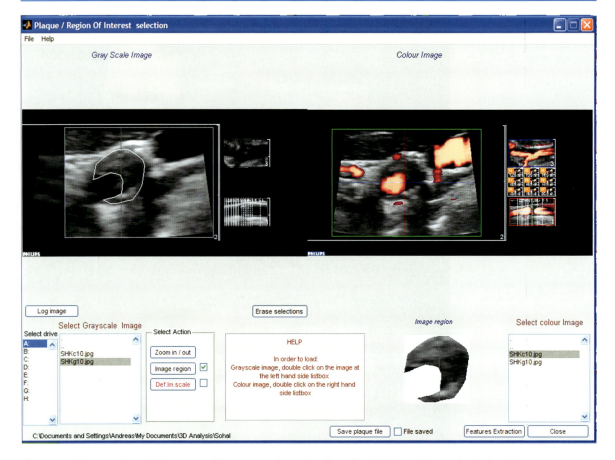

Fig. 18.11 Segmentation of plaque area with corresponding color slice using the Plaque Texture Analysis software

has resulted in the following features: type 3, discrete white areas (DWA) present, GSM 50, JBA 2.36 mm^2 (Fig. 18.16b), gray level dependence matrix (GLDM) difference entropy of 2.52, plaque area of 43 mm^2.

Image analysis of the second conventional 2D grayscale longitudinal image taken at a slightly different plane missed the echogenic area at the apex of the posterior component of the plaque (Fig. 18.17a) and produced similar texture features except for the size of the JBA: type 3, DWA present, GSM 46, JBA 8.16 mm^2 (Fig. 18.17b), GLDM difference entropy of 2.54, plaque area of 42.8 mm^2. The findings of the first image would classify the plaque as stable, while the finding of a JBA of 8.16 mm^2 would classify the plaque as unstable (Chap. 12). This type of discrepancy is expected to be avoided by 3D volume imaging that deals with the whole of the plaque rather than an ultrasonic longitudinal image which may not be representative.

18.5.1.2 Analysis of the 3D Image

Using the *iSlice* facility of the QLAB on the volume data set as described above produced 12 transverse sections at 1 mm intervals (Fig. 18.18). The values of GSM, plaque area, JBA, and SGLDM difference entropy are shown in Table 18.1. Using Eqs. 18.1 and 18.2, GSM$_w$ was 15.2, plaque volume was 482 mm^3 or 0.482 mL, JBV was 85 mm^3, and SGLDM difference entropy$_w$ was 2.12.

Inspection of the data in Table 18.1 indicates a great variation in GSM. It appears that proximal sections 1–5 are hyperechoic while distal sections are hypoechoic. Also, the GSM$_w$ of 15.2 is very different from the GSM of 50 or 46 obtained from the conventional longitudinal images. This is because the bulk of the hypoechoic area was lateral to and outside the planes of the longitudinal images. Also, there is no JBA in the proximal transverse sections of the plaque (numbered 1–5), but there is one in the distal seven sections (numbered 6–12). If the JBV

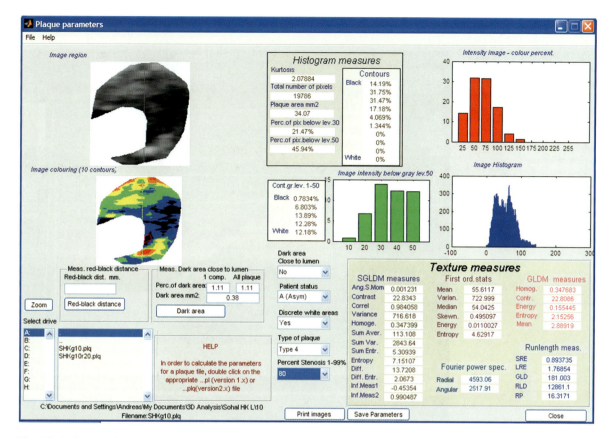

Fig. 18.12 Texture feature extraction

*SHK tran. sections.sav [DataSet1] - PASW Statistics Data Editor

1 : median 29.0327103

	mean	varian	median	area_mm2	mode	skew	energ	entr	gldm_hom
1	36.156822	9.1151394...	29.032710	16.68	0	.8355613	.0171317	4.4675980	.3199817
2	38.039049	5.5740521...	37.407143	12.61	0	.1310767	.0151288	4.3829259	.2831532
3	40.002739	6.9244275...	39.840278	13.69	0	.3826904	.0121564	4.5294187	.2859528
4	47.407049	8.3113785...	46.529412	21.42	0	.1084366	.0114950	4.6139060	.3075283
5	34.840010	6.1349786...	32.936047	20.41	0	.6632710	.0140317	4.4211878	.3039531
6	56.104525	7.7117320...	52.760563	23.87	50	.6439391	.0109436	4.6642189	.2353216
7	64.685828	7.4646459...	62.516129	38.32	52	.3102666	.0103436	4.6863491	.2390586
8	30.793824	7.1055741...	24.617241	26.30	7	1.1075203	.0161173	4.3871470	.3587814
9	63.307824	1.9599321...	53.432692	13.13	5	.6201769	.0078399	4.9920781	.2497786
10	54.627827	6.3440952...	54.462406	19.68	71	.2105292	.0113834	4.5987058	.2417985
11	58.113673	9.5156912...	57.718182	18.65	38	.1908984	.0094748	4.7489699	.2234938
12	40.139888	9.8112686...	34.642857	10.71	0	.7869947	.0133651	4.5831589	.2761713
13	40.869439	1.0205376...	34.020000	10.34	0	.4905607	.0136947	4.5605859	.2585522
14	45.454482	1.0032917...	38.380952	7.20	13	.6031020	.0105763	4.6799979	.2153259

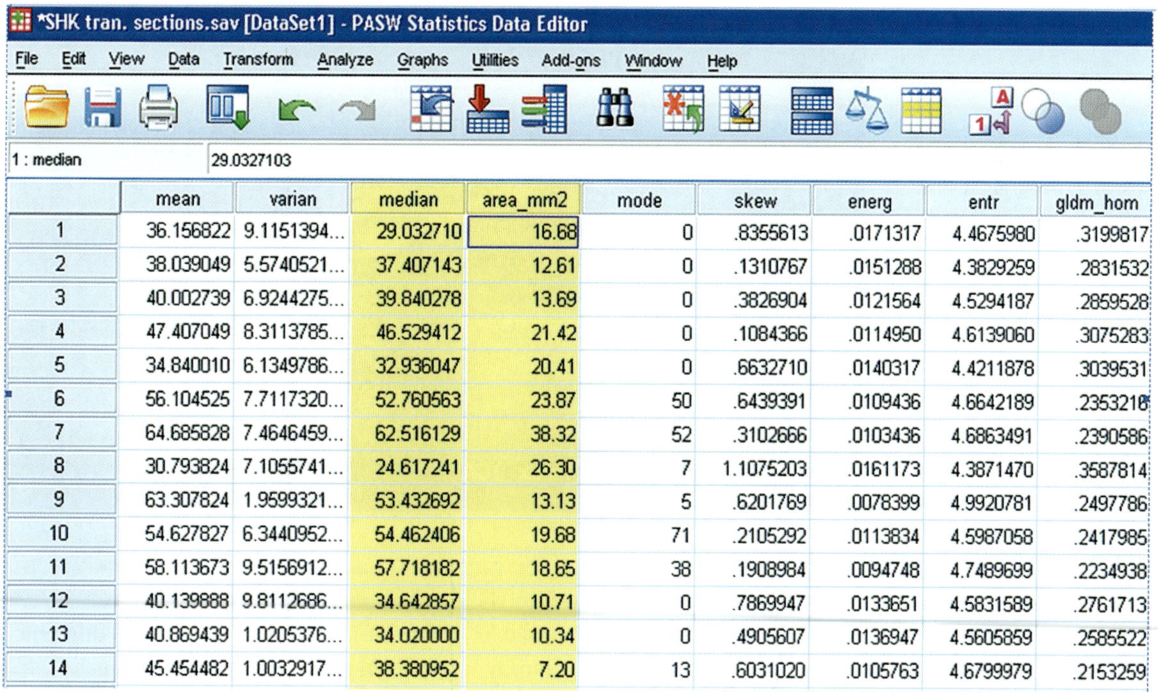

Fig. 18.13 Texture features from the 14 plaque slices as seen in the database. Grayscale median (GSM) and plaque area are shown in yellow

Fig. 18.14 (**a**) and (**b**) are two conventional 2D color views of the same highly stenotic plaque. (**b**) has been obtained by slight movement of the L9-3 vascular probe (approximately 1–2 mm laterally)

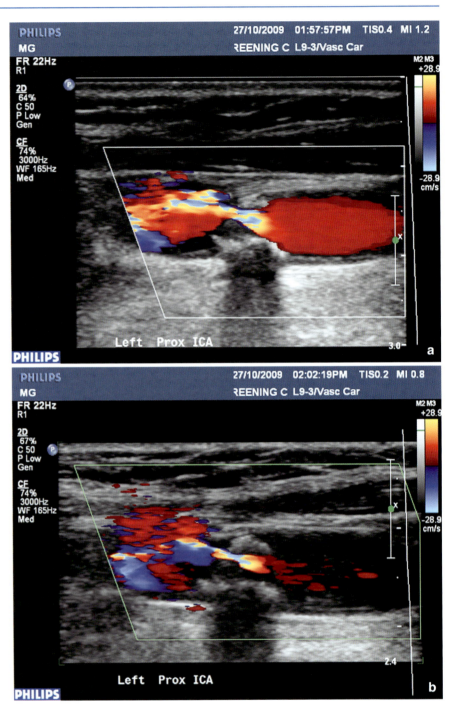

of 85 mm^3 is divided by 7, there is an average JBA of 12.3 mm^2 which should be visible in an appropriate longitudinal plane (not possible in the plane of the handheld probe) that would classify this plaque as unstable (Chap. 36). Finally, the SGLDM difference entropy is higher in the proximal sections (mean 2.52; standard deviation [SD] 0.161) than in the distal sections (mean 1.93; SD 0.156) ($P < 0.001$).

Fig. 18.15 (**a**) Plaque producing 90–95% stenosis as shown by the high peak systolic velocity of 625 cm/s and end diastolic velocity of 336 cm/s. (**b**) The severity of stenosis and shape of the residual lumen in transverse section. Note that the right half of the plaque is more hypoechoic than the rest of the plaque

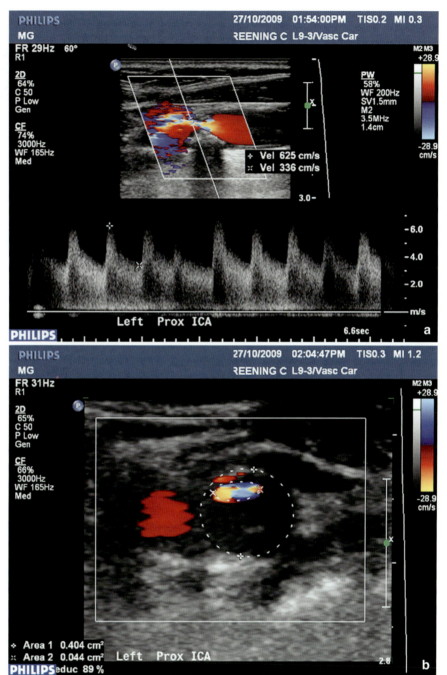

Fig. 18.16 (a) First conventional B-mode image. (b) Image analysis has resulted in the following features: type 3, DWA present, GSM 50, JBA 2.36 mm^2, GLDM difference entropy of 2.52, plaque area of 43 mm^2. These are characteristics of a "stable" plaque (see text)

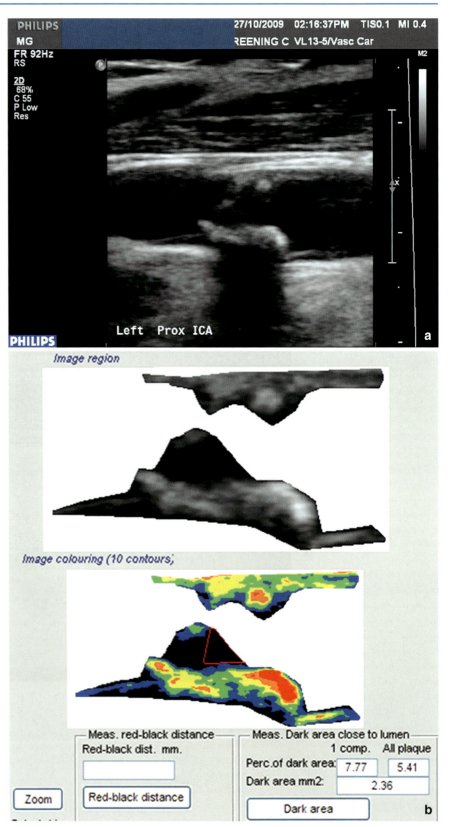

Fig. 18.17 (**a**) Second conventional B-mode image of the same plaque as in Fig. 18.17. (**b**) Image analysis has resulted in the following features: type 3, DWA present, GSM 46, JBA 8.16 mm^2 (Fig. 18.17b), GLDM difference entropy of 2.54, plaque area of 42.8 mm^2. The JBA of 8.16 mm^2 is a characteristic of an "unstable" plaque

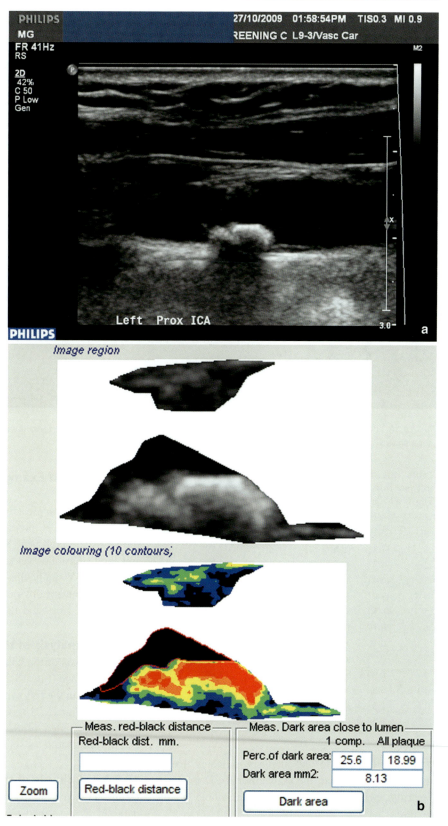

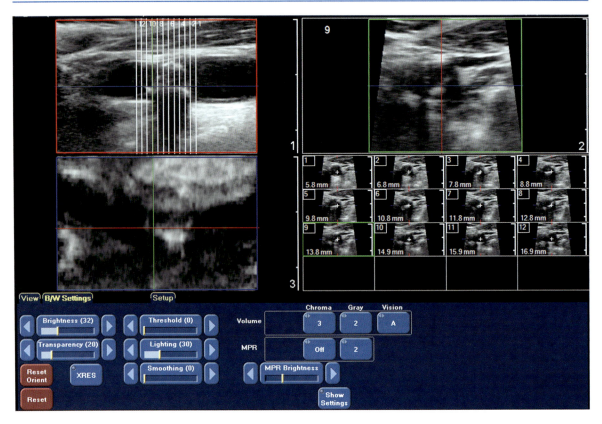

Fig. 18.18 Twelve transverse slices of the plaque at 1 mm intervals. The same was performed with the color flow 3D image which is not shown

Table 18.1 Features produced by the carotid image analysis software from the 12 slices of the plaque shown in Fig. 18.18. This is a heterogenous plaque

Slice	GSM	Plaque area (mm^2)	JBA (mm^2)	SGLDM_DEN
1	47.52	15.67	0	2.49
2	35.77	22.19	0	2.29
3	46.44	26.13	0	2.7
4	41.92	33.84	0	2.57
5	49.54	33.43	0	2.68
6	20.17	48.61	7	2.39
7	0.30	92.62	17	1.66
8	0.73	63.79	24	1.96
9	0.99	67.14	16	1.98
10	5.58	35.66	5	2.14
11	2.51	31.14	13	1.93
12	7.58	12.12	3	1.91

Thus, 3D imaging and analysis indicates that in this particular plaque, the conventional 2D image is far from being representative of the whole plaque texture.

18.5.2 Second Example

This is a large volume asymptomatic plaque, 27 mm in length (Fig. 18.19), producing an 80–85% stenosis as shown by the high peak systolic velocity of 547 cm/s and end diastolic velocity of 244 cm/s detected (Fig. 18.20). Visually, this is a predominantly echogenic plaque without any obvious hypoechoic area close to the lumen (Figs. 18.19 and 18.21a).

18.5.2.1 Analysis of the 2D Image

Image analysis of the conventional 2D grayscale longitudinal image (Fig. 18.21a) as described in Chap. 12 has resulted in the following features: type 4, GSM 50, JBA 1.69 (Fig. 18.21b), GLDM difference entropy of 2.35, plaque area of 82 mm^2. The findings would classify the plaque as stable.

18.5.2.2 Analysis of the 3D Volume Image

Using the *iSlice* facility of the QLAB on the volume data set as described above produced 26 transverse

Fig. 18.19 Asymptomatic plaque, 27 mm in length, with 80–85% stenosis

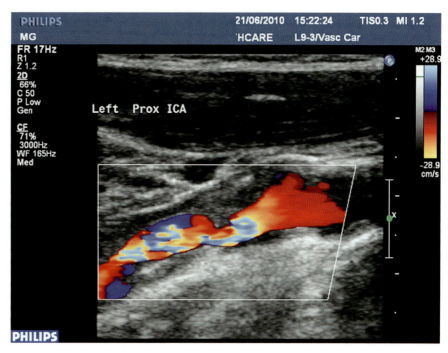

Fig. 18.20 The same plaque as Fig. 18.19. Peak systolic velocity of 547 cm/s and end diastolic velocity of 244 cm/s

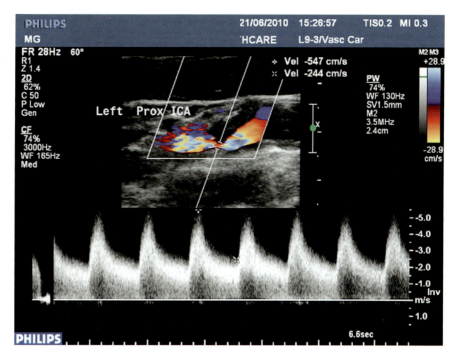

slices at 1 mm intervals (Fig. 18.22). The values of GSM, plaque area, JBA, and SGLDM difference entropy for slices 1–26 are shown in Table 18.2. Using Eqs. 18.1 and 18.2, GSM_w was 54, plaque volume was 1,312 mm^3 or 1.312 mL, JBV 9.7 mm^3 (largest of the two present), and SGLDM difference entropy$_w$ of 2.66.

Inspection of the data in Table 18.2 indicates relatively little variation in GSM. The GSM_w of 54 is close to the GSM of 50 obtained from the conventional

Fig. 18.21 (**a**) Conventional B-mode image. (**b**) Image analysis has resulted in the following features: type 4, GSM 50, JBA 1.69 (Fig. 18.21b), GLDM difference entropy of 2.35, plaque area of 82 mm^2. The findings would classify the plaque as stable

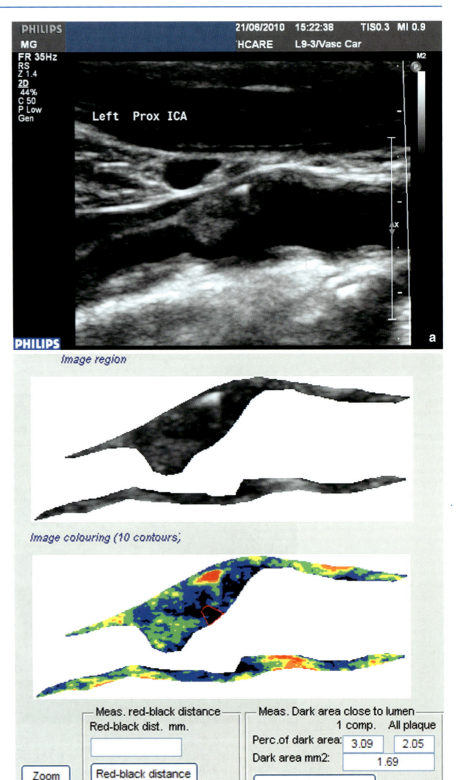

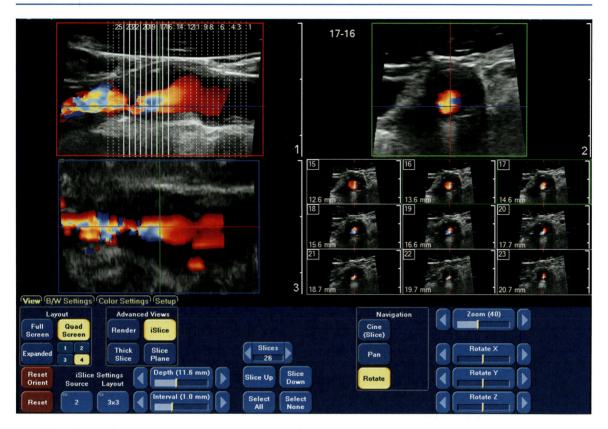

Fig. 18.22 Plaque from Fig. 18.21 with 26 transverse slices at 1 mm intervals

Table 18.2 Features produced by the carotid image analysis software from the 26 slices of the plaque shown in Fig. 18.22. This is a homogenous plaque

Slices	GSM	Plaque area (mm^2)	JBA (mm^2)	SGLDM-DEN
1	46.31	16.14	0	2.6
2	48.26	23.53	0	2.63
3	51.54	23.49	0	2.58
4	53.34	22.19	0	2.73
5	37.86	32.28	0	2.44
6	73.63	49.22	0	2.65
7	91.96	39.77	0	2.87
8	48.59	68.38	2.7	2.37
9	55.72	59.74	1.1	2.57
10	44.83	59.58	1.5	2.42
11	49.74	38.80	0	2.64
12	64.21	39.61	0	2.7
13	43.40	60.71	5.4	2.57
14	68.40	88.51	0.6	2.8
15	51.68	69.53	1.4	2.76
16	44.88	67.14	2.3	2.71

Table 18.2 (continued)

Slices	GSM	Plaque area (mm^2)	JBA (mm^2)	SGLDM-DEN
17	54.25	73.69	0	2.96
18	57.38	114.94	0	2.74
19	42.89	61.74	0	2.56
20	48.94	65.26	0	2.81
21	58.31	78.03	0	2.55
22	52.76	74.74	0	2.55
23	49.45	36.22	0	2.70
24	63.54	22.87	0	2.89
25	59.20	16.22	0	2.95
26	44.34	9.97	0	2.63

longitudinal image. There is a small JBA in transverse sections 8–10 and 13–16 of the plaque. The volumes of these are 5.3 mm^3 and 9.7 mm^3. The largest would produce an area of 2.4 mm^2 which should be visible in an appropriate longitudinal plane (not possible in the plane of the handheld probe) that would be of no significance. Finally, the SGLDM difference entropy$_w$ of 2.66 is close to the value obtained from the conventional longitudinal image.

Thus, volume imaging and analysis of this plaque indicate that apart from the plaque volume measurement, texture features obtained are similar to the ones obtained from the conventional longitudinal image and do not result in a reclassification of the plaque in terms of stability or instability. This is because this particular plaque consists of uniform texture, and, in contrast to the first example above, the conventional longitudinal image is representative of the plaque as a whole.

18.5.3 Texture Features from 2D and Corresponding 3D Images

A pilot study has been performed to determine (a) the correlation between 2D texture features and corresponding 3D texture features in a series of 12 carotid bifurcation plaques and (b) the magnitude of 3D texture measurement in symptomatic and asymptomatic plaques.

A series of six consecutive patients with symptomatic plaques (TIA or stroke) were studied. The diameter stenosis ranged from 50% to 90% NASCET (North American Symptomatic Carotid Endarterectomy Trial method of measuring stenosis). A further six patients with asymptomatic plaques matched for diameter stenosis with the symptomatic patients were also selected. For all patients, images were obtained in 2D grayscale and color as described in Chap. 12, followed by a 3D capture as described above.

Grayscale median (GSM), JBA, plaque area, and SGLDM difference entropy (SGLDM-DE) were obtained from the 2D images after image normalization and standardization for pixel density. Grayscale median weighted (GSMw), juxtaluminal plaque volume (JPV), plaque volume, and SGLDM difference entropy weighted (SGLDM-DEw) were obtained from the 3D image.

There was not any significant difference in the severity of stenosis between the symptomatic and the asymptomatic plaques (Mann–Whitney U test, $P = 0.57$). The mean stenosis was 70% in the asymptomatic and 73% in the symptomatic patients.

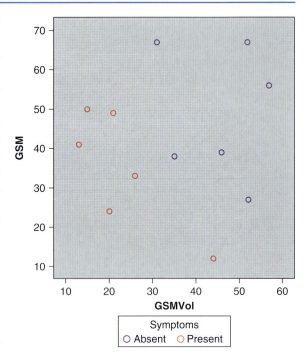

Fig. 18.23 Lack of correlation between GSM and GSMw

There was a lack of linear relationship between the GSM from the 2D images and the GSMw from the corresponding 3D images (Fig. 18.23). There was a trend (as expected) for the GSM to be lower in the symptomatic plaques, but this was not significant ($P = 0.24$). However, the GSMw was significantly lower in the symptomatic plaques ($P = 0.009$) (Fig. 18.24).

There was a moderate linear relationship ($r = 0.70$) between JBA from the 2D images and JBV from the corresponding 3D images (Fig. 18.25). The values of both JBA and JBV were higher in symptomatic than in asymptomatic plaques ($P = 0.004$ and $P = 0.002$, respectively) (Fig. 18.26).

There was a good linear relationship ($r = 0.79$) between plaque area from the 2D images and plaque volume from the corresponding 3D images (Fig. 18.27). There was a trend for higher values of plaque area in the symptomatic plaques ($P = 0.18$), but this was not present when plaque volume was measured ($P = 1.00$) (Fig. 18.28).

There was a poor linear relationship between SGLDM-DE from 2D images and SGLDM-DEw from 3D images ($r = 0.19$) (Fig. 18.29). There was a trend for lower values of SGLDM-DE, but this was not significant ($P = 0.18$). However, the SGLDM-DEw

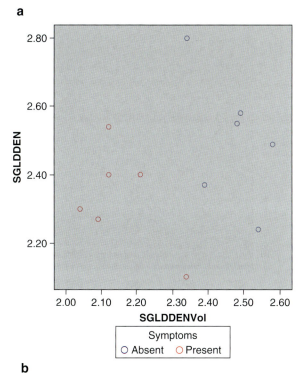

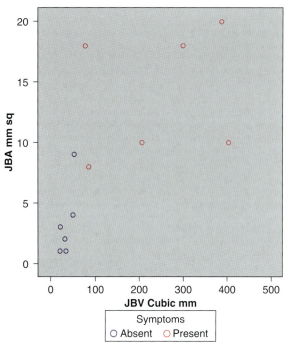

Fig. 18.25 Correlation between juxtaluminal black area (*JBA*) and juxtaluminal black volume (*JBV*)

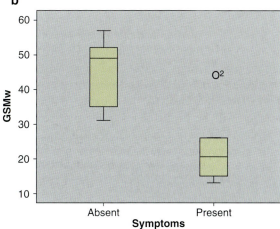

Fig. 18.24 (**a**) GSM and (**b**) GSMw in asymptomatic and symptomatic patients

was significantly lower in the symptomatic plaques ($P = 0.002$) (Fig. 18.30).

The results indicate that values of texture features based on volume data are often different and that they have the potential to improve plaque characterization. Larger studies are needed to verify this.

18.6 Implications for Future Research and Potential for Clinical Applications

The material presented in this chapter indicates that although currently tedious, 3D texture analysis is possible with the available technology and software. It demonstrates the potential to improve the precision of plaque characterization and classification in terms of plaque stability.

Much work has been done in terms of hardware and software to achieve what is currently the beginning of 3D image acquisition and texture analysis, but more is needed in terms of semi-automation to overcome some of the difficulties. Currently, mechanical acquisition probes are limited by the speed at which the scanning plane can be changed mechanically. This, in turn, leads to frequently incomplete color filling of the vessel lumen as a result of incompatibility between the speed of the cardiac cycle and the acquisition of the volume data set. However, because there are no

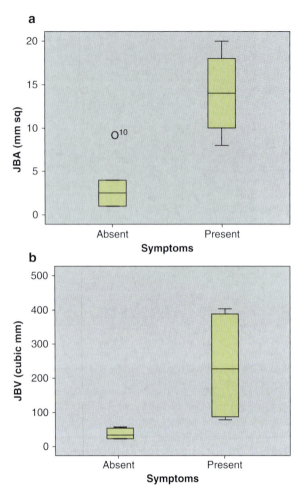

Fig. 18.26 Juxtaluminal black area (*JBA*) and juxtaluminal black volume (*JBV*) in asymptomatic and symptomatic patients

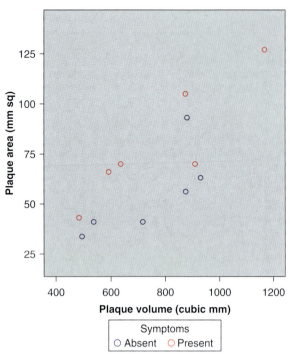

Fig. 18.27 Correlation between plaque area and plaque volume

moving parts, the new electronic acquisition probes known as matrix array transducers allow for the ultrasonic scanning plane to be moved or angled almost instantaneously, limited only by the finite speed of sound in the body. This makes this type of transducer ideal for applications where higher frame rates are necessary as in the case of live volume sonography or instantaneous 3D.

The intraobserver and interobserver reproducibilities need to be determined not only for volume but also for texture features. Training courses need to be organized that will allow vascular technologists to achieve high reproducibility. The person who is scanning needs to be familiar with the methodology of image analysis in order to know what is essentially required in the capture of volume data sets of images.

Once the expertise and high reproducibility are available, the ability of different texture features to differentiate between stable and unstable plaques should be determined. Based on the authors' experience with 2D texture analysis, it is expected that some features will be highly reproducible and some not. It is also expected that some features will be associated with symptomatic plaques and some not. What is needed is to determine which of these highly reproducible texture features are associated with symptomatic and, by definition, unstable plaques. Also, the changes in these features that occur in time as a result of therapy will need to be determined. This should result in the widespread use of 3D carotid image as a research tool.

Finally, 3D carotid imaging with plaque texture feature analysis should be used on baseline images of prospective studies similar to the asymptomatic carotid stenosis and risk of stroke study (ACSRS)[15] (Chap. 37) in order to determine the ability to stratify risk. When this is achieved, then 3D carotid imaging should enter into the clinical arena. By then, the technology and available software should be much improved. The impetus and motivation for further technological improvement have already been achieved and presented in this book.

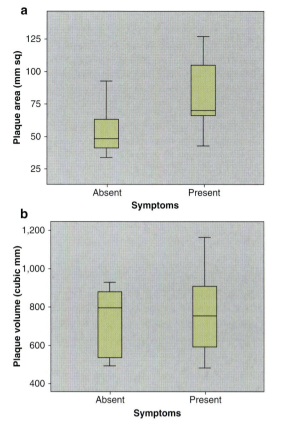

Fig. 18.28 Plaque area and plaque volume in asymptomatic and symptomatic patients

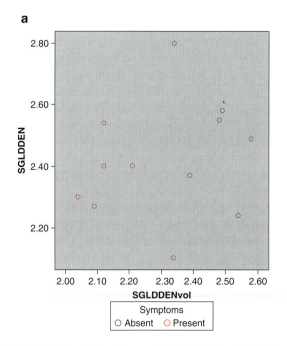

Fig. 18.29 Correlation between SGLDM-DEN and SGLDM-DENw

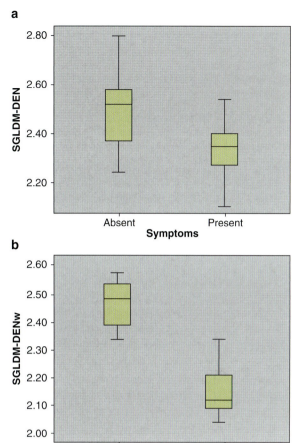

Fig. 18.30 SGLDM-DEN and SGLDM-DENw in asymptomatic and symptomatic patients

References

1. Zukowski AJ et al. The correlation between carotid plaque ulceration and cerebral infarction seen on CT scan. *J Vasc Surg*. 1984;1:782–786.
2. Carr S, Farb A, Pearce WH, Virmani R, Yao JS. Atherosclerotic plaque rupture in symptomatic carotid artery stenosis. *J Vasc Surg*. 1996;23:755–765.
3. Bassiouny HS et al. Juxtalumenal location of plaque necrosis and neoformation in symptomatic carotid stenosis. *J Vasc Surg*. 1997;26:585–594.
4. McCarthy MJ et al. Angiogenesis and the atherosclerotic carotid plaque: an association between symptomatology and plaque morphology. *J Vasc Surg*. 1999;30:261–268.
5. Redgrave JN, Gallagher P, Lovett JK, Rothwell PM. Critical cap thickness and rupture in symptomatic carotid plaques: the oxford plaque study. *Stroke*. 2008;39:1722–1729.
6. Griffin MB et al. Juxtaluminal hypoechoic area in ultrasonic images of carotid plaques and hemispheric symptoms. *J Vasc Surg*. 2010;52:69–76.
7. Shah F et al. Contrast-enhanced ultrasound imaging of atherosclerotic carotid plaque neovascularization: a new

surrogate marker of atherosclerosis? *Vasc Med*. 2007;12: 291–297.
8. Vince DG, Dixon KJ, Cothren RM, Cornhill JF. Comparison of texture analysis methods for the characterization of coronary plaques in intravascular ultrasound images. *Comput Med Imaging Graph*. 2000;24:221–229.
9. Murray SW, Stables RH, Palmer ND. Virtual histology imaging in acute coronary syndromes: useful or just a research tool? *J Invasive Cardiol*. 2010;22:84–91.
10. Nair A, Margolis MP, Kuban BD, Vince DG. Automated coronary plaque characterization with intravascular ultrasound backscatter: ex vivo validation. *EuroIntervention*. 2007;3:113–120.
11. Diethrich EB et al. Virtual histology intravascular ultrasound assessment of carotid artery disease: the Carotid Artery Plaque Virtual Histology Evaluation (CAPITAL) study. *J Endovasc Ther*. 2007;14:676–686.
12. Heliopoulos J et al. A three-dimensional ultrasonographic quantitative analysis of non-ulcerated carotid plaque morphology in symptomatic and asymptomatic carotid stenosis. *Atherosclerosis*. 2008;198:129–135.
13. Awad J, Krasinski A, Parraga G, Fenster A. Texture analysis of carotid artery atherosclerosis from three-dimensional ultrasound images. *Med Phys*. 2010;37:1382–1391.
14. Sztajzel R et al. Stratified gray-scale median analysis and color mapping of the carotid plaque. *Stroke*. 2005; 36:741–745.
15. Nicolaides AN et al. Asymptomatic internal carotid stenosis and cerebrovascular risk stratification. *J Vasc Surg*. 2010;52 (6):1486–1496.

Wall Motion Analysis

Peter R. Hoskins and Andrew W. Bradbury

19.1 Introduction

The walls of arteries move due to the changes in blood pressure and flow during the cardiac cycle. The largest and most obvious component of motion is radial, in that the diameter increases and decreases during the cardiac cycle. However, there are other important components of motion. It is increasingly apparent that arteries move longitudinally to some degree, and there is flexion and extension of the carotid arteries due to movement of the skeleton.

Movement of arteries is a natural function associated with their elasticity. The arteries expand during systole in order to accommodate the increase in blood volume following ejection from the heart, and contract during diastole as blood passes down the arterial tree. This simple reservoir effect gave rise to one of the oldest models of the arterial tree, the Windkessel. The arterial system is modelled as a simple elastic chamber which empties at a rate dependent on the wall elasticity and the downstream resistance.[1]

Movement of the arteries causes cyclic changes in the strain and stress distribution within the wall. The normal arterial system easily copes with the changes in stress. However, during the development and progression of aneurysmal or occlusive atherosclerotic disease, the arterial wall may weaken to the point where the local stress exceeds the local strength, in which case tearing or rupture of part or all of the wall will occur. In the case of the carotid arteries, plaque rupture can lead to stroke.

Measurements derived from wall motion, such as elastic modulus, strain, and stress, therefore offer the possibility of providing clinically useful diagnostic, therapeutic, and predictive (prognostic) information which cannot currently be obtained from other types of ultrasound imaging.

This chapter considers methods for estimating carotid arterial wall motion and strain ultrasound, and the estimation of quantities such as elastic modulus. A brief summary of clinical studies is provided. The first section describes the underlying mechanical principles of the arterial system.

19.2 Arterial Mechanics

In order to interpret wall motion data from the carotid artery, the general principles of the elastic behaviour of arteries and of the propagation of pressure and flow waves are described.

19.2.1 Arterial Structure

As indicated in previous chapters, arteries are composed of three layers, the intima, media, and adventitia. The innermost layer, the intima, is composed of a layer of endothelial cells which is adjacent to the flowing blood and is responsive to changes in wall shear stress and to stretching. The media is composed of smooth muscle cells, elastin fibers, collagen fibres, and ground

P.R. Hoskins (✉)
Department of Medical Physics, University of Edinburgh, Edinburgh, UK

A.W. Bradbury
Department of Vascular Surgery, University of Birmingham, Birmingham, UK

substance. The outermost layer, the adventitia, is mostly composed of collagen fibres, with smaller amounts of ground substance and fibroblasts.

From a mechanical point of view, the two main constituents of a healthy artery are the elastin and the collagen. Elastin is capable of large deformations, has a low stiffness, and the degree of stretch with increasing load is roughly linear. Collagen is stiffer, with a stiffness index that increases with the degree of stretch, due to unraveling of the collagen fibers with increased stretch.

As blood pressure increases, the load bearing is initially taken up by elastin, whereas at higher pressure, the load bearing is mainly taken up by the collagen. The overall relationship between stress and strain within an artery is elastin-like at low pressure and collagen-like at higher pressures. This leads to a nonlinear relationship between pressure and diameter, or stress and strain.[2]

19.2.2 The Arterial Pulse

The flow and pressure waves created in the systemic circulation by ejection of blood from the left ventricle travel down the aorta, and then through the distributive arterial system. Both waves are reflected by regions where there is a change in arterial impedance. Forward and reverse pressure waves combine in an additive manner resulting in increased pressure, while forward- and reverse-flow waves combine in a subtractive manner.[3-5]

Identification and separation of forward- and reverse-flow waves is possible using "wave intensity analysis."[5-7] A typical wave intensity plot from the common carotid artery is shown in Fig. 19.1, and decomposed pressure and flow waveforms in Fig. 19.2. This shows several peaks of wave intensity marked S, X, D, and R. The peak S is the early systolic wave originating from the heart associated with a rapid rise in pressure and flow. The small reverse-peak R is associated with reflected waves, probably from the distal arteriolar bed, leading to pressure augmentation and a reduction in flow. The forward-peak D is associated with a second wave originating from the heart, which is an expansion (suction) wave arising from closure of the aortic valve resulting in decrease of pressure and blood velocity within the carotid artery. There is a small forward-peak X that is not observed in the aorta, and has been hypothesised to be associated with reflection of the R-wave from a proximal site such as a bifurcation.[8]

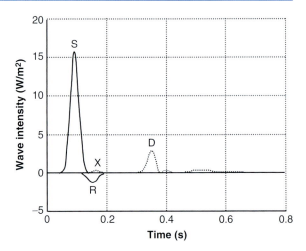

Fig. 19.1 Wave intensity plot in the common carotid artery showing a forward-traveling compression wave (*S*), backward-traveling compression wave (*R*), and two forward traveling expansion waves (*X*, *D*) (Used with permission of the American Physiological Society from Zambanini et al.[8]; permission conveyed through the Copyright Clearance Center, Inc.)

19.3 Measurement of Wall Motion

The measurement of wall motion involves detection of the movement of echoes from the wall with time, using various forms of tracking or by measurement of the wall velocity through Doppler techniques. In all cases below, ultrasound acquisition is undertaken transcutaneously using linear array transducers.

19.3.1 Motion in the Direction of the Ultrasound Beam

19.3.1.1 Single-Line Methods

Most literature on wall motion is devoted to the measurement of movement along the ultrasound beam axis. Provided that the artery lies parallel to the face of the transducer, which is usually attainable, such a measurement corresponds to the radial wall motion. Published studies have used the B-mode image, the M-mode trace, and the raw radiofrequency (RF) data. Best accuracy is obtained using the raw RF data, where movements of a fraction of a wavelength can easily be detected, in principle less than 10 μm. Early

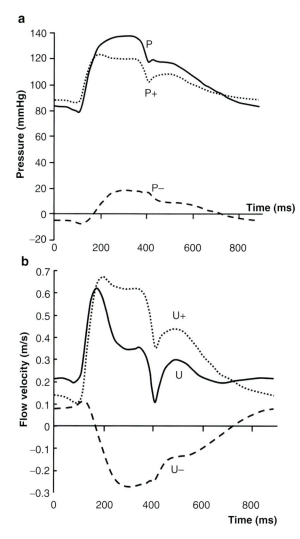

Fig. 19.2 Pressure and flow waveforms and their decomposition into forwards and backwards components using wave intensity analysis (Reprinted from Rakebrandt et al.,[9] with permission from Elsevier)

studies on processing of the RF data relied on the tracking of zero-crossings, that is the position where the RF signal passes from a positive to a negative half cycle.[10-13] A disadvantage of this approach was the need for the operator to manually position the tracking window on the vessel wall, as seen on the B-mode image. This method also suffered from loss of tracking, where slight movements of the transducer resulted in tracking "jumps" by one or more wavelengths. Other methods have relied on more sophisticated tracking of the echoes.[14-18] Further details are provided in review articles.[19]

Doppler-based methods in which the tissue velocity in the direction of the beam is estimated have been described in several papers.[20-24] Distension is provided by integration of velocity. The use of Doppler techniques to measure tissue motion is referred to as Tissue Doppler Imaging (TDI).

Both echo-tracking/correlation and Doppler methods provide distension-time waveforms. If separate tracking is performed on the near and far walls then the diameter-time waveform may be estimated. Figure 19.3 shows waveforms from the common carotid artery for a young subject and an old subject. TDI data is obtained at the near and the far wall. Figure 19.3 shows reduced velocities at the far wall, possibly as a result of restriction of movement due to the proximity of the cervical vertebrae.

From radial distension, a number of quantities can be derived, including circumferential elastic modulus, pressure, and pulse wave velocity, as described in Sect. 19.4 below.

19.3.1.2 Multi-Line Methods

Linear array scanners capable of measuring wall motion using several parallel scan lines provide information on the radial distension as a function of distance along the artery.

A system was developed which used two parallel lines to measure distension.[25] This allowed measurement of the time of travel of the distension waveform along the artery (from the foot of the waveform); hence with the known distance between the lines, pulse wave velocity (PWV) could be estimated. An improved system was able to track 16 parallel lines simultaneously.[26] Later work from the same group questioned the validity of this approach to PWV measurement,[27] stating that there was interference from a forward-going reflected wave from elsewhere within the cardiovascular system. The measurement of local PWV is further considered in a subsequent section.

Multi-line methods based on TDI were developed.[28,29] In healthy arteries, the distension pattern was relatively uniform as a function of distance along the axis. In diseased arteries, the distension pattern was complex and changed with time. Adjacent regions of the wall exhibited different motions, which would result in the creation of a strain gradient within the wall in the longitudinal direction. Figure 19.4 shows examples of wall-motion patterns in healthy and diseased arteries. It was shown that type 2 diabetes and dyslipidemia were

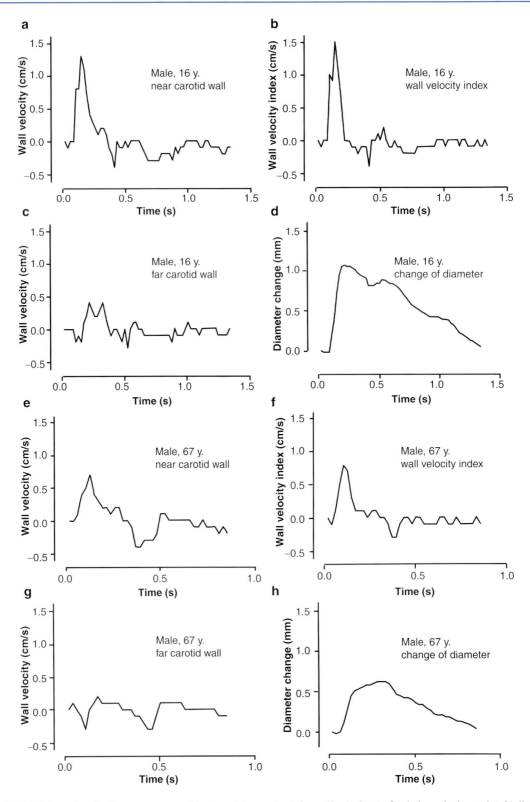

Fig. 19.3 Wall motion in the common carotid artery taken using TDI for a young and an old subject. Shown are variation with time over the cardiac cycle for; (**a**, **b**) near-wall velocity, (**c**, **d**) far-wall velocity, (**e**, **f**) relative velocity, and (**g**, **h**) diameter (Reprinted from Schmidt-Trucksass et al.,[22] with permission from Elsevier)

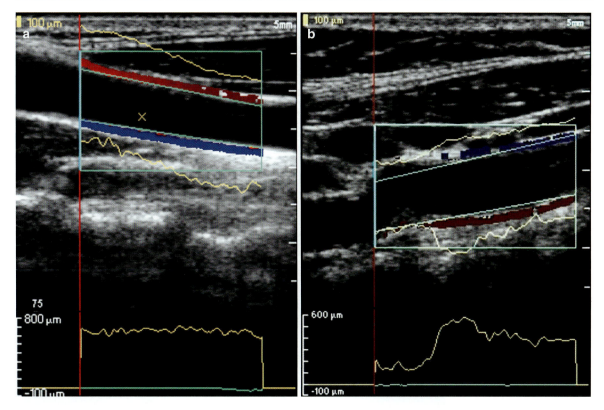

Fig. 19.4 Multi-line wall motion. *Top*: TDI images and instantaneous wall displacement (magnified). *Bottom*: maximum wall distension. (**a**) Healthy carotid showing no change in maximum distension with position along the vessel axis. (**b**) Stenosed artery showing restriction of movement within the region of the stenosis (Reprinted with permission from Dineley[30])

associated with a stiffer carotid at the level of the plaque than in an adjacent region of the common carotid, leading to an inward bending stress.[31] It was hypothesised that the repeated longitudinal bending stress may give rise to increased rupture risk.

19.3.2 Motion Transverse to the Beam

The assumption of radial-only motion in arteries is over-simplistic. Longitudinal motion of arteries had been concluded to be negligible or occurring as a result of respiration or cardiac motion. However, implanted transducers have been used to show that the carotid artery in a pig shortened and extended by 2.7% during the cardiac cycle.[32]

Quantification of motion transverse to the beam direction can be performed using speckle-tracking algorithms applied to the B-mode image.[33-36] In healthy volunteers, average longitudinal motion of the common carotid artery was 0.48–0.52 mm which was comparable to the radial motion of 0.47–0.65 mm.[35,36] These studies noted the differential longitudinal motion within the wall, with the inner (intima-medial) part of the wall demonstrating a larger displacement than the outer (adventitial) part. It was also shown that the differential displacement increased with adrenaline, and it was hypothesised that the shear stress induced between adjacent layers of the wall may be relevant in the development of a disease.[37]

19.3.3 2D Motion

Investigation of motion within the 2D plane has been performed in respect of atherosclerotic plaque. The motion may be analysed qualitatively by simple observation of the B-mode video sequence, or image processing methods involving frame to frame cross-correlation may be used to estimate displacement vectors. Observations using real-time B-mode imaging showed that some plaques moved with respect to the vessel wall during the cardiac cycle.[38] It was hypothesised that cyclic motion of the plaque would

Fig. 19.5 Surface motion calculated from consecutive frames, (**a**) asymptomatic plaque showing little motion, (**b**) symptomatic plaque showing greater motion (From Meairs.[42] Reprinted with permission)

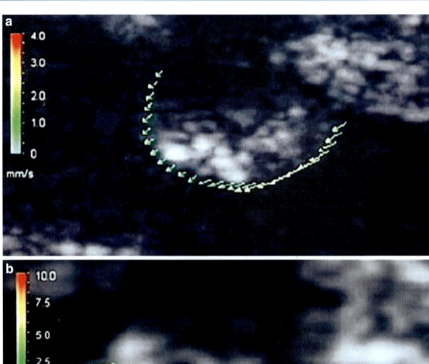
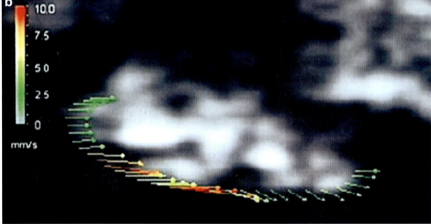

produce fissuring and rupture of the vasa-vasorum.[39,40] Subsequent studies have confirmed plaque motion in some patients.[41-45] Initial quantification suggested reduced surface velocity in asymptomatic compared to symptomatic plaque as shown in Fig. 19.5.[42]

advanced disease such as atherosclerotic plaque. Though the formulae below may be applied in advanced disease, the quantities estimated will be in error to some degree as the model assumptions are not valid. For advanced disease, allowance must be made of the 3D nature of the disease.

19.4 Quantities Derived from Radial Motion

The estimation of quantities derived from radial wall motion is described in this section. Derivations of the equations are provided in the Appendix. The underpinning assumptions are that the artery is uniform in wall thickness and elasticity, which is true in healthy arteries and possibly in early atherosclerosis and diseases which lead to generalised wall stiffening. However, these assumptions will not be true in

19.4.1 Distension

In ultrasound studies, the approach generally taken is to measure the diameter at peak systole and end diastole. The absolute distension then may be estimated:

$$\delta d = d_s - d_d \quad (19.1)$$

where d is diameter, and subscripts s and d are systole and diastole.

Alternatively, the relative distension may be estimated:

$$\delta d/d = \frac{d_s - d_d}{d_d} \quad (19.2)$$

19.4.2 Elastic Moduli

The elastic modulus E, or Young's modulus, describes the stiffness of a material. It is a fundamental property of a material, which has a single value provided that the material is homogeneous. Its calculation requires the relative distension, the wall thickness, and the diastolic and systolic blood pressure. It is common practice to measure pressure noninvasively using an arm cuff, with the assumption that brachial systolic and diastolic pressures are equal to those in the carotid arteries.[46]

$$E = \frac{d_d}{2h} \frac{(P_s - P_d)}{(d_s - d_d)/d_d} \quad (19.3)$$

where P is pressure and h is wall thickness.

Using modern ultrasound systems, the intima-media thickness (IMT) may be used as a measure of wall thickness. Older systems did not have the spatial resolution to measure wall thickness, and in deeper arteries, the wall is not easily resolved. Most studies, including those in the carotid artery, report a different index, the pressure–strain elastic modulus E_p. This was originally formulated to provide an index of arterial stiffness in circumstances where the wall thickness was difficult to measure.[47]

$$E_p = \frac{p_s - p_d}{(d_s - d_d)/d_d} \quad (19.4)$$

The pressure–strain elastic modulus is an example of an index of "structural stiffness" which describes the overall stiffness of the artery, as opposed to "material stiffness" as exemplified by elastic modulus E.[2] The value of E_p increases as wall thickness increases, due to the reduced distension which results.

Elastic modulus E and pressure–strain elastic modulus E_p are related by:

$$E = \frac{d_d}{2h} E_p \quad (19.5)$$

it was noted above that the pressure-diameter (stress/stain) behaviour of arteries is not linear, so that E and E_p provide an average value of the elastic moduli over the range of diastolic to systolic pressures.

The stiffness index β was formulated to account for the nonlinear stress–strain behavior of arteries.[48] In principle, the index should be independent of the exact pressure range over which it is measured. The stiffness index β, like the pressure–strain elastic modulus E_p, is an index of structural stiffness, as wall thickness is not accounted for.

$$\beta = \frac{ln(P_s/P_d)}{(d_s - d_d)/d_d} \quad (19.6)$$

19.4.3 Blood Pressure

The diameter and pressure waveforms in the carotid artery are similar. This has led to the diameter waveform being used as a surrogate for the pressure waveform. Calibration of the minimum and maximum diameters is performed against the systolic and diastolic pressures measured at the brachial artery using an arm cuff.[49] This approach assumes a linear relationship between diameter and pressure. It is also possible to scale the diameter waveforms to account for the nonlinear dependence of pressure on diameter.[50] The estimation of the blood pressure waveform from diameter is especially useful in the estimation of pulse wave velocity, as discussed in the next section.

19.4.4 Pulse Wave Velocity

The PWV in arteries may be measured from the "water hammer" equation:[51]

$$\frac{dP}{dV} = \rho c \quad (19.7)$$

where V is blood velocity, c is PWV, and ρ is density of blood. This equation, which is valid in the absence of reverse waves, states that the slope of the graph of pressure against blood velocity is proportional to the speed of pressure wave propagation. Early studies using this technique involved invasive flow meters and pressure transducers.[7] More recent noninvasive methods have involved estimation of blood velocity

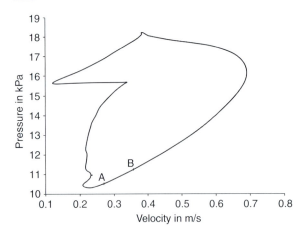

Fig. 19.6 Measurement of PWV from a diameter–velocity loop. (**a**) and (**b**) Are the start and end points of the linear portions used for the calculation of wave speed (Reprinted from Rakebrandt et al.,[9] with permission from Elsevier)

using Doppler ultrasound, with the pressure waveform measured using tonometry,[8] or the diameter waveform used as a surrogate for pressure.[9,52,53] Figure 19.6 shows a pressure–velocity loop, pressure obtained from the diameter. The linear part of the curve (marked AB) corresponds to the region in early systole where there are no reflected waves present from which the PWV is measured.

19.5 Applications

This section briefly describes wall motion and related quantities in health and disease. Details of the methods used to estimate wall motion are provided under the Sect. 19.3.

19.5.1 Healthy Arteries

Distension waveforms are shown in Fig. 19.3, using a TDI method. The overall shape indicates positive distension during systole followed by negative distension during diastole. There are minor deviations in diastole due to reflected waves, as discussed above. For a cylinder with a wall whose density does not change with stretch, it would be expected that the wall thickness would decrease with increase in diameter. Reduction in the intima-media thickness during the expansion phase in systole has been demonstrated.[54,55]

With increasing age, intima-media thickness, structural stiffness (E_p and β), and material stiffness (E) all increase. Distension decreases and diameter increases with age which is thought to be compensation for the reduced distension.

19.5.2 Atherosclerosis

Studies on subjects with carotid arterial disease demonstrated increases in several quantities when compared with healthy subjects. Diameter, intima-media thickness, and stiffness (E and E_p) were increased, for data obtained using TDI,[21] and using RF tracking.[56] However, it does not automatically follow that atherosclerosis in the individual patient is associated with increase in local stiffness[57] and previous reviews have noted contradictory findings concerning stiffness in atherosclerotic plaques.[2]

Plaque is generally associated with altered distension when compared to a (more) healthy proximal and distal artery. These differences in motion between adjacent regions may induce high strain and stress within the wall, which may be associated with disease progression and increased risk of rupture.

19.5.3 Diabetes and Blood Glucose

In a large population study, increase in fasting blood glucose was associated with increase in common carotid stiffness (elastic modulus E and pressure–strain elastic modulus E_p) in diabetic patients and in those in the pre-diabetic state.[58] Wall distension was measured using RF echo tracking. Reviews of this area[57-59] indicate that most studies show an increased stiffness in both insulin-dependent and non-insulin-dependent diabetes, and that stiffening is an early marker of the disease.

19.5.4 Other Diseases and Risk Factors

Changes in distension and elastic moduli have also been observed in hypertension, hypercholesterolemia, aortic valve disease, renal disease, and with smoking.[2,57,59]

19.6 Strain, Stress, and Elastic Modulus

The work described above has concentrated on the measurement of distension and the calculation of mechanical properties, assuming that the artery is a uniform cylinder, using simple equations. However, even in healthy arteries the uniform cylinder model is a considerable simplification and does not account for many of the known features of arteries, such as multiple layers (intima, media, and adventitia) or the presence of pre-stressing within the wall.

The uniform cylinder model is not useful in advanced disease especially with atherosclerotic plaques, which exhibit complex three-dimensional (3D) changes in geometry and mechanical properties. This section describes recent work which uses more realistic models of mechanical behavior, 3D geometry, and 3D changes in mechanical properties. These methods may offer the potential to deliver more clinically useful information based on estimated strain, elastic moduli, and stress. It will be seen below that the key to patient-specific estimation is the measurement of strain.

In order to highlight opportunities for ultrasound, this section draws on some literature from other arteries and other imaging modalities.

19.6.1 Stress Estimation in Non-diseased Arteries

The circumferential or hoop stress may be calculated using a simple equation if it is assumed that the artery consists of a uniform cylinder. Equation 19.8 assumes that the artery is thin-walled,[60] and Eq. 19.9 assumes that the artery is thick-walled.[61] For the thick-walled model, the stress σ varies with position within the wall, with the maximum value at the inner wall and minimum value at the outer wall, and Eq. 19.9 relates to the maximum stress. When the wall thickness is very small the two equations become equal.

$$\sigma = \frac{Pd}{2h} \tag{19.8}$$

$$\sigma = \frac{Pd}{2h}\left(\frac{d+2h}{d+h}\right) \tag{19.9}$$

A more complex model was developed which incorporated many of the known features of arteries – axial pre-stretching, thick-wall, nonlinear, hyperelastic, anisotropic, incompressible material with smooth muscle activity and residual stresses, with also incorporation of the mechanical contribution of individual constituents (elastin, matrix, collagen, and smooth muscle) through equations describing the stress–strain tensor.[62] Ultrasonic imaging was used to acquire data on the diameter and intima-media thickness, with pressure data acquired from pressure tonometry. It was shown that the predicted radial, circumferential and axial distension, and stress fields were similar to those found in vivo.

19.6.2 Strain Measurement

The techniques so far described have used signal processing methods which estimate displacement. The presence of high-strain regions, in the case of radial or longitudinal motion of the artery, could then be deduced from the differential displacement of adjacent regions of tissue (see Sect. 19.3 for details of ultrasound measurement methods). The measurement of the degree of strain *within* the interrogation region requires signal processing estimators which are able to measure both the displacement of tissues *and* the change in their dimension (degree of stretch or compression).

Techniques which measured strain, originally developed for use in the heart,[63] have been applied to arteries.[64] The method developed by Kanai is based on analysis of the RF data with correlation between successive received RF echoes. By assuming that the waveforms are identical, but their phase alters, changes in thickness of as little as 0.5 μm could be detected.[16]

Two-D strain estimators, which operate in both the axial and transverse directions, have been described.[65–68] For the details of the signal processing, the reader is referred to the individual papers. All of these use variations of a correlation-based approach, which search along the axial and lateral directions. Figure 19.7 shows an example of the strain image estimated from a normal carotid artery. The strain image is of interest in its own right, on the basis that stiff regions may be identified as they have low strain. The strain image may also be used in conjunction with

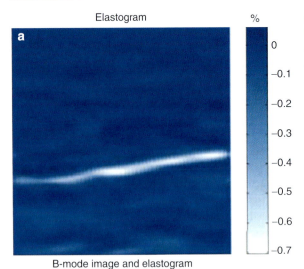

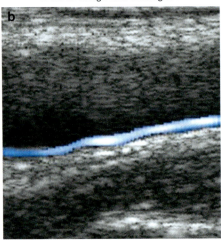

Fig. 19.7 2D strain images from the carotid artery. (**a**) Strain (%), (**b**) strain superimposed on B-mode image (Reprinted with permission from Maurice et al.[66])

computational modeling of the mechanical behavior of the artery in order to estimate the stress field and the local elastic moduli, as described in the next section.

19.6.3 Elastic Modulus and Stress Estimation in Plaque

The estimations of elastic moduli and stress have been considered, under the assumption that the artery can be modelled as a uniform cylinder or concentric series of cylinders. A more realistic model, capable of being used in focal disease, ideally, would take into account spatial variations in geometry and mechanical properties. Work in this area has involved computational modelling of the mechanical behaviour of the arterial wall (called "solid modelling"), in which variations in the elastic modulus, strain, and stress with position in space may be accounted for.

Estimation of stress in plaque has been performed using 2D cross-sectional data from magnetic resonance imaging (MRI)[69,70] and 3D data using MRI also.[71-73] This has involved identification of relevant features of the plaque (such as the lumen, lipid pool, wall, and fibrous cap), imposition of elastic modulus values from the literature and use of solid modelling to estimate the tissue stress. This approach is called "forward modelling" in which the geometry and elastic moduli are used as input to the computational model, and the output is the deformation, strain, and the stress distribution.

A more challenging method is called "inverse modelling," where the input is the geometry and the strain data from imaging, and the output is the elastic modulus. This approach has compared the strain predicted by solid modelling with the strain measured from imaging. The difference in strain is used to adjust the values of elastic moduli in the model, followed by iteration of the process until the predicted and measured strain agree to within limits set by the operator. To date, the only published work in this area has been performed using intravascular ultrasound.[74,75]

Forward and inverse modelling may in time become used in the carotid arteries for the estimation of stress and elastic modulus from ultrasound strain data. Further details of these methods can be found in review articles.[76]

19.7 Induced Vibration and Wall Motion

The final class of wall motions that is considered is induced vibrations and wall motion induced by non-physiologic means. Clinical medicine has used the sound of "bruits" from carotid arteries as evidence of disease. This is thought to be vibration of the wall in the post-stenotic region arising from turbulence. Direct evaluation of this effect using ultrasound recorded a wall displacement of 100 μm, and the production of audio frequencies in the range 100–145 Hz at peak systole.[77]

Radiation force has been used to induce wall movement. When combined with imaging pulses to estimate wall movement an image of strain may be produced as

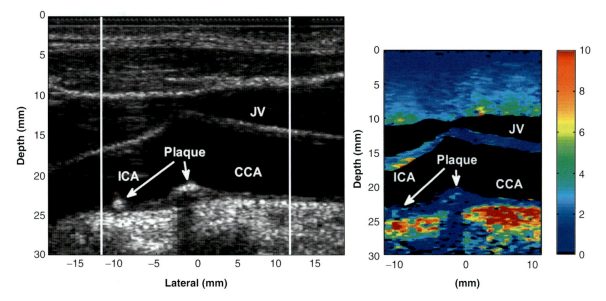

Fig. 19.8 B-mode and corresponding acoustic radiation force imaging (ARFI) strain image of a heterogeneous plaque. The plaque contains small, compliant regions in the largest portions of the plaque (indicated by the *arrows* in the right image, located in the bifurcation and internal carotid artery [ICA]). The size of these regions is approximately 0.5 mm (Reprinted from Dahl et al.,[78] with permission from Elsevier)

shown in Fig. 19.8.[78] The wall moves over a period of about 10–20 ms, during which time the artery is virtually stationary. An external vibrator has been used to induce vibrations in the carotid wall[79] which attenuate after a few cm. An ultrasound system may then be used to measure the local pulse wave velocity.

19.8 Conclusion

It has been shown that wall motion in health and disease is complex and that measurements may be made, of distension, stress, and elastic modulus, which may have diagnostic use. Most of the literature to date has involved radial wall motion, with elastic moduli estimated using an assumed model which treats the artery as a uniform cylinder. This has restricted the applicability of quantitative analysis, mostly to healthy arteries and early disease. Recent techniques have been introduced for tracking transverse motions, estimation of 2D strain, and of integration with solid modelling. These offer potential for exploiting more complex wall motions and for being applicable in focal disease such as atherosclerosis.

Appendix Derivation of Formulae

The derivation of several quantities which may be estimated from the measured radial distension is presented. The underlying model is that the artery is a uniform cylinder. Further details of relevant equations (Moens–Korteweg, Bramwell–Hill) are provided in a review article.[51]

Pulse Wave Velocity, Elastic Modulus and Pressure–Strain Elastic Modulus

The distension coefficient DC describes the change in cross sectional area of the artery which occurs as a result of the local increase in pressure:

$$\mathrm{DC} = \frac{\Delta A / A}{\Delta P}$$

where A is cross-sectional area, ΔA is the change in area occurring as a result of change in blood pressure ΔP.

The distension coefficient may also be written in terms of diameter d and change in diameter Δd:

$$DC = \frac{2\Delta d/d}{\Delta P} \quad (19.10)$$

The Moens-Korteweg equation describes the propagation of pressure waves down a thin-walled elastic tube. This relates the speed of propagation c to the elastic modulus E:

$$c = \sqrt{\frac{Eh}{\rho d}} \quad (19.11)$$

where h is wall thickness, ρ is density of blood and d is diameter.

The speed of propagation of the arterial pressure wave, known as the "pulse wave velocity" (PWV) may also be related to the distension coefficient by the Bramwell-Hill equation:

$$c = \sqrt{\frac{1}{\rho \times DC}} \quad (19.12)$$

Rearranging Eqs. 19.11 and 19.12 gives:

$$E = \frac{d}{h \times DC} \quad (19.13)$$

Incorporating DC from Eq. 19.10 gives:

$$E = \frac{d}{2h} \cdot \frac{\Delta P}{\Delta d/d}$$

The pressure–strain elastic modulus[47] E_p is defined by:

$$E_p = \frac{\Delta p}{\Delta d/d} \quad (19.14)$$

In terms of distension coefficient this gives:

$$E_p = \frac{2}{DC}$$

Elastic modulus E and pressure–strain elastic modulus E are related by the equation:

$$E = \frac{d}{2h} E_p \quad (19.15)$$

Incorporation of Finite Wall Thickness

In the literature, slightly different versions of these equations may be found. Equations 19.11 and 19.12 relate to a thin-walled model. Allowing for the thickness of the wall in arteries leads to a modified equation for PWV[80]:

$$c = \sqrt{\frac{Eh}{\rho d(1-v^2)}}$$

where v is the Poisson's ratio of the artery. The Poisson's ratio describes the extent to which the density of a material changes when it is compressed or stretched. Arteries can be considered to be incompressible in which case the Poisson's ratio is 0.5. Equations 19.11, 19.13, and 19.15 then become:

$$c = \sqrt{\frac{Eh}{0.75\rho d}}$$

$$E = \frac{0.75d}{h \times DC}$$

$$E = \frac{0.375d}{h} E_p$$

The inclusion of Poisson's ratio increases PWV by 15%, and reduces E by 25%. When comparing values of E from different papers, the reader should look carefully which equation for E has been used.

The approach taken above calculates a single value of E, essentially assuming that there is a linear relationship between applied pressure and distension. In practice, the relationship is nonlinear, so that the value of E depends on the pressure. In this case, the elastic modulus is termed the "incremental elastic modulus" or E_{inc}. Thus, a full description of the behavior of the artery would require specification of the incremental elastic modulus as a function of pressure from diastole to systole.

Stiffness Index

It was shown[48] for a number of different arteries (vertebral, carotid, femoral) that there was an exponential relationship between diameter and intraluminal pressure, so that Eq. 19.16 below provides a good description of behaviour.

$$P = P_o \bullet e^{\beta\left(\frac{d_s - d_o}{d_o}\right)} \qquad (19.16)$$

where subscript s refers to the standard pressure, and β is a constant.

Rearranging Eq. 19.16 provides a definition for the stiffness index β which, unlike incremental elastic modulus, should not vary within the cardiac cycle:

$$\beta = \frac{ln(P_0/P)}{(d - d_o)/d} \qquad (19.17)$$

References

1. Westerhof N, Lankhaar JW, Westerhof BE. The arterial windkessel. *Med Biol Eng Comput.* 2009;47:131–141.
2. Hayashi K. Experimental approaches on measuring the mechanical-properties and constitutive laws of arterial-walls. *J Biomech Eng.* 1993;115:481–488.
3. Westerhof N, Sipkema P, Bos GC, van den Elzinga G. Forward and backward waves in arterial system. *Cardiovasc Res.* 1972;6:648–656.
4. Murgo JP, Col MC, Westerhof N, Giolma JP, Altobelli SA. Manipulation of ascending aortic pressure and flow waveform reflections with the valsalva manoeuvre: relationship to input impedance. *Circulation.* 1981;63:122–132.
5. Parker KH, Jones CJH. Forward and backward running waves in the arteries – analysis using the method of characteristics. *J Biomech Eng.* 1990;112:322–326.
6. Parker KH. An introduction to wave intensity analysis. *Med Biol Eng Comput.* 2009;47:175–188.
7. Khir AW, O'Brien A, Gibbs JSR, Parker KH. Determination of wave speed and wave separation in the arteries. *J Biomech.* 2001;34:1145–1155.
8. Zambanini A, Cunningham SL, Parker KH, Khir AW, Thom SAM, Hughes AD. Wave-energy patterns in carotid, brachial, and radial arteries: a noninvasive approach using wave-intensity analysis. *Am J Physiol-Heart Circ Physiol.* 2005;289:H270-H276.
9. Rakebrandt F, Palombo C, Swampillai J, Schon F, Donald A, Kozakova M, Kato K, Fraser AG. Arterial wave intensity and ventricular-arterial coupling by vascular ultrasound: rationale and methods for the automated analysis of forwards and backwards running waves. *Ultrasound Med Biol.* 2009;35: 266–277.
10. Hokanson DE, Strandness DE, Sumner DS, Mozersky DJ. Phase-locked echo tracking system for recording arterial diameter changes in-vivo. *J Appl Physiol.* 1972;32:728–733.
11. Groves DH, Powalowski T, White DN. A digital technique for tracking moving interfaces. *Ultrasound Med Biol.* 1982;8:185–190.
12. Kawasaki T, Sasayama S, Yagi S, Asakawa T, Hirai T. Non-invasive assessment of the age related changes in stiffness of major branches of the human arteries. *Cardiovasc Res.* 1987;21:678–687.
13. Benthin M, Dahl P, Ruzicka R, Lindstrom K. Calculation of pulse-wave velocity using cross correlation – effects of reflexes in the arterial tree. *Ultrasound Med Biol.* 1991;17:461–469.
14. Hoeks APG, Brands PJ, Smeets FAM, Reneman RS. Assessment of the distensibility of superficial arteries. *Ultrasound Med Biol.* 1990;16:121–128.
15. de Jong PGM, Arts T, Hoeks APG, Reneman RS. Determination of tissue motion velocity by correlation interpolation of pulsed ultrasonic echo signals. *Ultrason Imaging.* 1990;12:84–98.
16. Kanai H, Koiwa Y, Zhang JP. Real-time measurements of local myocardium motion and arterial wall thickening. *IEEE Trans Ultrason Ferroelectr Freq Control.* 1999;46: 1229–1241.
17. Tortoli P, Bettarini R, Guidi F, Andreuccetti F, Righi D. A simplified approach for real-time detection of arterial wall velocity and distension. *IEEE Trans Ultrason Ferroelectr Freq Control.* 2001;48:1005–1012.
18. Rabben SI, Bjaerum S, Sorhus V, Torp H. Ultrasound-based vessel wall tracking: an auto-correlation technique with RF center frequency estimation. *Ultrasound Med Biol.* 2002;28:507–517.
19. Hoeks APG, Brands PJ, Willigers JM, Reneman RS. Non-invasive measurement of mechanical properties of arteries in health and disease. *J Eng Med.* 1999;213:195–202.
20. Claridge MW et al. A reproducibility study of a novel ultrasound-based system to calculate indices of arterial stiffness. *Ultrasound Med Biol.* 2008;34:215–220.
21. Claridge MW et al. Measurement of arterial stiffness in patients with peripheral arterial disease: are changes in vessel wall more sensitive than intima-media thickness? *Atherosclerosis.* 2009;205:477–480.
22. Schmidt-Trucksass A et al. Assessment of carotid wall motion and stiffness with tissue Doppler imaging. *Ultrasound Med Biol.* 1998;24:639–646.
23. Schmidt-Trucksass A et al. Relation of leisure-time physical activity to structural and functional arterial properties of the common carotid artery in male subjects. *Atherosclerosis.* 1999;145:107–114.
24. Schmidt-Trucksass A et al. Structural, functional, and hemodynamic changes of the common carotid artery with age in male subjects. *Arterioscler Thromb Vasc Biol.* 1999;19: 1091–1097.
25. Brands PJ, Willigers JM, Ledoux LAF, Reneman RS, Hoeks APG. A noninvasive method to estimate pulse wave velocity in arteries locally by means of ultrasound. *Ultrasound Med Biol.* 1998;23:1325–1335.
26. Meinders JM, Kornet L, Brands PJ, Hoeks APG. Assessment of local pulse wave velocity in arteries using 2D distension waveforms. *Ultrason Imaging.* 2001;23:199–215.
27. Hermeling E, Reesink KD, Reneman RS, Hoeks APG. Confluence of incident and reflected waves interferes with systolic foot detection of the carotid artery distension waveform. *J Hypertens.* 2008;26:2374–2380.
28. Bonnefous O. Stenoses dynamics with ultrasonic wall motion images. *Proc IEEE Ultrason Symp.* 1994;3: 1709–1712.

29. Bonnefous O, Montaudon M, Sananes JC, Denis E. Non invasive echographic techniques for arterial wall characterization. *Proc IEEE Ultrason Symp.* 1996;3:1059–1064.
30. Dineley JA. *Doppler Ultrasound Measurement of Arterial Wall Motion (AWM)* [Ph.D. thesis]. Edinburgh: Edinburgh University Library; 2005.
31. Paini A et al. Multiaxial mechanical characteristics of carotid plaque – analysis by multiarray echotracking system. *Stroke.* 2007;38:117–123.
32. Tozzi P, Hayoz D, Oedman C, Mallabiabarrena I, Von Segesser LK. Systolic axial artery length reduction: an overlooked phenomenon in vivo. *Am J Physiol Heart Circ Physiol.* 2001;280:H2300-H2305.
33. Persson M et al. A new non-invasive ultrasonic method for simultaneous measurements of longitudinal and radial arterial watt movements: first in vivo trial. *Clin Physiol Funct Imaging.* 2003;23:247–251.
34. Cinthio M et al. Evaluation of an ultrasonic echo-tracking method for measurements of arterial wall movements in two dimensions. *IEEE Trans Ultrason Ferroelectr Freq Control.* 2005;52:1300–1311.
35. Cinthio M et al. Longitudinal movements and resulting shear strain of the arterial wall. *Am J Physiol Heart Circ Physiol.* 2006;291:H394-H402.
36. Golemati S et al. Carotid artery wall motion estimated from B-mode ultrasound using region tracking and block matching. *Ultrasound Med Biol.* 2003;29:387–399.
37. Ahlgren AR et al. Effects of adrenaline on longitudinal arterial wall movements and resulting intramural shear strain: a first report. *Clin Physiol Funct Imaging.* 2009;29:353–359.
38. White A, Mccarty K, Morgan R, Wilkins P, Woodcock JP. Investigation of carotid plaque motility. In: Price R, Evans JA, eds. *Blood Flow Measurement in Clinical Diagnosis.* London: Biological Engineering Society; 1988:109–115.
39. Woodcock JP. Characterisation of the atheromatous plaque in the carotid. *Clin Phys Physiol Meas.* 1989;10(Suppl A):45–49.
40. Falk E. Why do plaque rupture? *Circulation.* 1992;86:30–42.
41. Iannuzzi A et al. Ultrasonographic correlates of carotid atherosclerosis in transient ischemic attack and stroke. *Stroke.* 1995;26:614–619.
42. Meairs S, Hennerici M. Four-dimensional ultrasonographic characterization of plaque surface motion in patients with symptomatic and asymptomatic carotid artery stenosis. *Stroke.* 1999;30:1807–1813.
43. Chan KL. 2 Approaches to motion analysis of the ultrasound image sequence of carotid atheromatous plaque. *Ultrasonics.* 1993;31:117–123.
44. Bang J et al. A new method for analysis of motion of carotid plaques from RF ultrasound images. *Ultrasound Med Biol.* 2003;29:967–976.
45. Dahl T, Bang J, Ushakova A, Lydersen S, Myhre HO. Parameters describing motion in carotid artery plaques from ultrasound examination: a reproducibility study. *Ultrasound Med Biol.* 2004;30:1133–1143.
46. Segers P et al. Carotid tonometry versus synthesized aorta pressure waves for the estimation of central systolic blood pressure and augmentation index. *Am J Hypertens.* 2005;18:1168–1173.
47. Peterson LH, Jensen RE, Parnell J. Mechanical properties of arteries in vivo. *Circ Res.* 1960;8:622–639.
48. Hayashi K, Handa H, Nagasawa S, Okumura A, Moritake K. Stiffness and elastic behavior of human intra-cranial and extra-cranial arteries. *J Biomech.* 1980;13:175–184.
49. Sugawara M, Niki K, Furuhata H, Ohnishi S, Suzuki S. Relationship between the pressure and diameter of the carotid artery in humans. *Heart Vessels.* 2000;15:49–51.
50. Meinders JM, Hoeks APG. Simultaneous assessment of diameter and pressure waveforms in the carotid artery. *Ultrasound Med Biol.* 2004;30:147–154.
51. Parker KH. A brief history of arterial wave mechanics. *Med Biol Eng Comput.* 2009;47:111–118.
52. Ohte N et al. Clinical usefulness of carotid arterial wave intensity in assessing left ventricular systolic and early diastolic performance. *Heart Vessels.* 2003;18:107–111.
53. Rabben SI et al. An ultrasound-based method for determining pulse wave velocity in superficial arteries. *J Biomech.* 2004;37:1615–1622.
54. Meinders JM, Kornet L, Hoeks APG. Assessment of spatial inhomogeneities in intima media thickness along an arterial segment using its dynamic behaviour. *Am J Physiol Heart Circ Physiol.* 2003;285:H384-H391.
55. Segers P et al. Functional analysis of the common carotid artery: relative distension differences over the vessel wall measured in vivo. *J Hypertens.* 2004;22:973–981.
56. van Popele NM et al. Association between arterial stiffness and atherosclerosis - the Rotterdam study. *Stroke.* 2001;32:454–460.
57. Reneman RS, Meinders JM, Hoeks APG. Non-invasive ultrasound in arterial wall dynamics in humans: what have we learned and what remains to be solved. *Eur Heart J.* 2005;26:960–966.
58. Salomaa V, Riley W, Kark JD, Nardo C, Folsom AR. Non-insulin-dependent diabetes-mellitus and fasting glucose and insulin concentrations are associated with arterial stiffness indexes – the ARIC study. *Circulation.* 1995;91:1432–1443.
59. Cheng KS, Baker CR, Hamilton G, Hoeks APG, Seifalian AM. Arterial elastic properties and cardiovascular risk/event. *Eur J Vasc Endovasc Surg.* 2002;24:383–397.
60. Williams MJA, Stewart RAH, Low CJS, Wilkins GT. Assessment of the mechanical properties of coronary arteries using intravascular ultrasound: an in vivo study. *Int J Cardiovasc Imaging.* 1999;15:287–294.
61. Tajaddini A et al. Impact of age and hyperglycemia on the mechanical behavior of intact human coronary arteries: an ex vivo intravascular ultrasound study. *Am J Physiol Heart Circ Physiol.* 2005;288:H250-H255.
62. Masson I, Boutouyrie P, Laurent S, Humphrey JD, Zidi M. Characterization of arterial wall mechanical behavior and stresses from human clinical data. *J Biomech.* 2008;41:2618–2627.
63. Kanai H, Hasegawa H, Chubachi N, Koiwa Y, Tanaka M. Noninvasive evaluation of local myocardial thickening and its color coded imaging. *IEEE Trans Ultrason Ferroelectr Freq Control.* 1997;44:752–768.
64. Kanai H, Hasegawa H, Ichiki M, Tezuka F, Koiwa Y. Elasticity imaging of atheroma with transcutaneous ultrasound preliminary study. *Circulation.* 2003;107:3018–3021.

65. Shi HR et al. Preliminary in vivo atherosclerotic carotid plaque characterization using the accumulated axial strain and relative lateral shift strain indices. *Phys Med Biol.* 2008;53:6377–6394.
66. Maurice RL et al. Non-invasive high-frequency vascular ultrasound elastography. *Phys Med Biol.* 2005;50:1611–1628.
67. Schmitt C, Soulez G, Maurice RL, Giroux MF, Cloutier G. Noninvasive vascular elastography: toward a complementary characterization tool of atherosclerosis in carotid arteries. *Ultrasound Med Biol.* 2007;33:1841–1858.
68. Maurice RL, Soulez G, Giroux MF, Cloutier G. Noninvasive vascular elastography for carotid artery characterization on subjects without previous history of atherosclerosis. *Med Phys.* 2008;35:3436–3443.
69. Li ZY et al. Stress analysis of carotid plaque rupture based on in vivo high resolution MRI. *J Biomech.* 2006;39:2611–2622.
70. Tang TY et al. Correlation of carotid atheromatous plaque inflammation with biomechanical stress: utility of USPIO enhanced MR imaging and finite element analysis. *Atherosclerosis.* 2008;196:879–887.
71. Tang DL et al. A negative correlation between human carotid atherosclerotic plaque progression and plaque wall stress: in vivo MRI-based 2D/3D FSI models. *J Biomech.* 2008;41:727–736.
72. Kock SA et al. Mechanical stresses in carotid plaques using MRI-based fluid-structure interaction models. *J Biomech.* 2008;41:1651–1658.
73. Gao H, Long Q, Graves M, Gillard JH, Li ZY. Carotid arterial plaque stress analysis using fluid-structure interactive simulation based on in-vivo magnetic resonance images of four patients. *J Biomech.* 2009;42:1416–1423.
74. Chandran KB et al. A method for in-vivo analysis for regional arterial wall material property alterations with atherosclerosis: preliminary results. *Med Eng Phys.* 2003;25:289–298.
75. Baldewsing RA et al. An inverse method for imaging the local elasticity of atherosclerotic coronary plaques. *IEEE Trans Inf Technol Biomed.* 2008;12:277–289.
76. Hoskins PR, Hardman D. 3D imaging and computational modelling for estimation of wall stress in diseased arteries. *Brit J Radiol* 2009;82:S3–S17
77. Plett MI et al. In vivo ultrasonic measurement of tissue vibration at a stenosis: a case study. *Ultrasound Med Biol.* 2007;27:1049–1058.
78. Dahl JJ, Dumont DM, Allen JD, Miller EM, Trahey GE. Acoustic radiation force impulse imaging for non-invasive characterization of carotid artery atherosclerotic plaques: a feasibility study. *Ultrasound Med Biol.* 2009;35:707–716.
79. Zhang XM, Kinnick RR, Fatemi M, Greenleaf JF. Noninvasive method for estimation of complex elastic modulus of arterial vessels. *IEEE Trans Ultrason Ferroelectr Freq Control.* 2005;52:642–652.
80. Bergel DH. The static elastic properties of the arterial wall. *J Physiol (Lond).* 1961;156:445–457.

Noninvasive Carotid Elastography

Hendrik H.G. Hansen and Chris L. de Korte

20.1 Introduction

As indicated in Chaps. 1 and 2, atherosclerosis is a systemic disease in which lipid-rich content is deposited in the arterial vessel wall. The accumulations of the lipid-rich material in the vessel wall are referred to as plaques. Usually, plaques start of as so-called fatty streaks, small accumulations of atherogenic lipoproteins, macrophages, white blood cells, and smooth muscle cells in the intima. Over time, these fatty streaks can disappear or develop into either stable or vulnerable plaques.[1] The differences in composition and geometry of stable and vulnerable plaques are illustrated in Fig. 20.1. A stable plaque has a small lipid pool that contains few macrophages and is separated from the blood by a thick fibrous cap. Vulnerable plaques are characterized by a large lipid pool rich with macrophages that are covered by a thin fibrous cap.[2] Another difference between both plaque types is that stable plaques slowly tend to grow into the luminal area, whereas most of the lumen area is maintained for vulnerable plaques.[3,4] The slow decrease in lumen area during growth of stable plaques, which decreases oxygen supply to tissue, is often recognized from clinical symptoms such as angina pectoris or intermittent claudication. Although severe occlusion of arteries will eventually result in ischemia and tissue necrosis, the aforementioned clinical symptoms can often be used as a warning and give a surgeon time to perform catheterization, stenting, or bypass surgery before it is too late. Based on the schematic representation of Fig. 20.1, vulnerable plaques seem less dangerous since the luminal area is not reduced. However, forces exerted by the pulsating blood flow can lead to rupture of the thin cap, leading to exposure of the lipid pool content to the blood flow. When this happens, a thrombus (blood clot) is formed.[5] In turn, this thrombus can break loose and cause a complete occlusion of a smaller artery downstream. This sudden occlusion of arteries often without preceding clinical symptoms is exactly what happens during a myocardial infarction or stroke. The majority of myocardial infarctions and strokes are caused by rupture of plaques in the coronary and carotid arteries, respectively.[6–8] Early identification of vulnerable plaques is therefore of crucial importance to prevent morbidity andmortality and a well-addressed topic in literature.[9–14]

A promising technique for vulnerable plaque detection is ultrasound strain imaging. Ultrasound strain imaging was first described by J. Ophir et al. in 1991.[15] The technique enables assessing the local strain in tissue by ultrasound. At first, the technique was mainly applied to detect hard and soft tumors within breast, prostate, thyroid, and liver tissue. The tissue was strained by application of an external force. Given its power to differentiate between various tissues, the technique was also applied for atherosclerotic plaque detection. de Korte et al. were one of the first groups to apply the technique intravascularly to distinguish stable from vulnerable plaques in coronary arteries.[16,17] Instead of applying an external force to deform the tissue, the strains caused by the blood flow pulsations were used. Although the intravascular

H.H.G. Hansen (✉) • C.L. de Korte
Clinical Physics Laboratory, Department of Pediatrics, Radboud University Nijmegen Medical Centre, Njimegen, The Netherlands

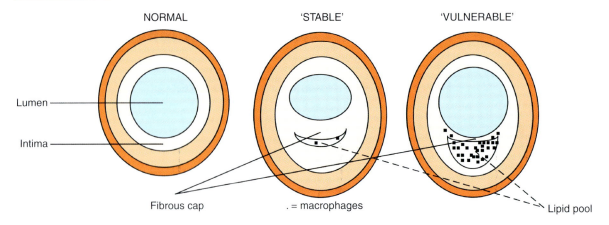

Fig. 20.1 Schematic representations of a healthy vessel, a vessel with a stable plaque, and a vessel with a vulnerable plaque

results were convincing, its intravascular nature restricts the technique to the cath-lab and prevents the technique from being applied as a screening tool. However, as equipment and strain imaging techniques improved, the concept of noninvasive strain imaging also became technically feasible. At this moment, multiple approaches for noninvasive ultrasound strain imaging have already been developed,[10,18–21] and preliminary in vivo results have just been published. The availability of noninvasive ultrasound strain imaging promises to enable early screening of populations at risk for vulnerable plaques, albeit no longer in coronary arteries, but for superficial arteries like the carotid artery and the femoral artery.

This chapter will first explain the basics of ultrasonic strain imaging. Next, a summary of the achievements obtained with intravascular ultrasound strain imaging will be given. Afterward, various methods for noninvasive ultrasound strain imaging will be presented together with an overview of the results obtained so far.

20.2 Principles of Ultrasound Strain Imaging

Strain imaging is based on the principle that soft tissue deforms more than hard tissue when an external force is applied (Fig. 20.2). To measure strain, a registration of a tissue is made before applying a force, the pre-deformation state, and after applying a force, the post-deformation state. From a comparison of the pre- and post-deformation registration, the local tissue displacements are obtained, which can be converted into tissue strains by first-order spatial derivation.

J. Ophir and coworkers were first to describe the concept of strain imaging using ultrasound data.[15] Ultrasound data is very suitable for strain imaging, due to the periodicity of ultrasound. Figure 20.3 shows simulated ultrasound signals for the tissue in Fig. 20.2 in pre- and post-deformation states. Ophir and coworkers determined the local tissue displacements by cross-correlating one-dimensional windows of pre- and post-deformation radio-frequency data. An example of the cross-correlation function for the marked windows is shown also in Fig. 20.3. The location of the peak of the normalized cross-correlation corresponds to the time shift in the radio-frequency (rf) signal, δt, caused by the displacement of the tissue. Since time corresponds to depth in ultrasound, the time shift can be translated into a local tissue displacement for the tissue in the window of interest. By repeating this cross-correlation procedure for multiple depths, the displacement field in the direction of the ultrasound beam can be estimated. In the next step, spatial derivation can be applied to obtain strains. Instead of direct point-to-point spatial derivation, often a least-squares strain estimator (LSQSE) is applied.[22] An LSQSE calculates a least-squares linear fit through the displacement values. The slope of this fit then corresponds to the strain. This is done to reduce the error in displacement estimates caused by high frequent noise.

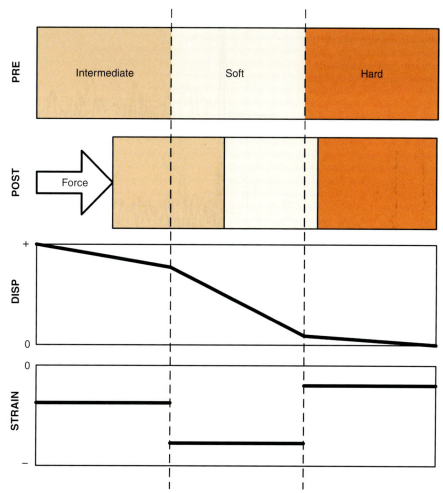

Fig. 20.2 Principle of strain imaging: the softer the tissue, the higher the strain. Strain can be calculated by comparing the registration of a tissue before and after an external force is applied (note that strain is negative since the tissue is "compressed")

20.3 Intravascular Ultrasound Strain Imaging

In the subsequent couple of years, ultrasound strain imaging techniques improved, and the range of applications increased. Since plaque vulnerability is mainly determined by its morphology and composition, and the fatty contents of the lipid pool and fibrotic tissue have different mechanical properties, strain imaging also became interesting for unstable plaque detection.

20.3.1 Methods and Results

The first reports on intravascular ultrasound (IVUS) strain imaging came from three different research groups.[23–25] The main principle of the technique is summarized in Fig. 20.4. An IVUS catheter was inserted in a diseased coronary artery, and rf A-line data were recorded for the full circumference for a low and a high intraluminal pressure, the pre- and post-deformation images, respectively. Next, radial strains were calculated by applying the aforementioned cross-correlation technique to each separate A-line. The strain image was plotted next to the IVUS echograms. A different way of visualization is by plotting only the inner ring of strain values (the rupture-prone region) on top of the brightness mode (B-mode) data.[26] Such an image is referred to as a palpogram.

The performance of the technique was first tested on homogeneous vessel-mimicking phantoms and vessel-mimicking phantoms with layers representing soft or hard plaques. The strain in the homogeneous vessel was in accordance with theory. Furthermore,

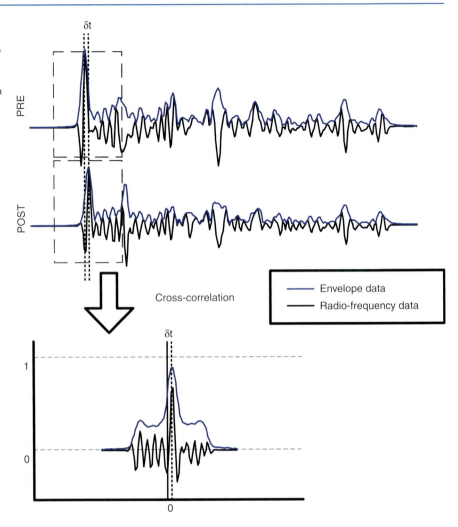

Fig. 20.3 Traditionally, displacements and strains were calculated locally by 1D cross-correlation of pre- and post-deformation ultrasound radio-frequency/envelope data

the harder and softer plaques were correctly identified.[23] Next, the technique was tested in vitro on excised coronary and femoral arteries. The obtained radial strain maps were locally compared with corresponding histology. It was shown that IVUS strain imaging enabled differentiation between fibrous, fatty, and fibro-fatty plaques based on their strain values.[16] Then, the step toward in vivo imaging was taken. IVUS strain imaging also proved to be successful for differentiating between fibrous and fatty materials using data from atherosclerotic iliac and femoral arteries of a Yucatan minipig.[27] In a later study, its ability to correctly classify vulnerable and stable plaques was investigated. IVUS strain data from 54 cross-sectional recordings of excised coronary arteries were compared with vulnerable plaque classification based on histology. It was shown that the technique identified vulnerable plaques in vitro with a sensitivity of 88% and specificity of 89%.[28] Next, the correlation between three-dimensional IVUS strain imaging and clinical symptoms was investigated.[29] Three-dimensional IVUS palpograms were estimated from rf data obtained during catheter pullback for 55 patients. A high correlation was found between the number of high-strain spots and the clinical symptoms of the patients. Patients suffering from unstable angina or from an acute myocardial infarction had significantly more high-strain spots than patients with stable angina.

The number of studies that confirm the usefulness of intravascular ultrasound strain imaging of the coronary arteries for vulnerable plaque detection is still increasing. However, a major drawback of IVUS elastography that will always remain is its invasive

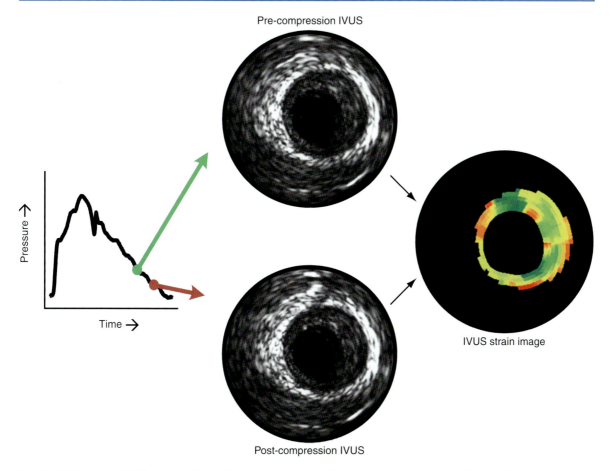

Fig. 20.4 Principle of IVUS elastography: radio-frequency (rf) data of a coronary artery are recorded at two different intraluminal pressure levels. From these recordings, a radial strain image is obtained

nature, which implies that the technique can only be applied to patients who are already in the cath-lab for catheterization. In other words, the technique can only be applied to people that already have clinical symptoms. As explained before, most people who are at risk of having a myocardial infarction or a stroke are asymptomatic.[30] Since ultrasound is relatively cheap and harmless compared with other imaging modalities like magnetic resonance imaging (MRI) and computerized tomography (CT), a noninvasive variant for vascular ultrasound strain imaging would be ideal for preventive screening of these populations as well. The imaging depth of coronary arteries is too great for noninvasive imaging with ultrasound while still having adequate resolution. Furthermore, it is located at the periphery of the beating heart which complicates accurate strain assessment even more. Noninvasive ultrasound strain imaging therefore focuses on superficial arteries, like carotid or femoral arteries. Since atherosclerosis is a systemic disease, the local findings in the carotid artery may also serve as a surrogate marker for overall disease in certain patients.[31]

20.4 Noninvasive Carotid Ultrasound Elastography

20.4.1 Introduction

One of the differences between the intravascular and the transcutaneous approach is the change from coronary to carotid artery. Using an intravascular catheter, Brusseau et al.[32] acquired rf data of a single excised human carotid artery at several intraluminal pressure steps. A one-dimensional (1D) cross-correlation-based

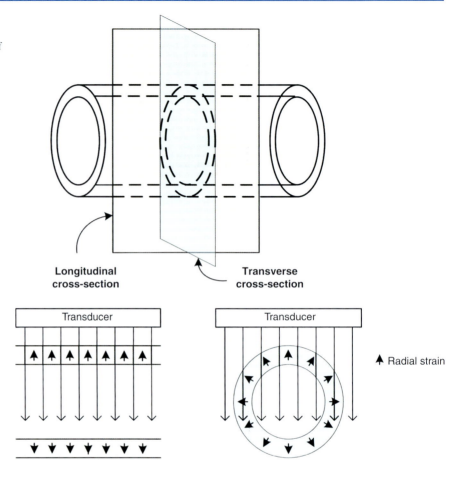

Fig. 20.5 Schematic overview of imaging planes used for ultrasonic imaging of the carotid artery. The orientation of the ultrasound beams with respect to the radial strains in the cross-section are shown

technique was applied to derive radial strain maps. A low-strain spot was observed at all pressure levels which corresponded well to the site of a collagen-rich region observed from histology data. This result supports that in principle strain imaging of the carotid arteries instead of the coronary arteries is possible. However, two major difficulties of strain imaging were not taken into account in this study. Firstly, the center frequency of the used ultrasound signal was 30–40 MHz. Center frequencies cannot be this high due to the attenuation of ultrasound that occurs when the signal travels through the skin, fat, and muscle tissue in between the transducer and the artery. Consequently, the spatial resolution of the ultrasonic signal and the strain images is also lower. Typically, center frequencies for strain imaging are around 7–10 MHz. The second difficulty with vascular strain imaging is that (at least for transverse vessel cross-sections) the ultrasound beams are not always aligned with the radial direction, as shown in Fig. 20.5. To circumvent this problem, usually the transducer is placed in the direction of the vessel axis. In this longitudinal imaging plane, the ultrasound beam direction (axial direction) corresponds to the radial strain direction. Methods and results with longitudinal strain imaging will be described first. Subsequently, other methods and results that are dedicated to radial and circumferential strain imaging for transverse vessel cross-sections will be discussed.

20.4.2 Strain Imaging for Longitudinal Cross-sections

20.4.2.1 Doppler-Based Method

Bonnefous and coworkers were first to describe a noninvasive strain imaging method for assessing vascular atherosclerosis. The technique was based on Doppler blood flow velocity imaging.[33] Using cross-correlation, the radial motion of a human carotid artery was estimated from in vivo recorded echo data. The technique was also applied to determine strain for cadaverous human arterial samples. The samples were placed in a temperature-regulated conservation bath and perfused with blood. Anti-coagulation drugs were added to prevent the formation of blood clots. A peristaltic pump and a frequency generator were used to generate a controlled pulsating blood flow through the arterial segments. During pulsations, intraluminal pressure and longitudinal echo data were recorded. Radial strain images were derived and compared to histology data. A high correlation was found between "hard" and "soft" lesions and low and high strains.

A different method that also originates from the field of Doppler-based blood flow velocity imaging is the method developed by Kanai et al. They developed a phase tracking method.[34] The technique is based on the principle that tissue displacement between a pre- and post-deformation situation induces a change in the phase of the echo signal. As long as the center frequency of the ultrasound beam is known, the technique can provide very accurate displacement and strain estimates.[18] The method was experimentally validated using a homogeneous vessel phantom. Compared with the theoretical strain profile, the error and the standard deviation in radial strain were 12.0% and 14.1%, respectively. The technique was also applied to in vitro recordings of a femoral artery. Low-strain regions corresponded well with calcified regions, and higher strains were observed for smooth muscle cells and collagen regions. A possible drawback of the phase tracking method is that it can only be applied to determine motion along the ultrasound beam, since it makes use of phase information. Another drawback might be that the technique does not take into account lateral motion, i.e., in plane motion in the direction perpendicular to the ultrasound beam. For tissue that has a lot of lateral motion between frames, it can be expected that the technique is not applicable. However, in their most recent paper,[35] the authors demonstrate a plane wave imaging sequence that enables recording rf data at frame rates of 3,500 Hz. For such high frame rates, the lateral interframe motion is negligible.

20.4.2.2 Lagrangian Speckle Motion Estimator

In 1999, Maurice et al. published a theoretical framework for a registration-based strain imaging method called the Lagrangian speckle motion estimator (LSME).[36] Later, the technique was adapted for noninvasive vascular strain imaging.[19] Basically, the method functions as follows: a pre-deformation image is deformed in multiple iterations until it matches a post-deformation image best. The translations and deformations of the pre-compression image that are required to find the optimal match correspond to the 2D displacements and strains that occurred between pre- and post-deformation situation. The method was first tested for simulated rf data of transverse cross-sections of cylindrical tissue. A homogeneous cylindrical blood vessel and a blood vessel with soft and hard regions were simulated. The results demonstrated the potential of the technique to detect "hard" and "soft" vascular tissue. Furthermore, it was shown that the technique allowed estimation of all 2D components of the strain tensor, which is useful for deriving strain components in other directions, like the radial and circumferential directions. In a later study, Maurice et al. showed that the LSME can also be used intravascularly.[37] Rf data of an excised human carotid artery were obtained for various intraluminal pressures, and radial strains were estimated. A low-strain region was found to correspond to a collagen-rich region as observed by histology. Although these publications report strain images for transverse vessel cross-sections, in vivo work of Maurice et al. mainly focuses on longitudinal recordings. The first in vivo results for the LSME method in human subjects were published in 2007.[13] Axial strains were determined for longitudinal cross-sections of two healthy subjects and two 75-year-old asymptomatic patients with severe carotid stenosis. It was shown that axial strains could be reproducibly measured for the healthy subjects over 5–7 heart cycles using an adapted version of the LSME. Cumulated axial strain curves for a region of interest (ROI) in the plaque region and an ROI in the wall region showed that the hard calcified plaque tissue strained less than the wall tissue. Furthermore, it was found that the strain pattern in the stenotic region was much more heterogeneous than the strain pattern for the vessel walls of the healthy subjects. In the most recent study, Maurice et al. applied the LSME to measure axial strains for healthy female and male subjects in four age categories.[38] Left and right common and internal carotid arteries were imaged longitudinally. Measurements were performed in duplicate by two different radiologists. The authors reported a good correlation between the measurements of both radiologists for the strain measurements for the common carotid arteries, whereas less consistency was observed for the internal carotid arteries. The correlation between measurements of the left and the right common carotid arteries was also larger than the correlation between the left and right internal carotid arteries. Axial strains for male common carotid arteries were less than for female common carotid arteries of the same age.

20.4.2.3 Cross-Correlation-Based Methods

The next group of methods that will be discussed are the coarse-to-fine or multi-level cross-correlation-based approaches.[21,39,40] Instead of cross-correlating the pre- and post-deformation data once for fixed window sizes, cross-correlation is repeated iteratively with decreasing window sizes. This is performed to be able to estimate large as well as small displacements and strains with high accuracy. The "coarser" displacement estimates from a preceding iteration are used to guide the algorithm in following iterations to find displacements on a finer scale. Since envelope-based cross-correlation is more robust when large translational motion occurs, often the first iteration is carried out on the B-mode/envelope signal, whereas in following iterations, rf data is used.

Several research groups have reported results on strain imaging of carotid arteries using a coarse-to-fine approach. In a study by Shi and coworkers,[21] the performance of a two-dimensional multi-step coarse-to-fine algorithm was compared with a single-step 1D cross-correlation method and a single-step 2D block-matching algorithm. It was shown from simulated data that whereas the other two techniques failed to provide correct displacement estimates in discontinuous displacement fields, the coarse-to-fine algorithm performs successfully. At the end of that paper, it is demonstrated that the technique also outperforms the other two techniques for in vivo recorded data of a carotid artery. In 2008, the technique was applied in a more clinical study.[41] Based on echo intensity and percentage of stenosis, 16 atherosclerotic plaques were classified as being "soft" or "calcified." Maximum axial strains were calculated for a certain region within each plaque and cumulated over time for three or more subsequent heartbeats. Furthermore, the relative lateral shift of the plaque compared to the vessel wall was calculated by comparing the lateral displacements for an ROI in the plaque with the lateral displacements for an ROI in the wall. It was observed that calcified plaques deformed less than soft plaques. The relative lateral shift was also less for the calcified plaques.

In the work by Kim et al., a multi-step strain imaging method is applied to in vivo images of a healthy volunteer and a diseased subject.[42] Axial strains were shown for two points of the brachial artery wall separated by 0.2 mm during 5 s. During the acquisition, the external compression applied with the transducer was increased. A nice cyclic pattern was observed. With increasing external pressure, the variations between the peak systolic and diastolic pressure increased up to a strain difference of 20%. The peak strain rate was reported to be 100%/s during diastole and −250%/s during systole. For the diseased vessel, the strain rate was about three times lower. Recently, the group applied the method to examine peripheral artery–vein bypass grafts.[43] Strain images were estimated before and after a stenosis developed for a 78-year-old subject who had a femoro-popliteal artery in situ bypass. Significantly, lower strain values were observed in the stenotic region compared with the normal tissue. Strain values were about four times lower than those of an 81-year-old subject who did not develop stenosis after bypass surgery. In another study,[44] the technique was applied to evaluate dialysis fistula stenosis in two subjects. Again, strain values in the stenotic regions were lower than in the "normal" regions of fistula.

20.4.3 Strain Imaging for Transverse Cross-sections

Analogous to the LSME, the cross-correlation-based algorithms can also be extended to two dimensions to derive the full 2D strain tensor. As explained above, extension to 2D enables the estimation of radial and circumferential strains for recordings of transverse vessel cross-sections. In a study by Ribbers et al.,[20] 2D strain data for both longitudinal and transverse cross-sections of a homogeneous vessel phantom with a concentric lumen were presented. The data were obtained using a 2D coarse-to-fine algorithm. For the transverse cross-sections, radial and circumferential strain images were also constructed. The constructed

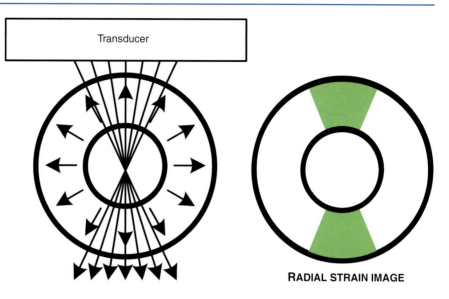

Fig. 20.6 Beam steering can be used to steer adjacent ultrasound beams through the center of a lumen. In this way, radial strains can be calculated for a small segment of the cross-section

radial strain images revealed a quadratic decay from the inner to the outer boundary, which corresponded to the strain profile predicted by theory. Next to the phantom results, axial strain images were derived for in vivo recordings of longitudinal and transverse cross-sections of 12 carotid arteries. A soft and a hard plaque were identified. The authors' conclusion was that noninvasive strain imaging of carotid arteries was feasible, but the quality of radial and circumferential strain images was severely deteriorated by the lateral strain contribution. Lateral strains cannot be estimated as accurate as axial strains, since no phase information is available in the lateral direction to enhance the cross-correlation procedure.

In the next two subsections, methods that require no or little lateral strain information for the estimation of radial strains in transverse cross-sections are presented.

20.4.3.1 A-Line-Based Beam Steering

Dedicated techniques for radial and circumferential strain imaging for transverse cross-sections are scarcely reported. As explained earlier, the radial direction does not correspond to the axial direction for transverse strain imaging. Although the phase tracking method of Kanai et al.[34] can only be applied to determine axial displacements, they found a way to circumvent the problem.[45] Adjacent ultrasound beams are all steered through the center of the lumen by changing the time delays of the transducer elements. By using this electronic steering, the ultrasound beams become aligned with the radial strains, and the phase tracking method can be applied to obtain radial strains for small segments of the cross-section (see also Fig. 20.6). A disadvantage of the technique is that only a partial strain image of the artery can be obtained since it is impossible to steer the ultrasound beam through the center for all 360°. Despite of the promising initial results for a rubber tube and in vivo acquisitions of a carotid artery, no further results on this technique have been presented.

20.4.3.2 Image-Based Beam Steering and Compounding

Another method dedicated to radial strain imaging for transverse cross-sections of superficial arteries is a method developed by Hansen and coworkers.[10] The technique also makes use of electronic beam steering. However, in this case, the beam steering is not performed separately for each rf line, but for the entire image plane, as shown in Fig. 20.7. Rf data are acquired at multiple beam steering angles in pre- and post-compression situations. For each angle, there are segments of the cross-section in which the ultrasound beam is (closely) aligned with the radial strain. For these segments, axial strains are calculated by a 2D coarse-to-fine cross-correlation algorithm. These axial strains, ε_{ax}, are converted into radial strains, ε_{rad}, by means of projection:

$$\varepsilon_{rad} = \frac{\varepsilon_{ax}}{2\cos^2\theta - 1}, \qquad (20.1)$$

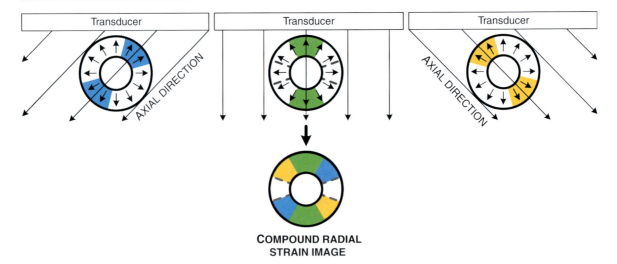

Fig. 20.7 Schematic overview of a beam steering approach for radial strain imaging of transverse cross-sections of a superficial artery. Acquisitions are performed at multiple beam steering angles. For each acquisition angle, radial strains are calculated for segments of the cross-section. The segments are added together to form a compound radial strain image

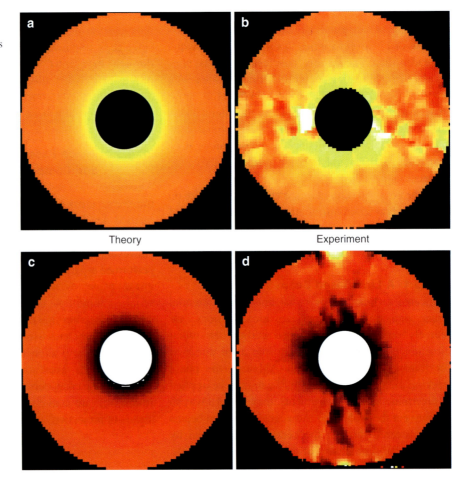

Fig. 20.8 (**a** and **c**) Theoretical radial and circumferential strain images for a homogeneous vessel, respectively. (**b** and **d**) Corresponding images obtained using the beam steering technique for acquisition angles of $-45°$, $-30°$, $-15°$, $0°$, $15°$, $30°$, and $45°$

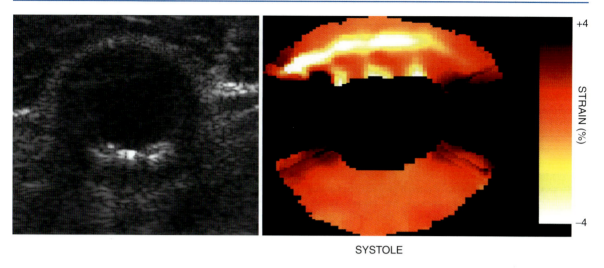

Fig. 20.9 An in vivo B-mode image (*left panel*) of a common carotid artery with a plaque and a compound radial strain image (*right panel*) are shown. The strain image was obtained in systolic phase, showing large radial compression for a certain region

where θ is the angle between the ultrasound beam and the radial direction. The segments with radial strain estimates from the various beam steering angles are compounded to form a radial strain image for the entire cross-section. The technique also enables estimation of circumferential strain images by selecting segments that are perpendicular to the segments selected for radial strain imaging.

The technique was first applied on a homogeneous vessel phantom made of gelatin with a concentric lumen. Rf data were recorded with a SONOS 7500 ultrasound machine (Philips Ultrasound, Andover, Massachusetts, USA), equipped with an 11–3L linear array transducer with a center frequency of 8.7 MHz. Data were recorded at beam steering angles ranging from −45° to 45° with an angular increment of 15°. Figure 20.8 shows the theoretical and the estimated radial and circumferential strain images. As can be observed, a good similarity was found between both images. Since the projection angles were limited to 30°, lateral strain information was required to complete the images at 3 and 9 o'clock. For the circumferential strain image, these are the 6- and 12-o'clock regions. This explains why the strains in these regions are noisy.

The method was also partially tested in vivo. Using the 3-angle SONO-CT mode of an iE33 ultrasound machine (Philips Ultrasound, Andover, Massachusetts, USA), recordings of a carotid artery with plaque were obtained. Figure 20.9 shows the B-mode image and the constructed compound radial strain images at several moments during the pressure cycle. At systole, large radial compression can be observed for a certain region within the plaque. This region might correspond to a soft lipid pool. However, since no histology data was available to confirm the presence of a lipid pool, in vivo validation of the technique is still required.

20.5 Conclusions

The potential of strain imaging for differentiation of vulnerable plaques from stable plaques has been confirmed using intravascular strain imaging techniques. In the past decade, multiple methods for noninvasive strain imaging of carotid arteries have been developed. The feasibility of most methods for clinical application has been shown using simulations and experimental data. The first in vivo pilot studies show that the technique enables differentiating between "soft" and "hard" tissue. Studies in which the in vivo acquisitions are compared with histology data are required to validate the developed methods, and patient studies will have to prove that noninvasive vulnerable plaque detection is possible.

References

1. Davies MJ. Stability and instability: two faces of coronary atherosclerosis. *Circulation*. 1996;94(8):2013–2020.
2. Schaar JA et al. Terminology for high-risk and vulnerable coronary artery plaques. *Eur Heart J*. 2004;25(12):1077–1082.
3. Glagov S, Weisenberg E, Zarins CK, Stankunavicius R, Kolettis GJ. Compensatory enlargement of human atherosclerotic coronary arteries. *N Engl J Med*. 1987;316(22):1371–1375.
4. Pasterkamp G et al. Relation of arterial geometry to luminal narrowing and histologic markers for plaque vulnerability: the remodeling paradox. *J Am Coll Cardiol*. 1998;32(3):655–662.
5. Richardson PD. Biomechanics of plaque rupture: progress, problems, and new frontiers. *Ann Biomed Eng*. 2002;30(4):524–536.
6. Carr S, Farb A, Pearce WH, Virmani R, Yao JS. Atherosclerotic plaque rupture in symptomatic carotid artery stenosis. *J Vasc Surg*. 1996;23(5):755–765.
7. Davies MJ, Thomas AC. Plaque fissuring – the cause of acute myocardial infarction, sudden ischaemic death, and crescendo angina. *Br Heart J*. 1985;53(4):363–373.
8. Falk E, Shah P, Fuster V. Coronary plaque disruption. *Circulation*. 1995;92(3):657–671.
9. Hurks R et al. Biobanks and the search for predictive biomarkers of local and systemic outcome in atherosclerotic disease. *Thromb Haemost*. 2009;101(1):48–54.
10. Hansen HHG, Lopata RGP, de Korte CL. Noninvasive carotid strain imaging using angular compounding at large beam steered angles: validation in vessel phantoms. *IEEE Trans Med Imaging*. 2009;28(6):872–880.
11. Lerakis S et al. Imaging of the vulnerable plaque: noninvasive and invasive techniques. *Am J Med Sci*. 2008;336(4):342–348.
12. Young JJ et al. Vulnerable plaque intervention: state of the art. *Catheter Cardiovasc Interv*. 2008;71(3):367–374.
13. Schmitt C, Soulez G, Maurice RL, Giroux MF, Cloutier G. Noninvasive vascular elastography: toward a complementary characterization tool of atherosclerosis in carotid arteries. *Ultrasound Med Biol*. 2007;33(12):1841–1858.
14. Behler RH, Nichols TC, Zhu H, Merricks EP, Gallippi CM. ARFI imaging for noninvasive material characterization of atherosclerosis. Part II: toward in vivo characterization. *Ultrasound Med Biol*. 2009;35(2):278–295.
15. Ophir J, Céspedes EI, Ponnekanti H, Yazdi Y, Li X. Elastography: a method for imaging the elasticity in biological tissues. *Ultrason Imaging*. 1991;13:111–134.
16. de Korte CL, Pasterkamp G, van der Steen AFW, Woutman HA, Bom N. Characterization of plaque components using intravascular ultrasound elastography in human femoral and coronary arteries in vitro. *Circulation*. 2000;102(6):617–623.
17. de Korte CL et al. Morphological and mechanical information of coronary arteries obtained with intravascular elastography: a feasibility study in vivo. *Eur Heart J*. 2002;23(5):405–413.
18. Hasegawa H, Kanai H. Reduction of influence of variation in center frequencies of RF echoes on estimation of artery-wall strain. *IEEE Trans Ultrason Ferroelectr Freq Control*. 2008;55(9):1921–1934.
19. Maurice RL et al. Noninvasive vascular elastography: theoretical framework. *IEEE Trans Med Imaging*. 2004;23(2):164–180.
20. Ribbers H et al. Noninvasive two-dimensional strain imaging of arteries: validation in phantoms and preliminary experience in carotid arteries in vivo. *Ultrasound Med Biol*. 2007;33(4):530–540.
21. Shi H, Varghese T. Two-dimensional multi-level strain estimation for discontinuous tissue. *Phys Med Biol*. 2007;52(2):389–401.
22. Kallel F, Ophir J. A least-squares strain estimator for elastography. *Ultrason Imaging*. 1997;19(3):195–208.
23. de Korte CL, Céspedes EI, van der Steen AFW, Lancée CT. Intravascular elasticity imaging using ultrasound: feasibility studies in phantoms. *Ultrasound Med Biol*. 1997;23(5):735–746.
24. Ryan LK, Foster FS. Ultrasonic measurement of differential displacement and strain in a vascular model. *Ultrason Imaging*. 1997;19:19–38.
25. Shapo BM et al. Strain imaging of coronary arteries with intraluminal ultrasound: experiments on an inhomogeneous phantom. *Ultrason Imaging*. 1996;18:173–191.
26. Céspedes EI, de Korte CL, van der Steen AFW. In: Intravascular Ultrasonic Palpation: Assessment of Local Wall Compliance; 1997; Toronto:1079–1082.
27. de Korte CL et al. Identification of atherosclerotic plaque components with intravascular ultrasound elastography in vivo: a Yucatan pig study. *Circulation*. 2002;105(14):1627–1630.
28. Schaar JA et al. Vulnerable plaque detection with intravascular elastography: a sensitivity and specificity study. *Circulation*. 2001;104(17):II-459.
29. Schaar JA et al. Incidence of high strain patterns in human coronary arteries: assessment with three-dimensional intravascular palpography and correlation with clinical presentation. *Circulation*. 2004;109(22):2716–2719.
30. Nicolaides A et al. The Asymptomatic Carotid Stenosis and Risk of Stroke (ACSRS) study. Aims and results of quality control. *Int Angiol*. 2003;22(3):263–272.
31. O'Leary DH, Polak JF, Kronmal RA. Carotid-artery intima and media thickness as a risk factor for myocardial infarction and stroke – reply. *N Engl J Med*. 1999;340(22):1763.
32. Brusseau E, Fromageau J, Finet G, Delachartre P, Vray D. Axial strain imaging of intravascular data: results on polyvinyl alcohol cryogel phantoms and carotid artery. *Ultrasound Med Biol*. 2001;27(12):1631–1642.
33. Bonnefous O et al. New noninvasive echographic technique for arterial wall characterization. *Radiology*. 1996;201:1129.
34. Kanai H, Sato M, Koiwa Y, Chubachi N. Transcutaneous measurement and spectrum analysis of heart wall vibrations. *IEEE Trans Ultrason Ferroelectr Freq Control*. 1996;43(5):791–810.
35. Hasegawa H, Kanai H. Simultaneous imaging of artery-wall strain and blood flow by high frame rate acquisition of RF

signals. *IEEE Trans Ultrason Ferroelectr Freq Control.* 2008;55(12):2626–2639.
36. Maurice RL, Bertrand M. Lagrangian speckle model and tissue-motion estimation – theory. *IEEE Trans Med Imaging.* 1999;18(7):593–603.
37. Maurice RL, Brusseau E, Finet G, Cloutier G. On the potential of the Lagrangian speckle model estimator to characterize atherosclerotic plaques in endovascular elastography: in vitro experiments using an excised human carotid artery. *Ultrasound Med Biol.* 2005;31(1):85–91.
38. Maurice RL, Soulez G, Giroux MF, Cloutier G. Noninvasive vascular elastography for carotid artery characterization on subjects without previous history of atherosclerosis. *Med Phys.* 2008;35(8):3436–3443.
39. Chen H, Shi H, Varghese T. Improvement of elastographic displacement estimation using a two-step cross-correlation method. *Ultrasound Med Biol.* 2007;33(1):48–56.
40. Lopata RG et al. Performance evaluation of methods for two-dimensional displacement and strain estimation using ultrasound radio frequency data. *Ultrasound Med Biol.* 2009;35(5):796–812.
41. Shi H et al. Preliminary in vivo atherosclerotic carotid plaque characterization using the accumulated axial strain and relative lateral shift strain indices. *Phys Med Biol.* 2008;53(22):6377–6394.
42. Kim K et al. Vascular intramural strain imaging using arterial pressure equalization. *Ultrasound Med Biol.* 2004;30(6): 761–771.
43. Weitzel WF, Kim K, Henke PK, Rubin JM. High-resolution ultrasound speckle tracking may detect vascular mechanical wall changes in peripheral artery bypass vein grafts. *Ann Vasc Surg.* 2009;23(2):201–206.
44. Weitzel WF et al. High-resolution ultrasound elasticity imaging to evaluate dialysis fistula stenosis. *Semin Dial.* 2009;22(1):84–89.
45. Nakagawa N, Hasegawa H, Kanai H. Cross-sectional elasticity imaging of carotid arterial wall in short-axis plane by transcutaneous ultrasound. *Jpn J Appl Phys.* 2004;43 (5B):3220–3226 (Part 1-Regular Papers Short Notes & Review Papers).

Motion Estimation of Carotid Artery Plaques

21

Sergio E. Murillo Amaya and Marios S. Pattichis

21.1 Introduction

Atherosclerosis is the primary cause of strokes and the third cause of death in the United States[1] with almost twice as many people dying from cardiovascular disease than from the combined deaths due to cancer. Plaque buildup is a characteristic of atherosclerosis, and a consequence of progressive intimal accumulation of lipid, protein, and cholesterol esters in the blood vessel wall[2] (Chap. 1) which results in a significant reduction of blood flow. Motion estimation of ultrasound videos of carotid artery plaques provides important information regarding plaque deformation and feature extraction to distinguish between stable and unstable plaques or symptomatic and asymptomatic plaques.[3]

In this chapter, the development of verifiable methods for the estimation of plaque motion and reconstruction of plaque trajectories is presented. The authors expect that plaque and wall motion analysis will provide additional information about plaque instability.

Previous studies[4,5] have assessed the accuracy of optical flow based techniques by generating ground truth video sequences that capture standard video motion characteristics like translational constant motion, non-deformable body motion, wide range of velocity values, diverging velocity fields, and occluding edges using a uniform light source. This prior research did not address some of the unique characteristics associated with ultrasound imaging of atherosclerotic plaque motion.

Here, it is noted that prior research did not address the need to account for realistic plaque motions under significant levels of ultrasound speckle. Ultrasound speckle can lead to large inaccuracies in the estimation. Realistic simulations corrupted by different levels of signal to noise ratios (SNR) are considered. A variety of realistic motions of the atherosclerotic plaque that undergoes periodic motions due to the cardiac cycle, with discontinuities that mimic sudden plaque and artery wall movements during systole and diastole, are also considered. Realistic simulations are used to estimate globally optimal method parameters that would be applicable to a wide variety of realistic conditions. Once the optimal parameters are found, they are used to calculate the motion of clinical ultrasound videos with special focus on the plaque which is segmented using an automated algorithm.[6] Finally, the estimated velocities are fed to a Kalman filter[7] that reconstructs pixel trajectories.

This chapter starts with a review of motion estimation techniques. Plaque motion analysis follows. Optimization techniques for choosing motion estimation input parameters are presented in the subsequent section followed by results and conclusions.

21.2 Motion Estimation and Optical Flow

This section presents an overview of optical flow based methods for motion estimation with special focus on optimization theory applied toward the minimization of energy functionals. Global and local

S.E.M. Amaya • M.S. Pattichis (✉)
Department of Electrical and Computer Engineering,
The University of New Mexico, Albuquerque, NM, USA

solutions are studied using the calculus of variations and least squares methods.

21.2.1 Overview of Motion Estimation and Optical Flow

Motion estimation from digital video assigns a velocity vector to each pixel of each frame in the video. Here, we are estimating motion associated with two-dimensional (2D) slices through the three-dimensional (3D) plaque anatomy. First, it is noted that there is no information to measure motion components that are orthogonal to the 2D slices. In addition to these constraints, there are also limits to what can be recovered from the projected motions.

In what follows, a brief overview of the area with more details given in subsequent sections will be provided. The work of Horn and Schunck[8] opened up the area of motion estimation using optical flow models with the classical assumption that the image intensity should be conserved under small displacements. At the same time, Lucas and Kanade[9] proposed a local solution to the conservation of image intensities using a weighted least squares fit. Five years later, Nagel and Enkelmann[10] proposed an oriented smoothness constraint for estimating the optical flow motion field. The conservation of the image intensities was applied to the image gradient by Uras et al.,[11] and Fleet and Jepson[12] were the first to use image phase information in the estimation of the motion field.

At this point, Barron et al.[13] published a comprehensive survey of optical flow techniques. This work gave quantitative comparisons among differential methods (e.g.,: Differential methods by Horn and Schunck, Lucas and Kanade, Nagel and Enkelmann, and Uras et al.[8-11]), block matching,[14] energy-based,[15] and phased-based techniques[12,16]. For the comparisons, Barron et al.[13] used synthetic images for which ground truth was available. Estimation performance was summarized in terms of the density of the flow field (percentage of the number of pixels with motion estimates as a fraction of all the pixels) and the angular error between ground truth and the estimated field.

Negahdaripour[17] modified the framework to allow changes in the pixel brightness intensities along their motion path. Subsequently, local and global solutions to motion estimation using optical flow models were merged by Bruhn. More recently, the intensity conservation assumption was assumed over multiple scales in conjunction with Amplitude Modulation-Frequency Modulation (AM-FM) image models.[18] A complete list of assumptions and energy functionals for each method is shown in Table 21.1. Table 21.2 shows the related motion parameters for each technique.

21.2.1.1 Constant Brightness Optical Flow Model for Motion Estimation

Beginning with the most basic assumption, let the image brightness intensity of a pixel with coordinates (x, y) at time t be denoted as $I(x, y, t)$. Optical flow techniques assume that the image brightness intensities remain constant along their motion path under a sufficiently small time interval δt giving:

$$I(x + \delta x, y + \delta y, t + \delta t) = I(x, y, t). \quad (21.1)$$

Expanding the left hand side of Eq. 21.1 into a first-order Taylor series, and neglecting high-order terms gives:

$$I(x, y, t) + \delta x \frac{\partial I}{\partial x} + \delta y \frac{\partial I}{\partial y} + \delta t \frac{\partial I}{\partial t} = I(x, y, t). \quad (21.2)$$

After subtracting $I(x, y, t)$ from both sides of Eq. 21.2, dividing by δt, and taking the limit as $\delta t \to 0$, we have the optical flow constraint (OFC):

$$I_x u + I_y v + I_t = 0. \quad (21.3)$$

Deviations from the OFC are measured using the following energy functional:

$$E_{\text{OFC}} = \iint_\Omega (I_x u + I_y v + I_t)^2 d\Omega \quad (21.4)$$

which is minimized over the entire image domain Ω. Alternatively, the OFC can be rewritten as:

$$\vec{\nabla I} \cdot \vec{v} = -I_t \quad (21.5)$$

where $\nabla I = (I_x, I_y)$ is the spatial intensity gradient, I_t is the first-order temporal derivative, and $\vec{v}$ is the optical flow field with components given by $u = dx/dt$ and $v = dy/dt$.

Table 21.1 List of model assumptions and energy functionals introduced by motion estimation techniques

Authors	Assumptions	Energy functionals	Comments
Horn and Schunck (1981)[8]	• Intensity conservation • Small displacements • Field smoothness	E_{OFC}, E_S	*Adv.*: Simple linear model. *Disadv.*: Intensity conservation often violated. Errors at object boundaries.
Lucas and Kanade (1981)[9]	• Weighted intensity conservation • Small displacements • Constant motion over blocks	E_{WOFC}	*Adv.*: Noise Robustness *Disadv.*: Low field density.
Nagel and Enkelmann (1986)[10]	• Intensity conservation • Small displacements • Oriented smoothness	E_{OFC}, E_{OS}	*Adv.*: Better handling of Occlusion. *Disadv.*: Approximation of second-order derivatives.
Uras et al. (1988)[11]	• Conservation of image gradient • No rotation or dilation of image intensities should be presen	E_G	*Adv.*: One constraint that provides two equations per pixel. *Disadv.*: Low field density. Requires approximation of second-order derivatives
Fleet and Jepson (1990)[12]	• Conservation of phase information • Small displacements	E_{Phase}	*Adv.*: Phase information is more robust than amplitude (intensity) information. *Disadv.*: Filter is tuned to only certain frequencies.
Negahdaripour (1998)[17]	• Non constant brightness • Small displacements • Field smoothness • Radiometric smoothness	E_{NCB} E_S E_{Srad}	*Adv.*: Realistic model *Disadv.*: Underdetermined model that requires smoothness across velocity and scene variation parameters.
Bruhn et al. (2002)[5]	• Local–global intensity conservation • Small displacements	E_{CLG}	*Adv.*: Combines global and local optical flow approaches *Disadv.* Integration scale of local–global region is chosen heuristically.
Murray et al. (2007)[18]	• Image intensity preservation translated into AM and FM constraints • Assumes motion continuity	E_{AM}, E_{FM}	*Adv.*: Three equations for each channel filter per pixel. *Disadv.*: Filterbank frequency should match the underlying motion to be estimated.

Table 21.2 Table of motion parameters associated with motion estimation techniques

Motion estimation parameters	
Authors	Parameter
Horn and Schunck (1981)[8]	• Spread of Gaussian smoothing filter σ • Weight of smoothness constraint α.
Lucas and Kanade (1981)[9]	• Spread of Gaussian smoothing filter σ
Nagel and Enkelmann (1986)[10]	• Spread of Gaussian smoothing filter σ • Weight of smoothness constraint α
Uras et al. (1988)[11]	• Spread of Gaussian smoothing filter σ
Fleet and Jepson (1990)[12]	• Spread of Gaussian smoothing filter σ • Threshold on local frequencies outside filter's tuning range
Negahdaripour (1998)[17]	• Spread of Gaussian smoothing filter σ • Weight of smoothness constraint λ • Weight of radiometric smoothness constraint β
Bruhn et al. (2002)[5]	• Noise scale ρ
Murray et al. (2007)[18]	• Weight of AM constraint α_{AM} • Weight of FM constraint β_{FM}

The solution to Eq. 21.5 is the velocity component in the direction of the spatial intensity gradient given by:

$$\vec{v}_n = \frac{-I_t \vec{\nabla} I}{\|\nabla I\|_2^2}. \qquad (21.6)$$

This introduces the aperture problem: Only the velocity component in the direction of the spatial intensity gradient can be estimated with the OFC. The component orthogonal to this direction, which is the component along contours of constant brightness intensity, cannot be determined. The velocity in the direction of the spatial gradient Eq. 21.6 is known as the normal velocity, i.e., the flow normal or orthogonal to local intensity structure, and only at locations where there is sufficient intensity structure, full image velocity can be estimated.[4]

The OFC is a single equation in two unknowns. The constraint can be expressed as a line in the velocity space and all the points (u, v) on that line are valid solutions. The normal velocity is the solution with the smallest magnitude on that line, and the problem of estimating full image velocity yields to introducing additional constraints.

21.2.1.2 Nonconstant Brightness Intensity Optical Flow Model for Motion Estimation

Geometric transformations provide only one set of changes that result in optical flow changes. Brightness changes induced by nonuniform light source, light source changes, shading, and surface reflection are present in time-varying images and all induce optical flow changes that violate the brightness constancy assumption. For ultrasound imaging, brightness variations are not due to lighting variations. Instead, they can arise from variable spatial gain levels or ultrasound imaging artifacts. To overcome the shortcomings of the image brightness constancy model, Negahdaripour[17] proposed a more general model for optical flow estimation that allows brightness intensity variations between successive time instants.

The brightness intensity change of a pixel after a small time interval can be modeled as:

$$\begin{aligned} m(x, y, t)I(x, y, t) + c(x, y, t) \\ = I(x + \delta x, y + \delta y, t + \delta t) \end{aligned} \qquad (21.7)$$

where the new terms $m(x, y, t)$ and $c(x, y, t)$ allow the approximation of brightness variations as a linear transformation of the intensity patterns using a multiplier $m(x, y, t)$ and offset $c(x, y, t)$ fields. Expanding the right hand side of Eq. 21.7 in a first-order Taylor series and neglecting high-order terms yields:

$$\begin{aligned} m(x, y, t)I(x, y, t) + c(x, y, t) \\ = I(x, y, t) + \delta x \frac{\partial I}{\partial x} + \delta y \frac{\partial I}{\partial y} + \delta t \frac{\partial I}{\partial t} \end{aligned} \qquad (21.8)$$

For small time intervals, δt, the multiplier field, is expected to be close to one, and the offset field is expected to be close to zero. This allows to approximate the multiplier and offset fields using $m(x, y, t) = 1 + \delta m$ and $c(x, y, t) = 0 + \delta c$. Equation 21.8 is reduced to:

$$I \delta m + \delta c = I_x \delta x + I_y \delta y + I_t \delta t. \qquad (21.9)$$

After dividing by δt, and taking the limit as $\delta t \rightarrow 0$ the Generalized Dynamic Image Model (GDIM) is expressed as:

$$I_x u + I_y v + I_t - I m_t - c_t = 0. \qquad (21.10)$$

Equation 21.10 reduces to the OFC when $m_t = c_t = 0$. Deviations from the GDIM are penalized using the following energy functional:

$$E_{\text{NCB}} = \iint_\Omega (I_x u + I_y v + I_t - m_t I - c_t)^2 d\Omega \qquad (21.11)$$

21.2.2 Global Solutions via Functional Optimization

Both the constant brightness model and the nonconstant brightness intensity model are underdetermined systems. Global methods assume that the motion field is continuous and differentiable in space and time[4] along with a global smoothness regularization term to compute dense optical flow estimates. If pixels in an image move independently, there is little hope to recover the flow field.[8] In what follows, the assumption is that velocity field of the image varies smoothly over the spatial support of the image.

21.2.2.1 Constant Brightness Model (CBM) Solution

The OFC Eq. 21.3 is not enough to fully estimate both components of the flow field (u, v) since it is a single equation with two unknowns per pixel. Additional constraints need to be introduced to the model formulation in order to calculate the optical flow field. Horn and Schunck measured the smoothness of the field by minimizing the square of the magnitude of the gradient of the velocity vector over the whole image in the following energy functional:

$$E_s = \iint_\Omega (u_x^2 + u_y^2 + v_x^2 + v_y^2)d\Omega \quad (21.12)$$

The solution to the CBM is the velocity field that minimizes the sum of the errors in the following combined functional:

$$E_{CBM} = E_{OFC} + \alpha^2 E_s$$
$$E_{OFC} = \iint_\Omega (I_x u + I_y v + I_t)^2 d\Omega \quad (21.13)$$
$$E_S = \iint_\Omega (u_x^2 + u_y^2 + v_x^2 + v_y^2)d\Omega$$

In Eq. 21.13, α is a parameter that weights the departure from the smoothness functional, E_S, relative to the optical flow constraint functional E_{OFC}. If brightness measures are accurate, this parameter should be small and large if they are noisy.[19]

Quantization error and noise affect the calculation of image intensity derivatives. Thus, the OFC will not be always equal to zero. Meanwhile, E_S only vanishes for constant velocities, i.e., $u_x = u_y = v_x = v_y = 0$. For nonconstant velocities, the smoothness functional is nonzero. The weight on the smoothness constraint is supposed to account for some of these errors. Clearly though, the choice of the correct regularization parameter is critical and optimizing for the best value is not a trivial task as shown in the authors' previous work.[18,20,21]

Minimizing a combined functional of the form of Eq. 21.13 is a problem for the calculus of variations.[22,23] The associated Euler-Lagrange equations are:

$$I_x^2 u + I_x I_y v = \alpha^2 \nabla^2 u - I_x I_t$$
$$I_x I_y u + I_y^2 v = \alpha^2 \nabla^2 v - I_y I_t \quad (21.14)$$

where finite differencing is used to approximate the Laplacian of the velocities. The equations Eq. 21.14 depend on the regularization parameter α, and a suitable value needs to be chosen in order to find a solution. The most common approach is a heuristic trial and error process that leads to inaccuracies in the estimated vector field.[10,20,24-26]

There are two equations per pixel and solving them Eq. 21.14 using one of the standard methods like Gauss-Jordan elimination will be very tedious. Alternatively, an iterative scheme[8] is used to calculate the new velocity values (u^{k+1}, v^{k+1}) from local velocity neighborhood averages at the previous iteration $(\bar{u}^k, \bar{v}^k)$ and brightness intensity derivatives using:

$$u^{k+1} = \bar{u}^k - \frac{I_x[I_x \bar{u}^k + I_y \bar{v}^k + I_t]}{\alpha^2 + I_x^2 + I_y^2}$$
$$v^{k+1} = \bar{v}^k - \frac{I_y[I_x \bar{u}^k + I_y \bar{v}^k + I_t]}{\alpha^2 + I_x^2 + I_y^2}. \quad (21.15)$$

Numerical differentiation is always a source of considerable error. Barron et al.[13] applied a spatiotemporal Gaussian pre-smoothing filter to enforce continuity of the image brightness patterns and attenuate the effects of noise. However, too much smoothing destroys local image structure, and some optimization will be needed in order to control the spread of the Gaussian filter.

21.2.2.2 Constant Brightness Model with Oriented Smoothness Constraint

In this model, as in the original approach by Horn and Schunck,[8] the OFC is combined with a smoothness constraint. Here, the smoothness constraint was modified to limit the variation of the motion field.[27] The variation of the motion field is captured in the first derivatives of the two velocity components.

Nagel accomplished this by minimizing the flow variation that is orthogonal to the image gradient ∇I. The oriented smoothness constraint is formulated as:

$$E_{os} = \iint \frac{\left[(u_x I_y - u_y I_x)^2 + (v_x I_y - v_y I_x)^2 + \delta(u_x^2 + u_y^2 + v_x^2 + v_y^2)\right]}{\|\nabla I\|^2 + 2\delta} dxdy. \quad (21.16)$$

The solution to the CBM with oriented smoothness constraint is the flow field that minimizes the combined functional:

$$E_{\text{CEMOS}} = E_{\text{OFC}} + \alpha^2 E_{\text{OS}},$$
$$E_{\text{OFC}} = \iint_\Omega (I_x u + I_y v + I_t)^2 d\Omega,$$
$$E_{\text{OS}} = \iint_\Omega \frac{\left[(u_x I_y - u_y I_x)^2 + (v_x I_y - v_y I_x)^2 + \delta(u_x^2 + u_y^2 + v_x^2 + v_y^2)\right]}{\|\nabla I\|^2 + 2\delta} dxdy.$$

(21.17)

The parameter α weights the departure from the oriented smoothness constraint relative to the error in the OFC, and δ was introduced for numerical stability and equals to 1.0.[13] Using Gauss-Seidel iterations, the solution can be computed using:

$$u^{k+1} = \xi(u^k) - \frac{I_x(I_x \xi(u^k) + I_y \xi(v^k) + I_t)}{I_x^2 + I_y^2 + \alpha^2},$$
$$v^{k+1} = \xi(v^k) - \frac{I_y(I_x \xi(u^k) + I_y \xi(v^k) + I_t)}{I_x^2 + I_y^2 + \alpha^2}.$$

(21.18)

In Eq. 21.18, k denotes the iteration number, while $\xi(u^k)$ and $\xi(v^k)$ are given by:

$$\xi(u^k) = \bar{u}^k - 2I_x I_y u_{xy}^k - q^T(\nabla u^k), \text{ and}$$
$$\xi(v^k) = \bar{v}^k - 2I_x I_y v_{xy}^k - q^T(\nabla v^k),$$

(21.19)

Where q and W are given by:

$$q = \frac{1}{I_x^2 + I_y^2 + 2\delta}$$
$$\times \nabla I^T \left[\begin{pmatrix} I_{yy} & -I_{xy} \\ -I_{xy} & I_{xx} \end{pmatrix} + 2 \begin{pmatrix} I_{xx} & I_{xy} \\ I_{xy} & I_{yy} \end{pmatrix} W \right] \text{ and}$$

(21.20)

$$W = (I_x^2 + I_y^2 + 2\delta)^{-1} \begin{pmatrix} I_y^2 + \delta & -I_x I_y \\ -I_x I_y & I_x^2 + \delta \end{pmatrix}.$$

(21.21)

Here, u_{xy}^k, v_{xy}^k denote estimates of the partial derivatives. Also, $\bar{u}^k$ and $\bar{v}^k$ denote local neighborhood averages of u^k and v^k.

21.2.2.3 Generalized Dynamic Image Model (GDIM) Solution

Conservation of image intensity is the basis of most optical flow techniques. When this assumption does not hold, true in most real video sequences, unreliable estimates can be obtained. To overcome the shortcomings of the image brightness constancy model, a generalized brightness variation model was proposed by Negahdaripour[17] where not only image geometric transformations are considered but also transformations of image brightness patterns Eq. 21.11. Originally, Negahdaripour[17] developed a local solution for the GDIM using a least square fit over block regions of 9×9 pixels. Such local solutions do not yield high-density fields because of regions where the least square system is ill-conditioned due to lack of or weak texture. In this paper, a global solution for the GDIM is computed using the calculus of variations.

Errors in the GDIM are penalized using the non-constant brightness energy functional E_{NCB}:

$$E_{\text{NCB}} = \iint_\Omega (I_x u + I_y v + I_t - m_t I - c_t)^2 d\Omega \quad (21.22)$$

Assuming that the unknowns (u, v, m_t, c_t) vary smoothly, the minimization problem can be formulated as one of estimating the functions u, v, m_t, c_t that minimize the combined energy functional:

$$E_{\text{GDIM}} = \lambda E_{\text{NCB}} + \beta E_{\text{Srad}} + E_{\text{S}}. \text{where}$$
$$E_{\text{NCB}} = \iint_\Omega (I_x u + I_y v + I_t - m_t I - c_t)^2 d\Omega,$$
$$E_{\text{Srad}} = \iint_\Omega (m_{tx}^2 + m_{ty}^2 + c_{tx}^2 + c_{ty}^2) d\Omega,$$
$$E_{\text{S}} = \iint_\Omega (u_x^2 + u_y^2 + v_x^2 + v_y^2) d\Omega.$$

(21.23)

The system of associated Euler-Lagrange differential equations is given by:

$$\lambda(I_x u + I_y v + I_t - m_t I - c_t) I_x = \nabla^2 u,$$
$$\lambda(I_x u + I_y v + I_t - m_t I - c_t) I_y = \nabla^2 v,$$
$$-\lambda(I_x u + I_y v + I_t - m_t I - c_t) I = \beta \nabla^2 m_t, \text{ and}$$
$$-\lambda(I_x u + I_y v + I_t - m_t I - c_t) = \beta \nabla^2 c_t.$$

(21.24)

The Laplacian of the velocities is approximated using finite differencing. The final system to solve can be written as:

$$\begin{bmatrix} \lambda I_x^2 + 1 & \lambda I_x I_y & -\lambda I_x I & -\lambda I_x \\ \lambda I_x I_y & \lambda I_y^2 + 1 & -\lambda I_y I & -\lambda I_y \\ -\lambda I_x I_y & -\lambda I_y I & \lambda I^2 + \beta & \lambda I \\ -\lambda I_x & -\lambda I_y & \lambda I & \beta + \lambda \end{bmatrix} \begin{bmatrix} u \\ v \\ m_t \\ c_t \end{bmatrix}$$

$$= \begin{bmatrix} \bar{u} - \lambda I_x I_t \\ \bar{v} - \lambda I_y I_t \\ \beta \bar{m}_t + \lambda I_t I \\ \beta \bar{c}_t + \lambda I_t \end{bmatrix}. \quad (21.25)$$

The Gauss-Seidel iteration scheme used by Horn and Schunck to solve system shown in Eq. 21.14 is applied to system in Eq. 21.25 to give:

$$u^{k+1} = \bar{u}^k - I_x \left[\frac{I_x \bar{u}^k + I_y \bar{v}^k + I_t - I \bar{m}_t^k - \bar{c}_t^k}{I_x^2 + I_y^2 + \beta'(I^2 + 1) + \lambda'} \right],$$

$$v^{k+1} = \bar{v}^k - I_y \left[\frac{I_x \bar{u}^k + I_y \bar{v}^k + I_t - I \bar{m}_t^k - \bar{c}_t^k}{I_x^2 + I_y^2 + \beta'(I^2 + 1) + \lambda'} \right],$$

$$m_t^{k+1} = \bar{m}_t^{k+1} - \beta' I \left[\frac{I_x \bar{u}^k + I_y \bar{v}^k + I_t - I \bar{m}_t^k - \bar{c}_t^k}{I_x^2 + I_y^2 + \beta'(I^2 + 1) + \lambda'} \right], \text{ and}$$

$$c_t^{k+1} = \bar{c}_t^{k+1} - \beta' \left[\frac{I_x \bar{u}^k + I_y \bar{v}^k + I_t - I \bar{m}_t^k - \bar{c}_t^k}{I_x^2 + I_y^2 + \beta'(I^2 + 1) + \lambda'} \right].$$

(21.26)

Here, note that β' and λ' are used and they are defined to be $1/\beta$ and $1/\lambda$ respectively. Then, when β' is large, m_t and c_t approach zero, the GDIM approximates the CBM method proposed by Horn.

21.2.2.4 Amplitude Modulation-Frequency Modulation Motion Estimation Model

The Amplitude Modulation-Frequency Modulation (AM-FM) motion estimation model was recently developed.[18] The interest for this method arises from the fact that motion vectors can be estimated independently using AM constraints alone, FM constraints alone, and the combination of both. The influence of the AM-FM constraints is controlled by weights on the energy functional formulation.

Amplitude Modulation-Frequency Modulation is a model that represents images in terms of amplitude and phase functions using:

$$I(x,y,t) \approx \sum_{n=1}^{M} a_n(x,y,t) \cos \varphi_n(x,y,t). \quad (21.27)$$

The idea is to let the amplitude modulated (AM) components $a_n(x,y)$ to capture slow-changing spatial variability in the image intensity, as well as the energy attributed to each component. The frequency modulation components (FM) come from the cosine terms. The FM components are used to describe texture variations. For a single AM-FM component approximation to the input video, we have:

$$I(x,y,t) = a(x,y,t) \exp(j\varphi(x,y,t)). \quad (21.28)$$

Assuming the OFC, Murray et al.[18] used Eq. 21.28 to derive:

$$a_x u + a_y v + a_t = 0, \text{ and} \quad (21.29)$$

$$\varphi_x u + \varphi_y v + \varphi_t = 0. \quad (21.30)$$

Combining Eqs. 21.29 and 21.30 with a smoothness constraint on the velocity estimates, the problem of estimating the optical flow field (u,v) reduces to minimizing the following combined energy functional over the entire image:

$$E_{\text{AMFM}} = E_s + \alpha_{\text{AM}} E_{\text{AM}} + \beta_{\text{FM}} E_{\text{FM}},$$

$$E_s = \iint_\Omega (u_x^2 + u_y^2 + v_x^2 + v_y^2) d\Omega,$$

$$E_{\text{AM}} = \iint_\Omega (a_x u + a_y v + a_t)^2 d\Omega, \quad (21.31)$$

$$E_{\text{FM}} = \iint_\Omega (\varphi_x u + \varphi_y v + \varphi_t)^2 d\Omega.$$

As in the case of the CBM and the GDIM models, the solution to Eq. 21.31 is computed after approximating derivatives with finite difference methods, and using an iterative scheme. The iterative computational scheme is given by:

$$u^{k+1} = \bar{u}^k - \alpha_{AM}\frac{(\varphi_x + \beta_{FM}a_y^2\varphi_x - \beta_{FM}a_ya_x\varphi_y)\bar{u}^k + \varphi_y\bar{v}^k + (\beta a_y^2 + 1)\varphi_t - \beta_{FM}a_y\varphi_ya_t}{1 + \alpha_{AM}(\varphi_y^2 + \varphi_x^2) + \alpha_{AM}\beta_{FM}(a_y\varphi_x - a_x\varphi_y)^2 + \beta_{FM}(a_y^2 + a_x^2)}\varphi_x$$
$$- \beta_{FM}\frac{[\alpha_{AM}(a_x\varphi_y - a_y\varphi_x)\varphi_y + a_x]\bar{u}^k + a_y\bar{v}^k - \alpha_{AM}a_y\varphi_y\varphi_t + (\alpha_{AM}\varphi_y^2 + 1)a_t}{1 + \alpha_{AM}(\varphi_y^2 + \varphi_x^2) + \alpha_{AM}\beta_{FM}(a_y\varphi_x - a_x\varphi_y)^2 + \beta_{FM}(a_y^2 + a_x^2)} \quad (21.32)$$

$$v^{k+1} = \bar{v}^k - \alpha_{AM}\frac{\varphi_x\bar{u}^k + (\varphi_y + \beta_{FM}a_x^2\varphi_y - \beta_{FM}a_xa_y\varphi_x)\bar{v}^k + (\beta_{FM}a_x^2 + 1)\varphi_t - \beta_{FM}a_x\varphi_xa_t}{1 + \alpha_{AM}(\varphi_y^2 + \varphi_x^2) + \alpha_{AM}\beta_{FM}(\varphi_xa_y - \varphi_ya_x)^2 + \beta_{FM}(a_x^2 + a_y^2)}\varphi_y$$
$$- \beta_{FM}\frac{a_x\bar{u}^k + [\alpha_{AM}(a_y\varphi_x - a_x\varphi_y)\varphi_x + a_y]\bar{v}^k - \alpha_{AM}a_x\varphi_x\varphi_t + (\alpha_{AM}\varphi_x^2 + 1)a_t}{1 + \alpha_{AM}(\varphi_y^2 + \varphi_x^2) + \alpha_{AM}\beta_{FM}(\varphi_xa_y - \varphi_ya_x)^2 + \beta_{FM}(a_x^2 + a_y^2)}a_y. \quad (21.33)$$

21.2.3 Local Solutions via Least Squares

Local solutions assume a constant velocity model and use least squares (LS) fits over pixel neighborhoods. Local solutions have the advantage that are robust in the present of noise[5,13] but suffer from low-density field estimates wherever the system of equations to solve is ill-conditioned.

21.2.3.1 Lucas and Kanade Least Squares Solution

Instead of adding further constraints to the CBM, Lucas and Kanade[9] chose to minimize a weighted version of the OFC assuming that nearby pixels share the same 2D velocity:

$$E_{W_{OFC}} = \iint_\Gamma W(x,y)(I_xu + I_yv + I_t)^2 d\Gamma \quad (21.34)$$

where the weighted functional Eq. 21.34 is minimized over a local spatial neighborhood Γ. In discrete form, we need to minimize:

$$\sum_{x \in \Gamma}[W(x,y)(I_xu + I_yv + I_t)^2]. \quad (21.35)$$

The associated Euler-Lagrange equations associated with Eq. 21.34 are given by:

$$W(x)(I_x^2u + I_xI_yv + I_xI_t) = 0, \text{ and}$$
$$W(x)(I_xI_yu + I_y^2v + I_yI_t) = 0. \quad (21.36)$$

The weight function $W(x,y)$ is assumed to be separable $W(x,y) = W_1(x)W_2(y)$ and a function of distance from the center. The idea is to give more emphasis to measurements at the center of the window than at the periphery. The constraint errors are added over a 5×5 region, leading to

$$\sum_{x \in \Gamma} W(x,y)(I_x^2u + I_xI_yv + I_xI_t) = 0$$
$$\sum_{x \in \Gamma} W(x,y)(I_xI_yu + I_y^2v + I_yI_t) = 0 \quad (21.37)$$

The least square estimator that minimizes the sum of the squared errors in Eq. 21.35 gives the solution to Eq. 21.37 as:

$$\vec{v} = [A^TWA]^{-1}A^TWb \quad (21.38)$$

where:

$$A = [\nabla I(x_1), \ldots, \nabla I(x_n)]^T,$$
$$W = \bar{w} \times \bar{w}^T, \text{ and} \quad (21.39)$$
$$b = -[I_t(x_1), \ldots, I_t(x_n)]^T$$

and $\vec{v}$ denotes the velocity estimates for n points $(x_i, y_i) \in \Gamma$ at a single time t. There is a closed form solution to $\vec{v}$ when A^TWA is non-singular given by:

$$A^TWA = \begin{bmatrix} \sum W(x,y)I_x^2 & \sum W(x,y)I_xI_y \\ \sum W(x,y)I_xI_y & \sum W(x,y)I_y^2 \end{bmatrix} \quad (21.40)$$

with summations taken over the entire window. Here, matrix $A^T W A$ has to be full rank and depends on accurate image gradient calculations.[28] Pre-smoothing is applied to the image sequences to attenuate the effect of quantization noise and the amplitude of high-order terms in Eq. 21.2. For high levels of noise and significant values of the higher order terms, sufficient smoothing will be needed to ensure the accuracy of the estimation. On the other hand, too much smoothing will also lead to inaccurate estimates since it destroys local image structure. The smoothing is controlled by adjusting the spread, σ, of a spatial Gaussian filter.

21.2.3.2 Uras Second-Order Differential Technique

Uras et al.[11] used the Hessian of the image brightness intensity to locally constrain the image velocity assuming the conservation of the image intensity gradient. Locally, they solved an over-determined system of equations over regions where the Hessian is non-singular. The conservation of image gradient energy functional is given by:

$$E_G = \iint_\Gamma \| \nabla(I_x u + I_y v + I_t) \|^2 d\Gamma. \qquad (21.41)$$

The associated Euler-Lagrange equations are:

$$\begin{aligned} I_{xx} u + I_{xy} v + I_{xt} &= 0, \text{ and} \\ I_{xy} u + I_{yy} v + I_{yt} &= 0 \end{aligned} \qquad (21.42)$$

and can be solved wherever the Hessian of the image brightness intensities is non-singular. In practice, for robustness,[13] the authors divide the image into 8×8 pixel regions.

The main problem with the conservation of ∇I, $d\nabla I/dt = 0$ is that it is a far more restrictive assumption than the conservation of image intensities because first-order deformations of image intensities, e.g., rotations or dilations, should not be present in the permissible motion field. In addition, second-order derivatives cannot be approximated accurately.

21.2.3.3 Phase-Based Technique for Motion Estimation

The use of phase information for the computation of optical flow was first introduced in 1990.[12] The input image is decomposed into band-pass channels using complex Gabor filters to extract amplitude and phase information. Each filter output can be written as:

$$R(\vec{x}, t) = \rho(\vec{x}, t) \exp[i\phi(\vec{x}, t)] \qquad (21.43)$$

and space-time surfaces of constant phase, $\phi(\vec{x}, t) = c$, are used to estimate the velocity component normal to level phase contours. Differentiating these surfaces leads to the phase energy functional which is given by:

$$E_{\text{Phase}} = \iint_\Gamma (\phi_x u + \phi_y v + \phi_t) d\Gamma. \qquad (21.44)$$

The velocity that minimizes Eq. 21.44 is called component velocity and is the velocity normal to level phase contours, $\vec{v}_n = s\vec{n}$ given by:

$$s = \frac{-\phi_t(\vec{x}, t)}{\| \nabla \phi(\vec{x}, t) \|}, \text{ and } \vec{n} = \frac{\nabla \phi(\vec{x}, t)}{\| \nabla \phi(\vec{x}, t) \|}. \qquad (21.45)$$

The computation of optical flow from the conservation of phase information is a differential technique applied to phase rather than image intensity, and it is motivated from the claim that phase information is more stable under changes in mean intensity and contrast than amplitude information.[29] However, phase instabilities do occur and Fleet and Jepson[12] detect them using:

$$\| (k_0, w_0) - (k, w) \| \le \sigma_k \tau, \qquad (21.46)$$

where (k_0, w_0) denotes the spatiotemporal frequency to which each filter is tuned, σ_k denotes the standard deviation of the filter's amplitude spectrum, and τ is a threshold that can be used to reject local frequencies that are far from the nominal tuning range of the filter.[12] Finally, using the measurements of component velocities, a linear velocity model:

$$\tilde{v}(\vec{x}, t) = (\alpha_0 + \alpha_1 x + \alpha_2 y, \beta_0 + \beta_1 x + \beta_2 y)^T \qquad (21.47)$$

is fitted to 5×5 regions yielding a linear system $Ra = \vec{v}_n$ that is solved using least squares. The estimated full 2D velocity was taken to be the constant parameters $\vec{v} = (\alpha_0, \beta_0)^T$, in Eq. 21.47.

21.2.4 Combining Global and Local Optical Flow Solutions

The combination of global and local methods, known as the combined local–global method, has been studied in Bauer et al.[30] Here, the methods by Horn and Schunck[8] and Lucas and Kanade[9] are merged in a hybrid technique using a structural tensor at different integration scales creating the combined local–global functional which gives a robust solution on local neighborhoods. The approach also yields high-density fields.

To understand the approach, consider the image sequence $I(x, y, t)$ smoothed with a Gaussian $K_\sigma(x, y)$ of standard deviation σ:

$$f(x, y, t) = (K_\sigma * I)(x, y, t) \quad (21.48)$$

where σ can be tuned to the noise scale. Then, assuming the conservation of image brightness intensities for small displacements gives:

$$f_x u + f_y v + f_t = 0. \quad (21.49)$$

Now, recall that Lucas and Kanade assumed constant velocities within some neighborhood of size ρ. The Lucas and Kanade method is reformulated as one of using weighted least squares to solve:

$$E_{LK} = K_\rho * \left((f_x u + f_y v + f_t)^2 \right). \quad (21.50)$$

In Eq. 21.50, ρ serves as an integration scale over which the influence of the weighted least squares is controlled.[5] In order to develop the combined local–global method, the authors define:

$$\begin{aligned} w &= (u, v, 1)^T, \\ |\nabla w|^2 &= |\nabla u|^2 + |\nabla v|^2, \\ \nabla_3 f &= (f_x, f_y, f_t)^T, \\ J_\rho(\nabla_3 f) &= K_\rho * (\nabla_3 f \nabla_3 f^T). \end{aligned} \quad (21.51)$$

Then, Eq. 21.50 can be expressed as:

$$E_{LK}(w) = w^T J_\rho(\nabla_3 f) w. \quad (21.52)$$

The constant brightness model combined energy functional Eq. 21.52 E_{CBM} becomes:

$$E_{CBM} = \iint_\Omega (w^T J_0(\nabla_3 f) w + \alpha^2 |\nabla w|^2) dx dy. \quad (21.53)$$

By replacing the matrix $J_0(\nabla_3 f)$ in Eq. 21.53 with the structure tensor $J_\rho(\nabla_3 f)$ with some integration scale $\rho > 0$, we have the combined local–global energy function given by:

$$E_{CLG} = \iint_\Omega (\vec{w}^T J_\rho(\nabla_3 f) \vec{w} + \alpha^2 |\nabla w|^2) d\Omega, \quad (21.54)$$

and the associated Euler-Lagrange equations are:

$$\nabla^2 u - \frac{1}{\alpha^2}[K_\rho * (f_x^2)u + K_\rho * (f_x f_y)v + K_\rho * (f_x f_t)] = 0, \text{ and}$$
$$\nabla^2 v - \frac{1}{\alpha^2}[K_\rho * (f_x f_y)u + K_\rho * (f_y^2)v + K_\rho * (f_y f_t)] = 0.$$

$$(21.55)$$

The system Eq. 21.55 is solved iteratively using the successive over relaxation method (SOR) method with finite differences.

21.2.5 Research on Motion Estimation Parameter Selection

Optical flow models for motion estimation use a smoothing constraint to uniquely determine the velocity field components of the model solution. The weight of the smoothness constraint is controlled by the value of the regularization parameter in order to find an appropriate trade-off among the model energy functionals. With the exception of the approaches discussed in this section, the most commonly used method for choosing the correct value of the regularization parameter is based on a heuristic trial and error approach.

21.2.5.1 The Data-Driven Approach

Assuming that the image is a square of $n \times n$ pixels, the data-driven approach adds extra error terms to Eq. 21.3 that are modeled as independent Gaussian random variables yielding to:

$$-I_t = I_x u + I_y v + \delta, \quad (21.56)$$

where δ is $N(0, \sigma^2 \mathbf{I_n})$ with zero mean, variance noise of σ^2, and $\mathbf{I_n}$ denotes the identity matrix of $n \times n$ size. A suitable performance measure needs to be defined to assess the accuracy of the estimates. Here, Solo[26] used a weighted error norm or estimated risk defined by:

$$R_\alpha = n^{-2} E[\| W(\hat{f} - f) \|^2], \qquad (21.57)$$

where:

$$f = [u, v]^T, \quad W = [\mathrm{diag}(I_x) \; \mathrm{diag}(I_y)], \qquad (21.58)$$

and $\hat{f}$ is the optical flow estimate obtained by minimizing the combined constant brightness model energy functional proposed by Horn.[8] From Table 1, we have:

$$E_{\mathrm{CBM}} = \iint_\Omega \left[(I_x u + I_y v + I_t)^2 + \alpha (\| \nabla u \|^2 + \| \nabla v \|^2) \right] dxdy.$$
$$(21.59)$$

The unbiased estimator of R_α Eq. 21.57 is given by:

$$\hat{R}_\alpha = -\sigma^2 + \frac{1}{n^2} \| e \|^2 - \frac{2\sigma^2}{n^2} \mathrm{trace}(WA^{-1}W^T), \qquad (21.60)$$

where $A = n^2 (E_{\mathrm{CBM}})_{\hat{f}\hat{f}}/2$, and the matrix $(E_{\mathrm{CBM}})_{\hat{f}\hat{f}}$ can be computed by discretizing Eq. 21.59 and taking derivatives with respect to each component of $f = [u, v]^T$. If σ^2 is known, then $\hat{R}_\alpha$ can be directly calculated and the optimal regularization parameter according to Eq. 21.60 is the α that minimizes $\hat{R}_\alpha$. If σ^2 is not known, then it can be replaced by an estimate.[26]

21.2.5.2 The Maximum Likelihood Regularization Parameter Estimator Method

Developed by Krajsek and Mester,[25] a combined marginal maximum likelihood/maximum a posteriori (MML/MAP) estimator for choosing the regularization parameter value was proposed using a Bayesian framework for examining regularization or their equivalent hyper-parameters in the Bayesian framework.[24]

The conservation of image intensities is expressed in the equivalent form of:

$$\vec{g}^T \vec{v}_h = 0, \qquad (21.61)$$

where $\vec{g} = (I_x, I_y, I_t)^T$ and $\vec{v}_h = (u, v, 1)^T$. Since it is not possible to fully estimate $\vec{v}_h$ from a single equation with two unknowns, the necessary additional constraint is incorporated by a regularization term $\rho(\vec{v})$, where ρ is an operator acting on $\vec{v} = (u, v)^T$, that imposes a smoothing constraint on permissible motion fields. The optical flow field is estimated by minimizing:

$$E_{\mathrm{CBM}} = \iint_\Omega (\psi(\vec{g}^T \vec{v}_h) + \lambda \rho(\vec{v})) dxdy, \qquad (21.62)$$

where ψ is a real positive function and the regularization parameter λ controls the influence of the regularization term $\rho(\vec{v})$ relative to the data term $\psi(\vec{g}^T \vec{v}_h)$. In the Bayesian formulation, the optical flow is estimated using a probability density function (*pdf*). In order to design the *pdf*, a regular grid in space-time is assumed where image intensities and optical flow vectors are only considered if they lie on the knots of the grid. Then, for N knots, we define:

$$\begin{aligned}
\vec{I} &= (I(x_1), I(x_2), \dots, I(x_N)), \\
\vec{u}_c &= (u(x_1), u(x_2), \dots, u(x_N)), \\
\vec{v}_c &= (v(x_1), v(x_2), \dots, v(x_N)), \\
\vec{v} &= (u, v)^T.
\end{aligned} \qquad (21.63)$$

In this framework, not only the measured image gradients $\vec{g} = (g(x_1), g(x_2), \dots g(x_N))$, but also the estimated field $\vec{v}$ are considered random variables with pdfs $p(\vec{v})$ and $p(\vec{g})$. Prior knowledge about $\vec{v}$ is incorporated into the estimation via the prior pdf $p(\vec{v})$. The maximum a posteriori (MAP) estimator infers the optical flow field by maximizing the posterior $p(\vec{v}|\vec{g})$. Using Bayes law:

$$\begin{aligned}
\hat{\vec{v}} &= \arg\max_{\vec{v}} \left\{ \frac{p(\vec{g}|\vec{v}) p(\vec{v})}{p(\vec{g})} \right\}, \\
\hat{\vec{v}} &= \arg\max_{\vec{v}} \left\{ -\ln(p(\vec{g}|\vec{v})) - \ln(p(\vec{v})) \right\}.
\end{aligned} \qquad (21.64)$$

The errors ε in the brightness constancy assumption are attributed only to the temporal component of the image gradient by writing:

$$g_{sj}^T \vec{v}_{hj} = \varepsilon_{tj}, \qquad (21.65)$$

where $\vec{g}_{sj} = (I_{xj}, I_{yj})^T$ is the error-free vector of spatial image gradient components. Expressing each random variable ε_{tj} in the joint pdf $p(\vec{\varepsilon}) = \prod_{j=1}^{N} p(\varepsilon_{tj})$, the likelihood function $p(\vec{g}_t | \vec{v}, \vec{g}_s)$ is given by:

$$p(\vec{g}_t | \vec{v}, \vec{g}_s) = \frac{1}{Z_L(\alpha)} \exp\left[-\alpha \sum_{j=1}^{N} \psi_1(\vec{g}_j \vec{v}_{hj})\right]. \qquad (21.66)$$

The prior $p(\vec{v})$ encodes the prior information/assumptions about the optical flow, i.e., the smoothness of the field, and then the *pdf* corresponding to the smoothness assumption is given by:

$$p(\vec{v}) = \frac{1}{Z_p(\vec{\beta})} \exp\left[-\sum_{j=1}^{N} \beta_x \psi_2(u_x^2 + u_y^2) + \beta_y \psi_2(v_x^2 + v_y^2)\right] \qquad (21.67)$$

where $\vec{\beta} = (\beta_x, \beta_y)^T$ in the more general anisotropic case. After substituting Eq. 21.66 and Eq. 21.66 in Eq. 21.67, the objective function $E^{(N)}$ is given by:

$$E^{(N)} = E_L(\alpha) + E_p(\beta) + \ln(Z_L(\alpha) Z_p(\beta)). \qquad (21.68)$$

In the isotropic case $\beta = \beta_x = \beta_y$, the regularization parameter is given by $\lambda = \beta/\alpha$ expressed in terms of the hyper-parameters α, and β. Subtracting $\ln(Z_L(\alpha) Z_p(\beta))$ from Eq. 21.68, taking the limit and dividing by α gives:

$$\begin{aligned} E &= \lim_{N \to \infty} \left(E^{(N)} - \ln(Z_L(\alpha) Z_p(\beta)) \right) \\ &= \iint_\Omega (\alpha \psi_1(\vec{g}^T \vec{v}_h) + \beta \psi_2(\|\nabla u\|^2 + \|\nabla v\|^2)) dx dy \\ &= \iint_\Omega (\psi_1(\vec{g}^T \vec{v}_h) + \lambda \psi_2(\|\nabla u\|^2 + \|\nabla v\|^2)) dx dy. \end{aligned} \qquad (21.69)$$

When the objective function Eq. 21.68 is minimized, rather than choosing ad hoc values for α, and β these are inferred using prior knowledge of the flow field. For example, the ground truth is used to compute moments of functions of the motion field. Using the maximum entropy principle,[31] the hyper-parameters are calculated by constructing the prior $p(\vec{v})$ and incorporating all the constraints imposed on $\vec{v}$.

21.2.6 Summary of Emerging Techniques

Motion estimation for video tracking under variation of image illumination was studied in Hager and Belhumeur[32] using a parametric model. A target-dependent basis for illumination changes is computed *a priory* and used to project the image to a low dimensional linear sub-space. The models are later incorporated into the tracking algorithm which can handle object deformations, changes in geometry, occlusion, and illumination variations.

Following Nagahdaripour's work,[17] Haussecker and Fleet[33] parameterized physical brightness changes in an attempt to model high-order brightness variations. They created models for changes due to light diffusion, exponential brightness decay, nonuniform moving illumination envelopes, and surface rotation under directional illumination. Using an anisotropic diffusion approach for modeling illumination changes, Alvarez.[34] created an energy functional that is invariant to linear brightness changes with the additional claim that their method can handle the estimation of large motion fields up to 10 pixels per frame.

In order to improve numerical stability and robustness, many researchers have focused on using different operators to improve the robustness of the solution of optical flow. Robust statistical estimators were introduced in the computation of optical flow[27,35] in order to better handle outliers, pixels that violate the assumptions, and reduce the estimation error due to discontinuity of the flow at object boundaries. Structural tensor based methods combined with diffusion approaches[36-39] proved to be a reliable tool for noise reduction, and the use of total variation TV-L^1 [40] has been used to minimize the energy functionals by replacing quadratic norm penalties with a L^1 penalty norm that allows for discontinuities in the motion field.

21.3 Atherosclerotic Plaque Motion Analysis

The present study is motivated from a desire to extend traditional motion estimation methods into the development of reliable methods for validating the motion estimates and also allow for trajectory estimation. First, a realistic plaque motion model based on clinical experience was developed. This simulator is used to investigate the limits of traditional motion estimation methods in assessing plaque and artery wall motion.

The simulator can create different motion patterns so that the motion estimation (ME) algorithms can be tested under different conditions and used to find a set of motion parameters that estimate the most accurate velocity vectors from ultrasound videos. To accomplish this goal, a global optimization algorithm[41] is used to calculate the parameter ranges that minimize the mean squared error (MSE) for several realistic simulation cases. Then, this parameter set is applied to clinical ultrasound videos and the results are visually and qualitatively graded. For this purpose, the velocity estimates are fed to a Kalman filter that tracks individual pixels along the video sequence. The information conveyed by the reconstructed trajectories along with the visual assessment of the videos provides the means for validation of the velocity estimates.

Optical flow can fail to produce reliable velocity vectors due to violations of the model assumptions. A hindering factor is speckle noise. Speckle produces variations in image intensities and makes ME difficult. Thus, in order to be able to find the most accurate pixel velocities in the presence of speckle, ME was performed using simulated videos of poor signal to noise ratio (SNR). These parameter values were used on clinical video sequences that exhibited poor SNR.

21.3.1 Motion Model of Ultrasound Videos of Carotid Artery Plaques

Periodic motion in ultrasound videos of carotid plaque artery can be observed and it comes from the fact that the artery follows the cardiac cycle. The period of this motion can be determined from the videos, and motion discontinuities are expected from random motion events induced by, for example, lung motions. These periodic motions (including their discontinuities) are simulated using a Fourier Series expansion. Here, note that the Fourier Series is applicable to any periodic continuous or discontinuous function (finite number of discontinuities). These discontinuities produce Fourier harmonic coefficients that are inversely proportional to the fundamental frequency.[42] Clinical verification of this fact on atherosclerotic plaque videos was given in previous work published in Murillo et al.[21] and also reported by Lever et al.,[43] Golemati et al.,[44] and Stoitsis et al.[45] where a cyclical pattern along with its discontinuities was observed.

A realistic motion model is created by taking the first frame of the video sequence and applying a set of coordinate transformation equations in order to displace the pixel intensity values to new coordinates. The coordinate transformation creates image pixel displacements in the axial and lateral directions governed by the following set of equations:

$$a(x, y, t) = A_a \sin\left(\frac{2\pi}{N} f_a t\right) + \frac{A_a}{2} \sin\left(\frac{2\pi}{N}(2f_a)t\right)$$
$$+ \frac{A_a}{3} \sin\left(\frac{2\pi}{N}(3f_a)t\right) + \eta_a(x, y, t), \text{ and}$$
$$l(x, y, t) = A_l \sin\left(\frac{2\pi}{N} f_l t\right) + \frac{A_l}{2} \sin\left(\frac{2\pi}{N}(2f_l)t\right)$$
$$+ \frac{A_l}{3} \sin\left(\frac{2\pi}{N}(3f_l)t\right) + \eta_l(x, y, t),$$

(21.70)

where N is the number of simulated video frames. The simulation parameters are given in Table 21.3 and Fig. 21.1 shows an ultrasound video frame with the axial and lateral directions. Here, f_a refers to the axial frequency and f_l refers to the lateral frequency. Similarly, A_a refers to the axial frequency amplitude, and A_l refers to the lateral frequency amplitude. The number of cycles was estimated from video observation so that the simulated motion had approximately the same fundamental frequency as the clinical videos. Periodic motions up to three harmonics are assumed in order to simulate the cardiac cycle. Also, the harmonic amplitudes were made inversely proportional to the harmonic frequencies. This is consistent with a

Table 21.3 Table of simulation parameters

Synthetic motion parameters				
Video number	#1	#2	#3	#4
Stenosis (%)	73%	60%	52%	26%
Axial frequency (cycles per video length)	5	3	5	5
Lateral frequency (cycles per video length)	6	2.5	4	4.5
Axial motion amplitude (pixels)	1.5	1	3.5	5.5
Lateral amplitude (pixels)	2	2	2.5	3.0
Frame dimensions (pixels × pixels)	100 × 240	221 × 251	125 × 250	125 × 250
Number of frames	300	200	300	300
Maximum velocity magnitude (pixels/frame)	0.5	0.3	1.1	1.8

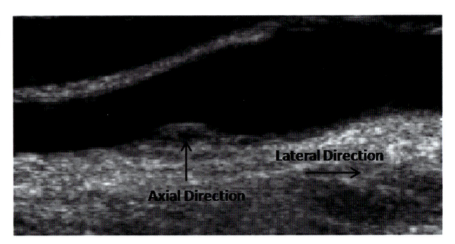

Fig. 21.1 Single frame of carotid ultrasound image. This figure illustrates the axial and lateral directions

discontinuity in the motion and has also been observed in the power spectra of the estimated trajectories published in 2006.[21]

For generating realistic plaque motion velocities, an automated segmentation method was used to separate the plaque from the rest of the video image.[6] The plaque and non-plaque regions were first assumed to move independently (using different Fourier Series expansions). To provide for continuity between the plaque and the carotid artery, a convolution with a low-pass filter was used to provide for a smooth transition from the plaque to the artery. Simulations for different degrees of stenosis are also provided. For larger degrees of stenosis, less smoothing between the artery and the plaque was also applied. For smaller degrees of stenosis, more smoothing was applied.

21.4 Optimal Motion Parameter Selection Using Global Optimization

The accuracy of the ME algorithms is affected by the selection of the parameter values used to weight their constraints and also for the spread of the Gaussian pre-smoother filter applied to the image sequence prior differentiation. Thus, optimization is necessary to find the parameter values that produce the most accurate velocity vectors. Moreover, when estimating motion of clinical videos, there is no ground truth or reference to compare and quantitatively evaluate the accuracy of the estimates. Using the realistic synthetic motions and a global optimization algorithm, a set of parameters that produces the smallest MSE of the velocity estimates is found. This process is equivalent to tuning up the ME algorithms to the motion present in the clinical videos.

The objective function is set to be the MSE of the estimated velocity magnitudes Eq. 21.72 with respect to the ground truth motion Eq. 21.71 for every pixel in the image:

$$GTMag = \| \vec{v}_{gt} \| = \sqrt{u_{gt}^2 + v_{gt}^2} \quad (21.71)$$

$$ESTMag(\vec{p}) = \| \vec{v}_{est}(\vec{p}) \| = \sqrt{u_{est}^2(\vec{p}) + v_{est}^2(\vec{p})}$$

$$f(\vec{p}) = \frac{1}{MN} \sum_{i=0}^{M-1} \sum_{j=0}^{N-1} (ESTMag_{ij}(\vec{p}) - GTMag_{ij})^2$$

$$(21.72)$$

The vector $\vec{p}$ is composed of the motion estimation parameters that govern the optical flow models and it varies for each method. In the case of Horn and Schunck method,[8] optimization was carried out for the spread of the spatiotemporal Gaussian pre-smoothing filter (σ), and the value of the weight α that controls the influence of the smoothness constraint E_s in the optical flow model Eq. 21.13. Thus, a closed set of possible values must be considered: $P = \{\vec{p} \in \Re^2 : \vec{a} \leq \vec{p} \leq \vec{b}\}$ where $\vec{a} = (0, 0.5)^T$, $\vec{b} = (100, 1.75)^T$, and $\vec{p} = (\alpha, \sigma)^T$.

For optimization, a branch and bound strategy is applied where the feasible set is partitioned into more and more refined parts (branching), over which lower and upper bounds of the minimum objective function value are determined (bounding). Parts of the feasible set with lower bounds higher than the best upper bound found at a certain stage are deleted from further consideration (pruning). This is due to the fact that these parts of the domain cannot contain an optimal point that is better of what is already in the best upper bound.

21.5 Results of Motion Estimation Parameter Optimization

The parameter optimization results are shown as contour plots and tables of the relative error. The relative error is measured with respect to the maximum velocity magnitude: *Relative Error = Magnitude Error/Max. Vel. Magnitude.* Figure 21.2 shows optimization for simulated videos #1 and #3.

Here, the simulator works under the assumption that low stenosis implies that there is room for motion and it allows the simulation of larger motion components. On the other hand, high degrees of stenosis do not leave much room for motion. Therefore, in these cases, smaller motion components were simulated. Thus, for video #1, a smooth velocity field of small amplitude was imposed. The maximum velocity of this video was $v_{GT(max)} = 0.5$ pix/frame.

For video #3, the simulated motion was allowed to have higher amplitudes and velocities. The maximum velocity of the video was $v_{GT(max)} = 1.1$ pix/frame. Tables 21.4 and 21.5 show the accuracy of the estimation for simulated cases #1 and #3. The values are expressed as percentages of the maximum velocity. For example, a value of 0.1 means that on average, the error is 10% of the maximum ground truth velocity.

The parameter values that returned the smallest error among all simulation were $\alpha = 1.0$ and $\sigma = 1.25$. This set was later used to estimate pixel velocities of clinical cases.

21.5.1 Speckle Simulation Results

The simulated examples were corrupted with speckle noise following the model proposed in Loizou et al.[46] This model assumes that speckle can be modeled as independent and identically distributed (i.i.d.) additive white Gaussian noise (AWGN) after logarithmic compression of the envelop detected signal. The goal is to use the global optimization algorithm to find a set of input parameters able to calculate the best possible velocity estimates. Contour levels of the relative error are shown in Fig. 21.3 for two SNRs of 10dbs and 30dbs.

21.5.2 Motion Estimation Results of Clinical Ultrasound Videos

Pixel motion estimation was computed for regions of interest (ROI) centered around the plaque using the Horn and Schunck technique.[8] The optimal motion parameter values calculated using the global optimization algorithm are used to estimate the motion of clinical video cases.

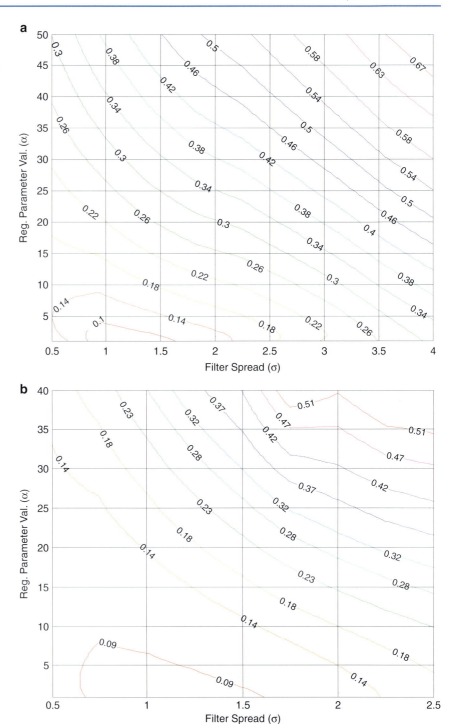

Fig. 21.2 Contour plots of relative error for simulated videos #1 (**a**) and #3 (**b**). The optimal motion parameters are the ones that produce the smallest error among all simulations

Table 21.4 Relative velocity estimation error for simulation #1. Relative errors up to 10% are considered acceptable

	Spread smoothing filter			
Reg. Par.	0.5	1.37	2.25	4
1.0	0.17	0.08	0.15	0.31
1.7	0.15	0.09	0.15	0.31
2.5.	0.15	0.10	0.15	0.32
4.0.5	0.86	0.12	0.17	0.33

Relative Velocity Error of Simulated Video # 1. Max Vgt = 0.5 pix/frame

Table 21.5 Relative velocity estimation error for simulation #3. Relative errors up to 10% are considered acceptable

	Spread smoothing filter				
Reg. Par.	0.75	1.0	1.5	1.75	2.0
1.0	0.13	0.07	0.09	0.10	0.12
2.5	0.11	0.08	0.09	0.11	0.13
8.6	0.11	0.10	0.13	0.15	0.17
11.6	0.11	0.11	0.15	0.17	0.20

Relative Velocity Error of Simulated Video #3. Max Vgt = 1.1 pix/frame

The evaluation of the estimated velocities is done visually by feeding the flow field to a Kalman filter that reconstructs pixel trajectories. Then, the clinical video is then played back with the trajectories over the plaque. This process identifies if the current motion parameters are doing a good job at estimating the true displacement field. When the trajectories lose track of the plaque, a new set of input parameters are used. Speckle is the cause that the parameters cannot track certain plaque regions; thus, for these cases, the motion parameters are changed to the ones found in the speckle simulation.

Figure 21.4 shows two clinical ultrasound frames of an atherosclerotic plaque during systole and diastole. The velocity vectors are overlaid on top of the plaque and artery with the arrows pointing in the direction of the motion.

Figure 21.5 shows four selected points located at different locations over the plaque. The axial and lateral trajectories are shown in Fig. 21.6. The reconstructed trajectories show that the lateral motion is in sync for all the points, while the axial motion exhibits more variability indicating the presence of different motion components over the plaque. The resolution of the clinical video is 0.15 mm/pixel.

For a second clinical video, the technique of Lucas and Kanade was also used to estimate video motion. The results of both methods show consistency in the reconstructed trajectories, see Fig. 21.7. This is evidence that when two different motion estimation algorithms produce almost the same estimates, they are most likely correctly estimating the true video motion. When the incorrect input parameters are used on two different methods, it is easy for the methods to produce different and wrong answers, but when the correct parameters are used, both methods will most likely converge close to the true velocity field.

21.6 Conclusions

The accuracy of the motion estimation is significantly affected by the selection of the model parameters. When working with clinical videos, i.e., no ground truth, it is very important to select the correct parameter value in order to achieve accurate estimation. Global optimization finds a range of parameter values that can be used on a variety of clinical videos producing accurate velocity estimates. In particular, the authors have found that a single set of optimal values can produce accurate results for a variety of motions and relatively low noise levels.

When noisy levels increase, another set of parameters is able to correctly estimate video motion. The velocities estimates can be used to estimate pixel trajectories and analyze the motion of the artery wall and plaque regions which provides important information on how the plaque moves during the cardiac cycle.

When estimating velocities of clinical videos, it is important to obtain high-density fields because it means that the algorithms are working correctly and are able to estimate the velocities for most of the video length. Moreover, the more dense the estimated field more information can be assessed from the video. Thus, global techniques are preferred to local methods because higher densities are obtained.

Fig. 21.3 Contour plots of the relative error for speckle simulations of SNR = 10 dB (**a**) and 30 dB (**b**). Compared to noise-free cases, higher regularization parameters and filter spreads are necessary to obtain reliable velocity estimates

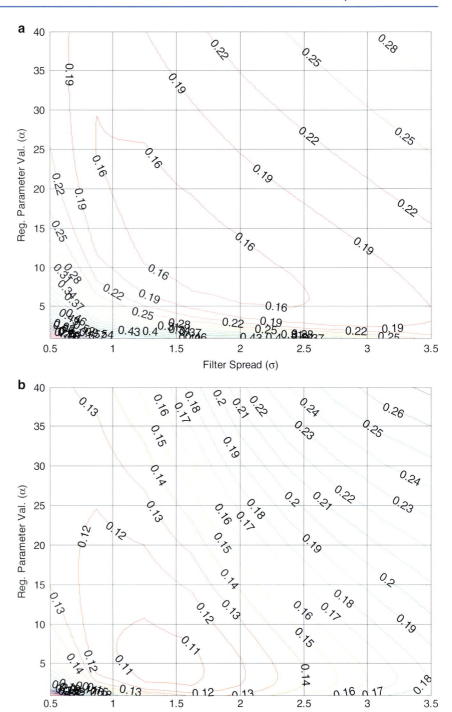

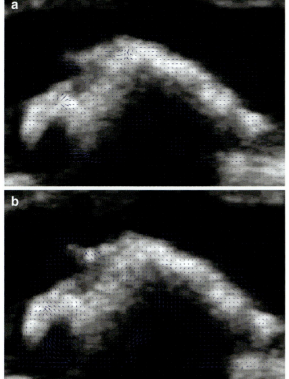

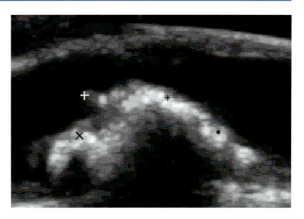

Fig. 21.5 Four selected points at different locations over the plaque

Fig. 21.4 Estimated motion vectors overlaid on top of the ultrasound frames during systole (**a**) and diastole (**b**) cardiac cycles

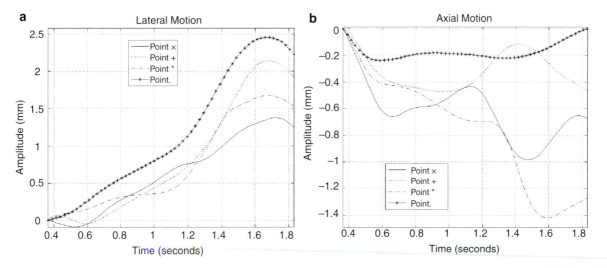

Fig. 21.6 Lateral (**a**) and axial (**b**) motions of the four selected points. Lateral motions are similar for the points while the axial motion exhibits more variability indicating different motion components over the plaque

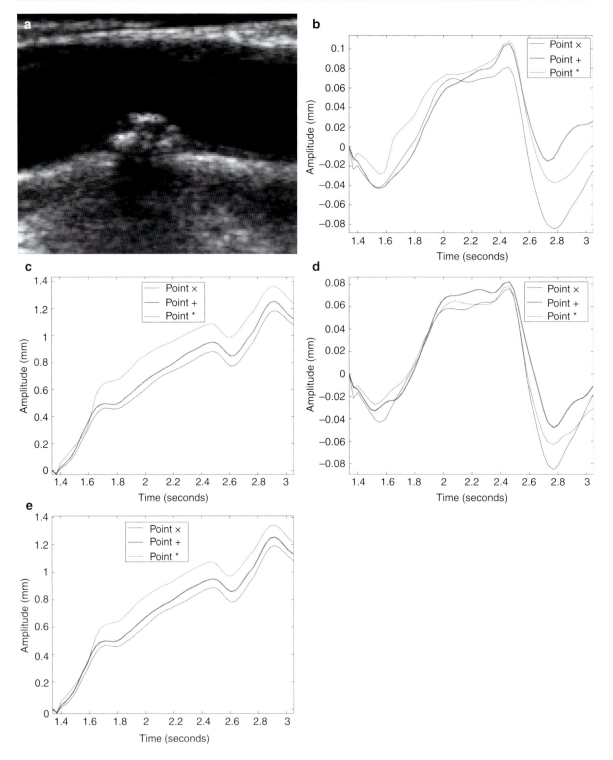

Fig. 21.7 Reconstructed trajectories of three plaque points using Horn's and Lucas's techniques. (**a**) Plaque points. (**b**) Horn axial motion. (**c**) Horn lateral motion. (**d**) Lucas axial motion. (**e**) Lucas lateral motion. Similar trajectories produced with two different methods indicate that the correct pixel velocities are being calculated

References

1. AHA Statistical Update Heart Disease and Stroke Statistics–2008 Update A Report From the American Heart Association Statistics Committee and Stroke Statistics Subcommittee, website: http://circ.ahajournals.org/content/117/4/e25.full, accessed September 9th, 2011.
2. Zarins CK, Xu C, Glagov S. Atherosclerotic enlargement of the human abdominal aorta. *Atherosclerosis*. 2001;155(1):157–164.
3. Meairs S, Hennerici M. Four-dimensional ultrasonographic characterization of plaque surface motion in patients with symptomatic and asymptomatic carotid artery stenosis. *Stroke*. 1999;30(9):1807–1813.
4. Beauchemin SS, Barron JL. The computation of optical flow. *ACM Comput Surv*. 1995;27(3):433–466.
5. Bruhn A, Weickert J, Schnorr C. Combining the advantages of local and global optic flow methods. In: *Pattern Recognition*. Berlin: Springer; 2002:454–462 (Lecture notes in computer science; vol 2449).
6. Loizou C, Pattichis C, Pantziaris M, Nicolaides A. An integrated system for the segmentation of atherosclerotic carotid plaque. *IEEE Trans Inf Technol Biomed*. 2007;11(6):661–667.
7. Haykin S. *Adaptive Filter Theory*. 4th ed. Upper Saddle River: Prentice Hall; 2002.
8. Horn B, Schunck B. Determining optical flow. *Artif Intell*. 1981;17(2):185–204.
9. Lucas BD, Kanade T. An iterative image registration technique with an application to stereo vision. In: International Joint Conference on Artificial Intelligence; August 24–28,1981; Vancouver: 674–679.
10. Nagel HH, Enkelmann W. An investigation of smoothness constraints for the estimation of displacement vector fields from image sequences. *IEEE Trans Pattern Anal Mach Intell*. 1986;8:565–593.
11. Uras S, Girosi F, Verri A, Torre V. A computational approach to motion perception. *Biol Cybern*. 1988;60(2): 79–87.
12. Fleet DJ, Jepson AD. Computation of component image velocity from local phase information. *Int J Comput Vis*. 1990;5(1):77–104.
13. Barron JL, Fleet DJ, Beauchemin SS. Performance of optical flow techniques. *Int J Comput Vis*. 1994;12(1):43–77.
14. Anandan P. A computational framework and an algorithm for the measurement of visual motion. *Int J Comput Vis*. 1989;2(3):283–310.
15. Heeger DJ. Model for the extraction of image flow. *J Opt Soc Am A*. 1987;4(8):1455–1471.
16. Waxman AM, Wu J, Bergholm F. Convected activation profiles and the measurement of visual motion. In: Proceedings of the Computer Society Conference on Computer Vision and Pattern Recognition; June 5–9, 1988; Ann Arbor:717 723.
17. Negahdaripour S. Revised definition of optical flow: integration of radiometric and geometric cues for dynamic scene analysis. *IEEE Trans Pattern Anal Mach Intell*. 1998;20(9): 961–979.
18. Murray V, et al. An AM-FM model for motion estimation in atherosclerotic plaque videos. In: 41st Asilomar Conference on Signals, Systems and Computers; November 4–7, 2007; Monterey:746–750.
19. Horn B. *Robot Vision*. Cambridge/New York: MIT/McGraw-Hill; 1986.
20. Murillo S, et al. Atherosclerotic plaque motion analysis from ultrasound videos. In: 40th Asilomar Conference on Signals, Systems and Computers; October 29–November 1, 2006; Monterey:836–840.
21. Murillo S, et al. Atherosclerotic plaque motion trajectory analysis from ultrasound videos. In: IEEE International Special Topic Conference on Information Technology Applications in Biomedicine; October 26–28, 2006; Ioannina:1–5.
22. Courant R, Hilbert D. *Methods for Mathematical Physics*. New York: Wiley-Interscience; 1989.
23. Strang G. *Introduction to Applied Mathematics*. Wellesley: Wellesley-Cambridge; 1986.
24. Krajsek K, Mester R. On the equivalence of variational and statistical differential motion estimation. In: IEEE Southwest Symposium on Image Analysis and Interpretation; 2006; Denver:11–15.
25. Krajsek K, Mester R. A maximum likelihood estimator for choosing the regularization parameters in global optical flow methods. In: IEEE International Conference on Image Processing; October 8–11, 2006; Atlanta:1081–1084.
26. Ng L, Solo V. A data-driven method for choosing smoothing parameters in optical flow problems. In: International Conference on Image Processing; October 26–29, 1997; Washington DC:360–363.
27. Teng C-H, Lai S-H, Chen Y-S, Hsu W-H. Accurate optical flow computation under non-uniform brightness variations. *Comput Vis Image Underst*. 2005;97(3):315–346.
28. Fleet DJ, Wiess Y. Optical flow estimation. In: Paragios N, Chen Y, Faugeras O, eds. *Handbook of Mathematical Models in Computer Vision*. New York: Springer; 2005:239–258.
29. Fleet DJ, Jepson AD. Stability of phase information. *IEEE Trans Pattern Anal Mach Intell*. 1993;15(12):1253–1268.
30. Bauer N, Pathirana P, Hodgson P. Robust optical flow with combined Lucas-Kanade/Horn-Schunck and automatic neighborhood selection. In: International Conference on Information and Automation; December 15–17, 2006; Shandong:378–383.
31. Thomas C. *Elements of Information Theory*. New York: Wiley; 1991.
32. Hager GD, Belhumeur PN. Efficient region tracking with parametric models of geometry and illumination. *IEEE Trans Pattern Anal Mach Intell*. 1998;20(10):1025–1039.
33. Haussecker HW, Fleet DJ. Computing optical flow with physical models of brightness variation. *IEEE Trans Pattern Anal Mach Intell*. 2001;23(6):661–673.
34. Alvarez L. Reliable estimation of dense optical flow fields with large displacements. *Int J Comput Vis*. 2000;39(1):41–56.
35. Kim Y-H, Martínez AM, Kak AC. Robust motion estimation under varying illumination. *Image Vis Comput*. 2005;23(4):365–375.
36. Beghdadi A, Auclair-fortier M-f, Monteil J. Tracking of image intensities based on optical flow: an evaluation of nonlinear diffusion process. In: 2nd IEEE International Symposium on Signal Processing and Information Technology; December 18–2, 2002; Marrakech:691–696.

37. Brox T, Weickert J. Nonlinear matrix diffusion for optic flow estimation. In: *Pattern Recognition Berlin*. Germany: Springer; 2002:446–453 (Lecture notes in computer science, vol. 2449).
38. Spies H, Scharr H. Accurate optical flow in noisy image sequences. In: Proceedings on 8th IEEE International Conference on Computer Vision, Vol. 1; July 7–14, 2001; Vancouver:587–592.
39. Xiao J, Cheng H, Sawhney H, Rao C, Isnardi M. Bilateral Filtering-Based Optical Flow Estimation with Occlusion Detection Lecture Notes in Computer Science. 2006;3951/2006:211–224.
40. Pock T, Urschler M, Zach C, Beichel R, Bischof H. A duality based algorithm for TV-L1-optical-flow image registration. In: Ayache N, Ourselin S, Maeder A, eds. *Medical Imaging and Computer-Assisted Intervention: MICCAI 2007*. Berlin: Springer; 2007:511–518 (Lecture notes in computer science, vol. 4792).
41. Horst R, Pardalos PM, Thoai NV. *Introduction to Global Optimization*. 2nd ed. Dordrecht: Kluwer Academic Publishers; 2000.
42. Kreyszig E. *Advance Engineering Mathematics*. New York: Wiley; 1988.
43. Lever MJ, Dimaki M, Bharath AA, Otawara M, Fujiwara H. Investigation of human carotid artery wall and atherosclerotic plaque mechanics using B-mode ultrasound. In: Summer Bioengineering Conference; June 25–29, 2003; Key Biscayne.
44. Golemati S, Sassano A, Lever JM, Bharath AA. Carotid artery wall motion estimated from B-mode ultrasound using region tracking and block matching. *Ultrasound Med Biol*. 2003;29(3):387–399.
45. Stoitsis J, Golemati S, Dimopoulos AK, Nikita KS. Analysis and quantification of arterial wall motion from B-mode ultrasound images - comparison of block-matching and optical flow. In: Proceedings of the 27th Annual International Conference of the Engineering in Medicine and Biology Society (IEEE-EMBS); January 17–18, 2005; Shanghai:4469–4472.
46. Loizou CP et al. Comparative evaluation of despeckle filtering in ultrasound imaging of the carotid artery. *IEEE Trans Ultrason Ferroelectr Freq Control*. 2005;52(10):1653–1668.

Part IV
Early Atherosclerosis

Carotid Intima-Media Thickness Measurement: A Suitable Alternative for Cardiovascular Risk?

Michiel L. Bots, Sanne A.E. Peters, and Diederick E. Grobbee

22.1 Introduction

Carotid intima-media thickness (IMT) measurements have been widely used in observational studies and randomized trials as exemplified in an increasing number of publications (Fig. 22.1). In observational (cohort) studies, IMT measurements are used as a primary outcome in studies relating risk factors to increased IMT in a similar manner as in studies into determinants of occurrence of cardiovascular events. Moreover, in these cohort studies, IMT measurements have also been used as determinants of prognosis, i.e., does increased IMT value predict an increased risk of coronary heart disease or stroke? More recently, the rate of change in IMT over time has been introduced as a primary outcome in intervention studies into the efficacy of lipid-lowering,[1] glucose-lowering,[3] or blood-pressure-lowering drugs.[2] In these trials, change in IMT over time was the primary outcome as an alternative for cardiovascular events. The basic assumption underlying IMT measurements is that an IMT measurement captures information on the process of atherosclerosis at an early or more advanced stage. As such IMT can be considered a biomarker. A biomarker is generally a measurement used as an indicator of a biological state. A biomarker is also a characteristic that can be objectively measured and evaluated as an indicator of normal biological or pathogenic processes. When IMT as a biomarker is used as a primary end point in intervention studies, it is regarded as a "surrogate" or "alternative end point". Based on the definition of the Food & Drug Administration (FDA) of the United States of America, "a surrogate endpoint is a laboratory measurement that is used in therapeutic trials as a substitute for a clinically meaningful endpoint that is a direct measure of how a patient feels, functions, or survives and is expected to predict the effect of the therapy." It represents a possible alternative end point that could allow more expedient trials, thus potentially reducing sample size requirements and the cost of conducting the study. It must represent quickly to the treatment relative to disease progression, must be prognostic for the true end point, and must explain most of the effect of the treatment on the clinical endpoint.

A "biomarker" as carotid IMT may be of great importance in cardiovascular research and in clinical practice. A noninvasively measurable reliable marker of the atherosclerotic disease process may facilitate etiologic and prognostic studies in the young, a group in which vascular events will not occur for decades.[4] Furthermore, an atherosclerotic biomarker may be of help to improve identification of high-risk asymptomatic subjects beyond information provided by the established risk factors.[5,6] Also, IMT measurements may provide new and important information on studies into diseases where a priori involvement of atherosclerosis has not been thought of, e.g., atherosclerosis as a cause of dementia[7] or as a consequence of human immunodeficiency (HIV) treatment.[8] Finally, a good atherosclerotic biomarker may facilitate the conduct of trials using change in biomarker as primary outcome instead of vascular events. An event trial will need thousands of participants and several years of follow-up, whereas a biomarker trial may need several hundreds of participants and several months of follow-up.[9]

M.L. Bots (✉) • S.A.E. Peters • D.E. Grobbee
Julius Center for Health Sciences and Primary Care, University Medical Center Utrecht, Utrecht, The Netherlands

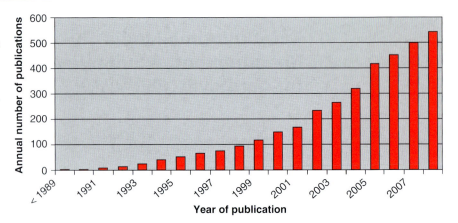

Fig. 22.1 The number of publications using "carotid intima-media thickness" in the title or abstract as assessed using PubMed database (Adapted from U.S. National Library of Medicine. PubMed. Available from http://www.ncbi.nlm.nih.gov/sites/entrez. Accessed August 21, 2009)

Table 22.1 Issues to be addressed to define IMT as a "validated" biomarker of atherosclerosis and cardiovascular risk

- Ultrasound measurement comparison with a "gold standard"
- Adequate reproducibility
- Cross-sectional relations with established risk factors and prevalent disease
- Relations with severity of atherosclerosis elsewhere in the arterial system
- Relations with the occurrence with future events
- Ability to change over time (natural history)
- Ability to be affected by interventions over time
- Relations between change over time and change in risk

However, the use of a biomarker depends on the evidence that indeed confirms the validity of the marker.[10] The concept of a "validated" biomarker comprises several aspects including comparison with a "gold standard", adequate reproducibility, cross-sectional relations with established risk factors and prevalent disease, relations with severity of atherosclerosis elsewhere in the arterial system, relations with the occurrence of future events, ability for a biomarker to change over time, ability to be affected by interventions over time, and relations between change over time in biomarker level and change in risk (Table 22.1). This chapter provides evidence for the validity of these aspects of IMT measurement.

22.2 Comparison with Gold Standard and IMT Reproducibility

Several studies have compared the IMT measurement obtained by ultrasound, measured as the distance between the typical "double-line pattern" with the actual histological measurement of the intima-media thickness of the carotid artery wall[11,12] (Chap. 10). These studies showed that a "far wall" IMT measurement closely relates to the true biological thickness of the vessel wall, whereas the "near wall" IMT measurement systematically overestimates the true value.[13–18] Although the near wall IMT ultrasound measurement may be off by a fixed value of certain tenths of a millimeter, the ranking of subjects based on near wall thickness into those with true thick and thin intima-media thickness walls is correct.[19]

A good reproducibility of a biomarker is a prerequisite for its use.[20] Although the measurement of IMT seems relatively simple to perform, considerable technical expertise is required to obtain reliable measurements. This is particularly essential when the aim of a study is to obtain a change over time estimate. Reproducibility has been studied in great detail for the IMT measurement in studies in which measurements were repeated in the same individual some weeks apart. Such designs capture all aspects that may affect the reproducibility of the measurement. Reproducibility data for change over time in IMT estimates are, however, not available. To appreciate the reproducibility study results, an understanding of the various ways to measure IMT is needed. In short, IMT measurements have been reported as a mean IMT from a single predefined site (usually the common carotid artery, proximal to the bulb), as a mean maximum IMT using the mean of the maximum thickness of 12 carotid segments (two walls (near and far wall), two sides (left and right carotid artery), and three segments (common carotid artery segment, carotid bifurcation, and the internal carotid artery segment)), or as a mean (or maximum) of segment specific measurements. Over the years the reproducibility of the IMT measurements has improved considerably. In studies during the late eighties, the intraclass correlation coefficient (ICC), a measure of reproducibility, ranged from 0.60 to 0.75,[21–24] whereas more recent studies have generated an ICC of between 0.80 and 0.95.[25–27] An ICC of 90% indicates that 90% of the variance in the CIMT measurements is due to patient differences, whereas 10% can be attributed to differences between visits (measurement aspects).

IMT is measured using an ultrasound device. The theoretical axial resolution of a 7.0 MHz transducer is approximately 0.3 mm. This means that if the IMT is thinner than 0.3 mm, the two echo interfaces cannot be separated, and thus IMT cannot be measured reliably. This is important particularly in the young.[28] However, in a recent review, the physics of measurement of change over time has been explained and indicated that indeed it is possible to obtain a change in IMT measurement over time which is below the axial resolution of one image.[28]

Despite a good comparison with the gold standard and excellent reproducibility, one should realize that atherosclerosis is a disorder which is restricted to the intimal layer of the arterial vessel wall. Carotid ultrasound imaging cannot discriminate between the intima layer and the media layer of vessel wall, and so a combined intima-media thickness is always measured, of which the media comprises a large part. When plaque is included in an IMT measurement, the proportion of the thickness due to an increased intima layer is much larger. This aspect has been addressed in the topic on whether IMT reflects atherosclerosis or whether it can be regarded as an adaptive response to blood pressure[29] (Chaps. 23 and 25).

22.3 IMT Relations with Established Risk Factors and Prevalent Disease in Cross-Sectional Studies

There is a wealth of data relating established risk factors to increased IMT. These studies have been performed among hospital-based populations, among groups of subjects who were selected based on presence or absence of a prevalent condition, or in studies performed in populations at large.[30–48] Graded direct relations with increased IMT have consistently been described for age, male gender, systolic blood pressure, hypertension, increased body mass index, increased low-density lipoprotein (LDL) cholesterol, decreased high-density lipoprotein (HDL) cholesterol, and smoking (Table 22.2). The direction of the associations is generally similar in women and men. Also, subjects with previous symptomatic cardiovascular events have increased IMT as compared to subjects free of cardiovascular disease. The relation between diastolic blood pressure and IMT appears to differ by age. In the young, generally a positive relationship is found, whereas in subjects of higher age an inverse relationship has been observed. This counterintuitive finding has been explained by increased stiffening of the central arteries with aging, partly due to development of atherosclerosis, leading to a decrease in diastolic pressure. Subjects with a history of cardiovascular disease have higher IMT measurements compared with those without a history of cardiovascular disease, independent of established risk factors.[49–51] In addition to established risk factors, inflammation is of critical importance in the pathogenesis of atherosclerosis. Elevated levels of C-reactive protein (CRP) have been associated with increased IMT.[52,53]

The consistent findings in a large number of studies and populations on the relation between risk factors and IMT strengthen the notion that the measurement reflects atherosclerosis and increased risk.

22.4 IMT and Severity of Atherosclerosis Elsewhere in the Arterial System

When IMT reflects atherosclerosis, the measurement should relate to atherosclerotic abnormalities elsewhere in the arterial system. This has been the main topic of a variety of studies in which carotid IMT measurements were related to atherosclerotic vessel wall disease in other arteries that were at high risk of development of atherosclerosis, such as the carotid bifurcation, the internal carotid artery,[54–56] the abdominal aorta,[57] the arteries of the lower extremities,[58,59] and the coronary arteries.[60]

A strong association between maximum common carotid IMT(IMTcc) and severity of internal carotid atherosclerosis has been reported in the Cardiovascular Health Study.[54] Results from the Atherosclerosis Risk In Communities (ARIC) study have demonstrated positive but modest associations between IMTcc

Table 22.2 Characteristics and results from a number of selected studies on the association of cardiovascular risk factors and carotid atherosclerosis, based on ultrasonographically assessed carotid intima-media thickness (IMT)

First author	Type	Prevalent condition	Number (M/F)	Age	D[a]	Association present[b]	Association absent[c]
Carotid atherosclerosis: IMT as a continuous variable from measurements at the common carotid only							
Bots	S	Asymptomatic, ISH	33/66[d]	≥55	a	ISH	
Haapanen	P	None	88/10[f]	31–77	b	Current smoking	LDL, HDL, glucose, insulin, fibrinogen
Markussis	S	Hypopituitarism	31/42[e]	26–75	c	Age, SBP, smoking (pack years), hypopituitarism	DBP, Obesity
O'Leary	P	None	2,255/2,946	≥65	d	Age, male, SBP, HT, LDL, HDL, TG, smoking (current, former), CHD, stroke, LVH, diabetes, glucose, insulin, left ventricular mass	
Poli	S	Hypercholesterolemia	38/29[e]	NR	e	Age, total cholesterol	
Psaty	S	Asymptomatic, ISH	867/1322[e]	≥65	d	ISH, SBP, DBP (inverse)	DBP, HDL, BMI, fibrinogen
Salonen	P	None	1,224 men	42–60	f	Age, PP, SBP, LDL, CHD, diabetes, pack years	Male, diabetes, race
Tell	H	Cerebrovascular symptoms	775/806	≥20	g	Age, HT, smoking (former, current)	
Wendelhag	S	Hypercholesterolemia	60/42[e]	20–72	h	Age, total cholesterol, LDL, apoB, smoking (pack years)	Pack years among controls
Carotid atherosclerosis: IMT as an average or summary score from measurements obtained at several sites of the carotid artery							
Crouse	H	Coronary stenosis (y/n)	182/194	NR	i	Age, HT, HDL, uric acid, smoking (pack years), LVH	Total cholesterol, BMI
Dempsey	H	Referred for any reason	790 NR	17–94	j	Age, HT, smoking (pack years)	Diabetes
Handa	H	Cerebrovascular disease	164/68	24–74	i	Age, male, total cholesterol, diabetes, stroke	Ht, smoking, obesity
Kawamori	S	Diabetes (y/n)	170/125	20–89	k	Age, LDL, smoking (pack years), diabetes	HDL, HT, SBP, DBP, HT, BMI

Rubens	H	Coronary stenosis (y/n)	183/199	NR	i	CHD, age, HT, HDL, LVH, smoking, uric acid, diabetes, race, HT	Gender, LDL, obesity, LVH
Ruy	S	Hypercholesterolemia	47 men	...	l	TG response, smoking	LDL, HDL, BMI
Carotid atherosclerosis: based on cutoff points from IMT measurements at several sites of the carotid artery							
Bonithon	P	Asymptomatic	517 women	45–54	m	Age, SBP, DBP, total cholesterol, LDL, HDL, current smoking, TG, apolipoprotein B	TG, BMI, fibrinogen, apo A-I
Heiss, Wu	P	Asymptomatic	772[d]	45–64	n	Age, SBP, DBP, HT, LDL, HDL, TG, BMI, smoking (current, former pack years), fibrinogen	Factor VII activity, factor VIII activity, antithrombin III
Prati	P	None	630/718	18–99	o	Age, male, SBP, HDL, smoking (pack years), alcohol use	DBP, LDL, fibrinogen, diabetes, cholesterol, Lp(a)

BMI body mass index, *CHD* coronary heart disease, *DBP* diastolic blood pressure, *HDL* high density lipoprotein cholesterol, *ISH* isolated systolic hypertension, *HT* hypertension, *LDL* low density lipoprotein cholesterol, *LVH* left ventricular hypertrophy, *M/F* male/female, *NR* not reported, *PP* pulse pressure, *SBP* systolic blood pressure, *TG* triglyceride, *H* hospital-based study, *P* population-based study, *S* otherwise selected populations

[a] Definition described in Table 5.1.4
[b] Refers to significant positive associations or, with respect to HDL cholesterol, a significant inverse association in a multivariate analysis
[c] Refers to no significant associations in a multivariate analysis
[d] Case–control study among subjects with and without carotid atherosclerosis
[e] Case–control study among subjects with and without prevalent condition
[f] Case–control study among twins discordant for smoking

and IMT at other sites of the carotid artery.[55] The magnitude of the association between ipsi- and contralateral abnormalities with left and right IMTcc was considerably reduced compared with the association found for the average of left and right far wall IMT.[56]

Presence of calcification of the abdominal aorta was associated with 18% increase in IMTcc.[57] A gradual increase in IMTcc with decrease in ankle-arm index, as an indicator of atherosclerosis in the arteries of the lower extremities, has been reported.[58,59] Subjects with peripheral arterial disease, defined as an ankle-brachial index < 0.90, had a significantly increased IMTcc compared with those without peripheral arterial disease (ankle-arm index ≥ 0.90). The age and gender adjusted difference was 0.107 mm [95% CI 0.071–0.143], reflecting a 15% increase.

Several reports have pointed to the weak correlation between increased IMT and coronary atherosclerosis as assessed using coronary angiography.[60] In a recent systematic review of the published literature (33 studies on this topic), it was shown that most of the studies (29 out of 33) showed a graded positive relationship, with correlation coefficients in the order of 0.3–0.4, although some reported lower or higher correlation coefficients and some studies showed no relationship at all. In addition, studies using intravascular coronary ultrasound to assess coronary atherosclerosis rather than coronary angiography reported that IMT was significantly related with left main coronary atherosclerosis, as measured by both mean and maximal plaque areas with correlation coefficients between 0.39 and 0.41.[61] The magnitude of the relationship between IMT and coronary atherosclerosis did not depend on sample size, and there seemed to be no evidence for publication bias. Of note is that the associations between carotid atherosclerosis and coronary atherosclerosis are of a similar magnitude to those shown in autopsy studies.

22.5 IMT and the Occurrence of Future Events

When IMT is used in studies as a primary outcome parameter as alternative for cardiovascular events, data should indicate that an increased IMT measurement relates to increased risk of future vascular events.

A number of observational studies demonstrated a strong relationship between increased IMT measurements of subclinical atherosclerosis and increased risk of cardiovascular events, as reviewed in detail elsewhere (Table 22.3).[62–81]

In the Kuopio Ischemic Heart Disease Risk Factor (KIHD) study, 1,288 Finnish men were followed for up to 2.5 years: An increased IMT (>1 mm) at baseline was related to a 2.2-fold (95% confidence interval [CI] 0.7–6.74) increased risk of myocardial infarction (MI).[80] In the Rotterdam Study in over 5,800 subjects, increased IMT was related to an increased risk of stroke and MI. An increase in IMT of one standard deviation (0.163 mm) resulted in an increased risk of 41% (95% CI 25–82) for stroke and 43% (95% CI 16–78) for MI over 2.7 years.[64] In the ARIC study, involving more than 12,000 men and women, a mean CIMT of ≥1 mm at baseline was associated with a 1.85-fold (95% CI 1.28–2.69) risk in men and a 5.07-fold (95% CI 3.08–8.36) increased risk in women compared with a mean IMT of ≤1 mm. Baseline IMT was related to new stroke events, with IMT ≥1 mm associated with a 3.6-fold (95% CI 1.5–9.2) increased risk of stroke in men and 8.5-fold (95% CI 3.5–20.7) increased risk in women compared with an IMT <0.6 mm.[65,66] The Cardiovascular Health Study (CHS), a 6-year follow-up of 5,858 older adults without a history of cardiovascular disease (CVD), showed that individuals in the highest quintile for IMT at baseline had a relative risk of MI or stroke of 3.9 (95% CI 2.72–5.51) compared with those in the lowest quintile.[74] Furthermore, recent data from the Carotid Atherosclerosis Progression Study (CAPS) indicate that baseline IMT predicts future vascular risk in younger (<50 years) as well as older (>50 years) individuals.[75] Finally, findings from the Second Manifestations of Arterial Disease (SMART) study and others support the view that increased IMT is related to an increased risk of vascular death and vascular events also in patients with manifest arterial disease.[82]

22.6 Ability for IMT to Change Over Time

For studies into natural history and determinants of development of atherosclerosis, it is important to be able to measure IMT over time in an adequate and

Table 22.3 Selection of prospective studies examining the relationship between IMT and vascular events

Reference	First author	IMT measurement	Clinical events associated with IMT	FU	Patient details Type of patient and (n)	Age at entry	Male, %	Unit of IMT	Adjusted RR (95% CI)
62	Aboyans	CCA	MI, stroke, CV death, coronary revascularization and peripheral arterial surgery	3.5	CABG patients (609)	67	82	<0.9 vs. >0.9	No independent predictor
63	Benedetto	CCA	CV death	2.5	ESRD (138)	60	59	0.1	1.24 (1.06–1.44)
64	Bots	CCA	MI and stroke	2.7	≥55 years (7,983)	~71	~64	0.16	Stroke 1.41 (1.25–1.82) MI 1.43 (1.16–1.78)
65	Chambless	CCA, ICA and BIF	MI and coronary death	5.2	General population	45–64	43	0.19 CCA	M 1.32 (1.13–1.54) F 1.92 (1.66–2.22)
66	Chambless	CCA, ICA and BIF	Non-fatal and fatal stroke	7.2	General population	45–64	45	0.18 CCA	M 1.52 (1.28–1.80) F 1.72 (1.49–1.99)
67	Folsom	CCA, ICA and BIF	MI, coronary revascularization and CHD death	10.2	DM (1,500)	45–64	43	1	M 2.3 (not given) F 4.7 (not given)
68	Held	CCA, ICA and BIF	Non-fatal MI and CV death	3.0	Angina pectoris (558)	60	67	>1.02 vs. <0.81	1.28 (0.59–2.78)
69	Hodis	CCA	Coronary death and non-fatal MI	8.8	CABG patients (146)	54	100	0.13	1.4 (1.1–1.8)
70	Hollander	CCA	Stroke	6.1	≥55 years (7,983)	70	40	0.16	1.28 (1.15–1.44)
71	Kato	CCA	CV mortality	~5	ESRD (219)	~58	66	0.1	1.41 (1.12–1.78)
72	Kitamura	CCA, ICA and BIF	Stroke	4.5	60–74 years (1,289)	~66	100	≤0.77 vs. >1.08	3.0 (1.1–8.3)
73	Lacroix	CCA	Worsening or recurrence of cardiac symptoms	0.9	PTCA patients (123)	62	22	≤0.7 vs. >0.7	No independent Predictor
74	O'Leary	CCA, ICA	MI and stroke	6.2	≥65 years (4,476)	73	39	0.2 CCA	1.35 (1.25–1.45)
75	Lorenz	CCA, ICA and BIF	MI, stroke and mortality	4.2	19–90 years (5,056)	50	49	0.16 CCA	Stroke 1.11 (0.97–1.28) MI 1.16 (1.05–1.27)

(continued)

Table 22.3 (continued)

Reference	First author	IMT measurement	Clinical events associated with IMT	FU	Patient details Type of patient and (n)	Age at entry	Male, %	Unit of IMT	Adjusted RR (95% CI)
76	Murakami	CCA, ICA and BIF	All-cause and vascular mortality	3.2	>75 years (298)			0.2	Left 1.40 (1.05–1.85) Right 2.23 (1.27–3.91)
77	Nishizawa	Carotid, location	CV mortality	2.5	ESRD (438)	60	60	1.0–2.0 vs. <1.0	3.17 (1.41–7.17)
78	Rosvall	CCA	MI or coronary death	7	46–68 years (5,163)	54		1.36	1.36 (1.21–1.54)
79	Rosvall	CCA	Stroke	7	46–68 years (5,163)	~58	~41	≤69 vs. >0.80	2.54 (1.20–5.40)
80	Salonen	CCA and BIF	Fatal and non-fatal MI	0.08	General population	42–60	100	0.1	1.11 (1.06–1.16)
81	Yamasaki	CCA, ICA and BIF	Angina pectoris and MI	3.1	DM type (287)	62	43	1	4.9 (1.7–14.1)

Follow-up and age at entry are given as mean median or range. Population in the studies of Bots and Hollander and on both studies by Chambless and Rosvall are overlapping *IMT* carotid intima-media thickness, *FU* follow-up, *RR* relative risk, *95% CI* 95% confidence interval, *CCA* common carotid artery, *ICA* internal carotid artery, *BIF* bifurcation, *MI* myocardial infarction, *CABG* coronary artery bypass graft, *CV* cardiovascular, *ESRD* end stage renal disease, *PTCA* percutaneous transluminal coronary angioplasty, *CHD* coronary heart disease, *DM* diabetes mellitus, *M* males, *F* females
Source: Dijk et al.[82] by permission of Oxford University Press

precise manner. Data on this issue mainly comes from control groups in randomized controlled trials. In these trials, IMT was measured in each individual at regular intervals, e.g., 6 months, during a period of several years, e.g., 2, 3, or 4. The change in IMT has usually been reported as rate of change in mean IMTcc or in mean maximum IMT in millimeter per year. A recent review has detailed the rates of change from placebo-controlled groups participating in randomized controlled trials (Table 22.4).[9] Although absolute estimates across populations differ, part of these differences will be due to the studied populations (differences across populations in main determinants of IMT), whereas part of the differences may be attributed to difference in IMT measurement approach. In the placebo-treated patients participating in the trial, IMT progressed on average. Estimated rates of change in IMT were 0.0147 mm/year [95% CI 0.0122–0.0173] for IMTcc and 0.0176 mm/year [95% CI 0.0149–0.0203] for mean maximum IMT.[9] As these estimates reflect group averages, it means that some participants progress more rapidly than others, and that some even may not change at all.

Information available on rate of change in IMT from cohort studies is much less. Furthermore, observational studies usually have only two IMT measurements over time, and the first ones initiated around 1990 were not a priori setup for assessment of change over time. Due to lower reproducibility of the IMT measurement in these early studies (intraclass correlation of repeated measurement of IMT of 0.59–0.75 in observational studies) and a higher measurement error, the reported associations likely underestimate the true relationships. One of the first reports on rate of change in IMT showed that increasing age, LDL cholesterol, and pack years of smoking were strongly related to 2-year progression of IMT. In contrast, in this sample of 100 participants, blood pressure levels and HDL cholesterol were apparently not related to progression of IMT.[83] Zureik and coworkers reported on the relations of pulse pressure and 4-year change in IMTcc among 957 healthy 59–71-year-old French men and women in the Étude du Vieillissement Artériel (EVA) study.[84] The AtheroGene Study among 502 subjects with suspected coronary artery disease indicated that age, male gender, and current smoking were determinants of IMTcc progression over a period of 2.5 years.[85] The ARIC study among 12,644 middle-aged men and women reported diabetes, current smoking, HDL cholesterol (in white men), and pulse pressure to be positively related to increased progression of IMT from 1987 to 1998.[86] In addition, increase from baseline from 1987 to 1998 in LDL cholesterol and triglycerides and onset of hypertension and diabetes were positively related to increased IMT progression.[86] In contrast, results from the CHS among 65-year-old men and women revealed no relations between established risk factors and 3-year progression of IMT.[87] Data from the Rotterdam study among 3,409 men and women aged 55 years or over, with second measurement after 6.5 years, indicated that moderate to severe progression of IMTcc was related to age, body mass index, male gender, current smoking, systolic blood pressure, and hypertension.[88] Lipid levels however were not related to increased progression of IMTcc. Recent information from the CAPS among 3,383 men and women, with a second IMT measurement after 3 years, showed that age, male gender, hypertension, diabetes, and smoking were related to increased progression of internal carotid IMT, whereas no relation was found for IMTcc.[89]

These findings from observational and intervention studies[90] show clearly that change over time in IMT can be assessed readily, and change in IMT relates to elevated levels of established risk factors.

22.7 Ability for IMT to be Affected by Interventions Over Time

Modification of risk factors is a proven way to reduce atherosclerosis progression and cardiovascular risk. When IMT is of use in evaluation of (new) non-pharmacological and pharmacological treatments, evidence should become available that the rate of change in IMT is affected by these treatments. In the past decades, there have been a large number of trials into the effect of treatment on the rate of change in IMT as primary outcome. These trials looked, for example, into the effect of lipid lowering,[1,91–120] of blood pressure lowering,[2,121–129] of glucose lowering,[3] of hormone replacement therapy,[130–134] or other interventions[135–140] on rate of change in IMT.[92]

The majority of the lipid lowering trials showed a reduced progression or a regression of IMT related to lipid-lowering statin treatment. Several reviews have summarized the data. Espeland and coworkers

Table 22.4 Estimates of annual rate of change in IMT (mm) among control groups from selected number of randomized placebo controlled trials

Publication year	Acronym	Ref	# Controls	CCA (mm)	CCA SD	BIF (mm)	BIF SD	Mean-max (mm)	Mean-max SD	Comments
1993	CLAS	91	39	0.02	0.06	n.a.	n.a.			Mean fw cca
1994	ACAPS	93	230	n.g.		n.g.		0.006	0.0455	Mean-max (12 segments)
1995	PLAC-II	97	76	0.0456	0.0497	0.1042	0.1325	0.0675	0.0689	All segments given
	REGRESS	98	127	−0.015	0.11	n.g.		n.g.		Mean fw cca
	KAPS	94	212	0.0285	0.0626	0.0401	0.0626	0.0309	0.0510	Mean Max based on cca and bif
		96	50	0.00767	0.125	n.a.		n.a.		Mean fw cca
1996	CAIUS	101	154	0.0077	0.0335	0.0036	0.0496	0.0089	0.0335	All segments given
	MARS	99	89	0.0095	0.0377	n.a.		n.a.		Mean cca
1998	LIPID	102	249	0.0195	0.1736	n.a.		n.a.		Far wall cca only
2000		126	309	0.010	n.g.	n.a.		n.a.		Far wall cca only
	ASAP	136	60	0.020	0.0258	n.a.		n.a.		Far wall cca only
	ASAP	136	60	0.016	0.0262	n.a.		n.a.		Far wall cca only
2001	Phorea	132	93	n.g.		n.g.		0.02	0.05	Mean-max 12 segments
	BCAPS	123	199	0.013	0.053	0.089	0.154	n.a.		Far wall only
	EPA	131	111	0.0036	0.04	n.a.		n.a.		Far wall cca only
	SECURE	127	227	n.g.		n.g.		0.0217	0.0407	Mean max 12 segments
	PREVENT	125	408	0.0038	0.242	0.0177	0.4484	0.011	0.242	All segments given
POOLED	All studies combined			0.0147	0.053 (median)			0.0176	0.050 (median)	
	Lipid lowering only			0.0147	0.06 (median)			0.0159	0.045 (median)	
	CHD patients only			0.0170	0.06 (median)			0.0258	0.068 (median)	

n.a. not assessed, *n.g.* not given in the report, *cca* common carotid artery, *bif* carotid bifurcation, *fw* far wall
Source: Bots et al.[9] reprinted with permission

Table 22.5 Clinical trials involving HMG-CoA reductase inhibitors and reporting both carotid IMT and cardiovascular event outcomes

Study	Relative impact on IMT progression (mm/year) Mean difference [95% CI]	Relative impact on reported vascular events Odds ratio [95% CI]
ACAPS	−0.015 [−0.023 to −0.007]	0.34 [0.12–0.69]
BCAPS	−0.008 [−0.013 to −0.003]	0.64 [0.24–1.66]
CAIUS	−0.014 [−0.021 to −0.005]	1.02 [0.14–7.33]
FAST	Significant benefit	0.32 [0.10–1.06]
KAPS	−0.014 [−0.022 to −0.006]	0.57 [0.22–1.47]
PLAC II	−0.009 [−0.031 to 0.013]	0.37 [0.11–1.24]
REGRESS	−0.030 [−0.056 to −0.004]	0.51 [0.24–1.07]

Source: Espeland et al.[141], reprinted with permission

conducted a meta-analysis that included seven statin trials (Table 22.5) and showed that lipid lowering led to an overall reduction rate of change in IMT of -0.012 mm/year (95% CI −0.015 to −0.007).[141] In addition, a larger LDL reduction seems to coincide with a larger attenuation of the rate of change in IMT.[142]

A recent review reported on the effects of blood pressure lowering on rate of change in IMT using data from randomized controlled trials (Fig. 22.2). Out of 22 trials identified through a PubMed search, 8 included 3,329 patients with diabetes or coronary heart disease. In these 8, blood-pressure-lowering treatment with an angiotensin-converting enzyme (ACE) inhibitor, a β-blocker, or a calcium-channel blocker (CCB) reduced the rate of change in IMT by 0.007 mm/year compared with placebo or no treatment. In 4,564 hypertensive patients participating in 9 trials, CCBs, ACE inhibitors, an angiotensin II receptor blocker, or a β-blocker, compared with diuretics or β-blockers, in the presence of similar blood pressure reductions, significantly decreased the rate of change in IMT by 0.003 mm/year.[2]

Similar finding have been reported for glucose-lowering treatment in subjects with diabetes mellitus.[3]

22.8 Change Over Time in IMT Level and Change in Risk

Data on change in IMT over time and future risk is very limited. One of the reasons is that for this type of data the time window required to perform baseline and follow-up measurements, and subsequently have cardiovascular events to occur, is considerable. To illustrate this point, manuscripts on the relation of baseline IMT and future cardiovascular events from large observational studies took between 5 and 12 years to be published after baseline examinations. Given that recent papers from such studies on determinants of progression have just been published, it is obvious that it may take some time before a sufficient number of events have been collected to allow estimation of relationships with sufficient precision. Another reason for lack of data on the relation between rate of change in IMT and events is that many randomized controlled trials with excellent rate of change in IMT data do not follow up participants for the occurrence of events after the trial has finished.

Only one study has provided information on the relation of change in IMT and the risk of future events.[143] In a population of 146 men with coronary artery disease, aged 40–59 years with a follow-up of 8.8 years, Hodis and coworkers showed that a 0.03 mm/year increase in IMTcc was related to a 2.2-fold increased risk of coronary events. Recently, Espeland and coworkers performed a meta-analysis showing that across the trials, statin therapy was associated with an average decrease of IMT progression of 0.012 mm/year [95% CI −0.016 to −0.007], and using the same studies, the meta-analysis yielded a risk reduction of 52% [95% CI 22–70] for cardiovascular events associated with statin therapy.[141] In this approach, the authors linked the IMT benefit to the reduction of events.

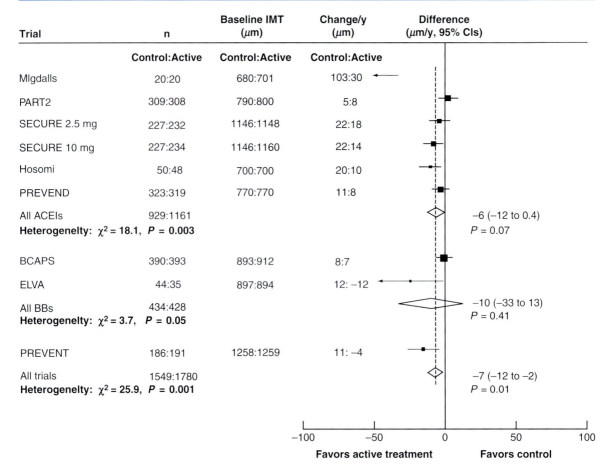

Fig. 22.2 Effects of antihypertensive treatment on changes in IMT compared with placebo or no treatment. *Solid squares* represent the difference in individual trials between study groups (active minus placebo) in changes over follow-up in IMT and have a size proportional to the total number of analyzed patients. The 95% CIs for individual trials are denoted by *lines*, and those for the pooled results by *diamonds*. *Dotted line* indicates the mean difference between randomized groups in all trials. BB and ACEIs indicate β-blockers and angiotensin-converting enzyme inhibitors, respectively. PART2 indicate Prevention of Atherosclerosis with Ramipril Trial2; SECURE, Study to Evaluate Carotid Ultrasound changes patients treated with Ramipril and vitamin E3; PREVEND, the Prevention of Renal and Vascular Endstage Disease intervention trial. (From Wang et al.,[2] reprinted with permission)

22.9 Conclusions

The current review provides information on whether IMT can be regarded as a validated marker of atherosclerosis and cardiovascular risk. The IMT measurement, as indicated above, complies with all criteria that Boisell[143] and Prentice[144] have suggested to be relevant for validated biomarkers. Furthermore, the FDA has approved IMT measurements as a primary outcome in drug trials as a valid and adequate alternative for cardiovascular events.

References

1. Revkin JH, Shear CL, Pouleur HG, Ryder SW, Orloff DG. Biomarkers in the prevention and treatment of atherosclerosis: need, validation, and future. *Pharmacol Rev*. 2007;59(1):40–53.
2. Wang JG et al. Carotid intima-media thickness and antihypertensive treatment: a meta-analysis of randomized controlled trials. *Stroke*. 2006;37:1933–1940.
3. Yokoyama H, Katakami N, Yamasaki Y. Recent advances of intervention to inhibit progression of carotid intima-media thickness in patients with type 2 diabetes mellitus. *Stroke*. 2006;37(9):2420–2427.

4. Geerts CC, Bots ML, Grobbee DE, Uiterwaal CS. Parental smoking and vascular damage in young adult offspring: is early life exposure critical? The atherosclerosis risk in young adults study. *Arterioscler Thromb Vasc Biol.* 2008;28(12):2296–2302.
5. Simon A, Gariepy J, Chironi G, Megnien JL, Levenson J. Intima-media thickness: a new tool for diagnosis and treatment of cardiovascular risk. *J Hypertens.* 2002;20:159–169.
6. Plantinga Y, Dogan S, Grobbee DE, Bots ML. Carotid intima-media thickness measurements in cardiovascular screening programmes. *Eur J Cardiovasc Prev Rehabil.* 2009;16(6):639–644.
7. Hofman A et al. Atherosclerosis, apolipoprotein E, and prevalence of dementia and Alzheimer's disease in the Rotterdam Study. *Lancet.* 1997;349(9046):151–154.
8. Hulten E, Mitchell J, Scally J, Gibbs B, Villines T. HIV positivity, protease inhibitor exposure, and subclinical atherosclerosis: a systematic review and meta-analysis of observational studies. *Heart.* 2009;95(22):1826–1835.
9. Bots ML, Evans GW, Riley W, Grobbee DE. Carotid intima-media thickness measurements in intervention studies. Designs options, progression rates and sample size considerations: a point of view. *Stroke.* 2003;34:2985–2994.
10. Tardif JC, Heinonen T, Orloff D, Libby P. Vascular biomarkers and surrogates in cardiovascular disease. *Circulation.* 2006;113(25):2936–2942.
11. Pignoli P, Tremoli E, Poli A, Oreste P, Paoletti R. Intimal plus medial thickness of the arterial wall: a direct measurement with ultrasound imaging. *Circulation.* 1986;74:1399–1406.
12. Bond MG, Ball M. Assessment of ultrasound B-mode imaging for detection and quantification of atherosclerotic lesions in arteries of animals. Bethesda, Maryland: National Heart, Lung, and Blood Institute; 1986. Report No.: NHLBI No1-HV-12916.
13. Wendelhag I, Gustavsson T, Suurküla M, Berglund G, Wikstrand J. Ultrasound measurement of wall thickness in the carotid artery: fundamental principles, and description of a computerized analyzing system. *Clin Physiol.* 1991;11:565–577.
14. Wong M, Edelstein J, Wollman J, Bond MG. Ultrasonic-pathological comparison of the human arterial wall. Verification of intima-media thickness. *Arterioscler Thromb.* 1993;13:482–486.
15. Gamble G et al. B-mode ultrasound images of the carotid artery wall: correlation of ultrasound with histological measurements. *Atherosclerosis.* 1993;102:163–173.
16. Gussenhoven EJ et al. Arterial wall characteristics determined by intravascular ultrasound imaging: an in vitro study. *J Am Coll Cardiol.* 1989;14(4):947–952.
17. Persson J, Formgren J, Israelsson B, Berglund G. Ultrasound-determined intima-media thickness and atherosclerosis. Direct and indirect validation. *Arterioscler Thromb Vasc Biol.* 1994;14:261–264.
18. Montauban van Swijndregt AD, De Lange EE, de Groot E, Ackerstaff RG. An in vivo evaluation of the reproducibility of intima-media thickness measurements of the carotid artery segments using B-mode ultrasound. *Ultrasound Med Biol.* 1999;25:323–330.
19. Bots ML, de Jong PT, Hofman A, Grobbee DE. Left, right, near or far wall common carotid intima-media thickness measurements: associations with cardiovascular disease and lower extremity arterial atherosclerosis. *J Clin Epidemiol.* 1997;50:801–807.
20. Kanters SD, Algra A, van Leeuwen MS, Banga JD. Reproducibility of in vivo carotid intima-media thickness measurements: a review. *Stroke.* 1997;28:665–671.
21. Salonen R, Haapanen A, Salonen JT. Measurement of intima-media thickness of common carotid arteries with high resolution B-mode ultrasonography: inter- and intra-observer variability. *Ultrasound Med Biol.* 1991;17:225–230.
22. O'Leary DH, Polak JF, Wolfson SK Jr, et al. Use of sonography to evaluate carotid atherosclerosis in the elderly. The Cardiovascular Health Study. *Stroke.* 1991;22:1155–1163.
23. Riley WA. Reproducibility of noninvasive ultrasonic measurement of carotid atherosclerosis. The Asymptomatic Carotid Artery Plaque Study. *Stroke.* 1992;23:1062–1068.
24. Bots ML, Mulder PGH, Hofman A, van Es GA, Grobbee DE. Reproducibility of carotid vessel wall thickness measurements. The Rotterdam Study. *J Clin Epidemiol.* 1994;47:921–930.
25. Bots ML, Evans GW, Riley W, et al. The Osteoporosis Prevention and Arterial effects of TiboLone (OPAL) study: design and baseline characteristics. *Controlled Clinical Trials.* 2003;24:752–775.
26. Crouse JR III et al. Carotid intima-media thickness in low-risk individuals with asymptomatic atherosclerosis: baseline data from the METEOR study. *Curr Med Res Opin.* 2007;23:641–648.
27. Kastelein JJ et al. The RADIANCE 1 and 2 Study Investigators. Designs of RADIANCE 1 and 2: carotid ultrasound studies comparing the effects of torcetrapib/atorvastatin with atorvastatin alone on atherosclerosis. *Curr Med Res Opin.* 2007;23(4):885–894.
28. Wikstrand J. Methodological considerations of ultrasound measurement of carotid artery intima-media thickness and lumen diameter. *Clin Physiol Funct Imaging.* 2007;27(6):341–345.
29. Chironi GN, Simon A, Bokov P, Levenson J. Correction of carotid intima-media thickness for adaptive dependence on tensile stress: implication for cardiovascular risk assessment. *J Clin Ultrasound.* 2009;37(5):270–275.
30. Handa N, Matsumoto M, Meada H, et al. Ultrasonic evaluation of early carotid atherosclerosis. *Stroke.* 1990;21:1567–1572.
31. Dempsey RJ, Moore RW. Amount of smoking independently predicts carotid artery atherosclerosis severity. *Stroke.* 1992;23:693–696.
32. Rubens J et al. Individual variation in susceptibility to extracranial carotid atherosclerosis. *Arteriosclerosis.* 1988;8:389–397.
33. Crouse JR et al. Risk factors for extracranial carotid artery atherosclerosis. *Stroke.* 1987;18:990–996.
34. Tell GS, Howard GH, McKinney WM. Risk factors for site specific extracranial carotid artery plaque distribution as measured by B-mode ultrasound. *J Clin Epidemiol.* 1989;42:551–559.
35. Wendelhag I, Olov G, Wikstrand J. Arterial wall thickness in familial hypercholesterolemia. Ultrasound measurements of intima-media thickness in the common carotid artery. *Arterioscler Thromb.* 1992;12:70–77.

36. Poli A et al. Ultrasonographic measurement of the common carotid artery wall thickness in hypercholesterolemic patients. *Atherosclerosis*. 1988;70:253–261.
37. Ryu J et al. Postprandial triglyceridemia and carotid atherosclerosis in middle-aged subjects. *Stroke*. 1992;23:823–828.
38. Bots ML, Hofman A, de Bruyn AM, de Jong PT, Grobbee DE. Isolated systolic hypertension and vessel wall thickness of the carotid artery: The Rotterdam Elderly Study. *Arterioscler Thromb*. 1993;13:64–69.
39. Psaty BM et al. Isolated systolic hypertension and subclinical cardiovascular disease in the elderly. Initial findings from the Cardiovascular Health Study. *JAMA*. 1992;268:1287–1291.
40. Kawamori R et al. Prevalence of carotid atherosclerosis in diabetic patients. *Diabetes Care*. 1992;15:1290–1294.
41. Markussis V et al. Detection of premature atherosclerosis by high-resolution ultrasonography in symptom-free hypopituitary adults. *Lancet*. 1992;ii:1188–1192.
42. Heiss G et al. Carotid atherosclerosis measured by B-mode ultrasound in populations: associations with cardiovascular risk factors in the ARIC study. *Am J Epidemiol*. 1991;134:250–256.
43. Wu KK et al. Association of coagulation factors and inhibitors with carotid artery atherosclerosis. Early results of the Atherosclerosis Risk in Communities (ARIC) study. *Ann Epidemiol*. 1992;2:471–480.
44. Salonen R, Salonen JT. Determinants of carotid intima-media thickness: a population-based ultrasonography study in eastern Finnish men. *J Intern Med*. 1991;229:225–231.
45. Haapanen A, Koskenvuo M, Kaprio J, Kesäniemi YA, Heikkilä K. Carotid arteriosclerosis in identical twins discordant for cigarette smoking. *Circulation*. 1989;80:10–16.
46. Bonithon-Kopp C et al. Risk factors for early carotid atherosclerosis in middle-aged French women. *Arterioscler Thromb*. 1991;11:966–972.
47. Prati P et al. Prevalence and determinants of carotid atherosclerosis in a general population. *Stroke*. 1992;23:1705–1711.
48. O'Leary DH et al. Distribution and correlates of sonographically detected carotid artery disease in the Cardiovascular Health Study. *Stroke*. 1992;23:1752–1760.
49. el-Barghouti N et al. The ultrasonic evaluation of the carotid intima-media thickness and its relation to risk factors of atherosclerosis in normal and diabetic population. *Int Angiol*. 1997;16(1):50–54.
50. Geroulakos G, O'Gorman DJ, Kalodiki E, Sheridan DJ, Nicolaides AN. The carotid intima-media thickness as a marker of the presence of severe symptomatic coronary artery disease. *Eur Heart J*. 1994;15(6):781–785.
51. Ebrahim S et al. Carotid plaque, intima media thickness, cardiovascular risk factors, and prevalent cardiovascular disease in men and women: the British Regional Heart Study. *Stroke*. 1999;30(4):841–850.
52. Sakurai S et al. Relationships of soluble e-selectin and high-sensitivity c-reactive protein with carotid atherosclerosis in Japanese men. *J Atheroscler Thromb*. 2009;16(4):339–345.
53. Baldassarre D et al. Carotid intima-media thickness and markers of inflammation, endothelial damage and hemostasis. *Ann Med*. 2008;40(1):21–44.
54. Polak JF et al. Sonographic evaluation of the carotid artery atherosclerosis in the elderly: relationship of disease severity to stroke and transient ischemic attack. *Radiology*. 1993;188:363–370.
55. Howard G, Burke GL, Evans GW, et al. Relations of intimal-medial thickness among sites within the carotid artery as evaluated by B-mode ultrasound. *Stroke*. 1994;25:1581–1587.
56. Bots ML, Hofman A, De Jong PT, Grobbee DE. Common carotid intima-media thickness as an indicator of atherosclerosis at other sites of the carotid artery. The Rotterdam Study. *Ann Epidemiol*. 1996;6:147–153.
57. Bots ML, Witteman JC, Grobbee DE. Carotid intima-media wall thickness in elderly women with and without atherosclerosis of the abdominal aorta. *Atherosclerosis*. 1993;102:99–105.
58. Allan PL, Lee PI, Grobbee AJ, Fowkes FG. Relationship between carotid intima-media thickness and symptomatic and asymptomatic peripheral arterial disease. The Edinburgh Artery Study. *Stroke*. 1997;28:348–353.
59. Bots ML, Hofman A, Grobbee DE. Common carotid intima-media thickness and lower extremity arterial atherosclerosis. The Rotterdam Study. *Arterioscler Thromb*. 1994;14:1885–1891.
60. Bots ML et al. Carotid intima-media thickness and coronary atherosclerosis: weak or strong relations? *Eur Heart J*. 2007;28(4):398–406.
61. Ogata T et al. Atherosclerosis found on carotid ultrasonography is associated with atherosclerosis on coronary intravascular ultrasonography. *J Ultrasound Med*. 2005;24(4):469–474.
62. Aboyans V et al. Common carotid intima-media thickness measurement is not a pertinent predictor for secondary cardiovascular events after coronary bypass surgery. A prospective study. *Eur J Cardiothorac Surg*. 2005;28:415–419.
63. Benedetto FA, Mallamaci F, Tripepi G, Zoccali C. Prognostic value of ultrasonographic measurement of carotid intima media thickness in dialysis patients. *J Am Soc Nephrol*. 2001;12:2458–2464.
64. Bots ML, Hoes AW, Koudstaal PJ, Hofman A, Grobbee DE. Common carotid intima-media thickness and risk of stroke and myocardial infarction: the Rotterdam Study. *Circulation*. 1997;96:1432–1437.
65. Chambless LE et al. Association of coronary heart disease incidence with carotid arterial wall thickness and major risk factors: the Atherosclerosis Risk in Communities (ARIC) Study, 1987–1993. *Am J Epidemiol*. 1997;146:483–494.
66. Chambless LE et al. Carotid wall thickness is predictive of incident clinical stroke: the Atherosclerosis Risk in Communities (ARIC) study. *Am J Epidemiol*. 2000;151:478–487.
67. Folsom AR, Chambless LE, Duncan BB, Gilbert AC, Pankow JS. Prediction of coronary heart disease in middle-aged adults with diabetes. *Diabetes Care*. 2003;26:2777–2784.

68. Held C et al. Prognostic implications of intima-media thickness and plaques in the carotid and femoral arteries in patients with stable angina pectoris. *Eur Heart J.* 2001;22:62–72.
69. Hodis HN et al. The role of carotid arterial intima-media thickness in predicting clinical coronary events. *Ann Intern Med.* 1998;128:262–269.
70. Hollander M et al. Comparison between measures of atherosclerosis and risk of stroke: the Rotterdam Study. *Stroke.* 2003;34:2367–2372.
71. Kato A, Takita T, Maruyama Y, Kumagai H, Hishida A. Impact of carotid atherosclerosis on long-term mortality in chronic hemodialysis patients. *Kidney Int.* 2003;64:1472–1479.
72. Kitamura A et al. Carotid intima-media thickness and plaque characteristics as a risk factor for stroke in Japanese elderly men. *Stroke.* 2004;35:2788–2794.
73. Lacroix P et al. Carotid intima-media thickness as predictor of secondary events after coronary angioplasty. *Int Angiol.* 2003;22:279–283.
74. O'Leary DH et al. Carotid-artery intima and media thickness as a risk factor for myocardial infarction and stroke in older adults. Cardiovascular Health Study Collaborative Research Group. *N Engl J Med.* 1999;340:14–22.
75. Lorenz MW, von Kegler S, Steinmetz H, Markus HS, Sitzer M. Carotid intima-media thickening indicates a higher vascular risk across a wide age range: prospective data from the Carotid Atherosclerosis Progression Study (CAPS). *Stroke.* 2006;37:87–92.
76. Murakami S et al. Common carotid intima-media thickness is predictive of all-cause and cardiovascular mortality in elderly community-dwelling people: Longitudinal Investigation for the Longevity and Aging in Hokkaido County (LILAC) study. *Biomed Pharmacother.* 2005;59(Suppl 1):S49–S53.
77. Nishizawa Y et al. Intima-media thickness of carotid artery predicts cardiovascular mortality in hemodialysis patients. *Am J Kidney Dis.* 2003;41:S76–S79.
78. Rosvall M, Janzon L, Berglund G, Engstrom G, Hedblad B. Incident coronary events and case fatality in relation to common carotid intima-media thickness. *J Intern Med.* 2005;257:430–437.
79. Rosvall M, Janzon L, Berglund G, Engstrom G, Hedblad B. Incidence of stroke is related to carotid IMT even in the absence of plaque. *Atherosclerosis.* 2005;179:325–331.
80. Salonen JT, Salonen R. Ultrasonographically assessed carotid morphology and the risk of coronary heart disease. *Arterioscler Thromb.* 1991;11:1245–1249.
81. Yamasaki Y et al. Carotid intima-media thickness in Japanese type 2 diabetic subjects: predictors of progression and relationship with incident coronary heart disease. *Diabetes Care.* 2000;23:1310–1315.
82. Dijk JM, van der Graaf Y, Bots ML, Grobbee DE, Algra A. Carotid intima-media thickness and the risk of new vascular events in patients with manifest atherosclerotic disease: the SMART study. *Eur Heart J.* 2006;27(16):1971–1978.
83. Salonen R, Salonen JT. Progression of carotid atherosclerosis and its determinants: a population-based ultrasonography study. *Atherosclerosis.* 1990;81(1):33–40.
84. Zureik M et al. Cross-sectional and 4-year longitudinal associations between brachial pulse pressure and common carotid intima-media thickness in a general population. The EVA study. *Stroke.* 1999;30(3):550–555.
85. Espinola-Klein C et al. Impact of infectious burden on progression of carotid atherosclerosis. *Stroke.* 2002;33(11):2581–2586.
86. Chambless LE et al. Risk factors for progression of common carotid atherosclerosis: the Atherosclerosis Risk in Communities Study, 1987–1998. *Am J Epidemiol.* 2002;155(1):38–47.
87. Yanez ND 3rd, Kronmal RA, Shemanski LR, Psaty BM, Cardiovascular Health Study. A regression model for longitudinal change in the presence of measurement error. *Ann Epidemiol.* 2002;12(1):34–38.
88. van der Meer IM. Risk factors for progression of atherosclerosis measured at multiple sites in the arterial tree: the Rotterdam Study. *Stroke.* 2003;34(10):2374–2379.
89. Mackinnon AD et al. Rates and determinants of site-specific progression of carotid artery intima-media thickness: the carotid atherosclerosis progression study. *Stroke.* 2004;35(9):2150–2154.
90. Vergeer M et al. Cholesteryl ester transfer protein inhibitor torcetrapib and off-target toxicity. A pooled analysis of the rating atherosclerotic disease change by imaging with a new CETP inhibitor (RADIANCE) trials. *Circulation.* 2008;118(24):2515–2522.
91. Blankenhorn DH et al. Beneficial effects of colestipol-niacin therapy on the common carotid artery. Two- and four-year reduction of intima-media thickness measured by ultrasound. *Circulation.* 1993;88:20–28.
92. Mack WJ et al. One-year reduction and longitudinal analysis of carotid intima-media thickness associated with colestipol/niacin therapy. *Stroke.* 1993;24:1779–1783.
93. Furberg CD et al. Effect of lovastatin on early carotid atherosclerosis and cardiovascular events. Asymptomatic Carotid Artery Progression Study (ACAPS) Research Group. *Circulation.* 1994;90:1679–1687.
94. Salonen R et al. Kuopio Atherosclerosis Prevention Study (KAPS). A population-based primary preventive trial of the effect of LDL lowering on atherosclerotic progression in carotid and femoral arteries. *Circulation.* 1995;92:1758–1764.
95. Byington RP, Furberg CD, Crouse JR III, Espeland MA, Bond MG. Pravastatin, lipids, and atherosclerosis in the carotid arteries (PLAC-II). *Am J Cardiol.* 1995;76:54C–59C.
96. Wendelhag I, Wiklund O, Wikstrand J. Intima-media thickness after cholesterol lowering in familial hypercholesterolemia. A three-year ultrasound study of common carotid and femoral arteries. *Atherosclerosis.* 1995;117:225–236.
97. Crouse JR III et al. Pravastatin, lipids, and atherosclerosis in the carotid arteries (PLAC-II). *Am J Cardiol.* 1995;75:455–459.
98. de Groot E et al. Effect of pravastatin on progression and regression of coronary atherosclerosis and vessel wall changes in carotid and femoral arteries: a report from the Regression Growth Evaluation Statin Study. *Am J Cardiol.* 1995;76:40C–46C.

99. Hodis HN et al. Reduction in carotid arterial wall thickness using lovastatin and dietary therapy: a randomized controlled clinical trial. *Ann Intern Med.* 1996;124:548–556.
100. Forbat SM et al. The effect of cholesterol reduction with fluvastatin on aortic compliance, coronary calcification and carotid intimal-medial thickness: a pilot study. *J Cardiovasc Risk.* 1998;5:1–10.
101. Mercuri M et al. Pravastatin reduces carotid intima-media thickness progression in an asymptomatic hypercholesterolemic mediterranean population: the Carotid Atherosclerosis Italian Ultrasound Study. *Am J Med.* 1996;101:627–634.
102. MacMahon S et al. Effects of lowering average of below-average cholesterol levels on the progression of carotid atherosclerosis: results of the LIPID Atherosclerosis Substudy. LIPID Trial Research Group. *Circulation.* 1998;97:1784–1790.
103. Byington RP et al. Effects of lovastatin and warfarin on early carotid atherosclerosis: sex-specific analyses. Asymptomatic Carotid Artery Progression Study (ACAPS) Research Group. *Circulation.* 1999;100: e14–e17.
104. Smilde TJ et al. Effect of aggressive versus conventional lipid lowering on atherosclerosis progression in familial hypercholesterolaemia (ASAP): a prospective, randomised, double-blind trial. *Lancet.* 2001;357:577–581.
105. Markwood TT et al. Design and rationale of the ARBITER trial (Arterial Biology for the Investigation of the Treatment Effects of Reducing Cholesterol) – a randomized trial comparing the effects of atorvastatin and pravastatin on carotid artery intima-media thickness. *Am Heart J.* 2001;141:342–347.
106. Kastelein JJ et al. Effect of torcetrapib on carotid atherosclerosis in familial hypercholesterolemia. *N Engl J Med.* 2007;356:1620–1630.
107. Bots ML et al. Torcetrapib and carotid intima-media thickness in mixed dyslipidaemia (Radiance II): a randomised double-blind trial. *Lancet.* 2007;370:153–160.
108. Crouse JR 3rd et al. Effect of rosuvastatin on progression of carotid intima-media thickness in low-risk individuals with subclinical atherosclerosis: the METEOR trial. *JAMA.* 2007;297:1344–1353.
109. Devine PJ, Turco MA, Taylor AJ. Design and Rationale of the ARBITER 6 Trial (Arterial Biology for the Investigation of the Treatment Effects of Reducing Cholesterol)-6-HDL and LDL Treatment Strategies in Atherosclerosis (HALTS). *Cardiovasc Drugs Ther.* 2007;21:221–225.
110. Sawayama Y et al. Effects of probucol and pravastatin on common carotid atherosclerosis in patients with asymptomatic hypercholesterolemia. Fukuoka Atherosclerosis Trial (FAST). *J Am Coll Cardiol.* 2002;39:610–616.
111. Shukla A, Sharma MK, Jain A, Goel PK. Prevention of atherosclerosis progression using atorvastatin in normolipidemic coronary artery disease patients – a controlled randomized trial. *Indian Heart J.* 2005;57:675–680.
112. Takahashi T et al. HMG-CoA reductase inhibitors suppress the development and progression of carotid artery intimal-medial thickening in hypercholesterolemic type 2 diabetic patients. *J Atheroscler Thromb.* 2005;12:149-153.
113. Taylor AJ, Sullenberger LE, Lee HJ, Lee JK, Grace KA. Arterial Biology for the Investigation of the Treatment Effects of Reducing Cholesterol (ARBITER) 2: a double-blind, placebo-controlled study of extended-release niacin on atherosclerosis progression in secondary prevention patients treated with statins. *Circulation.* 2004;110: 3512–3517.
114. Taylor AJ, Lee HJ, Sullenberger LE. The effect of 24 months of combination statin and extended-release niacin on carotid intima-media thickness: ARBITER 3. *Curr Med Res Opin.* 2006;22:2243–2250.
115. Yamanaka Y et al. Effects of combined estriol/pravastatin therapy on intima-media thickness of common carotid artery in hyperlipidemic postmenopausal women. *Gynecol Obstet Invest.* 2005;59:67–69.
116. Yu CM et al. Comparison of intensive and low-dose atorvastatin therapy in the reduction of carotid intimal-medial thickness in patients with coronary heart disease. *Heart.* 2007;93:933–999.
117. Anderssen SA, Hjelstuen AK, Hjermann I, Bjerkan K, Holme I. Fluvastatin and lifestyle modification for reduction of carotid intima-media thickness and left ventricular mass progression in drug-treated hypertensives. *Atherosclerosis.* 2005;178:387–397.
118. Kastelein JJ et al. Simvastatin with and without ezetimibe in familial hypercholesterolemia. *N Engl J Med.* 2008;358:1431–1443.
119. Fleg JL et al. Effect of statins alone versus statins plus ezetimibe on carotid atherosclerosis in type 2 diabetes: the SANDS (Stop Atherosclerosis in Native Diabetics Study) trial. *J Am Coll Cardiol.* 2008;52(25):2198–2205.
120. Howard BV et al. Effect of lower targets for blood pressure and LDL cholesterol on atherosclerosis in diabetes: the SANDS randomized trial. *JAMA.* 2008;299 (14):1678–1689.
121. Zanchetti A et al. Different effects of antihypertensive regimens based on fosinopril or hydrochlorothiazide with or without lipid lowering by pravastatin on progression of asymptomatic carotid atherosclerosis: principal results of PHYLLIS- – a randomized double-blind tria. *Stroke.* 2004;35:2807–2812.
122. Simon A, Gariepy J, Moyse D, Levenson J. Differential effects of nifedipine and co-amilozide on the progression of early carotid wall changes. *Circulation.* 2001;103: 2949–2954.
123. Hedblad B, Wikstrand J, Janzon L, Wedel H, Berglund G. Low-dose metoprolol CR/XL and fluvastatin slow progression of carotid intima-media thickness: main results from the Beta-Blocker Cholesterol-Lowering Asymptomatic Plaque Study (BCAPS). *Circulation.* 2001;103: 1721–1726.
124. Stanton AV et al. Effects of blood pressure lowering with amlodipine or lisinopril on vascular structure of the common carotid artery. *Clin Sci (Lond).* 2001;101:455–464.
125. Pitt B et al. Effect of amlodipine on the progression of atherosclerosis and the occurrence of clinical events. PREVENT Investigators. *Circulation.* 2000;102:1503–1510.
126. MacMahon S et al. Randomised placebo controlled trial of the angiotensin converting enzyme ramipril in patients with coronary or other occlusive arterial disease. *J Am Coll Cardiol.* 2000;36:438–443.
127. Lonn E et al. Effects of ramipril and vitamin E on atherosclerosis: the study to evaluate carotid ultrasound changes

in patients treated with ramipril and vitamin E (SECURE). *Circulation*. 2001;103:919–925.
128. Borhani NO et al. Final outcome results of the Multicenter Isradipine Diuretic Atherosclerosis Study (MIDAS). A randomized controlled trial. *JAMA*. 1996;276:785–791.
129. Stumpe KO et al. Vascular wall thickness in hypertension: the Perindopril Regression of Vascular Thickening European Community Trial: PROTECT. *Am J Cardiol*. 1995;76:50E–54E.
130. de Kleijn MJ et al. Hormone replacement therapy in perimenopausal women and 2-year change of carotid intima-media thickness. *Maturitas*. 1999;32:195–204.
131. Hodis HN et al. Estrogen in the prevention of atherosclerosis. A randomized, double-blind, placebo-controlled trial. *Ann Intern Med*. 2001;135:939–953.
132. Angerer P, Stork S, Kothny W, Schmitt P, von Schacky C. Effect of oral postmenopausal hormone replacement on progression of atherosclerosis: a randomized, controlled trial. *Arterioscler Thromb Vasc Biol*. 2001;21:262–268.
133. Bots ML et al. The effect of tibolone and continuous combined conjugated equine oestrogens plus medroxyprogesterone acetate on progression of carotid intima-media thickness: the Osteoporosis Prevention and Arterial effects of tiboLone (OPAL) study. *Eur Heart J*. 2006;27:746–755.
134. Ntaios G et al. The effect of folic acid supplementation on carotid intima-media thickness in patients with cardiovascular risk: a randomized, placebo-controlled trial. *Int J Cardiol*. 2009;134(3):322–329.
135. Nanayakkara PW et al. Effect of a treatment strategy consisting of pravastatin, vitamin E, and homocysteine lowering on carotid intima-media thickness, endothelial function, and renal function in patients with mild to moderate chronic kidney disease: results from the Anti-Oxidant Therapy in Chronic Renal Insufficiency (ATIC) Study. *Arch Intern Med*. 2007;167(12):1262–1270.
136. Salonen JT et al. Antioxidant Supplementation in Atherosclerosis Prevention (ASAP) study: a randomized trial of the effect of vitamins E and C on 3-year progression of carotid atherosclerosis. *J Intern Med*. 2000;248: 377–386.
137. Azen SP et al. Effect of supplementary antioxidant vitamin intake on carotid arterial wall intima-media thickness in a controlled clinical trial of cholesterol lowering. *Circulation*. 1996;94:2369–2372.
138. Agewall S et al. Multiple risk intervention trial in high risk hypertensive men: comparison of ultrasound intima-media thickness and clinical outcome during 6 years of follow-up. *J Intern Med*. 2001;249:305–314.
139. Persson J, Israelsson B, Stavenow L, Holmstrom E, Berglund G. Progression of atherosclerosis in middle-aged men: effects of multifactorial intervention. *J Intern Med*. 1996;239:425–433.
140. Suurkula M, Agewall S, Fagerberg B, Wendelhag I, Wikstrand J. Multiple risk intervention in high-risk hypertensive patients. A 3-year ultrasound study of intima-media thickness and plaques in the carotid artery. Risk Intervention Study (RIS) Group. *Arterioscler Thromb Vasc Biol*. 1996;16:462–470.
141. Espeland MA et al. Carotid intimal-media thickness as a surrogate for cardiovascular disease events in trials of HMG-CoA reductase inhibitors. *Curr Control Trials Cardiovasc Med*. 2005;6(1):3.
142. Amarenco P, Labreuche J, Lavallée P, Touboul PJ. Statins in stroke prevention and carotid atherosclerosis: systematic review and up-to-date meta-analysis. *Stroke*. 2004;35 (12):2902–2909.
143. Boissel JP, Collet JP, Moleur P, Haugh M. Surrogate endpoints: a basis for a rational approach. *Eur J Clin Pharmacol*. 1992;43:235–244.
144. Prentice RL. Surrogate endpoints in clinical trials: definition and operational criteria. *Stat Med*. 1989;8:431–440.

Intima-Media Thickness and Carotid Plaques in Cardiovascular Risk Assessment

Thomas-Duythuc To and Tasneem Z. Naqvi

23.1 Introduction

Coronary artery disease is the number one cause of morbidity and mortality in developed nations. Its clinical course ranges from an asymptomatic state to chronic stable angina or to a life-changing event of acute coronary syndrome and subsequent related complications. The type of presentation is related to the progression of atherosclerosis within the arterial vasculature, spanning a spectrum of reducing arterial flow to thrombus formation and ruptured plaques.[1] The complexity of the pathogenesis of coronary artery disease as discussed in Chap. 1 involves a variety of environmental and genetic factors, resulting in endothelial dysfunction, increased expression of endothelial adhesive and permeability factors, quantitative alteration in procoagulant and in vasoconstrictive and inflammatory molecules, a rise in cytokines and chemokines, elevated oxidative stress, and proliferation and migration of smooth muscle cells.[2,3] However, the common final endpoint is atherosclerosis affecting nearly all arterial vascular beds. Thus, identification of asymptomatic coronary artery disease patients with subclinical atherosclerosis is important for the prevention of complications of atherosclerosis.

Currently, several equations, such as Framingham,[4,5] Prospective Cardiovascular Münster (PROCAM),[6] the Sheffield table system,[7] and the British Regional Heart Study (BRHS) scoring systems,[8] are commonly used to predict cardiovascular events. These equations are limited by very low sensitivity and specificity due to their exclusion of several emerging, genetic, and unknown risk factors. Thus, although these scoring systems identify high-risk populations (greater than 20% events over 10 years), they fail to detect the majority of patients who develop cardiovascular events, despite being classified as "low risk" by the same criteria. For instance, the Framingham risk score heavily accounts for age and gender, thereby underestimating the risk of coronary artery disease in young women. Optimizing medical treatment of risk factors has been shown to reduce cardiovascular events in symptomatic[9] and asymptomatic subjects.[10] Similar effects may benefit individuals with diseased vessels or subclinical atherosclerosis who have not yet developed signs and symptoms of clinical atherosclerosis. B-mode ultrasound evaluation of the carotid artery vessel wall in the form of intima-media thickness (IMT) has been identified as a sensitive, noninvasive, reproducible imaging study to detect atherosclerosis, predict its clinical complications, and monitor its progression and regression. This technique offers direct visualization of systemic arterial vasculature. B-mode ultrasound is able to measure the thickness of the arterial wall as well as detect the presence, size, and nature of plaques, each of which has a strong positive correlation with relative risk for cardiovascular events. Carotid IMT has been shown to be linked to several known[11] and unknown[12] cardiovascular risk factors, predicting the prevalence and incidence of cardiovascular disease[12-16] (Chap. 22).

T.-D. To
Department of Internal Medicine, University of Southern California, Los Angeles, CA, USA

T.Z. Naqvi (✉)
Department of Cardiology, University of Southern California, Los Angeles, CA, USA

Thus far, the American Heart Association (AHA) Prevention Conference V has recommended that "in asymptomatic persons older than 45 years, carefully performed carotid ultrasound examination with IMT measurement can add incremental information to traditional risk factor assessment and that in experienced laboratories, this test can now be considered for further clarification of coronary artery disease risk assessment at the request of a physician".[17] In 2001, the National Cholesterol Education Program (NCEP) advised "if carried out under proper conditions, carotid IMT could be used to identify persons at higher risk than that revealed by the major risk factors alone".[18] Similarly, the 2003 European Society of Hypertension–European Society of Cardiology guidelines suggest carotid IMT assessment particularly for patients without damage to target organs based on routine screenings, such as an electrocardiogram.[19]

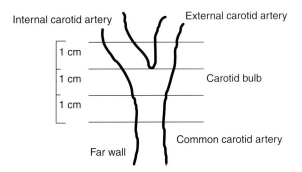

Fig. 23.1 This schematic diagram delineates extracranial carotid anatomical sites that are commonly associated with IMT progression and plaque formation. Thus, as depicted, B-mode ultrasound is employed to scan areas approximately 10 mm above and below the bulb as well as the bifurcation

23.2 Intima-Media Thickness

23.2.1 IMT Parameters and Location of Measurement

Ultrasonographic measurement of carotid IMT can be verified reliably via autopsy.[20] Likewise, the severity of carotid and coronary atherosclerosis also has been well correlated based on autopsy results.[21-23] There is variability in IMT thickness and measurement reproducibility in different segments: common carotid artery (IMTcc), bulb (IMTbulb) or bifurcation, and internal carotid artery (IMTic), near or far wall. Because of the maximum reproducibility of IMTcc at the distal 1–2 cm of the common carotid artery, most studies have consistently measured the far-wall IMTcc. The mean and maximum IMT are commonly calculated, of which the mean IMT of the right and left CCA is more commonly reported (Fig. 23.1) (Chap. 22).

In healthy adults, the normal range of mean IMTcc is from 0.25 to 1.5 mm,[24] and values of 1.0 mm are often regarded as abnormal. For instance, in the Community Health Study with a population age greater than 65 years, the 80th percentile of IMTcc was found to be 1.18 mm.[25] Overall, carotid bifurcations or bulbs appear to have a larger wall thickness than that of common carotid artery. There is much variability in internal carotid values. Arterial wall thickness in men is uniformly larger than in women, and IMTic increases progressively with age. Cross-sectional analysis of the ARIC study demonstrated that age-related wall thickness advances, on average, an annual rate of 0.015 mm in women and 0.018 mm in men in the carotid bulb, 0.010 mm for women and 0.014 mm for men in the internal carotid, and 0.010 mm for both genders in the common carotid.[26] In older populations, IMTcc progression is estimated at 0.008–0.010 mm/year in males and females[27] (Fig. 23.2). On average, common carotid wall thickness of a healthy person reaches an IMT of 0.78 mm at 76 years of age. The presence of risk factors for atherosclerosis, particularly high blood pressure, promotes and accelerates IMT. In familial hypercholesterolemia patients, pathological IMT is already reached at the age of 40 years.[28] Thus, IMT is a useful tool to investigate normal ageing and preclinical atherosclerosis.

23.2.2 Predictive Value of IMT in Primary Risk Stratification

The correlation between increased carotid IMT and increased cardiovascular risk was first established with clinical evidence in the Kuopio Ischemic Heart Disease Risk Factor Study (KIHD).[29] The study prospectively showed patients with a diseased carotid artery to have an increased risk for cardiovascular events. The comparison was made between the maximum IMTcc in the far wall of control and study subjects. In this study, 1 mm of IMTcc was determined to be a useful cutoff value for assessment of cardiovascular event occurrence.

Fig. 23.2 Illustration of (**a**) a normal carotid segment appearance and (**b**) evidence of thickened IMT at CCA

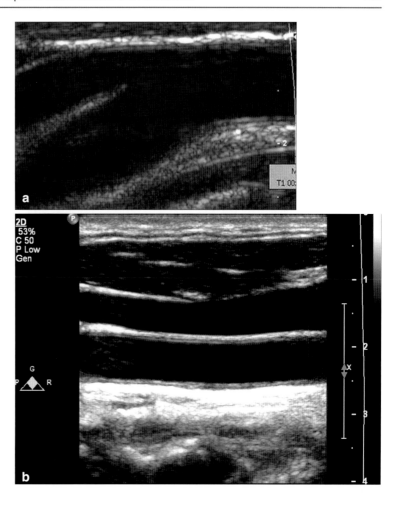

Subsequently, several other prospective studies followed KIHD to further validate the link between IMT and cardiovascular (CV) events.[26,30-39] In the Cardiovascular Health Study, a prospective study of 4,476 patients aged greater than 65 years, combined IMTcc and IMTic predicted both prevalence and incidence of disease after 6.2 years of follow-up.[40] The association for both IMTcc and IMTic was demonstrated after adjustment of traditional cardiovascular risk factors. The relative risk of combined thickness, adjusted for age, gender, and traditional risk factors of cardiovascular disease, was 3.15 (95% confidence interval [CI], 2.19–4.52).

Lorenz et al. conducted a meta-analysis and found IMT to have high predictive value for future cardiovascular events.[41] After adjustment for age and gender, for every increase in IMT by 1 standard deviation [SD] shifting toward the right on the bell curve, the overall estimated relative risk of myocardial infarction (MI) was 1.26 (95% CI, 1.21–1.30) and 1.32 (95% CI, 1.27–1.38) for stroke. Likewise, for every 0.10 mm increment in IMT, the relative risk was 1.15 (95% CI, 1.12–1.17) for acute coronary syndrome and 1.18 (95% CI, 1.16–1.21) for stroke.

As the progression of atherosclerotic vascular disease starts in childhood and spans a spectrum of adulthood,[42] increasing carotid IMT has been found to correlate with incident cardiovascular disease events across a wide age range. Similar results among multiple large prospective studies have shown the strongest association from age 42 to 74 years (Table 23.1). Several other studies have also noted a relationship between increasing risk factor burden, emerging risk factors, and IMT in young adults (18–42 years old).[45-52] Specifically, the Carotid Atherosclerosis Progression Study (CAPS) showed IMT to have

Table 23.1 Carotid IMT as prognostic indicator of acute coronary events and complications

Study	N (% female)	Age (years)	Follow-up (years)	Carotid US parameters	Endpoint	IMT RR (95% CI)
KIHD[29]	1,257 (0)	42–60	1 month to 2½ years	Normal IMTcc >1.0 mm	MI	IMTcc >1.0 mm: 2.17 (0.7–6.74)
CHS[40]	4,476 (39)	>65	6.2	Quintiles or SD of maximum CCA and/or ICA IMT	MI	IMTcc – fifth quintile: 3.15 (2.19–4.52) IMTic – fifth quintile: 3.00 (1.80–5.01)
ARIC[39]	12,841 (57)	45–64	5.2	Mean IMT of 6 sites (CCA, bulb, ICA)	MI, cardiac death	IMT < 1.0 mm vs. IMT ≥ 1.0 mm Women: HRR: 2.62 (1.55–4.46) Men: HRR: 1.20 (0.81–1.77)
CAPS[43]	5,056 (50)	19–90	4.2	Quartiles or SD of mean IMTcc	MI	Fourth quartile: 1.83 (0.97–3.45)
MDCS[44]	5,163 (60)	46–68	7	Tertile of SD of maximum IMTcc	MI, cardiac death	Third tertile: 1.50 (0.81–2.59)

N number of subjects, *IMT* intima-media thickness, *RR* relative risk, *CI* confidence interval, *KIHD* Kuopio Ischemic Heart Disease Study, *IMTcc* common carotid artery intima-media thickness, *MI* myocardial infarction, *CHS* Cardiovascular Health Study, *IMTic* internal carotid artery intima-media thickness, *ARIC* Atherosclerosis Risk in Communities Study, *CAPS* Carotid Atherosclerosis Progression Study, *MDCS* Malmö Diet and Cancer Study

significant predictive value for cardiovascular events among 2,436 subjects with mean age of 38.7 years.[43] The carotid IMT relative risk appeared to be higher among the younger adults in the study.

While several studies have defined a predictive role of IMTcc for cardiovascular events, others have found that IMTcc has a weak predictive role. In the Rotterdam Elderly Study, the role of IMTcc to predict stroke and acute myocardial infarction was examined.[37] Significant relationships were found between disease events and IMTcc, but after adjustment for other risk factors, these fell to insignificant levels for myocardial infarction and were of only borderline significance for stroke. However, in this study, history of previous cardiovascular disease was used as a variable in the multivariate analysis. This may explain why the Rotterdam investigators were unable to show a strong association between IMTcc and the risk of myocardial infarction.[53]

In the Tromsø study, a population-based prospective study of 2,971 and 3,208 Norwegian men and women, respectively, Johnsen et al. investigated the relationship between increased IMT and the presence of plaques as predictors for a first acute coronary syndrome event[54] (Chap. 24). Overall, this study provides further evidence to suggest that IMTcc alone might not be adequate, and multiple carotid segments should be evaluated along with the inclusion of plaque when IMT assessment is performed for cardiovascular risk stratification. The importance of carotid plaque as a predictor for cardiovascular risks will be further discussed in subsequent sections.

23.2.3 Utility of IMT in Youth

A number of studies have shown an associated relationship between increased carotid IMT and exposure to risk factors, such as low-density lipoprotein (LDL) and high-density lipoprotein (HDL) cholesterol,[46] body mass index (BMI),[55] triglycerides in females,[49] and children with familial hypercholesterolemia.[56] Children with hypercholesterolemia and diabetes show increased IMT compared to healthy controls, with a relatively greater increase in the aortic IMT than in the carotid IMT.[57] Four other studies measured carotid IMT in children and young adults.[58-61]

de Giorgis et al. examined carotid IMT in prepubertal children with a positive family history of premature cardiovascular disease (PFHPCD) in addition to the relationship between IMT and other conventional risk factors involved in morphologic alteration of the vascular wall, such as insulin resistance, oxidant status, and lipid profile.[62] The study showed children with PFHPCD to have higher carotid IMT ($P = 0.001$) compared to the control group. Based on multiple linear regression analysis and adjustment for age, gender, and body mass index, increased IMT and levels of prostaglandin F-2alpha were found to be directly correlated ($\beta = 0.905$; $P = 0.002$; $r = 2$, 0.63). Thus, subclinical atherosclerosis was already present in prepubertal children with PFHPCD.

Furthermore, increased IMT in obese children and children with type 2 diabetes mellitus was documented in 446 subjects (age range from 10 to 24 years) by Urbina et al.[63] The mean IMTcc, IMTbulb, and IMTic were measured and compared among three groups of lean, obese, and diabetic participants. Relative to lean and obese youths, the IMTcc and the IMTbulb were found to be greater in subjects with type 2 diabetes mellitus. The internal carotid artery (ICA) IMTic and carotid arterial stiffness were also higher in obese and type 2 diabetes mellitus youths compared to the lean group.

23.2.4 IMT in Established Coronary Artery Disease

The presence of increased carotid IMT in individuals with established coronary artery disease has been postulated and shown to predict risk for a clinical presentation of acute coronary syndromes (Table 23.2). In a prospective study, Hodis et al. examined the relationship between IMTcc in 146 men, 40–59 years old, all with history of coronary artery bypass graft surgery.[64] After 2 years of follow-up, the study found that an annual rate of each 0.03-mm increment in IMTcc was associated with a relative risk of 2.2 (95% CI, 1.4–3.6) and 3.1 (95% CI, 2.1–4.5) for nonfatal myocardial infarction or coronary death and any coronary events (including indication for coronary artery revascularization secondary to recurrence of unstable angina), respectively.

Table 23.2 Carotid IMT as acute coronary events and related complications risk assessment in patients with established CAD

Study	N (% woman)	Age (years)	Follow-up (years)	Carotid US parameters	Endpoint	Results
Hodis et al.[64]	146 (0)	40–59	2	IMTcc	MI, CAD death	Annual rate increment of 0.3 mm: 3.1 (2.1–4.5)$^{\Sigma \text{ (sigma)}, \Omega \text{ (omega)}}$
Zielinski et al.[65]	297 (29)	31–82	1 month–6.6 years	Mean of bulb, IMTcc, and 5-year-survival rate. Low IMTcc: ($\leq$1.13 mm; high IMTcc: >1.13 mm)	Primary: death from all causes	Low IMTcc vs. high IMTcc: 99% vs. 78% survival rate
					Secondary: MI or stroke or death from all causes	Low IMTcc vs. high IMTcc: 95% vs. 74% survival rate
Held et al. (APSIS)[66]	558 (33)	<70	3	Maximal IMTcc	MI, CAD death	IMTcc 0·81–1·02 mm: 0·62 (0·27–1·45)$^{\Sigma \text{ (sigma)} \Omega \text{ (omega)}}$
						IMTcc >1·02 mm: 0·78 (0·36–1·70)$^{\Sigma \text{ (sigma)} \Omega \text{ (omega)}}$

N number of subjects, MI myocardial infarction, CAD coronary artery disease, N/A not applied, IMTcc common carotid intima-media thickness, APSIS Angina Prognosis Study in Stockholm
Σ (sigma)Relative risk (95% CI)
Ω (omega)Adjusted for age, gender, and conventional risk factors

Zielinsk et al. conducted a prospective study of 297 hypertensive subjects with coronary artery disease to evaluate the value of IMTmax measured in the common carotid artery (CCA) and carotid bulb (i.e., including plaques) as an independent prognostic indicator of future cardiovascular events.[65] After a follow-up period ranging from 1 to 79 months, with the main and secondary endpoints defined as death from all causes and myocardial infarction, stroke, or death from all causes, respectively, survival rates between the study groups were compared. For the main endpoint, a 5-year survival rate was calculated to be close to 99% and 78% in patients with "low carotid artery intima-media thickness (CIMT)" (≤ 1.13 mm) and "high CIMT" (>1.13 mm) (log-rank test; $P < 0.001$), respectively. For the secondary endpoint, the 5-year event-free survival rate was 95% and 74% in individuals with low and high IMTmax ($P < 0.008$), respectively. After adjustments for age, gender, history of tobacco use, diabetes mellitus, hyperlipidemia, and other risk factors, the odds ratio of increased IMTmax in relation to the primary endpoint was 1.38 (95% CI, 1.15–1.67).

In the Angina Prognosis Study in Stockholm (APSIS), a prospective study of 558 subjects with clinical diagnosis of stable angina pectoris and a follow-up period of 3 years, univariate Cox regression analyses showed that IMTcc and plaques were related to the risk of cardiovascular death or myocardial infarction. Femoral IMT was related to cardiovascular death or myocardial infarction, as well as to revascularization, whereas femoral plaques were only related to the latter. After adjustment for age, sex, smoking, previous cardiovascular disease, and lipid status, IMTcc failed to predict any cardiovascular events, whereas carotid plaques tended ($P = 0.056$) (relative risk of 1.83 with 95% CI, 0.96–3.51) to predict the risk of cardiovascular death or myocardial infarction. Femoral IMT ($P < 0.01$) and plaques ($P < 0.05$) were also related to the risk of revascularization after adjustments.[66] The authors concluded that carotid and femoral vascular changes were differently related to cardiovascular events and that evaluations of plaques provided better prediction than assessments of IMT in patients with stable angina.

Thus, carotid plaques are shown to a have strong predictive value for cardiovascular events, even in high risk patients independent of other conventional risk factors.

23.3 IMT and CAD Prevalence

Increased carotid IMT also has been shown to strongly correlate with the prevalence of coronary artery disease (CAD). Several studies have looked at that relationship especially in type 1[67] and type 2 diabetes mellitus[68] and hypertension.[69] Cicorella et al. retrospectively (over a period of 10 years) compared carotid wall changes with coronary angiographic findings in 1,337 patients and reported odds ratios for coronary artery stenosis greater than 50% in at least one coronary artery. The markers of carotid atherosclerosis increased proportionally in patients with one-, two-, or three-vessel coronary artery disease. At univariate analysis, intima-media thickness more than 0.90 mm was associated with an odds ratio of coronary artery disease of 2.28 (95% CI, 1.8–2.9) ($P < 0.0001$), unstable plaque of 3.6 (95% CI 2.3–5.7) ($P < 0.001$), and severe carotid stenosis of 4.2 (95% CI, 2.0–8.7) ($P = 0.0001$). At multivariate analysis, the three markers mentioned above were independent risk factors for coronary artery disease even after adjusting for other risk factors.[70]

23.4 Predictive Role of IMT Versus Plaque

23.4.1 Basic Considerations

23.4.1.1 Risk Factor Association

Carotid IMT has been shown to strongly correlate with traditional risk factors, such as systolic blood pressure,[71] familial hypercholesterolemia,[72] dyslipidemia,[73] type 1 diabetes mellitus,[57] BMI,[74] and active and passive smoking,[75] most of which are, to a certain extent, genetically determined. Research is currently active in the field of genomics to further identify specific genes associating with increased IMT.[76] Carotid plaques, however, appear to be more influenced by the conventional risk factors of age, gender, hypertension, diabetes mellitus, hypercholesterolemia, amount of nicotine consumed, factor VIII, and von Willebrand factor (not genetic inheritance).[77]

23.4.1.2 Pathophysiology

The difference of pathophysiology between carotid IMT and carotid plaque development helps to explain their variations in risk factor association. Intimal thickening, in addition to smooth muscle hyperplasia and intimal fibrocellular hypertrophy, contribute to IMT progression. Such characteristics appear to be influenced by age-related sclerosis and pressure overload against the arterial wall with increased blood pressure.[78,79] Thus, arteriosclerosis may be the underlying cause of increased IMT. On the contrary, carotid plaque formation occurs at the internal carotid artery and the carotid bulb, representing an early manifestation of the atherosclerosis process.[80] Plaque is less commonly present at the common carotid artery, likely a result of the laminar blood flow profile at such a location. In addition, the intrinsically thinner medial layer of carotid bulb compared to that of the smooth portion of the common carotid artery appears to indicate a true atherosclerosis process in carotid plaque formation. Such a process is juxtaposed to plaque development in coronary artery disease.

23.4.1.3 Mechanism of Plaque Development

As indicated in Chap. 1, inflammation plays pivotal role in the transition from a nascent fatty streak to a mature atheromatous plaque with a lipid-laden core embedded within a collagen-rich matrix. Early in the process of plaque formation, oxidation of increased levels of circulating LDL-cholesterol particles causes systemic endothelial dysfunction, which induces expression of adhesion receptors and factors. This results in enhanced adhesion of leukocytes, monocytes, and T-lymphocytes to the arterial wall.[81] When endothelial adhesion is secured, cellular migration into the arterial intima takes place by a process termed "diapedesis". Early atherosclerotic lesions are defined by the presence of foam cells, which are formed by macrophages (derived from mature monocytes) and intracellular uptake of oxidized lipoproteins. Secretion of growth factors and cytokines from activated macrophages recruit additional monocytes and induce smooth muscle proliferation, thus promoting plaque progression. The immune response further enhances plaque development when imbalance occurs between pro- and anti-atherosclerotic lymphocytes. This process involves a complex and intricate interrelationship between humoral and cellular components of the immune system, such as T-lymphocytes, B-lymphocytes, dendritic cells, interferons, tumor necrosis factors, and interleukins.[82,83]

Platelets also significantly contribute to the process of atherothrombosis through signaling pathways between inflammation and thrombosis, which propagate atherosclerosis by positive feedback loops.[84] In response to inflammatory influence, arterial endothelium releases abundant amounts of von Willebrand factor, which sends a signal to recruit platelets to corresponding plaque sites. Binding of platelets to endothelial cells is induced by the interaction between von Willebrand factor and glycoprotein Ib. Subsequently, expression of several platelet surface proteins and molecules, such as thromboxane A_2, adenosine diphosphate, and thrombin, and their mutual interaction positively activate platelets. Other proinflammatory mediators, such as platelet-derived growth factor and platelet factor-4,[85] are then released and stimulate monocytes, macrophages, endothelial cells, and platelets to produce cellular mediators of plaque progression.

Angiogenesis is another important contributor to atherothrombosis. The process is defined by neovascularization, and it originates from the *vasa vasorum* in atheromatous plaques, involving chemokines such as vascular endothelial growth factor and hypoxia-inducible transcription factor.[86] Hypoxia is believed to serve as a stimulating factor for angiogenesis when neovessels are observed to be surrounded by neutrophil-rich hypoxic areas. These neovessels possess leaky endothelial gap junctions and are associated with the development of plaque hemorrhage.[87] A tendency toward plaque rupture is related to stability of the fibrous cap, which is influenced by inflammatory response and degradation of the plaque's collagen matrix through the action of cytokines and interleukins, such as collagenases, elastases, and matrix metalloproteinases.[88] In addition, formation and expansion of necrotic cores in advanced atheromatous plaques by similar enzyme-mediated-cellular processes play a critical role in advancement toward plaque rupture and acute thrombosis.[89]

23.4.2 Predictive Value of Plaque in Primary Risk Stratification

According to the Mannheim Carotid IMT Consensus, a carotid plaque is defined as a focal structure of at least 0.5 mm, or 50% of the surrounding IMT value, that encroaches into the arterial lumen or demonstrates a thickness greater than 1.5 mm as measured from the media-adventitia interface to the intima lumen

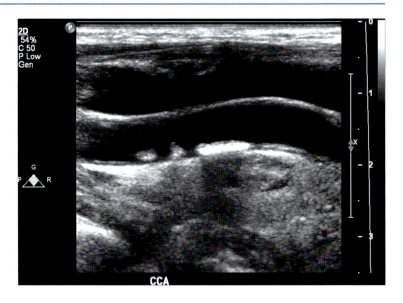

Fig. 23.3 An example of carotid plaque located in left CCA. Note the bright echogenicity, the rugged borders, and inconsistency in the structural boundary

interface.[90,91] Other common criteria for plaque identification are shadowing in wall texture, roughness, and inconsistency in the visualization of structural boundaries along with bright echogenicity (Fig. 23.3).

As mentioned above, based on variation in the pathophysiology of carotid IMT and plaque development, their predictive value of cardiac and cerebral events appears to differ. For instance, due to the relatively low occurrence rate of plaques in the common carotid artery, investigation of atherosclerosis and risk assessment in individual patients at such a location is less likely to yield optimal results compared to carotid bifurcation and internal segments. A number of studies have reported on the high predictive value of plaque as an independent predictor of cardiovascular events,[92] whereas association of IMT with future events is not very strong. Discrepancy among different studies is partly explained by the inclusion or exclusion of plaque in the experimental protocol for assessing IMT values.

The correlation among IMTcc, IMTbulb, and plaque varies in patterns of association with risk factors and prevalent disease. IMTcc is strongly associated with risk factors for cerebrovascular events and stroke prevalence, whereas the IMTbulb and plaque are more directly linked to coronary artery disease risk factors and prevalence.[31] The inclusion of plaque thickness in IMT measurements may therefore confound two qualitatively different pathological processes: arteriosclerosis and atherosclerosis.

On the other hand, the appearance of increased carotid IMT has been demonstrated to develop as a precursor for plaque formation through several cross-sectional and prospective epidemiologic studies of carotid atherosclerosis.[93,94] Specifically, age, hypertension, history of smoking, and brightness mode (B-mode) ultrasound detection in asymptomatic individuals may have predictive value for the occurrence of carotid atherosclerotic plaque. Currently, more prospective studies are needed to further evaluate the pathological relationship between advanced carotid IMT and plaque. Such determination perhaps might better define the clinical application of carotid plaque and IMT as independent risk factors for specific cardiovascular events.

23.4.3 Studies Evaluating the Predictive Role of Carotid Plaque (Table 23.3)

In the KIHD study, carotid plaque was defined based on altered morphology of the arterial wall secondary to calcification or focal protrusion into the arterial lumen.[95] After a follow-up period of 1–30 months, in comparison to men free of any structural changes in the carotid artery wall at baseline, the risk of having an acute

Table 23.3 Carotid plaques as prognostic indicator for acute coronary events and complications

Study	N (% woman)	Age (years)	Follow-up (years)	Carotid US parameters	Endpoint	Plaque HR (95% CI)$^\Omega$
The Tromsø study[54]	6,226 (52)	25–84	6	PAT at CCA, bulb, and ICA	MI	Women: Highest PAT vs. no plaque: 3.95 (2.16–7.19)$^\Sigma$ Men: Highest PAT vs. no plaque: 1.56 (1.04–2.36)$^\Sigma$
APSIS[66]	558 (33)	60 ±7 $^\mu$ (mu)	3	Presence of plaque at CCA, bulb, ICA, ECA, FA	MI, CAD death	Grade 1: 2·00 (0·97–4·12)$^\Sigma$ Grade 2–3: 1·85 (0·77–4·46)$^\Sigma$ Any type: 1·83 (0·96–3·51)$^\Sigma$
KIHD[95]	1,288 (0)	42–60	1 month to 2½ years	Normal Non-stenotic plaque Stenotic plaque	MI	Non-stenotic: 4.15 (1.51–11.47) Stenotic: 6.71 (1.33–33.91)
ARIC[96]	12,375 (54)	45–64	5.2	Presence of plaque at CCA, bulb, and ICA	MI, CAD death	Women: Without AS vs. no plaque: 1.78 (1.22, 2.60) With AS vs. non-AS: 1.73 (1.07, 2.80) Men: Without AS vs. no plaque: 1.59 (1.22, 2.07) With AS vs. non-AS: 1.04 (0.72, 1.51)
Rotterdam study[97]	6,389 (62)	≥55	7–10	Presence of plaque at CCA, bulb, and ICA	MI	Severe: 1.83 (1.27–2.62)

N number of subjects, *HR* hazard ratio, *CI* confidence interval, *APSIS* Angina Prognosis Study in Stockholm, *CCA* common carotid artery, *MI* myocardial infarction, *CAD* coronary artery disease, *ICA* internal carotid artery, *ECA* external carotid artery, *FA* femoral artery, *ARIC* Atherosclerosis Risk in Communities Study, *KIHD* Kuopio Ischemic Heart Disease Study, *PAT* plaque area tertile
$^\Omega$Adjusted for age, gender, and conventional risk factors
$^\Sigma$Relative risk
$^{\mu \text{ (mu)}}$Mean age

coronary syndrome event increased 3.29-fold (95% CI, 1.31–8.29; $P = 0.0074$) with the presence of any structural changes in the common carotid artery or carotid bulb, 4.15-fold (95% CI, 1.51–11.47; $P < 0.01$) with carotid plaques, 6.71-fold (95% CI, 1.33–33.91; $P < 0.01$) with stenotic plaques, and 2.17-fold (95% CI, 0.70–6.74; $P = $ NS) with IMTcc greater than 1.0 mm. In addition, the KIHD study also estimated that the risk for an ACS event rose to 2.14-fold (95% CI, 1.08–4.26) for every 1-mm increment in IMTcc.

Belcaro et al. conducted important studies to assess the predictive value of plaque in cardiovascular events. In their studies, severity of atherosclerosis was determined on a grading system that ranged from normal IMTcc to intima-media granulation (or increased IMT > 1 mm) to non-stenotic and stenotic plaque. The first study[98] included asymptomatic, healthy subjects without prior history of diabetes mellitus, hypercholesterolemia, hypertension, renal disease, or cardiovascular events. High-resolution ultrasound was used to examine carotid and femoral arterial bifurcations. After 6 years of follow-up, the results of 2,000 (1,124 males, 876 females) showed that individuals with no plaque or increased IMTcc had a cardiovascular event rate of 0.56% compared to 27% in those with at least one plaque in the carotid bifurcation and common femoral bifurcation. Among those with plaques, the event rate was 18% for small plaques (class III, defined as focal increase in IMT greater than 2.0 mm without hemodynamic disturbance on color Doppler)

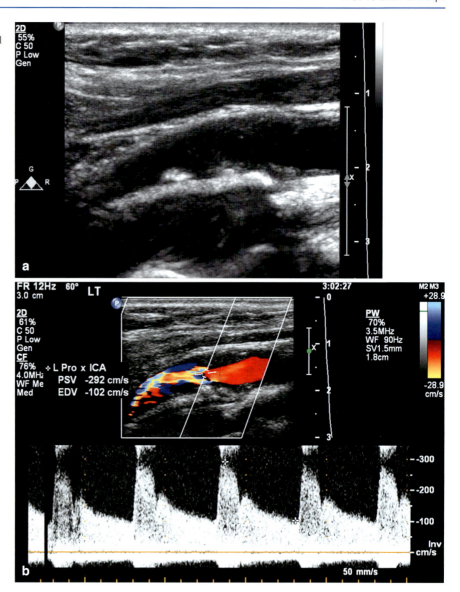

Fig. 23.4 (**a**) Left ICA is showing 80–99% intraluminal stenosis with (**b**) evidence of hemodynamic disturbance detected by color Doppler

and 42% for large stenotic plaques (class IV, defined as diameter stenosis greater than 50% and with hemodynamic alteration on duplex imaging) (Fig. 23.4). In another prospective study with a 10-year follow-up,[99] both common carotid and common femoral bifurcations of 10,000 low-risk healthy subjects were examined by B-mode ultrasound to measure IMTcc and evaluate the presence of plaques in relation to a cardiovascular event endpoint. The results showed that only 1.4% of total cardiovascular events occurred in patients with class I (considered to be normal) arterial morphology. The event rate was calculated to be 0.12%, 9%, 39%, and 81% in subjects with class I, class II (increased IMT > 1.0 mm), class III, and class IV morphology, respectively. The study also discovered that a normal IMTcc was found in 74%, 54%, and 44% in subjects with class II, class III, and class IV morphology, suggesting that the presence of plaques in the bifurcation in the absence of abnormal IMTcc still has a high predictive value for a cardiovascular event.

The correlation of the Framingham risk score (FRS) with IMTcc, carotid plaques, and their predictive power of cerebrovascular events were studied by Touboul et al.[100] The presence and absence of carotid plaques significantly altered the relationship between IMTcc and FRS. Subjects with carotid plaques and increased IMTcc showed an incremental value between 10% and 20% in the 10-year FRS. Absence of carotid plaques in this population was associated with a decrease between 5% and 20% in the 10-year FRS. In addition, IMTcc, Framingham cerebrovascular risk score, and carotid plaques were found, by multiple conditional logistic regression for matched sets, to be independently associated with cerebrovascular event risk, with an odds ratio of 1.68 (1.25–2.26; $P = 0.0006$), 2.16 (1.57–2.98; $P < 0.0001$), and 2.73 (1.68–4.44; $P < 0.0001$), respectively.

The Northern Manhattan Study, a prospective clinical trial with 1939 subjects, further assessed the risk of ischemic strokes in relation to carotid plaques.[101] After a mean follow-up period of 6.2 years, presence of morphologically altered plaques detected by B-mode ultrasound at any segments of common carotid artery, carotid bulb, and internal carotid artery carried a statistically significant hazard ratio (adjusted for demographics, traditional vascular risk factors, variation in plaque thickness, and stenosis) of 3.1 (95% CI, 1.1–8.5) associated with an ischemic cerebrovascular event.

The EVA study, a longitudinal study in western France that included 1,040 subjects aged 59–71 years with a family history of premature coronary artery disease, focused on carotid IMT in a risk assessment for a genetically inherent pattern of cardiovascular events. The study found that subjects with a history of premature death from coronary artery disease had a higher prevalence of atheromatous plaques in the common carotid, carotid bifurcation, and internal carotid artery compared with those without plaques. In contrast, IMTcc was not associated with parental history of premature death from coronary artery disease.[102] The odds ratio of atheromatous plaques associated with a parental history of premature death from coronary artery disease after adjustment for age and gender was 2.85 (95% CI, 1.60–5.08; $P < 0.001$). Several other observational studies with at least 1,000 subjects demonstrated equal or higher relative risks of cardiovascular events for plaque compared to increased carotid IMT.[44,96,97,103-105] Thus, carotid plaques indeed appear to have significant predictive power in the risk assessment of cardiovascular events.

In the Tromsø study, a population-based prospective study of 2,971 and 3,208 Norwegian men and women (age range from 25 to 84 years), respectively, Johnsen et al. investigated the relationship between increased IMT and the presence of plaques as predictors for a first acute coronary event.[54] Ultrasonographic measurements were performed at the far and near walls of the right common carotid artery, bulb, and internal carotid artery. The endpoint was determined by occurrence of the first acute coronary event, which was documented by clinical signs and symptoms, changes in electrocardiogram, and levels of cardiac biomarkers. After 6 years of follow-up, the study showed a myocardial infarction rate of 6.6% and 3.0% in men and women, respectively. Compared to subjects without carotid plaques, individuals with the highest plaque area tertile carried an adjusted relative risk (RR) (95% CI) of 1.56 (1.04–2.36) in men and 3.95 (2.16–7.19) in women. The increased plaque echolucency in women especially correlated with a significantly higher risk for acute coronary events. The adjusted RR (95% CI) in the highest versus lowest IMT quartile was 1.73 (0.98–3.06) in men and 2.86 (1.07–7.65) in women. Interestingly, exclusion of carotid bulb measurements from analyses did not validate IMTcc as a predictor for acute coronary events in either gender (Chap. 24).

23.5 Carotid Plaque Features

23.5.1 Carotid Plaque Area as Predictor of Cardiovascular Events

In relation to directional blood flow within the arterial wall, development of plaques progresses longitudinally and grows along the vessel wall at a faster rate than luminal thickening.[106] In addition to assessment of carotid plaque thickness, a few recent studies with compelling data have shown a high predictive power of carotid plaque area within the arterial wall for cardiovascular events.[54,105] In a prospective study of 1,686 patients, Spence et al. examined the value of employing carotid plaque area measurements to identify patients with an increased risk for cardiovascular events.[105] A cross-sectional area of longitudinal views of all plaques in the common carotid, internal carotid, and external carotid arteries was repeatedly scanned using ultrasound and recorded in association with clinical presentation at 1-year intervals. After 5 years of follow-up, the study found the adjusted relative risk of combined stroke and acute coronary events in subjects with the highest carotid plaque area quartile to be 2.9 (95% CI, 1.4–5.8) (Chap. 25). Based on these findings and the study protocol, they suggested that inclusion of carotid plaque area to be a powerful risk assessment tool to detect and prevent the progression of subclinical atherosclerosis in high risk patients.

23.5.2 Carotid Plaque Echogenicity and Associated Cardiovascular Risks

Based on ultrasonographic and histologic findings, classification of simple (echogenic with calcified, fibrous tissue) (Fig. 23.5) and complex (echolucent which have increased macrophage density and lipid content) plaques are commonly used to predict the relative risk of cardiovascular events (Fig. 23.6). A tendency toward rupture largely depends on the morphology of plaques. Echolucent carotid plaques appear to carry an association with elevated risk for future acute coronary events.[107] Several prospective studies[54,108] and cross-sectional studies[109,110] using gray scale median after image normalization or backscatter analysis have also illustrated the function of plaque echolucency as a predictor of cardiovascular risk. Furthermore, plaque lucency after image normalization

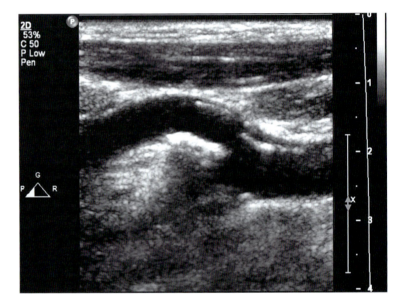

Fig. 23.5 An example of calcified plaque, which is mainly composed of calcified, fibrous tissue (note the associated location near the carotid bulb)

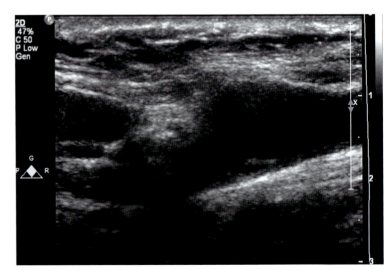

Fig. 23.6 Hypoechoic carotid plaque is shown here, located at carotid bulb. Structural composition is associated with increased macrophage density and lipid content

(Chap. 12) is more reproducible than measurement of plaque thickness.[111] Honda et al. investigated the predictive power of carotid plaque echolucency for the development of acute coronary syndromes in patients with a clinical diagnosis of stable angina.[108] Through a prospective study of 215 subjects and a follow-up period up to 30 months, the predictive power was calculated to be 83%. After adjustment for age, gender, and traditional risk factors, echolucent carotid plaques, in patients with stable angina, independently predicted the occurrence of acute coronary events, with a hazard ratio of 7.0 (95% CI, 2.3–21.4).

23.6 Effects of Lipid-Lowering Therapy

23.6.1 Effects of Lipid-Lowering Therapy on IMT Progression and Cardiovascular Events

Statins have been widely employed as important agents in primary and secondary prevention to treat patients with hyperlipidemia, dyslipidemia, coronary artery disease, acute coronary syndromes, stroke, and transient ischemic attack. Thus far, the relationship between lipid profile and IMT progression has been examined in a number of clinical trials based on specific therapeutic agents and cholesterol composition. Many studies have been conducted to investigate the effect of statin-induced LDL-cholesterol reduction rather than HDL-cholesterol improvement in relation to IMT evolution. These studies are discussed in detail below (Table 23.4).

Based on the underlying complex mechanisms of vascular changes, in general, statin therapy-induced lipid profile alterations did not show the same degree of morphological changes in arterial wall form and function. Therapeutic treatment with various lipid profiles altering medical regimens has been shown with considerable evidence to depress and/or regress the progression of carotid IMT. Espeland et al. conducted a meta-analysis of several HMG-CoA reductase inhibitor trials, which analyzed IMT changes in relation to cardiovascular event occurrence. The study found an annual mean change in IMT progression of -0.012 mm/year (95% CI, -0.016 to -0.007 mm), which was associated with an odds ratio of 0.48 (95% CI, 0.30–0.78) for the reduction in cardiovascular events.[124]

Variation in carotid location measurements and parameters, statistical analysis, and technological methods provide challenges to compare IMT data from different statin intervention trials. Overall, however, the utility of IMT as a surrogate endpoint for lipid-altering drug trials is well supported with clinical evidence, suggesting a beneficial influence of plasma LDL reduction in relation to atherosclerotic regression. An increase in HDL and further lowering of LDL in therapies did not significantly alter the course of IMT progression. The findings of the Measuring Effects on Intima-Media Thickness: An Evaluation of Rosuvastatin (METEOR) study (which is discussed in detail below) validated the predictive value of carotid IMT as a detection and monitoring tool of subclinical atherosclerosis in patients with low Framingham risk score. Aggressive LDL lowering in such a low-cardiovascular-risk population has been shown to effectively hinder advancement of atherosclerosis.[123]

23.6.2 LDL Reduction Therapies and IMT Progression

In the Regression Growth Evaluation Statin Study (REGRESS), a double-blind, placebo-controlled clinical trial of 255 men with angiographic evidence of coronary artery disease, de Groot et al. examined the influence of pravastatin (daily dose of 40 mg) on IMTcc and femoral IMT (IMTfem) structural alteration.[112] After 2 years of follow-up with sequential ultrasound measurements at 6-monthly intervals, pravastatin therapy reduced the mean IMTcc/IMTfem and maximal IMT by 0.05 and 0.005 mm, respectively ($P < 0.01$).

Crouse et al. conducted the first randomized, double-blind clinical study called the Pravastatin, Lipids and Atherosclerosis in the Carotid Arteries (PLACII trial). They further examined the therapeutic benefit of the lipid-lowering drug on progression of subclinical atherosclerosis.[113] The daily dose of 10–40 mg of pravastatin was randomly given to 151 subjects with a previous diagnosis of coronary artery disease and an IMT value greater than 1.3 mm in at least one of the extracranial carotid segments. After 3 years of sequential ultrasound measurements at 6-monthly intervals,

Table 23.4 Overview of clinical studies that examined the effects of lipid-lowering therapy on carotid IMT progression (subclinical atherosclerosis)

Study	N (% woman)	Age (years)	Follow-up (years)	US parameters	Agent(s) (mg/day)	% LDL reduction	Results
REGRESS[112]	255 (0)	<70	2	Mean IMTcc/FA	Pravastatin (40)	−29	−0.05 mm in mean FA-IMTcc/FA
PLAC II[113]	150 (NR)	NR	3	Mean max of CCA/CB/ICA-IMT	Pravastatin (10–40)	−28	NS 12% reduction in mean Max IMT
							Significant 35% reduction in IMTcc
KAPS[114]	424 (0)	44–65	3	Mean max CCA/CB/FA-IMT	Pravastatin (40)	−27	CCA treatment effect: 66% (95% CI, 30–95%, $P < 0.002$)
							CB treatment effect of 30% (95% CI, −1 to 54%, $P = 0.056$)
							No significant treatment effect at FA
CAIUS[115]	305 (47)	45–65	3	Mean max CCA/CB/ICA-IMT	Pravastatin (40)	−22	Annual rate of progression: ($P < 0.0007$)
							Study group: −0.0043 mm/year
							Placebo: 0.009 mm/year
LIPID[116]	522 (12)	61 $\mu_{(mu)}$	4	Mean IMTcc	Pravastatin (40)	−27	Study group: −0.014 mm.
							Placebo group: 0.048 mm
MARS[117]	188 (8)	37–67	4	Mean IMTcc	Lovastatin (80)	−45	Annual rate of progression: ($P < 0.001$)
							Study group: −0.028 ± 0.003 mm/year
							Placebo: 0.015 ± 0.005 mm/year
ACAPS[118,119]	919 (48)	40–79	3	Mean max of CCA/CB/ICA-IMT	Lovastatin (20–40)	−28	Annual rate of progression: ($P = 0.001$)
							Study group: −0.009 ± 0.003 mm/year
							Placebo: 0.006 ± 0.003 mm/year
BCAPS[120]	793 (62)	49–70	3	Mean IMTcc	Fluvastatin (40)	−23	Annual rate of progression: ($P = 0.002$)
							−0.009 (95% CI, −0.015 to −0.003 mm/year)
ARBITER I[121]	161 (29)	60 $\mu_{(mu)}$	1	Mean IMTcc	Atorvastatin (80)	−49	−0.034 ± 0.021 mm, $P = 0.03$
					Pravastatin (40)	−27	0.025 ± 0.017 mm; $P = 0.03$
ASAP[122]	325 (61)	30–70	2	Mean CCA/CB/ICA-IMT	Atorvastatin (80)	−41	−0.031 mm (95% CI, −0.007 to −0.055, $P = 0.0017$)
					Simvastatin (40)	−51	0.036 mm (95% CI, 0.014–0.058, $P = 0.0005$)

(continued)

Table 23.4 (continued)

Study	N (% woman)	Age (years)	Follow-up (years)	US parameters	Agent(s) (mg/day)	% LDL reduction	Results
METEOR[123]	984 (40)	β (beta)	2	Mean max of CCA/CB/ICA-IMT	Rosuvastatin (80)	−49	Annual rate of progression: ($P < 0.001$)
							Study group: −0.0014 mm/year (95% CI, −0.0041 to 0.0014 mm)
							Placebo: 0.0131 mm/year (95% CI, 0.0087–0.0174 mm)

N number of subjects, *Max* maximum, *NR* not reported, *CCA* common carotid artery, *FA* femoral artery, *CB* carotid bulb, *ICA* internal carotid artery, *IMT* intima-media thickness, *IMTcc* common carotid IMT, *NS* nonsignificant, *CI* confidence interval, *REGRESS* Regression Growth Evaluation Statin Study, *PLAC II* Pravastatin, Lipids and Atherosclerosis in the Carotid Arteries, *KAPS* Kuopio Atherosclerosis Prevention Study, *CAIUS* Carotid Atherosclerosis Italian Ultrasound Study, *LIPID* Long-term Intervention with Pravastatin in Ischemic Disease, *MARS* Monitored Atherosclerosis Regression study, *ACAPS* Asymptomatic Carotid Artery Progression Study, *BCAPS* β(BETA)-Blocker Cholesterol-lowering Asymptomatic Plaque Study, *ARBITER I* Arterial Biology for the Investigation of the Treatment Effects of Reducing Cholesterol, *ASAP* Atherosclerosis Progression in Familial Hypercholesterolemia, *METEOR* Measuring Effects on Intima-Media Thickness: An Evaluation of Rosuvastatin

$^{\mu\ (mu)}$Mean age
$^{\beta\ (beta)}$45–70 years in men and 55–70 years in women

the mean IMTmax of the carotid bifurcation showed a nonsignificant annual 12% reduction in the pravastatin treatment group. Regression of atherosclerosis, however, was indicated by IMTcc alone with a significant reduction in thickness (35%) in the study group ($P = 0.03$).

The Kuopio Atherosclerosis Prevention Study (KAPS) was the first prospective study that explored the effects of statin therapy as a primary prevention of the advancement of carotid and femoral atherosclerosis. Salonen et al. enrolled 447 men who were randomized to be treated with either pravastatin (daily dose of 40 mg) or a placebo.[114] After 3 years of follow-up, the pravastatin-treated individuals showed a 45% (95% CI, 16–69%) reduction in carotid atherosclerosis progression rate (0.017 mm/year) compared to the control group (0.031 mm/year) ($P = 0.005$). The treatment effect on the common carotid artery was documented as 66% (95% CI, 30–95%; pravastatin 0.010 mm/year; placebo 0.029 mm/year; $P < 0.002$). Statistical analysis of the femoral arteries did not show any significant treatment effect. Two other studies also showed the clinical benefits of pravastatin therapy in light of inducing carotid IMT regression. The Carotid Atherosclerosis Italian Ultrasound Study (CAIUS) documented an annual rate of IMT reduction (mean of 12 maximum thickness measurements in each carotid bifurcation) of −0.0043 mm/year in the pravastatin groups in contrast to an annual rate of increase of 0.009 mm/year in the placebo population. Divergence of IMT progression slopes between control and study groups were observed after 6 months of medical intervention.[115] In the Long-term Intervention with Pravastatin in Ischemic Disease (LIPID) study, after 4 years of follow-up, pravastatin therapy (daily dose of 40 mg) reduced the average IMTcc by 0.014 mm, while the placebo group experienced a 0.048-mm increase.[116]

The beneficial clinical effects of statin therapy other than pravastatin on IMTcc progression were reported in the Monitored Atherosclerosis Regression Study (MARS), another randomized, double-blind, placebo-controlled trial of 188 subjects with angiographically diagnosed coronary artery disease.[117] In this study, Hodis et al. prescribed lovastatin (daily dose of 80 mg) to study individuals and serially measured their IMTcc for a follow-up period of 4 years. Control subjects were given a placebo in addition to a cholesterol-lowering diet. At 2 and 4 years, the lovastatin study group showed statistically significant reduction in the annual rate of IMTcc regression compared to the placebo group, which demonstrated annual atherosclerosis advancement based on their increased IMTcc ($P < 0.001$). The mean IMTcc reduction rate was 0.038 mm and 0.028 mm/year at 2 and 4 years, respectively. In the control population, the mean IMTcc progressed at an annual rate of 0.019 mm and 0.015 mm/year at 2 and 4 years, respectively.

The therapeutic benefits of lovastatin alone and lovastatin in combination with warfarin therapy were investigated in the Asymptomatic Carotid Artery Progression Study (ACAPS), which involved 919 asymptomatic men and women (age range from 40 to 79 years) with ultrasonographic carotid evidence of early atherosclerosis. IMT (mean of 12 maximum measurements in each carotid bifurcation) was measured every 6 months for a total of 3 years.[118,119] The final results showed overall annual IMT reduction rates of -0.009 mm/year for the lovastatin group and an annual IMT increased rate of 0.006 mm/year for the placebo group ($P = 0.001$). In a subsequent analysis related to gender, combination therapy of lovastatin and warfarin showed the most significant overall disease regression in women ($P = 0.02$); however, data for lovastatin alone in women also had a trend toward a reversed disease progression ($P = 0.09$). In men, therapy with lovastatin alone offered the greatest reduction ($P = 0.02$), although warfarin alone also showed clinical benefits.[125] Evidence from a separate non-placebo controlled trial also found that a high daily dose (80 mg) of another lipid-lowering agent, simvastatin, to effectively reverse IMT progression in subjects with familial hypercholesterolemia.[118]

In a placebo-controlled, randomized, clinical trial study called the β-Blocker Cholesterol-lowering Asymptomatic Plaque Study (BCAPS),[120] Hedblad et al. tested the effects of a beta-blocker and statin on IMT advancement in the presence of carotid plaques. In this study, 793 asymptomatic subjects (age range from 49 to 70 years) were enrolled and given metoprolol XL (daily dose of 25 mg) or fluvastatin (daily dose of 40 mg) at random assignments along with placebo control groups. After a follow-up period of 3 years, the observed annual IMTcc progression rate in the placebo group was 0.013 ± 0.053 mm/year. The annual IMTmax progression rate in the bifurcation in the placebo group was 0.089 ± 0.154 mm/year. Fluvastatin but not metoprolol CR/XL reduced the rate of progression of IMTcc compared with placebo mean difference between groups, -0.009 mm/year (95% CI, -0.015 to -0.003; $P = 0.002$); ultrasonographic assessment of maximum IMT in the carotid bulb area showed an annual reduction rate of -0.058 mm (95% CI, -0.094 to -0.023; $P = 0.004$) and -0.023 mm (95% CI, -0.044 to -0.003; $P = 0.014$) at 18 months and 36 months, respectively.

Taylor et al. directly compared the clinical efficacy of atorvastatin (daily dose of 80 mg) and pravastatin (daily dose of 40 mg) on IMTcc progression in a randomized clinical trial of 161 subjects (46% of whom had a history of cardiovascular disease), known as the Arterial Biology for the Investigation of the Treatment Effects of Reducing Cholesterol (the ARBITER 1) study.[121] After 1 year of medical therapy, a significant regression of IMTcc (-0.034 ± 0.021 mm) was recorded in the atorvastatin group while IMTcc did not change (0.025 ± 0.017 mm) in patients who received pravastatin therapy.

In the Atherosclerosis Progression in Familial Hypercholesterolemia study (ASAP), Smilde et al. compared the influence of high-dose statin therapy using atorvastatin (daily dose of 80 mg) to the conventional simvastatin therapy (daily dose of 40 mg) on IMT progression.[122] The common carotid, carotid bulb, and internal carotid along with femoral IMT were combined in 325 subjects (age range from 30 to 70 years) who had a diagnosis of familial hypercholesterolemia. After a treatment period of 2 years, atorvastatin-treated patients showed an IMT reduction of -0.031 mm (95% CI, -0.007 to -0.055; $P = 0.0017$) compared to an overall IMT increase of 0.036 mm (95% CI, 0.014–0.058; $P = 0.0005$) in the simvastatin-treated group. In conjunction with IMT regression, high-dose treatment of atorvastatin also reduced LDL concentration to a greater extent compared to therapy with the conventional dose of simvastatin. In a subsequent study, the prevention of atherosclerosis progression in a low Framingham risk score, asymptomatic population but who had IMT-detected subclinical atherosclerosis was shown to be effective with aggressive lipid-lowering therapy.[126]

Another subclass of statins was used in the METEOR study. This randomized, placebo-controlled, double-blinded study examined the effect of rosuvastatin on carotid IMT progression in 984 asymptomatic individuals (age range of 45–70 years in men and 55–70 years in women) who had moderately elevated LDL (>120 to <160 mg/dl), a 10-year Framingham risk score of less than 10%, and subclinical atherosclerosis based on an IMTmax of 1.2–3.5 mm.[123] These criteria indicate that most of the subjects in this study had plaques. Patients were randomized to receive either rosuvastatin (daily dose of 40 mg) or a placebo. The IMTs of the CCA, carotid bulb, and ICA were ultrasonographically measured at 6-month intervals, and the IMTmax values were analyzed. After 2 years of follow-up, LDL and triglycerides reduction, and HDL elevation were reported in the rosuvastatin study group. Overall, rosuvastatin reduced the annual IMTmax progression rate for the 12 carotid sites at a rate of -0.0014 mm/year (95% CI, -0.0041 to 0.0014 mm) compared to an increase of 0.0131 mm/year (95% CI, 0.0087–0.0174 mm) in the control group ($P < 0.001$). At individual sites, rosuvastatin reduced the annual rate of IMT progression to -0.0038 mm/year (95% CI, -0.0064 to -0.0013 mm, $P < 0.001$), -0.0040 mm/year (95% CI, -0.0090 to 0.0010 mm, $P < 0.001$), and an increase of 0.0039 mm/year (95% CI, -0.0009 to 0.0088 mm, $P = 0.02$) for the common carotid, the carotid bulb, and the internal carotid sites, respectively. The change in the mean IMTcc for the rosuvastatin group was 0.0004 (95% CI, -0.0011 to 0.0019; $P < 0.001$) mm/year. Based on the final results, this study was the first clinical trial to substantiate the preventive benefits of HDL elevation on the advancement of atherosclerosis. Although rosuvastatin significantly depressed IMT progression, at the primary endpoints, such therapy did not induce IMT regression.

23.7 Effects of Inducing HDL Elevation and IMT

Blankenhorn et al. conducted the Cholesterol-Lowering Atherosclerosis Study (CLAS), which was the first study to show a correlation between carotid IMT reduction and change in subclinical atherosclerosis during lipid-lowering intervention.[127] In this randomized, placebo-controlled clinical trial, serial ultrasound measurements of the IMTcc in nonsmoking men with a previous history of coronary bypass surgery were examined in relation to colestipol-niacin plus dietary therapy. At 2- and 4-year intervals, study individuals exhibited a mean IMTcc reduction of 0.05 mm in contrast to an increase of 0.04 mm and 0.05 mm in the IMTcc of the placebo group, respectively ($P < 0.001$). CLAS is also the only study to look at the therapeutic value of medical intervention in relation to changes in IMT and the rate of cardiovascular events. Patients who had completed the CLAS study were followed for an average of 8.8 years, and the final results demonstrated an annual 0.03-mm IMTcc increment to be associated with a threefold elevation in relative risk for any coronary event. Angiographic coronary anatomy and atherosclerosis and lipid profiles were shown to be less indicative of risk for coronary events than IMTcc.

Fewer studies have been conducted to examine the clinical benefits of HDL elevation in relation to atherosclerosis progression. The Arterial Biology for the Investigation of the Treatment Effects of Reducing Cholesterol (ARBITER) 2[128] and ARBITER 3[129] studies both investigated secondary preventive effects of niacin therapy (in addition to statin monotherapy) on IMTcc progression in patients with a diagnosis of coronary artery disease along with low levels of HDL. At the 12-month follow-up, niacin therapy only significantly reduced the IMTcc progression rate in non-insulin-resistant subjects. After 24 months of treatment, the niacin study group showed IMTcc regression of 59.6% compared to the placebo study group.

Kastelein et al. investigated the effects of the cholesteryl ester transfer protein (CETP) inhibitor, torcetrapib, on atherosclerosis progression within carotid and coronary vasculature in the Rating Atherosclerotic Disease Change by Imaging with a New CETP Inhibitor 1 (RADIANCE 1) study.[130] Torcetrapib increases plasma HDL concentration by negatively interfering with the CETP-mediated transfer of cholesterol esters from HDL particles to LDL molecules and triglycerides transport.[131,132] In this prospective, double-blind, randomized, multicenter, parallel-group study, 850 patients with a diagnosis of familial heterozygous hypercholesterolemia were randomly given monotherapy of atorvastatin or combination therapy of torcetrapib (daily dose of 60 mg) and atorvastatin. The CCA, carotid bulb, and ICA IMTs were ultrasonographically scanned at 6-month intervals for a total of 24 months. After a 2-year period of follow-up, a 54% increase in HDL from 52 to 82 mg/dl in the combination therapy (torcetrapib-atorvastatin) group did not translate into a greater reduction of atherosclerosis progression compared to the control group receiving mono-atorvastatin therapy. IMT progression (mean of maximum thickness in the near and far wall of the common carotid, bulb, and internal carotid on both sides) was found to have an annual rate of increase of 0.0053 ± 0.0028 mm/year and 0.0047 ± 0.0028 mm/year in the control monotherapy and the combined therapy groups, respectively ($P = 0.87$). Calculation of the mean IMTcc as a secondary efficacy measure found an annual rate of increase of 0.0038 mm/year in the torcetrapib-atorvastatin group in contrast to a decreased annual rate of -0.0014 mm/year in the atorvastatin-only group ($P < 0.005$). Subjects in the combination study group were also discovered to have a mean increase of 2.9 mmHg in systolic blood pressure.

The RADIANCE 2 study provided more unfavorable data on treatment using a CEPT inhibitor in 752 patients with mixed dyslipidemia. Subjects were randomly assigned to a control group of atorvastatin monotherapy or a combination therapy of torcetrapib-atorvastatin (torcetrapib daily dose of 60 mg). The CCA, carotid bulb, and ICA-IMT were ultrasonographically measured at sequential 6-month intervals, with the primary endpoint defined as the annual rate of change in the maximum IMT of 12 carotid segments. After 2 years of treatment, the torcetrapib-atorvastatin study group and the atorvastatin monotherapy control arm both showed an annual rate of increase in IMT of 0.025 mm/year and 0.030 mm/year ($P = 0.46$), respectively. Subjects in the combination therapy group experienced a mean rise of 5.4 mmHg in systolic blood pressure compared to monotherapy patients. A substantial elevation of 63% in plasma HDL concentration and an 18% reduction of LDL were reported in patients who received CETP inhibitor therapy. The findings in this study did not show torcetrapib therapy to be clinically beneficial in the treatment of atherosclerosis progression. In another study of patients with a diagnosis of coronary artery disease, similar results were illustrated through intravascular ultrasound examination of coronary atheroma volume.[133]

23.8 Summary

Ultrasonographic assessment of carotid arterial wall structure as IMT is a powerful tool for cardiovascular risk stratification because it detects subclinical atherosclerosis. Its predictive power specifically in the presence of plaque has been shown to have greater value than the traditional Framingham risk score. This test has been recommended by the AHA to be performed for further risk stratification in individual patients. Carotid IMT and carotid plaque examination provide an accurate and noninvasive screening test, which could be employed in a wide spectrum of age ranges, from childhood to old age, for detailed evaluation of cardiovascular risk.

References

1. Virmani R, Burke AP, Farb A, Kolodgie FD. Pathology of the vulnerable plaque. *J Am Coll Cardiol*. 2006;47: C13–C18.
2. Li Z, Froehlich J, Galis ZS, Lakatta EG. Increased expression of matrix metalloproteinase-2 in the thickened intima of aged rats. *Hypertension*. 1999;33:116–123.
3. Asai K, Kudej RK, Shen YT, et al. Peripheral vascular endothelial dysfunction and apoptosis in old monkeys. *Arterioscler Thromb Vasc Biol*. 2000;20:1493–1499.
4. Anderson KM, Odell PM, Wilson PW, Kannel WB. Cardiovascular disease risk profiles. *Am Heart J*. 1990;121:293–298.
5. Wilson PW, D'Agostino RB, Levy D, Belanger AM, Silbershatz H, Kannel WB. Prediction of coronary heart disease using risk factor categories. *Circulation*. 1998;97:1837–1847.
6. Assmann G, Cullen P, Schulte H. Simple scoring scheme for calculating the risk of acute coronary events based on the 10-year follow-up of the Prospective Cardiovascular Münster (PROCAM) Study. *Circulation*. 2002;105:310–315.
7. Haq IU, Jackson PR, Yeo WW, Ramsay LE. Sheffield risk and treatment table for cholesterol lowering for primary prevention of coronary heart disease. *Lancet*. 1995;346:1467–1471.
8. Shaper AG, Pocock SJ, Phillips AN, Walker M. A scoring system to identify men at high risk of a heart attack. *Health Trends*. 1987;19:37–39.
9. Pedersen TR, Kjekshus J, Berg K, et al. Scandinavian Simvastatin Survival Study group: randomised trial of cholesterol lowering in 4,444 patients with coronary heart disease: the Scandinavian Simvastatin Survival Study (4S). *Lancet*. 1994;344:1383–1389.
10. Downs JR, Clearfield M, Weis S, et al. Primary prevention of acute coronary events with lovastatin in men and women with average cholesterol levels: results of AFCAPS/TexCAPS. Air Force/Texas Coronary Atherosclerosis Prevention Study. *JAMA*. 1998;279:1615–1622.
11. Ebrahim S, Papacosta O, Whincup P, et al. Carotid plaque, intima media thickness, cardiovascular risk factors, and prevalent cardiovascular disease in men and women: the British Regional Heart Study. *Stroke*. 1999;30:841–850.
12. Simon A, Gariepy J, Chironi F, Megnien JL, Levenson J. Intima-media thickness: a new tool for diagnosis and treatment of cardiovascular risk. *J Hypertens*. 2002;20:159–169.

13. Aminbakhsh A, Mancini CBJ. Carotid intima-media thickness measurements: what defines an abnormality? A systemic review. *Clin Invest Med*. 1999;22:149–157.
14. Van Bortel LM. What does intima–media thickness tell us? *J Hypertens*. 2005;23:37–39.
15. O'Leary DH, Polak JK. Intima-media thickness: a tool for atherosclerosis imaging and event prediction. *Am J Cardiol*. 2002;90(suppl):18L-21L.
16. Touboul PJ. Clinical impact of carotid intima-media measurement. *Eur J Ultrasound*. 2002;16:105–113.
17. Greenland P, Abrams J, Aurigemma M, et al. Prevention conference V: beyond secondary prevention: identifying the high-risk patient for primary prevention: noninvasive tests of atherosclerosis burden: writing group III. *Circulation*. 2000;101:e16-e22.
18. National Cholesterol Education Program (NCEP) Expert Panel (ATP III). Third report of the National Cholesterol Education Program (NCEP) expert panel on detection, evaluation, and treatment of high blood cholesterol in adults (adult treatment panel III) final report. *Circulation*. 2002;106:3143–3421.
19. Guidelines committee. 2003 European Society of Hypertension– European Society of Cardiology guidelines for the management of arterial hypertension. *J Hypertens*. 2003;21:1011–1053.
20. Pignoli P, Tremoli E, Poli A, Oreste P, Paoletti R. Intimal plus medial thickness of the arterial wall: a direct measurement with ultrasound imaging. *Circulation*. 1986;6:1399–1406.
21. Young W, Gofman JW, Tandy R, Malamud N, Waters ESG. The quantitation of atherosclerosis, III: the extent of correlation of degrees of atherosclerosis within and between the coronary and cerebral vascular beds. *Am J Cardiol*. 1960;6:300–308.
22. Mitchell JRA, Schwartz CJ. Relationship between arterial disease in different sites: a study of the aorta and coronary, carotid, and iliac arteries. *Br Med J*. 1963;1:1293–1301.
23. Mathur KS, Kashyap SK, Kumar V. Correlation of the extent and severity of atherosclerosis in the coronary and cerebral arteries. *Circulation*. 1963;27:929–934.
24. Veller MG, Fisher CM, Nicolaides AN. Measurement of the ultrasonic intima-media complex thickness in normal subjects. *J Vasc Surg*. 1993;17:719–725.
25. Kuller L, Borhani N, Furberg CD, et al. Prevalence of subclinical atherosclerosis and cardiovascular disease and association with risk factors in the Cardiovascular Health Study. *Am J Epidemiol*. 1994;139:1164–1179.
26. Howard G, Sharrett AR, Heiss G, et al. Carotid artery intimal-medial thickness distribution in general populations as evaluated by B-mode ultrasound. ARIC Investigators. *Stroke*. 1993;24(9):1297–1304.
27. O'Leary DH, Polak JF, Kronmal RA, et al. Distribution and correlates of detected carotid artery disease in the cardiovascular health study. *Stroke*. 1992;23:1752–1760.
28. de Groot E, Hovingh GK, Wiegman A, et al. Measurement of arterial wall thickness as a surrogate marker for atherosclerosis. *Circulation*. 2004;109(suppl III):III-33–III-38.
29. Salonen JT, Salonen R. Ultrasound B-mode imaging in observational studies of atherosclerotic progression. *Circulation*. 1993;87:II56-II65.
30. Bots ML, Hoes AW, Koudstaal PJ, Hofman A, Grobbee DE. Common carotid intima-media thickness and risk of stroke and myocardial infarction: the Rotterdam Study. *Circulation*. 1997;96:1432–1437.
31. Allan PL, Mowbray PI, Lee AJ, Fowkes GR. Relationship between carotid intima-media thickness and asymptomatic peripheral arterial disease. The Edinburgh artery study. *Stroke*. 1997;28:348–353.
32. Bonithon-Kopp C, Toubout PI, Berr C, Magne C, Ducimetiere P. Factors of carotid arterial enlargement in a population aged 59 to 71 years. *Stroke*. 1996;27:654–660.
33. Salonen R, Seppanen K, Rauramaa R, Salonen IT. Prevalence of carotid atherosclerosis and serum cholesterol levels in eastern Finland. *Arteriosclerosis*. 1988;8:788–792.
34. Salonen R, Salonen IT. Determinants of carotid intimamedia thickness: a population-based ultrasonography study in eastern Finnish men. *J Intern Med*. 1991;229:225–231.
35. O'Leary DH, Polak JF, Kronmal RA, et al. Thickening of carotid wall. A marker for atherosclerosis in the elderly? *Stroke*. 1996;27:224–231.
36. Bots ML, Hofman A, Grobbee DE. Common carotid intima-media thickness and lower extremity arterial atherosclerosis. *Arterioscler Thromb*. 1994;14:1885–1891.
37. Hofman A, Grobbee DE, de Jong PT, van den Ouweland FA. Determinants of disease and disability in the elderly: the Rotterdam elderly study. *Eur J Epidemiol*. 1991;7:403–422.
38. Bots ML, Witteman JC, Hofman A, de Jong PT, Grobbee DE. Low diastolic blood pressure and atherosclerosis in elderly subjects. *Arch Intern Med*. 1996;156:843–848.
39. Chambless LE, Heiss G, Folsom AR, et al. Association of coronary heart disease incidence with carotid arterial wall thickness and major risk factors: the Atherosclerosis Risk in Communities (ARIC) study, 1987–1993. *Am J Epidemiol*. 1997;146:483–494.
40. O'Leary DH, Polak JF, Kronmal RA, Manolio TA, Burke GL, Wolfson SK Jr. Carotid artery intima and media thickness as a risk factor for myocardial infarction and stroke in older adults. Cardiovascular Health Study Collaborative Research Group. *N Engl J Med*. 1999;340:14–22.
41. Lorenz MW, Markus HS, Bots ML, Rosvall M, Sitzer M. Prediction of clinical cardiovascular events with carotid intima-media thickness: a systematic review and meta-analysis. *Circulation*. 2007;115:459–467.
42. McGill HC Jr, McMahan CA, Herderick EE, et al. Effects of coronary heart disease risk factors on atherosclerosis of selected regions of the aorta and right coronary artery: PDAY research group, Pathobiological Determinants of Atherosclerosis in Youth. *Arterioscler Thromb Vasc Biol*. 2000;20:836–845.
43. Lorenz MW, von Kegler S, Steinmetz H, Markus HS, Sitzer M. Carotid intima-media thickening indicates a higher vascular risk across a wide age range: prospective data from the Carotid Atherosclerosis Progression Study (CAPS). *Stroke*. 2006;37:87–92.
44. Rosvall M, Janzon L, Berglund G, Engstrom G, Hedblad B. Incident coronary events and case fatality in relation to common carotid intimamedia thickness. *J Intern Med*. 2005;257:430–437.
45. Urbina EM, Srinivasan SR, Tang R, Bond MG, Kieltyka L, Berenson GS. Impact of multiple coronary risk factors on

the intima-media thickness of different segments of carotid artery in healthy young adults (the Bogalusa heart study). *Am J Cardiol*. 2002;90:953–958.
46. Li S, Chen W, Srinivasan SR, et al. Childhood cardiovascular risk factors and carotid vascular changes in adulthood: the Bogalusa heart study. *JAMA*. 2003;290:2271–2276.
47. Tzou WS, Douglas PS, Srinivasan SR, et al. Increased subclinical atherosclerosis in young adults with metabolic syndrome: the Bogalusa Heart Study. *J Am Coll Cardiol*. 2005;46:457–463.
48. Davis PH, Dawson JD, Mahoney LT, Lauer RM. Increased carotid intimal-medial thickness and coronary calcification are related in young and middle-aged adults: the Muscatine study. *Circulation*. 1999;100:838–842.
49. Davis PH, Dawson JD, Riley WA, Lauer RM. Carotid intimal-medial thickness is related to cardiovascular risk factors measured from childhood through middle age: the Muscatine study. *Circulation*. 2001;104:2815–2819.
50. Oren A, Vos LE, Uiterwaal CS, Grobbee DE, Bots ML. Cardiovascular risk factors and increased carotid intima-media thickness in healthy young adults: the Atherosclerosis Risk in Young Adults (ARYA) study. *Arch Intern Med*. 2003;163:1787–1792.
51. Knoflach M, Kiechl S, Kind M, et al. Cardiovascular risk factors and atherosclerosis in young males: ARMY study (Atherosclerosis Risk factors in Male Youngsters). *Circulation*. 2003;108:1064–1069.
52. Raitakari OT, Juonala M, Kahonen M, et al. Cardiovascular risk factors in childhood and carotid artery intima-media thickness in adulthood: the Cardiovascular Risk in Young Finns Study. *JAMA*. 2003;290:2277–2283.
53. del Sol AI, Moons KG, Hollander M, et al. Is carotid intima-media thickness useful in cardiovascular disease risk assessment? The Rotterdam Study. *Stroke*. 2001;32:1532–1538.
54. Johnsen SH, Mathiesen EB, Joakimsen O, et al. Carotid atherosclerosis is a stronger predictor of myocardial infarction in women than in men: a 6-year follow-up study of 6226 persons: the Tromsø Study. *Stroke*. 2007;38(11):2873–2880.
55. Stein JH, Fraizer MC, Aeschlimann SE, Nelson-Worel J, McBride PE, Douglas PS. Vascular age: integrating carotid intima-media thickness measurements with global coronary risk assessment. *Clin Cardiol*. 2004;27:388–392.
56. Wiegman A, de Groot E, Hutten BA, et al. Arterial intima-media thickness in children heterozygous for familial hypercholesterolaemia. *Lancet*. 2004;363:369–370.
57. Järvisalo MJ, Jartti L, Näntö-Salonen K, et al. Increased aortic intima-media thickness a marker of preclinical atherosclerosis in high-risk children. *Circulation*. 2001;104:2943–2947.
58. Pauciullo P, Iannuzzi A, Sartorio R, Irace C, Di Costanzo A, Rubba P. Increased intima-media thickness of common carotid artery in hypercholesterolemic children. *Arterioscler Thromb*. 1994;14:1075–1079.
59. Tonstad S, Joakimsen O, Stensland-Bugge E, et al. Risk factors related to carotid intima-media thickness and plaque in children with familial hypercholesterolemia and control subjects. *Arterioscler Thromb Vasc Biol*. 1996;16:984–991.
60. Lavrencic A, Kosmina B, Keber I, Videcnik V, Keber D. Carotid intima-media thickness in young patients with familial hypercholesterolemia. *Heart*. 1996;76:321–325.
61. Tonstad S, Joakimsen O, Stensland-Bugge E, Ose L, Bonaa KH, Leren TP. Carotid intima-media thickness and plaque in patients with familial hypercholesterolemia mutations and control subjects. *Eur J Clin Invest*. 1998;28:971–979.
62. de Giorgis T, Giannini C, Scarinci A, et al. Family history of premature cardiovascular disease as a sole and independent risk factor for increased carotid intima-media thickness. *J Hypertens*. 2009;27(4):822–828.
63. Urbina EM, Kimball TR, McCoy CE, Khoury PR, Daniels SR, Dolan LM. Youth with obesity and obesity-related type 2 diabetes mellitus demonstrate abnormalities in carotid structure and function. *Circulation*. 2009;119(22):2913–2919.
64. Hodis HN, Mack WJ, LaBree L, et al. The role of carotid arterial intima-media thickness in predicting clinical coronary events. *Ann Intern Med*. 1998;128(4):262–269.
65. Zielinski T, Dzielinska Z, Januszewicz A, et al. Carotid intima-media thickness as a marker of cardiovascular risk in hypertensive patients with coronary artery disease. *Am J Hypertens*. 2007;20(10):1058–1064.
66. Held C, Hjemdahl P, Eriksson SV, Björkander I, Forslund L, Rehnqvist N. Prognostic implications of intima-media thickness and plaques in the carotid and femoral arteries in patients with stable angina pectoris. *Eur Heart J*. 2001;22(1):62–72.
67. Ogawa Y, Uchigata Y, Iwamoto Y. Progression factors of carotid intima-media thickness and plaque in patients with long-term, early- onset type 1 diabetes mellitus in Japan: simultaneous comparison with diabetic retinopathy. *J Atheroscler Thromb*. 2009;16:821–828.
68. Lee E, Emoto M, Teramura M, et al. The combination of IMT and stiffness parameter beta is highly associated with concurrent coronary artery disease in type 2 diabetes. *J Atheroscler Thromb*. 2009;16(1):33–39.
69. Baroncini LA, de Oliveira A, Vidal EA, et al. Appropriateness of carotid plaque and intima-media thickness assessment in routine clinical practice. *Cardiovasc Ultrasound*. 2008;6:52.
70. Cicorella N, Zanolla L, Franceschini L, et al. Usefulness of ultrasonographic markers of carotid atherosclerosis (intima-media thickness, unstable carotid plaques and severe carotid stenosis) for predicting presence and extent of coronary artery disease. *J Cardiovasc Med (Hagerstown)*. 2009;10:906–912.
71. Psaty BM, Furberg CD, Kuller LH, et al. Isolated systolic hypertension and subclinical cardiovascular disease in the elderly. Initial findings from the Cardiovascular Health Study. *JAMA*. 1992;268:1287–1291.
72. Wendelhag I, Wiklund O, Wikstrand J. Arterial wall thickness in familial hypercholesterolemia. Ultrasound measurement of intima-media thickness in the common carotid artery. *Arterioscler Thromb*. 1992;12:70–77.
73. Gnasso A, Pujia A, Irace C, Mattioli PL. Increased carotid arterial wall thickness in common hyperlipidemia. *Coron Artery Dis*. 1995;6:57–63.
74. Honzikova N, Labrova R, Fiser B, et al. Influence of age, body mass index, and blood pressure on the carotid

intimamedia thickness in normotensive and hypertensive patients. *Biomed Tech (Berl)*. 2006;51:159–162.
75. Howard G, Burke GL, Szklo M, et al. Active and passive smoking are associated with increased carotid wall thickness. The Atherosclerosis Risk in Communities Study. *Arch Intern Med*. 1994;154:1277–1282.
76. Lanktree MB, Hegele RA, Yusuf S, Anand SS. Multi-ethnic genetic association study of carotid intima-media thickness using a targeted cardiovascular SNP microarray. *Stroke*. 2009;40(10):3173–3179.
77. Moskau S, Golla A, Grothe C, Boes M, Pohl C, Klockgether T. Heritability of carotid artery atherosclerotic lesions. An ultrasound study in 154 families. *Stroke*. 2005;36:5–8.
78. Roman MJ, Saba PS, Pini R, et al. Parallel cardiac and vascular adaptation in hypertension. *Circulation*. 1992;86:1909–1918.
79. Glagov S, Zarins CK. Is intimal hyperplasia an adaptive response or a pathological process? Observations on the nature of nonatherosclerotic intimal thickening. *J Vasc Surg*. 1989;10:571–573.
80. Li R, Duncan BB, Metcalf PA, et al. B-Mode-detected carotid artery plaque in a general population. *Stroke*. 1994;25:2377–2383.
81. Schönbeck U, Libby P. The CD40/CD154 receptor/ligand dyad. *Cell Mol Life Sci*. 2001;58:4–43.
82. Hansson GK. Immune mechanisms in atherosclerosis. *Arterioscler Thromb Vasc Biol*. 2001;21:1876–1890.
83. Libby P, Ridker PM, Maseri A. Inflammation and atherosclerosis. *Circulation*. 2002;105:1135–1143.
84. Croce K, Libby P. Intertwining of thrombosis and inflammation in atherosclerosis. *Curr Opin Hematol*. 2007;14:55–61.
85. Mach F, Schönbeck U, Libby P. CD40 signaling in vascular cells: a key role in atherosclerosis? *Atherosclerosis*. 1998;137(Suppl):S89-S95.
86. Bayer IM, Caniggia I, Adamson SL, Langille BL. Experimental angiogenesis of arterial vasa vasorum. *Cell Tissue Res*. 2002;307:303–313.
87. Ribatti D, Levi-Schaffer F, Kovanen PT. Inflammatory angiogenesis in atherogenesis—a double-edged sword. *Ann Med*. 2008;40:606–621.
88. Libby P. Inflammation in atherosclerosis. *Nature*. 2002;420:868–874.
89. Virmani R, Kolodgie FD, Burke AP, Farb A, Schwartz SM. Lessons from sudden coronary death: a comprehensive morphological classification scheme for atherosclerotic lesions. *Arterioscler Thromb Vasc Biol*. 2000;20:1262–1275.
90. Touboul PJ, Hennerici MG, Meairs S, et al. Mannheim intima-media thickness consensus. *Cerebrovasc Dis*. 2004;18:346–349.
91. Touboul PJ, Hennerici MG, Meairs S, et al. Mannheim Carotid Intima-media Thickness Consensus (2004–2006): an update on behalf of the advisory board of the 3 rd and 4th watching the risk symposium, 13th and 15th European stroke conferences, Mannheim, Germany, 2004, and Brussels, Belgium, 2006. *Cerebrovasc Dis*. 2007;23:75–80.
92. Griffin M, Nicolaides AN, Belcaro G, Shah E. Cardiovascular risk assessment using ultrasound: the value of arterial wall changes including the presence, severity and character of plaques. *Pathophysiol Haemost Thromb*. 2002;32:367–370.
93. Bonithon-Kopp C, Touboul PJ, Berr C, Leroux C, Mainard F, Courbon D. Relation of intima-media thickness to atherosclerotic plaques in carotid arteries. The Vascular Aging (EVA) Study. *Arterioscler Thromb Vasc Biol*. 1996;16:310–316.
94. Prati P, Vanuzzo D, Casaroli M, et al. Determinants of carotid plaque occurrence. A long-term prospective population study: the San Daniele project. *Cerebrovasc Dis*. 2006;22:416–422.
95. Salonen IT, Salonen R. Ultrasonographically assessed carotid morphology and the risk of coronary heart disease. *Arterioscler Thromb*. 1991;11:1245–1249.
96. Hunt KJ, Sharrett AR, Chambless LE, Folsom AR, Evans GW, Heiss G. Acoustic shadowing on B-mode ultrasound of the carotid artery predicts CHD. *Ultrasound Med Biol*. 2001;27:357–365.
97. van der Meer I, Bots ML, Hofman A, del Sol AI, van der Kuip DA, Witteman JC. Predictive value of noninvasive measures of atherosclerosis for incident myocardial infarction: the Rotterdam study. *Circulation*. 2004;109:1089–1094.
98. Belcaro G, Nicolaides AN, Laurora G, et al. Ultrasound morphology classification of the arterial wall and cardiovascular events in a 6-year follow-up study. *Arterioscler Thromb Vasc Biol*. 1996;16(7):851–856.
99. Belcaro G, Nicolaides AN, Ramaswami G, et al. Carotid and femoral ultrasound morphology screening and cardiovascular events in low risk subjects: a 10-year follow-up study (the CAFES-CAVE study(1)). *Atherosclerosis*. 2001;156(2):379–387.
100. Touboul PJ, Labreuche J, Vicaut E, Amarenco P. GENIC Investigators. Carotid intimamedia thickness, plaques, and Framingham risk score as independent determinants of stroke risk. *Stroke*. 1745;36:1741–1745.
101. Prabhakaran S, Rundek T, Ramas R, et al. Carotid plaque surface irregularity predicts ischemic stroke: the northern Manhattan study. *Stroke*. 2006;37(11):2696–2701.
102. Zureik M, Touboul PJ, Bonithon-Kopp C, Courbon D, Ruelland I, Ducimetiére P. Differential association of common carotid intima-media thickness and carotid atherosclerotic plaques with parental history of premature death from coronary heart disease the EVA Study. *Arterioscler Thromb Vasc Biol*. 1999;19:366–371.
103. Kitamura A, Iso H, Imano H, et al. Carotid intima-media thickness and plaque characteristics as a risk factor for stroke in Japanese elderly men. *Stroke*. 2004;35:2788–2794.
104. Stork S, van den Beld AW, von Schacky C, et al. Carotid artery plaque burden, stiffness, and mortality risk in elderly men: a prospective, population-based cohort study. *Circulation*. 2004;110:344–348.
105. Spence JD, Eliasziw M, DiCicco M, Hackam DG, Galil R, Lohmann T. Carotid plaque area: a tool for targeting and evaluating vascular preventive therapy. *Stroke*. 2002;33.2916–2922.
106. Barnett PA, Spence JD, Manuck SB, Jennings JR. Psychological stress and the progression of carotid artery disease. *J Hypertens*. 1997;15:49–55.
107. Saito D, Shiraki T, Oka T, Kajiyama A, Doi M, Masaka T. Morphologic correlation between atherosclerotic lesions of

108. Honda O, Sugiyama S, Kugiyama K, et al. Echolucent carotid plaques predict future coronary events in patients with coronary artery disease. *J Am Coll Cardiol*. 2004;43:1177–1184.
109. Triposkiadis F, Sitafidis G, Kostoulas J, Skoularigis J, Zintzaras E, Fezoulidis I. Carotid plaque composition in stable and unstable coronary artery disease. *Am Heart J*. 2005;150:782–789.
110. Seo Y, Watanabe S, Ishizu T, et al. Echolucent carotid plaques as a feature in patients with acute coronary syndrome. *Circ J*. 2006;70:1629–1634.
111. Joakimsen O, Bønaa KH, Stensland-Bugge E. Reproducibility of ultrasound assessment of carotid plaque occurrence, thickness and morphology: the Tromso Study. *Stroke*. 1997;28:2201–2207.
112. de Groot E, Jukema JW, van Boven AJ, et al. Effect of pravastatin on progression and regression of coronary atherosclerosis and vessel wall changes in carotid and femoral arteries: A report from the Regression Growth Evaluation Statin Study. *Am J Cardiol*. 1995;76(9):40C–46C.
113. Crouse JR 3rd, Byington RP, Bond MG, et al. Pravastatin, lipids and atherosclerosis in the carotid arteries (PLAC II). *Am J Cardiol*. 1995;75(7):455–459.
114. Salonen R, Nyyssönen K, Porkkala E, et al. Kuopio Atherosclerosis Prevention Study (KAPS). A population-based primary preventive trial of the effect of LDL lowering on atherosclerotic progression in carotid and femoral arteries. *Circulation*. 1995;92(7):1758–1764.
115. Mercuri M, Bond MG, Sirtori CR, et al. Pravastatin reduces carotid intima-media thickness progression in an asymptomatic hypercholesterolemic mediterranean population: The Carotid Atherosclerosis Italian Ultrasound Study. *Am J Med*. 1996;101(6):627–634.
116. MacMahon S, Sharpe N, Gamble G, et al. Effects of lowering average of below-average cholesterol levels on the progression of carotid atherosclerosis: Results of the LIPID Atherosclerosis Substudy. LIPID Trial Research Group. *Circulation*. 1998;97(18):1784–1790.
117. Hodis HN, Mack WJ, LaBree L, et al. Reduction in carotid arterial wall thickness using lovastatin and dietary therapy: a randomized controlled clinical trial. *Ann Intern Med*. 1996;124(6):548–556.
118. Nolting PR, de Groot E, Zwinderman AH, Buirma RJ, Trip MD, Kastelein JJ. Regression of carotid and femoral artery intima-media thickness in familial hypercholesterolemia: treatment with simvastatin. *Arch Intern Med*. 2003;163(15):1837–1841.
119. Furberg CD, Adams HP Jr, Applegate WB, et al. Effect of lovastatin on early carotid atherosclerosis and cardiovascular events. Asymptomatic Carotid Artery Progression Study (ACAPS) Research Group. *Circulation*. 1994;90(4):1679–1687.
120. Hedblad B, Wikstrand J, Janzon L, Wedel H, Berglund G. Low-dose metoprolol CR/XL and fluvastatin slow progression of carotid intima-media thickness: Main results from the β-Blocker Cholesterol-Lowering Asymptomatic Plaque Study (BCAPS). *Circulation*. 2001;103(13):1721–1726.
121. Taylor AJ, Kent SM, Flaherty PJ, Coyle LC, Markwood TT, Vernalis MN. ARBITER: Arterial Biology for the Investigation of the Treatment Effects of Reducing Cholesterol: a randomized trial comparing the effects of atorvastatin and pravastatin on carotid intima medial thickness. *Circulation*. 2002;106(16):2055–2060.
122. Smilde TJ, van Wissen S, Wollersheim H, Trip MD, Kastelein JJ, Stalenhoef AF. Effect of aggressive versus conventional lipid lowering on atherosclerosis progression in familial hypercholesterolaemia (ASAP): a prospective, randomised, double-blind trial. *Lancet*. 2001;357(9256):577–581.
123. Crouse JR 3rd, Raichlen JS, Riley WA, et al. Effect of rosuvastatin on progression of carotid intima-media thickness in low-risk individuals with subclinical atherosclerosis: The METEOR trial. *J Am Med Assoc*. 2007;297(12):1344–1353.
124. Espeland MA, O'Leary DH, Terry JG, Morgan T, Evans G, Mudra H. Carotid intimal-media thickness as a surrogate for cardiovascular disease events in trials of HMG-CoA reductase inhibitors. *Curr Control Trials Cardiovasc Med*. 2005;6(1):3.
125. Byington RP, Evans GW, Espeland MA, et al. Effects of lovastatin and warfarin on early carotid atherosclerosis: sex specific analyses. Asymptomatic Carotid Artery Progression Study (ACAPS) Research Group. *Circulation*. 1999;100(3):e14-e17.
126. van Wissen S, Smilde TJ, Trip MD, Stalenhoef AF, Kastelein JJ. Longterm safety and efficacy of high-dose atorvastatin treatment in patients with familial hypercholesterolemia. *Am J Cardiol*. 2005;95(2):264–266.
127. Blankenhorn DH, Selzer RH, Crawford DW, et al. Beneficial effects of colestipol-niacin therapy on the common carotid artery. Two- and four-year reduction of intima-media thickness measured by ultrasound. *Circulation*. 1993;88(1):20–28.
128. Taylor AJ, Sullenberger LE, Lee HJ, Lee JK, Grace KA. Arterial Biology for the Investigation of the Treatment Effects of Reducing Cholesterol (ARBITER) 2: a double-blind, placebocontrolled study of extended-release niacin on atherosclerosis progression in secondary prevention patients treated with statins. *Circulation*. 2004;110(23):3512–3517.
129. Taylor AJ, Lee HJ, Sullenberger LE. The effect of 24 months of combination statin and extended-release niacin on carotid intima-media thickness: ARBITER 3. *Curr Med Res Opin*. 2006;22(11):2243–2250.
130. Kastelein JJ, van Leuven SI, Burgess L, et al. Effect of torcetrapib on carotid atherosclerosis in familial hypercholesterolemia. *N Engl J Med*. 2007;356(16):1620–1630.
131. Brousseau ME, Schaefer EJ, Wolfe ML, et al. Effects of an inhibitor of cholesteryl ester transfer protein on HDL cholesterol. *N Engl J Med*. 2004;350:1505–1515.
132. Lewis GF, Rader DJ. New insights into the regulation of HDL metabolism and reverse cholesterol transport. *Circ Res*. 2005;96(12):1221–1232.
133. Nissen SE, Tardif JC, Nicholls SJ, et al. Effect of torcetrapib on the progression of coronary atherosclerosis. *N Engl J Med*. 2007;356(13):1304–1316.

Plaque Size, Growth, Echogenicity and Cardiovascular Risk: The Tromsø Study

24

Ellisiv B. Mathiesen and Stein H. Johnsen

24.1 Introduction

In the late 1980s, ultrasound measurements of atherosclerosis in the carotid arteries were introduced in epidemiological population studies on cardiovascular disease[1-4] (Chaps. 23 and 24). Ultrasonography is an excellent tool for longitudinal epidemiological studies of atherosclerosis as it is suitable for out-of-clinic settings, swift, painless, and free from risk, and may be repeated as often as preferred. In epidemiological studies, ultrasound-assessed atherosclerosis is often treated as a risk factor as well as an endpoint, as it can be regarded as intermediate endpoint for genetic and environmental exposure for cardiovascular risk factors and as a predictor for clinical cardiovascular disease. In the Tromsø Study, the authors have since 1994 repeatedly measured total plaque area, plaque echogenicity, intima-media thickness (IMT), and other measures of carotid atherosclerosis in a large sample from the general population. In this chapter, an overview of some of the results from the study is presented.

The Tromsø Study was initiated in 1974 as a result of the high mortality from cardiovascular disease in Norway at that time. The primary aim was to determine the etiological factors for cardiovascular disease and to develop efficient preventive measures. The study design included repeated population health surveys to which total birth cohorts and random samples were invited. In all cross-sectional surveys, emphasis has been placed on the registration of risk factors that can be of importance in revealing causal factors. Six surveys have been performed so far. Each survey has collected extensive information on exposure variables by use of questionnaires, interviews, physiological measurements, and analyses of blood and urine samples. The population is being followed up on an individual level with registration of disease (myocardial infarction, stroke, atrial fibrillation, diabetes, and fractures) and cause-specific death.

Ultrasound examination of the carotid arteries was included in the fourth (1994–1995), fifth (2001–2002), and sixth (2007–2008) surveys and comprises assessment of IMT, number of plaques, plaque area, plaque thickness, and plaque echogenicity. IMT has been measured in the near and far wall of the right distal common carotid and the far wall of the bifurcation. Plaque measurements were performed in the near and far walls of the common carotid, bifurcation, and proximal internal carotid artery. A total of 6,727 individuals participated in the fourth, 5,453 in the fifth, and 7,084 in the sixth survey. Of these, 10,934 persons have participated at least once, 5,478 twice, and 2,781 thrice.

24.2 Prevalence of and Predictors of Carotid Plaques, Carotid Stenosis, and Plaque Echogenicity

24.2.1 Prevalence of Carotid Plaques

Plaques, defined as a focal protrusion of more than 50% of the surrounding IMT value,[5] are advanced manifestations of atherosclerosis and may progress

E.B. Mathiesen (✉)
Department of Clinical Medicine, University of Tromsø, Tromsø, Norway

S.H. Johnsen
Department of Neurology, University Hospital of North Norway, Tromsø, Norway

from small protrusions without hemodynamic significance to high-grade stenosis and occlusion of the vessel lumen. It is well established through large clinical trials that the risk of stroke increases with the degree of carotid stenosis and is highest in patients with high-grade stenosis. Progression of carotid plaque size and stenosis is associated with higher risk of stroke and major adverse cardiovascular events in other vascular territories compared to plaques that do not increase in size.[6–8] Measurement of carotid plaque area is a sensitive tool in the assessment of plaque evolution and progression and may play an important role in risk stratification, in monitoring treatment, and prevention in individual patients.[9]

Carotid plaque is a common finding in middle-aged and elderly in Western populations.[10,11] In Tromsø, 55% of men and 46% of women aged 55–84 years had carotid plaques.[12] A linear increase in plaque prevalence with age was observed in men, whereas the relationship was curvilinear in women, with an inflection at approximately 50 years of age, suggesting an adverse effect of menopause on atherosclerosis. The sex difference in atherosclerosis prevalence declined after the age of 50, with similar plaque prevalence in elderly men and women. In contrast, men had a larger proportion of plaques with low echogenicity, and the sex difference in plaque echogenicity increased significantly with age. As lower plaque echogenicity was associated with higher risk of ischemic coronary and cerebral vascular events,[13–18] the excess risk of cardiovascular disease in elderly men may partly be attributed to a higher proportion of low-echogenic, rupture-prone plaques in men compared to women, despite a similar prevalence of atherosclerosis.[19]

24.2.2 Risk Factors Associated with Novel Plaque Formation, Plaque Progression, and Plaque Echogenicity

Numerous studies have shown consistent associations between established cardiovascular risk factors and presence of carotid plaque and carotid stenosis.[2,20–23] However, prospective data on predictors of novel plaque formation and plaque progression in general populations are limited as this requires repeated ultrasound measurements years apart in a large number of people. Population studies are well suited for this

Table 24.1 Predictors of novel plaque formation: the Tromsø Study

	χ^2	OR (95% CI)
Monocyte count × 10^9/L	14.1	1.18 (1.08–1.29)
Age, years	58.2	1.61 (1.42–1.81)
Male sex	9.2	1.33 (1.11–1.59)
Total cholesterol, mmol/L	25.2	1.26 (1.15–1.38)
Current smoking	28.4	1.73 (1.41–2.11)
Systolic blood pressure, mmHg	23.2	1.25 (1.14–1.37)
Intima-media thickness, mm	46.8	1.43 (1.29–1.58)
R^2		0.19

The multivariate-adjusted odds ratio predicts the probability of being in a higher category (more plaques) for 1-SD increase in the independent continuous variable or for being a male or current smoker
Source: From Johnsen et al.[24], reprinted with permission

and make it possible to study the development of atherosclerosis both the initial formation of novel plaques and the progression of plaque size and number in persons with already established atherosclerosis.

In a prospective design, the authors examined predictors of novel plaque formation in 2,610 plaque-free men and women who had no plaque at baseline. In multivariate models, monocyte count, age, sex, total cholesterol, current smoking, systolic blood pressure, and IMT were independent predictors of novel plaque formation.[24] The odds ratio for having plaque after 7 years was 1.85 (95% CI 1.41–2.24) in the highest quartile of monocyte count compared to the lowest quartile (Table 24.1). This fits well with the biological model of atherogenesis where activation of monocytes and differentiation into lipid-laden macrophages are fundamental events in the generation of atherosclerotic lesions. In persons who remained plaque-free, monocytes were not associated with carotid artery intima-media thickness (CIMT), suggesting that monocyte activity is a determining factor for plaque formation but not for diffuse intima thickening.

Predictors for plaque progression after 7 years were evaluated in 1,952 persons with preexisting plaque at baseline. Progression of plaque size was assessed as increase in total plaque area, a summation of the areas of all plaques in the distal common carotid, bifurcation, and proximal internal carotid artery. Plaque area increased in 70% of cases, and most plaques became more echogenic over the follow-up interval. Higher

Table 24.2 Predictors of plaque area progression: the Tromsø Study

Risk factor	Model I β^a (SE)	P	Model II β^a (SE)	P	Model III β^a (SE)	P	Model IV β^a (SE)	P
HDL cholesterol	−0.95 (0.43)	0.02	−0.98 (0.44)	0.03	−0.93 (0.44)	0.03	−1.46 (0.48)	0.002
Age	...	...	1.47 (0.43)	0.0006	1.46 (0.45)	0.001	1.34 (0.48)	0.005
Male sex	...	...	1.07 (0.89)	0.2	1.13 (0.91)	0.2	1.25 (0.99)	0.2
Total cholesterol	...	...	...	...	−0.28 (0.44)	0.5	0.73 (0.51)	0.2
Systolic blood pressure	...	...	...	...	1.21 (0.44)	0.006	1.07 (0.48)	0.03
Smoking, yes vs no	...	...	...	...	3.18 (0.92)	0.0005	3.20 (1.00)	0.001

Model I was unadjusted
Model II was adjusted for age and sex
Model III was adjusted for age, sex, total cholesterol, systolic blood pressure, and smoking
Model IV excluded persons who had ever used lipid-lowering drugs (n = 442)
a Values are regression coefficients (SE) expressed in mm² for a 1-SD change in continuous variables and for presence vs absence of categorical variables
Source: From Johnsen et al.[25], reprinted with permission

levels of high-density lipoprotein (HDL) cholesterol were protective against plaque growth, while higher systolic blood pressure and current smoking promoted plaque growth (Table 24.2).[25] For a 1 standard deviation (SD) (0.41 mmol/L) lower HDL cholesterol level, mean plaque area increased by 0.93 mm² ($P = 0.03$). Exclusion of users of lipid-lowering drugs from analysis strengthened the HDL estimate. A possible explanation is that HDL cholesterol stabilizes plaques and counteracts their growth by reducing their lipid content and inflammation. No association between baseline echogenicity and later plaque growth. However, the plaques that increased most in echogenicity had the lowest growth rate and the highest proportion with regressed lesions. The association between change in echogenicity and plaque growth suggests that plaques that remain echolucent may have a higher growth potential than plaques that remain echogenic. HDL cholesterol may stabilize plaques and counteract their growth by reducing their lipid content and inflammation. This is plausible if one mechanism of plaque growth and plaque regression is accumulation and removal of lipids. Accumulation of lipids within a plaque will increase the echolucent proportion of the plaque as it grows. Conversely, removal of lipids may increase the echogenic proportion, so the regressed plaque will appear more echogenic.

In subjects with carotid stenosis, low levels of HDL cholesterol, higher systolic blood pressure, younger age, and more severe stenosis were independently associated with an increased risk of having an echolucent, rupture-prone atherosclerotic plaque. For 1-SD increase in HDL cholesterol, the risk of having lower plaque echogenicity decreased by approximately 30% (OR 0.69, 95% CI 0.52–0.93).[26] In a cross-sectional study on 57 persons with and 38 persons without carotid plaques, the association between postprandial clearance of triglyceride-rich lipoproteins and lipoprotein lipase activity 4 h after a standardized high fat meal was examined.[27] Low plasma lipoprotein lipase activity promotes a proatherogenic lipid profile, and delayed chylomicron clearance is a risk factor for atherosclerosis. Lipoprotein lipase activity and mass was determined before and after heparin administration. Subjects with echolucent plaques had delayed postprandial clearance of chylomicron triglycerides compared to controls. Postheparin lipoprotein lipase activity was decreased in subjects with echolucent plaques compared to subjects with echogenic plaques and to controls. Plaque echogenicity increased linearly with increasing levels of postheparin lipoprotein lipase activity and mass. Low lipoprotein lipase activity (LPL) due to attenuated mobilization of LPL from capillary endothelium may play an important role in the formation of echolucent plaques by modulation of postprandial lipids and subsequent fat accumulation in the arterial wall. The apolipoprotein C-I (apoC-I) content of very low density lipoprotein (VLDL) particles was associated with plaque size in persons with carotid atherosclerosis,[28] supporting the concept that the number of apoC-I per VLDL particle may be of importance for the development of atherosclerosis. Furthermore, a significant inverse relationship was observed between higher plasma tissue-plasminogen activator antigen t-PA and plaque echogenicity.[29] Also, echogenic plaques were associated with higher levels of thrombin-antithrombin complexes (TAT) and prothrombin fragment 1 + 2 (F1 + 2). TAT and F1 + 2 increased linearly with plaque echogenicity, indicating that increasing plaque echogenicity is associated with thrombin generation in persons with carotid stenosis.[30]

The role of sex hormones in the development of atherosclerosis and cardiovascular disease is not fully understood. In cross-sectional analysis, women with late menopause and ever-users of estrogens had significantly less plaques than women with early menopause and never-users of estrogen[31] indicating a protective effect of estrogen against cardiovascular disease in women. However, hormone replacement therapy has failed to protect against cardiovascular disease in large randomized trials.[32–35]

Several studies have indicated a role of endogenous sex hormones in the development of atherosclerosis in aging men. Low free testosterone levels and higher estradiol levels were predictive of progression of IMT in middle-aged and elderly men.[36,37] In a cross-sectional study, an inverse relationship between total testosterone level and intima-media thickness was observed in middle-aged men.[38] However, no prospective associations was found between sex hormone levels at baseline and change in plaque area or IMT from 1994 to 2001.[39]

Markers of inflammation are consistently associated with atherosclerosis and cardiovascular disease.[40,41] The authors found significantly elevated levels of white blood cell count (WBC) and fibrinogen, but not C-reactive protein (CRP), in both men and women with carotid plaque as compared to subjects without plaques.[42] All three inflammatory markers were significantly associated with plaque area in men. WBC was significantly associated with plaque echogenicity in women, whereas no association was found between fibrinogen and CRP and plaque echogenicity in either gender.

The role of novel, less well established risk factors have also been explored. Microalbuminuria predicts cardiovascular events, especially in persons with diabetes and hypertension,[43] and is also associated with early signs of atherosclerosis.[44,45] The authors found that albumin-to-creatinine ratio (ACR) was positively related to both plaque initiation and plaque growth.[46] This relationship was substantially modified by fibrinogen in previously plaque-free subjects. Subjects with high levels of both ACR and fibrinogen developed plaques with the largest area. In subjects with preexisting plaques, ACR was related to plaque progression. In these individuals, the interaction between fibrinogen and ACR on plaque growth appeared only in those with minimal atherosclerosis at baseline. Thus, the joint effect of microalbuminuria and fibrinogen on plaque growth was most pronounced in the earliest phase of atherosclerosis development.

Proinsulin is increased in persons at cardiovascular risk, and it has been suggested that proinsulin has more of a proatherogenic effect than insulin.[47,48] Whether the proinsulin:insulin ratio or insulin:glucose ratio (an insulin resistance surrogate) predicted carotid plaque size was assessed in nondiabetic participants of the Tromsø Study. The proinsulin-to-insulin ratio was associated with progression of plaque size in women, but not in men.[49] The study lends support to the hypothesis that proinsulin has atherogenic properties, at least in women. In nondiabetic individuals who participated in the fourth survey, glycated hemoglobin levels were strongly related to the presence of carotid artery plaques with high echogenicity.[50]

Osteoprotegerin (OPG) and receptor activator of nuclear factor-κ B ligand (RANKL) are parts of a cytokine network involved in the regulation of bone metabolism and vascular calcification.[51] Intervention studies in animal models suggest that osteoprotegerin functions as an inhibitor of atherosclerosis,[52] whereas studies on humans indicate the opposite. Several clinical studies found higher levels of OPG in patients with cardiovascular disease.[52–54] Results from a prospective epidemiological study in humans indicated that OPG was an independent risk factor for progression of atherosclerosis and onset of cardiovascular disease.[55] In a sample of 100 Tromsø Study participants without cardiovascular disease, persons with echogenic carotid plaques had significantly lower serum OPG level compared to persons with echolucent plaques and persons without plaques.[56] In a study of 2,191 men and 2,329 women, OPG predicted novel plaque formation after 7 years in crude analysis in both women and men, but not after adjustment for age and other atherosclerotic risk factors. OPG predicted plaque growth in women, whereas no associations were demonstrated in men. Soluble RANKL did not predict plaque formation or plaque growth.[57] In a study on the relationship between OPG and CIMT, CIMT increased significantly across tertiles of OPG after adjustment for cardiovascular risk factors. However, there was a significant interaction between age and OPG, with an inverse relationship between OPG and CIMT in subjects younger than 45 years, whereas a positive relationship was observed in subjects aged 55 years and above.[58] These results of the studies from the Tromsø Study support the concept that OPG may play an important role in arterial calcification. However, increased serum OPG does not seem to promote early atherosclerosis in younger subjects. One might speculate whether the increased levels observed at later stages of atherosclerosis and in clinical cardiovascular disease may reflect compensatory mechanisms.

24.2.3 Prevalence and Risk Factors of Carotid Stenosis

Whereas plaque occurs in approximately half of the general middle-aged and elderly population, significant carotid stenosis is less frequent. The overall prevalence of carotid stenosis in the Tromsø Study was 3.8% (95% confidence interval [CI] 3.2–4.6%) in men and 2.7% (95% CI 2.2–3.3%) in women.[23] The prevalence increased by age in both genders. In an individual participant data meta-analysis of 23,706 participants of 4 population-based studies (the Malmö Diet and Cancer Study, the Tromsø Study, the Carotid Atherosclerosis Progression Study, and the Cardiovascular Health Study), the prevalence of moderate asymptomatic carotid stenosis ($\geq$50%) ranged from 0.2% in men aged <50 years to 7.5% in men aged $\geq$80 years. For women, this prevalence increased from 0% to 5.0%. Prevalence of severe asymptomatic carotid stenosis ($\geq$70%) ranged from 0.1% in men aged <50 years to 3.1% in men aged $\geq$80.[59] The low prevalence implies that screening of the general population for asymptomatic stenosis will hardly be cost-effective. However, high-risk groups may benefit from screening. In addition to age and sex, total cholesterol, HDL cholesterol (inverse), systolic and diastolic blood pressure, markers of inflammation, smoking, diabetes, and cardiovascular disease are associated with presence of carotid stenosis.[2,21,23] Using individual data from the four population studies, prediction rules for identification of high-risk individuals with a high probability of having carotid stenosis were developed. In models with easily obtainable predictors (age, sex, lipids, blood pressure, body mass index [BMI], and smoking), subgroups with a high risk of having moderate and severe stenosis were easily identified (area under the receiver operating characteristics (ROC) curve of 0.815 and 0.793 for moderate and severe stenosis, respectively).[60]

24.3 Carotid Plaque Size as Predictor of Cardiovascular Disease and Mortality

Carotid plaque burden can be measured as plaque presence (yes/no), the number of plaques, plaque thickness, plaque area, and plaque volume, and all these modalities have been shown to be predictive of future ischemic cerebral events. Measurement of total plaque seems to be a powerful tool for risk assessment. In 2002, David Spence and coworkers found that total plaque area predicted cardiovascular disease in a study of 1,686 patients recruited from an atherosclerosis clinic (Chap. 25). The 5-year multivariate-adjusted relative risk for the combined endpoint stroke, myocardial infarction (MI), and vascular death was 3.5 (95% CI, 1.8–6.7; $P < 0.001$) in the highest quartile of plaque area compared to the lowest quartile.[6] The 5-year adjusted risk of the combined outcome was 9.4%, 7.6%, and 15.7% for patients with carotid plaque area regression, no change, and progression, respectively ($P = 0.003$). In the Tromsø Study, the authors followed 6,226 men and women aged 25–84 years at baseline for 6 years and found that carotid plaque area was a stronger predictor of first-ever MI than IMT.[61] During follow-up, MI occurred in 6.6% of men and 3.0% of women. The adjusted relative risk (RR; 95% CI) between the highest plaque area tertile versus no plaque was 1.56 (1.04–2.36) in men and 3.95 (2.16–7.19) in women (Fig. 24.1). IMT measured in the distal common carotid (CCA-IMT) was not associated with MI in either sex. This is in line with previous findings[20] and probably reflects the differences in the pathological processes leading to intima-media thickening of the distal part of CCA and plaque formation in the coronary arteries, whereas plaque formation in the carotid and coronary arteries is more closely related.[62]

In a longitudinal study on 3,240 men and 3,344 women, plaque area predicted first-ever stroke after 10 years of follow-up.[63] The multivariable-adjusted hazards ratio (HR) for ischemic stroke for 1-SD increase

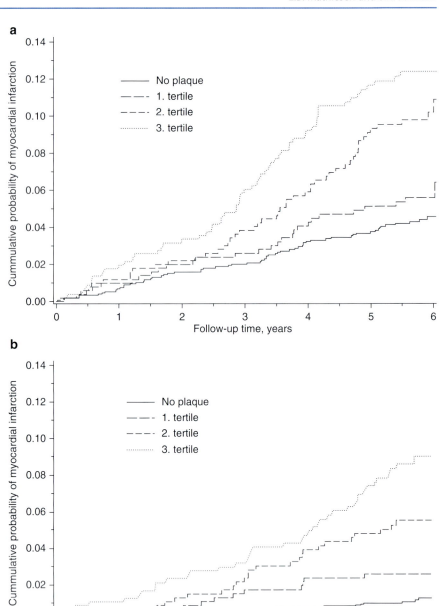

Fig. 24.1 Proportion of myocardial infarction in men (**a**) and women (**b**) according to total plaque area (From Johnsen et al.[61] reproduced with permission)

in the square root transformed total plaque area was 1.23 (95% CI 1.09–1.38) in men and 1.19 (95% CI 1.01–1.41) in women. The HR in the highest quartile of total carotid plaque area compared to no plaque was 1.73 (95% CI 1.19–2.52) in men and 1.62 (95% CI 1.04–2.53) in women. The multivariable-adjusted HR for 1-SD increase in IMT was 1.08 (95% CI 0.95–1.22) in men and 1.24 (95% CI 1.05–1.48) in women. There were no differences in stroke risk across quartiles of IMT. The results suggest that total plaque area is a stronger predictor of ischemic stroke than IMT. This is further supported in a cross-sectional population-based study, where total plaque area appeared to be more strongly associated with the prevalence of cardiovascular disease than IMT.[64]

Previous studies have found that repeated assessments of total plaque area are useful tools for monitoring the effect of preventive measures in patients with known risk factors for cardiovascular disease[9] and that plaque measurement can improve stroke risk prediction in high-risk individuals. In models with established cardiovascular risk factors (age, total cholesterol, HDL cholesterol, systolic blood pressure, use of blood pressure-lowering drugs, current smoking, prevalent diabetes, and coronary heart disease), the authors tested whether adding total plaque area or IMT improved stroke risk prediction. The area under the receiver operating characteristics curve did not increase substantially when total plaque area, IMT, or both were added to the model.[63] This finding is in line with previous results from the Rotterdam Study on IMT in risk prediction of myocardial infarction and stroke[65] and indicates that neither IMT nor total plaque area is useful as a screening tool in a stroke-free population-based cohort. However, Prati et al. found that IMT and plaque presence added little to individual risk prediction by the Framingham stroke risk score (FSRS), but improved risk prediction in high-risk subjects.[66] In the Northern Manhattan Study, those in the highest quartile of plaque thickness and with high Framingham risk score (FRS) had a 10-year risk of combined vascular events of 30.7%, whereas the risk was 25% in those with low FRS and plaque.[67]

Randomized controlled trials have shown that the degree of carotid stenosis is a strong risk factor for cardiovascular mortality in both symptomatic and asymptomatic patients,[68–71] but information from the general population has been scarce. In 248 subjects with large carotid plaques causing at least 35% lumen reduction and 496 age- and sex-matched control subjects who were followed up for 4.2 years, the stenosis group had increased relative risk of all-cause mortality of 3.47 (95% CI 1.47–8.19). The adjusted relative risk in persons with stenosis and no cardiovascular disease or diabetes was 5.66 (95% CI 1.53–20.90). There was a significant dose–response relationship between degree of stenosis and risk of death.

24.4 Plaque Echogenicity and Cardiovascular Risk

The first prospective study showing an association between plaque echogenicity and stroke was published by Johnson and coworkers in 1985.[72] Numerous

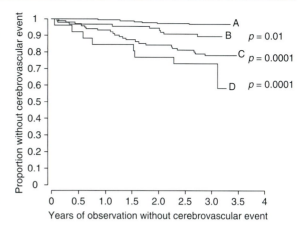

Fig. 24.2 Proportion of ischemic cerebrovascular events according to plaque echogenicity. (*A*) Subjects without stenosis, (*B*) subjects with echogenic and predominantly echogenic plaques, (*C*) subjects with predominantly echolucent plaques, and (*D*) subjects with echolucent plaques. Probability values refer to comparison between group *B*, *C*, or *D* versus control subjects *A* (From Mathiesen et al.[14] reproduced with permission)

studies have subsequently confirmed that presence of echolucent (or hypoechoic) plaques is highly predictive of stroke and other cardiovascular events.[6,13,73,74] In the Tromsø Study, plaque echogenicity was initially graded according to a modified version of the Gray-Weale classification.[75] As computer-assisted measurements of echogenicity were reported to have lower measurement variability and were highly predictive for stroke,[15,76,77] all carotid plaque images from the three screening surveys were later reassessed with computer-assisted measurements of gray scale median (GSM).[78] In a prospective study, almost 30% of subjects with echolucent stenotic plaques experienced one or more ischemic cerebrovascular events in the 3.6 years follow-up period as compared to 9.5% with echogenic plaques and 3% in a control group with no stenosis (Fig. 24.2).[14] The adjusted relative risk for cerebrovascular events was 4.56 (95% CI 1.10–18.93) in subjects with echolucent stenotic plaques as compared to subjects without stenotic plaques, and there was a significant linear trend for higher risk with lower plaque echogenicity. The relationship was independent of the degree of stenosis.

Studies have shown that the presence of echolucent carotid plaques predicts future coronary events in patients with stable coronary artery disease.[6,17] In the

Tromsø population, there was a significant trend toward a higher MI risk with increasing plaque echolucency (measured as GSM) in women, but not in men. When adjusted for other cardiovascular risk factors, the HR for MI in women in the lowest tertile of GSM was 2.79 (95% CI 1.45–5.37) compared to the highest tertile.[61]

As mentioned above, atherosclerosis and osteoporosis appear to be related, possibly by involvement of the OPG/RANKL system. In order to examine whether carotid artery plaques with different morphology predict nonvertebral fractures in women, 2,733 women aged 55–74 years (75% of the eligible population) were followed for 6 years. Plaques were categorized into three groups based on overall GSM value of the total plaque mass at baseline. The age-adjusted relative risk (RR) of fracture was significantly higher among women with echogenic plaques than among women without plaques (RR 1.6, 95% CI 1.1–2.5).[79] Further adjustment for bone mineral density at baseline, BMI, body height, HDL cholesterol, smoking status, and muscle strength did not influence the association. Subjects with other plaque types were not at an increased risk compared to subjects without plaques.

24.5 Summary

In conclusion, evidence from several prospective epidemiological and clinical studies has shown that measurements of plaque size and echogenicity are closely associated with traditional cardiovascular risk factors and are predictive of future stroke, MI, and cardiovascular disease. Measurement of total plaque area seems to be a powerful tool for risk assessment. In the general population, addition of plaque measurements to risk prediction models is of limited value, but in high-risk patients, assessments of plaque size and morphology can be useful as tools for individual stratification and could be included in decision-making algorithms for the selection of prevention and treatment strategies.

References

1. Salonen JT, Seppänen K, Rauramaa R, Salonen R. Risk factors for carotid atherosclerosis: the Kuopio Ischaemic Heart Disease Risk Factor Study. *Ann Med.* 1989;21:227–229.
2. Bots ML, Breslau PJ, Briët E, et al. Cardiovascular determinants of carotid artery disease. The Rotterdam Elderly Study. *Hypertension.* 1992;19:717–720.
3. The ARIC investigators. The atherosclerosis risk in communities (ARIC) study: design and objectives. *Am J Epidemiol.* 1989;129:687–702.
4. Fried LP, Borhani NO, Enright P, et al. The Cardiovascular Health Study: design and rationale. *Ann Epidemiol.* 1991;1:263–276.
5. Touboul P-J, Hennerici MG, Meairs S, et al. Mannheim carotid intima-media thickness consensus (2004–2006): an update on behalf of the Advisory Board of the 3 rd and 4th watching the risk symposium, 13th and 15th European stroke conferences, Mannheim, Germany, 2004, and Brussels, Belgium, 2006. *Cerebrovasc Dis.* 2007;23:75–80.
6. Spence JD, Eliasziw M, DiCicco M, Hackam DG, Galil R, Lohmann T. Carotid plaque area: a tool for targeting and evaluating vascular preventive therapy. *Stroke.* 2002;33:2916–2922.
7. Bertges DJ, Muluk V, Whittle J, et al. Relevance of carotid stenosis progression as a predictor of ischemic neurological outcomes. *Arch Intern Med.* 2003;163:2285–2289.
8. Sabeti S, Schlager O, Exner M, et al. Progression of carotid stenosis detected by duplex ultrasonography predicts adverse outcomes in cardiovascular high-risk patients. *Stroke.* 2007;38:2887–2894.
9. Spence JD, Hackam DG. Treating arteries instead of risk factors: a paradigm change in management of atherosclerosis. *Stroke.* 2010;41:1193–1199.
10. Li R, Duncan BB, Metcalf PA, et al. B-mode-detected carotid artery plaque in a general population. Atherosclerosis Risk in Communities (ARIC) Study Investigators. *Stroke.* 1994;25:2377–2383.
11. Polak JF, O'Leary DH, Kronmal RA, et al. Sonographic evaluation of carotid artery atherosclerosis in the elderly: relationship of disease severity to stroke and transient ischemic attack. *Radiology.* 1993;188:363–370.
12. Joakimsen O, Bønaa KH, Stensland-Bugge E, Jacobsen BK. Age and sex differences in the distribution and ultrasound morphology of carotid atherosclerosis. The Tromsø Study. *Arterioscler Thromb Vasc Biol.* 1999;19:3007–3013.
13. Polak JF, Shemanski L, O'Leary D, et al. Hypoechoic plaque at US of the carotid artery: an independent risk factor for incident stroke in adults aged 65 years or older. *Radiology.* 1998;208:649–654.
14. Mathiesen EB, Bønaa KH, Joakimsen O. Echolucent plaques are associated with high risk of ischemic cerebrovascular events in carotid stenosis. The Tromsø Study. *Circulation.* 2001;103:2171–2175.
15. Grønholdt M-LM, Nordestgaard BG, Schroeder TV, Vorstrup S, Sillesen H. Ultrasonic echolucent carotid plaques predict future strokes. *Circulation.* 2001;104:68–73.
16. Sabetai MM, Tegos TJ, Nicolaides AN, et al. Hemisperic symptoms and carotid plaque echomorphology. *J Vasc Surg.* 2000;31:39–49.
17. Honda O, Sugiyama S, Kugiyama K, et al. Echolucent carotid plaques predict future coronary events in patients with coronary artery disease. *J Am Coll Cardiol.* 2004;43:1177–1184.
18. Hirano M, Nakamura T, Kitta Y, et al. Assessment of carotid plaque echolucency in addition to plaque size increases the

predictive value of carotid ultrasound for coronary events in patients with coronary artery disease and mild carotid atherosclerosis. *Atherosclerosis*. 2010;211:451–455.
19. Johnsen SH, Joakimsen O, Fosse E, Arnesen E. Sex difference in carotid plaque morphology may explain the higher male prevalence of myocardial infarction compared to angina pectoris. The Tromsø Study. *Scand Cardiovasc J*. 2005;39:36–41.
20. Ebrahim SB, Papacosta O, Whincup P, et al. Carotid plaque, intima media thickness, cardiovascular risk factors, and prevalent cardiovascular disease in men and women. The British Regional Heart Study. *Stroke*. 1999;30:841–850.
21. O'Leary DH, Polak JF, Kronmal RA, et al. Distribution and correlates of sonographically detected carotid artery disease in the Cardiovascular Health Study. *Stroke*. 1992;23: 1752–1760.
22. Nieto FJ, Diez-Roux A, Szklo M, Comstock GW, Sharrett AR. Short- and long-term prediction of clinical and subclinical atherosclerosis by traditional risk factors. *J Clin Epidemiol*. 1999;52:559–567.
23. Mathiesen EB, Joakimsen O, Bønaa KH. Prevalence of and risk factors associated with carotid artery stenosis. The Tromsø Study. *Cerebrovasc Dis*. 2001;12:44–50.
24. Johnsen SH, Fosse E, Joakimsen O, et al. Monocyte count is a predictor of novel plaque formation. A 7-year follow-up study of 2610 persons without carotid plaque at baseline. The Tromsø Study. *Stroke*. 2005;36:715–719.
25. Johnsen SH, Mathiesen EB, Fosse E, et al. Elevated high-density lipoprotein cholesterol levels are protective against plaque progression. A follow-up study of 1952 persons with carotid atherosclerosis. The Tromsø Study. *Circulation*. 2005;112:498–504.
26. Mathiesen EB, Bønaa KH, Joakimsen O. Low high-density lipoprotein is associated with echolucent, soft carotid artery plaques. The Tromsø Study. *Stroke*. 2001;32: 1960–1965.
27. Notø ATW, Mathiesen EB, Brox J, Björkegren J, Hansen JB. Delayed metabolism of postprandial triglyceride-rich lipoproteins in subjects with echolucent carotid plaques. *Lipids*. 2008;43:353–360.
28. Notø ATW, Mathiesen EB, Brox J, Björkegren J, Hansen JB. The ApoC-I content of VLDL particles is associated with plaque size in persons with carotid atherosclerosis. *Lipids*. 2008;43:673–679.
29. Notø ATW, Mathiesen EB, Amiral J, Vissac AM, Hansen JB. Endothelial dysfunction and systemic inflammation in persons with echolucent carotid plaques. *Thromb Haemost*. 2006;96:53–59.
30. Notø ATW, Mathiesen EB, Østerud B, Amiral J, Vissac AM, Hansen JB. Increased thrombin generation in persons with echogenic carotid plaques. *Thromb Haemost*. 2008;99:602–608.
31. Joakimsen O, Bønaa KH, Stensland-Bugge E, Jacobsen BK. Population-based study of age at menopause and ultrasound assessed carotid atherosclerosis. The Tromsø Study. *J Clin Epidemiol*. 2000;53:525–530.
32. Hulley S, Grady D, Bush T, et al. Randomized trial of estrogen plus progestin for secondary prevention of coronary heart disease in postmenopausal women. *JAMA*. 1998;280:605–613.
33. Simon JA, Hsia J, Cauley JA, et al. Postmenopausal hormone therapy and risk of stroke. The Heart and Estrogen-progestin Replacement Study (HERS). *Circulation*. 2001;103:638–642.
34. Writing Group for the Women's Health Initiative Investigators. Risks and Benefits of Estrogen Plus Progestin in Healthy Postmenopausal Women: Principal Results From the Women's Health Initiative Randomized Controlled Trial. *JAMA*. 2002;288:321–333.
35. Wassertheil-Smoller S, Hendrix S, Limacher M, et al. Effect of estrogen plus progestin on stroke in postmenopausal women: the women's health initiative: a randomized trial. *JAMA*. 2003;289:2673–2684.
36. Muller M, van den Beld AW, Bots ML, Grobbee DE, Lamberts SW, van der Schouw YT. Endogenous sex hormones and progression of carotid atherosclerosis in elderly men. *Circulation*. 2004;109:2074–2079.
37. Tivesten A, Hulthe J, Wallenfeldt K, Wikstrand J, Ohlsson C, Fagerberg B. Circulating estradiol is an independent predictor of progression of carotid artery intima-media thickness in middle-aged men. *J Clin Endocrinol Metab*. 2006;91: 4433–4437.
38. Svartberg J, von Mühlen D, Mathiesen EB, Joakimsen O, Bønaa KH, Stensland-Bugge E. Low testosterone levels are associated with carotid atherosclerosis in men. *J Intern Med*. 2006;259:576–582.
39. Vikan T, Johnsen SH, Schirmer H, Njølstad I, Svartberg J. Endogenous testosterone and the prospective association with carotid atherosclerosis in men: the Tromsø study. *Eur J Epidemiol*. 2009;24:289–295.
40. Emerging Risk Factors Collaboration, Kaptoge S, Di Angelantonio E, et al. C-reactive protein concentration and risk of coronary heart disease, stroke, and mortality: an individual participant meta-analysis. *Lancet*. 2010;375: 132–140.
41. Fibrinogen Studies Collaboration, Kaptoge S, White IR, et al. Associations of plasma fibrinogen levels with established cardiovascular disease risk factors, inflammatory markers, and other characteristics: individual participant meta-analysis of 154,211 adults in 31 prospective studies. *Am J Epidemiol*. 2007;166:867–879.
42. Halvorsen DS, Johnsen SH, Mathiesen EB, Njølstad I. The association between inflammatory markers and carotid atherosclerosis is sex dependent: the Tromsø Study. *Cerebrovasc Dis*. 2009;27:392–397.
43. Sarnak MJ, Levey AS, Schoolwerth AC, et al. Kidney disease as a risk factor for development of cardiovascular disease: a statement from the American Heart Association Councils on kidney in cardiovascular disease, high blood pressure research, clinical cardiology, and epidemiology and prevention. *Circulation*. 2003;108:2154–2169.
44. Furtner M, Kiechl S, Mair A, et al. Urinary albumin excretion is independently associated with carotid and femoral artery atherosclerosis in the general population. *Eur Heart J*. 2005;26:279–287.
45. Mykkänen L, Zaccaro DJ, O'Leary DH, Howard G, Robbins DC, Haffner SM. Microalbuminuria and carotid artery intima-media thickness in nondiabetic and NIDDM subjects: the Insulin Resistance Atherosclerosis Study (IRAS). *Stroke*. 1997;28:1710–1716.
46. Jørgensen L, Jenssen T, Johnsen SH, et al. Albuminuria as risk factor for initiation and progression of carotid

47. Perry IJ, Wannamethee SG, Whincup PH, Shaper AG, Walker MK, Alberti KG. Serum insulin and incident coronary heart disease in middle-aged British men. *Am J Epidemiol*. 1996;144:224–234.
48. Yudkin JS, May M, Elwood P, et al. Concentrations of proinsulin like molecules predict coronary heart disease independently of insulin: prospective data from the Caerphilly Study. *Diabetologia*. 2002;45:327–336.
49. Kronborg J, Johnsen SH, Njølstad I, Toft I, Eriksen BO, Jenssen T. Proinsulin:insulin and insulin:glucose ratios as predictors of carotid plaque growth: a population-based 7 year follow-up of the Tromsø Study. *Diabetologia*. 2007;50:1607–1614.
50. Jørgensen L, Jenssen T, Joakimsen O, Heuch I, Ingebretson OC, Jacobsen BK. Glycated hemoglobin level is strongly related to the prevalence of carotid artery plaques with high echogenicity in nondiabetic individuals: the Tromsø Study. *Circulation*. 2004;110:466–470.
51. Hofbauer LC, Schoppet M. Clinical implications of the osteoprotegerin/RANKL/RANK system for bone and vascular diseases. *JAMA*. 2004;292:490–495.
52. Price PA, June HH, Buckley JR, Williamson MK. Osteoprotegerin inhibits artery calcification induced by warfarin and by vitamin D. *Arterioscler Thromb Vasc Biol*. 2001;21:1610–1616.
53. Jono S, Ikari Y, Shioi A, et al. Serum osteoprotegerin levels are associated with the presence and severity of coronary artery disease. *Circulation*. 2002;106:1192–1194.
54. Schoppet M, Sattler AM, Schaefer JR, Herzum M, Haisch B, Hofbauer LC. Increased osteoprotegerin serum levels in men with coronary artery disease. *J Clin Endocrinol Metab*. 2003;88:1024–1028.
55. Kiechl S, Schett G, Wenning G, et al. Osteoprotegerin is a risk factor for progressive atherosclerosis and cardiovascular disease. *Circulation*. 2004;109(18):2175–2180.
56. Vik A, Mathiesen EB, Notø ATW, Sveinbjørnsson B, Brox J, Hansen JB. Serum osteoprotegerin is inversely associated with carotid plaque echogenicity in humans. *Atherosclerosis*. 2006;191:128–134.
57. Vik A, Mathiesen EB, Johnsen SH, et al. Serum osteoprotegerin, sRANKL and carotid plaque formation and growth in a general population – the Tromsø study. *J Thromb Haemost*. 2010;8:898–905.
58. Vik A, Mathiesen EB, Brox J, et al. Relation between serum osteoprotegerin and carotid intima media thickness in a general population – the Tromsø Study. *J Thromb Haemost*. 2010;8:2133–2139.
59. de Weerd M, Greving JP, Hedblad B, et al. Prevalence of asymptomatic carotid artery stenosis in the general population: an individual participant data meta-analysis. *Stroke*. 2010;41:1294–1297.
60. de Weerd M. *Asymptomatic Carotid Artery Stenosis [PhD thesis]*. Utrecht: University of Utrecht; 2010.
61. Johnsen SH, Mathiesen EB, Joakimsen O, et al. Carotid atherosclerosis is a stronger predictor of myocardial infarction in women than in men. A 6-year follow-up study of 6226 persons: the Tromso Study. *Stroke*. 2007;38:2873–2880.
62. Spence JD, Hegele RA. Noninvasive phenotypes of atherosclerosis: similar windows but different views. *Stroke*. 2004;35:649–653.
63. Mathiesen EB, Johnsen SH, Wilsgaard T, et al. Carotid plaque area and intima-media thickness in prediction of first-ever ischemic stroke. A 10-year follow-up of 6584 men and women. The Tromsø Study. *Stroke*. 2011;42:972–978.
64. Griffin M, Nicolaides A, Tyllis T, et al. Plaque area at carotid and common femoral bifurcations and prevalence of clinical cardiovascular disease. *Int Angiol*. 2010;29:216–225.
65. del Sol AI, Moons KGM, Hollander M, et al. Is carotid intima-media thickness useful in cardiovascular disease risk assessment? The Rotterdam Study. *Stroke*. 2001;32:1532–1538.
66. Prati P, Tosetto A, Vanuzzo D, et al. Carotid intima media thickness and plaques can predict the occurrence of ischemic cerebrovascular events. *Stroke*. 2008;39:2470–2476.
67. Rundek T, Arif H, Boden-Albala B, Elkind MS, Paik MC, Sacco RL. Carotid plaque, a subclinical precursor of vascular events: the Northern Manhattan Study. *Neurology*. 2008;70:1200–1207.
68. Barnett HJM, Taylor DW, Eliasziw M, et al. Benefit of carotid endarterectomy in patients with symptomatic moderate or severe stenosis. *N Engl J Med*. 1998;339:1415–1425.
69. European Carotid Surgery Trialists' Collaborative Group. Randomised trial of endarterectomy for recently symptomatic carotid stenosis: final results of the MCR European Carotid Surgery Trial (ECST). *Lancet*. 1998;351:1379–1387.
70. The Executive Committee for the Asymptomatic Carotid Atherosclerosis Study. Endarterectomy for asymptomatic carotid artery stenosis. *JAMA*. 1995;273:1421–1428.
71. MRC ACST Collaborative Group. Prevention of disabling and fatal strokes by successful carotid endarterectomy in patients without recent neurological symptoms: randomised controlled trial. *Lancet*. 2004;363:1491–1502.
72. Johnson JM, Kennelly MM, Desecare D, Morgan D, Sparrow A. Natural history of asymptomatic carotid plaque. *Arch Surg*. 1985;120:1010–1012.
73. Sterpetti AV, Schultz RD, Feldhaus RJ, et al. Ultrasonographic features of carotid plaque and the risk of subsequent neurologic deficits. *Surgery*. 1988;104:652–660.
74. Geroulakos G, Hobson RW, Nicolaides A. Ultrasonographic carotid plaque morphology in predicting stroke risk. *Br J Surg*. 1996;83:582–587.
75. Gray-Weale AC, Graham JC, Burnett JR, Byrne K, Lusby RJ. Carotid artery atheroma: comparison of preoperative B-mode ultrasound appearance with carotid endarterectomy specimen pathology. *J Cardiovasc Surg (Torino)*. 1988;29:676–681.
76. El-Barghouty NM, Geroulakos G, Nicolaides A, Androulakis A, Bahal V. Computer-assisted carotid plaque characterization. *Eur J Vasc Endovasc Surg*. 1995;9:389–393.

77. Biasi GM, Sampaolo A, Mingazzini P, et al. Computer analysis of ultrasonic plaque echolucency in identifying high risk carotid bifurcation lesions. *Eur J Vasc Endovasc Surg*. 1999;17:476–479.
78. Fosse E, Johnsen SH, Stensland-Bugge E, et al. Repeated visual and computer-assisted carotid plaque characterization in a longitudinal population-based ultrasound study. The Tromsø Study. *Ultrasound Med Biol*. 2006; 32:3–11.
79. Jørgensen L, Joakimsen O, Mathiesen EB, et al. Carotid plaque echogenicity and risk of nonvertebral fractures in women: a longitudinal population-based study. *Calcif Tissue Int*. 2006;79:207–213.

25 Toward Clinical Applications of Carotid Ultrasound: Intima-Media Thickness, Plaque Area, and Three-Dimensional Phenotypes

J. David Spence and Tatjana Rundek

25.1 Introduction

Atherosclerosis is the underlying process that causes the most death and disability worldwide.[1] It is the cause of myocardial infarctions, peripheral vascular disease, and a large proportion of strokes, and contributes to much of heart failure. There are several ways to quantify the burden of atherosclerosis, and quantifying change in atherosclerotic burden over time may be useful. These include risk stratification, evaluation of the contribution of risk factors (new and old) to atherosclerosis, evaluation of a patient's response to therapy, genetic research, and evaluation of potential new therapies for atherosclerosis.

There are a number of ways to calculate the future risk of cardiovascular events based on levels of risk factors such as age, sex, serum cholesterol, smoking, and blood pressure. The Framingham risk score[2] is the best known, but others include the Reynolds score,[3] Prospective Cardiovascular Münster (PROCAM) Score,[4] the European (EU) Score,[5] the NCEP III/ATP III [National Cholesterol Education Program (NCEP) Expert Panel on Detection, Evaluation, and Treatment of High Blood Cholesterol in Adults (Adult Treatment Panel III)] risk calculator,[6] and QRISK (University of Nottingham, Nottingham, United Kingdom, and EMIS, Rawdon, Leeds, United Kingdom).[7]

J.D. Spence (✉)
Stroke Prevention & Atherosclerosis Research Centre, Robarts Research Institute, University of Western Ontario, London, ON, Canada

T. Rundek
Department of Neurology, Miller School of Medicine, University of Miami, Miami, FL, USA

These scoring systems are useful, but will identify only about a third of those who will have events during follow-up. Imaging methods have been used to increase the sensitivity of risk prediction with such tools as coronary calcium scoring,[8] but the radiation exposure for such testing is substantial. Furthermore, in most studies, such quantification of atherosclerosis burden has not improved prediction of events; i.e., it has not added to the area under the curve of receiver-operator curves for prediction of events based on risk factors. Ultrasound methods for quantifying the burden of vascular disease have therefore been developed for this purpose. These methods include one-dimensional measurement of intima-media thickness (IMT) and plaque thickness, two-dimensional plaque area, and three-dimensional measurement of plaque volume and vessel wall volume. Romanens et al. have recently shown that total plaque area significantly increased the C-statistic for prediction of cardiovascular events among patients free of manifest atherosclerosis at baseline.[9]

25.2 Ultrasound Phenotypes of "Atherosclerosis"

At a genetics meeting in Honolulu organized by the American Heart Association about 10 years ago, there were presentations on genetics of "atherosclerosis" by various groups. Some presented results using IMT, others using coronary calcium, others with angiographic stenosis of femoral arteries, and the authors' group using carotid total plaque area measured by ultrasound. Contemplating the differences among these phenotypes, Spence came to the realization that intima-media thickness, plaque, and stenosis were very different phenotypes. This can be understood in the light of the concept of compensatory enlargement: as plaque develops, the artery enlarges to accommodate the plaque so that the lumen remains unchanged. Glagov et al. hypothesized that this resulted from responses to changes in shear, with the biological goal of maintaining a constant shear rate at the endothelium[10] (Chaps. 2 and 28). Spence hypothesized that arteries grow away from high shear via effects of nitric oxide and fill in at regions of low shear via effects of endothelin.[11] Figure 25.1 illustrates the principle.

An important issue in the understanding of IMT is that different protocols for measurement will lead to different phenotypes and different results (Chaps. 22 and 23). When measured according to the Mannheim consensus,[13] in the distal far wall of the common carotid artery where there is no plaque, it is a different phenotype from measurements that include plaque thickness, usually in the carotid bulb. IMT is approximately 20% intima and 80% media,[14] whereas atherosclerosis is primarily an intimal process.[15] IMT probably represents mostly hypertensive medial hypertrophy.[16,17] Plaque is influenced more by traditional coronary risk factors and likely represents effects of factors that impair endothelial function. Stenosis, on the other hand, is the result of plaque rupture with thrombosis,[18] so it is determined (a) by factors that predispose to rupture, such as inflammation, possibly infection,[19] matrix metalloproteinases, lipoprotein-associated phospholipase A2,[20] neovascularization of the plaque by vasa vasorum,[21] etc., (b) by factors that increase thrombosis, and (c) by factors that impair thrombolysis (Chap. 28). This is illustrated by the recent finding that lipoprotein (a), which increases thrombosis and impairs thrombolysis,[22] is not associated with plaque area, but strongly associated with stenosis and occlusion of the carotid arteries.[23]

The principle is also illustrated by the different relationships between ultrasound phenotypes of atherosclerosis and coronary risk factors. In multivariable regression, coronary risk factors (age, sex, cholesterol, systolic blood pressure, smoking, and diabetes) explain very different proportions of the ultrasound phenotypes: The R^2 (proportion of explained variance) for IMT is 0.15–0.17,[17,24] for total plaque area it is 0.52, but for stenosis,

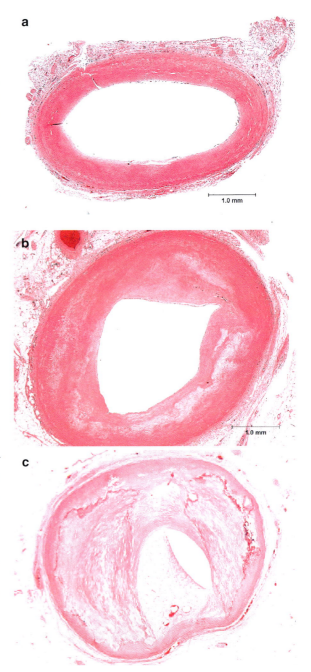

Fig. 25.1 Stages of atherosclerosis. The figure illustrates the concept of compensatory enlargement. When plaque forms, the artery enlarges to accommodate plaque so that the lumen remains patent. Stenosis and occlusion probably do not result from plaque growth, but from plaque rupture, with thrombosis. (**a**) Normal artery; (**b**) thickened wall with plaque but patent lumen; (**c**) severe stenosis resulting from plaque rupture and thrombosis (Courtesy of Dr. Edward Tweedie, Department of Pathology, University of Western Ontario. Reprinted from Spence et al.[12] copyright 2010, with permission from Elsevier)

it is only 0.13.[25] Although IMT (in the absence of plaque) is a predictor of cardiovascular risk, it should be understood that it is not truly atherosclerosis; this issue was reviewed recently by Finn et al.[26] An important consequence of this concept is that therapies for atherosclerosis would be expected to affect plaque and IMT differently.

25.3 Risk Stratification

25.3.1 One-Dimensional Measurements: IMT and Plaque Thickness

Measurement of carotid IMT began with the pioneering work of Dr. Eugene Bond at Winston-Salem in North Carolina. He and his colleagues were assessing atherosclerosis in monkey models.[27,28] The technique was subsequently adapted to human studies.[29] Baldassare et al.,[30] and many others, utilized measurement of IMT for risk stratification and for other purposes discussed below.

It is crucial to understand that two distinct approaches to measuring carotid IMT lead to different results with respect to risk stratification as well as response to therapy. These two approaches are shown in Fig. 25.2. One school, exemplified by the Mannheim consensus,[13] specifies that IMT should be measured in the distal common carotid artery in the far wall at a site where there is no plaque. This recommendation is made largely for technical reasons relating to reproducibility and reliability of the measurement. Another school of thought, exemplified by the work of Professor Michiel Bots[31] at Rotterdam and others including CHS[32] and Atherosclerosis Risk in Communities (ARIC)[33] studies, includes plaque thickness in the measurement of IMT (Chaps. 22 and 23). In addition, some studies have included subjects with the IMT measurement above a certain threshold level of IMT, which produced the effect of pooling subjects with plaques into the higher IMT level group because plaques tend to be more common in those with a thicker IMT.[34] These two approaches give significantly different results with respect to risk stratification, as illustrated in Table 25.1. These issues were recently reviewed by Simon et al.[36]

A meta-analysis[37] reported that the age and sex-adjusted overall estimates of the relative risk of myocardial infarction were 1.26 (95% confidence interval [CI], 1.21–1.30) per standard deviation common carotid artery IMT difference and 1.15 (95% CI, 1.12–1.17) per 0.10 mm common carotid artery IMT difference. The age and sex-adjusted relative risks of stroke were 1.32 (95% CI, 1.27–1.38) per standard deviation of common carotid artery IMT difference and 1.18 (95% CI, 1.16–1.21) per 0.10 mm common carotid artery IMT difference. The report concluded that IMT was a somewhat stronger predictor of stroke than that of myocardial infarction, and that major sources of heterogeneity were age distribution, carotid segment definition, and IMT measurement protocol.

Confusion about these differences and a paucity of data on progression of IMT may underlie perceptions that IMT is a relatively weak predictor of coronary artery disease.[14,38] However, there is substantial evidence that carotid plaque presence and carotid plaque area are more strongly predictive of coronary artery disease or coronary events than IMT.[34,39–41]

Rundek et al.[42] showed in the Northern Manhattan study that carotid plaque thickness strongly predicted ischemic stroke, myocardial infarction, or vascular death. Among participants with low Framingham risk scores, the 10-year risk of cardiovascular events was 5.8% in those without plaque, 18.3% in those with plaques <1.9 mm in thickness, and 24.7% among those with plaque 1.9 mm or greater in thickness. Among participants with Framingham risk scores in the moderate range, the 10-year risk of cardiovascular events was 11.5% with no plaque, 18.6% with plaques <1.9 mm in thickness, and 25.1% with plaques with 1.9 mm or more in thickness. These differences remained significant after adjustment (Cox proportional hazard) for hypertension, diabetes, any cardiac disease, alcohol consumption, current cigarette smoking, high-density lipoprotein, low-density lipoprotein, and body mass index levels, use of aspirin, and lipid-lowering medication. Over 30% of those with low or moderate Framingham risk scores could be reclassified to moderate to severe risk category if the information on the presence and size of carotid plaque was available. These patients could be treated more aggressively to lower lipid targets per NCEP ATPIII guidelines.

Fig. 25.2 Measurement of carotid intima-media thickness (IMT) and plaque thickness. The *green line* in the lumen is a reference line used by the software for density of blood. Measurements are shown in the *blue window*. (**a**) IMT in the common carotid, far wall; mean IMT is 0.656 mm; maximal IMT is 0.783 mm. (**b**) IMT in the common carotid, near wall; mean IMT is 0.766 mm; maximal IMT is 0.882 mm. (**c**) IMT in the bifurcation; mean IMT is 0.843 mm; maximal IMT is 0.993 mm. (**d**) Thickened IMT in the internal carotid; mean IMT is 0.883 mm; maximal IMT is 1.051 mm. (**e**) Plaque thickness and plaque area in the common carotid artery; mean thickness is 2.64 mm; maximal thickness is 3.74 mm; area is 51.04 mm^2

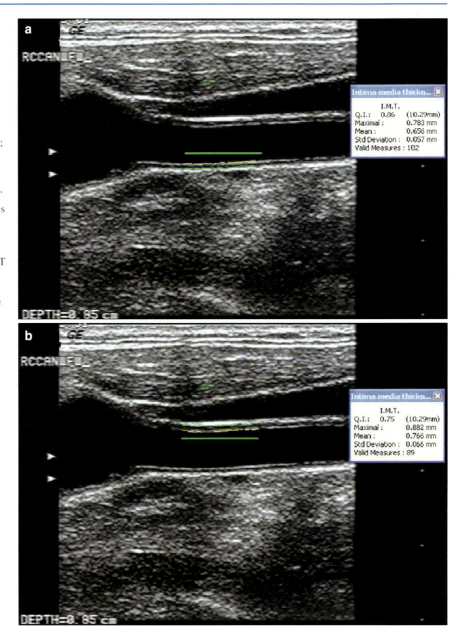

25.3.2 Two-Dimensional Measurements: Total Plaque Area

This method was developed in 1990 in the Spence's laboratory by Maria DiCicco, registered vascular technician (RVT). Previously, the burden of plaque and change over time had been tracked using drawings of the plaque on templates of the carotid bifurcation. One day in 1990, Spence asked Ms. DiCicco how he could rely on the drawings being consistent from year to year. Her reply was, "Well, there is software in the machine that I can use to measure the plaques, if you want." This led to the development of total plaque area. Every plaque seen between the clavicle and the angle of the jaw, in the common, internal and external carotid, and where visible, in the subclavian artery, is measured in a longitudinal view. The plane of measurement is selected for the largest view of the plaque. The cross-sectional area of each plaque is measured in the longitudinal view by tracing around the plaque on the screen

Fig. 25.2 (continued)

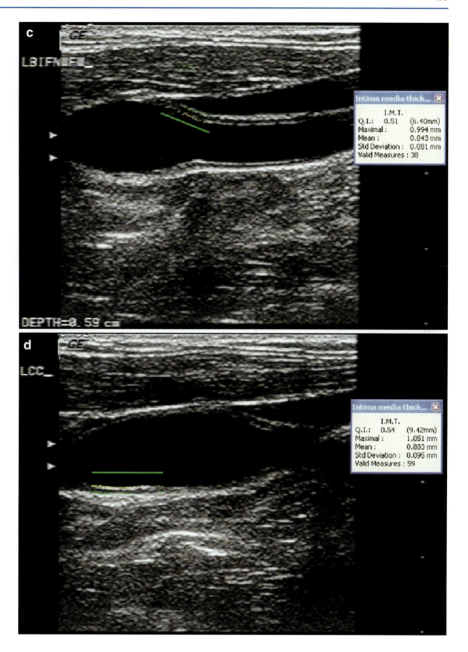

with a cursor; the area is computed by the software in the duplex scanner (Fig. 25.3). The sum of cross-sectional areas of all plaques seen is total plaque area.[43] The reliability of the method was tested by having two technologists repeat measurements of total plaque area on two occasions a week apart. The intraclass correlation coefficient for intraobserver reliability was 0.95 for repeat measurement by the senior technologist with the higher-resolution machine; interobserver reliability for exchange of videotapes between the two technologists was 0.99, but when the two technologists independently measured plaque in the same patients, the junior technologist with the lower-resolution machine systematically measured less plaque, and the intraclass correlation coefficient was 0.85. The difference between measurement from videotapes and patients suggests that most of the error was in the choice of the plane for the measurements. Wikstrand heard of this from Spence and published a version of the method in 1992.[44] Mancini et al.[45] also published a variant of the

Fig. 25.2 (continued)

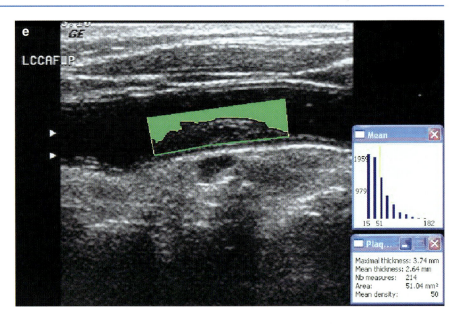

Table 25.1 IMT including or excluding plaque thickness

Maximal IMT including plaque thickness[32]:
4,476 subjects age 72.5 ± 5.5 years followed for a median of 6.2 years

	Quintiles	IMT
	1st (ref)	<0.09 mm
RR adjusted[a] (95% CI)	2nd 1.54 (1.04–2.28)	0.91–1.10
	3rd 1.84 (1.26–2.67)	1.11–1.39
	4th 2.01 (1.38–2.91)	1.40–1.80
	5th RR 3.15 (2.19–4.52)	≥ 1.81 mm

Mean CCA IMT without plaque thickness[35]:
5,056 patients age range 19–90 years; mean age 50.1 followed for a mean of 4.2 years

	Quartiles	IMT (mm)
	1st (ref)	<0.63
RR adjusted[b] (95% CI)	2nd 1.22 (0.68–2.16)	0.63–0.69
	3rd 0.89 (0.48–1.64)	0.70–0.79
	4th 1.83 (0.97–3.45)	> 0.79

[a]For age, sex, blood pressure, cholesterol, smoking
[b]Age, sex, BMI, systolic and diastolic blood pressure, antihypertensive medication, LDL cholesterol, lipid-lowering medication, nicotine consumption, history of diabetes

method, including a new approach to taking the sum of IMT and plaque area. The Tromsø Study group published their variant of the method, developed independently, in 2006[46] (Chap. 24).

The Spence et al. reported in 2002[47] that among 1,686 patients being followed in the vascular prevention clinics at University Hospital in London, Canada, total plaque area strongly predicted the 5-year risk of stroke, vascular death, or myocardial infarction. After adjusting for age, sex, cholesterol, systolic blood pressure, smoking (pack–years) diabetes, total homocysteine, and treatment of blood pressure and cholesterol, patients in the top quartile of plaque area had 3.4 times higher risk of events compared to the lowest quartile.

Fig. 25.3 Measurement of carotid plaque area. Each plaque is measured in the longitudinal axis, in the plane in which it is biggest, by tracing around the perimeter of the plaque with a cursor. The boundaries are the same as for IMT, but instead of measuring only the thickness, the area is measured. All plaques seen between the clavicle and the angle of the jaw area are measured; the sum of all plaque areas is Total Plaque Area. *Panel* (**a**) shows a plaque with some soft areas not well seen; *Panel* (**b**) shows Doppler color flow around the plaque so that the soft areas are seen; *Panel* (**c**) shows the plaque outlined, with an area of 0.74 mm^2

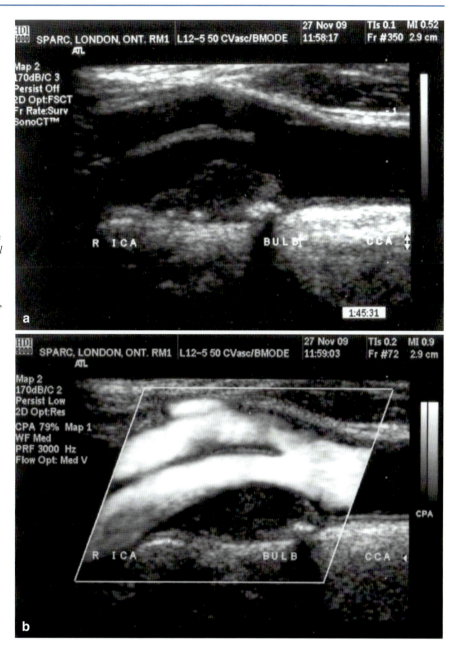

In the first year of follow-up, 26% of patients had regression of plaque by more than 5 mm^2 (the median change), 15% had no change in plaque area, and 59% had progression of carotid plaque area in the first year of follow-up, despite treatment according to consensus guidelines. Patients with plaque progression had twice the risk of those with stable plaque or regression after adjustment for the same panel of risk factors. This study has been criticized as a "small study," but the population was high-risk, with as many events in 2.5 ± 1.3 years of follow-up (range 1–5 years) as in the first 10 years of the Framingham study: a total of 45 strokes, 94 myocardial infarctions, and 41 deaths (27 vascular, 12 cancer, and 2 other).

The above study was validated by the Trømso study,[48] a population-based study in which 6,226

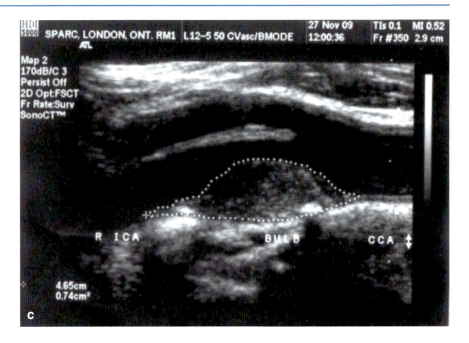

Fig. 25.3 (continued)

men and women aged 25–84 were followed for 6 years after carotid ultrasound measurements at baseline (Chap. 24). During follow-up, myocardial infarction (MI) occurred in 6.6% of men and 3.0% of women. The relative risk of MI was strongly predicted by total plaque area in men, with a relative risk (RR) of 1.56 (95% CI, 1.04–2.36), and more strongly in women with an RR of 3.95 (95% CI, 2.16–7.19). IMT that included plaque thickness in the carotid bulb also predicted coronary events RR 1.73 (95% CI, 0.98–3.06) in men, and in women RR 2.86 (1.07–7.65), but IMT as measured in the distal common excluding plaque did not predict MI in either sex.

25.3.3 Three-Dimensional Measurements: Plaque Volume, Vessel Wall Volume

Studies are underway to compare IMT, total plaque area, plaque volume (Fig. 25.4), vessel wall volume (VWV) (Fig. 25.5), and other three-dimensional (3D) ultrasound parameters of atherosclerosis (ulceration, plaque roughness, plaque texture) (Chaps. 16–18) as predictors of cardiovascular events; no results have yet been published.

25.4 Evaluation of Vascular Risk Factors

25.4.1 One-Dimensional Measurements: IMT and Plaque Thickness

Traditional vascular risk factors have been associated with carotid IMT and plaque thickness in many large epidemiological studies[51-55] (Chaps. 22 and 23).

Carotid IMT is consistently associated with age, hypertension, low-density lipoprotein cholesterol, and smoking. However, it seems that there are some carotid segment specific differences. A greater proportion of the variability in common carotid IMT can be explained by traditional cardiovascular risk factors than for the carotid artery bulb and internal carotid IMT.

In a large cohort of 3,258 individuals, a large proportion of the variability of common carotid artery IMT was explained by cardiovascular risk factors (27%) but less so for the bulb (11%) and internal carotid artery (8%). Associations with diastolic blood pressure and fasting glucose may be important for common carotid IMT while hypertension, diabetes, and current smoking for bulb IMT and low-density lipoprotein (LDL) cholesterol for internal carotid artery IMT.[56]

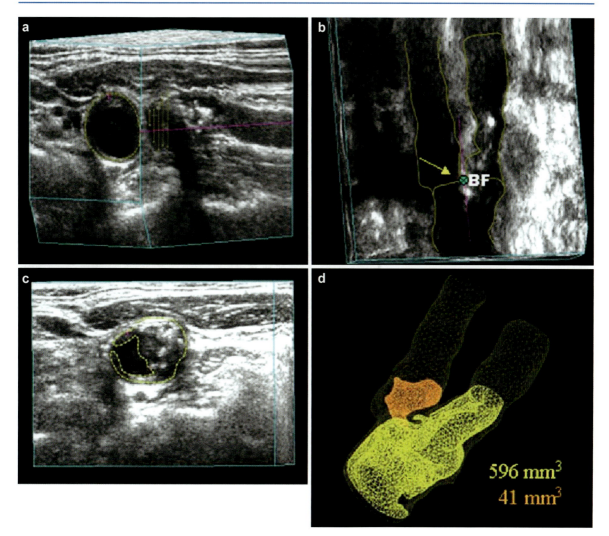

Fig. 25.4 Measurement of carotid plaque volume. Procedure for determining plaque volumes from 3D US images. (**a**) An approximate axis of the vessel is selected in a longitudinal view (*colored line*), and the internal elastic lamina and lumen boundary are outlined (*yellow*). (**b**) Using the surfaces generated by the vessel contours and the 3D ultrasound (US) image, the position of the bifurcation (*BF*; *yellow arrow*) is determined and marked. The axis of the vessel is selected based on the bifurcation point, and marked along the branch as far as the plaque can be measured (*colored line*). This axis will be used as a reference for distance measurements. (**c**) All plaques within the measurable distance are outlined; different colors are being used for each separate plaque to aid in identification. (**d**) Volumes are calculated for each plaque, and surfaces of the vessel wall and plaques are generated to better visualize the plaques in relation to the carotid arteries (Reprinted from Ainsworth et al.[49])

Some novel vascular risk factors including homocysteine,[57] the metabolic syndrome,[58] inflammatory markers,[59] and infectious agents such as *C. pneumoniae*[60] have recently been associated with IMT.

Although in the past some studies have used IMT measurements that had included plaque, carotid IMT and carotid plaque have different relationships to risk factors and vascular outcomes as they are considered separate phenotypes.[61] Plaque measured in the carotid bulb or internal carotid artery is more strongly related to hyperlipidemia and smoking and is a stronger predictor for MI, whereas common carotid artery intima-media thickness (CCA-IMT) has a stronger relation to hypertension and ischemic stroke.

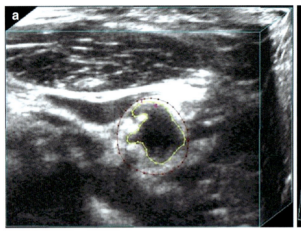 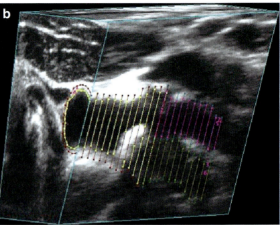

Fig. 25.5 Measurement of carotid vessel wall volume. (**a**) The lumen and media/adventitia boundary are traced in cross-sectional views of the artery; (**b**) the volume of the lumen and vessel wall is computed using the interslice distance (1 mm) (Reprinted from Egger et al.[50] copyright 2007, with permission from Elsevier)

25.4.2 Two-Dimensional Measurements: Total Plaque Area

Total plaque area has been used to study a number of potential risk factors, beginning with a study published in 1997[43] that evaluated the rise in pressure during mental stress. Barnett et al. showed that blood pressure during mental stress was a stronger predictor of plaque progression than any of the Framingham risk factors. Since then total plaque area has been used to show that plasma total homocysteine (but not a polymorphism of methylene-tetrahydrofolate reductase),[62] a polymorphism of mannose-binding lectin that predisposes to chlamydia infection,[63] von Willebrand factor and fibrinolytic factors,[64] and keloid scars[65] are independently predictive of carotid plaque in multivariable regression.

The Tromsø Study group has also used plaque area measurements to study a number of risk factors including proinsulin/insulin ratio,[66] insulin/glucose ratio,[66] the protective effect of high levels of high-density lipoprotein (HDL) cholesterol,[67] and sex differences in inflammatory markers[68] (Chap. 24).

25.4.3 Three-Dimensional Measurements: Plaque Volume, Vessel Wall Volume

As 3D ultrasound is newer, less work has been done on evaluation of risk factors. Al-Shali et al.[17] found in a comparison of one-dimensional (1D), two-dimensional (2D), and 3D ultrasound phenotypes that IMT was more strongly associated with hypertension, plaque area with smoking, and serum cholesterol, whereas plaque volume was most closely associated with diabetes. Pollex et al.[69] found that 3D plaque volume was significantly higher among diabetics, whereas IMT was not, in a small case-control study (49 in each group) emphasizing that required sample sizes for such studies were much smaller for plaque volume than for IMT. In contrast, metabolic syndrome was more closely related to IMT than to plaque volume.

25.5 Genetic Research

A key issue for studies of genetics is that IMT, plaque area, stenosis, plaque volume, and probably vessel wall volume are biologically and genetically distinct phenotypes. As discussed above in the introduction, genes related to IMT are likely to be genes affecting blood pressure, plaque area by genes affecting lipids and endothelial function, and stenosis by genes affecting plaque rupture, thrombosis, and fibrinolysis.[16,25]

25.5.1 One-Dimensional Measurements: IMT and Plaque Thickness

Carotid IMT and plaque have a significant genetic *heritability*, ranging from 0.30 to 0.60.[70-73] In the

National Heart, Lung, and Blood Institute (NHLBI) Framingham Offspring cohort, heritability of carotid IMT among whites was about 0.40. Among type II diabetics, the heritability of carotid IMT was 0.41. It was 0.64 in a study of Latino families in California and between 0.44 and 0.54 in Caribbean Hispanics from Northern Manhattan Family Study. Significant genetic correlations between carotid IMT and systolic blood pressure (BP) and renal function have been observed among Hispanic American families ascertained via a hypertensive parent.[74]

25.5.1.1 Carotid IMT and Genes

Several studies have evaluated candidate genes for carotid IMT; however, the results have been inconsistent.[75] Of the many candidate gene studies reviewed, only one variant that was previously linked to clinical disease, the 5A/6A polymorphism of the MMP3 gene, showed consistently positive associations with carotid IMT.[76] The paraoxonase 1 (PON1) Leu55met variant was weakly associated with IMT in certain subgroups. Modest associations for variants in Apolipoprotein E (APOE), Angiotensin-Converting Enzyme (ACE), and NOS3 candidate gene with carotid IMT have been reported. Carotid IMT was associated with allelic variants of stromelysin-1, interleukin 6, and hepatic lipase.[76]

Genome-wide association studies (GWAS) provide a more comprehensive approach, unconstrained by existing knowledge, to test common genetic variation across the genome using high-throughput genotyping. In the NHLBI Offspring Cohort of the Framingham Study among 1,345 subjects from 310 families, there was no association for carotid IMT meeting criteria for genome-wide significance.[77] However, 11 single nucleotide polymorphisms (SNPs) with $P < 10^{-5}$ were identified for maximum internal carotid IMT and 5 SNPs with $P < 10^{-5}$ by family-based association testing (FBAT) for mean common carotid IMT. In addition, several regions of linkage to internal carotid IMT were identified on chromosome 12, confirming previous results from the same population.[78]

However, the 100K SNP chip used in Framingham may not be sufficiently dense to identify associations with a complex subclinical atherosclerosis phenotype such as carotid IMT.

In the Mexican–American Coronary Artery Disease family study, a genome-wide scan using data from 91 two-generation families, the strongest evidence of IMT linkage was on chromosome 2 at D2S2944 and an only modest linkage on chromosomes 6 and 13.[79] In the Family Study of Stroke Risk and Carotid Atherosclerosis study among 1,390 subjects from 100 Dominican families, several quantitative trait loci (QTLs) for IMT are reported on chromosomes 7p and 14q.[80] The QTL on 14q replicates a suggestive linkage peak delimited in the Framingham Heart Study. These QTLs accounted for a substantial amount of trait heritability and therefore warrant further fine mapping. The important observation was that Dominican families with a higher prevalence of hypertension significantly contributed to the IMT linkage signal on chromosome 14q. This suggests that loci in chromosome 14q may interact with hypertension to determine carotid IMT variations and may have an implication for future fine mapping or association studies which should consider this interaction to avoid potential confounding on phenotype–genotype correlation.

Multiple genes are likely to influence carotid IMT. As previously discussed, candidate genes related to hypertension and inflammation are most likely to be related to IMT. In contrast, those related to the lipid metabolism, diabetes, and coagulation are most likely to be related to plaque.

25.5.1.2 Carotid Plaque and Genes

A variety of candidate genes have been suggested to play a role in plaque formation. They include genes involved in control of lipids, monocytes, smooth muscle cells, and factors affecting endothelial function such as oxidative stress, homocysteine, and inflammation.[81,82]

The alpha2-Heremans-Schmid glycoprotein (AHSG) gene which was associated with serum fetuin A levels, free phosphate levels, and cardiovascular death was reported to be associated with calcified carotid plaque in 829 European–American subjects with type 2 diabetes from the Diabetes Heart Study.[83] In the NHLBI Family Heart Study, a GWAS revealed no regions of significant linkage for plaque. However, in the stratified analysis of the subset with the youngest age ($\leq$55), suggestive linkage (logarithm of the odds ratio [LOD] of 2.13) was found on chromosome 2p11.2 (D2S1790).[84]

Considering candidate gene, GWAS or family study design, information on the genes associated with carotid IMT and plaque is still limited, particularly among different race-ethnic populations.

Table 25.2 Linear multiple regression of total carotid plaque area with coronary risk factors (Forced entry; $n = 2{,}634$)

Model		Unstandardized coefficients		Standardized coefficients		
		B	Std. error	Beta	t	Sig.
1	(Constant)	−.593	.053		−11.247	.000
	Age at first visit	.017	.000	.558	36.495	.000
	Sex	−.143	.014	−.153	−10.552	.000
	Total cholesterol	.016	.006	.040	2.839	.005
	HDL cholesterol	−.042	.015	−.039	−2.703	.007
	Systolic blood pressure	.002	.000	.099	6.930	.000
	Taking lipid medication	.109	.014	.115	8.013	.000
	Smoking (pack–years)	.005	.000	.206	15.088	.000
	Taking BP medication	.069	.013	.074	5.218	.000

$R^2 = 0.538$ Dependent variable: cube root transformation of total plaque area to normalize the distribution

25.5.2 Two-Dimensional Measurements: Total Plaque Area

Not many studies have used plaque area measurements for genetic research. Spence et al. studied the association of total plaque area with polymorphisms of methylene-tetrahydrofolate reductase,[62] mannose-binding lectin,[63] and lipoprotein lipase.[85] An interesting approach to the use of plaque area measurements is to use multivariable regression to quantify the extent to which atherosclerosis is more severe or less severe than would be predicted by traditional risk factors. The quantitative trait is the residual score in a multivariable regression model.[86,87] Table 25.2 shows an example of such a model, and Fig. 25.6 shows the distribution of residual scores. Schork et al.[88,89] have shown that by using extremes of the distribution of such quantitative traits, genome-wide association studies can be done with much smaller samples than with such discrete traits as myocardial infarction in case-control studies.

25.5.3 Three-Dimensional Measurements: Plaque Volume, Vessel Wall Volume

Few studies as yet have assessed genetic contributions to plaque volume or vessel wall volume.

Al-Shali et al.[90] studied the relationship between ultrasound phenotypes and polymorphisms of peroxisome proliferator-activated receptor gamma (PPARγ), an important molecule in atherogenesis, associated with insulin resistance, diabetes, and atherosclerosis (Table 25.3). They found different associations of

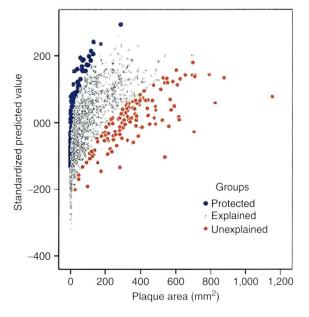

Fig. 25.6 Unexplained atherosclerosis: a quantitative trait. The quantitative trait is the residual score in the multivariable regression model shown in Table 25.2; $n = 1{,}305$. (The residual score represents the distance off the regression line, similar to a standard deviation). The *red circles* represent patients with unexplained atherosclerosis, i.e., those with residual scores in the highest 10% (>1.226); the *gray circles* are those with as much atherosclerosis as would be expected from their risk factors; the *blue dots* are patients who are protected by some genetic factor as they have much less atherosclerosis than would be predicted, with residual scores in the lowest 10% (<-1.321)

alleles of PPARγ with carotid IMT and total plaque volume (TPV). Subjects with more than 1 PPARγ A12 allele had less carotid IMT than others (0.72 ± 0.03 versus 0.80 ± 0.02 mm; $P = 0.0045$), with no between-genotype difference in TPV.

Table 25.3 Sample size and duration of studies required to show effects of therapy on ultrasound phenotypes

Modality	Duration of study	N per group
IMT[91]	2 years	468
2D plaque area[92]	2 years	144
3D VWV[93]	6 months	140
3D VWV[93]	1 year	35

Effect size of 30% and statistical power of 0.80 were assumed for all calculations, with a two-sided significance of $P < 0.05$, using the calculator at http://www.stat.ubc.ca/~rollin/stats/ssize/n2.html. Sources of data used in the sample size calculations are referenced

In contrast, subjects with the PPARγ c.1431T allele had greater TPV than others (124 + 18.4 versus 65.1 + 23.3 mm^3; $P = 0.0079$), with no between-genotype difference in IMT.[90]

Hegele et al.[94] studied SNPs of a promoter governing transcription of the *PCK1* gene. The −232G-containing promoter was associated with a doubling of diabetes compared with the −232C promoter, and in vitro showed marked increased in expression of its product (cytosolic phosphoenolpyruvate carboxykinase, PEPCK; EC 4.1.1.32).[95] They studied the relation of these polymorphisms to carotid IMT and 3D TPV. The subjects with the *PCK1*−232G/G genotype had more carotid IMT (0.80 ± 0.02 versus 0.73 ± 0.03 mm; $P = 0.007$) but less TPV (10 ± 9 versus 38 ± 13 mm^3; $P = 0.03$) than subjects with other genotypes.[94]

These distinct relationships of alleles to IMT versus plaque volume highlight the biological and genetic differences between IMT and plaque. These genetic differences have been reviewed by Pollex and Hegele.[96]

25.6 Evaluation of Response to Therapy

25.6.1 One-Dimensional Measurements: IMT and Plaque Thickness

IMT has been used in many studies to evaluate effects of therapies for hypertension and lipid-lowering. A meta-analysis of studies of antihypertensive drugs using IMT[97] indicated that newer therapies (ACE inhibitors, calcium channel antagonists, angiotensin receptor blockers, and alpha blockers) reduced IMT by 3 μm/year, given the same blood pressure reduction. Calcium channel antagonists reduced IMT compared to ACE inhibitors, at the same blood pressure, by 23 μm/year. However, in the ELSA study,[98] baseline IMT rather than change in IMT with lacidipine predicted cardiovascular events. Effects of lipid-lowering therapies on IMT have in part been confounded by whether the method included plaque thickness.

25.6.2 Two-Dimensional Measurements: Total Plaque Area

Few studies have used 2D plaque area to assess effects of therapy. The effect of vitamin therapy on progression of carotid plaque was studied by the Spence's group.[92,99] The Hackam et al. studied 101 patients with vascular disease, 51 with initial plasma levels of total homocysteine (tHcy) above, and 50 below 14 mmol/L. Among patients with a tHcy of 14 mmol/L or more, the rate of progression of plaque area was 21 ± 41 mm^2/year before vitamin therapy and −4.9 ± 24 mm^2/year after vitamin therapy ($P < 0.0001$). Among patients with a tHcy level of <14 mmol/L, the rate of progression of plaque was 13 ± 24 cm^2/year before vitamin therapy and −2.4 ± 29 mm^2/year after vitamin therapy ($P = 0.022$). The change in rate of progression was −15 ± 44 mm^2/year in those with tHcy <14 mmol/L, and −26.5 ± 46 mm^2/year above 14 mmol/L ($P = 0.20$).[92]

Ranke et al.[100] studied the effect of aspirin on carotid plaque progression.[100] Their approach was different from that of the Spence's; rather than analyzing total plaque area, they analyzed the effects of therapy on individual plaques; some of which progressed, while other plaques regressed. They showed that high-dose aspirin (900 mg/day) was associated with greater regression of plaques compared to low-dose aspirin (50 mg/day); they postulated that this was due to an anti-inflammatory effect rather than to an effect on platelet function.

25.6.3 Three-Dimensional Measurements: Plaque Volume, Vessel Wall Volume

Because plaques not only progress along the artery 2.4 times faster than they thicken,[43] but also progress and regress circumferentially, three-dimensional measurement of carotid plaque volume or vessel wall volume is even more sensitive to the effects of therapy than 2D plaque area, and much more sensitive than measuring only thickness: each dimension added, from IMT to plaque area, to plaque volume, reduces by an order of magnitude the sample size and duration required to study the effects of anti-atherosclerotic therapy.

In order to assess how quickly and in how small a sample size effects of therapy could be detected by 3D plaque volume, Ainsworth et al.[49] randomized patients with asymptomatic carotid stenosis to atorvastatin 80 mg versus placebo. The duration of the study was limited by ethical concerns; even though patients with known coronary artery disease were excluded because it would not have been ethical at that time to randomize them to placebo since patients with asymptomatic carotid stenosis have a high risk of coronary artery disease. The duration of the study was therefore limited to 3 months. Thirty-eight participants completed the study; 21 randomized to placebo and 17 to atorvastatin. Plaque volume progressed on placebo by 16.81 ± 74.10 mm^3, and regressed on atorvastatin by -90.25 ± 5.12 mm^3 ($P < 0.0001$).

Egger et al. described measurement of 3D vessel wall volume, which has some advantages over measurement of plaque volume, with regard to ease of measurement and reproducibility.[50] This method has been used to evaluate the effect of diet on progression of atherosclerosis and was also evaluated on the images from the atorvastatin study of Ainsworth et al., as described above. In 3 months, atorvastatin also significantly reduced vessel wall volume compared to placebo.[93]

A recent controversy regarding effects of ezetimibe on "atherosclerosis" is instructive. Ezetimibe, which blocks cholesterol absorption, lowers LDL cholesterol synergistically with statins. In a study of ezetimibe versus placebo added to simvastatin, there was no improvement of IMT with ezetimibe, despite lowering of serum LDL cholesterol.[101] In another study,[102] in which niacin or ezetimibe was added to statin, niacin was more effective than ezetimibe at improving carotid IMT. This study population was older, with already low levels of LDL cholesterol, and rather low levels of HDL cholesterol, which were markedly raised by niacin. These studies led to speculation that ezetimibe might be harmful to the arteries.[103] However, in the first study, the arteries were normal, with a mean IMT ~0.8 mm; normal arteries cannot be made "more normal." Furthermore, this speculation fails to recognize that carotid IMT is not really atherosclerosis.[26,104] The Spence and Hackam have reported that intensive lipid-lowering therapy guided by carotid imaging resulted in regression of atherosclerosis burden (assessed as total plaque area) in half of their patients attending vascular prevention clinics.[105] This regression led to a marked reduction in risk of stroke and myocardial infarction among patients with asymptomatic carotid stenosis.[106] Much of this improvement was due to administration of ezetimibe to patients whose plaque was progressing, despite already low levels of LDL.[107]

25.7 Summary and Conclusions

Carotid ultrasound measurement of IMT and plaque can be used for risk stratification, genetic research, and evaluation of new therapies. For management of patients, plaque measurement is more useful, because changes can be measured over shorter time frames than with IMT.

Carotid ultrasound phenotypes of atherosclerosis are biologically and genetically distinct. It is crucial in interpreting studies of IMT to understand whether the measurements excluded or included plaque thickness. Carotid plaque area is a stronger predictor of coronary events than IMT. For evaluation of new therapies, 3D ultrasound measurement of plaque volume and vessel wall volume permits much smaller sample sizes, and much shorter duration of follow-up, than studies relying on IMT. Furthermore, as plaque and IMT are biologically distinct, therapies directed against atherosclerosis should be evaluated by measurement of plaque.

References

1. Bonow RO, Smaha LA, Smith SC Jr, Mensah GA, Lenfant C. World Heart Day 2002: the international burden of cardiovascular disease: responding to the emerging global epidemic. *Circulation*. 2002;106(13):1602–1605.
2. D'Agostino RB Sr et al. General cardiovascular risk profile for use in primary care: the Framingham Heart study. *Circulation*. 2008;117(6):743–753.
3. Ridker PM, Paynter NP, Rifai N, Gaziano JM, Cook NR. C-reactive protein and parental history improve global cardiovascular risk prediction: the Reynolds Risk Score for men. *Circulation*. 2008;118(22):2243–2251, 4p.
4. Assmann G, Cullen P, Schulte H. Simple scoring scheme for calculating the risk of acute coronary events based on

the 10-year follow-up of the prospective cardiovascular Munster (PROCAM) study. *Circulation*. 2002;105(3): 310–315.
5. De BG et al. European guidelines on cardiovascular disease prevention in clinical practice: third joint task force of European and other societies on cardiovascular disease prevention in clinical practice (constituted by representatives of eight societies and by invited experts). *Eur J Cardiovasc Prev Rehabil*. 2003;10(4):S1-S10.
6. D'Agostino RB Sr et al. Executive summary of the third report of the National Cholesterol Education Program (NCEP) expert panel on detection, evaluation, and treatment of high blood cholesterol in adults (Adult Treatment Panel III) General cardiovascular risk profile for use in primary care: the Framingham Heart study. *JAMA*. 2001;285(19):2486–2497.
7. Hippisley-Cox J et al. Predicting cardiovascular risk in England and Wales: prospective derivation and validation of QRISK2. *BMJ*. 2008;336(7659):1475–1482.
8. Alexopoulos N, Raggi P. Calcification in atherosclerosis. *Nat Rev Cardiol*. 2009;6(11):681–688.
9. Romanens M et al. Imaging as a cardiovascular risk modifier in primary care patients using predictor models of the European and international atherosclerosis societies. *Kardiovaskuläre Medizin*. 2007;10:139–150.
10. Glagov S, Weisenberg E, Zarins CK, Stankunavicius R, Kolettis GJ. Compensatory enlargement of human atherosclerotic coronary arteries. *N Engl J Med*. 1987;316(22): 1371–1375.
11. Spence JD. Advances in atherosclerosis: new understanding based on endothelial function. In: Fisher M, Bogousslavsky J, eds. *Current Review of Cerebrovascular Disease*. 3rd ed. Philadelphia: Current Medicine; 1999:1–13.
12. Spence JD. The role of lipoprotein(a) in the formation of arterial plaques, stenoses and occlusions. *Can J Cardiol*. 2010;26:37A-40A.
13. Touboul PJ et al. Mannheim intima-media thickness consensus. *Cerebrovasc Dis*. 2004;18(4):346–349.
14. Adams MR et al. Carotid intimal-media thickness is only weakly correlated with the extent and severity of coronary artery disease. *Circulation*. 1995;92:2127–2134.
15. Kolodgie FD, Burke AP, Nakazawa G, Virmani R. Is pathologic intimal thickening the key to understanding early plaque progression in human atherosclerotic disease? *Arterioscler Thromb Vasc Biol*. 2007;27(5):986–989.
16. Spence JD, Hegele RA. Noninvasive phenotypes of atherosclerosis. *Arterioscler Thromb Vasc Biol*. 2004;24(11): e188-e189.
17. Al Shali K et al. Differences between carotid wall morphological phenotypes measured by ultrasound in one, two and three dimensions. *Atherosclerosis*. 2005;178(2):319–325.
18. Kolodgie FD et al. Intraplaque hemorrhage and progression of coronary atheroma. *N Engl J Med*. 2003;349(24): 2316–2325.
19. Spence JD, Norris J. Infection, inflammation, and atherosclerosis. *Stroke*. 2003;34(2):333–334.
20. Kolodgie FD et al. Lipoprotein-associated phospholipase A2 protein expression in the natural progression of human coronary atherosclerosis. *Arterioscler Thromb Vasc Biol*. 2006;26(11):2523–2529.
21. Virmani R et al. Atherosclerotic plaque progression and vulnerability to rupture: angiogenesis as a source of intraplaque hemorrhage. *Arterioscler Thromb Vasc Biol*. 2005;25(10):2054–2061.
22. Feric NT, Boffa MB, Johnston SM, Koschinsky ML. Apolipoprotein(a) inhibits the conversion of Glu-plasminogen to Lys-plasminogen: a novel mechanism for lipoprotein(a)-mediated inhibition of plasminogen activation. *J Thromb Haemost*. 2008;6(12):2113–2120.
23. Klein JH et al. Lipoprotein(a) is associated differentially with carotid stenosis, occlusion, and total plaque area. *Arterioscler Thromb Vasc Biol*. 2008;28:1851–1856.
24. O'Leary DH et al. Thickening of the carotid wall. A marker for atherosclerosis in the elderly? Cardiovascular Health Study Collaborative Research Group. *Stroke*. 1996;27(2): 224–231.
25. Spence JD, Hegele RA. Noninvasive phenotypes of atherosclerosis: similar windows but different views. *Stroke*. 2004;35:649–653.
26. Finn AV, Kolodgie FD, Virmani R. Correlation between carotid intimal/medial thickness and atherosclerosis: a point of view from pathology. *Arterioscler Thromb Vasc Biol*. 2010;30(2):177–181.
27. Clarkson TB, Bond MG, Bullock BC, McLaughlin KJ, Sawyer JK. A study of atherosclerosis regression in *Macaca mulatta*. V. Changes in abdominal aorta and carotid and coronary arteries from animals with atherosclerosis induced for 38 months and then regressed for 24 or 48 months at plasma cholesterol concentrations of 300 or 200 mg/dl. *Exp Mol Pathol*. 1984;41(1):96–118.
28. Bond MG, Wilmoth SK, Gardin JF, Barnes RW, Sawyer JK. Noninvasive assessment of atherosclerosis in nonhuman primates. *Adv Exp Med Biol*. 1985;183:189–195.
29. Bond MG, Wilmoth SK, Enevold GL, Strickland HL. Detection and monitoring of asymptomatic atherosclerosis in clinical trials. *Am J Med*. 1989;86(4A):33–36.
30. Baldassarre D et al. Measurement of carotid artery intima-media thickness in dyslipidemic patients increases the power of traditional risk factors to predict cardiovascular events. *Atherosclerosis*. 2007;191(2):403–408.
31. Bots ML, Hoes AW, Koudstaal PJ, Hofman A, Grobbee DE. Common carotid intima-media thickness and risk of stroke and myocardial infarction: the Rotterdam study. *Circulation*. 1997;96(5):1432–1437.
32. O'Leary DH et al. Carotid-artery intima and media thickness as a risk factor for myocardial infarction and stroke in older adults. *N Engl J Med*. 1999;340:14–22.
33. Chambless LE et al. Carotid wall thickness is predictive of incident clinical stroke: the Atherosclerosis Risk in Communities (ARIC) study. *Am J Epidemiol*. 2000;151 (5):478–487.
34. Ebrahim S et al. Carotid plaque, intima media thickness, cardiovascular risk factors, and prevalent cardiovascular disease in men and women: the British Regional Heart study. *Stroke*. 1999;30(4):841–850.
35. Lorenz MW, von Kegler J, Steinmetz H, Markus H, Sitzer M. Carotid intima-media thickening indicates a higher vascular risk across a wide range: prospective data from the Carotid Atherosclerosis Progression Study (CAPS). *Stroke*. 2006;37:87–92.

36. Simon A, Megnien JL, Chironi G. The value of carotid intima-media thickness for predicting cardiovascular risk. *Arterioscler Thromb Vasc Biol*. 2009;30(2):182–185.
37. Lorenz MW, Markus HS, Bots ML, Rosvall M, Sitzer M. Prediction of clinical cardiovascular events with carotid intima-media thickness: a systematic review and meta-analysis. *Circulation*. 2007;115:459–467.
38. Bots ML et al. Carotid intima-media thickness and coronary atherosclerosis: weak or strong relations? *Eur Heart J*. 2007;28(4):398–406.
39. Prati P et al. Carotid intima media thickness and plaques can predict the occurrence of ischemic cerebrovascular events. *Stroke*. 2008;39(9):2470–2476.
40. Brook RD et al. A negative carotid plaque area test is superior to other non-invasive atherosclerosis studies for reducing the likelihood of having significant coronary artery disease. *Arterioscler Thromb Vasc Biol*. 2006;26:656–662.
41. Chan SY et al. The prognostic importance of endothelial dysfunction and carotid atheroma burden in patients with coronary artery disease. *J Am Coll Cardiol*. 2003;42(6):1037–1043.
42. Rundek T et al. Carotid plaque, a subclinical precursor of vascular events: the Northern Manhattan study. *Neurology*. 2008;70:1200–1207.
43. Barnett PA, Spence JD, Manuck SB, Jennings JR. Psychological stress and the progression of carotid artery disease. *J Hypertens*. 1997;15(1):49–55.
44. Persson J et al. Noninvasive quantification of atherosclerotic lesions. Reproducibility of ultrasonographic measurement of arterial wall thickness and plaque size. *Arterioscler Thromb*. 1992;12(2):261–266.
45. Mancini GB, Abbott D, Kamimura C, Yeoh E. Validation of a new ultrasound method for the measurement of carotid artery intima medial thickness and plaque dimensions. *Can J Cardiol*. 2004;20(13):1355–1359.
46. Fosse E et al. Repeated visual and computer-assisted carotid plaque characterization in a longitudinal population-based ultrasound study: the Tromso study. *Ultrasound Med Biol*. 2006;32(1):3–11.
47. Spence JD et al. Carotid plaque area: a tool for targeting and evaluating vascular preventive therapy. *Stroke*. 2002;33:2916–2922.
48. Johnsen SH et al. Carotid atherosclerosis is a stronger predictor of myocardial infarction in women than in men: a 6-year follow-up study of 6226 persons: the Tromso study. *Stroke*. 2007;38(11):2873–2880.
49. Ainsworth CD et al. 3D ultrasound measurement of change in carotid plaque volume: a tool for rapid evaluation of new therapies. *Stroke*. 2005;36(9):1904–1909.
50. Egger M, Spence JD, Fenster A, Parraga G. Validation of 3D ultrasound vessel wall volume: an imaging phenotype of carotid atherosclerosis. *Ultrasound Med Biol*. 2007;33(6):905–914.
51. Kuller L et al. Prevalence of subclinical atherosclerosis and cardiovascular disease and association with risk factors in the Cardiovascular Health study. *Am J Epidemiol*. 1994;139(12):1164–1179.
52. Sharrett AR et al. Smoking, diabetes and blood cholesterol differ in their associations with subclinical atherosclerosis: the Multiethnic Study of Atherosclerosis (MESA). *Atherosclerosis*. 2005;186:441–447.
53. Heiss G et al. Carotid atherosclerosis measured by B-mode ultrasound in populations: associations with cardiovascular risk factors in the ARIC study. *Am J Epidemiol*. 1991;134(3):250–256.
54. Salonen R, Seppanen K, Rauramaa R, Salonen JT. Prevalence of carotid atherosclerosis and serum cholesterol levels in eastern Finland. *Arteriosclerosis*. 1988;8(6):788–792.
55. Fine-Edelstein JS et al. Precursors of extracranial carotid atherosclerosis in the Framingham study. *Neurology*. 1994;44(6):1046–1050.
56. Polak JF et al. Segment-specific associations of carotid intima-media thickness with cardiovascular risk factors: the Coronary Artery Risk Development in Young Adults (CARDIA) study. *Stroke*. 2010;41(1):9–15.
57. Malinow MR, Nieto FJ, Szklo M, Chambless LE, Bond G. Carotid artery intimal-medial wall thickening and plasma homocyst(e)ine in asymptomatic adults. The Atherosclerosis Risk in Communities study. *Circulation*. 1993;87(4):1107–1113.
58. Rundek T et al. The metabolic syndrome and subclinical carotid atherosclerosis: the northern Manhattan study. *J Cardiometab Syndr*. 2007;2(1):24–29.
59. Elkind MS et al. Interleukin-2 levels are associated with carotid artery intima-media thickness. *Atherosclerosis*. 2005;180(1):181–187.
60. Melnick SL et al. Past infection by *Chlamydia pneumoniae* strain TWAR and asymptomatic carotid atherosclerosis. Atherosclerosis Risk in Communities (ARIC) study investigators. *Am J Med*. 1993;5:499–504.
61. Johnsen SH, Mathiesen EB. Carotid plaque compared with intima-media thickness as a predictor of coronary and cerebrovascular disease. *Curr Cardiol Rep*. 2009;11(1):21–27.
62. Spence JD et al. Plasma homocyst(e)ine, but not MTHFR genotype, is associated with variation in carotid plaque area. *Stroke*. 1999;30:969–973.
63. Hegele RA, Ban MR, Anderson CM, Spence JD. Infection-susceptibility alleles of mannose-binding lectin are associated with increased carotid plaque area. *J Investig Med*. 2003;48:198–202.
64. Nilsson TK et al. Quantitative measurement of carotid atherosclerosis in relation to levels of von Willebrand factor and fibrinolytic variables in plasma – a 2-year follow-up study. *J Cardiovasc Risk*. 2002;9(4):215–221.
65. Bhavsar S et al. Keloid scarring, but not Dupuytren's contracture, is associated with unexplained carotid atherosclerosis. *Clin Invest Med*. 2009;32(2):E95-E102.
66. Kronborg J et al. Proinsulin:insulin and insulin:glucose ratios as predictors of carotid plaque growth: a population-based 7 year follow-up of the Tromso study. *Diabetologia*. 2007;50(8):1607–1614.
67. Johnsen SH et al. Elevated high-density lipoprotein cholesterol levels are protective against plaque progression: a follow-up study of 1952 persons with carotid atherosclerosis the Tromso study. *Circulation*. 2005;112(4):498–504.
68. Halvorsen DS, Johnsen SH, Mathiesen EB, Njolstad I. The association between inflammatory markers and carotid

atherosclerosis is sex dependent: the Tromso study. *Cerebrovasc Dis*. 2009;27(4):392–397.
69. Pollex RL et al. A comparison of ultrasound measurements to assess carotid atherosclerosis development in subjects with and without type 2 diabetes. *Cardiovasc Ultrasound*. 2005;3:15.
70. Lange LA et al. Heritability of carotid artery intima-medial thickness in type 2 diabetes. *Stroke*. 2002;33(7):1876–1881.
71. Juo SH et al. Genetic and environmental contributions to carotid intima-media thickness and obesity phenotypes in the Northern Manhattan Family study. *Stroke*. 2004;35(10):2243–2247.
72. Xiang AH et al. Heritability of subclinical atherosclerosis in Latino families ascertained through a hypertensive parent. *Arterioscler Thromb Vasc Biol*. 2002;22(5):843–848.
73. Fox CS et al. Genetic and environmental contributions to atherosclerosis phenotypes in men and women: heritability of carotid intima-media thickness in the Framingham Heart study. *Stroke*. 2003;34(2):397–401.
74. Chen YC et al. Carotid intima-media thickness (cIMT) cosegregates with blood pressure and renal function in hypertensive Hispanic families. *Atherosclerosis*. 2008;198(1):160–165.
75. Manolio TA, Boerwinkle E, O'Donnell CJ, Wilson AF. Genetics of ultrasonographic carotid atherosclerosis. *Arterioscler Thromb Vasc Biol*. 2004;24(9):1567–1577.
76. Rundek T et al. Carotid intima-media thickness is associated with allelic variants of stromelysin-1, interleukin-6, and hepatic lipase genes: the Northern Manhattan Prospective Cohort study. *Stroke*. 2002;33(5):1420–1423.
77. O'Donnell CJ et al. Genome-wide association study for subclinical atherosclerosis in major arterial territories in the NHLBI's Framingham Heart study. *BMC Med Genet*. 2007;8(suppl 1):S4.
78. Fox CS et al. Genomewide linkage analysis for internal carotid artery intimal medial thickness: evidence for linkage to chromosome 12. *Am J Hum Genet*. 2004;74(2):253–261.
79. Wang D et al. A genome-wide scan for carotid artery intima-media thickness: the Mexican-American Coronary Artery Disease family study. *Stroke*. 2005;36(3):540–545.
80. Sacco RL et al. Heritability and linkage analysis for carotid intima-media thickness: the family study of stroke risk and carotid atherosclerosis. *Stroke*. 2009;40(7):2307–2312.
81. Pollex RL, Hegele R. Genetic determinants of carotid ultrasound traits. *Curr Atheroscler Rep*. 2006;8(3):206–215.
82. Yasuda H et al. Association of single nucleotide polymorphisms in endothelin family genes with the progression of atherosclerosis in patients with essential hypertension. *J Hum Hypertens*. 2007;21(11):883–892.
83. Lehtinen AB et al. Association of alpha2-Heremans-Schmid glycoprotein polymorphisms with subclinical atherosclerosis. *J Clin Endocrinol Metab*. 2007;92(1):345–352.
84. Pankow JS et al. Familial aggregation and genome-wide linkage analysis of carotid artery plaque: the NHLBI family heart study. *Hum Hered*. 2004;57(2):80–89.
85. Spence JD, Ban MR, Hegele RA. Lipoprotein lipase (LPL) gene variation and progression of carotid artery plaque. *Stroke*. 2003;34:1178–1182.
86. Spence JD, Barnett PA, Bulman DE, Hegele RA. An approach to ascertain probands with a non traditional risk factor for carotid atherosclerosis. *Atherosclerosis*. 1999;144:429–434.
87. Spence JD. Technology Insight: ultrasound measurement of carotid plaque – patient management, genetic research, and therapy evaluation. *Nat Clin Pract Neurol*. 2006;2(11):611–619.
88. Schork NJ, Nath SK, Fallin D, Chakravarti A. Linkage disequilibrium analysis of biallelic DNA markers, human. *Am J Hum Genet*. 2000;67(5):1208–1218.
89. Malo N, Libiger O, Schork NJ. Accommodating linkage disequilibrium in genetic-association analyses via ridge regression. *Am J Hum Genet*. 2008;82(2):375–385.
90. Al Shali KZ et al. Genetic variation in PPARG encoding peroxisome proliferator-activated receptor gamma associated with carotid atherosclerosis. *Stroke*. 2004;35(9):2036–2040.
91. Bots ML, Evans GW, Riley WA, Grobbee DE. Carotid intima-media thickness measurements in intervention studies: design options, progression rates, and sample size considerations: a point of view. *Stroke*. 2003;34(12):2985–2994.
92. Hackam DG, Peterson JC, Spence JD. What level of plasma homocyst(e)ine should be treated? Effects of vitamin therapy on progression of carotid atherosclerosis in patients with homocyst(e)ine levels above and below 14 mol/L. *Am J Hypertens*. 2000;13:105–110.
93. Krasinski A, Chiu B, Spence JD, Fenster A, Parraga G. Three-dimensional ultrasound quantification of intensive statin treatment of carotid atherosclerosis. *Ultrasound Med Biol*. 2009;35:1763–1772.
94. Hegele RA et al. Disparate associations of a functional promoter polymorphism in PCK1 with carotid wall ultrasound traits. *Stroke*. 2005;36(12):2566–2570.
95. Cao H et al. Promoter polymorphism in PCK1 (phosphoenolpyruvate carboxykinase gene) associated with type 2 diabetes mellitus. *J Clin Endocrinol Metab*. 2004;89(2):898–903.
96. Pollex RL, Hegele RA. Genetic determinants of carotid ultrasound traits. *Curr Atheroscler Rep*. 2006;8:206–215.
97. Wang JG et al. Carotid intima-media thickness and antihypertensive treatment: a meta-analysis of randomized controlled trials. *Stroke*. 2006;37(7):1933–1940.
98. Zanchetti A et al. Baseline values but not treatment-induced changes in carotid intima-media thickness predict incident cardiovascular events in treated hypertensive patients: findings in the European Lacidipine Study on Atherosclerosis (ELSA). *Circulation*. 2009;120(12):1084–1090.
99. Peterson JC, Spence JD. Vitamins and progression of atherosclerosis in hyper-homocyst(e)inaemia [letter]. *Lancet*. 1998;351(9098):263.
100. Ranke C, Hecker H, Creutzig A, Alexander K. Dose-dependent effect of aspirin on carotid atherosclerosis. *Circulation*. 1993;87:1873–1879.
101. Kastelein JJ et al. Simvastatin with or without ezetimibe in familial hypercholesterolemia. *N Engl J Med*. 2008;358(14):1431–1443.
102. Taylor AJ et al. Extended-release niacin or ezetimibe and carotid intima-media thickness. *N Engl J Med*. 2009;361(22):2113–2122.

103. Spence JD. Is carotid intima-media thickness a reliable clinical predictor? *Mayo Clin Proc*. 2008;83(11):1299–1300.
104. Spence JD. The importance of distinguishing between diffuse carotid intima medial thickening and focal plaque. *Can J Cardiol*. 2008;24(suppl C):61C-64C.
105. Spence JD, Hackam DG. Treating arteries instead of risk factors: a paradigm change in management of atherosclerosis. *Stroke*. 2010;41(6):1193–1199.
106. Spence JD et al. Effects of intensive medical therapy on microemboli and cardiovascular risk in asymptomatic carotid stenosis. *Arch Neurol*. 2010;67(2):180–186.
107. Spence JD. Adding ezetimibe to statin halts progression of carotid plaque. *Basic Clin Pharmacol Toxicol*. 2010;107 (suppl 1):2194.

26. Arterial Wall, Plaque Measurements, Biomarkers, and Metabolic Syndrome: Results from the Gothenburg Studies

Björn O. Fagerberg

26.1 Introduction

The rising incidence of obesity, accompanied by the cluster of cardiovascular risk factors constituting the metabolic syndrome and type 2 diabetes, is a serious threat to public health by increasing the risk of cardiovascular diseases such as myocardial infarction and stroke. The major underlying cause is atherosclerosis, a silent process that in general takes many years to develop into overt clinical disease. Today we know that both the initiation of atherosclerotic lesions and the progression to vulnerable plaques leading to complicated lesions and symptomatic cardiovascular disease are closely linked to inflammation. The rupture-prone vulnerable plaque, with its large lipid core, thin fibrous cap, and abundance of inflammatory cells, is not only the most common atherosclerotic lesion leading to acute coronary syndromes but also occurring as a frequent cause of symptomatic carotid disease. Atherosclerosis is to a large extent a manifestation of aging, and as an example, the majority of subjects above the age of 70 years have carotid plaques. Most of these will never cause any cardiovascular disease. Consequently, there is a need to find methods to identify plaques at high cardiovascular risk and, in the end, to develop therapies to stabilize such plaques. Methods for identification of high-risk plaques include imaging techniques and circulating biomarkers. A growing body of data indicates that plaque vulnerability may be a widespread phenomenon within the individual and that it is not limited to a singular plaque in an individual artery.

Ultrasound can be used to study the vascular wall in the carotid and femoral arteries (Chaps. 22–25). The overall objective was to use this technique to examine the occurrence and development of atherosclerotic disease in population samples of men and women with the metabolic syndrome and type 2 diabetes, to examine underlying mechanisms, and to search for biomarkers of atherosclerosis. Biomarker is defined as a characteristic that is objectively measured and evaluated as an indicator of normal biologic processes, pathogenic processes, or responses to a therapeutic intervention (Chap. 27). The author also conducted a randomized, controlled multi-factorial intervention study in a cohort at high cardiovascular risk, and the experiences from that study have provided insight in the relationship between clinical events and noninvasively assessed intima-media thickness and plaque occurrence.

26.2 Gothenburg Studies

26.2.1 Atherosclerosis in Insulin Resistance (AIR) Study

The Atherosclerosis in Insulin Resistance (AIR) study is a prospective cohort study with re-examinations after 3 and 9 years.[1] Prior to the design of this study, a population-based pilot study was undertaken to explore the occurrence of subclinical carotid atherosclerosis in different age strata in the population, showing that among men at age 55–60 years, carotid plaques were

B.O. Fagerberg
Wallenberg Laboratory for Cardiovascular Research,
Department of Molecular and Clinical Medicine,
Institute of Medicine, Sahlgrenska University Hospital,
Gothenburg, Sweden

increasing in prevalence with still relatively few subjects being on cardiovascular medication. Hence, male sex and age 58 years were chosen for the AIR study that started as a population-based cross-sectional study with stratified sampling.[1,2] Exclusion criteria were cardiovascular or other clinically overt disease, or treatment with cardiovascular drugs that might modify the measurements in the study. Stratified sampling was used to increase the power to examine if insulin resistance was associated with carotid atherosclerosis by using the following approach: In all 852 screened men, insulin sensitivity was estimated by using an algorithm that was based on body mass index and fasting glucose. This algorithm was validated by using the euglycemic, hyperinsulinemic clamp method. All screened men were divided by insulin sensitivity in quintiles, and all men in the lowest and highest quintiles, as well as a random sample of 20% of the men in quintiles 2–4, were included in the study ($n = 391$). The rationale for using this approach was to accumulate more data points in the two ends of the distribution of insulin sensitivity. The underlying power calculation was based on a previous pilot study where the author's group was first to show that insulin resistance, assessed with the gold standard clamp technique, was associated with increased carotid intima-media thickness (IMT).[3]

As mentioned above, re-examinations were performed in the AIR study after 3 and 9 years. At the 3-year re-examination, 237 men with known diabetes, hypertension, or cardiovascular disease who were identified at the screening examination were also included.[4] National registers were used to obtain information on vitality status, causes of death, and diagnoses for in-hospital care.

26.2.2 Diabetes, Impaired Glucose Tolerance in Women, and Atherosclerosis (DIWA) Study

The Diabetes, Impaired Glucose Tolerance in Women and Atherosclerosis (DIWA) study is a prospective cohort study with a re-examination after 6 years. In this study, the author's group invited all 64-year-old women born during the same years as the men included in the AIR study.[5] More than 2,500 women were screened with oral glucose tolerance tests, which were repeated if the glucose tolerance was abnormal. The definitions of diabetes and impaired glucose tolerance were based on World Health Organization (WHO) criteria. The women with diabetes were included, as well as similarly sized random samples of those with impaired glucose tolerance and normal glucose tolerance, resulting in a total group of 612 women. Type 1 diabetes was defined as very early onset insulin-treated diabetes or elevated serum levels of glutamic acid decarboxylase antibodies. National registers were used to obtain the same information on vitality status and diagnoses as was obtained in the AIR study.

26.2.3 Risk Factor Intervention (RIS) Study

This was a randomized, open, parallel group trial examining the effect of multiple risk factor intervention compared with usual care with a mean follow-up time of almost 7 years that ran between 1987 and 1995.[6] Treated hypertensive men, aged 50–72 years, with at least one of the following: serum cholesterol 5.5 mmol/L or higher, diabetes, and smoking were randomized to an intervention group ($n = 253$) or a usual care group ($n = 255$). The specific intervention was based on group meetings to encourage lipid lower diet, weight reduction, improved diabetes control, and smoking cessation. Additional medication was used if necessary to reach treatment goals. Relative to the usual care group, the special intervention lowered mean-in-trial low-density lipoprotein (LDL) cholesterol, triglycerides, blood glucose, body weight, and proportion of smokers. Sixty-four patients (25.1%) died in the usual care group and 41 patients (16.2%) in the intervention group ($p = 0.016$). There was a 44% reduction in risk of cardiovascular death ($p = 0.021$).

A randomized sample of 164 patients was also included in ultrasound examinations of the right carotid artery at entry and during follow-up. After almost 7 years follow-up, baseline and follow-up examinations were available in 97 patients.[7]

26.2.4 Ultrasound Methods

The carotid arteries were examined bilaterally in the AIR and DIWA studies using established techniques with measurements as described in Chap. 10. In brief, the ultrasound images were analyzed in an automated analyzing system based on automatic detection of the echo structures in the image but with the option to make manual corrections by the operator. IMT was defined as the distance from the leading edge of the lumen–intima interface of the far wall to the leading edge of the media–adventitia interface of the far wall. The measurement of IMT was made in two separate segments: along a 10-mm-long segment in the common carotid artery and along a 10-mm-long segment distal to the beginning of the carotid artery bulb (i.e., where the echoes from the near and far walls are no longer parallel). The computer program calculated the mean thickness of the intima–media complex of the far wall. Lumen diameter was defined by the distance between the leading edges of the intima–lumen interface of the near wall and the lumen–intima interface of the far wall. A composite measure of IMT in the carotid artery was calculated as the mean IMT in the common carotid artery (CCA) and the carotid bulb from the right and left side. The inter-observer variability for measurement of IMT in the CCA and the carotid artery bulb was 5.3% and 6.0%, respectively, and 7.6% for the composite measure.

A plaque was defined as a distinct area with an IMT 50% greater than neighboring sites (visually judged). This analysis included plaques in the near wall as well as the far wall in both the carotid arteries. The computer program was used to calculate the area of each plaque. Assessment of plaque echogenicity was based on the version of classification proposed by Gray-Weale et al., modified in the present study to two classes: (1) dominantly or substantially echolucent plaques, or (2) dominantly or uniformly echogenic lesions. Recently a new semi-automated method to assess plaque echogenicity has been developed with a new feature, percentage white, which seems to provide other information than the established gray scale median.[8]

The right femoral artery was also examined in each subject using similar techniques.[2]

26.3 Intima-Media Thickness, Plaque Occurrence, Intervention Effects, and Cardiovascular Disease

26.3.1 Observational Study

It is well known that carotid IMT is an independent predictor of cardiovascular disease. In regards to plaque occurrence, the author's group already found in the RIS study that prevalent carotid plaques were associated with increased cardiovascular risk.[6] In the AIR study, occurrence of plaques in either the carotid or femoral arteries was associated with statistically significant twofold increases in odds ratio for cardiovascular disease during 10 years of follow-up, independently of other risk factors.[9] Plaque burden, calculated as the number of arteries with plaques, was accompanied by a parallel increase in cardiovascular risk.

26.3.2 Interventional Study

In the RIS study, good quality carotid ultrasound examinations were available at study entry in 142 patients, and re-examinations were performed after 3 years ($n = 119$) and 7 years ($n = 97$).[7] After almost 7 years of follow-up, total mortality was lower in the comprehensive risk factor intervention group ($n = 69$) compared with the usual care group ($n = 73$) (13% vs 29%; 95% confidence interval [CI] for relative risk = 0.19–0.91). However, there was no difference in carotid IMT progression during follow-up between the two groups. The explanation to this unexpected finding was that patients with plaques more often survived and were available for examination in the intervention group (Fig. 26.1) and that patients with plaques at baseline had much larger increase in IMT over time than those with no plaques (Fig. 26.2). Among patients with no plaques, there was no difference in treatment effects between intervention and usual care (Fig. 26.1). The author's group hypothesized that the comprehensive intervention may have stabilized vulnerable plaques, being the mechanism underlying the reduced cardiovascular morbidity. In a post hoc analysis, they observed that intervention only reduced cardiovascular risk among patients with echolucent carotid plaques and not in those with echogenic plaques when comparisons were made with the usual care group.[10] However, this finding remains to be confirmed in a larger study with pre-calculated sample size.

The interpretation of the author's group was that in high-risk populations, long-term studies with changes of carotid IMT as a surrogate endpoint of atherosclerosis may be misleading. The reason is that many patients with potentially large increases in IMT are lost to follow-up due to death or severe morbidity. Furthermore, treatment leading to stabilizing of vulnerable plaques may reduce cardiovascular risk without necessarily affecting intima-media thickness.

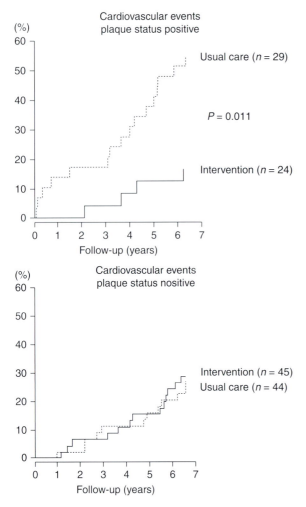

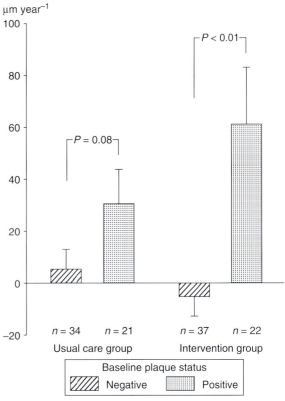

Fig. 26.1 Effects of a comprehensive cardiovascular risk factor intervention compared with usual care on incidence of cardiovascular events in middle-aged men with treated hypertension and at least one further risk factor (hypercholesterolemia, diabetes, smoking). *Upper panel*: Patients with carotid plaques at entry. *Lower panel*: Patients with no plaques at entry (Reprinted with permission from Agewall et al.[7])

Fig. 26.2 Effects of a comprehensive cardiovascular risk factor intervention compared with usual care on progression rate of intima-media thickness in the common carotid artery after 3 years of follow-up in patients subdivided by plaque status at baseline (Reprinted with permission from Agewall et al.[7])

26.4 Arterial Wall, Insulin Resistance, Metabolic Syndrome, Impaired Glucose Tolerance, and Type 2 Diabetes

26.4.1 Insulin Resistance

Insulin resistance is defined by an abnormally low response of target cells to insulin, and this phenomenon is associated with the cluster of cardiovascular risk factors that has lead to the concept of the metabolic syndrome. It has been suggested that insulin resistance is the central component in the metabolic syndrome and that it may have pro-atherogenic effects directly or indirectly by promoting the development of cardiovascular risk factors such as dyslipidemia and diabetes. The author's group measured insulin sensitivity in a randomly selected subgroup of men in the AIR study ($n = 104$) by using the best available method, i.e., the euglycemic, hyperinsulinemic clamp and adjusted the glucose infusion rate for fat-free mass. They found that insulin sensitivity showed a weak negative correlation to common carotid artery IMT and no associations with mean carotid bulb IMT or common femoral artery IMT.[2] The association between insulin sensitivity and common carotid IMT did not remain after adjustment for other covariates.

Insulin resistance is accompanied by an increased demand of insulin, resulting in hyperinsulinemia, as long as the pancreatic beta-cells have the ability to increase the insulin production. The beta-cells co-secrete insulin metabolites such as C-peptide, intact proinsulin, and intermediates together with specific insulin, and this co-secretion increases in parallel with increasing insulin resistance. Hence, both hyperinsulinemia and increased circulating levels for C-peptide and proinsulin are associated with insulin resistance. It has been suggested that proinsulin has a more pro-atherogenic effect than specific insulin. In the AIR study, we found in a cross-sectional analysis that fasting plasma proinsulin and C-peptide were associated with common carotid artery IMT, independent of conventional risk factors for atherosclerosis.[1] The multicollinearity between the insulin peptides and propeptides makes it difficult to clarify the exact role of each peptide. However, a later finding in the AIR showing that serum proinsulin was more directly related to small LDL particle size than insulin lend support to the concept that proinsulin is more pro-atherogenic[11] (see below).

In a follow-up study of the AIR cohort, cardiovascular events occurring during 10 years of follow-up were obtained from official registers.[9] The analyses showed that baseline insulin levels were not associated with these future cardiovascular events.

26.4.2 Metabolic Syndrome

In the AIR study, the author's group examined the association between the metabolic syndrome according to the definition proposed by WHO and carotid atherosclerosis. It was found that the occurrence of the metabolic syndrome was associated with increased IMT in the common carotid arteries and in the carotid bulbs.[12] Similar findings were also made in the femoral arteries.[12]

In the 3-year follow-up study of the AIR cohort, it was found that more than 10% of the men had the metabolic syndrome (WHO definition) both at baseline and after 3 years, and this was associated with increasing carotid artery IMT.[13]

26.4.3 Impaired Glucose Tolerance

Impaired glucose tolerance is a consequence of insulin resistance and is also related to increased risk of developing type 2 diabetes. Subjects with impaired glucose tolerance are at increased cardiovascular risk, but it is not clear if hyperglycemia per se causes atherosclerosis or if impaired glucose tolerance is merely a predictor of future type 2 diabetes and the associated high cardiovascular risk. Only a few of previously published studies, examining if impaired glucose tolerance is associated with increased carotid IMT, have shown statistically significant differences.[14] This lack of consistent findings may be explained by the low precision of oral glucose tolerance test (OGTT) to diagnose impaired glucose tolerance. It is well known that half of subjects with impaired glucose tolerance at a first OGTT have normal glucose tolerance at a repeated test. In a population-based DIWA study, the author's group sharpened the diagnosis of impaired glucose tolerance by demanding two repeated oral glucose tolerance tests showing impaired glucose tolerance. Still, they did not find that in comparison with women with normal glucose tolerance, those with impaired glucose tolerance had larger carotid IMT or increased occurrence of carotid plaques.[15] The author's group also performed a meta-analysis of the 12 available studies in the literature and found that overall impaired glucose tolerance is associated with a 0.030-mm-larger (95% confidence interval 0.012–0.048) carotid IMT than those with normal glucose tolerance.[15]

26.4.4 Type 2 Diabetes

Type 2 diabetes is an established strong risk factor for macrovascular atherosclerotic disease. The author's group performed a meta-analysis of 21 published or unpublished studies showing that overall type 2 diabetes is associated with a 0.134-mm-larger (95% CI 0.123–0.144) carotid artery IMT than those with normal glucose tolerance.[14] In the DIWA study, 10% of the screened women suffered from diabetes, and half of those were detected by the screening procedure.[5] Carotid IMT was, in comparison with the normal control group, enlarged in both women with newly detected and previously known diabetes.[16] In the AIR study, the author's group observed that there was a linear trend in carotid IMT, ranging from men with normal glucose tolerance, to those with newly detected, and to those with known type 2 diabetes.[4] Similar findings were obtained for common carotid IMT and carotid bulb IMT. Similarly, the occurrence of moderate to large plaques gradually increased across the same groups.

26.5 Arterial Wall, Lipids, Oxidation, and Metabolic Syndrome

The typical dyslipidemia associated with the metabolic syndrome and type 2 diabetes is characterized by hypertriglyceridemia and low circulating high-density lipoprotein (HDL) cholesterol levels. During the last decade, a further insight has been that this dyslipidemia, related to the metabolic syndrome, is also characterized by an abundance of small LDL particles. Small LDL particles seem to be associated with an increased risk of cardiovascular disease. It has been hypothesized that small LDL particles may be easily retained and oxidized in the arterial wall and that oxidized LDL may be an important antigen, triggering the inflammatory response in atherosclerosis. Serum level of apolipoproteinA-I (apoA-I) is a measure of the number of anti-atherogenic HDL particles in the circulation as each such particle is covered by one apoA-I molecule. Correspondingly, each very low-density lipoprotein, intermediate-density lipoprotein, and LDL particle is covered by an apolipoproteinB (apoB) molecule. Hence, the serum concentration of apoB is a measure of the total number of pro-atherogenic lipoprotein particles. Consequently, the apoB/apoA-I ratio is a composite measure of all pro- and anti-atherogenic lipoproteins, and it has been shown to be superior to LDL cholesterol in predicting future cardiovascular disease. It has been unclear whether it also predicts subclinical carotid atherosclerosis.

A further aim in the AIR and DIWA studies has been to examine if subclinical, ultrasound-assessed atherosclerosis in the carotid and femoral arteries can be explained by the mechanisms that have been postulated in the hypothesis described above and if the apoB/apoA-I ratio can be used as a marker of atherosclerosis.

26.5.1 Arterial Wall, ApolipoproteinB/ApolipoproteinA-I Ratio, and the Metabolic Syndrome

Among men in the cross-sectional part of the AIR study, apolipoproteinB (apoB) correlated positively and apolipoproteinA-I (apoA-I) negatively to common carotid artery IMT.[2] In the 3-year prospective part of the AIR study, the men with apolipoproteinB/apolipoproteinA-I ratio (apoB/apoA-I) above the first tertile (0.73) had a 20-μm-higher (95% CI 7–30 μm) annual increase in IMT compared with those below this apoB/apoA-I level.[17] A similar multivariate analysis performed after 9 years of follow-up showed that an apoB/apoA-I ratio above 0.74 was associated with a significantly higher annual increase in composite carotid IMT than those below this level (5.1 μm, 95% CI 1.5–8.6 μm).[18] Analyses of AIR data performed after 6.6 years of follow-up of clinical events showed in addition that apoB/apoA-I ratio >0.9 predicted cardiovascular disease in contrast to LDL cholesterol levels.[19] After a follow-up time of 9 years in the AIR study, it was found that apoB/apoA-I ratio equal or >0.63 at baseline was associated with a threefold increase in risk of peripheral occlusive arterial disease.[20] Among women in the DIWA study, apoB/apoA-I was associated with enlarged IMT in the common carotid artery, the carotid bulb, and the femoral artery, in a cross-sectional analysis.[21]

In the AIR study, the apoB/A-I ratio showed strong and consistent correlations to the major components of the metabolic syndrome: body mass index, waist-to-hip ratio, insulin, serum triglycerides, diastolic blood pressure, and reversely to HDL cholesterol and LDL particle size.[17] Circulating oxidized LDL levels (see below) correlated positively to apoB and negatively to apoA-I.[22] With an increasing occurrence of factors constituting the metabolic syndrome in a subject, there was a parallel increase in the apoB/apoA-I ratio. In subjects with an apoB/apoA-I ratio above 0.90, two-thirds of the men had metabolic syndrome according to several of the most used definitions. In men with apoB/apoA-I ratio equal or <0.90, only one-third fulfilled the criteria for the metabolic syndrome.[17]

26.5.2 Arterial Wall, Small LDL Particles, and Metabolic Syndrome

In the AIR study, the author's group measured LDL particle size on commercially available nondenaturing polyacrylamide gradient gels and found that LDL particle size correlated negatively to common carotid artery IMT, carotid bulb IMT, and femoral artery IMT.[12] In addition, both in the carotid and femoral arteries, the occurrence of plaques was inversely associated with LDL particle size.[12]

In the AIR study, the men with metabolic syndrome had on average much smaller LDL particles than those without the metabolic syndrome.[12] Small LDL particle size was associated with components constituting the metabolic syndrome such as hyperinsulinemia, hypertriglyceridemia, low HDL concentration, hypertension, and obesity.[12] Insulin resistance, as assessed by clamp technique, was also associated with small LDL particle size.[11] Serum proinsulin was more directly related to small LDL particle size than insulin.[11] LDL particle size showed high negative correlations with oxidized LDL (see below).

26.5.3 Arterial Wall, Oxidized LDL, and the Metabolic Syndrome

Inflammation plays an important role in atherosclerosis, and retained oxidized LDL particles may be a key antigen in this inflammatory response, which largely drives the atherosclerotic process. Oxidized LDL (ox-LDL) as well as antibodies against epitopes of ox-LDL have been found in human plasma and in atherosclerotic lesions. Now it is possible to measure one type of circulating ox-LDL. The author's group used enzyme-linked immunosorbent assay (ELISA) with a specific monoclonal antibody mAb-4E6 directed towards a conformational epitope in the apolipoproteinB-100 moiety of LDL.[23]

In a cross-sectional analysis of the AIR-study, the author's group observed that increasing circulating ox-LDL concentrations were associated with increasing intima-media thickness in the common carotid artery, carotid bulb, and femoral artery.[23] Ox-LDL and LDL cholesterol were independently associated with occurrence of atherosclerotic plaques in the carotid or femoral arteries taken together.

In the prospective part of the AIR study with 3 years of follow-up, plasma ox-LDL concentrations were associated with the annual change in carotid IMT.[24] This was independent of other cardiovascular risk factors. Plasma ox-LDL but not LDL cholesterol levels at baseline were associated with the occurrence and size of carotid plaques after 3 years.[24] Only ox-LDL and systolic blood pressure at baseline were associated with plaque status at the follow-up examination. Neither serum concentrations of LDL, or HDL cholesterol, or triglycerides showed such associations.

The degree of echogenicity has emerged as an alternative modality in the ultrasound assessment of plaques. High echogenicity is found in fibrotic and calcified carotid plaques, whereas echolucent plaques contain more hemorrhage, inflammation, and lipids. The latter type of plaque is related to the concept of plaque vulnerability, and the author's group and others have observed that plaque echolucency is associated with cardiovascular events.[10,25] In a cross-sectional analysis of AIR data, that author's group has reported that a higher frequency of echolucent carotid plaques was observed with increasing levels of ox-LDL and systolic blood pressure.[26] In a multiple logistic regression analysis, ox-LDL was independently associated with echolucent plaques.

As also shown in the AIR study, the metabolic syndrome was characterized by high plasma ox-LDL levels, which correlated to many factors in the metabolic syndrome: central obesity, plasma insulin, serum concentrations of triglycerides, apoB, and reversely LDL particle size, HDL cholesterol, and apoA-I.[22] Circulating ox-LDL also correlated to cell adhesion molecule and high-sensitivity C-reactive protein (hsCRP) in the AIR study.[23,27]

26.6 Arterial Wall, Inflammation, and the Metabolic Syndrome

The inflammatory pathways in both the fast, unspecific response and the slower but more specific adaptive response play important roles in atherosclerosis. Oxidation and other modifications of LDL particles result in antigens evoking an immunological response. Acute phase reactants, representing the innate inflammatory response, are mainly produced by the liver after stimulation of pro-inflammatory cytokines that are expressed by inflammatory cells in plaques.

26.6.1 Arterial Wall, Autoantibodies to LDL, and the Metabolic Syndrome

The concept that oxidized LDL (Ox-LDL) plays an important role in atherosclerosis is supported by the observation that T-cell clones responsive to Ox-LDL have been isolated from human atherosclerotic lesions. The author's group used ELISA to measure circulating concentrations of IgG and IgM antibodies to Ox-LDL in the baseline examination of the AIR cohort.[28] The results showed that IgG antibodies to Ox-LDL correlated to common carotid artery IMT, but this was not independently of other covariates such as measures of obesity, abdominal obesity, blood pressure, serum triglycerides, and smoking. Circulating Ox-LDL antibody titers were associated with hsCRP, independent of other factors.[29]

26.6.2 Arterial Wall, hsCRP, and the Metabolic Syndrome

High-sensitivity C-reactive protein (hsCRP) has emerged as a predictor of cardiovascular disease, although the underlying mechanisms are largely unknown. In the AIR cohort, there were no associations between C-reactive protein (CRP) and ultrasound-assessed atherosclerosis in the carotid arteries. This was examined both in the cross-sectional analyses at baseline, as well as after 3 years, and in the longitudinal part of the study with almost 9 years of follow-up.[4,18,29] Neither was the occurrence of echolucent carotid plaques associated with hsCRP.[26] However, hsCRP was associated with IMT and plaque occurrence in the femoral artery in the AIR cohort,[29] but this seems largely mediated by smoking. As a contrast, among women in the DIWA study, hsCRP was associated with carotid bulb IMT.

CRP was associated with the metabolic syndrome and the factors constituting the syndrome: insulin resistance, total body fat mass, truncal fat mass, plasma insulin and insulin metabolites, hypertriclyceridema, LDL lipid size, low HDL cholesterol, and smoking.[30] Both newly detected and established diabetes were accompanied by increased hsCRP in relation to healthy control men.[4] hsCRP was also associated with circulating antibody titers to Ox-LDL.[29]

26.6.3 Arterial Wall, Cell Adhesion Molecules, and the Metabolic Syndrome

Recruitment of inflammatory cells from the circulation and their transendothelial migration is an important step in the atherosclerotic process. This mechanism is largely mediated by cellular adhesion molecules, which are expressed in the vascular endothelium and on leucocytes in response to inflammatory stimuli. Intercellular adhesion molecule-1 (ICAM-1), but not vascular cellular adhesion molecule-1 (VCAM-1), has been associated with cardiovascular disease.

The author's group examined serum concentrations of those cell adhesion molecules in the AIR cohort and found that, at baseline, ICAM-1 was associated with the occurrence of atherosclerotic plaques in the carotid and femoral arteries.[31] VCAM-1 showed no such associations. After almost 7 years of follow-up, serum levels at baseline of both ICAM-1 and VCAM-1 differed between those who experienced cardiovascular events and those who did not.[32] Using these cut-off levels, it was found that both ICAM-1 and VCAM-1 were associated by an increased occurrence of plaques in the femoral, but not in the carotid arteries, at the baseline examination.[32]

Serum ICAM-1, but not VCAM-I concentrations, correlated to circulating oxidized LDL, independently of covariates such as smoking, LDL cholesterol, and apolipoproteinA-I and B.[27] Serum ICAM-1 was also associated with hsCRP.[31]

26.6.4 Arterial Wall, Other Factors in Relation to Inflammation, and Metabolic Syndrome

Metalloproteinase 9 (MMP-9) is an extracellular matrix-degrading enzyme that is expressed by inflammatory cells in atherosclerotic lesions. This molecule seems to play an important role in plaque rupture by proteolytic weakening of the cap. Circulating levels of MMP-9 have been associated with cardiovascular disease. At the 3-year follow-up examination of the AIR cohort, previously screened men with known cardiovascular risk factors and prevalent diseases were also included in addition to the subjects with varying degrees of insulin sensitivity. All these men were included in a study when plasma MMP-9 levels were related to ultrasound-assessed atherosclerosis.[33] Prior to that, a methodological study of pre-analytical sources of variations was performed, showing that plasma samples were requested in order to avoid the very high variability accompanying the use of serum.[33] It was found that plasma MMP-9 levels were associated with femoral artery IMT and plaque occurrence, whereas no such findings were made for the carotid arteries.[33]

Plasma MMP-9 levels were not related to obesity per se and showed weak associations with the metabolic syndrome and circulating insulin.[34] Plasma MMP-9 covariated with white blood cell count and hsCRP.

Adiponectin is produced by adipocytes and is associated with anti-inflammatory effects, improved insulin sensitivity, and anti-atherosclerotic mechanisms. Serum adiponectin levels are lower among patients with diabetes mellitus, obesity, and metabolic syndrome compared to healthy subjects. In the DIWA cohort, low serum adiponectin levels were associated with increased carotid artery IMT and several risk factors for cardiovascular disease, mainly type 2 diabetes and those constituting the metabolic syndrome.[35,36] In a subgroup of men from the AIR study who had undergone a euglycemic, hyperinsulinemic clamp examination, adiponectin was associated with the metabolic syndrome and related factors, including LDL particle size.[37] There was an inverse relationship between adiponectin and hsCRP.[38] The close covariability between circulating adiponectin and the factors constituting the metabolic syndrome made it impossible to find whether adiponectin was independently associated with carotid artery IMT in this cross-sectional study.

Circulating CD44 is a cell surface glycoprotein expressed on inflammatory and vascular cells. CD44 is involved in inflammation, immunoactivation, and also in atherosclerosis by mechanisms such as adhesion of activated lymphocytes to inflamed endothelium, and cell activation. CD44 deficiency reduces the development of atherosclerosis in mice. Macrophages from subjects with atherosclerosis were found to have elevated levels of CD44 transcript and protein in comparison with macrophages from healthy subjects.[39] Soluble CD44 is believed to be generated through cleavage of cell surface CD44 or alternative splicing. The author's group examined whether soluble CD44, in similarity with other pro-inflammatory cytokines such as ICAM-1, were associated with cardiovascular risk factors or atherosclerosis. Men and women from the AIR and DIWA studies were included in a cross-sectional study, which showed that soluble CD44 levels were higher among women than men. There were, however, no findings indicating that soluble CD44 was associated with either any cardiovascular risk factors or carotid artery IMT.[40]

26.7 Conclusions

The author's group has examined the development of atherosclerotic disease in population based cohorts of middle-aged men and women with varying degrees of obesity, insulin sensitivity, and glucose tolerance in cross-sectional and prospective studies lasting for up to 10 years. They have also performed a randomized controlled multi-factorial risk factor intervention study with a follow-up of 7 years, examining the use of carotid IMT and plaque occurrence as surrogate variables for cardiovascular disease. The results can be summarized as follows.

Ultrasound-assessed plaques in the carotid and femoral arteries predicted cardiovascular events in men during up to 10 years follow-up, and the risk increased with total plaque burden.

The risk factor intervention study in men at high cardiovascular risk showed that mortality and clinical events decreased without any corresponding change in carotid IMT. This was explained by the fact that patients with plaques more often survived in the intervention group and that patients with plaques at baseline had much larger increase in IMT over time than those with no plaques. Tentatively, the intervention may have stabilized plaques as the major treatment effect since only patients with echolucent plaques showed significant effects of such treatment. Further studies are needed to examine this issue.

Type 2 diabetes and metabolic syndrome were associated with increases in carotid IMT and plaque occurrence. Impaired glucose tolerance was associated with a small increase in carotid IMT in a meta-analysis of published studies. Insulin resistance and hyperinsulinemia were not strong determinants of carotid atherosclerosis in the AIR cohort.

The apoB/apoA-I ratio was closely associated with the factors constituting the metabolic syndrome and is a valuable biomarker of both increases in carotid artery IMT in men and future cardiovascular events.

Circulating ox-LDL was associated with IMT and plaque status in both cross-sectional and prospective studies, indicating a causal effect. Ox-LDL was also related to plaque echolucency. The consistent association between the metabolic syndrome, small LDL particle size, ox-LDL concentrations, and subclinical atherosclerosis lend support to the concept of retention and oxidation of LDL-particles as important mechanisms in the atherosclerotic process occurring in this category of subjects.

Among cell adhesion molecules, ICAM-1 was more consistently associated with cardiovascular events, subclinical atherosclerosis, and cardiovascular risk factors than VCAM-1 among men. The data also indicate that the role of endothelial adhesion molecules is more discernable as regards atherosclerosis in the femoral compared with the carotid arteries.

Despite consistent associations between hsCRP and most of the components constituting the metabolic syndrome and other cardiovascular risk factors such as smoking, hsCRP was not associated with carotid IMT in either cross-sectional or prospective studies among the men in the AIR study. In women, however, hsCRP was associated with carotid IMT.

Circulating plasma MMP-9 must be measured in plasma, and not in serum, to avoid large pre-analytical variation. Plasma MMP-9 was associated with femoral artery IMT and plaque occurrence, whereas no such findings were made for the carotid arteries. Plasma MMP-9 was weakly associated with circulating insulin.

In women, low serum adiponectin levels were associated with increased carotid artery IMT and several risk factors for cardiovascular disease, mainly type 2 diabetes and those constituting the metabolic syndrome[12]. In men, adiponectin was associated with the metabolic syndrome and related factors, including LDL particle size.

The overall experience is that the ultrasound technique is a very effective method to use in longitudinal epidemiological and intervention studies in order to better understand the complicated etiology of atherosclerosis.

References

1. Bokemark L, Wikstrand J, Wedel H, Fagerberg B. Insulin, insulin propeptides and intima-media thickness in the carotid artery in 58-year-old clinically healthy men. The Atherosclerosis and Insulin Resistance study (AIR). *Diabet Med*. 2002;19:144–151.
2. Bokemark L et al. Insulin resistance and intima-media thickness in the carotid and femoral arteries in clinically healthy 58-year-old men. The Atherosclerosis and Insulin Resistance Study (AIR). *J Intern Med*. 2001;249:59–67.
3. Agewall S et al. Carotid artery wall intima-media thickness is associated with insulin-mediated glucose disposal in men at high and low coronary risk. *Stroke*. 1995;26:956–960.
4. Sigurdardottir V, Fagerberg B, Hulthe J. Preclinical atherosclerosis and inflammation in 61-year old men with newly diagnosed diabetes and established diabetes. *Diabetes Care*. 2004;27:880–884.
5. Brohall G, Behre CJ, Hulthe J, Wikstrand J, Fagerberg B. Prevalence of diabetes mellitus and impaired glucose tolerance in 64-year old Swedish women. Experiences of using repeated oral glucose tolerance tests. *Diabetes Care*. 2006;29:363–367.
6. Fagerberg B et al. Mortality rates in treated hypertensive men with additional risk factors are high but can be reduced. A randomized intervention study. *Am J Hypertens*. 1998;11:14–22.
7. Agewall S, Fagerberg B, Schmidt C, Wendelhag I, Wikstrand J. Multiple risk factor intervention in high risk hypertensive men: comparison of ultrasound intima-media thickness and clinical outcome during six years of follow-up. *J Intern Med*. 2001;249:305–314.
8. Prahl U et al. Percentage white: a new feature for ultrasound classification of plaque echogenicity in carotid artery atherosclerosis. *Ultrasound Med Biol*. 2010;36(2):218–226.
9. Davidsson L, Fagerberg B, Bergström G, Schmidt C. Ultrasound-assessed plaque occurrence in the carotid and femoral arteries are independent predictors of cardiovascular events in middle-aged men during 10 years of follow-up. *Atherosclerosis*. 2010;209(2):469–473.
10. Schmidt C, Fagerberg B, Wikstrand J, Hulthe J, RIS Study Group. Multiple risk factor intervention reduces cardiovascular risk in hypertensive patients with echolucent plaques in the carotid artery. *J Intern Med*. 2003;253:430–438.
11. Fagerberg B, Hulthe J, Bokemark L, Wikstrand J. Low density lipoprotein particle size, insulin resistance and proinsulin in a population sample of 58-year old men. *Metabolism*. 2001;50:120–124.
12. Hulthe J, Bokemark L, Wikstrand J, Fagerberg B. The metabolic syndrome, LDL particle size and atherosclerosis. The Atherosclerosis and Insulin Resistance study (AIR). *Arterioscler Thromb Vasc Biol*. 2000;20:2140–2147.
13. Wallenfeldt K, Hulthe J, Fagerberg B. The metabolic syndrome in middle-aged men according to different definitions and related changes in carotid artery IMT during 3 years of follow-up. *J Intern Med*. 2005;258:28–37.
14. Brohall G, Odén A, Fagerberg B. Carotid artery intima-media thickness in patients with type 2 diabetes mellitus and impaired glucose tolerance: a systematic review. *Diabet Med*. 2006;23:609–616.
15. Brohall G et al. Association between impaired glucose tolerance and carotid atherosclerosis: a study in 64-year-old women and a meta-analysis. *Nutr Metab Cardiovasc Dis*. 2009;19:327–333.
16. Brohall G. *Atherosclerosis in 64-Year Old Women with Diabetes Mellitus and Impaired Glucose Tolerance* [Ph.D. thesis]. Gothenburg: Gothenburg University; 2007.
17. Wallenfeldt K, Bokemark L, Wikstrand J, Hulthe J, Fagerberg B. Apolipoprotein B/apolipoprotein A-I in relation to the metabolic syndrome and change in carotid artery

intima-media thickness during three years in middle-aged men. *Stroke*. 2004;35:2248–2252.
18. Schmidt C, Wikstrand J. High apoB/apoA-I ratio is associated with increased progression rate of carotid artery intima-media thickness in clinically healthy 58-year-old men: experiences from very long-term follow-up in the AIR study. *Atherosclerosis*. 2009;205:284–289.
19. Schmidt C, Fagerberg B, Wikstrand J, Hulthe J. ApoB/ApoA-I ratio is related to femoral artery plaques and is predictive for future cardiovascular events in healthy men. *Atherosclerosis*. 2006;189:178–185.
20. Johansson L, Schmidt C. Increased apoB/apoA-I ratio is predictive of peripheral arterial disease in initially healthy 58-year-old men during 8.9 years of follow-up. *Angiology*. 2009;60:539–545.
21. Schmidt C, Fagerberg B. ApoB/apoA-I ratio is related to femoral artery plaques in 64-year-old women also in cases with low LDL cholesterol. *Atherosclerosis*. 2007;196:817–822.
22. Sigurdardottir V, Fagerberg B, Hulthe J. Circulating oxidized low–density lipoprotein (LDL) is associated with risk factors of the metabolic syndrome and LDL size in clinically healthy 58-year-old (AIR study). *J Intern Med*. 2002;252:440–447.
23. Hulthe J, Fagerberg B. Circulating oxidized LDL is associated with subclinical atherosclerosis development and inflammatory cytokines (AIR Study). *Arterioscler Thromb Vasc Biol*. 2002;22:1162–1167.
24. Wallenfeldt K, Wikstrand J, Fagerberg B, Hulthe J. Oxidized low density lipoprotein in plasma is a prognostic marker of subclinical atherosclerosis development in clinically healthy men. *J Intern Med*. 2004;256:413–420.
25. Schmidt C, Fagerberg B, Hulthe J. Non-stenotic echolucent ultrasound-assessed femoral artery plaques are predictive for future cardiovascular events in middle-aged men. *Atherosclerosis*. 2005;181:125–130.
26. Sigurdardottir V, Fagerberg B, Wikstrand J, Schmidt C, Hulthe J. Circulating oxidized LDL is associated with the occurrence of echolucent plaques in the carotid artery in 61-year-old men. *Scand J Clin Lab Invest*. 2008;68:292–297.
27. Hulthe J, Fagerberg B. Circulating oxidized LDL is associated with increased levels of cell-adhesion molecules in clinically healthy 58-year old men (AIR study). *Med Sci Monit*. 2002;8:CR148-CR152.
28. Hulthe J, Bokemark L, Fagerberg B. Antibodies to oxidized LDL in relation to intima-media thickness in carotid arteries in 58-year-old subjectively clinically healthy men. *Arterioscler Thromb Vasc Biol*. 2001;21:101–107.
29. Hulthe J, Wikstrand J, Fagerberg B. Relationship between C-reactive protein and intima media thickness in the femoral arteries and to antibodies against oxidized low density lipoprotein in men: the Atherosclerosis and Insulin Resistance (AIR) study. *Clin Sci*. 2001;100:371–378.
30. Fagerberg B, Behre CJ, Wikstrand J, Hulten LM, Hulthe J. C-reactive protein and tumor necrosis factor-alpha in relation to insulin-mediated glucose uptake, smoking and atherosclerosis. *Scand J Clin Lab Invest*. 2008;18:1–8.
31. Hulthe J, Wikstrand J, Mattsson-Hultén L, Fagerberg B. Circulating ICAM-1 (intercellular cell-adhesion molecule 1) is associated with early stages of atherosclerosis development and with inflammatory cytokines in healthy 58-year-old men (AIR study). *Clin Sci*. 2002;103:23–129.
32. Schmidt C, Hulthe J, Fagerberg B. Baseline ICAM-1 and VCAM-1 are increased in initially healthy middle-aged men who develop cardiovascular disease during 6.6 years of follow-up. *Angiology*. 2009;60:108–114.
33. Olson FJ et al. Circulating matrix metalloproteinase 9 levels in relation to sampling methods, femoral and carotid atherosclerosis. *J Intern Med*. 2008;263:626–635.
34. Gummesson A et al. Adipose tissue is not an important source for matrix metalloproteinase-9 in the circulation. *Scand J Clin Lab Invest*. 2009;69:636–642.
35. Behre CJ, Brohall G, Hulthe J, Wikstrand J, Fagerberg B. Are serum adiponectin concentrations in a population sample of 64 year-old Caucasian women with varying glucose tolerance associated with ultrasound assessed atherosclerosis? *J Intern Med*. 2006;260:238–244.
36. Behre CJ, Brohall G, Hulthe J, Fagerberg B. Serum adiponectin in a population sample of 64-year-old women in relation to glucose tolerance, family history of diabetes, autoimmunity, insulin sensitivity, C-peptide, and inflammation. *Metabolism*. 2006;55:188–194.
37. Hulthe J, Hultén L, Fagerberg B. Low adipocyte-derived plasma protein adiponectin concentrations are associated with the metabolic syndrome and small dense low-density lipoprotein particles: atherosclerosis and insulin resistance study. *Metabolism*. 2003;52:1612–1614.
38. Behre CJ, Fagerberg B, Mattsson Hultén L, Hulthe J. The reciprocal association of adipocytokines with insulin resistance and CRP in clinically healthy men. *Metabolism*. 2005;54:439–444.
39. Hagg D et al. Augmented levels of CD44 in macrophages from atherosclerotic subjects: a possible IL-6-CD44 feedback loop? *Atherosclerosis*. 2007;190:291–297.
40. Sjöberg S, Svensson L, Hulthe J, Fagerberg B, Krettek A. Circulating sCD44 is higher among women than men and is not associated with cardiovascular risk factors or subclinical atherosclerosis. *Metabolism*. 2005;54:139–141.

Novel Biomarkers and Subclinical Atherosclerosis

27

Andrie G. Panayiotou, Debra Ann Hoppensteadt, Andrew Nicolaides, and Jawed Fareed

27.1 Introduction

More than 50 years ago, William Kannel[1] first popularized the concept of cardiovascular disease risk factors for clinicians and clinical epidemiologists.[2] The word "factor" derives from Latin (meaning doer) which implies causality. However, from the time of its initial use in 1961, the term "risk factor" included both causal and predictive factors. Typically, risk factors are surrogates for deeper causes (and better predictors) of cardiovascular disease and atherosclerosis.[3]

More recently, the National Institutes of Health (NIH) Definition Working Group established definitions for both risk factor and biomarker in order to help end their arbitrary use.[4] According to their definition, a *Risk Factor* is "an environmental, behavioral, or biologic factor confirmed by temporal sequence, usually in longitudinal studies, which if present directly increases the probability of a disease occurring, and if absent or removed reduces the probability. Risk factors are part of the causal chain, or expose the host to the causal chain. Once disease occurs, removal of a risk factor may not result in a cure." Likewise, a *Biomarker* is "a characteristic that is objectively measured and evaluated as an indicator of normal biological processes, pathogenic processes, or pharmacological responses to a therapeutic intervention." Changes in the biomarker that result from therapy are expected to reflect changes in clinically meaningful end points.[5]

Genes that are consistently overexpressed or suppressed in a certain clinical context may also be considered as biomarkers. A genetic marker, therefore, is defined as variations in the DNA (genetic polymorphisms) that, alone or in combination with others, are associated with a specific disease phenotype. Markers whose presence (or absence) confers a high level of probability of disease (high predictive value) would be most useful as diagnostic tools, predictors of prognosis or response to therapy. Even markers with modest effects may provide us with important clues to disease pathophysiology or suggest new ways of therapeutic intervention.[6]

Most clinical and biochemical risk factors identified thus far and that are associated with the development and progression of atherosclerosis and are used in daily practice have demonstrated a consistent dose–response effect and are substantiated by large series of consistent prospective studies in large populations, usually in association with a clinical end point. The relationship between conventional risk factors and subclinical atherosclerosis has been dealt with in Chaps. 22 and 23.

In recent years, a number of ultrasonic measurements of the arterial wall, described in

---

A.G. Panayiotou (✉)
Cyprus International institute of Environmental and Public Health, Cyprus University of Technology, Limassol

D.A. Hoppensteadt
Department of Pathology, Loyola University Chicago, Maywood, IL, USA

A. Nicolaides
Imperial College and Vascular Screening and Diagnostic Centre, London, UK

J. Fareed
Department of Pathology and Pharmacology, Loyola University Medical Center, Maywood, IL, USA

previous chapters, have been increasingly used in research on subclinical atherosclerosis and as surrogate end points for cardiovascular disease. These measurements have provided us with the ability to study early subclinical atherosclerosis in vivo. In addition, a plethora of biochemical and genetic biomarkers have recently emerged. Existing evidence on their associations with intima-media thickness (IMT) and atherosclerotic plaques (both carotid and femoral) will be discussed in this chapter (and summarized in Tables 27.1 and 27.2). They are presented in alphabetic order. Where relevant, results are presented from the authors' own data derived from the Cyprus Epidemiological Study in which ultrasonic arterial measurements involved common carotid IMT (IMTcc) and maximum IMT (IMTmax), which includes plaques in the carotid bifurcation and plaque features (presence, thickness, area, and echodensity).

27.2 Heritability of Ultrasonic Features

Before conducting genetic studies for IMT and plaque features, it is important to know how much of the variability seen is due to heritable factors (i.e., genes) and therefore whether use of such intermediate phenotypes is valid in genetic studies. Heritability (H^2) can be calculated by statistical packages, such as SOLAR (Sequential Oligogenic Linkage Analysis Routines, Southwest Foundation for Biomedical Research, San Antonio, Texas, USA), that use information from families. Twin studies are a classic example of obtaining such information, although difficult to recruit for.

The heritability of carotid IMT has been calculated in several studies and has been found to range considerably according to the population used. In the Vietnam Era Twin Registry, the heritability of carotid IMT in 98 male pairs was found to be 59% after adjusting for coronary risk factors.[34] However, when twin pairs cannot be ascertained, information from families (siblings and parents) can be used, such as in the case of the Framingham Offspring cohort where the multivariable-adjusted heritability of the internal carotid artery (ICA) IMT was estimated to be 35% and of the common carotid artery (CCA) IMT, 38%.[35] In other population-based studies, the adjusted heritability of IMT has been found to range from 21% in American Indians[36] to 35% in a Dutch isolate population,[37] to 61% in an unspecified German population selected through a parent with atherosclerosis,[38] to 65% in Caribbean Hispanics.[39] The variation in the heritability reported for IMT is most probably attributable to variations in the methodology and site of IMT measurements as well as to selection of study populations. Using data from pedigrees of Cypriot origin, the authors estimated the adjusted heritability of IMT to be around 36%, whereas the heritability of the presence of plaques in any of the four bifurcations scanned was 32% and that of plaque area, 39%. In other studies, IMT was shown to have the strongest heritability compared to vascular wall mass (27%) or arterial stiffness (24%)[36]; in the authors' study, plaque area in all four bifurcations and plaque presence had an equally large percentage variability attributable to genetic factors.

These results suggest that ultrasonic features, such as IMT and plaque measurements, can be used as intermediate phenotypes in genetic studies, which may help provide information on the pathophysiology of early and subclinical atherosclerosis.

27.3 Biomarkers and Subclinical Atherosclerosis

27.3.1 Angiotensinogen-Converting Enzyme (ACE) I/D Polymorphism

Angiotensinogen-converting enzyme (ACE) converts inactive angiotensin I to the vasoconstrictor angiotensin II, and it also inactivates the vasodilator bradykinin, leading to increased vascular tone, vascular smooth muscle cell growth, neointimal proliferation, and extracellular matrix deposition.[40,41] Genetic variants associated with higher ACE activity may be related with increased carotid wall thickness and plaque formation. An example of such genetic variability is the insertion (I) or deletion (D) of a 287-bp alu-repeat sequence in intron 16 of the Angiotensinogen-Converting gene, associated with substantially different levels of plasma ACE activity in a codominant fashion, with DD homozygotes having the highest levels.[42] Results from association studies for the I/D polymorphism have proved, however, to be inconsistent, with the majority of studies showing no association,[9,43-46] whereas several show higher carotid IMT and plaque frequency in DD homozygotes or D allele carriers. Only two studies reported possible interactions of the D allele in relation to IMT in that IMT increased more steeply with increasing systolic

Table 27.1 Characteristics and results from a number of selected studies on the association of biomarkers and atherosclerosis based on ultrasonographically assessed carotid intima-media thickness (*CIMT*)

First author	Prevalent condition	Number	Age (mean or range)	Association present	Association absent
Hulthe[7]	Asymptomatic (only men)	391	58	CRP (femoral IMT)	CRP (carotid IMT)
Brohall[8]	Asymptomatic (only women)	393	64		Impaired glucose tolerance (IGT)
Mannami[9]	Asymptomatic	4,031	30–68		*ACE* (I/D)
Wallenfeldt[10]	None (only men)	326	58	Ox-LDL (change in IMT)	LDL (change in IMT)
Langlois[11]	None	2,524	35–55		Ox-LDL (carotid IMT or femoral IMT)
Furuki[12]	Asymptomatic	575	62.6	Plasma ADMA levels at baseline (IMT) Plasma ADMA levels (predictor of IMT after 6-year follow-up)	
Orbe[13]	Asymptomatic	400	54.3	sMMP10	sMMP1, sMMP9
Olson[14]	Asymptomatic (only men)	473	61	Plasma total and active MMP9 (femoral IMT)	
Juonala[15]	None	879	10.9 at baseline and 31.9 at follow-up	ApoA1, apoB/apoA1 (IMT in adulthood)	ApoB (IMT in adulthood)
Schmidt[16]	Asymptomatic (only men)	305	58	ApoB/apoA1, serum insulin (IMT progression rate after 8.9 years)	hsCRP, LDL particle size, BP, smoking, fasting glucose, insulin
Paramo[17]	Asymptomatic	519	55.5	Fibrinogen	CRP
Chen[18]	Asymptomatic	810	>39	MetS (in women)	MetS (in men)
Andersson[19]	Asymptomatic	1,016	70	BMI, TNF-α (IM-GSM)	
Lind[20]	Asymptomatic	1,016	70	HDL-C, fasting glucose, Ox-LDL	LDL-C, TG, Hcy
Schmidt[21]	Asymptomatic (only women)	646	64	Serum apoB/apoA1 (IMT and femoral IMT)	
Maas[22]	None	2,958	58	ADMA levels (ICA/bulb IMT)	ADMA levels (IMTcc)
Panayiotou[23]	None	767	60.5	Serum apoB/A1 ratio	
Slooter[24]	None	5,401	>55	*ApoE* (E2/E3/E4) genotype	
Panayiotou[25]	None	767	60.5	Serum homocysteine	*MTHFR* (677C > T)
Jerrard-Dunne[26]	None	1,000	50–65	IL-6 (−174C > G) (IMTcc) in those drinking >30 g/day of alcohol	
Kronenberg[27]	None	826	40–79	Plasma Lp(a)	

blood pressure and age in D allele carriers than in II homozygotes.[47] Another study showed an association of the DD genotype with echolucent (high-risk) plaques despite lack of association with IMT or stenosis in diabetic subjects.[45] Of interest are the findings by Balkestein et al., reporting that the number of *ACE* D alleles was associated with increased IMT of the femoral, but not of the carotid, arteries and that the effect was confined to carriers of two other polymorphisms in the aldosterone synthase and α-adducin genes.[48] A meta-analysis of 46 studies (32,715 subjects) in Caucasians concluded that although the I/D polymorphism affects plasma ACE activity, it is not associated with neither blood pressure nor increased risk of myocardial infarction, ischemic heart disease, or ischemic cerebrovascular disease.[49] The authors' own data support the lack of an association between the *ACE* I/D polymorphism and subclinical atherosclerosis.

Table 27.2 Characteristics and results from a number of selected studies on the association of biomarkers and subclinical atherosclerosis based on ultrasonographically assessed carotid and femoral plaques

First author	Prevalent condition	Number	Age (mean or range)	Association present	Association absent
Hulthe[7]	Asymptomatic (only men)	391	58		CRP (femoral plaques)
Halvorsen[28]	Asymptomatic	5,341	66	Fibrinogen (carotid plaques)	CRP
Brohall[8]	Asymptomatic (only women)	393	64		Impaired glucose tolerance (IGT) (carotid plaques)
Sigurdardottir[29]	Asymptomatic (only men)	513	61	Ox-LDL and smoking (echolucent femoral plaques)	CRP
Wallenfeldt[10]	None (only men)	326	58	Ox-LDL (number and size of carotid plaques at follow-up)	LDL (number and size of carotid plaques at follow-up)
Langlois[11]	None	2,524	35–55	Ox-LDL (femoral plaques)	
Zureik[30]	Free of CHD (only men)	238	56.5	sTIMP-1 (carotid plaques)	
Orbe[13]	Asymptomatic	400	54.3	sMMP10	sMMP1, sMMP9
Olson[14]	Asymptomatic (only men)	473	61	Plasma total and active MMP9 (femoral plaques)	
Lembo[31]	Hypertension	375	22–78	eNOS (Gly298Asp) (carotid plaques)	
Kronenberg[27]	None	826	40–79	Plasma Lp(a) at baseline (development of new carotid plaques at 5-year follow-up)	
Schmidt[32]	Asymptomatic (only men)	391	58	ApoB/apoA1 (femoral plaques)	
Schmidt[21]	Asymptomatic (only women)	646	64	ApoB/apoA1 (femoral plaques)	ApoB/apoA1 (carotid plaques)
Chen[18]	Asymptomatic	810	>39	CRP (in men) (carotid plaques)	CRP (in women) (carotid plaques)
Ebrahim[33]	Asymptomatic	800	56–77	Fibrinogen (carotid plaques)	

27.3.2 Asymmetric Dimethylarginine (ADMA)

Asymmetric dimethylarginine (ADMA) is one of the most important endogenous inhibitors of nitric oxide synthase (NOS), derived from the catabolism of proteins containing methylated arginine residues. When these proteins undergo hydrolysis, their methylated arginine residues are released and excreted in the urine. This explains the increase in plasma ADMA levels in patients with renal insufficiency. The major metabolic pathway for ADMA is regulated by dimethylarginine dimethylaminohydrolase (DDAH). Both isoforms of DDAH have been found in every cell type examined. ADMA is constantly being produced in the course of normal protein turnover, and its production is balanced by its metabolism by DDAH. Accordingly, inhibition of DDAH activity causes a gradual accumulation of ADMA sufficient to induce vasoconstriction.[50]

The hypothesis that endogenous ADMA accelerates atherosclerosis originated from animal studies that showed that supplemental dietary arginine enhanced NO synthesis in the rabbit aorta.[51] There are, some, similar data from humans. In two Japanese studies, in subjects with varying levels of risk factors[52] and without overt cardiovascular disease,[53] plasma levels of ADMA were shown to be an independent determinant of IMT of the carotid artery. In a prospective second study with 6-year follow-up, which was better suited to test any temporal effect, ADMA levels were also found to be the only independent predictor of IMT progression in addition to hyperuricacidemia.[12] ADMA was also associated with cerebral small vessel disease in a small case–control study.[54]

More evidence comes from the Framingham study which reported an association between higher plasma ADMA concentrations and greater ICA/bulb IMT, but not for common carotid IMT (IMTcc).[22] Maas et al. argue that their data are consistent with the notion that ADMA promotes subclinical atherosclerosis in a site-specific manner, with a greater proatherogenic influence at known vulnerable sites in the arterial tree. Other studies looking at ADMA levels are mostly in patients with renal disease, but on the cumulative results seem to point toward a positive role of ADMA for atherosclerosis development and progression.

27.3.3 ApoB/apoA1 Ratio

Apolipoprotein A1 (apoA1) is the major protein constituent of plasma HDL (high-density lipoprotein) and plays a crucial role in lipid transport and metabolism, whereas apolipoprotein B100 (apoB), a large, hydrophobic protein synthesized in the liver, comprises 30–40% of the protein content of plasma very-low-density lipoprotein (VLDL) and more than 95% of the protein in low-density lipoprotein (LDL). apoB is required for the assembly and secretion of apoB-containing lipoproteins (i.e., LDL) which transport hydrophobic lipids, cholesteryl ester, and triglycerides in their cores.[55] Thus, apoB serum concentration is a measure of the number of LDL, intermediate-density lipoprotein, and VLDL athero-sclerotic particles,[56] and studies have shown that apoB is a better candidate for risk parameter than non-HDL cholesterol for identifying subgroups of individuals with elevated cardiovascular risk as well as predicting IMT.[57]

The ratio of apoB/apoA1 is, therefore, a better measure of proatherogenic versus antiatherogenic particles and would be a more informative marker for atherosclerosis than the commonly used TChol/HDL-C (high-density lipoprotein cholesterol) ratio. Most studies have correlated apoB/apoA1 ratio with late atherosclerosis, mainly clinical events, but the authors and others have suggested that the apoB/apoA1 ratio is also associated with subclinical atherosclerosis and may be a key factor in the early formation of stable and unstable plaques. In the Prospective Investigation of the Vasculature in Uppsala Seniors (PIVUS) study, apoB/apoA1 ratio was associated with increased plaque size in the carotids,[58] whereas in the Cyprus study, it was associated with hypoechoic (echolucent) plaques in both carotid and femoral arteries.[23] In the Gothenburg cohort, the apoB/apoA1 ratio was associated with carotid and femoral IMT, but not with presence of carotid plaques in 64-year-old women with various degrees of glucose intolerance[21] and with atherosclerosis in the femoral artery in 58-year-old men[32] (Chap. 26). In the prospective follow-up of the Gothenburg study, apoB/apoA1 ratio at baseline was found to be independently associated with a more rapid increase in carotid IMT after 3 years of follow-up[59] as well as after 8.9 years of follow-up.[16] This finding, coupled with reports for an association between apoB/apoA1 ratio in childhood and increased CIMT in adulthood in young Finns,[15] further strengthens the evidence toward a causal role of apoB/apoA1 in subclinical atherosclerosis and of its use in risk determination.

27.3.4 Apolipoprotein E (apoE) E2/E3/E4 Polymorphism

A much-studied gene in relation to carotid atherosclerosis is the apolipoprotein E (*apoE*) gene, which codes for apolipoprotein E. Three common alleles (designated E2, E3, and E4) produce 3 protein isoforms differing at amino acid positions 112 and 158 on the mature polypeptide. The most common allele, E3, produces the apoE E3 isoform with cysteine at position 112 and arginine at position 158, whereas the least common E2 allele produces the apoE E2 isoform with cysteine at both positions and apoE E4 has arginine at both positions. Apolipoprotein levels vary by allele, with the E2 allele associated with higher and E4 associated with lower plasma apoE levels.[60] In the Rotterdam study, which measured common carotid IMT and plaque presence in 5,401 subjects, the *apoE* E2/E3 genotype was found to be associated with a lower IMT and fewer plaques than the E3/E3 genotype. The E4 allele was not found to be an important risk factor for carotid atherosclerosis.[24] The same was true for another population study of middle-aged men, with the E2 allele being associated with lower carotid IMT.[61] In the Perth Carotid Ultrasound Disease Assessment Study (CUDAS), apoE genotype was found to be associated with carotid plaque formation, with the risk increasing from E2 to E4, but not with IMT, and the associations were sex-dependent.[62] In the Cyprus study, apoE genotype was strongly associated with presence of any plaque in four bifurcations scanned, with an adjusted OR of 2.76 ($P = 0.005$) for the E2/E2, E2/E3 versus E3/E3, E3/E4 genotypes. A recent meta-analysis of 22 studies on apoE genotype and carotid IMT presents positive evidence of an association and suggests a possible specific association with large-artery ischemic stroke.[63]

27.3.5 CD40 Ligand

CD40 ligand (CD40L) is a transmembrane protein, member of the tumor necrosis factor (TNF) superfamily, expressed on the surface of lymphocytes as well as on the cells of the vascular system, such as endothelial cells, smooth muscle cells (SMCs), and macrophages.[64] It exists in two forms: the 39-kDa, cell-associated form and the soluble, biologically active form (sCD40L).[65] The sCD40L is cleaved from the platelet-bound CD40L, which is expressed upon agonist stimulation on platelet surface.[66] In circulation, sCD40L may pass through damaged atherosclerotic endothelium and come into direct contact with cells inside the lesion. More importantly, sCD40L may activate circulating leukocytes or platelets to enhance the release of metalloproteinases (MMPs) and increase the likelihood of rupture of the plaques. Recently, studies have demonstrated that the interaction of CD40L with its receptor (CD40), forming the CD40–CD40L complex, is associated with formation of atherosclerosis and the long-term atherosclerotic process.[67,68] The binding of CD40L with CD40 mediates many inflammatory responses important in atherosclerosis. A wide variety of inflammatory cells express CD40L, and stimulation by other proinflammatory cytokines increases endothelial cell expression of the latter.[69] Ligation of CD40 induces the expression of leukocyte adhesion molecules and triggers the release of chemoattractants, such as monocyte chemoattractant protein 1 (MCP1), overexpressed in human atheroma.[70-72] Furthermore, CD40 ligation potently induces the expression of tissue factor (TF),[73,74] an important prothrombotic component of the intraplaque lipid pool (TF converts factor X to Xa). In addition to proinflammatory and prothrombotic properties, recent studies also suggest a potent metabolic function of CD40L.[75] Thus, the spectrum of functions of CD40L appears to span a wide range from early atherogenesis to late thrombotic complications.[76]

Not many studies have been conducted, looking at the association between sCD40L and early atherosclerosis in populations. In a small Japanese study of type I diabetes patients, higher serum sCD40L levels were found in diabetics and were associated with increased carotid IMT.[77] However, in newly diagnosed hypertensive men, sCD40L levels were not found to correlate with the degree of subclinical atherosclerosis as measured by IMT,[78] and in the Multi-Ethnic Study of Atherosclerosis (MESA), they were not associated with coronary artery calcium.[79] In the Firefighters and Their Endothelium (FATE) study, sCD40L levels correlated poorly with the Framingham Coronary Heart Disease Risk score but correlated well with cross-reactive protein (CRP) levels.[80] Somewhat surprisingly, lower plasma levels of sCD40L were found to be associated with greater plaque area in both common carotid and common femoral arteries in asymptomatic individuals over 40 years of age in the authors' own cohort. Reports from the MIAMI (Markers of Inflammation and Atorvastatin effect in previous Myocardial Infarction) study showing an increase in sCD40L levels after treatment with atorvastatin for 2 years[81] further support an inverse relationship, a possible result of CD40L being consumed in complicating thrombi and thus being depleted from the circulation.

Further data are needed in order to gain a better perspective on the role of sCD40L in early atherosclerosis and to decide on its prognostic capabilities.

27.3.6 Cholesterylester transfer Protein (CETP)

Cholesterylester transfer protein (CETP) is a hydrophobic glycoprotein that is secreted mainly from the liver and circulates in plasma, mainly bound to HDL. It promotes the redistribution of cholesteryl esters (CE), triglycerides (TG), and, to a lesser extent, phospholipids between plasma lipoproteins. CETP transfers lipids from one lipoprotein particle to another in a process that results in equilibration of lipids between lipoprotein fractions.[82]

CETP appears to have both proatherogenic and antiatherogenic effects; CETP-mediated transfer of cholesteryl esters (CE) decreases HDL levels and increases CE in VLDL–IDL–LDL (very-low-density lipoproteins–intermediate-density lipoproteins–high-density lipoproteins). The decreased HDL levels would reduce the atheroprotective functions of HDL and thus would be proatherogenic. If the increased CE in LDL is taken up by vessel wall macrophages to increase foam cell formation, then this activity would also be proatherogenic. However, if the increased CE transfer to VLDL–IDL–LDL results instead in transport of CE back to the liver via the LDL receptor, then CETP would facilitate reverse cholesterol transport (RCT) and would act in an atheroprotective way. Finally, CETP-mediated HDL remodeling during CE transfer results in the production of lipid-poor apoA1, which can be used for ABCA1-mediated cholesterol efflux, an atheroprotective process.[82,83] The ultimate outcome of this combination of CETP activities, in terms of atherosclerosis, is not easy or simple to predict. The available clinical data in humans are incomplete and do not allow for a definite conclusion about the relation of CETP deficiency to the risk of coronary heart disease to be reached, whereas data on subclinical atherosclerosis are even more sparse.

Animal studies of CETP in several rabbit models of atherosclerosis have shown that inhibiting CETP results in a marked reduction in atherosclerosis. A recent study[84] in cholesterol-fed rabbits, using a chemical inhibitor of CETP that reduced CETP activity by more than 90%, doubled the levels of HDL cholesterol and decreased the non-HDL cholesterol by approximately 50%, with an accompanying 70% reduction in atherosclerotic lesions. It was then speculated that short-term treatment of humans with the same CETP inhibitor would result in a 40–45% increase in HDL cholesterol and a 15–20% decrease in LDL cholesterol. Three CETP inhibitors have been tested on humans to date: torcetrapib (Pfizer, New York, NY, USA), which although did lead to HDL-C increase (study outcome) also led to blood pressure increase, resulting to a failure of phase III trials; anacetrapib, which was shown to double HDL-C while not affecting blood pressure and aldosterone levels, in phase III trials[85]; and dalcetrapib, which is less potent than anacetrapib but also with no obvious off-target side effects so far.[86] Although results from phase II trials for anacetrapib and dalcetrapib are encouraging, the long-term safety of the drugs is still unknown. Given the complexity of CETP functions on lipid metabolism, it was debated whether the increased cardiovascular disease (CVD) risk seen with torcetrapib was due to only off-target side effects or to the complexity of CETP-mediated increase of HDL. However, a meta-analysis of the effect of *CETP* single-nucleotide polymorphisms (SNPs) and torcetrapib treatment on lipids and blood pressure indicated that the hypertensive action of torcetrapib was unlikely to be due to CETP inhibition or shared by chemically dissimilar CETP inhibitors.[87] Research on the beneficial effects of CETP inhibition for atherosclerosis is ongoing.

27.3.6.1 CETP Gene Polymorphisms

Several mutations of the *CETP* gene have been identified as a cause of CETP deficiency and elevated levels of HDL cholesterol. These include the I405V, R451Q, A373P, -629C>A, -2505C>A, and TaqIB.

The I405V polymorphism has been associated with carotid IMT in men, with the 405VV genotype being associated with increased carotid IMT, especially in men who were heavy drinkers,[88] whereas in the men of the Stanislas Cohort, the I405V polymorphism explained 3.8% of the variability of carotid IMT.[89] On the other hand, in the MESA study, which included 855 people of different ethnicities, only the R451Q polymorphism was found to be associated with presence of carotid plaques, whereas none of the aforementioned polymorphisms was associated with IMT.[90] In the Cyprus study, the TaqIB polymorphism was associated with IMTmax (including plaques) and plaque echogenicity, and the I405V was associated with total plaque thickness in two common carotid and two common femoral arteries.

Genetic homogeneity (or heterogeneity) of the populations studied may have played some part in studies reporting conflicting results. A recent genome-wide analysis including data from more than 18,000 initially healthy women followed for 10 years reported that SNPs in the *CETP* locus were associated with both HDL levels and risk for future myocardial infarction (MI), supporting a causal role of CETP in atherosclerosis via an HDL-mediated mechanism.[91]

27.3.7 Cross-reactive Protein (CRP)

Cross-reactive protein (CRP) is a 110-kDa protein produced in response to acute injury, infection, or other inflammatory stimuli.[92] While its exact role remains unclear, CRP can stimulate mononuclear cells to release tissue factor (TF), activate the complementary pathway, and neutralize platelet-activating factor. It is found not only in plasma but also in the intimal and medial layers of human atherosclerotic arteries,[93] as well as on the surface of foam cells.[94]

Several studies have suggested CRP to be involved in atherosclerosis and development of CVD.[95-97] Ridker et al., demonstrated that CRP levels predict the risk of cardiovascular events in apparently healthy men and women in the Physicians' Health Study,[98] whereas the very recent Justification for the Use of Statins in Prevention: an Interventional Trial Evaluating Rosuvastatin (JUPITER) randomized controlled study showed a beneficial effect of statins on apparently healthy men and women with low levels of LDL but high levels of CRP.[99,100] Elevated serum levels of CRP were also associated with abnormal endothelial vascular reactivity in patients with carotid artery disease (CAD).[101] The American Heart Association had stated that it is reasonable to measure CRP as an adjunct to the measurement of established risk factors in order to assess the risk of coronary heart disease.[102] The report acknowledged, however, that the epidemiologic data to support this view were not entirely consistent and recommended that larger prospective studies be undertaken to improve the reliability of the evidence. Since then at least one large case–control study has been published,[103] and their results indicate that CRP is a moderate predictor of cardiovascular heart disease (CHD), with the authors suggesting that recommendations regarding use of CRP in predicting the likelihood of CHD need to be reviewed. Supporting their argument are the results of a recent, large systematic review of 31 prospective cohort studies that showed only a moderate and not consistent improvement of risk discrimination for coronary heart disease.[104] Although CRP may not be causally related to atherosclerosis, it seems to be a useful marker of risk and will most likely continue to be studied for some time.

27.3.8 Endothelium Nitric Oxide Synthase (eNOS)

Evidence suggests that loss of endothelium-dependent vasodilation by nitric oxide (NO) is characteristic throughout the development of atherosclerosis and has adverse consequences, specifically vasoconstriction.[105] In the vessel, the endothelial isoform of NO synthase (eNOS) is responsible for the production of NO, and substantial *in vitro* evidence suggests that eNOS-derived NO acts as an antiatherogenic molecule.[106,107] Nitric oxide from eNOS inhibits leukocyte-endothelial adhesion, vascular smooth muscle cell (VSMC) migration and proliferation, and platelet aggregation, all of which are important steps in atherogenesis. It is now being widely recognized that eNOS becomes dysfunctional and produces superoxide rather than NO in hyperlipidemia and atherosclerosis. Dysfunctional eNOS is closely implicated to the endothelial dysfunction in atherosclerotic vessels.[108] Soluble plasma NO was not associated with any of the markers of subclinical atherosclerosis in our data.

27.3.8.1 eNOS Gene Glu298Asp Polymorphism

A common polymorphism of the eNOS gene, the Glu298Asp (894G > T) has been considered to involve a genetic risk of coronary artery disease in one study,[109] but results from other studies remain conflicting. Lembo et al. have demonstrated an association between the Glu298Asp polymorphism and presence of carotid plaques defined as IMT greater than 1.5 mm; in their study, the risk of having carotid plaques increased to threefold in 298Asp homozygotes compared to 298Glu homozygotes, independently of age, blood pressure, or smoking.[31] The same was also true for an Italian population of 375 hypertensive patients where the 298Asp homozygotes were found to be associated with presence of atherosclerotic plaques.[31] However, an association between the Glu298Asp polymorphism and blood pressure, left ventricular mass, and carotid IMT was not demonstrated in the OPERA (Observatoire sur la Prise en charge hospitalière, l'Evolution à un an et les caRactéristiques de patients présentant un infArctus du myocarde avec ou sans onde Q) population study, including 1,024 subjects that had greater power to detect a possible relationship.[110] The authors of the

Finnish study argue that although the *eNOS* Glu298Asp polymorphism is likely to alter the function of the eNOS protein, this altered function does not affect endothelium-dependent vasodilatation in Caucasian subjects. The NO production catalyzed by *eNOS* Glu298Asp protein may be sufficient to relax the endothelial vascular smooth muscle cells, or other mechanisms regulating the blood pressure might compensate for the shortness of the action of NO. It also seems likely that this polymorphism has a greater effect on Japanese than Caucasian, e.g., Finnish subjects and the Finnish are likely to be genetically more homogeneous.[110] In 210 patients with type 2 diabetes mellitus (T2DM), the 4a allele of a 27-bp repeat intronic polymorphism of the eNOS gene was also found to be associated with total mean IMT and plaque score (sum of diameter of each plaque).[111]

27.3.9 Fibrinogen (Fb)

Fibrinogen (Fb) is a glycoprotein that circulates largely inactively in the bloodstream. It is produced from hepatocytes after activation from interleukin-6 and consists of six polypeptide chains held together by disulphide bonds in a molecule with bilateral symmetry.[112] Fibrinogen is involved in primary hemostasis, platelet aggregation, and leukocyte-endothelial cell interactions and is the major determinant of whole blood and plasma viscosity.[113] It has mostly been associated with clinical disease, but elevated fibrinogen levels have also been demonstrated to be significantly associated with IMT in 519 asymptomatic subjects[17] as well as with carotid plaque presence and size but not with plaque echogenicity in the Trømso study.[28] Results from our own study are in accordance, with increased fibrinogen being associated with IMT and plaque presence but not with sum of plaque area in four bifurcations after adjustment for confounding.

Whether fibrinogen is just a marker of the inflammation related to vascular disease or whether it is involved in actively mediating the vascular disease process is not entirely known. Recent studies have suggested that it is a true modifier of vascular disease, augmenting fibrin deposition in certain organs and regulating fibrin turnover,[114] but more prospective studies are needed on the topic.

27.3.10 Homocysteine

Homocysteine is a sulphuric amino acid present in dietary proteins, which is rapidly metabolized during the methylation process back to methionine or catabolized to cysteine. Both pathways are catalyzed by group B vitamins – folic acid and B12 or B6, respectively.[115] In vascular cells, homocysteine metabolism is limited to the B12–folate-dependent remethylation pathway catalyzed by methionine synthase.[116] Several studies have suggested that elevated plasma homocysteine levels have both atherogenic and thrombogenic effects. Hyperhomocysteinemia causes endothelial dysfunction by increasing oxidant stress[117] and decreases the release of NO, impairing vasodilation.[118] Excess of homocysteine stimulates smooth muscle cell proliferation and collagen synthesis, promoting intima-media thickening[119,120] and causing increased platelet aggregation and coagulation abnormalities.[121] High homocysteine is also associated with increased lipid peroxidation.[122,123]

Most studies performed so far, involving subclinical atherosclerosis, have investigated the role of homocysteine and carotid IMT in different patient groups, especially renal patients. A few studies[46,124-131] have done so in general population groups and have found a weak or often absent association between homocysteine and carotid IMT.[132] The authors have shown that higher levels of homocysteine were associated with both IMT (Fig. 27.1) and plaques (Fig. 27.2) in both carotid and femoral arteries in a general population and that the association was

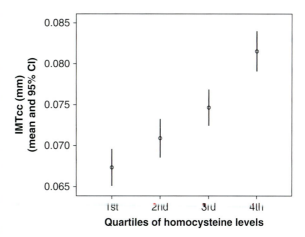

Fig. 27.1 Association between IMTcc (mm) and quartiles of serum homocysteine levels (ANOVA; P for trend < 0.001)

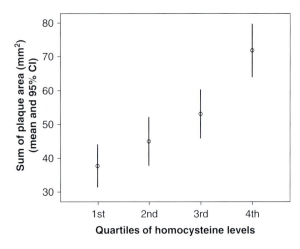

Fig. 27.2 Association between sum of plaque area (*SPA*) (mm^2) in four arteries and quartiles of serum homocysteine levels (ANOVA; P for trend < 0.001)

acute phase proteins from hepatocytes, such as CRP and fibrinogen, and could lead to insulin resistance.[134] In addition, it can affect platelet function, regulate the accumulation of leukocytes, and possibly be the link between obesity and insulin resistance.[113] Despite the proatherosclerotic role of higher levels of IL6 and its association with CVD,[135] experimental studies have been controversial. It appears that physiological levels of IL6 are essential in keeping inflammatory reactions in check and regulate glucose and lipid metabolism.[134]

In the Cyprus study, circulating levels of IL6 were not associated with plaque area in four bifurcations in 350 asymptomatic individuals, but they were associated with presence of plaques, number of bifurcations with plaque, and plaque echogenicity with a relatively large effect size.

graded. The 5,10-methylenetetrahydrofolate reductase (MTHFR) 677C > T genotype, despite strong associations with homocysteine levels, was not associated with subclinical atherosclerosis and the presence of plaques in the Cypriot population studied; using the principle of Mendelian randomization, this absence could indicate that the association of homocysteine with atherosclerosis arose either via residual confounding or via reverse causality.[25] A large meta-analysis also using data on the MTHFR C > T polymorphism and covering 111 studies up to 2003 concluded that there was evidence for a causal association between homocysteine levels and stroke.[133] The latter was better powered to test such an association, albeit with a different outcome.

27.3.11 Interleukin-6 (IL6)

Interleukin-6 (IL6) is a 26-kDa cytokine that plays a central part in the inflammatory response, being the only cytokine that can stimulate the synthesis of all the acute phase proteins involved in the inflammatory response. It is produced by a variety of cells, such as macrophages, monocytes, B and T cells, adipocytes, endothelial cells, and skeletal muscle cells, linking obesity to low-grade systemic inflammation as a possible mechanism for cardiovascular and metabolic disease. Among others, it stimulates platelet production from megakaryocytes, migration, and proliferation of smooth muscle cells and mediates the production of

27.3.11.1 IL6 Gene-174G>C Polymorphism

One of the most studied polymorphisms in the IL6-coding gene lies in the promoter region and has been found to be associated with IL-6 levels. It involves a single-base change from guanine to cytosine at position -174 ($-174G > C$), and the G allele is associated with higher IL-6 production than the C allele; this has been demonstrated both *in vitro* and *in vivo*.[113] A study on the effect of this polymorphism on carotid IMT reported that the risk of elevated IMT was confined to CC homozygotes with no clear heterozygote effect. This suggests that there may be a threshold effect, with only very high levels of interleukin-6 predisposing to disease. The same study demonstrated that the interleukin-6 $-174G > C$ polymorphism may modulate the effect of alcohol on carotid atherosclerosis, with the CC genotype associated with higher interleukin-6 levels, elevated IMTcc, and increased risk of carotid plaque in heavy drinkers.[26] In the Northern Prospective Cohort study, subjects with the -174GG genotype had 11% greater carotid IMT compared to the CC and CG genotypes combined.[136] Ethnicity might play a part as the -174GG genotype was reported as an independent predictor of angiographically assessed coronary artery disease after adjustment in African-Brazilians, but not Caucasian-Brazilians, who underwent coronary angiography.[137] In the Cyprus study, the $-174G > C$ polymorphism was not associated with plaque area in those with plaques but was associated with having a plaque present.

27.3.12 Lipoprotein (a)

Lipoprotein(a) is a cholesteryl ester–rich lipoprotein that resembles LDL but has distinctive structural, epidemiological, and genetic properties. It is believed to contribute to lipid-induced atherogenesis, similarly to LDL particles[138]; however, compared to LDL, it contains lower amounts of antioxidants and exhibits a high affinity to extracellular matrix and fibrinogen,[139-141] which prolongs residence time in the subintima. Both properties of lipoprotein(a) facilitate its oxidative modification and may enhance its capacity to cause injury. It has been suggested that lipoprotein(a) exhibits both atherogenic and thrombogenic properties and may thus promote both early and advanced stages of atherosclerosis.[27]

Not much data have been published on the association between lipoprotein(a) and subclinical atherosclerosis in the general population, and its role still remains controversial. In the Bruneck Study, the risk of early atherogenesis (incident nonstenotic) in the high-LDL group (> 3.3 mmol/L) increased gradually with increasing lipoprotein(a) concentration (Chap. 28). In this study, which involved 826 random population individuals with 5-year follow-up on progression of carotid atherosclerosis, lipoprotein(a) plasma concentration predicted the risk of early atherogenesis synergistically with high LDL-C (low-density lipoprotein cholesterol).[27] A cross-sectional evaluation of the Atherosclerosis Risk in Communities (ARIC) study yielded analogous results in that lipoprotein(a) was significantly elevated in subjects with increased IMT.[142] Whether the assessment of lipoprotein(a) adds prognostic information to overall risk in primary prevention remains uncertain mainly due to the fact that lipoprotein(a) appears to be an important marker primarily in individuals with markedly elevated risk caused either by diabetes or by hyperlepidemia.[27,143,144] Other comparative studies have found lipoprotein(a) to predict risk but to have a modest magnitude compared with several other novel markers. Some of this effect is caused by the nonlinearity of lipoprotein(a) in that risk primarily increases in those with very high levels.[145]

27.3.13 Metabolic Syndrome (MetS)

There are currently three common definitions of the MetS, the World Health Organization (WHO),[146]

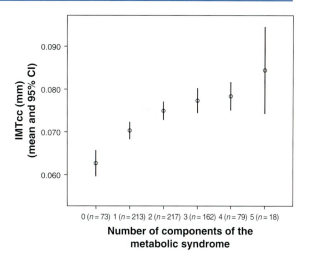

Fig. 27.3 Association between IMTcc (mm) and number of components of MetS (ANOVA; P for trend < 0.001)

the National Cholesterol Education Program Expert Panel (NCEP),[147] and the International Diabetes Federation (IDF).[148] These definitions are in general agreement on the essential components of MetS but differ in their cutoffs and methods of combining the individual components. A study done by Paras et al., on the relationship of these three definitions with subclinical atherosclerosis demonstrated that although all three definitions were associated with increased IMT and sum of plaque area after adjustment, the WHO definition was the only one associated with all three measures of atherosclerosis (IMT, sum of plaque area, and prevalence of focal lesions).[149] The WHO definition also appeared to be associated with an increase in IMT during the 3-year follow-up of the Gothenburg study compared with the NCEP definition,[150] but the study wasn't powered for such a comparison.

Individuals with the MetS had significantly greater IMT values compared with individuals without the MetS in two studies,[150,151] the first of which demonstrated this with a 3-year follow-up as well as with total plaque volume, another measurement of subclinical atherosclerosis. However, after adjustment for age and sex, the difference remained significant only for IMT. A strong trend was also observed toward increased common carotid IMT (Fig. 27.3) and plaque area (Fig. 27.4) in four bifurcations in the Cyprus study and increasing numbers of MetS components after adjustment. These results suggest that measurements of subclinical atherosclerosis are associated with the

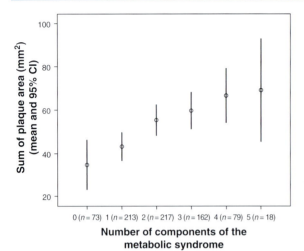

Fig. 27.4 Association between sum of plaque area (*SPA*) (mm²) in four arteries and number of components of MetS (ANOVA; *P* for trend < 0.001)

MetS and that the individual's risk increases from having even one component of the MetS.

27.3.14 Metalloproteinases (MMPs)

Integrity of the extracellular matrix constitutes a critical determinant in the stability of coronary atheroma. In particular, degradation of fibrillar collagen may decrease the ability of the fibrous cap to withstand mechanical stress. Several members of the metalloproteinase (MMP) family contribute to collagen degradation.[152]

Dysregulation of MMPs is thought to play a part in both atherogenesis and precipitation of acute coronary syndromes by regulating connective tissue remodeling, thus determining the volume expansion of the atherosclerotic plaque, its stability, and the potential for smooth muscle cell proliferation. Indeed, both smooth muscle cells and macrophages synthesize and secrete a range of MMPs, and MMP expression has been demonstrated in human atherosclerotic plaques,[153] especially in rupture-prone areas of plaques.[154-156] Several MMPs have been studied in relation to atherosclerosis, mostly at the site of plaques.

Induction of MMP-9, as well as MMP-1, expression has been shown in both vascular smooth muscle cells and accumulating macrophages in atherosclerotic plaques, particularly in the shoulder and core of plaques prone to rupture. These observations raised the possibility that these MMPs are strongly associated with the molecular mechanism of the onset and development of acute coronary syndromes. In addition, the expression of MMP-1, MMP-3, and MMP-9 was shown to be augmented in plaques compared to the adjacent control regions.[157] In the same study, upregulation of MMPs in plaques was disproportional to that of tissue inhibitors of MMPs (TIMPs), suggesting that imbalanced degradation and synthesis of extracellular matrix persist in advanced lesions, particularly in plaques with disruption.[157] In another study, by measuring mRNA transcript levels of MMP-1, -3, -7, -9, and -12 in carotid atherosclerotic plaques with different histopathological characteristics, it was shown that plaques with a thin fibrous cap (prone to rupture) had significantly higher levels of MMP-1 transcripts compared to plaques with a thick fibrous cap. MMP-3, -7, and -12 levels showed a trend for increased levels. In ruptured plaques, MMP-12 transcript levels were significantly higher compared to lesions without cap disruption.[158]

MMP-3 levels have also been associated with positive coronary arterial remodeling as shown by intravascular ultrasound.[159] In a histochemical study looking at presence of MMPs in atherosclerotic plaques, both MMP-7 mRNA and protein were expressed primarily at the border between the fibrous cap and the lipid core.[160] Others have reported similar findings, noting that the degradation by MMP-7, particularly of versican (a large matrix proteoglycan), in the border area facilitates the separation of the fibrous cap from the lipid core.[161] MMP-12 mRNA and protein were found in macrophages, particularly at the border between the fibrous cap and the lipid core.[160] These data further support a role of MMPs in determining atherosclerotic plaque stability. Plasma levels of both total and active MMP-9 were independently associated with femoral IMT and echolucent femoral plaques in 473 men of the Gothenburg study, but no such association was shown for carotid IMT or plaques.[14] In a recent study of 400 individuals without cardiovascular disease, circulating levels of MMP-10 were independently associated with carotid IMT and with presence of carotid plaques,[13] whereas levels of tissue inhibitor MMP 1 (TIMP-1) were also associated with carotid plaques in 238 men with no CHD.[30] Circulating levels of MMP1, MMP2, MMP8, MMP9, and TIMP1 and 2 were not associated with carotid IMT or plaques in the carotid and femoral arteries in a Cypriot population, although levels of MMP1 were inversely associated with clinical CVD at baseline (unpublished data). In a British prospective study on MI and stroke, baseline levels of MMP9, although univariably associated with risk of MI and stroke, were not a strong independent predictor of risk.[162]

27.3.14.1 MMP Genes Polymorphisms

Polymorphisms in the genes coding for MMPs have also been implicated in atherosclerosis. An association between the *MMP3* 5A/6A genotype and carotid IMT has been demonstrated in at least three independent studies, which have shown that individuals with the 6A/6A genotype have greater IMT values compared with 5A/6A or 5A/5A individuals.[136,163,164] In one of these studies, the 6A/6A genotype was also associated with enlarged arterial lumen and local reduction of wall shear stress, which might predispose to atherosclerotic plaque localization.[163] In the Cyprus study, the *MMP3* 5A/6A genotype was not associated with increased IMT or plaque presence in neither men nor women. However, associations between *MMP* genotypes and subclinical atherosclerosis were shown to be sex-dependent, with the MMP1 1G/2G polymorphism associated with presence of plaques in the femoral arteries in women only (unpublished data). In a Spanish case–control study, the MMP1 2G/2G genotype was associated with the risk of MI.[165] In women of the Cyprus study, the *MMP12*-82AA genotype was associated with higher IMT and plaque presence in the femoral arteries, whereas the biggest effect was shown by the *MMP9* R279Q polymorphism, with the RR genotype being associated with a threefold increase in risk for presence of plaques – especially in the carotid arteries – in men (unpublished data). An association between MMP9 haplotypes (279R and −1562C haplotype) and presence of carotid plaques in men was also shown in a large prospective study in Austria.[166]

27.3.15 Monocyte Chemoattractor Protein-1 (MCP-1)

Monocyte chemoattractor protein-1 (MCP-1) is a chemokine widely expressed in endothelial cells, smooth muscle cells, and monocytes in response to stimuli by several molecules, such as CD40L and IL-1β, through the NF-κB pathway.[167] It has been implicated in promoting atherosclerosis, especially in animal models; overexpression of MCP-1 in the leukocytes of susceptible mice results in increased plaque size.[168] MCP-1 is expressed in human lesions, and CCR2 (its receptor) is expressed on leukocytes.[169-171] It induces arrest and transmigration from the circulation of CCR2+ monocytes under conditions of physiological shear stress and promotes monocyte differentiation to lipid-laden macrophages (foam cells).[172,173] It also contributes to the proliferation of arterial smooth muscle cells,[174] which, along with macrophages, constitute the key cellular components of plaques.

MCP-1 has been implicated in atherosclerosis mostly in animal models, while data from humans are contradictory. Studies have suggested links between circulating MCP-1 levels and atherosclerosis, with higher MCP-1 levels being associated with increased risks of myocardial infarction, sudden death, coronary angioplasty, and stent restenosis.[175-178] However, little is known about the role of MCP-1 levels in cardiovascular disease in the general population,[179] and data are lacking on the association between MCP1 and early atherosclerosis. In the Cyprus study, plasma MCP1 levels were associated with all measurements of subclinical atherosclerosis (IMT, plaques, plaque area, and plaque type) invariably. However, the observed associations did not hold after adjustment for conventional risk factors and were mostly explained by age and sex.

27.3.16 Oxidized LDL (Ox-LDL)

The hypothesis that oxidized LDL (Ox-LDL) is necessary, if not obligatory, in the development of atherosclerotic lesions was formulated more than 25 years ago with the seminal observation that uptake of native LDL by macrophages did not result in foam cell formation. In contrast, uptake of Ox-LDL via scavenger receptors resulted in the upregulated accumulation of lipids.[180,181] There is substantial evidence that Ox-LDL is present in vivo within atherosclerotic, but not normal, blood vessels. Ox-LDL (*in vivo*) has a wide range of atherogenic properties from early lesion formation to plaque rupture. These include: inducing expression of adhesion molecules on endothelial cells, monocyte chemotaxis and adhesion, cytotoxicity, upregulating inflammatory genes and growth factors, endothelial dysfunction, platelet aggregation and thrombus formation, and destabilizing plaques through mechanisms including increased expression of metalloproteinases (MMPs).[181-183]

The origins of plasma Ox-LDL as well as its determinants are unknown, but high plasma and plaque levels of Ox-LDL have been associated with plaque instability, i.e., high number of macrophages.[184] The characteristics of Ox-LDL isolated from the plasma of patients with coronary artery disease are comparable to those of Ox-LDL isolated from lesions.[185] The potential origin of circulating Ox-LDL may be the direct release of modified LDL from ruptured or permeable plaques or ischemic injury.[181,184] Plasma Ox-LDL has been associated with subclinical atherosclerosis in clinically healthy populations in the Gothenburg/AIR (Atherosclerosis and Insulin Resistance) study,[10,29,186] where Ox-LDL levels at baseline were associated with change in carotid IMT as well as with occurrence and size of plaques in the carotid and femoral arteries at follow-up. In contrast, in the Asklepios study of 2,524 asymptomatic subjects, circulating Ox-LDL was associated with femoral plaques but not with femoral or carotid IMT and carotid plaques after adjustment.[11] The authors argue that femoral plaques confound the association of Ox-LDL with carotid atherosclerosis, which further strengthens the argument of different factors acting in different vascular beds. In the multiethnic MESA study, Ox-LDL levels were associated with stenotic plaques in the carotid arteries,[187] whereas in the ATTICA (association between prehypertension status and oxidative stress markers related to atherosclerotic disease) study, they were associated with prehypertension.[188] Although Ox-LDL is essential in the transformation of monocytes to macrophages, a necessary component of plaques, more studies are needed before circulating Ox-LDL can be considered for addition in risk algorithms.

27.3.17 Tumor Necrosis Factor-α (TNF-α)

Tumor necrosis factor-α (TNF-α) is a proinflammatory cytokine with a wide range of proinflammatory activities. It is primarily produced by monocytes/macrophages, although significant amounts are also secreted by other cell types.[189] TNF-α elicits the expression of the messenger cytokine IL-6, which in turn induces expression of cell adhesion molecules from leukocytes and hepatocytes. Adhesion of circulating leukocytes to endothelial cells with ensuing transendothelial migration is considered an important step in atherogenesis, and increased expression of cell adhesion molecules may represent one mechanism by which TNF-α is implicated in atherothrombotic disease.[189] TNF-α plasma levels have been associated with common carotid IMT in healthy middle-aged men;[189] however, it remains unclear whether elevated serum TNF-α in patients with atherosclerosis is derived from plaques or from nonvascular sources.[189] In a large case–control Swedish study of MI, higher serum levels of TNF-α were associated with an increased MI risk in men, and the risk was even greater in obese subjects.[190]

27.3.17.1 TNF-α Gene −308G>A Polymorphism

While many factors can affect TNF-α production (i.e., infection), genetic regulation also plays a significant role.[191] Among many variants in the *TNF-α* gene, a G to A transition at the −308-bp position of the promoter was shown to be associated with increased promoter activity[192] and elevated TNF-α plasma levels.[193] However, findings from the Helsinki Sudden Death study in 700 autopsy cases do not support an association between the *TNF-α* −308G > A genotype (increasing TNF-α levels) and coronary atherosclerosis.[194] In accordance, the −308G > A polymorphism was not associated with any measure of subclinical atherosclerosis in the Cyprus study after adjustment for conventional risk factors.

More data are needed before any solid argument can be made either in favor or against the value of measuring TNF-α levels or polymorphisms in atherosclerosis, especially since the potential effect of the −308A > G polymorphism on stroke has been shown to be dependent on race in a large meta-analysis.[195]

27.4 Gene Expression in Echolucent and Echogenic Atherosclerotic Plaques

In addition to genetic polymorphisms that may or may not affect gene expression, gene expression profiles themselves can represent markers of activation/deactivation of specific pathways and give further insight into the pathophysiology of disease.

Gene expression is the process by which information from a gene (DNA) is used to synthesize a product, usually a protein, via synthesis of RNA. The genetic code (DNA) is "decoded" via gene expression, and the products of this process give rise to the organism's phenotype. Gene expression is, therefore, a central process via which the number and/or type of genes, as well as the percentage of expression in each cell, are determined. There are many levels of modulation/control between DNA and protein, such as transcription, RNA splicing, translation, and post-translational modification, giving the cell control over its structure and function.

Technological advances of the past few years have allowed us to explore gene expression profiles of different tissues using several techniques, the most effective being quantitative reverse transcription polymerase chain reaction (qRT-PCR) and the more high-throughput microarrays. One of the advantages of microarrays is that they can be hypothesis-free, i.e., no previous knowledge is necessary. In this way, results are not hypothesis-driven and can be entirely novel and sometimes even surprising. These can in turn be confirmed (or refuted) with the use of targeted qRT-PCR and Western/Northern blots preferably in new, independent samples.

Only a limited number of studies have looked at gene expression profiles in atherosclerosis. Those that have done usually compare different tissues that may differ in many other aspects that affect expression. This section will review studies that have used microarrays in order to study expression profiles in atherosclerosis. Gene expression profiles in these studies have been compared in symptomatic versus asymptomatic patients, in different parts of plaques versus nonatherosclerotic tissue or cells, as well as in different types of plaques and advanced atherosclerosis from autopsies.

27.4.1 Gene Expression Profiles in Symptomatic Versus Asymptomatic Patients/Plaques

Two studies have compared gene expression profiles in symptomatic versus asymptomatic plaques, though using different arrays and methodologies, as well as sample selection. The first used endarterectomy plaques from patients presenting with stroke (symptomatic) ($n = 6$) versus asymptomatic patients ($n = 4$) matching for degree of stenosis and risk factors and found increased expression of metabolic, signal transduction, and ionic homeostasis genes in plaques from symptomatic patients.[196] The authors of this study argue that increased metabolic activity and second-messenger signaling could promote faster plaque growth predisposing to rupture and stroke.

The second study included samples from the Helsinki Carotid Endarterectomy Study and used symptomatic and asymptomatic plaques from the same patients ($n = 4$) to identify differentially expressed genes and gene clusters and then confirmed those results in 40 new plaques.[197] They reported an – albeit small – overexpression of two genes involved in iron–heme homeostasis (CD163 and HO-1) in symptomatic plaques and suggested that this might be in response to plaque hemorrhages. Though this approach minimizes background noise by comparing different plaques from the same patient, as the study's authors themselves acknowledge, coming across such patients with bilateral stenotic plaques with only one producing symptoms [stroke, transient ischemic attack (TIA), or amaurosis fugax (AF)] is quite rare, and results would be difficult to replicate.

27.4.2 Gene Expression Profiles in Different Areas of the Atherosclerotic Plaque

Studies of the difference in expression between several segments of atherosclerotic plaques from the same patients have been designed in order to reduce interspecimen variability.

Papaspyridonos et al. have classified segments of plaques ($n = 79$) into stable and unstable according to their histological characteristics and analyzed their gene expression using both an intraplaque and an interplaque analysis.[198] Consistently differentially expressed genes from both analyses were further validated at the mRNA and protein level, thus using a whole transcriptome approach in their study and giving their results more validity. Eighteen out of the 27 confirmed genes in their study had not been previously associated with plaque instability, highlighting the potential of hypothesis-free microarray analysis for the identification of novel targets for atherosclerosis. These included the metalloproteinase ADAMDEC1 and the metalloproteinases -1 and -9, as well as cathepsin B and legumain, a potential activator of MMPs and cathepsins.[198] Matrix metalloproteinase-9 (MMP-9), cathepsin B, and legumain (a novel gene) were also confirmed at the protein level.

In a more complicated study design, Adams et al. chose to compare the expression profiles of the plaque's fibrous cap versus normal media versus nonatherosclerotic adjacent intima versus whole plaque using 26,000 gene UniGene clusters in pooled endarterectomy samples from men.[199] Their results indicate a unique expression profile for the fibrous cap, distinguishable from that of the underlying intima and of the adjacent nonatherosclerotic intima. The cap phenotype included 11 genes that were consistently upregulated in the cap versus the intima and 43 downregulated genes. The expression of versican (a proteoglycan implicated in accumulation of LDL in intima and plaques), nonmuscle myosin heavy chain-B (NMMHC-B – a marker of human intima), connective tissue growth factor (CTGF – implicated in endothelial cell function and angiogenesis), and most importantly RG55 (a differential marker of arteries versus veins), whose expression is lost in the fibrous cap, was verified in additional samples.[199]

27.4.3 Gene Expression Profiles in Primary Versus Restenotic Plaques

Neointimal thickening is the major cause of restenosis after stenting or carotid endarterectomy. Not all carotid arteries undergo restenosis after surgery, and the factors determining which ones will remain plaque-free are not well known. To answer this question, studies have looked at gene expression profiles in primary versus restenotic plaques[200-202] with mixed results.

Murillo et al. used microarrays to identify altered expression of 13 out of 96 genes in 3 primary and 3 restenotic plaque samples containing reference tissue, transition zone, and plaque. These included genes for metalloproteinases (MMP2 and MMP9) and their tissue inhibitors (TIMP1, TIMP2, and TIMP2), as well as genes coding for integrins ($\alpha 2$, $\alpha 6$, and $\beta 1$) that mediate adhesion to the extracellular matrix, a process necessary for proliferation, differentiation, and cell survival. Some discordance between microarray data and Western blot analysis and zymography highlights the importance of the multiple levels of control of MMPs and TIMPs as well as pointing to possible confounding from stage of disease and presence of atherosclerosis from the reference tissue.[200]

An older study comparing cultured normal human medial VSMCs and cells from primary plaques or stent-stenosis sites revealed a stable gene expression profile of stent-stenotic VSMCs that had intermediate features between normal medial and primary plaque. Genes overexpressed in primary versus normal medial VSMCs ($n = 8$) included IGF-BP2, laminin $\beta 1$, skeletal muscle α-tropomyosin, etc., whereas genes overexpressed in stent-stenotic versus normal medial VSMCs ($n = 36$) included genes associated with cell proliferation, contractile machinery, and cell-matrix signaling.[201]

A third study using microscopic tissue from symptomatic in-stent restenosis and controls from gastrointestinal and coronary arteries reported overexpression of FKBP12 at both the mRNA and protein level of human neointima and underexpression of MDGI.[202] FKBP12 controls TGF-β (tissue growth factor-beta) receptor I signaling and may therefore inhibit TGF-β-mediated cell-cycle arrest. It is also the receptor for rapamycin (sirolimus), an immunosuppressant and antiproliferative drug known to prolong the life of mice and reduce neointima formation, suggesting even a possible therapeutic target.

27.4.4 Gene Expression in Plaques with Different Pathological Grades

One of the most comprehensive studies of gene expression in plaques so far was done by Al-Shali et al., They used 32 coronary artery segments from 22 cardiac transplant patients that were graded histologically according to the American Heart Association grading system (type I to V) and a custom-made 22K oligonucleotide microarray in a system-based approach that included pathway development analysis based on connectivity, thus identifying genes that are possible candidates for therapeutic targeting.[203] Most differentially expressed genes were found when comparing grade I versus grade V ($n = 168$) and grade III versus grade V ($n = 169$). Pathway analysis revealed that inflammatory, cell-cycle regulatory, and lipid metabolism genes were overexpressed in grade V

Table 27.3 Differentially expressed pathways for comparisons between plaque types (Geroulakos classification 1–5) using the Kyoto Encyclopedia of Genes and Genomes (KEGG) bioinformatics resource

Type of plaques compared	Enriched pathways using KEGG (number of differentially expressed genes)
Type 1 versus type 2	Focal adhesion pathway (32 genes) Adherence junction pathway (15 genes) Leukocyte transendothelial migration pathway (18 genes) T cell receptor signaling pathway (15 genes) Regulation of actin cytoskeleton pathway (26 genes) TGF-β signaling pathway (13 genes) Hematopoietic cell lineage pathway (13 genes) High-mannose-type N-glycan biosynthesis pathway (4 genes) Gap junction pathway (14 genes) N-glycan biosynthesis pathway (8 genes) ECM-receptor interaction pathway (13 genes) Epithelial cell signaling in *Helicobacter pylori* pathway (8 genes)
Type 1 versus type 3	Cell cycle pathway (14 genes) Neurodegenerative disorder pathway (6 genes) Phosphatidylinositol signaling system pathway (10 genes) MAPK signaling pathway (20 genes) Nucleotide sugar metabolism pathway (4 genes) Inositol phosphate metabolism (8 genes) Ubiquitin-mediated proteolysis pathway (6 genes)
Type 1 versus type 4	WNT signaling pathway (14 genes) Focal adhesion pathway (16 genes) Epithelial cell signaling in Helicobacter pylori infection pathway (7 genes) Tight junction pathway (10 genes) ECM-receptor interaction pathway (8 genes) Regulation of actin cytoskeleton pathway (13 genes)
Type 2 versus type 3	Adherens junction pathway (21 genes) TGF-β signaling pathway (18 genes) Phosphatidylinositol signaling system pathway (19 genes) Leukocyte transendothelial migration pathway (21 genes) Inositol phosphate metabolism (14 genes) JAK-STAT signaling pathway (24 genes) Tight junction pathway (19 genes) SNARE interactions in vesicular transport pathway (8 genes)
Type 3 versus type 4	Gap junction pathway (7 genes)
Type 1 and 2 versus type 3 and 4	Inositol phosphate metabolism pathway (8 genes) Cell cycle pathway (10 genes) Phosphatidylinositol signaling system pathway (9 genes) MAPK signaling pathway (18 genes)

Source: Pathway analysis was performed using Database for Annotation, Visualization and Integrated Discovery (DAVID) software from the National Institute of Allergy and Infectious Diseases (NIAID), National Institutes of Health. Available from: http://david.abcc.ncifcrf.gov/home.jsp. Accessed February 17–24, 2008

when compared to grade I. Cell proliferation and growth, apoptosis, and cell–cell and cell–matrix interaction genes were downregulated when compared to grade III. Cytoskeleton organization and cell-growth genes were overexpressed in grade I. No significantly differentiated genes were found when comparing grade I with III in accordance to the fact that it is the presence of lipid pools rather than cell type changes that distinguishes grade III plaques from grade I.

In a similar approach by the authors' group, tissue from 24 ultrasonically characterized plaques (Geroulakos classification 1–5) was analyzed using the Affymetrix U133A 2.0 array (Affymetrix, Santa Clara, California, USA) and subsequent pathway analysis. Results from each comparison between plaque types are shown in Table 27.3. The authors' data also suggest changes in pathways involved in cell cycle growth, cell signaling, focal adhesion, and adherence,

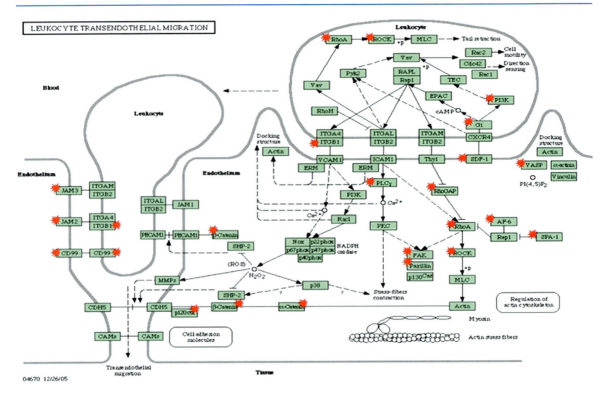

Fig. 27.5 Leukocyte transendothelial migration pathway using the Kyoto Encyclopedia of Genes and Genomes (*KEGG*). Differentially expressed genes when comparing plaque types 2 versus 3 are marked with a star

as well as in leukocyte transendothelial migration, MAPK signaling, and TGF-β signaling, with several genes in these pathways interacting with genes from other differentially expressed pathways. Examples of pathway analysis results are shown in Figs. 27.5 and 27.6.

27.4.5 Summary

In spite of the differences in study design and variability of results presented here, a common theme has emerged. Genes found to be differentially expressed mostly originated from basic cell processes, such as cell–cell interactions and cell cycle, as well as basic inflammatory, pathways.

As described in previous chapters, not all atherosclerotic plaques carry the same risk of an event, with vulnerable, complex plaques carrying the highest. Gene expression studies using microarrays are mostly hypothesis-free and have the potential of discovering a distinct gene expression profile between low- and high-risk plaques which will contribute to both elucidating the pathophysiological mechanisms of disease as well as offering insight into novel therapeutic targets.

The variability of results reported thus far points to the difficulties in performing such studies. The variability in study design and sample composition/selection, as well as selection of control tissue, presents the researcher with many practical difficulties, as depicted in the studies reviewed here. Furthermore, the variability in analysis strategies makes study comparability even harder. Development of more advanced software for statistical and pathway analysis and a systems-biology approach that can account for gene interactions are already on the way and will further help future studies to answer the question of what drives a plaque into complications/events and of whether we can identify such plaques early on based on their gene expression profile.

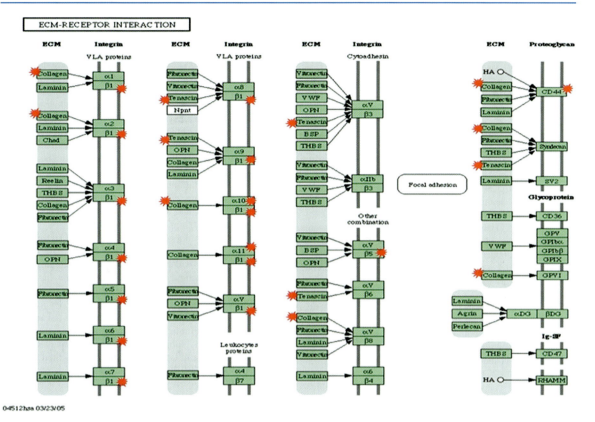

Fig. 27.6 ECM-receptor interaction pathway using the Kyoto Encyclopedia of Genes and Genomes. Differentially expressed genes when comparing plaque types 1 versus 4 are marked with a star

27.5 Conclusion

A plethora of novel markers with suggested involvement in atherosclerosis and cardiovascular disease have emerged in the past few years, and some have been presented here. For the remaining, not many studies (if any) have been conducted using subclinical atherosclerosis as an outcome, and these have been omitted. Indicatively, some are mentioned here: myeloperoxidase (MPO), microparticles (MP), uncoupling proteins (UCP-2 and UCP-3), tissue factor (TF), and tissue factor pathway inhibitor (TFPI).

In a recent review of studies addressing the association between carotid IMT and soluble markers and investigating whether the observed inconsistencies could be explained by the characteristics of the patients included in different studies, only CRP and fibrinogen seemed to be unequivocally related to IMT. For all other soluble markers considered, no clear-cut conclusions could be drawn by the authors.[204]

Most studies conducted to date, investigating markers and early atherosclerosis, have done so in relatively small patient groups, thus further confounding for disease status – often other than atherosclerosis – and late epiphenomena, and have often excluded plaques. Few are large, and more importantly prospective, population studies that have data on IMT and/or plaques and are therefore better equipped to look at the use of such soluble and genetic markers in risk models. Meta-analyses, including several small studies as well as better designed larger-scale studies that include plaques, are needed in order to further elucidate the mechanisms behind atherosclerosis initiation and progression. The inclusion of hypothesis-free results from genomic arrays of well-defined tissue and their subsequent confirmation or refutal using a more systematic approach will hopefully improve the predictive capabilities of risk equations, especially for those at intermediate risk.

References

1. Kannel W, Dawber T, Kagan A. Factors of risk in the development of coronary heart disease: 6-year follow-up experience. The Framingham Study. *Ann Intern Med.* 1961;55:33–50.
2. Dzau VJ. Markers of malign across the cardiovascular continuum interpretation and application. *Circulation.* 2004;109(suppl IV):IV-1-IV-2.
3. Stampfer MJ, Ridker PM PM, Dzau VJ. Risk factor criteria. *Circulation.* 2004;109(suppl IV):IV-3-IV-5.
4. Atkinson AJ et al. Biomarkers and surrogate endpoints: preferred definitions and conceptual framework. *Clin Pharmacol Ther.* 2001;69(3):89–95.
5. Tardif JC, Heinonen T, Orloff D, Libby P. Vascular biomarkers and surrogates in cardiovascular disease. *Circulation.* 2006;113(25):2936–2942.
6. Gibbons GH et al. Genetic markers progress and potential for cardiovascular disease. *Circulation.* 2004;109(25 suppl 1):47–58.
7. Hulthe J, Wikstrand J, Fagerberg B. Relationship between C-reactive protein and intima-media thickness in the carotid and femoral arteries and to antibodies against oxidized low-density lipoprotein in healthy men: the Atherosclerosis and Insulin Resistance (AIR) study. *Clin Sci.* 2001;100(4):371–378.
8. Brohall G et al. Association between impaired glucose tolerance and carotid atherosclerosis: a study in 64-year-old women and a meta-analysis. *Nutr Metab Cardiovasc Dis.* 2009;19(5):327–333.
9. Mannami T et al. Low potentiality of angiotensin-converting enzyme gene insertion/deletion polymorphism as a useful predictive marker for carotid atherogenesis in a large general population of a Japanese city: the Suita study. *Stroke.* 2001;32(6):1250–1256.
10. Wallenfeldt K, Fagerberg B, Wikstrand J, Hulthe J. Oxidized low-density lipoprotein in plasma is a prognostic marker of subclinical atherosclerosis development in clinically healthy men. *J Intern Med.* 2004;256(5):413–420.
11. Langlois MR et al. Femoral plaques confound the association of circulating oxidized low-density lipoprotein with carotid atherosclerosis in a general population aged 35–55 years: the Asklepios Study. *Arterioscler Thromb Vasc Biol.* 2008;28(8):1563–1568.
12. Furuki K et al. Plasma level of asymmetric dimethylarginine (ADMA) as a predictor of carotid intima-media thickness progression: six-year prospective study using carotid ultrasonography. *Hypertens Res.* 2008;31(6):1185–1189.
13. Orbe J et al. Independent association of matrix metalloproteinase-10, cardiovascular risk factors and subclinical atherosclerosis. *J Thromb Haemost.* 2007;5(1):91–97.
14. Olson FJ et al. Circulating matrix metalloproteinase 9 levels in relation to sampling methods, femoral and carotid atherosclerosis. *J Intern Med.* 2008;263(6):626–635.
15. Juonala M et al. Childhood levels of serum apolipoproteins B and A-I predict carotid intima-media thickness and brachial endothelial function in adulthood: the cardiovascular risk in young finns study. *J Am Coll Cardiol.* 2008;52(4):293–299.
16. Schmidt C, Wikstrand J. High apoB/apoA-I ratio is associated with increased progression rate of carotid artery intima-media thickness in clinically healthy 58-year-old men: experiences from very long-term follow-up in the AIR study. *Atherosclerosis.* 2009;205(1):284–289.
17. Paramo J, Beloqui O, Roncal C, Benito A, Orbe J. Validation of plasma fibrinogen as a marker of carotid atherosclerosis in subjects free of clinical cardiovascular disease. *Haematologica.* 2004;89(10):1226–1231.
18. Chen PC et al. C-reactive protein and the metabolic syndrome correlate differently with carotid atherosclerosis between men and women in a Taiwanese community. *Metabolism.* 2008;57(8):1023–1028.
19. Andersson J et al. Echogenicity of the carotid intima media complex is related to cardiovascular risk factors, dyslipidemia, oxidative stress and inflammation: the Prospective Investigation of the Vasculature in Uppsala Seniors (PIVUS) study. *Atherosclerosis.* 2009;204(2):612–618.
20. Lind L et al. Brachial artery intima-media thickness and echogenicity in relation to lipids and markers of oxidative stress in elderly subjects:–the prospective investigation of the vasculature in Uppsala Seniors (PIVUS) Study. *Lipids.* 2008;43(2):133–141.
21. Schmidt C, Fagerberg B. ApoB/apoA-I ratio is related to femoral artery plaques in 64-year-old women also in cases with low LDL cholesterol. *Atherosclerosis.* 2008;196(2):817–822.
22. Maas R et al. Association of the endogenous nitric oxide synthase inhibitor ADMA with carotid artery intimal media thickness in the Framingham Heart Study Offspring cohort. *Stroke.* 2009;40(8):2715–2719.
23. Panayiotou A et al. ApoB/ApoA1 ratio and subclinical atherosclerosis. *Int Angiol.* 2008;27(1):74–80.
24. Slooter AJ et al. Apolipoprotein E and carotid artery atherosclerosis: the Rotterdam study. *Stroke.* 2001;32(9):1947–1952.
25. Panayiotou A et al. Serum total homocysteine, folate, 5,10-methylenetetrahydrofolate reductase (MTHFR) 677C − >T genotype and subclinical atherosclerosis. *Expert Opin Ther Targets.* 2009;13(1):1–11.
26. Jerrard-Dunne P et al. Interleukin-6 promoter polymorphism modulates the effects of heavy alcohol consumption on early carotid artery atherosclerosis: the Carotid Atherosclerosis Progression Study (CAPS). *Stroke.* 2003;34:402–407.
27. Kronenberg F et al. Role of lipoprotein(a) and apolipoprotein(a) phenotype in atherogenesis: prospective results from the Bruneck Study. *Circulation.* 1999;100(11):1154–1160.
28. Halvorsen DS, Johnsen SH, Mathiesen EB, Njølstad I. The association between inflammatory markers and carotid atherosclerosis is sex dependent: the Tromsø study. *Cerebrovasc Dis.* 2009;27(4):392–397.
29. Sigurdardottir V, Fagerberg B, Wikstrand J, Schmidt C, Hulthe J. Circulating oxidized low-density lipoprotein is associated with echolucent plaques in the femoral artery

independently of hsCRP in 61-year-old men. *Atherosclerosis*. 2007;190(1):187–193.
30. Zureik M, Beaudeux JL, Courbon D, Bénétos A, Ducimetière P. Serum tissue inhibitors of metalloproteinases 1 (TIMP-1) and carotid atherosclerosis and aortic arterial stiffness. *J Hypertens*. 2005;23(12):2263–2268.
31. Lembo G et al. A common variant of endothelial nitric oxide synthase (Glu298Asp) is an independent risk factor for carotid atherosclerosis. *Stroke*. 2001;32(3):735–740.
32. Schmidt C, Fagerberg B, Wikstrand J, Hulthe J. apoB/apoA-I ratio is related to femoral artery plaques and is predictive for future cardiovascular events in healthy men. *Atherosclerosis*. 2006;189(1):178–185.
33. Ebrahim S et al. Carotid plaque, intima media thickness, cardiovascular risk factors, and prevalent cardiovascular disease in men and women: the British Regional Heart Study. *Stroke*. 1999;30(4):841–850.
34. Zhao J et al. Heritability of carotid intima-media thickness: a twin study. *Atherosclerosis*. 2008;197(2):814–820.
35. Fox CS et al. Genetic and environmental contributions to atherosclerosis phenotypes in men and women: heritability of carotid intima-media thickness in the Framingham Heart Study. *Stroke*. 2003;34(2):397–401.
36. North KE et al. Heritability of carotid artery structure and function: the Strong Heart Family Study. *Arterioscler Thromb Vasc Biol*. 2002;22(10):1698–1703.
37. Sayed-Tabatabaei FA et al. Heritability of the function and structure of the arterial wall: findings of the Erasmus Rucphen Family (ERF) study. *Stroke*. 2005;36(11):2351–2356.
38. Moskau S et al. Heritability of carotid artery atherosclerotic lesions: an ultrasound study in 154 families. *Stroke*. 2005;36(1):5–8.
39. Sacco RL et al. Heritability and linkage analysis for carotid intima-media thickness. The family study of stroke risk and carotid atherosclerosis. *Stroke*. 2009;40(7):2307–2312.
40. Jeng J. Carotid thickening, cardiac hypertrophy, and angiotensin converting enzyme gene polymorphism in patients with hypertension. *Am J Hypertens*. 2000;13:111–119.
41. Sass C et al. Apolipoprotein E4, lipoprotein lipase C447 and angiotensin-I converting enzyme deletion alleles were not associated with increased wall thickness of carotid and femoral arteries in healthy subjects from the Stanislas cohort. *Atherosclerosis*. 1998;140:89–95.
42. Rigat B et al. An insertion/deletion polymorphism in the angiotensin I-converting enzyme gene accounting for half the variance of serum enzyme levels. *J Clin Invest*. 1990;86(4):1343–1346.
43. Zannad F et al. Genetics strongly determines the wall thickness of the left and right carotid arteries. *Hum Genet*. 1998;103:183–188.
44. Dessì-Fulgheri P et al. Angiotensin converting enzyme gene polymorphism and carotid atherosclerosis in a low-risk population. *J Hypertens*. 1995;13:1593–1596.
45. Diamantopoulos E et al. Atherosclerosis of carotid arteries and the ace insertion/deletion polymorphism in subjects with diabetes mellitus type 2. *Int Angiol*. 2002;21(1):63–69.
46. Markus H et al. Increased common carotid intima-media thickness in UK African Caribbeans and its relation to chronic inflammation and vascular candidate gene polymorphisms. *Stroke*. 2001;32(11):2465–2471.
47. Manolio TA, Boerwinkle E, O'Donnell CJ, Wilson AF. Genetics of ultrasonographic carotid atherosclerosis. *Arterioscler Thromb Vasc Biol*. 2004;24:1567–1577.
48. Balkestein EJ et al. Carotid and femoral intima-media thickness in relation to three candidate genes in a Caucasian population. *J Hypertens*. 2002;20(8):1551–1561.
49. Agerholm-Larsen B, Nordestgaard BG, Tybjærg-Hansen A. ACE gene polymorphism in cardiovascular disease meta-analyses of small and large studies in whites. *Arterioscler Thromb Vasc Biol*. 2000;20:484–492.
50. Cooke JP. Does ADMA cause endothelial dysfunction? *Arterioscler Thromb Vasc Biol*. 2000;20(9):2032–2037.
51. Tsao PS, McEvoy LM, Drexler H, Butcher EC, Cooke JP. Enhanced endothelial adhesiveness in hypercholesterolemia is attenuated by L-arginine. *Circulation*. 1994;89(5):2176–2182.
52. Miyazaki H et al. Endogenous nitric oxide synthase inhibitor: a novel marker of atherosclerosis. *Circulation*. 1999;99(9):1141–1146.
53. Furuki K et al. Plasma levels of asymmetric dimethylarginine (ADMA) are related to intima-media thickness of the carotid artery: an epidemiological study. *Atherosclerosis*. 2007;191(1):206–210.
54. Khan U, Hassan A, Vallance P, Markus HS. Asymmetric dimethylarginine in cerebral small vessel disease. *Stroke*. 2007;38:411–413.
55. Loscalzo J, ed. *Molecular Mechanisms of Atherosclerosis*. Abingdon: Taylor & Francis Group; 2005.
56. Sniderman A, Scantlebury T, Cianflone K. Hypertriglyceridemic hyperapoB: the unappreciated atherogenic dyslipoproteinemia in type 2 diabetes mellitus. *Ann Intern Med*. 2001;135(6):447–459.
57. Sniderman A et al. Apolipoproteins versus lipids as indices of coronary risk and as targets for statin treatment. *Lancet*. 2003;361(9359):777–780.
58. Andersson J et al. The carotid artery plaque size and echogenicity are related to different cardiovascular risk factors in the elderly: the Prospective Investigation of the Vasculature in Uppsala Seniors (PIVUS) study. *Lipids*. 2009;44(5):397–403.
59. Wallenfeldt K, Bokemark L, Wikstrand J, Hulthe J, Fagerberg B. Apolipoprotein B/apolipoprotein A-I in relation to the metabolic syndrome and change in carotid artery intima-media thickness during 3 years in middle-aged men. *Stroke*. 2004;35:2248–2252.
60. Eichner JE et al. Apolipoprotein E polymorphism and cardiovascular disease: a HuGE review. *Am J Epidemiol*. 2002;155(6):487–495.
61. Ilveskoski E et al. Apolipoprotein E polymorphism and carotid artery intima-media thickness in a random sample of middle-aged men. *Atherosclerosis*. 2000;153:147–153.
62. Beilby JP et al. Apolipoprotein E gene polymorphisms are associated with carotid plaque formation but not with intima-media wall thickening: results from the Perth Carotid Ultrasound Disease Assessment Study (CUDAS). *Stroke*. 2003;34(4):869–874.
63. Paternoster L, Martínez González NA, Lewis S, Sudlow C. Association between apolipoprotein E genotype and

carotid intima-media thickness may suggest a specific effect on large artery atherothrombotic stroke. *Stroke.* 2008;39(1):48–54.
64. Schönbeck U, Libby P. The CD40/CD154 receptor/ligand dyad. *Cell Mol Life Sci.* 2001;58(1):4–43.
65. Schönbeck U, Varo N, Libby P, Buring J, Ridker PM. Soluble CD40L and cardiovascular risk in women. *Circulation.* 2001;104:2266–2268.
66. Henn V et al. CD40 ligand on activated platelets triggers an inflammatory reaction of endothelial cells. *Nature.* 1998;391:591–594.
67. Phipps R et al. The CD40-CD40 ligand system: a potential therapeutic target in atherosclerosis. *Curr Opin Investig Drugs.* 2001;2:773–777.
68. Ozmen J, Bobryshev YV, Lord R. CD40 co-stimulatory molecule expression by dendritic cells in primary atherosclerotic lesions in carotid arteries and in stenotic saphenous vein coronary artery grafts. *Cardiovasc Surg.* 2001;9:329–333.
69. Karmann K, Hughes CC, Schechner J, Fanslow WC, Pober JS. CD40 on human endothelial cells: inducibility by cytokines and functional regulation of adhesion molecule expression. *Proc Natl Acad Sci USA.* 1995;92:4342–4346.
70. Kornbluth R, Kee K, Richman D. CD40 ligand (CD154) stimulation of macrophages to produce HIV-1-suppressive b-chemokines. *Proc Natl Acad Sci USA.* 1998;95:5205–5210.
71. Mach F et al. Differential expression of three T lymphocyte-activating CXC chemokines by human atheroma-associated cells. *J Clin Invest.* 1999;104:1041–1050.
72. Denger S et al. Expression of monocyte chemoattractant protein-1 cDNA in vascular smooth muscle cells: induction of the synthetic phenotype: a possible clue to SMC differentiation in the process of atherogenesis. *Atherosclerosis.* 1999;144:15–23.
73. Mach F, Schönbeck U, Bonnefoy JY, Pober JS, Libby P. Activation of monocyte/macrophage functions related to acute atheroma complication by ligation of CD40: induction of collagenase, stromelysin, and tissue factor. *Circulation.* 1997;96:396–399.
74. Schönbeck U et al. CD40 ligation induces tissue factor expression in human vascular smooth muscle cells. *Am J Pathol.* 2000;156:7–14.
75. Missiou A et al. CD40L induces inflammation and adipogenesis in adipose cells – a potential link between metabolic and cardiovascular disease. *Thromb Haemost.* 2010;103(4):788–796.
76. Blake GJ et al. Soluble CD40 ligand levels indicate lipid accumulation in carotid atheroma an in vivo study with high-resolution MRI. *Arterioscler Thromb Vasc Biol.* 2003;23:e11-e14.
77. Katakami N et al. Association of soluble CD40 ligand with carotid atherosclerosis in Japanese type 1 diabetic patients. *Diabetologia.* 2006;49(7):1670–1676.
78. Penno G et al. Soluble CD40 ligand levels in essential hypertensive men: evidence of a possible role of insulin resistance. *Am J Hypertens.* 2009;22(9):1007–1013.
79. de Lemos JA et al. Associations between soluble CD40ligand, atherosclerosis risk factors, and subclinical atherosclerosis: results from the Dallas Heart study. *Arterioscler Thromb Vasc Biol.* 2005;25(10):2192–2196.
80. Verma S et al. The relationship between soluble CD40 ligand levels and Framingham coronary heart disease risk score in healthy volunteers. *Atherosclerosis.* 2005;182(2):361–365.
81. Baldassarre D et al. Markers of inflammation, thrombosis and endothelial activation correlate with carotid IMT regression in stable coronary disease after atorvastatin treatment. *Nutr Metab Cardiovasc Dis.* 2009;19(7):481–490.
82. Barter PJ et al. Cholesterol ester transfer protein a novel target for raising HDL and inhibiting atherosclerosis. *Arterioscler Thromb Vasc Biol.* 2003;23:160–167.
83. Brewer HB. High-density lipoproteins: a new potential therapeutic target for the prevention of cardiovascular disease. *Arterioscler Thromb Vasc Biol.* 2004;24:387–391.
84. Okamoto H et al. A cholesteryl ester transfer protein inhibitor attenuates atherosclerosis in rabbits. *Nature.* 2000;406(6792):203–207.
85. Masson D. Anacetrapib, a cholesterol ester transfer protein (CETP) inhibitor for the treatment of atherosclerosis. *Curr Opin Investig Drugs.* 2009;10(9):980–987.
86. Joy T, Hegele RA. The end of the road for CETP inhibitors after torcetrapib? *Curr Opin Cardiol.* 2009;24(4):364–371.
87. Sofat R et al. Separating the mechanism-based and off-target actions of cholesteryl ester transfer protein inhibitors with CETP gene polymorphisms. *Circulation.* 2010;121(1):52–62.
88. Kakko S et al. Cholesteryl ester transfer protein gene polymorphisms are associated with carotid atherosclerosis in men. *Eur J Clin Invest.* 2000;30:18–25.
89. Pallaud C, Sass C, Zannad F, Siest G, Visvikis S. APOC3, CETP, fibrinogen, and MTHFR are genetic determinants of carotid intima-media thickness in healthy men (the Stanislas Cohort). *Clin Genet.* 2001;59:316–324.
90. Tsai MY et al. Cholesteryl ester transfer protein genetic polymorphisms, HDL cholesterol, and subclinical cardiovascular disease in the multi-ethnic study of atherosclerosis. *Atherosclerosis.* 2008;200(2):359–367.
91. Ridker PM et al. Polymorphism in the CETP gene region, HDL cholesterol, and risk of future myocardial infarction: genomewide analysis among 18,245 initially healthy women from the Women's Genome Health Study. *Circ Cardiovasc Genet.* 2009;2(1):26–33.
92. Ballantyne C, Nambi V. Markers of inflammation and their clinical significance. *Atheroscler Suppl.* 2005;6(2):21–29.
93. Torzewski M et al. C-reactive protein in the arterial intima: role of C-reactive protein receptor-dependent monocyte recruitment in atherogenesis. *Arterioscler Thromb Vasc Biol.* 2000;20(9):2094–2099.
94. Torzewski J et al. C-reactive protein frequently colocalizes with the terminal complement complex in the intima of early atherosclerotic lesions of human coronary arteries. *Arterioscler Thromb Vasc Biol.* 1998;18(9):1386–1392.
95. Mendall MA, Patel P, Ballam L, Strachan D, Northfield TC. C-reactive protein and its relation to cardiovascular risk factors: a population based cross sectional study. *BMJ.* 1996;312(7038):1061–1065.

96. Haverkate E, Thompson SG, Pyke SD, Gallimore JR, Pepys MB. Production of C-reactive protein and risk of coronary events in stable and unstable angina. *Lancet.* 1997;349:462–466.
97. Rifai N, Ridker PM. High-sensitivity C-reactive protein: a novel and promising marker of coronary heart disease. *Clin Chem.* 2001;47(3):403–411.
98. Ridker PM, Cushman M, Stampfer MJ, Tracy RP, Hennekens CH. Inflammation, aspirin and the risk of cardiovascular disease in apparently healthy men. *N Engl J Med.* 1997;336(14):973–979.
99. Mora S et al. Statins for the primary prevention of cardiovascular events in women with elevated high-sensitivity C-reactive protein or dyslipidemia: results from the Justification for the Use of Statins in Prevention: an Intervention Trial Evaluating Rosuvastatin (JUPITER) and meta-analysis of women from primary prevention trials. *Circulation.* 2010;121(9):1069–1077.
100. Ridker PM et al. Rosuvastatin to prevent vascular events in men and women with elevated C-reactive protein. *N Engl J Med.* 2008;359(21):2195–2207.
101. Fichtlscherer S et al. Elevated C-reactive protein levels and impaired endothelial vasoreactivity in patients with coronary artery disease. *Circulation.* 2000;102 (9):1000–1006.
102. Pearson TA et al. Markers of inflammation and cardiovascular disease: application to clinical and public health practice: a statement for healthcare professionals from the Centers for Disease Control and Prevention and the American Heart Association. *Circulation.* 2003;107(3):499–511.
103. Danesh J et al. C-reactive protein and other circulating markers of inflammation in the prediction of coronary heart disease. *N Engl J Med.* 2004;350(14):1387–1397.
104. Shah T et al. Critical appraisal of CRP measurement for the prediction of coronary heart disease events: new data and systematic review of 31 prospective cohorts. *Int J Epidemiol.* 2009;38(1):217–231.
105. Gonzalez M, Selwyn A. Endothelial function, inflammation, and prognosis in cardiovascular disease. *Am J Med.* 2003;115(8A):99S-106S.
106. Sarkar R, Meinberg EG, Stanley JC, Gordon D, Webb RC. Nitric oxide reversibly inhibits the migration of cultured vascular smooth muscle cells. *Circ Res.* 1996;78 (2):225–230.
107. \De Caterina R et al. Nitric oxide decreases cytokine-induced endothelial activation. Nitric oxide selectively reduces endothelial expression of adhesion molecules and proinflammatory cytokines. *J Clin Invest.* 1995;96(1):60–68.
108. Kawashima S, Yokoyama M. Dysfunction of endothelial nitric oxide synthase and atherosclerosis. *Arterioscler Thromb Vasc Biol.* 2004;24:998–1005.
109. Colombo MG et al. Endothelial nitric oxide synthase gene polymorphisms and risk of coronary artery disease. *Clin Chem.* 2003;49(3):389–395.
110. Karvonen J et al. Endothelial nitric oxide synthase gene Glu298Asp polymorphism and blood pressure, left ventricular mass and carotid artery atherosclerosis in a population-based cohort. *J Intern Med.* 2002;251:102–110.
111. Park JH et al. Association of the endothelial nitric oxide synthase (ecNOS) gene polymorphism with carotid atherosclerosis in type 2 diabetes. *Diabetes Res Clin Pract.* 2006;72(3):322–327.
112. Scott EM, Ariens RAS, Grant PJ. Genetic and environmental determinants of fibrin structure and function relevance to clinical disease. *Arterioscler Thromb Vasc Biol.* 2004;24:1558–1566.
113. Woods A, Brull DJ, Humphries SE, Montgomery HE. Genetics of inflammation and risk of coronary artery disease: the central role of interleukin-6. *Eur Heart J.* 2000;21:1574–1583.
114. Kerlin B et al. Cause-effect relation between hyperfibrinogenemia and vascular disease. *Blood.* 2004;103 (5):1728–1734.
115. Skibińska E et al. Homocysteine and progression of coronary artery disease. *Kardiol Pol.* 2004;60(3):197–205.
116. Carmel R, Jacobsen D, eds. *Homocysteine in Health and Disease.* Cambridge: Cambridge University Press; 2001.
117. Kanani PM et al. Role of oxidant stress in endothelial dysfunction produced by experimental hyperhomocyst(e)inemia in humans. *Circulation.* 1999;100:1161–1168.
118. Stühlinger MC et al. Homocysteine impairs the nitric oxide synthase pathway: role of asymmetric dimethylarginine. *Circulation.* 2001;104:2569–2575.
119. Majors A, Ehrhart L, Pezacka E. Homocysteine as a risk factor for vascular disease. Enhanced collagen production and accumulation by smooth muscle cells. *Arterioscler Thromb Vasc Biol.* 1997;17:2074–2081.
120. Voutilainen S, Alfthan G, Nyyssönen K, Salonen R, Salonen JT. Association between elevated plasma total homocysteine and increased common carotid artery wall thickness. *Ann Med.* 1998;30:300–306.
121. Khajuria A, Houston D. Induction of monocyte tissue factor expression by homocysteine; a possible mechanism for thrombosis. *Blood.* 2000;96:966–972.
122. Voutilainen S et al. Enhanced in vivo lipid peroxidation at elevated plasma total homocysteine levels. *Arterioscler Thromb Vasc Biol.* 1999;19(5):1263–1266.
123. Soinio M, Marniemi J, Laakso M, Lehto S, Rönnemaa T. Elevated plasma homocysteine level is an independent predictor of coronary heart disease events in patients with type 2 diabetes mellitus. *Ann Intern Med.* 2004; 140:94–100.
124. Malinow M, Nieto FJ, Szklo M, Chambless LE, Bond G. Carotid artery intimal-media wall thickening and plasma homocyst(e)ine in asymptomatic adults. The Atherosclerosis Risk in Communities Study. *Circulation.* 1993;87: 1107–1113.
125. McQuillan BM, Beillby JP, Nidorf M, Thompson PL, Hung J. Hyperhomocysteinemia but not the C677T mutation of methylenetetrahydrofolate reductase is an independent risk determinant of carotid wall thickening: the Perth Carotid Ultrasound Disease Assessment Study (CUDAS). *Circulation.* 1999;99:2383–2388.
126. Bots M, Launer LJ, Lindemans J, Hofman A, Grobbee DE. Homocysteine, atherosclerosis and prevalent cardiovascular disease in the elderly: the Rotterdam Study. *J Intern Med.* 1997;242:339–347.
127. Adachi H et al. Plasma homocysteine levels and atherosclerosis in Japan: epidemiological study by use of carotid ultrasonography. *Stroke.* 2002;33:2177–2181.

128. Inamoto N, Katsuya T, Kokubo YEA. Association of methylenetetrahydrofolate reductase gene polymorphism with carotid atherosclerosis depending on smoking status in a Japanese general population. *Stroke*. 2003; 34:1628–1633.
129. de Bree A et al. Relation between homocysteine concentrations and structural and functional arterial parameters in a French general population. *J Inherit Metab Dis*. 2003;26(suppl):24.
130. Durga J et al. Homocysteine not associated with intima-media thickness. *J Inherit Metab Dis*. 2003;26(suppl):25.
131. Vermeer SE et al. Homocysteine, silent brain infarcts and white matter lesions: the Rotterdam Scan Study. *Ann Neurol*. 2002;51:285–289.
132. Durga J, Verhoef P, Bots ML, Schouten E. Homocysteine and carotid intima-media thickness: a critical appraisal of the evidence. *Atherosclerosis*. 2004;176:1–19.
133. Casas JP, Bautista LE, Smeeth L, Sharma P, Hingorani AD. Homocysteine and stroke: evidence on a causal link from mendelian randomisation. *Lancet*. 2005;365 (9455):224–232.
134. Schuett H, Luchtefeld M, Grothusen C, Grote K, Schieffer B. How much is too much? Interleukin-6 and its signalling in atherosclerosis. *Thromb Haemost*. 2009;102 (2):215–222.
135. Harris TB et al. Associations of elevated interleukin-6 and C-reactive protein levels with mortality in the elderly. *Am J Med*. 1999;106(5):506–512.
136. Rundek T et al. Carotid intima-media thickness is associated with allelic variants of stromelysin-1, interleukin-6, and hepatic lipase genes: the Northern Manhattan Prospective Cohort Study. *Stroke*. 2002;33:1420–1423.
137. Rios DL et al. Interleukin-1 beta and interleukin-6 gene polymorphism associations with angiographically assessed coronary artery disease in Brazilians. *Cytokine*. 2010;50 (3):292–296.
138. Kronenberg F, Steinmetz A, Kostner GM, Dieplinger H. Lipoprotein(a) in health and disease. *Crit Rev Clin Lab Sci*. 1996;33:495–543.
139. Pillarisetti S, Paka L, Obunike JC, Berglund L, Goldberg IJ. Subendothelial retention of lipoprotein (a): evidence that reduced heparan sulfate promotes lipoprotein binding to subendothelial matrix. *J Clin Invest*. 1997;100:867–874.
140. Harpel P, Gordon B, Parker T. Plasmin catalyzes binding of lipoprotein(a) to immobilized fibrinogen and fibrin. *Proc Natl Acad Sci USA*. 1989;86:3847–3851.
141. Loscalzo J, Weinfeld M, Fless GM, Scanu AM. Lipoprotein(a), fibrin binding, and plasminogen activation. *Arteriosclerosis*. 1990;10:240–245.
142. Brown S, Morrissett JD, Boerwinkle E, Hutchinson R, Patsch W. The relation of lipoprotein(a) concentrations and apolipoprotein(a) phenotypes with asymptomatic atherosclerosis in subjects of the Atherosclerosis Risk in Communities (ARIC) Study. *Arterioscler Thromb*. 1993;13:1558–1566.
143. Luc G et al. Lipoprotein (a) as a predictor of coronary heart disease: the PRIME Study. *Atherosclerosis*. 2002;163 (2):377–384.
144. von Eckardstein A, Schulte H, Cullen P, Assmann G. Lipoprotein(a) further increases the risk of coronary events in men with high global cardiovascular risk. *J Am Coll Cardiol*. 2001;37(2):434–439.
145. Sharrett A et al. Coronary heart disease prediction from lipoprotein cholesterol levels, triglycerides, lipoprotein(a), apolipoproteins A-I and B, and HDL density subfractions: the Atherosclerosis Risk in Communities (ARIC) Study. *Circulation*. 2001;104(10):1108–1113.
146. Alberti K, Zimmet P. Definition, diagnosis and classification of diabetes mellitus and its complications. Part 1: diagnosis and classification of diabetes mellitus provisional report of a WHO consultation. *Diabet Med*. 1998;15 (7):539–553.
147. Adult Treatment Panel III. Executive summary of the third report of the National Cholesterol Education Program (NCEP) expert panel on detection, evaluation, and treatment of high blood cholesterol in adults. *JAMA*. 2001;285:2486–2497.
148. International Diabetes Federation. *The IDF Consensus Worldwide Definition of the Metabolic Syndrome*. Brussels: IDF; 2005.
149. Paras E, Mancini GBJ, Lear SA. The relationship of three common definitions of the metabolic syndrome with subclinical carotid atherosclerosis. *Atherosclerosis*. 2008;198 (1):228–236.
150. Wallenfeldt K, Hulthe J, Fagerberg B. The metabolic syndrome in middle-aged men according to different definitions and related changes in carotid artery intima-media thickness (IMT) during 3 years of follow-up. *J Intern Med*. 2005;258(1):28–37.
151. Pollex RL et al. Relationship of the metabolic syndrome to carotid ultrasound traits. *Cardiovasc Ultrasound*. 2006;4:28.
152. Yan JC, Wu ZG, Kong XT, Zong RQ, Zhan LZ. Relation between upregulation of CD40 system and complex stenosis morphology in patients with acute coronary syndrome. *Acta Pharmacol Sin*. 2004;25(2):251–256.
153. Jormsjö S et al. Allele-specific regulation of matrix metalloproteinase-12 gene activity is associated with coronary artery luminal dimensions in diabetic patients with manifest coronary artery disease. *Circ Res*. 2000;86 (9):998–1003.
154. Galis ZS, Sukhova GK, Lark MW, Libby P. Increased expression of matrix metalloproteinases and matrix degrading activity in vulnerable regions of human atherosclerotic plaques. *J Clin Invest*. 1994;94:2493–2503.
155. Shah P et al. Human monocyte-derived macrophages induce collagen breakdown in fibrous caps of atherosclerotic plaques: potential role of matrix-degrading metalloproteinases and implications for plaque rupture. *Circulation*. 1995;92:1565–1569.
156. Brown DL, Hibbs MS, Kearney M, Loushin C, Isner JM. Identification of 92-kD gelatinase in human coronary atherosclerotic lesions: association of active enzyme synthesis with unstable angina. *Circulation*. 1995;91(8):2125–2131.
157. Higashikata T et al. Altered expression balance of matrix metalloproteinases and their inhibitors in human carotid plaque disruption: results of quantitative tissue analysis using real-time RT-PCR method. *Atherosclerosis*. 2006;185(1):165–172.
158. Morgan AR et al. Differences in matrix metalloproteinase-1 and matrix metalloproteinase-12 transcript levels among carotid atherosclerotic plaques with different

159. Schoenhagen P et al. Relation of matrix-metalloproteinase 3 found in coronary lesion samples retrieved by directional coronary atherectomy to intravascular ultrasound observations on coronary remodeling. *Am J Cardiol.* 2002;89(12):1354–1359.
160. Katsuda S, Kaji T. Atherosclerosis and extracellular matrix. *J Atheroscler Thromb.* 2003;10(5):267–274.
161. Halpert I et al. Matrilysin is expressed by lipid-laden macrophages at sites of potential rupture in atherosclerotic lesions and localizes to areas of versican deposition, a proteoglycan substrate for the enzyme. *Proc Natl Acad Sci USA.* 1996;93(18):9748–9753.
162. Jefferis BJ et al. Prospective study of matrix metalloproteinase-9 and risk of myocardial infarction and stroke in older men and women. *Atherosclerosis.* 2010;208(2):557–563.
163. Gnasso A et al. Genetic variation in human stromelysin gene promoter and common carotid geometry in healthy male subjects. *Arterioscler Thromb Vasc Biol.* 2000;20:1600–1605.
164. Rauramaa R et al. Stromelysin-1 and interleukin-6 gene promoter polymorphisms are determinants of asymptomatic carotid artery atherosclerosis. *Arterioscler Thromb Vasc Biol.* 2000;20:2657–2662.
165. Román-García P et al. Matrix metalloproteinase 1 promoter polymorphisms and risk of myocardial infarction: a case-control study in a Spanish population. *Coron Artery Dis.* 2009;20(6):383–386.
166. Rauch I, Iglseder B, Paulweber B, Ladurner G, Strasser P. MMP-9 haplotypes and carotid artery atherosclerosis: an association study introducing a novel multicolour multiplex RealTime PCR protocol. *Eur J Clin Invest.* 2008;38(1):24–33.
167. Lim J, Um HJ, Park JW, Lee IK, Kwon TK. Interleukin-1beta promotes the expression of monocyte chemoattractant protein-1 in human aorta smooth muscle cells via multiple signaling pathways. *Exp Mol Med.* 2009;41(10):757–764.
168. Aiello R et al. Monocyte chemoattractant protein-1 accelerates atherosclerosis in apolipoprotein E-deficient mice. *Arterioscler Thromb Vasc Biol.* 1999;19:1518–1525.
169. Ylä-Herttuala S et al. Expression of monocyte chemoattractant protein 1 in macrophage-rich areas of human and rabbit atherosclerotic lesions. *Proc Natl Acad Sci USA.* 1991;88:5252–5256.
170. Nelken N, Coughlin SR, Gordon D, Wilcox JN. Monocyte chemoattractant protein-1 in human atheromatous plaques. *J Clin Invest.* 1991;88:1121–1127.
171. Takeya M, Yoshimura T, Leonard EJ, Takahashi K. Detection of monocyte chemoattractant protein-1 in human atherosclerotic lesions by an anti-monocyte chemoattractant protein-1 monoclonal antibody. *Hum Pathol.* 1993;24:534–539.
172. Gersztén R et al. MCP-1 and IL-8 trigger firm adhesion of monocytes to vascular endothelium under flow conditions. *Nature.* 1999;398:718–723.
173. Tabata T, Mine S, Kawahara C, Okada Y, Tanaka Y. Monocyte chemoattractant protein-1 induces scavenger receptor expression and monocyte differentiation into foam cells. *Biochem Biophys Res Commun.* 2003;305:380–385.
174. Viedt C et al. Monocyte chemoattractant protein-1 induces proliferation and interleukin-6 production in human smooth muscle cells by differential activation of nuclear factor-kB and activator protein-1. *Arterioscler Thromb Vasc Biol.* 2002;22:914–920.
175. de Lemos JA et al. Association between plasma levels of monocyte chemoattractant protein-1 and long-term clinical outcomes in patients with acute coronary syndromes. *Circulation.* 2003;107:690–695.
176. Cipollone F et al. Elevated circulating levels of monocyte chemoattractant protein-1 in patients with restenosis after coronary angioplasty. *Arterioscler Thromb Vasc Biol.* 2001;21:327–334.
177. Oshima S et al. Plasma monocyte chemoattractant protein-1 antigen levels and the risk of restenosis after coronary stent implantation. *Jpn Circ J.* 2001;65:261–264.
178. Deo R et al. Association among plasma levels of monocyte chemoattractant protein-1, traditional cardiovascular risk factors, and subclinical atherosclerosis. *J Am Coll Cardiol.* 2004;44:1812–1818.
179. McDermott DH et al. CCL2 polymorphisms are associated with serum monocyte chemoattractant protein-1 levels and myocardial infarction in the Framingham Heart Study. *Circulation.* 2005;112(8):1113–1120.
180. Steinberg D, Parthasarathy S, Carew TE, Khoo JC, Witztum JL. Beyond cholesterol: modifications of low-density lipoprotein that increase its atherogenicity. *N Engl J Med.* 1989;320:915–924.
181. Tsimikas S, Witztum JL. Measuring circulating oxidized low-density lipoprotein to evaluate coronary risk. *Circulation.* 2001;103:1930–1932.
182. Berliner JA et al. Atherosclerosis: basic mechanisms: oxidation, inflammation, and genetics. *Circulation.* 1995;91(9):2488–2496.
183. Aikawa M et al. Lipid lowering by diet reduces matrix metalloproteinase activity and increases collagen content of rabbit atheroma: a potential mechanism of lesion stabilization. *Circulation.* 1998;97(24):2433–2444.
184. Nishi K et al. Oxidized LDL in carotid plaques and plasma associates with plaque instability. *Arterioscler Thromb Vasc Biol.* 2002;22:1649–1654.
185. Holvoet P, Collen D. Oxidation of low density lipoproteins in the pathogenesis of atherosclerosis. *Atherosclerosis.* 1998;137:S33-S38.
186. Hulthe J, Fagerberg B. Circulating oxidized LDL is associated with subclinical atherosclerosis development and inflammatory cytokines (AIR Study). *Arterioscler Thromb Vasc Biol.* 2002;22:1162–1167.
187. Holvoet P et al. The relationship between oxidized LDL and other cardiovascular risk factors and subclinical CVD in different ethnic groups: the Multi-Ethnic Study of Atherosclerosis (MESA). *Atherosclerosis.* 2007;194(1):245–252.
188. Chrysohoou C et al. The association between pre-hypertension status and oxidative stress markers related to atherosclerotic disease: the ATTICA study. *Atherosclerosis.* 2007;192(1):169–176.

189. Skoog T et al. Plasma tumour necrosis factor-alpha and early carotid atherosclerosis in healthy middle-aged men. *Eur Heart J*. 2002;23:376–383.
190. Bennet AM et al. Association of TNF-(alpha) serum levels and TNFA promoter polymorphisms with risk of myocardial infarction. *Atherosclerosis*. 2006;187(2):408–414.
191. Wang XL, Oosterhof J. Tumour necrosis factor alpha G-308 – >A polymorphism and risk for coronary artery disease. *Clin Sci*. 2000;98(4):435–437.
192. Wilson AG, Symons JA, McDowell TL, McDevitt HO, Duff GW. Effects of a polymorphism in the human tumor necrosis factor alpha promoter on transcriptional activation. *Proc Natl Acad Sci USA*. 1997;94(7):3195–3199.
193. Louis E et al. Tumour necrosis factor (TNF) polymorphism influences TNF-a production in lipopolysaccharide (LPS)-stimulated whole blood cell culture in healthy humans. *Clin Exp Immunol*. 1998;113:401–406.
194. Keso T et al. Polymorphisms within the tumor necrosis factor locus and prevalence of coronary artery disease in middle-aged men. *Atherosclerosis*. 2001;154(3):691–697.
195. Pereira TV, Rudnicki M, Franco RF, Pereira AC, Krieger JE. Effect of the G-308A polymorphism of the tumor necrosis factor alpha gene on the risk of ischemic heart disease and ischemic stroke: a meta-analysis. *Am Heart J*. 2007;153(5):821–830.
196. Raghu V, Robert JD. Increased expression of genes that control ionic homeostasis, second messenger signaling and metabolism in the carotid plaques from patients with symptomatic stroke. *J Neurochem*. 2006;97(s1):92–96.
197. Ijäs P et al. Microarray analysis reveals overexpression of CD163 and HO-1 in symptomatic carotid plaques. *Arterioscler Thromb Vasc Biol*. 2007;27(1):154–160.
198. Papaspyridonos M et al. Novel candidate genes in unstable areas of human atherosclerotic plaques. *Arterioscler Thromb Vasc Biol*. 2006;26(8):1837–1844.
199. Adams LD, Geary RL, Li J, Rossini A, Schwartz SM. Expression profiling identifies smooth muscle cell diversity within human intima and plaque fibrous cap: loss of RGS5 distinguishes the cap. *Arterioscler Thromb Vasc Biol*. 2006;26(2):319–325.
200. Murillo CA et al. Integrin and matrix metalloproteinase expression in human carotid plaque. *J Surg Res*. 2009;155(1):157–164.
201. Zhang QJ, Goddard M, Shanahan C, Shapiro L, Bennett M. Differential gene expression in vascular smooth muscle cells in primary atherosclerosis and in stent stenosis in humans. *Arterioscler Thromb Vasc Biol*. 2002;22(12):2030–2036.
202. Zohlnhöfer D et al. Gene expression profiling of human stent-induced neointima by cDNA array analysis of microscopic specimens retrieved by helix cutter atherectomy: detection of FK506-binding protein 12 upregulation. *Circulation*. 2001;103(10):1396–1402.
203. Al-Shali K et al. Differences between carotid wall morphological phenotypes measured by ultrasound in one, two and three dimensions. *Atherosclerosis*. 2005;178(2):319–325.
204. Baldassarre D et al. Carotid intima-media thickness and markers of inflammation, endothelial damage and hemostasis. *Ann Med*. 2008;40(1):21–44.

28 Subclinical Atherosclerosis, Markers of Inflammation, and Oxidative Stress

Stefan Kiechl, Philipp Werner, Michael Knoflach, and Johann Willeit

28.1 The Inflammatory Background of Atherosclerosis

The concept that atherosclerosis is an inflammatory disease goes back to the middle of the nineteenth century when Rudolf Virchow stated that "he felt no hesitation in admitting an inflammation of the inner arterial coat to be the starting point of the so-called atheromatous degeneration"[1] and Carl von Rokitansky considered "chronic inflammation of the cellular sheet of the diseased vessel to be a secondary consecutive appearance which associated itself with the already established deposit."[2] Both scientists agreed in that there are infiltrations of chronic inflammatory cells in all stages of human atherosclerosis including precursor lesions (fatty streaks) but were uncertain whether inflammation is a primary or secondary phenomenon. In the 1970s, Russell Ross has coined the now generally accepted response-to-injury hypothesis assuming atherosclerosis to emerge as a consequence of the adaptive and innate immune defense against numerous pro-atherogenic stimuli such as lipid retention in the vessel wall, oxidative modification of lipoproteins, and endothelial stress and dysfunction.[3,4] Meanwhile, there has been substantial progress in our recognition of key inflammatory pathways and processes featuring the inflammatory environment of atherosclerotic tissue.

Atherosclerotic lesions contain a variety of immune cells, mostly T-cells and macrophages, but also mast cells, B cells, and temporary neutrophils.[5] Endothelial activation elicited by bioactive lipids retained in the vasculature and other noxes contributes early on to atherosclerosis development (Fig. 28.1). Initial events are the over-expression of adhesion molecules especially vascular cell adhesion molecule-1 (VCAM-1) and chemokines mediating the attachment of inflammatory cells and their migration into the arterial wall (Fig. 28.1). Hemodynamic factors influence the distribution of adhesion molecules on the endothelial surface with sites of altered shear stress and disturbed flows near branching points becoming sites of predilection for atheroma formation. Monocytes trapped in the arterial wall differentiate to macrophages under the influence of monocyte colony-stimulating factor and express scavenger, toll-like, and other innate immune receptors. Accumulation of intracellular cholesterol via scavenger receptors leads to the characteristic appearance of foam cells, and ligation of toll-like receptors cause a release of inflammatory mediators (Fig. 28.1).

T-cells further amplify the inflammatory response once activated via antigen-presenting cells (dendritic cells, B cells, and macrophages) adopting a type 1 helper T-cell (Th-1) phenotype.[6] T-cell cytokines like interferon-γ cause a production of downstream components of the inflammation cascade, and C-reactive protein is detected in peripheral circulation. The so far best characterized T-cell antigens are heat-shock protein 60, Chlamydia proteins, and oxidatively modified low-density lipoprotein (LDL). While Th-1

S. Kiechl (✉) • M. Knoflach • J. Willeit
Department of Neurology, Medical University Innsbruck, Innsbruck, Tyrol, Austria

P. Werner
Neurovascular Disease and Stroke Center, State Hospital, Feldkirch, Vorarlberg, Austria

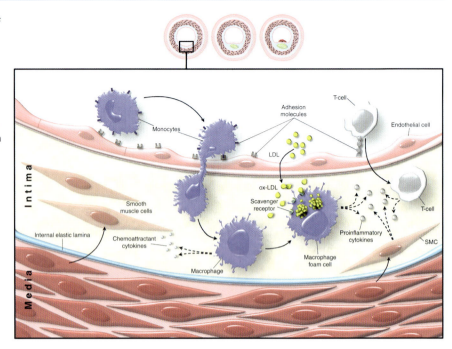

Fig. 28.1 Transition from the normal arterial wall to early atherosclerosis. Key mechanisms involved are the endothelial expression of adhesion molecules, monocyte and T cell chemotaxis, immune activation, formation of foam cells, and migration of smooth muscle cells (*SMCs*) from the tunica media into the intima

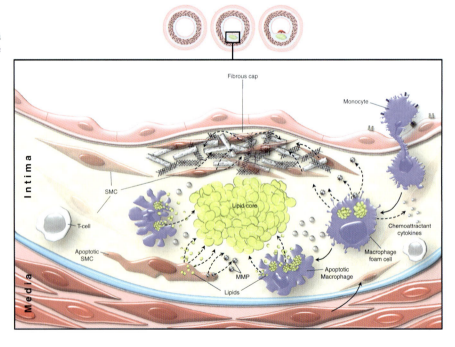

Fig. 28.2 Stable atheroma (fibrofatty plaque). Stable plaques are characterized by a high content of smooth muscle cells (*SMCs*), formation of extracellular matrix, ongoing but balanced immuno-inflammation, and formation of a lipid core

cells are pro-atherogenic, Th-2 cells show both pro- and anti-atherogenic properties, and special regulatory T-cell lines, the so-called CD4[+]FoxP3 T-cells, suppress injurious immune responses in a dominant manner.[6]

Plaques initially progress slowly and are composed of foam cells, extracellular lipid droplets, caps of smooth muscle cells that have immigrated from the tunica media, and extracellular matrix (fibrofatty plaque or stable atheroma – Figs. 28.1 and 28.2). Macrophages, T-cells, and mast cells that accumulate in more mature lesions may release considerable amounts of cytokines, proteases like metalloproteinase

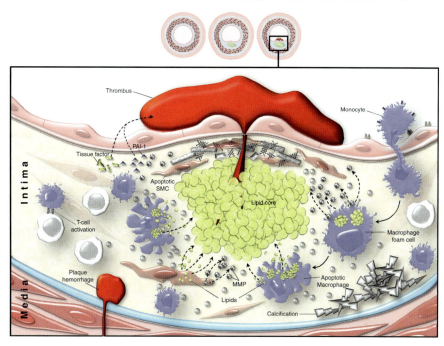

Fig. 28.3 Transition of a stable to an unstable plaque phenotype. Core features are a substantial up-regulation of plaque inflammation, formation of a large lipid core, matrix degradation, thinning of the fibrous cap, cell senescence and smooth muscle cell (*SMC*) apoptosis, neovascularization and plaque hemorrhage, calcification, plaque rupture, release of plasminogen activator inhibitor-1 (*PAI-1*) and tissue factor, and subsequent thrombus formation

8 and 9, prothrombotic molecules like tissue factor, and vasoactive compounds. Consequences are the breakdown of macromolecules and extracellular matrix, apoptosis and senescence of smooth muscle cells, necrosis and apoptosis of foam cells with a release of intracellular debris, further accumulation of immune cells, critical thinning of the fibrous cap, and, finally, plaque rupture and atheroma-associated thrombus formation (complicated plaque – Fig. 28.3). Most culprit lesions causing myocardial infarction or stroke are of moderate size not causing hemodynamic compromise prior to the event.

Apart from inflammation, there has been also substantial progress in the understanding of the mechanisms underlying arterial calcification. It is now broadly recognized that calcification represents a process that is subject to a complex positive and negative regulation involving specific vessel-derived calcification inhibitors – rather than a passive accumulation of mineral (Fig. 28.3).[7] Specifically, the non-collagenous proteins osteopontin, osteonectin, and osteoprotegerin regulate bone formation and mineralization in atherosclerotic tissue and in diabetic vasculopathy. Vascular calcification is assumed to stabilize atherosclerotic plaques, but under certain circumstances, calcium deposits in the intima layer may enhance shear stress forces rendering plaques susceptible to rupture.

In addition to the classic rupture of inflamed lesions with a thinned out fibrous cap and to endothelial denudation, intra-plaque hemorrhage based upon neovascularization significantly contributes to plaque destabilization (Fig. 28.3).

The phenomenon of atheroma-associated thrombus formation is determined by the balance between procoagulant factors and the activity of anti-thrombotic systems and endogenous fibrinolysis – as discussed subsequently in this chapter. Tissue factor is a particularly potent trigger of the coagulation cascade (Fig. 28.3). It originates from the complicated plaques and from tissue factor microparticles traveling with blood monocytes – thus closing the link between systemic inflammation and thrombogenicity.

28.2 Contributors to Systemic Inflammation in Patients with Atherosclerosis

Levels of inflammatory markers have consistently been linked to atherosclerosis in various vascular territories and to its main clinical sequelae stroke and myocardial infarction.[8,9] The sources of inflammation, mediators and triggers of the inflammatory process, and predisposing genetic background are less well established but are the subject of extensive current research efforts. All these issues will shortly be addressed below.

28.2.1 Sources of Inflammation

In brief, systemic inflammation associated with and predictive of atherosclerosis progression and cardiovascular disease is assumed to originate from (a) autoimmune disorders, (b) chronic infections, (c) chronic inflammatory and allergic diseases, (d) cardiovascular risk factors with a strong inflammatory component, and (e) active atherosclerosis itself.

28.2.1.1 Autoimmune Disorders

There is now compelling evidence of a relationship between autoimmune diseases including systemic lupus erythematosus and rheumatoid arthritis with vascular disease.[10] In all these disorders, premature atherosclerosis is the most common cause of stroke and myocardial infarction, surpassing the relevance of genuine vasculitis, associated coagulation disorders (anti-phospholipid antibody syndrome), and autoimmune endocarditis. In rheumatoid arthritis, cardiovascular disease risk is twofold to threefold that of normal, and cardiovascular disease drives much of the excess mortality in patients with rheumatoid arthritis. Adequate therapy with immunosuppressant drugs has been shown to reduce the risk of stroke and myocardial infarction. There is good reason to assume that the increased vascular risk extends to other autoimmune diseases and cancer alike, but the scientific evidence currently available is insufficient to draw firm conclusions.

Knowledge about the mechanisms linking autoimmune diseases with an enhanced burden of atherosclerosis is rapidly expanding.[10] Pro-inflammatory cytokines especially TNFα (tumor necrosis factor alpha) and IL-1 released from affected joints in rheumatoid arthritis act on other tissues at a distance. In particular, chronic systemic inflammation triggers endothelial dysfunction and promotes oxidative stress in the vasculature.

28.2.1.2 Chronic Infections

Other prominent sources of systemic inflammation are common chronic infections affecting a large segment of the adult population.[11] Chronic infection subsumes periodontitis, chronic sinusitis and bronchitis, and chronic urinary tract and skin infections including the classic diabetic foot. Most of these conditions have been linked to an amplified risk of cardiovascular disease and atherosclerosis as have been infections with specific pathogens (*C. pneumoniae* and virulent strains of *H. pylori*). Remarkably, the strength of association is modified by the extent of inflammation elicited by the infectious agents reflecting their virulence and the individual host–pathogen interaction.[11]

28.2.1.3 Chronic Inflammatory and Allergic Diseases

Two disorders of expanding frequency – chronic obstructive pulmonary disease and allergic asthma – were suggested to enhance the risk of stroke and myocardial infarction.[11,12] There is ample evidence that pulmonary inflammation in chronic obstructive pulmonary disease and localized allergic diseases give rise to a systemic inflammatory response mediated by the release of vasoactive peptides and cytokines into the circulation. Endothelial cells at locations distinct from the pulmonary circulation and site of allergen exposure have been found to enhance adhesion molecule expression, thus facilitating leukocyte trafficking into the vessel wall and promoting atherosclerosis. Furthermore, mast cells – the cellular hallmark of allergies and a frequent constituent of atherosclerotic tissue – participate in the local innate immune defense and exert various pro-atherogenic properties (Fig. 28.4).[12,13] Finally, up-regulation of pro-atherogenic leukotrienes may contribute to the coincidence of allergic and vascular diseases.

28.2.1.4 Cardiovascular Risk Factors

Several cardiovascular risk factors have an inflammatory basis and promote vascular disease in part through pro-inflammatory mechanisms as is firmly established for cigarette smoking, diabetes, insulin resistance, and adiposity. In current and ex-smokers and subjects exposed to environmental tobacco smoke, inflammation is an important intermediate component in the mediation of injurious effects of cigarette smoke on

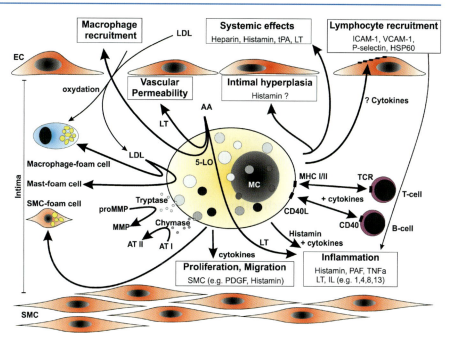

Fig. 28.4 Pro-atherogenic properties of mast cells (*MCs*). *AA* arachidonic acid, *5-LO* 5-lipoxygenase, *LT* leukotrienes, *PAF* platelet-activating factor, *PDGF* platelet-derived growth factor, *tPA* tissue plasminogen activator (Reprinted with permission from Knoflach et al.[12] Copyright © 2005 American Medical Association. All rights reserved)

the vasculature. The authors and others have shown that an excess burden of atherosclerosis and high risk of vascular disease are confined to smokers exhibiting elevated levels of C-reactive protein or suffering from chronic infections.[14] In diabetes, there is an ongoing dispute on whether low-grade inflammation triggers hepatic insulin resistance (e.g., by enhancing nuclear factor kappa B [NF-κB] activation) or whether inflammation develops as a component of the (pre)-diabetic milieu.[15] Regardless of its precise role in the manifestation of diabetes, chronic inflammation significantly contributes to the fate and prognosis of individual patients.[15]

28.2.2 The Genetic Background

The extent of inflammation elicited by pro-inflammatory risk conditions is assumed to be largely determined by the individual genetic background. Individuals can roughly be classified as high- versus low-cytokine responders. Analyses of gene–environment interactions are now in progress, and first promising data regarding vascular inflammation have become available and replicated in independent populations.[16] In spite of these advances and the availability of genome-wide association studies, the bulk of genetic predisposition for the development of atherosclerosis – related to

inflammation and oxidative stress – still remains to be characterized. Vice versa, key genetic contributors to cardiovascular disease discovered recently, like the common variant on chromosome 9p21 (rs1333049), have been linked to the cell cycle proteins *CDKN2A* and *CDKN2B* implicit in cell senescence rather than to inflammatory signaling pathways.[17,18]

28.2.3 Noxes, Pathways, and Mechanisms

As to the underlying pro-inflammatory signaling pathways, the innate immune system has moved into recent focus of attention.[5] As anticipated, atherosclerosis is viewed to emerge as a consequence of the local adaptive and innate immune defense against oxidized lipoproteins, heat-shock proteins, and microbial products critically involving scavenger receptors and toll-like receptors 2 and 4.

28.2.3.1 Noxes

Microbial products such as bacterial endotoxin, petidoglycan, and heat-shock proteins originate from chronic infection but also from bacteria continuously crossing the skin or mucosal barrier, from cigarette smoke, and from pollution.[19] Oxidative modification of lipoproteins with generation of reactive and pro-atherogenic oxidized phospholipid moieties is among the first events in the atherosclerosis process and starts with the retention of lipoproteins in the vessel wall and exhausting of anti-oxidant vitamins.[20] Heat-shock proteins in turn are expressed on the surface of activated endothelial cells and are released from necrotic cells and all types of bacteria.[21] A substantial number of activated T-cells in atherosclerotic tissues actually have specificity to one of these epitopes.

28.2.3.2 Pathways and Mechanisms

Inflammatory signaling and defense is highly complex and involves endocytic, secreted, and trans-membrane innate immune receptors; natural antibodies; and adaptive B and T-cell immunity.[3-5] Pathways, molecular mechanisms, and pro-atherogenic consequences are exemplified for toll-like receptors 2 and 4 – the two key signaling receptors of the innate immune system (Fig. 28.5).

In brief, innate immunity constitutes a first-line defense system against various stress factors, which can rapidly be mobilized within minutes to hours. In contrast to adaptive immunity, it recognizes not every possible antigen but a few highly conserved molecular patterns exposed by large groups of microorganisms but foreign to the host – the so-called pathogen-associated molecular patterns. Examples are bacterial lipopolysaccharide, peptidoglycan, flagellin, mannans, bacterial CpG-DNA repeats, and double-stranded RNA (Fig. 28.5). Of the toll family, toll-like receptors 4 and 2, which are expressed on virtually all human cells, may take a crucial position given the wide spectrum of potential exogenous and endogenous ligands.[22] Upon ligation of most toll-like receptors including type 4 and 2, the adapter protein MyD88 is recruited to the receptor complex, and the NF-κB and mitogen-activated protein kinase (MAPK) pathways are activated, ultimately leading to the expression of genes encoding for anti-microbial peptides, peptides inducing apoptosis, inflammatory cytokines, chemokines, proteins involved in the production of oxygen species and phagocytosis, and co-stimulatory molecules that provide a link to adaptive immunity (Fig. 28.5).[22] These inflammatory mediators can exert various pro-atherogenic effects involving the expression of adhesion molecules on endothelial cells, proliferation of smooth muscle cells, activation of immune cells, and stimulation of the acute-phase response (Fig. 28.5).[22] Relevancy of toll-like receptor pathways in atherogenesis derives support from both epidemiological studies and animal research.[23,24] For example, atherosclerosis-susceptible mice strains cross-bred with MyD88 knock-out mice enjoy near-complete protection against vessel pathology.[24] In line, inbred mouse strains with a mutated TLR4 gene (C3H/HeJ) are resistant to neointimal hyperplasia and cholesterol-induced atherosclerosis.

28.3 Early and Advanced Atherosclerosis

In spite of the particular strengths of carotid IMT like its high reproducibility and ease of assessment, it is a simplistic measure that fails to capture the complexity of plaque evolution and does not allow one to study changes of vessel status on an individual basis. This is because IMT growth over a practicable time period is relatively slow and beneath the detection limit of current ultrasound equipment. Moreover, IMT does not show linear growth kinetics, but kinetics that flatten in the upper range. For all these shortcomings, development of person-based progression models of atherosclerosis allowing to differentiate between early and advanced complicated stages of disease and to assess stage-specific risk profiles and pathomechanisms are required.[25,26] A simple model was set up and validated within the framework of the Bruneck study and showed excellent performance in a number of analyses. Methodological and practical details have been published in detail,[27-29] but a brief summary is given below.

28.3.1 Methodological and Practical Details of the Bruneck Study

28.3.1.1 Population Recruitment and Follow-up

The Bruneck study is a prospective population-based survey on the epidemiology and etiology of carotid atherosclerosis. The baseline examination was performed between July 1990 and November 1990 in the semi-urban mountainous area of Bruneck (Bolzano Province, Italy) in a random population of 1,000 individuals. To best utilize population size in terms of accurate sex- and age-specific rates of atherosclerosis

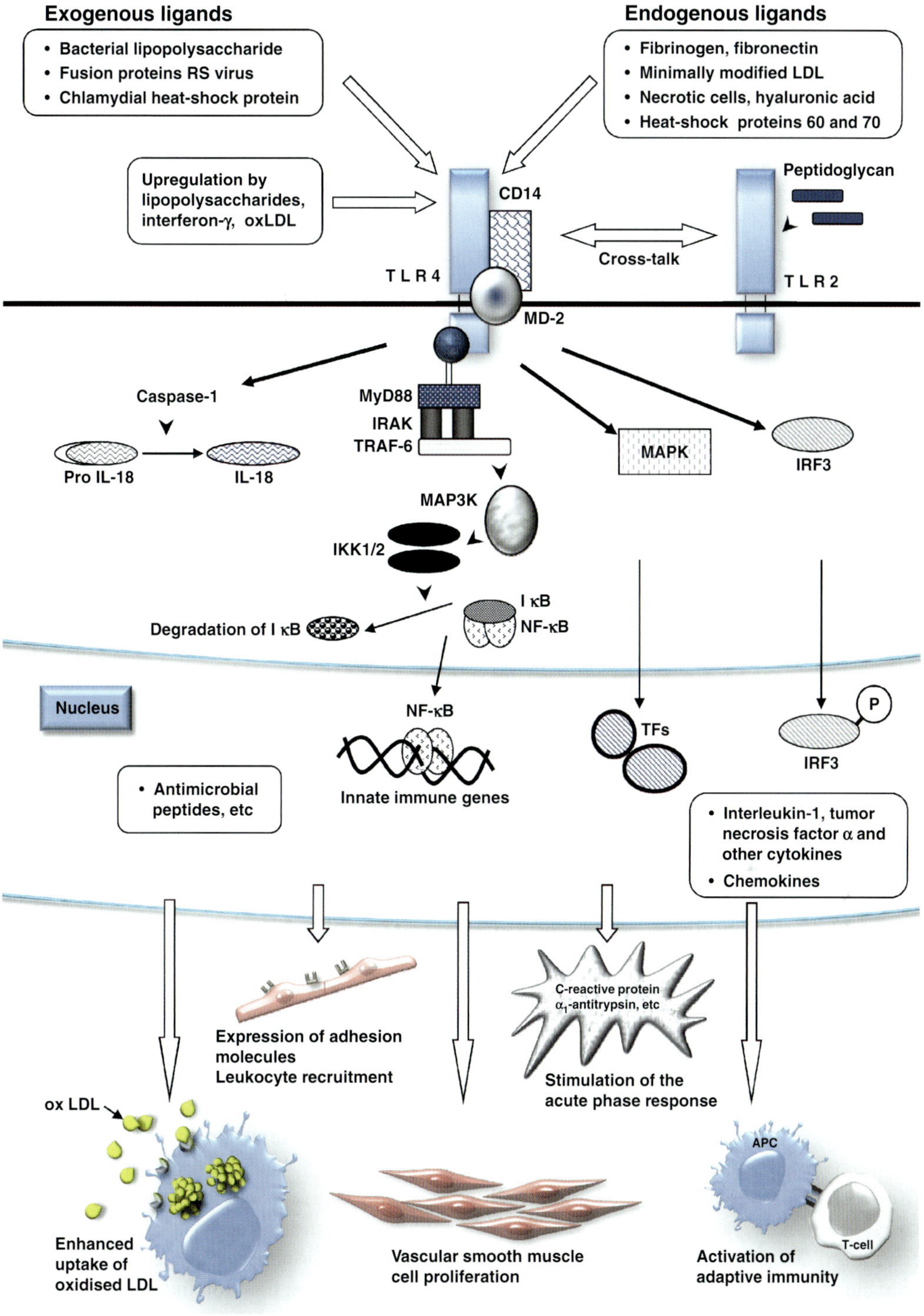

Fig. 28.5 Toll-like receptor (TLR) 2 and 4 signaling pathways – a schematic overview of ligands, regulation of receptor expression, and mechanisms of signal transduction. Activation of TLR2 and TLR4 recruits the adapter protein MyD88, which initiates a signaling cascade leading to activation of IκB kinases 1 and 2. These kinases trigger degradation of IκB and the release and nuclear translocation of NF-κB with a subsequent transcription of inflammatory- and immune-response genes. In addition, interferon regulatory factor 3 (IRF3), caspase-1, and mitogen-activated protein kinase (MAPK) are activated in a MyD88-independent manner. Pro-atherogenic consequences are visualized in the lower part of this graph

incidence and progression, equal contingents of men and women ($n = 125$) in each the fifth to eight decade were selected for inclusion. In the choice of the follow-up interval, the authors were mainly guided by the objective of ascertaining a sufficient number of incident carotid stenoses as the ultrasound endpoint with the lowest rate of occurrence. Extrapolation of cross-sectional data suggested that a follow-up period of 5 years was sufficient for this requirement. The first re-evaluation was scheduled for July 1995 to October 1995 when 826 individuals were available. Incident cardiovascular disease, defined as cardiovascular death, myocardial infarction, stroke, and transient ischemic attack, was assessed up to 2010.

28.3.1.2 Scanning Protocol

Sonographic assessment of the extracranial carotid arteries was performed using a duplex ultrasound system (ATL8, Advanced Technology Laboratories, Bothell, Washington, USA) with 10-MHz scanning frequency in brightness mode (B-mode) and 5-MHz scanning frequency in pulsed-Doppler mode. All subjects were examined in the supine position. The scanning protocol included imaging of the right and left common carotid arteries (CCA) and internal carotid arteries at the following locations: proximal CCA (15–30 mm proximal to the carotid bulb), distal CCA (<15 mm proximal to the carotid bulb), proximal internal carotid artery (ICA) (carotid bulb, identified by loss of the parallel wall present in the CCA and the initial 10 mm of the vessel above the flow divider between external and internal carotid arteries), and distal ICA (>10 mm above the flow divider). For each segment, the sonographer imaged the vessel in multiple longitudinal and transverse planes to identify the largest axial diameter of focal plaques and to adequately visualize the interface required to measure intima-media thickness (IMT). The maximum axial diameter of plaques was assessed in each of 16 vessel segments, and an atherosclerosis score was calculated by addition of diameters. Pulsed Doppler was used to provide information on blood flow velocity and to identify the various arteries.

Atherosclerotic lesions were defined by two ultrasound criteria: (1) wall surface (protrusion into the lumen or roughness of the arterial boundary) and (2) wall texture (echogenicity). The authors did not use an IMT cut-off to discriminate plaques from wall thickening. The maximum axial diameter of each plaque was measured as the distance from the leading edge of the lumen–intima interface to the leading edge of the media–adventitia interface. For the assessment of stenosis, Doppler criteria or, when no hemodynamic disturbances were detectable, the percentage of maximum diameter reduction in the B-mode images was applied. Peak systolic velocities exceeding 180 and 250 cm/s were considered indicative of stenosis greater than 60% and 80%, respectively. Scanning was performed every 5 years by the same experienced sonographer, who was unaware of the subjects' clinical and laboratory characteristics. For documentation purposes, short segments of real-time ultrasonography and frozen longitudinal and transversal images were recorded for each vessel segment.

28.3.1.3 Incidence of Carotid Atherosclerosis

Age-specific incidence/progression rates were assessed for age strata of 5 years each and detailed in Kiechl and Willeit[27]. Rates were calculated under the assumption of a consistent probability of incident/progressive atherosclerosis across the 5-year age intervals. Equal risks were allocated from the first to fifth year of follow-up; cases contributed, on average, 2.5 years of follow-up to the denominator of the incidence formula. Cumulative Λ rates were converted into cumulative risks by means of the formula $P = 1 - \exp(-\Lambda)$.

28.3.1.4 Risk Profiles at 5 Years

The risk profile of early atherogenesis consisted of traditional risk factors, such as hypertension, hyperlipidemia, and cigarette smoking (pack years), supplemented by a variety of less well-established risk conditions, including high body iron stores, hypothyroidism, microalbuminuria, and high alcohol consumption. In contrast, the risk profile of advanced atherogenesis included markers of enhanced prothrombotic capacity, attenuated fibrinolysis, and clinical conditions known to interfere with coagulation: high fibrinogen, low antithrombin, factor V Leiden mutation, lipoprotein(a) >0.32 g/L, high platelet count, cigarette smoking, and diabetes.[29] These findings, along with the epidemiological features of advanced atherogenesis and emergence of an elevated fibrin turnover (high D-dimer), suggest atherothrombosis to be a key mechanism in the development of advanced stenotic atherosclerosis.

Atherosclerosis is a heterogeneous process that subsumes etiologically and epidemiologically distinct disease entities. The multifactorial etiology of atherosclerosis, which goes far beyond the traditional risk factors, has not yet achieved adequate attention in clinical practice and disease prevention.

28.3.2 The Various Stages in Atherosclerosis

Most atherosclerotic lesions developed at sites with enhanced vessel wall thickness. Incidence of atherosclerosis in premenopausal women was less than half that observed in men of equal age. The sex difference disappeared within 5 years after menopause and was attributed to gender variations in body iron stores (Fig. 28.6)[30] and hormonal changes. Overall, incidence rates of carotid atherosclerosis range from near zero to 184 per 1,000 person-years dependent on age and sex.[27]

Based on the pathomechanisms outlined at the beginning of this chapter (Figs. 28.1–28.3) and elsewhere in the book, atherosclerosis is hallmarked by the dichotomy of (a) early conventional atherosclerosis causing continuous growth of plaques and ending up in what is commonly termed "diffuse dilative atherosclerosis" and (b) advanced complicated atherosclerosis featured by plaque rupture or endothelial denudation and atherothrombosis, and resulting in stenotic or occlusive vessel pathology.[25,26] From an ultrasound point of view, atherosclerotic lesions may experience two different fates according to this dichotomy.[27,28] (a) Non-stenotic progression was characterized by a slow and continuous plaque extension which usually affected several lesions simultaneously and did not primarily focus on the carotid bifurcation. This step-by-step process relies on a cumulative exposure to well-known risk factors supplemented by several promising less well-established risk conditions such as iron overload, hypothyroidism, microalbuminuria, chronic infections, and heavy alcohol drinking (Fig. 28.7). Compensatory enlargement of the artery at the site of active atherosclerosis effectively preserves a normal lumen (see below). (b) The second main type of plaque growth was characterized by occasional prominent increases in lesion size and failure in vascular remodeling (see below). This process was primarily manifest near branching points like at the initial segment of the internal carotid artery and was mediated by pro-coagulant risk factors in a way that peak levels were relevant rather than cumulative exposure.[29] The risk profile included markers of enhanced thrombotic activity, attenuated fibrinolysis, and clinical conditions known to interfere with coagulation (Fig. 28.7).[29]

Fighting the same standard risk factors in all patients – as is common clinical practice – ignores the complexity of atherogenesis and its multifactorial etiology. While there is substantial knowledge about mechanisms of and contributors to early atherogenesis, data on triggers of plaque destabilization and atherothrombosis are still sparse.

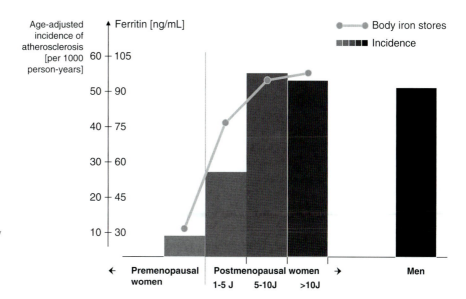

Fig. 28.6 Body iron stores reflected by serum ferritin levels in men and women prior, during, and after menopause in the Bruneck study. Accumulation of body iron is closely related to the loss of pre-menopausal protection against atherosclerosis

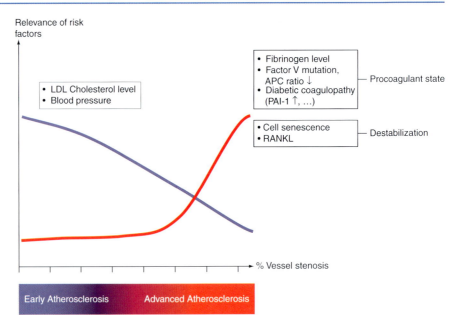

Fig. 28.7 Changes in the relevance of vascular risk factors according to the stage of vessel pathology

28.3.3 Vascular Remodeling

In animal-experimental research, various types of arteries have been shown to enlarge in response to diet-induced atherogenesis. Relevancy of such a process in the human vasculature was first proposed by Glagov based on post-mortem evaluations (Fig. 28.8).[31] He observed that coronary arteries enlarge in relation to plaque area, and functionally important lumen stenosis is delayed until the lesion occupies 40% of the internal elastic lamina area.[31] A limitation of autopsy evaluation is that only a static view of a dynamic process can be provided. A first large-scale proof-of-concept in vivo was performed in the prospective Bruneck study (Fig. 28.8).[28] Early atherosclerosis showed a slow and continuous type of plaque growth. This process was accompanied by a compensatory enlargement of the vessel at the site of active atherosclerosis which effectively maintained a normal lumen, even when plaques grew larger than 3–4 mm in diameter, or was overcompensatory (Fig. 28.8). Vascular remodeling apart from local compensation involved a generalized dilation response of vessel segments not primarily affected. A second main type of plaque growth was characterized by an episodic marked increase in lesion volume probably on the basis of plaque thrombosis. In this setting, there was not a maximum yet insufficient compensation but usually no compensation at all. Failure of vascular remodeling and marked expansion in plaque size acted synergistically in producing significant lumen compromise (Fig. 28.8).[28]

Interestingly, carotid arteries free of atherosclerosis and wall thickening preserved a normal size until high ages. In contrast, common and internal carotid arteries free of plaques but with elevated intima-media thickness experienced marked age-dependent dilation starting in the fifth decade and continuously accelerating thereafter.[28] These changes reflect the structural aging of the vasculature.

28.3.4 Atherosclerosis Progression

Pre-existing atherosclerosis strongly predicted the risk of further plaque development independent of the presence or absence of vascular risk factors (Fig. 28.9).[29] For example, individuals with the same three risk factors with and without pre-existing atherosclerosis differed in their probability of atherosclerosis progression (manifestation of new plaques and non-stenotic progression of prevalent lesions) by a factor of two to three (Fig. 28.9). This observation from prospective population studies provides solid evidence of an auto-catalytic component in atherogenesis and reinforces the necessity to intervene early in the disease process – preferable in the young before definite atherosclerosis has emerged. The mechanisms underlying this phenomenon are not precisely defined, but

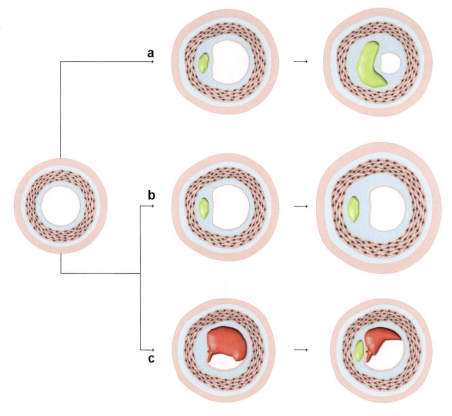

Fig. 28.8 Vascular remodeling concepts proposed by Glagov et al.[29] (**a**) and derived from the Bruneck study[25,26] (**b** and **c**). Efficacy of vascular remodeling primarily depends on the type of atherosclerosis progression (see text)

plaque inflammation and autoimmunity are likely to be of relevance.[21] Speculatively, inflammation and dysimmunity initiated by risk factors proceed even if the risk factors are tightly controlled.

28.4 Traditional Markers of Inflammation and Oxidative Stress

28.4.1 C-Reactive Protein & Co.

Atherosclerosis and its clinical presentations are closely linked to low-grade systemic inflammation. Apart from being involved in various key processes of plaque development, markers of inflammation have proven useful for the purposes of cardiovascular risk prediction and an individual tailoring of preventive measures especially statin medication. Among various acute-phase reactants relevant to this scenario, high-sensitivity C-reactive protein is the one most extensively studied and best established.[8] C-reactive protein is a member of a highly conserved pentraxin protein family and serves as a soluble innate immune receptor. Levels of C-reactive protein predict vascular risk in a broad variety of clinical settings as has been shown in various large studies and meta-analyses and, in some instances, allow reclassifications of individuals to a higher risk category.[8] In comparison to other acute-phase reactants, assessment of C-reactive protein bears several advantages including the high consistency of serum levels over time (in case blood samples are collected in periods free of infection, trauma, and surgery), availability of standardized assays, and excellent scientific basis. Additional promising markers of inflammation not yet recommended for clinical application are fibrinogen, serum amyloid A, and interleukin-6 as well as components of specific inflammation pathways such as CD40 ligand, vascular cell adhesion molecule-1 (VCAM-1), intracellular adhesion molecule-1 (ICAM-1), monocyte chemo-attractant protein-1 (MCP-1), or myeloperoxidase (MPO) (Chap. 27).

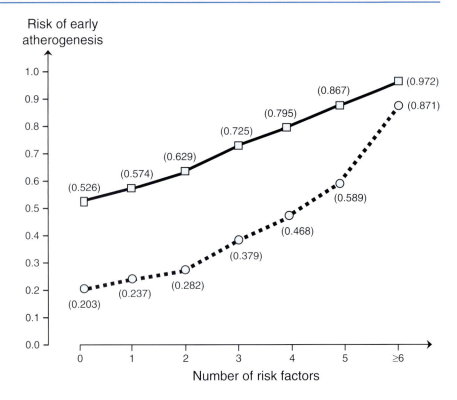

Fig. 28.9 Risks of atherosclerosis progression according to the number of vascular risk factors and presence or absence of baseline atherosclerosis in the Bruneck study. The lines symbolize subjects with (*upper line*) and without (*lower line*) baseline atherosclerosis

28.4.2 Oxidized Phospholipids

Oxidative stress is a key mechanism through which atherosclerosis and cardiovascular disease develop. It is mediated by reactive oxygen species that alter the fundamental properties of cholesterol, cholesterol esters, and phospholipids on lipoproteins, to make them dysfunctional, immunogenic, and pro-atherogenic.[20] Oxidative stress can be enhanced by non-enzymatic pathways, such as iron cations, as well as by enzymatic pathways involving lipoxygenases and myeloperoxidases. Pro-oxidant pathways are balanced by anti-oxidant vitamins present within lipoproteins (alpha-tocopherol and carotenoids) and various anti-oxidant enzymes (superoxide dismutase and glutathione peroxidase). Many of these enzymes and products of oxidation can be measured in the circulation (oxidized low-density lipoprotein, isoprostanes, lipoprotein-associated phospholipase A2, myeloperoxidases, etc.) and have been shown to predict the risk of cardiovascular disease. Of note, plasma level of oxidized phospholipids (OxPL) present on individual apolipoprotein B-100 particles and measured by the murine monoclonal antibody E06 has been reported to correlate with the extent of carotid and coronary atherosclerosis and manifestation of cardiovascular diseases.[32,33] The vast majority of pro-atherogenic OxPLs in circulation travel on Lp(a) particles, and the preferential binding of OxPL by Lp(a) may be part of an innate immune response to detoxify OxPL. This concept gives Lp(a) a new physiological meaning. Chronically elevated levels may be detrimental due to Lp(a)'s high content of pro-inflammatory OxPL and prolonged residence time in the arterial wall.[34] In support of this view, Lp(a) is highly enriched in lipoprotein-associated phospholipase A2 (sevenfold higher than LDL), an enzyme that degrades OxPL, and Lp(a) appears to increase in plasma in a manner similar to acute-phase proteins.

28.4.3 Iron Overload

Among the various pro-oxidant stimuli, tissue and especially macrophage iron deserves special attention. Experimentally, it is well established that iron catalyzes the formation of toxic hydroxyl radicals thereby contributing to a pro-oxidant and inflammatory stress environment. Human atherosclerotic tissue contains large amounts of iron (3- to 17-fold that of normal vasculature) capable of inducing lipid peroxidation in vitro. Main sources of iron are micro-hemorrhages within the plaque and inflammation-driven iron retention in macrophages. Iron facilitates macrophage uptake of lipids through stimulation of scavenger receptor expression, foam-cell formation, and macrophage apoptosis with a subsequent recruitment of new macrophages. In atherosclerosis-susceptible mice, this vicious circle can effectively be interrupted by iron restriction or chelation.

Iron overload has been linked to an increased risk of atherosclerosis and its clinical sequelae stroke and myocardial infarction even though current epidemiological evidence is not entirely consistent.[30] The hypothesis of a key role of iron in lipid-induced atherogenesis has attracted substantial interest given the availability of effective and well-tolerated measures to deplete body iron stores (regular blood donation), the common practice of alimentary iron fortification in industrialized countries, and the high frequency of the HFE C282Y genotype comprising a genetic predisposition to iron overload. Moreover, the iron hypothesis provides an intriguing explanation for the gender difference in cardiovascular disease and the loss of female protection against atherosclerosis after menopause when iron rapidly accumulates (Fig. 28.6). The ongoing debate about the validity of this concept recently intensified and peaked at the time of publication of the results from a large proof-of-concept intervention trial (NCT00032357) failing to demonstrate beneficial effects of iron depletion on new-onset cardiovascular disease among peripheral artery disease patients but showing a significant lowering in vascular risk among individuals younger than 69 years.[35]

28.5 Novel Markers of Inflammation and Oxidative Stress

In recent years, the understanding of the pathological processes involved in atherogenesis has been enriched by hypotheses on several novel risk conditions and effector pathways. An excerpt of particularly promising recent developments is outlined below.

28.5.1 Lipoprotein-Associated Phospholipase A$_2$ (Lp-PLA$_2$)

The lipoprotein-associated phospholipase A$_2$ (Lp-PLA$_2$) enzyme specifically hydrolyzes oxidized phospholipids on oxidatively modified lipoproteins thereby producing pro-atherogenic oxidized free fatty acids and lyosphosphatidylcholine.[32,33] These molecules stimulate monocyte chemotaxis and trapping in the vessel wall. Resident monocytes transform to macrophages and amplify the production and release of Lp-PLA$_2$ more than 100-fold. Lp-PLA$_2$ partly re-enters the bloodstream and preferentially attaches to LDL particles by protein–protein interaction with the apo-B100 moiety. Concentration of Lp-PLA$_2$ in lipoprotein particles is assumed to depend on the particles' turnover with highest levels seen in lipoproteins with low clearance rates like small dense LDL and Lp(a).

Lp-PLA$_2$ mass is a risk predictor of cardiovascular disease independent of and additive to conventional risk factors and has recently been cleared for clinical application.[36] Of note, high activity of Lp-PLA$_2$ (enzyme) and high levels of oxidized phospholipids (substrate) synergistically amplify the risk of myocardial infarction and stroke as shown in the Bruneck study based on the 10-year cardiovascular outcomes (Fig. 28.10).[33]

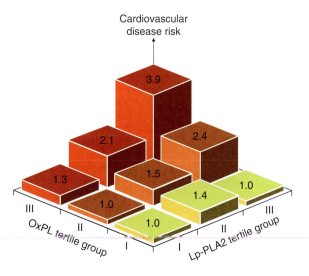

Fig. 28.10 Synergistic effects of oxidized phospholipids (OxPLs) and Lp-PLA$_2$ activity on cardiovascular disease risk (Reprinted with permission from Kiechl et al.[33])

Moreover, Lp-PLA$_2$ is assumed to actively contribute to plaque destabilization. Its expression is up-regulated in the shoulder region of lipid-rich plaques prone to rupture and co-localizes with foam cells, macrophages, T-cells, and mast cells. Statins lower LDL concentrations and by its close coupling with LDL also Lp-PLA$_2$ mass and activity. Selective inhibition of Lp-PLA$_2$ is feasible as well and currently tested for potential protective effects on acute vascular syndromes (STABILITY [Stabilization of Atherosclerotic Plaque by Initiation of Darapladib Therapy] phase III trial).

28.5.2 The OPG–RANK–RANKL System

The frequent coincidence between atherosclerosis and osteoporosis tempts speculations about common risk factors and pathways, and a shared genetic predisposition. The osteoprotegerin (OPG)/receptor activator of nuclear factor-κB (RANK)/receptor activator of nuclear factor-κB ligand (RANKL) system is a cytokine network crucially involved in the regulation of bone remodeling and recently implicated in arterial calcification, formation of aortic aneurysms, heart failure, and advanced atherosclerosis as well as its clinical consequences stroke and myocardial infarction.[37] OPG and RANKL are assumed to exert pleiotropic effects on vascular calcification and matrix integrity and proposed to be engaged in human immune defense and the regulation of vascular inflammation and apoptosis (Fig. 28.11).[38] Both members of the TNF and TNF receptor superfamily are expressed in vascular cells and immune cells harbored in the vessel wall (Fig. 28.11). Tissue concentrations of RANKL are substantially up-regulated in atherosclerotic plaques prone to rupture especially in border zones to calcifications and in lipid-rich vulnerable plaques. In line, RANKL expression on circulating T-cells is amplified in patients with an unstable plaque pheno-

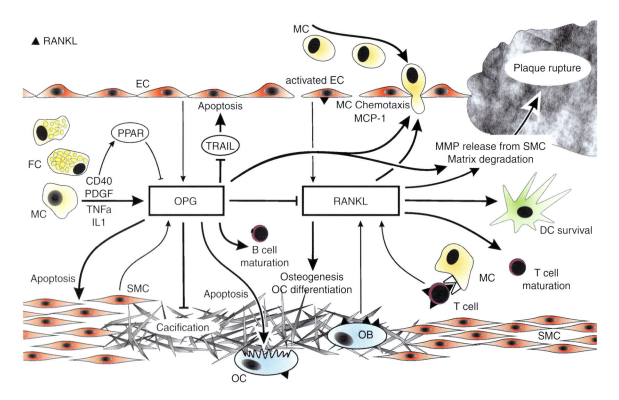

Fig. 28.11 Schematic overview of current knowledge about the role of OPG and RANKL in atherosclerosis. Both molecules are assumed to exert pleiotropic effects on vascular calcification, matrix integrity, vascular inflammation, and apoptosis (Adapted from Kiechl et al.[37] With permission of Expert Reviews)

type, and serum level of RANKL predicts acute vascular syndromes.[39] In the Bruneck study, baseline serum level of RANKL emerged as a highly significant predictor of vascular risk (adjusted hazard ratio per 1-unit increase in soluble RANKL, 1.27; 95% confidence interval, 1.16–1.40; $P < 0.001$). Predictive significance was independent of that afforded by the classic vascular risk factors, C-reactive protein, osteoprotegerin concentration, and severity of carotid atherosclerosis. Findings were internally consistent and robust in a variety of sensitivity analyses. Notably, soluble RANKL was not associated with carotid or femoral artery atherosclerosis. This study lends large-scale epidemiological support to a role for RANKL in cardiovascular disease. In the absence of a significant association between RANKL and atherosclerosis, the idea that RANKL promotes plaque destabilization and rupture is a highly appealing concept. Accordingly, RANKL is considered to be a promising target for therapeutical intervention. Pharmacological RANKL antagonism has recently been established as a novel approach in the therapy of osteoporosis. Serum level of OPG in turn is a reliable marker of the overall activity of the OPG/RANK/RANKL system and has been linked to advanced atherosclerosis, cardiovascular disease, and mortality with the predictive capacity surpassing that of most conventional risk factors and biomarkers.[40] It may well find future application in the routine estimation of vascular risk.

28.5.3 Chemokine Receptors and Impaired Fibrinolysis

Chemokines are soluble proteins produced by leukocytes that upon binding to their cognate receptors result in the initiation of G-protein-dependent intracellular signal and chemotaxis of T-cells and monocytes along a chemokine concentration gradient. CCR5 similar to other chemokine receptors is a trans-membrane-spanning α-helices structure with an extracellular N-terminal segment involved in chemokine binding and a cytoplasmic C-terminal tail involved in G protein signaling. CCR5 is expressed on various vascular cells and mediates the activities of pro-atherogenic ligands like RANTES, eotaxin, MIP-1α, and MIP-1β. Levels of chemokines and chemokine receptors are notoriously difficult to measure, but there are genetic variants that allow exploring functional consequences of chemokine action on atherogenesis. For example, the common 32-bp frameshift deletion mutation in the chemokine receptor CCR5 completely attenuates receptor function in a homozygous state, rendering individuals resistant against various infectious and inflammatory diseases like human immunodeficiency virus (HIV), hepatitis C, and rheumatoid arthritis.

In the Bruneck study, the authors have investigated the association of the functional 32-bp frameshift deletion mutation in chemokine receptor (CCR5) in relation to atherosclerosis. Genetic screening of this mutation was carried out using polymerase chain reaction in 810 subjects of whom 7 were homozygous, 102 were heterozygous, and 701 were normal. The mutation was associated with significantly lower levels of C-reactive protein in a dose-dependent manner. Moreover, CCR5-del32 was associated with a significantly lower carotid intima-media thickness in the common carotid artery (del32/del32, 837 ± 8 μm; wt/del32, 909 ± 21 μm; wt/wt, 958 ± 8 μm; $P = 0.007$ after multivariable adjustment). Furthermore, incident cardiovascular disease (1995–2005) was markedly reduced in del32 homozygote and heterozygote subjects compared with wild-type homozygotes (del32/del32 = 0%, wt/del32 = 7.8%, wt/wt = 14.8%, $P = 0.020$).

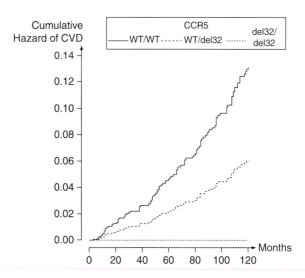

Fig. 28.12 Cumulative hazard curves of incident cardiovascular disease (CVD) by CCR5 genotype in the Bruneck study. The common 32-bp frameshift deletion mutation in a homozygous state confers excellent protection against cardiovascular disease

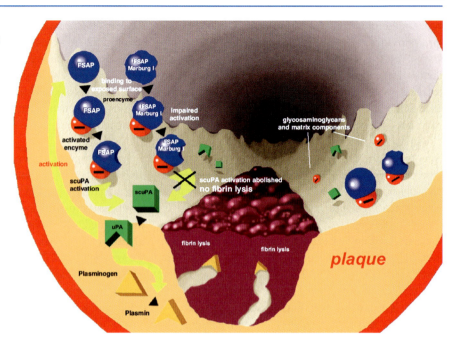

Fig. 28.13 FSAP – activation and potential role in endogenous fibrinolysis and atherothrombosis (see text)

Findings equally applied to coronary artery and cerebrovascular disease. The chemokine receptor CCR5-del32 association with low levels of C-reactive protein, decreased intima-media thickness, and cardiovascular disease risk is consistent with the hypothesis that the chemokine receptor CCR5 is involved in the mediation of low-grade systemic inflammation and may play a role in human atherosclerosis and cardiovascular disease (Fig. 28.12).[41]

Atherothrombosis is of outstanding relevance in the evolution and progression of vessel stenosis and counteracted by anti-thrombotic systems and endogenous fibrinolysis. The former include tissue factor inhibitor, antithrombin III, and the protein C/protein S pathways while tissue plasminogen activator cleaving plasminogen to plasmin and urokinase are the main constituents of endogenous fibrinolysis. The serine protease Factor Seven Activating Protease (FSAP) is a potent activator of prourokinase in vitro. In an analysis of the Bruneck study involving 810 men and women, the FSAP Marburg I polymorphism was found in 37 subjects (carriage rate 4.4%). Individuals with this genetic variant showed a prominently reduced in vitro capacity to activate prourokinase. No relation was found to exist between the Marburg I polymorphism and early atherogenesis. In contrast, it emerged as a strong and independent risk predictor of incident/progressive carotid stenosis (multivariate odds ratio [95%CI], 6.6 [1.6–27.7]). The risk profile of advanced atherogenesis further included cigarette smoking, high lipoprotein(a), the factor V Leiden mutation, low antithrombin III, high fibrinogen, and diabetes. Thus, in concert with other genetic and acquired conditions known to interfere with coagulation or fibrinolysis, the Marburg I polymorphism of FSAP, which attenuates its capacity to activate prourokinase and facilitates arterial thrombosis in vivo, is a significant risk predictor for the evolution and progression of carotid stenosis (Fig. 28.13).[42]

28.6 Inflammation and Early Vessel Pathology in the Young

28.6.1 General Remarks and Historical Notes

Traditionally, atherosclerosis has been viewed as a prototypic disease of the elderly. Over the past years, however, it became apparent that atherosclerosis already starts in early life and slowly progresses over decades until it manifests clinically as myocardial infarction, peripheral artery occlusive disease, or stroke. Most of the knowledge about vascular risk factors originates from data assessed in middle-aged and elderly populations. Vice versa, insights into the frequency and risk conditions of very early vessel pathology among young individuals are preliminary. In concert, current evidence suggests that (a) the atherosclerosis process starts in adolescence, (b) conventional risk factors of adult life are relevant to the initiating stages of vessel pathology but comparatively rare in this age group, and (c) nontraditional risk conditions reflecting systemic inflammation, oxidative stress, and dysimmunity have a considerable weight.

28.6.2 Assessment of Intima-Media Thickness (IMT) as a Surrogate of Atherosclerosis Applicable to Young Individuals

28.6.2.1 The Atherosclerosis Risk-Factors in Female Youngsters (ARFY) Study

The Atherosclerosis Risk-Factors in Female Youngsters (ARFY) study was designed by the authors' group to investigate the association between traditional and numerous nontraditional risk factors and carotid artery IMT in a population of women aged 18–22 years.[43] Special focus was put on inflammation markers, levels of humoral and cellular immune reactivity to heat-shock protein 60 (HSP60), metabolic abnormalities as well as environmental exposure to tobacco smoke, and exhaust gases as a main source of ambient air pollution. This cross-sectional study enrolled 205 18- to 22-year-old female students from the Educational Centre for Allied Health Professions.

The ultrasound protocol involved scanning of the common and internal carotid arteries (CCA and ICA, respectively) on both sides with a 10-MHz linear transducer on a General Electric Logic7 (Milwaukee, Wisconsin, USA). All scans were performed by two experienced sonographers unaware of subjects' characteristics. Different scanning angles (anterior and posterolateral) were used to identify the greatest wall thickness, and longitudinal images were recorded at multiple vessel segments with the ultrasound beam directed through the axis of the vessel. Measurements were made from stored digital images by a single highly experienced sonographer, who again was blinded to all characteristics of study participants. IMT was assessed as the distance between the interface of lumen and intima and the interface between media and adventitia. Maximum far wall IMT values were recorded for the CCA (segments 0–40 mm below the flow divider) and ICA (first 10 mm distal to the flow divider separating internal and external carotid arteries) and averaged for the left and right sides (mean maximum IMT). High IMT was considered given when at least one segment-specific IMT value exceeded the 90th percentile (≥ 0.70 mm in the CCA and ≥ 0.55 mm for the ICA).

In multivariable logistic regression analysis, systolic blood pressure, family history for hypertension, lipoprotein(a), homocysteine, T-cell immune reaction against human heat-shock protein 60, and exposure to environmental tobacco smoke and exhaust gases emerged as independent predictors of high IMT. Obesity, metabolic syndrome, and classical risk factors other than high blood pressure were rare and unrelated to IMT. Findings were similar once focusing on IMT as a continuous variable. It was concluded that in female youngsters displaying initiating stages of vascular pathology, blood pressure level and numerous nontraditional risk conditions showed a significant relation to high IMT. The authors' study indicated that (auto)immune processes, high lipoprotein(a), and environmental exposure to tobacco smoke and traffic exhaust may play a role in early atherogenesis.

28.6.2.2 The Atherosclerosis Risk-Factors in Male Youngsters (ARMY) Study

The Atherosclerosis Risk-Factors in Male Youngsters (ARMY) study was performed in order to evaluate the relation of traditional vascular risk factors, markers of inflammation, and levels of humoral and cellular immune reactivity to HSP60s with carotid and femoral artery IMT in a population of male youngsters.[44] A total of 159 individuals agreed to participate and were subjected to a B-mode ultrasound study of the carotid and femoral arteries. The ultrasound protocol involved scanning of the internal carotid artery, carotid bulb, common carotid artery, and superficial femoral artery on both sides with a 10- to 5-MHz broadband linear transducer on an HDI 3000 (ATL, Bothell, Washington, USA). All scans were performed by the same sonographer using different scanning angles (anterior and posterolateral) to identify the greatest wall thickness. Longitudinal images directed through the center of the artery were taken at each vessel site. Measurements were made from stored digital images by an experienced reader. The IMT was assessed at the far wall as the distance between the interface of the lumen and intima and the interface between the media and adventitia. The maximal IMT was recorded at each of the four vessel segments and averaged for the left and right sides. High IMT was considered to be present when at least one segment-specific IMT exceeded the 90th percentile. In a multivariate logistic regression analysis, cigarette smoking, high diastolic blood pressure, prominent immune reactivity to human and/or mycobacterial HSP60s, alcohol consumption (inverse), and low high-density lipoprotein (HDL) cholesterol levels (inverse) were all associated with high IMT. The prevalence of high IMT substantially increased from 0 to 60% when the number of risk conditions in a single individual increased from 0 to 4 ($P < 0.001$ for linear trend). The results of this study support the concept that atherosclerosis begins in the first decades of life and suggests a role of the immune system, especially immunoreactivity against HSP60s, in atherosclerosis of young individuals.

28.6.2.3 IMT in Young Individuals

In Fig. 28.14, the distribution of mean maximum IMT is presented, measured in the common carotid and internal carotid arteries, from three population samples of distinct age which were evaluated by the very same ultrasound methodology and research teams.[43,44] IMT curves for the young populations (ARFY and ARMY) clearly indicate that most definitions for an enhanced IMT (e.g., over 1 mm) would leave all young individuals in the normal range. Still, IMT in young men and women shows a substantial variability, and IMT values exceeding the 90th percentile of the distribution in one or more vessel segments were by far more frequent in individuals with a clustering of vascular risk conditions. A total of 64% of young men and 55% of young women with four or more risk factors already showed increased IMT according to this definition. In young age groups, the CCA exhibits a higher IMT variability than the ICA. Interestingly, IMT is very much similar in young men and women of identical age, suggesting that the well-established gender difference is not determined at birth or during puberty but develops later in life probably triggered by a more unfavorable risk profile in men and hormonal protection in women. In summary, although the prognostic

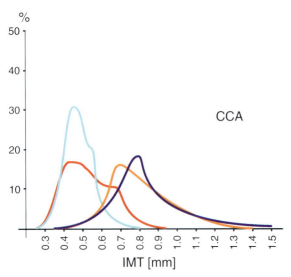
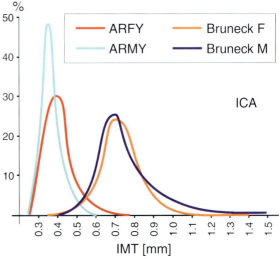

Fig. 28.14 Distribution of mean maximum common carotid artery (CCA) and internal carotid artery (ICA) IMT in young women aged 18–22 years (ARFY study – *red line*), young men aged 17–18 years (ARMY study – *light blue line*), and middle-aged men (*dark blue line*) and women (*orange line*) from the Bruneck study (age range 45–64 years)

value of IMT for the lifetime risk of cardiovascular disease and the cumulative burden of atherosclerosis remains to be elucidated for young individuals, IMT is associated with traditional and novel risk conditions in this age group.[43,44]

28.6.3 Immunity to Heat-Shock Proteins

Like in adults, inflammation is a driving force of early atherogenesis in the young. As a response to injurious noxes, vascular endothelium expresses adhesion molecules and increases its permeability. Mononuclear cells (T-lymphocytes and macrophages) attach to the activated endothelium and migrate into the intima. These cells interact with endogenous and microbial molecules via pattern-recognition receptors and specific T-cell receptors and induce a release of inflammatory cytokines, chemokines, and oxygen and nitrogen radicals leading to inflammation, tissue damage, and early atherosclerosis. A promising hypothesis links the immune reaction against heat-shock protein 60 (Hsp60) to human atherosclerosis.[21] Heat-shock proteins are chaperoning proteins that are expressed in reaction to various forms of stress. This protection system has been conserved during evolution from bacteria onward to mammals, and therefore different heat-shock proteins yield a high sequence homology (e.g., more than 50% between *E. coli* and human). As a consequence, antibodies and T-cells specifically detecting bacterial Hsp60 can cross-react with human Hsp60 that is expressed on stressed vascular endothelial cells (molecular mimicry) or with biochemically altered Hsp60 (bona fide autoimmunity) (Fig. 28.15). In the Bruneck study, levels of sHSP60 were significantly elevated in subjects with prevalent/incident carotid atherosclerosis and correlated with common carotid artery intima-media thickness. Multiple logistic regression analysis documented these associations as independent of age, sex, and other risk factors. Interestingly, sHSP60 was also correlated with anti-lipopolysaccharide, anti-*Chlamydia* and anti-HSP60 antibodies, various markers of inflammation, and the presence of chronic infections. The risk of

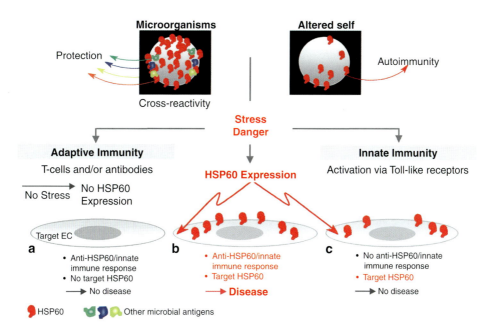

Fig. 28.15 The potential role of autoimmunity to heat-shock protein 60 (HSP60) in human atherosclerosis. Protection against microbial infection is in part mediated by innate and adaptive immunity directed against microbial HSP60. (**a**) Under physiological conditions, human vascular endothelial cells (EC) do not express HSP60. (**b**) The stress-induced expression of HSP60 on target ECs can result in cross-reactivity of the immune response between human and microbial HSP60 entailing dysfunction of ECs. (**c**) In some cases, autoimmunity might not develop, despite the presence of human HSP60 on ECs, because the MHC class I and II grooves of these individuals do not accommodate the atherogenic HSP60 epitopes (Reprinted with permission from Wick et al.[21] Permission conveyed through Copyright Clearance, Inc.)

atherosclerosis associated with high sHSP60 levels was amplified when subjects had clinical and/or laboratory evidence of chronic infections.[45,46] In line, T-cell reactivity to Hsp60 was significantly related to early atherosclerosis in cross-sectional studies of young men and women as well as in experimental animals, however, not in adults with more advanced atherosclerosis.[21]

28.6.4 Practical Notes

Given the exceptional occurrence of full-born atherosclerotic lesions in the young, a focus on definite plaques in epidemiological research would require very large population samples and put an inadequate weight to infrequent disorders of lipid metabolism and early-onset diabetes. In order to study effects of lifestyle factors as well as traditional and nontraditional risk factors on early vessel pathology, IMT is a useful target measure to be assessed. Given the modest variability of mean IMT values calculated from measurements in distinct vessel segments, the ARFY and ARMY studies gave preference to maximum IMT assessments detecting areas of focal wall thickening which are already prevalent at this age range and adequately model the focal nature of early atherosclerosis.[43,44]

28.7 A Short Digression on Cell Senescence

Telomeres are nucleoprotein complexes capping the extreme ends of chromosomes and contributing to the maintenance of the chromosomal integrity. Telomeres progressively shorten with each cell cycle, and telomere length accurately reflects the biological age at a cellular level. Excessive cell replication and telomere attrition lead to cell senescence featured by cell cycle arrest and changes in gene expression. A series of recent stimulating experimental investigations has suggested a tight interplay between cell senescence and atherosclerosis. In vitro studies on senescent endothelial cells revealed multiple pro-atherogenic changes in cell phenotype and yielded evidence of a decreased repair and vascular remodeling capacity, and impaired angiogenic properties (Fig. 28.16). In advanced plaques, senescence of various cell lines including vascular smooth muscle cells favors plaque rupture and atherothrombosis. Specifically, accumulation of aged cells due to high cell turnover and impaired phagocytic clearance elicits prominent tissue inflammation and matrix degradation which results in a thinning of the fibrous cap (Fig. 28.16). Accordingly, cell aging is assumed to promote the transition of a stable to an unstable plaque phenotype. Epidemiological studies to prove this concept are under way. So far, investigations have suggested a link between leukocyte telomere length – a surrogate for telomere length in the vasculature – and overall cardiovascular disease risk.[47]

Two recent population-based studies[48,49] tested the association of mean leukocyte telomere length with ultrasonic measures of subclinical atherosclerosis and cardiovascular disease. In both studies of similar size, the carotid and femoral bifurcations were scanned ($n = 762$ and $n = 800$). Mean leukocyte telomere length was determined with a quantitative real-time polymerase chain reaction (PCR)-based method. The studies agreed in that mean leukocyte telomere length was inversely and significantly related to new-onset cardiovascular disease and to subclinical atherosclerosis, and findings remained robust after correction for traditional risk factors. There was some heterogeneity in men and women,[48] different vascular beds and stages of atherosclerosis.[48,49] Leukocyte telomere length was also associated with age and sex-adjusted levels of high-sensitivity C-reactive protein (hsCRP), sCD40L, homocysteine, creatinine, HDL cholesterol and ApoA1, Lp(a), ferritin level, diabetes, and homeostatic model assessment of insulin resistance (HOMA-IR). The results support the telomere hypothesis and may provide insights into a novel treatment to prevent atherosclerosis.

28.8 Future Perspectives

How does all this rapidly expanding knowledge based on the study of subclinical atherosclerosis using ultrasound translate into clinical routine? Potential advances are threefold.

First, new insights into inflammatory and oxidative mechanisms in atherogenesis have offered new opportunities for the diagnosis and management of vascular diseases. Sophisticated imaging techniques

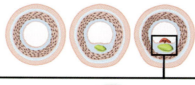
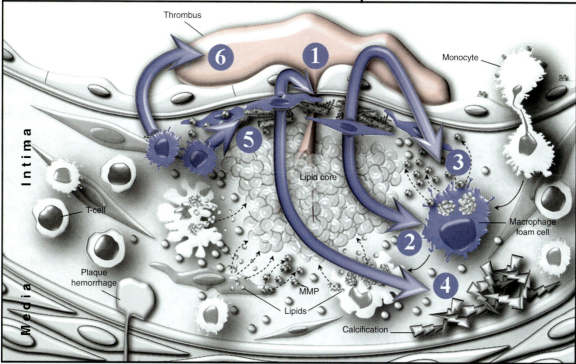

Fig. 28.16 Schematic overview of pathomechanisms linking telomere shortening, replicative cell senescence, and advanced atherosclerosis. Senescent smooth muscle cells (*SMCs*) and macrophages accumulate in advanced lesions (in *blue*) and undergo multiple pro-atherogenic changes in cell phenotype leading to an impaired healing of plaque fissures (1), prominent inflammation (2), matrix degeneration (3), calcification (4), thinning of the fibrous cap (5), and thrombus formation (6)

to accurately identify vulnerable plaques prone to rupture have recently been developed.[50] Promising examples are computed tomography–positron emission tomography (CT–PET) fusion techniques and magnetic resonance (MR) imaging with novel contrast agents like ultrasmall superparamagnetic iron oxide (USPIO) accumulating in macrophages and visualizing plaque zones with dense inflammatory infiltrates.

Second, assessment of inflammatory markers and in future also of an inflammatory gene load may assist in clinical risk stratification of individual patients and appropriate application of preventive drug regimes especially statins. Concentration of high-sensitivity C-reactive protein and level of Lp-PLA$_2$ have been recommended by the American Heart Association (AHA) and cleared by the Food and Drug Administration (FDA), respectively, for the estimation and classification of vascular risk. Other novel laboratory markers with a high discriminative potential have been discovered and are likely to enrich routine vascular risk prediction in near future. In analogy to other major health problems, detection of early disease stages by carotid ultrasound should find consideration in risk prediction as well, and algorithms composed of lifestyle characteristics, laboratory biomarkers, and ultrasound measures are currently being developed based on large prospective data sets.

Third, consequent treatment and prevention of pro-inflammatory risk conditions like chronic infection should be obligatory in the management of high-risk patients. Most of the drugs in use for vascular prevention have prominent anti-inflammatory properties such as statins or angiotensin receptor blockers. A better understanding of the molecular effector pathways will result in the development of new specific anti-inflammatory therapies. For example, testing of leukotriene antagonists and inhibitors of Lp-PLA$_2$ is under way, and several therapeutic regimes approved for non-vascular diseases like RANKL antagonism and CCR5 blockage may prove useful in advanced symptomatic atherosclerosis as well. There is a particular promise in the recent identification of risk conditions potentially involved in the transition of stable to unstable plaques rather than in conventional vessel pathology. Finally, vaccination against atherosclerosis and a therapeutic modulation of T-cell responses are intriguing research fields, but these strategies will not become clinical reality in the very next years.

References

1. Virchow RLK. *Cellular Pathology*. London: John Churchill; 1859.
2. Rokitansky C. *A Manual of Pathological Anatomy*. Philadelphia: Blanchard & Lea; 1855.
3. Ross R, Glomset JA. The pathogenesis of atherosclerosis. *N Engl J Med*. 1976;295:369–377.
4. Ross R, Glomset JA. The pathogenesis of atherosclerosis. *N Engl J Med*. 1976;295:420–425.
5. Hansson GK. Inflammation, atherosclerosis, and coronary artery disease. *N Engl J Med*. 2005;352:1685–1695.
6. Andersson J, Libby P, Hansson GK. Adaptive immunity and atherosclerosis. *Clin Immunol*. 2010;134(1):33–46.
7. Van Campenhout A, Golledge J. Osteoprotegerin, vascular calcification and atherosclerosis. *Atherosclerosis*. 2009;204: 321–329.
8. Danesh J et al. C-reactive protein and other circulating markers of inflammation in the prediction of coronary heart disease. *N Engl J Med*. 2004;350:1387–1397.
9. Fibrinogen Studies Collaboration et al. Plasma fibrinogen and the risk of major cardiovascular diseases and non-vascular mortality: meta-analysis of individual data for 151,649 adults in 31 prospective studies. *JAMA*. 2005;294:1799–1809.
10. Libby P. Role of inflammation in atherosclerosis associated with rheumatoid arthritis. *Am J Med*. 2008;121:S21-S31.
11. Kiechl S et al. Chronic infections and the risk of carotid atherosclerosis. Prospective results from a large population study. *Circulation*. 2001;103:1064–1070.
12. Knoflach M, Kiechl S, Mair A, Willeit J, Wick G. Allergic rhinitis, asthma and atherosclerosis in the Bruneck and ARMY Studies. *Arch Intern Med*. 2005;165:2521–2526.
13. Sun J et al. Mast cells promote atherosclerosis by releasing proinflammatory cytokines. *Nat Med*. 2007;13:719–724.
14. Kiechl S et al. Active and passive smoking, chronic infections and the risk of carotid atherosclerosis. Prospective results from the Bruneck Study. *Stroke*. 2002;33: 2170–2176.
15. Mazzone T, Chait A, Plutzky J. Cardiovascular disease risk in type 2 diabetes mellitus: insights from mechanistic studies. *Lancet*. 2008;371:1800–1809.
16. Markus H et al. Pro-inflammatory genes variants predispose to carotid and femoral artery atherosclerosis in the presence of pro-inflammatory risk factors and chronic infection. *Stroke*. 2006;37:2253–2259.
17. McPherson R et al. A common allele on chromosome 9 associated with coronary heart disease. *Science*. 2007;316:1488–1491.
18. Ye S, Willeit J, Kronenberg F, Xu Q, Kiechl S. Association of genetic variation on chromosome 9p21 with susceptibility and progression of atherosclerosis – a prospective study. *J Am Coll Cardiol*. 2008;52:378–384.
19. Wiedermann CI et al. Association of endotoxemia with carotid atherosclerosis and cardiovascular disease. Prospective results from the Bruneck study. *J Am Coll Cardiol*. 1999;34:1975–1981.
20. Steinberg D, Parthasarathy S, Carew TE, Khoo JC, Witztum JL. Beyond cholesterol. Modifications of low-density lipoprotein that increase its atherogenicity. *N Engl J Med*. 1989;320:915–924.
21. Wick G, Knoflach M, Xu Q. Autoimmune and inflammatory mechanisms in atherosclerosis. *Annu Rev Immunol*. 2004;22:361–403.
22. Kiechl S, Wiedermann CJ, Willeit J. TLR-4 and disease. *Ann Med*. 2003;35:165–171.
23. Kiechl S et al. Toll-like receptor 4 polymorphisms and atherogenesis in humans. *N Engl J Med*. 2002;347:185–192.
24. Björkbacka H et al. Reduced atherosclerosis in MyD88-null mice links elevated serum cholesterol levels to activation of innate immunity signaling pathways. *Nat Med*. 2004;10: 416–421.
25. Fuster V, Badimon L, Badimon JJ, Chesebro JH. The pathogenesis of coronary artery disease and the acute coronary syndromes (1). *N Engl J Med*. 1992;326:242–250.
26. Fuster V, Badimon L, Badimon JJ, Chesebro JH. The pathogenesis of coronary artery disease and the acute coronary syndromes (2). *N Engl J Med*. 1992;326:310–318.
27. Kiechl S, Willeit J. The natural course of atherosclerosis. Part I: incidence and progression. *Arterioscler Thromb Vasc Biol*. 1999;19:1484–1490.
28. Kiechl S, Willeit J. The natural course of atherosclerosis. Part II: vascular remodeling. *Arterioscler Thromb Vasc Biol*. 1999;19:1491–1498.
29. Willeit J et al. Distinct risk profiles of early and advanced atherosclerosis. Prospective results from the Bruneck study. *Arterioscler Thromb Vasc Biol*. 2000;20:529–537.
30. Kiechl S, Willeit J, Egger G, Poewe W, Oberhollenzer F. Body iron stores and the risk of carotid atherosclerosis. Prospective results from the Bruneck study. *Circulation*. 1997;96:3300–3307.
31. Glagov S, Weisenberg E, Zarins CK, Stankunavicius R, Kolettis GJ. Compensatory enlargement of human atherosclerotic coronary arteries. *N Engl J Med*. 1987;316:1371–1375.
32. Tsimikas S et al. Lipoprotein-associated phospholipase A2 activity, ferritin levels, metabolic syndrome and 10-year cardiovascular and non-cardiovascular mortality: results from the Bruneck study. *Eur Heart J*. 2009;30:107–115.

33. Kiechl S et al. Oxidized phospholipids, lipoprotein(a), lipoprotein-associated phospholipase A2 activity and 10-year cardiovascular outcomes: prospective results from the Bruneck study. *Arterioscler Thromb Vasc Biol*. 2007;27:1788–1795.
34. The Emerging Risk Factors Collaboration. Lipoprotein(a) concentration and the risk of coronary heart disease, stroke and nonvascular mortality. Individual data analysis of 121,944 participants from 34 cohorts. *JAMA*. 2009;302:412–423.
35. Zacharski LR et al. Reduction of iron stores and cardiovascular outcomes in patients with peripheral arterial disease: a randomized controlled trial. *JAMA*. 2007;297:603–610.
36. Davidson MH et al. Consensus panel recommendation for incorporating lipoprotein-associated phospholipase A2 testing into cardiovascular disease risk assessment guidelines. *Am J Cardiol*. 2008;101:51F-57F.
37. Kiechl S et al. The OPG/RANK/RANKL system – a bone key to vascular disease. *Expert Rev Cardiovasc Ther*. 2006;4:801–811.
38. Collin-Osdoby P. Regulation of vascular calcification by osteoclast regulatory factors RANKL and osteoprotegerin. *Circ Res*. 2004;95:1046–1057.
39. Kiechl S et al. Soluble receptor activator of nuclear factor-κB ligand (RANKL) and risk of cardiovascular disease. *Circulation*. 2007;116:385–391.
40. Kiechl S et al. Osteoprotegerin is a risk predictor of progressive atherosclerosis and cardiovascular disease. *Circulation*. 2004;109:2175–2180.
41. Afzal AR et al. Common CCR5-del32 frameshift mutation associated with serum levels of inflammatory markers and cardiovascular disease risk in the Bruneck population. *Stroke*. 2008;39:1972–1978.
42. Willeit J et al. The Marburg I polymorphism of factor VII activating protease: a prominent risk predictor of arterial thrombosis. *Circulation*. 2003;107:667–670.
43. Knoflach M et al. Cardiovascular risk factors and atherosclerosis in young women – ARFY study (Atherosclerosis Risk-Factors in Female Youngsters). *Stroke*. 2009;40:1063–1069.
44. Knoflach M et al. Vascular risk factors and atherosclerosis in young males – ARMY study (Atherosclerosis Risk-Factors in Male Youngsters). *Circulation*. 2003;108:1064–1069.
45. Xu Q et al. Serum soluble heat shock protein 60 is elevated in subjects with atherosclerosis in a general population. *Circulation*. 2000;102:14–20.
46. Xu Q et al. Association of serum antibodies to heat-shock protein 65 with carotid atherosclerosis. *Lancet*. 1993;341:255–259.
47. Brouilette SW et al. Telomere length, risk of coronary heart disease, and statin treatment in the West of Scotland primary prevention study: a nested case-control study. *Lancet*. 2007;369:107–114.
48. Panayiotou A et al. Leukocyte telomere length is associated with measures of subclinical atherosclerosis. *Atherosclerosis*. 2010;211(1):176–181.
49. Willeit P et al. Cellular aging reflected by leukocyte telomere length predicts advanced atherosclerosis and cardiovascular disease risk. *Arterioscler Thromb Vasc Biol*. 2010;30:1649–1656.
50. Jaffer FA, Libby P, Weissleder R. Optical and multimodality molecular imaging: insights into atherosclerosis. *Arterioscler Thromb Vasc Biol*. 2009;29:1017–1024.

29. Screening for Cardiovascular Risk Using Ultrasound: A Practical Approach

Andrew Nicolaides, Maura Griffin, Andrie G. Panayiotou, and Dawn Bond

29.1 Introduction

As indicated in previous chapters, cardiovascular disease (CVD) is one of the most common causes of death in the western world, and stroke, the most common cause of disability in women. Treatment is a major financial burden to health services, and effective prevention has now become a priority. The official aim in the UK is to reduce mortality from heart disease among men under 75 by 40%.[1]

Traditional methods of risk assessment for premature heart attacks and strokes using conventional risk factors such as smoking, high blood pressure, and high blood cholesterol to express the result as a 10-year Framingham Risk Score (FRS) or Prospective Cardiovascular Münster Heart Study (PROCAM) Risk Score (depending on the equation used) have produced moderate results. In the PROCAM study, 6.5% of the population were classified as high risk (10-year risk >20%), 14% as intermediate risk (10-year risk 10–20%), and 79.5% as low risk (10-year risk <10%).[2] At 10 years, 33%, 35%, and 32% of all the myocardial infarctions (MI) recorded occurred in the high-, the intermediate-, and the low-risk groups, respectively. This is because the low-risk group was very large, and at least 30% of those who developed MI did not have any of the conventional risk factors. Thus, such methods do identify high-risk groups, but if followed up, these high-risk groups contain at best only a fraction of the events that will occur in the subsequent 10 years. As a result of this, epidemiologists and health care providers have been trying to determine whether relatively simple tests can provide information over and above that obtained by conventional risk factors and be practical and effective enough to be adopted for general population screening.

Screening and improved selection of individuals for more effective prevention is now possible because of the following: (a) preclinical (silent) atherosclerotic plaques develop slowly over several decades before they rupture or obstruct an artery becoming clinically manifest, (b) screening methods are now available for detecting the presence and severity of such plaques, and (c) current prophylaxis with aggressive risk factor modification can reduce morbidity and mortality from heart attacks and strokes by 50%.

Three methods are currently available for cardiovascular risk screening: (a) measurement of ankle-brachial index (ABI), (b) coronary artery calcium scoring (CACS) using multislice computed tomography (CT) scanning known as Electron Beam Tomography (EBT), and (c) ultrasonic arterial scanning. Each method provides information that can improve the FRS to a lesser or greater extent, each having its own advantages and disadvantages. This is because the information obtained by each method is related to different characteristics of preclinical atherosclerosis

A. Nicolaides (✉)
Imperial College and Vascular Screening and Diagnostic Centre, London, UK

M. Griffin • D. Bond
Vascular Screening and Diagnostic Centre, London, UK

A.G. Panayiotou,
The Cyprus International Institute of Environmental and Public Health, Cyprus University of Technology, Cyprus

at different stages in time (earlier or later) in different vascular beds with different significance and associated costs. This chapter summarizes the efficacy of each method and associated advantages and disadvantages in an attempt to answer the questions of which method or combination of methods are relevant and when they should be used, and most importantly what advice should be given to individuals once the results become available.[3]

29.2 Measurement of ABI

Measurement of ABI consists of measurements of ankle and brachial systolic pressures with a handheld "pocket Doppler" and calculating the ratio of ankle pressure over brachial pressure. This is the oldest and least expensive method. It was introduced in 1969 by the vascular team at St. Mary's Hospital Medical School as a method of assessing the severity of lower limb ischemia and the response to medical or surgical therapy.[4] Subsequently, it became an epidemiological tool.

A recent meta-analysis has assessed the results of 16 general population cohort studies[5] involving 24,955 men and 23,339 women. Asymptomatic individuals without any history of cardiovascular disease had their ABI measured at baseline and followed up for the detection of cardiovascular events and mortality. The 10-year cardiovascular mortality in men with low (abnormal) ABI (≤ 0.90) was 18.7%, and in those with normal ABI (1.11–1.40), 4.4% (Hazard ratio [HR] 4.2; 95% CI 3.3–5.4). Corresponding mortalities in women were 12.6% and 4.1% (HR 3.5; 95% CI 2.4–5.1). The sensitivity and specificity of a low ABI (≤ 0.90) for predicting coronary heart disease were 16.5% and 92.7%; for stroke, 16.0% and 92.2%; and for cardiovascular mortality, 41.0% and 87.9%, respectively. It is important to note that a low ABI is found in only a small number in the younger groups, e.g., 1.4% in those less than 50 years and 3.5% in those 50–54 years. This is in contrast to older groups, e.g., 12.7% in those 75 years or older and 22.6% in those 80 years or older.[6]

It can be concluded that the ABI has the advantage of ease of use in general practice by a doctor or a trained nurse in asymptomatic individuals over the age of 70 without prior history of cardiovascular disease or older than 50 with one additional cardiovascular (CV) risk factor.[6] It is inexpensive and takes 10–15 min to perform. The finding of a low ABI (≤ 0.90) in an individual without a prior history of cardiovascular disease or diabetes is an indication for aggressive risk factor modification as in patients with established vascular disease. A disadvantage of the method is its low sensitivity and its low yield in individuals younger than 55 years. This is because a low ABI is the result of advanced lower limb occlusive arterial disease, albeit still asymptomatic, that occurs in older age groups. This is a major drawback of ABI because it is particularly in the younger groups (40s and 50s), when atherosclerosis is at its early stages, that prophylaxis is likely to be most effective.

29.3 Coronary Artery Calcium Score Using Multislice CT-Scanning

A recent meta-analysis of six prospective studies has demonstrated that coronary artery calcium score (CACS) obtained by CT is an independent predictor of future coronary events,[7] i.e., it provides information over and above that of the FRS. The risk of annual fatal myocardial infarction (MI) for CACS (Agatston score) less than 100 is low (<0.4%), for CACS 100–400 is moderate (1.3%), and for CACS 400 or higher is high (2.4%). When compared to individuals with CACS of zero, the corresponding relative risks (RR) and 95% confidence interval (CI) are 1.9 (1.3–2.8), 4.3 (3.1–6.1), and 7.8 (5.8–9.8), respectively. Although CACS is a good predictor of coronary artery disease, it cannot identify those with non-calcific unstable (vulnerable) plaques.[7] Also, the finding of a high CACS in the absence of any significant coronary artery stenosis (>50%) is common, indicating the need to improve predictive ability. Finally, CACS is related to atherosclerotic disease in the coronary arteries and does not provide information on stroke risk.

On the basis of the available data, the American College of Cardiology Foundation and American Heart Association have stated in their guidelines[7] that screening using the CACS is of limited clinical value in individuals who are at low risk for coronary events, i.e., 10-year FRS less than 10%. However, in individuals with a 10-year FRS of 10–20%, the finding of CACS of 400 or greater would increase the risk to that associated with diabetes or peripheral arterial disease. Thus, clinical decision making could be altered by CACS measurement in individuals with an intermediate FRS. Individuals with a high FRS (≥20%) should be treated aggressively according to the current National Cholesterol Education Program III (NCEP III) guidelines and do not require additional testing.[8] The current literature does not support the concept that high-risk asymptomatic individuals can be safely excluded from prophylaxis even if CACS is zero.

The disadvantage of CACS screening is that the method is expensive, and the high radiation dose associated with it does not allow frequent testing. Also, CACS does not provide information on stroke risk.

29.4 Screening with Ultrasound

29.4.1 Relevant Messages from Previous Chapters

High-resolution ultrasound can provide images of the arterial wall and plaques with measurements of intima-media thickness (IMT) (Chap. 22), plaque thickness, and plaque area (Chaps. 23–25) at a resolution of 0.2 mm. Several studies have indicated that IMT can be used to study the effect of risk factor modification in large groups and has become a validated biomarker[9] (Chaps. 22–25). However, it is only marginally better than conventional risk factors in identifying individuals at increased risk (Chaps. 23–25). Thus, IMT is not a helpful test for risk assessment in individuals. However, ultrasonic arterial wall measurements such as the presence and thickness of plaques[10-12] and plaque echolucency[12-14] (Chaps. 24 and 25) not only in the carotid but also in the common femoral have been shown to be stronger predictors of risk with an RR of 3.0–5.0.

Two prospective studies have shown that carotid plaque area is a better predictor of future myocardial infarction than IMT.[15,16] In the Tromsø study[15] (Chap. 24), IMT, total plaque area, and plaque echolucency were measured in 6,226 men and women aged 25–84 years with no previous MI followed for 6 years. The adjusted RR and 95% CI between the highest plaque area tertile versus no plaque was 1.56 (1.04–2.36) in men and 3.95 (2.16–7.19) in women.

The adjusted corresponding RR and 95% CI for IMT was 1.73 (0.98–3.06) in men and 2.86 (1.07–7.65) in women. Plaque echolucency (low collagen content) indicating plaque instability was also associated with increased risk of MI. In the study performed in Canada[16] (Chap. 25), carotid plaque areas from 1,686 patients followed for up to 5 years were categorized into four quartiles. The combined 5-year risk of stroke, myocardial infarction, and vascular death by quartiles of plaque area were: 5.6%, 10.7%, 13.9%, and 19.5%, respectively. These results place any individual with a plaque in the intermediate-risk (10-year risk: 10–20%) or high-Framingham-risk group (10-year risk ≥ 20%).

The authors' study performed in a subgroup of the ongoing British Regional Heart Study in the late 1990s (425 men and 375 women) has demonstrated that the presence and number of plaques in the carotid and common femoral bifurcations have a stronger association with prevalence of clinical cardiovascular disease than carotid IMT alone.[10]

29.4.2 Messages from the Cyprus Epidemiological Study

In an ongoing study performed by the authors, 2,000 individuals over the age of 40 are being screened for conventional risk factors and clinical and preclinical cardiovascular disease, and are followed-up for 5 years.[17,18] Both carotid and both common femoral bifurcations are scanned with ultrasound. The cohort consists of near total population (95%) of a number of randomly selected areas (villages). In the first 762 individuals, evidence of clinical cardiovascular disease was present in 113 (14.8%) at baseline. Scanning of both carotid and both common femoral bifurcations with ultrasound was performed. The following measurements were made with high ultrasound: IMT of both common carotid arteries (IMTcc), the maximum IMT in each carotid bifurcation (IMTmax) which included plaque thickness, the number of bifurcations (carotid or common femoral) with plaque which ranged from 0 to 4, the total plaque thickness (TPT) defined as the sum of the thicknesses of the largest plaque found in each bifurcation, plaque area of the largest plaque found in each bifurcation, and total plaque area (TPA) defined as the sum of all plaque areas measured.

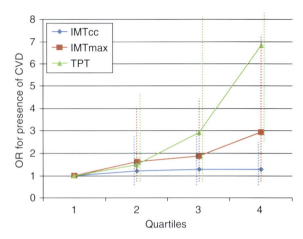

Fig. 29.1 Odds ratios (OR) and 95% CI of quartiles of common carotid IMT (IMTcc), maximum IMT (IMTmax), and total plaque thickness (TPT) for prevalence of clinical cardiovascular disease after adjustment for age, sex, pack years, systolic blood pressure, total cholesterol, diabetes, and administration of cholesterol-lowering therapy and antihypertensive therapy

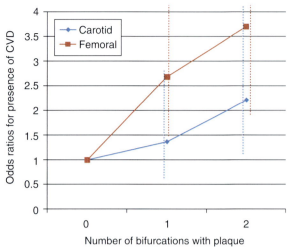

Fig. 29.2 Odds ratios and 95% CI of number of bifurcations with plaque (carotid or femoral) for prevalence of clinical cardiovascular disease after adjustment for age, sex, pack years, systolic blood pressure, total cholesterol, diabetes, and administration of cholesterol-lowering therapy and antihypertensive therapy

The baseline data from the first 762 individuals screened indicate that the presence, number, and size of plaques have a stronger association with prevalence of clinical cardiovascular disease than IMT. After adjustment for conventional risk factors, the association of total plaque thickness (TPT) with prevalence of clinical cardiovascular disease was high (Odds Ratio of upper to lower TPT quartile: 6.87; 95% CI 2.42–19.43) (Fig. 29.1). A cutoff point of TPT greater than 0.52 cm [maximum combined sensitivity and specificity (75.2%) derived from receiver operator characteristic (ROC) curve analysis] identified 247 (32%) of the population that contained 85/113 (75%) of the individuals with clinical cardiovascular disease. The positive predictive value was 34.4%; the negative predictive value, 94.6%; and the likelihood ratio for a positive test result, 3.03%.[18]

Presence and number of plaques of any size in the carotid or common femoral bifurcation were also associated with increased prevalence of clinical cardiovascular disease (Fig. 29.2), but the strongest association was found when the number of plaques in both carotid and common femoral bifurcations was considered (Fig. 29.3).[18]

After adjustment for conventional risk factors, the association of total plaque area (TPA) (sum of all plaque

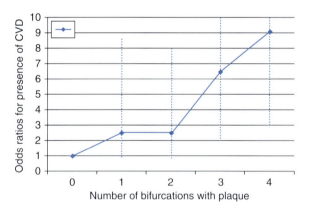

Fig. 29.3 Odds ratios and 95% CI of number of bifurcations with plaque (carotid and femoral) for prevalence of clinical cardiovascular disease after adjustment for age, sex, pack years, systolic blood pressure, total cholesterol, diabetes, and administration of cholesterol-lowering therapy and antihypertensive therapy

areas) with prevalence of clinical cardiovascular disease was also high (Odds Ratio of upper to lower TPA quintile: 8.38; 95% CI 2.57–27.32) (Fig. 29.4). TPA greater than 42 mm^2 (maximum combined sensitivity and specificity (75%) derived from ROC curve analysis) identified 266 (34.9%) of the population that contained

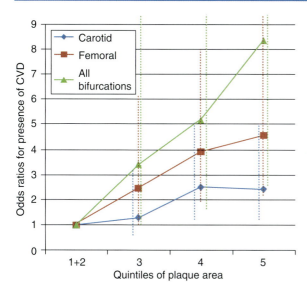

Fig. 29.4 Odds ratios and 95% CI of quintiles of plaque area (in carotid, femoral, and all four bifurcations) for prevalence of clinical cardiovascular disease after adjustment for age, sex, pack years, systolic blood pressure, total cholesterol, diabetes, and administration of cholesterol-lowering therapy and antihypertensive therapy

87/113 (76.9%) of the clinical events (positive predictive value: 33%; negative predictive value: 94%).[18]

Thus, the presence and size of preclinical plaques in both carotid and both common femoral arteries are emerging as having a strong association with coronary heart disease and stroke. The simplest measurement that is highly applicable to screening is the number of bifurcations that contain a plaque.

In the Cyprus epidemiological study, 42% of asymptomatic individuals in the low FRS group had atherosclerotic plaques present. In another recent study using ultrasound, carotid plaques were found in 34% of individuals at low FRS and having CACS of zero.[19]

Advantages of screening with ultrasound are that it is relatively inexpensive and devoid of ionizing radiation. High-resolution portable equipment is now available. A scan can be performed in 20 min. In addition, it can be repeated at six monthly intervals or annually providing information on plaque progression or regression. The availability of atherosclerotic plaque images provides an incentive to individuals to persevere with prophylactic therapy as compliance issues often contribute to the reduced effectiveness of such therapies. An added benefit of ultrasound is that with the addition of an extra 5 min, individuals over the age of 65 can be screened for the presence of abdominal aortic aneurysm as recently recommended by the National Institute for Health and Clinical Excellence (NICE).

29.5 A Rational Screening Plan

29.5.1 Individuals with Low FRS

Individuals with low FRS should be screened with ultrasound. Absence of plaques found in 60% of individuals in this low-risk group will confirm the low risk, and further follow-up with ultrasound will not be necessary for 3–4 years. However, the presence of plaques found in the other 40% will result in reclassification to a higher risk and will prompt the clinician to advise not only on risk factor modification but also to look for nonconventional risk factors such as elevated homocysteine. Two recent prospective randomized controlled trials in individuals with known cardiovascular disease have demonstrated that lowering homocysteine with vitamin supplements has reduced the risk of ischemic stroke by 25%.[20,21] The physician advising the individual on prevention should explain that any atherosclerotic plaques visualized are representative of what may be happening in the rest of the arterial tree; also that plaques are early deposits of cholesterol, and although the individual is now asymptomatic and in good health, these plaques if untreated are likely to grow and produce symptoms in the future.

29.5.2 Individuals with an Intermediate FRS

Individuals with an intermediate FRS should be initially screened with ultrasound. Those with plaques are advised to have aggressive risk factor modification as plaques should not be allowed to progress and that regression, which with treatment to target can occur in 28%, is associated with a 50% reduction in risk.[16] An annual electrocardiogram (ECG) stress test should also be advised. If plaques are absent, then CACS may be performed. The latter will allow reclassification to a lower or higher risk group with confidence.

29.5.3 Individuals with a High FRS

Individuals with a high FRS are advised to have aggressive risk factor modification according to the current guidelines. Screening with ultrasound in order to follow plaque progression or regression is optional. However, this and the associated plaque images provide a strong incentive to persevere with prophylactic therapy as compliance can be challenging.

29.5.4 Practical Aspects of Suggested Strategy

The strategy outlined above uses a combination of conventional risk factors with ultrasound which is in the forefront of noninvasive, inexpensive imaging modalities for screening asymptomatic individuals. It should go a long way towards achieving the target of reducing heart attacks and strokes by 40%[1] because it identifies many individuals at increased risk that would be missed by FRS.

Setting up cardiovascular screening services or centers should be seriously considered. The major investment would not be in the equipment, which is now relatively inexpensive and portable, but in trained staff. Asymptomatic individuals should be referred to such centers by their own physicians. This should avoid inappropriate use of the services. The referring doctor should be responsible for making the decisions on targeted preventive measures based on the individual's clinical and imaging assessment.

A final consideration is that ultrasound could prove a potent tool in lifestyle modification as there is nothing more powerful than asymptomatic individuals experiencing a real-time image of their arteries showing atherosclerotic deposits. Such deposits are the end result of all risk factors, known, emerging, and yet unknown including genetic.

References

1. Department of Health, United Kingdom. *National Service Frameworks for Coronary Heart Disease*. London: Department of Health; 2000.
2. Voss R, Cullen P, Schulte H, Assmann G. Prediction of risk of coronary events in middle-aged men in the prospective cardiovascular Münster study (PROCAM) using neural networks. *Int J Epidemiol*. 2002;31:1253–1262.
3. Nicolaides AN. Screening for cardiovascular risk. *Br J Cardiol*. 2010;17:105–107.
4. Yao ST, Hobbs JT, Irvine WT. Ankle systolic pressure measurements in arterial disease affecting the lower extremities. *Br J Surg*. 1969;56:676–679.
5. Ankle Brachial Index Collaboration et al. Ankle brachial index combined with Framingham risk score to predict cardiovascular events and mortality: a meta-analysis. *JAMA*. 2008;300:197–208.
6. Doobay AV, Anand SS. Sensitivity and specificity of ankle-brachial index to predict future cardiovascular outcomes: a systematic review. *Arterioscler Thromb Vasc Biol*. 2005;25:1463–1469.
7. Greenland P et al. ACCF/AHA 2007 clinical expert consensus document on coronary artery calcium scoring by computed tomography in global cardiovascular risk assessment and in evaluation of patients with chest pain. *Circulation*. 2007;115:402–426.
8. National Cholesterol Education Program (NCEP) Expert Panel on Detection, Evaluation, and Treatment of High Blood Cholesterol in Adults (Adult Treatment Panel III). Third report of the NCEP expert panel on detection, evaluation and treatment of high blood cholesterol in adults (Adult Treatment Panel III) final report. *Circulation*. 2002;106:3143–3421.
9. Lorenz MW, Marcus HS, Bots ML, Rosvall M, Sitzer M. Prediction of clinical cardiovascular events with carotid intima-media thickness. *Circulation*. 2007;115:459–467.
10. Ebrahim S et al. Carotid plaque, intima media thickness, cardiovascular risk factors, and prevalent cardiovascular disease in men and women: the British Regional Heart study. *Stroke*. 1999;30:841–850.
11. Hollander M et al. Carotid plaques increase the risk of stroke and subtypes of cerebral infarction in asymptomatic elderly: the Rotterdam study. *Circulation*. 2002;105: 2872–2877.
12. Schmidt C, Fagerberg B, Hulthe J. Non-stenotic echolucent ultrasound-assessed femoral artery plaques are predictive for future cardiovascular events in middle-aged men. *Atherosclerosis*. 2005;181:125–130.
13. Honda O et al. Echolucent carotid plaques predict future coronary events in patients with coronary artery disease. *J Am Coll Cardiol*. 2004;43:1177–1184.
14. Seo Y et al. Echolucent carotid plaques as a feature in patients with acute coronary syndrome. *Circ J*. 2006;70:1629–1634.
15. Johnsen SH et al. Carotid atherosclerosis is a stronger predictor of myocardial infarction in women than in men: a 6-year

15. follow up study of 6226 persons: the Trømso study. *Stroke*. 2007;38:2873–2880.
16. Spence JD et al. A tool for targeting and evaluating vascular preventive therapy. *Stroke*. 2002;33:2916–2922.
17. Griffin M et al. Carotid and femoral arterial wall changes and prevalence of clinical cardiovascular disease. *Vasc Med*. 2009;14:227–232.
18. Griffin M et al. Plaque area at carotid and common femoral bifurcation, and prevalence of clinical cardiovascular disease. *Int Angiol*. 2010;29:216–225.
19. Lester SJ, Eleid MF, Khandheria BK, Hurst RT. Carotid IMT thickness and coronary artery calcium score as indications of subclinical atherosclerosis. *Mayo Clin Proc*. 2009;84:229–233.
20. Lonn E et al. Homocysteine lowering with folic acid and b vitamins in vascular disease. *N Engl J Med*. 2006;354:1567–1777.
21. Saposnik G, Ray JG, Sheridan P, McQueen M, Lonn E. Homocysteine-lowering therapy and stroke risk, severity and disability. *Stroke*. 2009;40:1365–1372.

Part V

Late Atherosclerosis

Grading Internal Carotid Artery Stenosis

30

Kimon Bekelis, Nicos Labropoulos, Maura Griffin, and Andrew Nicolaides

30.1 Historical Introduction

In the 1970s and 1980s, angiography was the standard method used for grading internal carotid artery stenosis. With the introduction of ultrasound in the 1980s and early 1990s, angiography became the gold standard used for the development of duplex velocity criteria for different grades of stenosis.

Technological advances in the 1990s improved duplex scanners to such an extent that preoperative angiography was less frequently used. In centers where the accuracy of duplex scanning had been validated against angiography, patients without clinical evidence of lesions in the supra-aortic vessels could proceed to carotid endarterectomy without angiography, provided that computed tomography (CT) or magnetic resonance imaging (MRI) brain scan had excluded hemorrhage, tumor, or a large intracerebral aneurysm.[1,2] Another factor influencing the development of this approach has been the combined stroke and death rate of 1–4% associated with intra-arterial contrast injection.[3,4]

K. Bekelis
Department of Neurosurgery, Dartmouth-Hitchcock Medical Center, Hanover, NH, USA

N. Labropoulos (✉)
Department of Surgery, Stony Brook University Medical Center, Stony Brook, NY, USA

M. Griffin
Vascular Screening and Diagnostic Centre, London, UK

A. Nicolaides
Imperial College and Vascular Screening and Diagnostic Centre, London, UK

The results of the randomized multicenter trials of carotid endarterectomy for symptomatic[5,6] and asymptomatic[3,7] carotid lesions did not fulfill the expectations that the treatment decision process for defined stenotic categories would be clear-cut[8] with corresponding clear-cut duplex criteria. Several confounding factors are responsible for this: the different angiographic grading methods used, the imprecision of Doppler velocities in grading a stenosis, and the fact that the early duplex velocity criteria postulated by the University of Washington were in relation to diameter reduction in relation to the carotid bulb; also, the subsequently developed Doppler velocity criteria that were tailored for different sensitivities and specificities depending on whether duplex scanning was used for screening or a definitive diagnostic testing prior to surgery.

30.1.1 Angiographic Grading Methods

The first confounding factor was that two different angiographic grading systems for internal carotid artery stenosis were used (Fig. 30.1) in the multicenter randomized controlled studies producing considerable confusion to outcome interpretation.[3,5–7] One method defined the residual lumen as a percentage of the normal distal internal carotid artery. This method dates back to the 1970s when it was believed that most carotid territory symptoms were associated with hemodynamically significant flow reducing stenosis. It was used in the North American Symptomatic Carotid Endarterectomy Trial (NASCET)[5] and the Asymptomatic Carotid Atherosclerosis Study (ACAS)[4] and has become known as the North

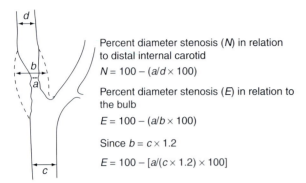

Fig. 30.1 The "N" and "E" methods used to calculate the degree of angiographic internal carotid stenosis (Reprinted with permission from Nicolaides et al.[8])

American or "N" method. The disadvantage of this method is that it underestimates the size of a plaque in the carotid bulb. For example, a plaque with a 44% diameter reduction that uniformly fills the bulb will produce a lumen measurement equal to the distal internal carotid.

Another technique expressed the residual lumen as a percentage of the diameter of the bulb and has been used in the European Carotid Surgery Trial (ECST)[6] becoming known as the European or "E" method. In contrast to the "N" approach, the "E" method could provide a good estimate of the size of plaques in the carotid bulb. However, the outline of the bulb was not often seen on angiography. In the 1970s and early 1980s, the University of Washington team used the presence of microcalcification on the unsubtracted film of digital subtraction angiograms to measure the size of the bulb. In contrast, the ECST authors "guessed" where the bulb boundaries should be. This problem was overcome when the authors' team studied a large series of normal intra-arterial selective angiograms performed as part of the investigation of intracranial disease in the 1960s and 1970s. A constant ratio of 1.19 ± 0.09 between the angiographic diameter of the proximal common carotid artery and that of the bulb was found.[9] This method allowed a more precise calculation of the diameter of the bulb based on the proximal common carotid artery, which is practically always seen on angiography and was adopted by several teams.[10,11] A disadvantage of the "E" method arises when the plaque does not involve the bulb. In this scenario, expressing the residual lumen as a percentage of the diameter of the bulb gives an erroneous impression of the size of the plaque.

A more accurate way of describing the degree of stenosis is to state the extent of the plaque and the site of maximum stenosis (whether in the proximal, middle, or distal bulb, or even distal to the bulb) and express the residual lumen both as a percentage of the diameter of the distal internal carotid and as a percentage of the diameter of the bulb.[8]

30.1.2 The Use of Velocities

The second confounding factor was the inability of duplex scanning to grade the severity of carotid stenosis with precision. In the 1980s and 1990s, because the resolution of brightness mode (B-mode) ultrasound was poor, the degree of stenosis was graded by the velocity at the point of maximum stenosis. It was soon realized that for the same degree of stenosis in different patients, there was a range of velocities. In other words, duplex scanning was not accurate enough to be used to predict a single percentage of stenosis.[12,13] This is because the Doppler velocity recorded at the site of maximum stenosis depends on the pressure gradient across the stenosis. This pressure gradient is a function of both the severity of the stenosis and the collateral circulation. Let us assume that three patients have a 70% diameter stenosis of the left internal carotid artery. The right carotid bifurcation is normal in the first patient, while in the second, it is occluded. In the third patient, the right carotid bifurcation is normal, but the circle of Willis is incomplete. In these three patients, the velocities at the stenosis in the left internal carotid will be different because the pressure gradients will not be the same. An overestimation of the degree of stenosis may result in the second and third patients if one adheres to absolute velocities. For these reasons, the use of defined stenotic strata was recommended, and duplex scanning was found to be more accurate when lesions were classified as being above or below a single level, such as 60% stenosis or 70% stenosis.[14] Vascular laboratories were encouraged to establish protocols for stratifying the degree of internal carotid artery (ICA) stenosis, and, once established, these criteria were consistently applied.

30.1.3 The University of Washington Duplex Criteria

The third confounding factor was that the early duplex velocity criteria postulated by the University of Washington in the 1980s were in relation to the "E" method of grading internal carotid stenosis.[15–17] These were based on peak systolic velocity (PSV) and end-diastolic velocity (EDV) at the point of maximum stenosis, and spectral broadening. Six grades were suggested: A = normal; B = 1–15% stenosis for PSV < 125 cm/s with minimal spectral broadening; C = 15–50% stenosis for PSV < 125 cm/s with marked spectral broadening; D = 50–79% stenosis for PSV > 125 cm/s with marked spectral broadening but still EDV < 140; D+ = 80–99% stenosis for PSV > 125 cm/s with marked spectral broadening and EDV > 140 cm/s; and E = occlusion for absence of any velocity signals (see Table 2.1). These velocities were subsequently modified by Zweibel in 1993[18] in order to correspond to stenosis expressed in relation to the distal internal carotid, i.e., the "N" method (see Table 2.1). Others produced normograms that allowed one to see at a glance the relationship between the velocity criteria of the University of Washington with both "E" and "N" methods of expressing stenosis (Fig. 30.2).

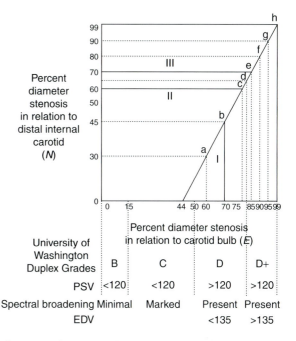

Fig. 30.2 The relationship between the two methods used to calculate the degree of angiographic stenosis and the University of Washington duplex criteria. Different size plaques (a–h) are shown in relation to the corresponding "N" and "E" degrees of stenosis. I, II, and III represent the cutoff points for considering carotid endarterectomy according to the ECST, ACAS, and NASCET studies, respectively. *EDV* end-diastolic velocity, *PSV* peak systolic velocity (Reprinted with permission from Nicolaides et al.[8])

30.1.4 The Introduction of Velocity Ratios

Velocity ratios were introduced following the realization that absolute velocity criteria could be inaccurate in a number of clinical conditions.[17] Cardiac arrhythmia, aortic valve disease, tandem plaques, recent hemispheric stroke, carotid dilatation, or aneurysm could result in underestimation of the degree of stenosis. Conversely, carotid coiling or kinking, arteriovenous malformations, carotid body tumors, and contralateral severe stenosis or occlusion could produce an overestimation of the stenosis.

The fourth confounding factor was that the criteria for different velocity ratios were initially tailored to screening and selecting patients for subsequent angiography. Thus, they had a high sensitivity at the expense of specificity. The aim was not to miss a patient with a stenosis greater than 60% "N". However, subsequently, with the need to make decisions to proceed to carotid endarterectomy without angiography, the criteria were tailored to have equal sensitivity and specificity. The criteria listed in Table 30.1 are based on the latter option with emphasis in obtaining the highest combined sensitivity and specificity for surgically important grades greater than 70% "E" as indicated by ECST, 60% "N" as indicated by ACAS trial, and 70% "N" as indicated by NASCET. This table was developed by the authors in the late 1990s[8] and has been used by all the centers taking part in the Asymptomatic Carotid Stenosis and Risk of Stroke Study (ACSRS)[19] (Chap. 37).

All the developments summarized above occurred over a period of 20 years, and unless the history described is appreciated, a novice in the field attempting to review the literature can be easily confused.

Considerable progress has been made in the quality of ultrasound examinations of the carotid arteries over the past two decades.[14] Ultrasound has undergone great advances, and the imaging community has gained

Table 30.1 Duplex velocity criteria selected for highest accuracy[a]

Angiographic diameter stenosis		Duplex velocity criteria				
N%	E%	PSV_{IC}[18,19]	EDV_{IC}[17-19]	PSV_{IC}/PSV_{CC}[20-22]	PSV_{IC}/EDV_{CC}[23,24]	EDV_{IC}/EDV_{CC}[b]
12	50	<125	<40	<1.5	<7	
30	60					<2.6
47	70	125–150	40–80	1.5–2	7–10	
60	77		80–130	2–3.2		
65	80	150–250				
70	83		>130	3.2–4	10–20	2.6–5.5
82	90	>250		>4	20–30	
90	95				>30	>5.5
99	99			Trickle flow		

Source: Reprinted with permission from Nicolaides et al, 1996[8]
N NASCET, *E* ECST, *PSV* peak systolic velocity, *EDV* end-diastolic velocity, *IC* internal carotid, *CC* common carotid
[a]Combined maximum sensitivity with maximum specificity
[b]Baker JD. Standardized imaging and Doppler criteria for cerebrovascular diagnosis using duplex sonography. Presented at AIUM, Las Vegas, NV, 1986

expertise in performance of carotid scans and interpretation of the results through the widespread use of technology, research, and continuing medical education. In addition, various accrediting bodies have been established, such as the Intersocietal Commission for Accreditation of Vascular Laboratories, the American Institute of Ultrasound in Medicine, and the American College of Radiology, in an attempt to improve and standardize the quality of vascular examinations. In an attempt to minimize the existing variability in the performed examination, an expert panel from various faculties has suggested a series of guidelines on grading carotid stenosis with ultrasound (see below).

30.2 Stratification of Stenosis

Grading of different degrees of stenosis which are less than 50% in relation to the normal distal internal carotid with velocity measurements is inaccurate[14] because such lesions are of no hemodynamic significance. These stenoses should be reported as less than 50%, and B-mode estimation in transverse section with the use of color flow when the plaque borders are not easily seen should be used to subcategorize them (see below). For practical surgical decision purposes, the degree of stenosis stratified on the basis of B-mode and Doppler velocity measurements results into the following strata: normal, less than 50% stenosis, 50–69% stenosis, 70–80% stenosis, 80–99% stenosis, and occlusion. This can be achieved using the criteria listed in Table 30.1. The threshold of 70% stenosis has been chosen because it is the threshold currently used by most centers for intervention in symptomatic patients[14] and 80% for asymptomatic patients.

The residual lumen (area or diameter reduction) can also be determined in transverse section using color flow for the majority of lesions producing higher grades of stenosis, provided there is no calcification that produces acoustic shadowing. Several studies[20-22] have produced sensitivities in the range of 85–87% and specificities in the range of 89–97% when compared to angiography.

The diagnosis of "trickle flow," i.e., 95–99% stenosis, often cannot be diagnosed by velocities because the flow is so low that it may not be detected by the Doppler ultrasound beam. These stenoses with a lumen reduction of greater than 95% are referred to as subtotal stenoses. The term pseudo-occlusion has also been used to describe the angiographic appearance of such stenotic lesions, which show a layer of contrast material along the posterior wall distal to the site of a high-grade stenosis of the ICA in the late venous phase.

Several criteria[23] have been used to correlate duplex sonographic findings with those of angiography for preocclusive stenosis. Some of the most commonly used ultrasound identifiers of high-grade stenosis or occlusion are: identification of echogenic plaque or thrombus filling the lumen and dampened ipsilateral common carotid artery flow velocity in comparison to the contralateral side.

By using color flow Doppler, Berman et al.[24] have recognized 94% of the pseudo-occlusions in their study. Mansour et al.[25] have shown similar results with color flow Doppler having a positive predictive value for total occlusion of 98%. Their color flow scanning prediction for preocclusive lesions was accurate in 84% of 31 cases. AbuRahma et al.,[26] in their series of 91 arteries, demonstrated that the accuracy of carotid duplex ultrasound in diagnosing total carotid occlusion was 97% with a positive predictive value (PPV) of 96%, negative predictive value (NPV) of 98%, sensitivity of 91%, and specificity of 99%. Sitzer et al.,[27] by using color flow duplex imaging, have demonstrated a 96% PPV in the diagnosis of carotid occlusion (95% confidence interval 94–98%) and 83% in the diagnosis of 95–99% stenosis (95% confidence interval 63–89%).

Color flow Doppler is superior to velocity measurements in differentiating complete occlusions from pseudo-occlusions because it offers the ability to detect low flow in difficult imaging situations since flow can be detected without the accurate placement of a sample volume. When occlusion is suspected based on the absence of velocity (complete absence of flow distal to the stenosis), color flow Doppler permits further evaluation of the proximal and distal internal carotid artery. However, in some instances, evaluation of such a condition even with the use of color flow may be hampered due to plaque composition, exceptionally narrowed residual lumen, and possibly a patient's clinical condition, such as low blood pressure or reduced cardiac output.

A method to overcome these difficulties aiming for a 100% accuracy is to inject brighter reflectors than blood into the vascular system. Gas-filled microbubbles are one such reflector. As indicated in Chap. 7, ultrasound microbubble contrast agents given intravenously were introduced in the early 1990s to enhance the echogenicity of blood and improve the ultrasound visualization of the residual lumen in patients with severe internal carotid stenosis.[27] It was soon found that they could detect the presence of "trickle flow" and identify falsely diagnosed carotid occlusions.[28,29] More recently, they have been used to improve the diagnosis of intracranial stenosis.[30,31] They are currently used in some laboratories and avoid the need of angiography in patients with suspected pseudo-occlusion.

30.2.1 Use of Above Criteria

Various laboratories are using some or all the velocity parameters for the evaluation of ICA stenosis, as listed in Table 30.1. There appears to be a consensus in favor of the use of peak systolic velocity in the internal carotid (PSVic) and the presence of plaque on grayscale and/or color imaging when diagnosing and grading stenosis.[14] The PSVic is easy to obtain, has good reproducibility, and should be used in conjunction with available grayscale and color Doppler information to ensure concordance of diagnostic information. The degree of stenosis estimated by using PSVic and the degree of narrowing of the internal carotid lumen on transverse images of grayscale and color Doppler images should be similar.

Published literature is replete with velocity thresholds for categorizing ICA stenosis.[8,17,18,32–40] Tremendous variation exists among these studies in the methods used to assess individual Doppler parameters and in the thresholds recommended for diagnosing ICA stenosis. Jahromi et al.,[41] in a systematic review and meta-analysis of 47 studies, concluded that a significant number of the studies were flawed by poor documentation of clinical features, variation in disease prevalence and severity, verification effects (the selection of patients to undergo the gold standard test after the results of the index test are known), clinical review effects (the knowledge of clinical information in the interpretation of test results), and lack of blinding (the knowledge of one test result in the interpretation of the other). Their meta-analysis has demonstrated that the threshold of PSVic above 130 cm/s is associated with a sensitivity of 98% and specificity of 88% in the detection of greater than 50% angiographic stenosis in relation to the distal internal carotid diameter. For the diagnosis of angiographic stenosis of greater than 70%, a PSVic greater than 200 cm/s has a sensitivity of 90% and a specificity of 94%.

The end-diastolic velocity in the internal carotid EDVic is a useful corroborative measurement, as shown in Table 30.1. However, EDVic parameters are inaccurate in the distinction of 95–99% ICA stenosis from occlusion. Low EDVic can be found in a number of patients with minor or no internal carotid artery disease, particularly in those with a stroke or silent cerebral infarct. The low EDVic can be used to assess distal ICA disease (plaque or dissection).

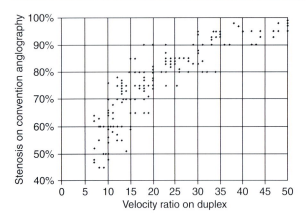

Fig. 30.3 The ratio of the peak systolic velocity of the internal carotid artery to the end-diastolic velocity of the common carotid artery (PSVic/EDVcc) plotted against the percentage stenosis in relation to the distal internal carotid [8]

It is important though to have significant asymmetry with the contralateral side.[27]

Three velocity ratios are also available, and anyone of them can be used to provide additional cutoff points or in cases of cardiac arrhythmias or other cardiac disease listed above that may make PSV inaccurate (Table 30.1). For example, in a patient with low cardiac output, the PSVic may be disproportionately low when compared to the PSVic/PSVcc (peak systolic velocity common carotid) ratio. This discrepancy should prompt the interpreter to consider all grayscale and color information when stratifying the degree of ICA stenosis. In particular, in such cases, the interpretation should be based more heavily on a velocity ratio than on absolute values.

The ratio of the peak systolic velocity of the internal carotid artery to the end-diastolic velocity of the common carotid artery (PSVic/EDVcc) has been correlated with angiographic stenosis in relation to the distal internal carotid based on 101 biplanar angiograms.[8] This criterion can be extremely useful for stenosis in the range of 60–99%, defining a percentage diameter stenosis with ±10% accuracy (Fig. 30.3). Different values correspond to different degrees of stenosis: a PSVic/EDVcc 10–15 corresponds to a 60–70% stenosis, a PSVic/EDVcc between 15 and 20 corresponds to a 70–80% stenosis, a PSVic/EDVcc 20–30 corresponds to a 80–90% stenosis, and a PSVic/EDVcc greater than 30 corresponds to 90–99% stenosis.

30.2.2 Guidelines of the Society of Radiologists in Ultrasound for Grading of the Degree of Stenosis in Relation to the Diameter of the Normal Distal Internal Carotid ("N" Method)

The analysis of numerous studies in this matter resulted in the following recommendations for ultrasonographic grading of the degree of stenosis[14]:

1. The ICA is considered normal when PSVic is less than 125 cm/s and no plaque or intimal thickening is visible sonographically. Additional criteria include PSVic/PSVcc ratio less than 2.0 and EDVic less than 40 cm/s.
2. A less than 50% ICA stenosis is diagnosed when PSVic is less than 125 cm/s and plaque or intimal thickening is visible sonographically. Additional criteria include PSVic/PSVcc ratio less than 2.0 and EDVic less than 40 cm/s.
3. A 50–69% ICA stenosis is diagnosed when PSVic is in the range of 125–230 cm/s and plaque is visible sonographically. Additional criteria include PSVic/PSVcc ratio of 2.0–4.0 and EDVic of 40–100 cm/s.
4. A greater than 70% stenosis but less than near occlusion of the ICA is diagnosed when the PSVic is greater than 230 cm/s and visible plaque and luminal narrowing are seen at grayscale and color Doppler ultrasound. Additional criteria include PSVic/PSVcc ratio greater than 4.0 and EDVic greater than 100 cm/s. The higher the PSVic above the threshold of 230 cm/s, the greater the likelihood of severe stenosis.
5. In cases of near occlusion of the ICA, the velocity parameters may not apply since velocities may be high, low, or undetectable. This diagnosis is established primarily by demonstrating a markedly narrowed lumen on color or power Doppler.[42]
6. Total occlusion of the ICA should be suspected when there is no detectable patent lumen on grayscale ultrasound and no flow with spectral, power, and color Doppler. Often, the "blue cap" of flow reversal is also seen at the origin of the affected ICA. Magnetic resonance angiography (MRA), computed tomographic angiography (CTA), or conventional selective angiography may be used for confirmation in this setting.[43]

In this consensus of guidelines, the cutoff values for 80% stenosis or greater were not analyzed. However, this cutoff point is important because, as mentioned earlier, many specialists treat asymptomatic carotid stenosis with surgery when greater than 80%. The EDVic has been shown to be the best criterion for identifying a greater than 80% stenosis. Initially, the cutoff value was set at 140 cm/s but later was reduced to 125 cm/s. Another useful criterion is a PSVic/EDVcc greater than 20.

Because of the rarity of correlative angiograms nowadays in most institutions, the establishment of internally validated Doppler cutoff criteria is difficult. As a result, the use of the proposed cutoff criteria has been developed and can be applied at laboratories that cannot validate their own Doppler thresholds on the basis of correlative imaging or clinical information. The use of CTA or MRA for validation has not yet been fully established.

30.2.3 Limitations of Duplex Velocity Criteria

The limitations and drawbacks of duplex velocity criteria in predicting arteriographic stenoses are thought to be attributed to several factors. These include variations in technique, such as insonation angle, sample volume, and machine type, as well as local anatomic factors, such as contralateral ICA stenosis and occlusion, carotid kinking, preocclusive ICA stenosis, ICA siphon stenosis or occlusion, and previous carotid patching. Systemic hemodynamic factors such as blood pressure and low cardiac output may greatly influence the velocity measurements independent of the extent of disease in the ICA.[17]

Errors can be introduced into the performance and interpretation of duplex ultrasonography in many ways. The Doppler angles or the angles of insonation of the vessel are very important, and small errors in their determination can lead to errors in the calculated stenosis. This problem is greater in vessels that are either tortuous or difficult to visualize. Calcification can hinder the assessment of a diseased vessel, especially when a thick calcified plaque obscures the degree of stenosis, which can lead to an underestimation of the disease. In the majority of the patients, calcification is not a problem for detecting the degree of stenosis as the highest velocities are found at the exit of the stenosis.

In order to minimize such pitfalls, vascular departments must apply recognized and agreed scanning protocols. Most high-end ultrasound systems have examination specific presets that can either be set by the manufacturer or the vascular department can customize according to local policies. Ideally, a 60° Doppler angle should be used to obtain velocity recordings, although for angles between 45% and 60%, the error is small.[44] Where this is not possible, an explanation and the Doppler angle used should be documented to aid with future follow-up examinations.

30.2.4 Joint Recommendations for Reporting Carotid Ultrasound Investigation in the United Kingdom

These guidelines were published in 2009 and have been endorsed by the British Medical Ultrasound Society, the Royal College of Physicians, the Society and College of Radiographers, the Society for Vascular Technology of Great Britain and Ireland, the United Kingdom Association of Sonographers, and the Vascular Society of Great Britain and Ireland.[44]

They have recommended that the NASCET method should be used for expressing the percentage of diameter stenosis as this is the method used by most surgeons. In addition, an advantage of this method is that a 50% stenosis corresponds to a 2.2 mm residual lumen and a 70% stenosis corresponds to a 1.3 mm residual lumen. Such measurements can be made by duplex ultrasound.

They have also suggested that "in order to best manage patients and monitor disease progression, it is desirable to measure the degree of stenosis in deciles" using velocity ratios (see below).

Another recommendation is the routine measurement of PSV and EDV in both the distal CCA and the ICA at the site of highest PSV found. The recommended indices may be calculated from these measurments.

The guidelines recommend that the Doppler angle should be in the range of 45–60° with proper correction applied using the angle correction cursor. For example, "in the case of an eccentric jet within a stenosis the angle cursor should be aligned to the jet."

Table 30.2 Duplex velocity criteria for different grades of internal carotid stenosis in the Joint Recommendations for Reporting Carotid Ultrasound Investigation in the United Kingdom[44]

Stenosis% NASCET	PSVic (cm/s)	PSVic/PSVcc	PSVic/EDVcc
<50	<125	<2	<8
50–59	>125	2–4	8–10
60–69	>125	2–4	11–13
70–79	>230	>4	14–21
80–89	>230	>4	22–34
>90 but less than near occlusion	>400	>5	>35
Near occlusion	High, low, or string flow	Variable	Variable
Occlusion	No flow	Not applicable	Not applicable

The diagnostic velocity criteria recommended for different grades of stenosis are summarized in Table 30.2.

A summary of the recommendations as published[44] is given below:

1. Carotid duplex should be a bilateral scan and includes a basic assessment of the vertebral arteries.
2. All results and calculations to refer to the NASCET method of measurement.
3. The following four velocities to be measured and recorded: PSVcc and EDVcc 1–2 cm below the bifurcation; PSVic and EDVic at point of highest velocity or distal to the bulb in the absence of significant disease.
4. Doppler velocities to be measured at an angle of 45–60° with proper correction using the angle correction cursor.
5. PSVic and PSVic/PSVcc to stratify 50% and 70% levels (Table 30.2).
6. PSVic/EDVcc (St. Mary's ratio)[8] to stratify in deciles.
7. In the case of a large plaque in a large bulb (>10 mm in diameter), measure and report the bulb diameter, plaque thickness, and residual lumen.
8. Qualitatively note the nature of the plaque (calcified, irregular, echo-poor, etc.).
9. Record length of longer stenoses.
10. Record distance of bifurcation below mastoid process in centimeters.
11. Note any cautions in diagnostic reliability of the report.

30.2.5 Other Methods of Grading ICA Stenosis with Ultrasound

B-mode image measurement of the carotid bifurcation is an attractive diagnostic modality because, unlike velocity parameters, B-mode imaging is a direct measure of carotid plaque dimensions and may therefore minimize the limitations of velocity criteria.[45] Current scanning technology provides excellent image resolution that facilitates the direct visualization of both the arterial lumen and the outer arterial wall. In the longitudinal view, B-mode measurements of a single dimension of the plaque shows large variations from one operator to another because of the difficulty of reproducing the direction of incidence and the often irregular stenosis of the lumen.[46] Therefore, the longitudinal view when used alone is not reliable enough to evaluate the degree of stenosis, and in many cases, this examination should be complemented by transverse views. Also, in some cases (hypoechoic atheroma, calcified plaque, and critical stenosis), the internal lumen of the artery cannot be correctly visualized and measured.[47]

Transverse views with color imaging are used to counteract the drawback of longitudinal views and to provide an accurate measurement of the anatomical degree of stenosis.[8] The use of multiplanar anatomical measurements can overcome the variability observed with this method (see Fig. 30.8 at the end of the chapter). In order to calculate the local area of stenosis with the planimetric method, the ECST method of expressing stenosis is used. In addition, color Doppler allows the operator to visualize blood flow, avoiding

Table 30.3 Table incorporating the guidelines of the Society of Radiologists in Ultrasound[14] and the Joint Recommendations for Reporting Carotid Ultrasound Investigation in the United Kingdom[44] as used by the authors. The ECST percent stenosis column has been added for ease of use for those who want to grade lesions in terms of stroke risk (see Chaps. 36 and 37) (ECST stenosis is linearly related to stroke risk, but NASCET stenosis is not)

Stenosis%		Duplex velocity criteria				
"NASCET"	"ECST"	PSVic	EDVic	PSVic/PSVic	PSVic/EDVcc	Plaque and lumen
Normal	Normal	<125	<40	<2	<8	Absent
<50	<70	<125	<40	<4	<8	Present
50–59	70–76	125–230	40–100	2–4	8–10	Narrowing
60–69	77–82	125–230	40–100	2–4	11–14	Narrowing
70–79	83–89	230–400	100–125	5–5	15–20	Narrowing
80–89	90–94	230–400	>125	>4.0	21–30	Narrowing
90–99	95–99	>400[a]	>125[a]	>4.0[a]	>30[a]	Narrowing

PSVic peak systolic velocity in internal carotid artery, *EDVic* end-diastolic velocity in internal carotid artery, *ic* internal carotid artery, *cc* common carotid artery
[a]In cases of "trickle flow," these velocities may not be detectable (see text)

most misinterpretations of the B-mode image. It provides a clear outline of the plaque contours, detects irregularities, facilitates the identification of the narrowest point of stenosis, and contributes to the diagnosis of occlusion.[48] The color with the longitudinal image provides an anatomic view, which can be easily interpreted by physicians without extensive knowledge of ultrasonography.

The efficacy of this method and its good correlation with angiography has been studied in investigations comparing this technique with angiographic data and pathology specimens.[49] Jmor et al.[45] have shown a good correlation of the planimetric degree of stenosis by ultrasound with specimen measurements. In addition, Eckstein et al.[49,50] have supported that planimetric measurements are valid in the quantification of high-grade ICA stenosis. Beebe et al.[51] have published their experience with the prospective evaluation of 713 carotid bifurcations with direct ultrasound scan imaging. In this series of arteries, decile percent groupings for stenoses greater than 50% identified with ultrasound were evaluated as to their predictive power for arteriographically defined carotid stenoses. In this study, stenoses of 60–69%, 70–79%, 80–99% had positive predictive values for arteriographic stenosis of 75%, 82%, and 94%, respectively. The addition of selected PSV or EDV criteria to these decile percent stenosis groupings improved the predictive power of ultrasound for 50–99%, 60–99%, and 70–99% arteriographic stenoses on average by 11%. Wardlaw and Lewis[52] have shown a good correlation of ultrasound planimetric measurements with angiography using the ECST method. Planimetric evaluation of the stenosis is accurate, and when used in combination with the velocity measurements, the diagnostic confidence is higher with a probable increase in the diagnostic accuracy as well.

Table 30.3 is a hybrid table that incorporates the guidelines of the Society of Radiologists in Ultrasound[14] and the Joint Recommendations for Reporting Carotid Ultrasound Investigation in the United Kingdom[44] as used by the authors. The ECST percent stenosis column has been added for ease of use (a) for those who want to grade lesions in terms of stroke risk (see Chaps. 36 and 37) (ECST stenosis is linearly related to stroke risk, but NASCET stenosis is not) and (b) for ease of conversion from ECST to NASCET when the planimetric method for plaques in the bulb is used.

30.2.6 Comparison of Ultrasound with MRA and CTA

The development of new imaging technologies has prompted their use in the diagnosis and grading of carotid stenosis. Several meta-analyses of the studies comparing MRA and ultrasound have shown similar discriminatory power or were slightly in favor of the MRA.[53] However, the cost-effectiveness, portability and repeatability of duplex scanning make it the test of choice in the vast majority of patients.

30.2.7 Effect of Contralateral Disease on Duplex Measurements of ICA

Ultrasound does not assess the presence of proximal (aortic arch) or distal (carotid siphon) lesions, intracerebral vascular abnormalities, trickle flow beyond a subocclusive arterial stenosis, and disease within heavily calcified vessels.[54] There is also a tendency for standard duplex velocity criteria to overestimate the severity of stenosis when it is compared with arteriography using the "N" method.[55–59] Hayes et al.[55] have demonstrated that this overestimation appears to be proportional to the severity of contralateral disease, with only 2.6% of carotid stenoses being overestimated if contralateral stenosis is less than 45% and 35% of scans being erroneously upgraded if there is a contralateral occlusion. These discrepancies are unlikely to be the result of observer variation as duplex underestimation of disease is relatively infrequent. Spadone et al.[56] have suggested that more reliance should be placed on the B-mode images when there is contralateral disease. However, of the 14 patients in whom the stenosis was reclassified following contralateral endarterectomy, seven had suboptimal ultrasound imaging as a consequence of mural calcification or complex plaque formation.

The importance of taking into account contralateral stenosis is underscored by Ray et al.[54] who demonstrated that bilateral carotid artery disease can cause overestimation of the stenosis by duplex ultrasonography. They have shown that in patients with bilateral carotid stenosis undergoing unilateral carotid endarterectomy, PSV and EDV were decreased in the unoperated site postoperatively. These changes were clinically relevant with six of nine patients reported to have 80–99% stenosis being reclassified to a lower category following contralateral surgery. Without preoperative arteriography or repeat ultrasonography, these patients could have been offered an inappropriate endarterectomy. More importantly, the velocity in the original operated artery was probably similarly increased by disease in the contralateral artery.

The increase in velocity in the contralateral artery may be a consequence of increased collateral flow through it, producing a jet effect and artificially high velocities.[54] Successful ipsilateral endarterectomy would lead to a reduction in contralateral flow and more accurate velocity measurement. The hypothesis is supported by van Everdingen et al.'s study,[60] which demonstrated that the distal PSVic was related to ICA flow measured by MRA. In this study, patients with ICA flow in excess of 274 ml/min on MRA were more than twice likely to have duplex overestimation of disease than those with smaller volume flows (46% versus 20%). The extent of the discrepancy between serial ultrasonography before and after contralateral endarterectomy presumably reflects the portion of blood passing through the imaged artery. It is possible that, where velocity changes are minimal, there are adequate ipsilateral periorbital and/or posterior circulatory collaterals.

30.2.8 Grading Restenosis in Stented Carotid Arteries

Although the current velocity criteria can fairly accurately predict the degree of stenosis in untreated patients and in those that have undergone carotid endarterectomy, this does not seem to be the case in patients with carotid stents[61] (see Fig. 30.9 at the end of the chapter). While it is not clear whether carotid restenosis in the setting of carotid stenting can give similar symptoms to primary stenosis, carotid restenosis in this population appeared to be higher in comparison to patients undergoing carotid endarterectomy (CEA) in the Carotid and Vertebral Artery Transluminal Angioplasty Study (CAVATAS) and Stent Protected Angioplasty versus Carotid Endarterectomy (SPACE) trials. Long-term follow-up data are needed in patients with stents to investigate the clinical consequences of in-stent restenosis. Prior to these analyses, we need reliable cutoff criteria to diagnose in-stent restenosis. Duplex ultrasound appears to be a good tool in the evaluation of restenosis.[61] It can readily image carotid bifurcation stents, and serial testing can identify stent-related abnormalities, including thrombosis, in-stent stenosis, stent deformity, lack of apposition to artery wall, and migration. Blood flow patterns within a nonstenotic stent are nondisturbed except at proximal and distal stent orifices where diameter/compliance mismatch exists.

PSV is the best predictor for the severity of the stenosis. However, the degree of restenosis in a stented carotid artery, measured according to the North American Symptomatic Carotid Endarterectomy Trial (NASCET) criteria on CTA or MRA, is usually less severe than expected based on the PSV measured with ultrasound. Possibly, blood turbulence and blood flow are different in an artificial rigid stent than in a normal vessel.[62] An artery without a stent is more likely to have a more elastic wall than a stented one, even if restenosis is present.

This discrepancy occurs across all degrees of stenoses and persists over a long follow-up period. Velocity criteria have developed for various degrees of stenosis based on their clinical applicability. Lal et al.[61] have proposed the use of greater than 20%, 50%, and 80% as the appropriate thresholds for identifying in-stent restenosis.

These degrees of stenosis are important for patients undergoing carotid stenting. Moderate degree of in-stent restenosis (50–79%) does not appear to progress, but its natural history is not well defined yet.[61] Current recommendations for patients with greater than 50% in-stent restenosis include close monitoring with ultrasound every 6 months.[63] Furthermore, this threshold is important for reporting purposes since a more than 50% stenosis (in relation to distal ICA) is the accepted definition of in-stent restenosis in the arterial bed of the carotid artery.[64,65] In fact, intervention has been recommended by some in symptomatic patients with a more than 50% restenosis.[66,67]

Asymptomatic restenosis is generally not treated unless the threshold of 80% stenosis has been reached.[64,66,67] In-stent residual stenosis immediately after stenting has been variously defined as lesions of greater than 20%,[62,64] 30%,[65] or even 50%,[66,67] depending on how strictly one chooses to define technical success of the procedure. The use of 20% as the threshold for residual stenosis is considered as the most conservative estimate of technical success to be reported on the first poststenting ultrasound examination. In addition, residual stenosis is a strong predictor of functional outcome[67–69] and of future high grade in-stent restenosis with need for reintervention. As such, patients with carotid stenting should be monitored aggressively until the natural history of their disease is better defined.

The early studies performed to determine cutoff criteria to characterize in-stent restenosis were biased by the lack of a reliable analysis of their velocities.[70–73] Furthermore, only patients with high velocities underwent carotid arteriography for comparison, which may lead to potential bias towards higher velocity thresholds and may impact the rate of false negative and false positive values. The more recent studies in the field have been methodologically sounder.[61,74–76] However, a clear consensus on the grading of internal carotid artery in-stent restenosis is lacking.

Lal et al.[61,62] support that a normal luminal diameter (<20% stenosis) can be recognized by a PSV of less than 150 cm/s with an ICA/CCA ratio of less than 2.15. This cutoff criterion confirms technical success in patients undergoing carotid artery stenting. In-stent restenosis greater than 50% can be identified with a PSV higher than 220 cm/s and an ICA/CCA ratio above 2.7. High-grade in-stent restenosis (>80%) is best identified with a PSV higher than 340 cm/s and an ICA/CCA ratio above 4.15. The combination of the PSV and the ICA/CCA thresholds results in a small improvement in accuracy. The main goal for identifying patients with residual stenoses greater than 20% and in-stent restenosis greater than 50% is to enhance monitoring, for identifying in-stent restenosis greater than 80% is to identify patients for potential reintervention.

Armstrong et al.,[74] in their series of 111 patients, suggest a surveillance protocol with ultrasound for patients undergoing internal carotid artery stenting. Their study has revealed a 5% risk of procedure failure due to the development of high in-stent restenosis. They concluded that testing individuals at intervals of 6 months is sufficient to detect stenting site stenosis and monitor 50–70% stenotic lesions for progression. However, surveillance is also important to detect contralateral ICA stenosis progression. Imaging of the stent site in less than a month is useful to exclude residual stenosis and reconfirm the severity of contralateral disease. If testing confirms less than 50% stenosis bilateral beyond the first 18 months, an annual scan is adequate for disease monitoring. Surveillance every 6 months is recommended in patients with greater than 50% ipsilateral or contralateral ICA stenosis. The development of hemispheric symptoms in the presence of greater than 50% stenosis, or asymptomatic disease progression to a high-grade stenosis should result in prompt surgical or endovascular reintervention in appropriate patients.

30.3 Clinical Cases

Several examples of ultrasound examinations are given to clarify grading of carotid stenosis in different patients and hemodynamic conditions Figs. 30.4–30.9.

Fig. 30.4 ICA stenosis grade 50–69%. Female patient who presented with amaurosis fugax in the left eye: duplex scanning as seen on (**a**) demonstrated a 50–69%. All criteria were present: PSVic greater than 125 cm/s, EDVic greater than 40 cm/s, and PSVic/PSVcc higher than 2.0. An irregular echolucent plaque was found at the posterior wall of the proximal ICA, as shown by the filling defect on color mode. EDVic was 42 cm/s, and the PSVic/PSVcc was 2.1, indicating that the stenosis was closer to the lower end of the stenosis grade. The scan findings shown in (**b**) are from a male patient who presented with an asymptomatic bruit on the right side from an irregular calcified plaque on the posterior wall. This patient is on the higher end of the stenosis grade as indicated by the higher velocities (PSVic 200 cm/s) and the PSVic/PSVcc ratio of 3.2

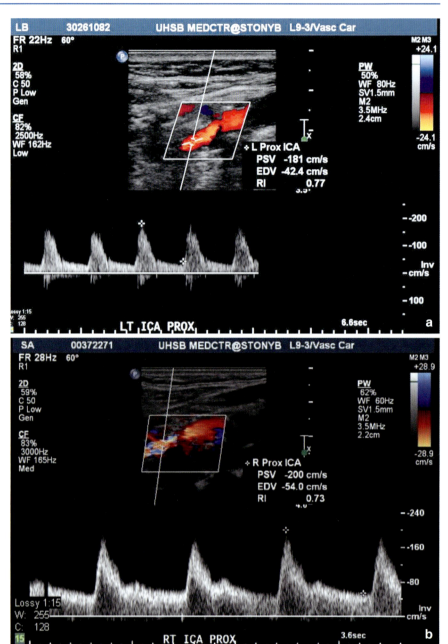

Fig. 30.5 ICA stenosis grade 70–95%. A male patient who presented with transient ischemic attack had an irregular plaque causing a greater than 70% ICA stenosis on the left side (**a**). The EDVic was greater than 100 cm/s, and the PSVic/PSVcc was 4.7 (259/55). In (**b**), a greater than 80% stenosis is shown in a male asymptomatic patient who had a carotid ultrasound because of a loud bruit on the left side. The EDVic was 210 cm/s well above the 125 cm/s cutoff value for 80% stenosis. The PSVic/PSVcc was 7.3 (443/61)

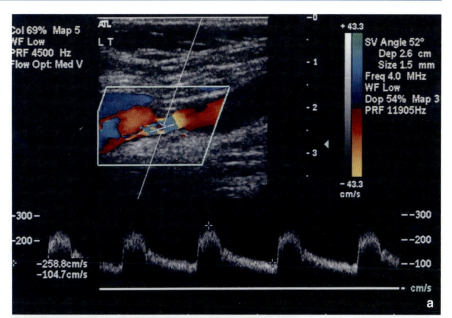

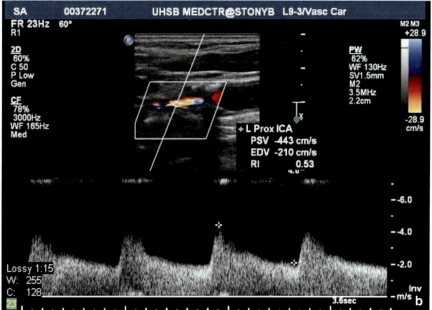

Fig. 30.6 ICA string sign stenosis. A male patient who had a previous stroke and a documented occlusion of the left ICA by ultrasound and angiography was followed up for a 50% right ICA stenosis. He was found to have an asymptomatic recanalization of his left ICA. Low EVDic was detected in the distal CCA indicating an ICA tight stenosis or occlusion (**a**). The ICA was patent with low amplitude flow (**b**). An irregular flow channel with a small diameter of 1.6 mm was found due to previous chronic occlusion (**c**). The cross-sectional view shows a string sign flow in the ICA and normal flow in the ECA confirming the findings (**d**)

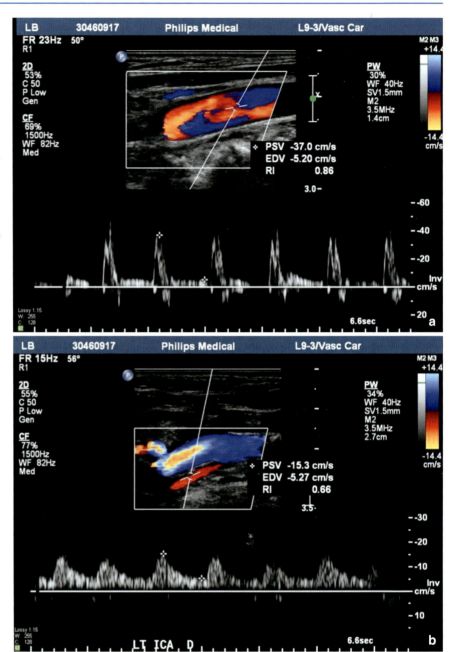

Fig. 30.6 (continued)

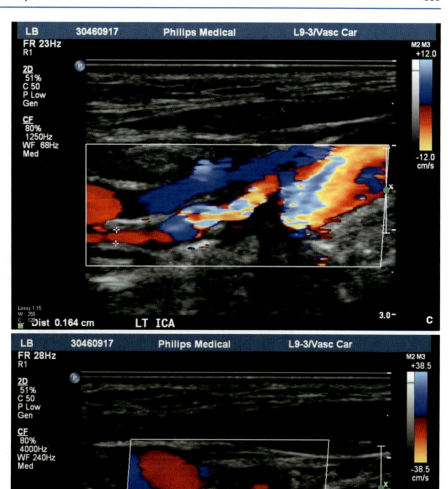

Fig. 30.7 ICA acute and chronic occlusion. A male asymptomatic patient who had a previous ICA occlusion and was followed up for the contralateral ICA stenosis. Power Doppler imaging demonstrated a chronic ICA occlusion as seen by the small diameter measuring 2 mm (**a**). Another male patient who came to the hospital with a stroke was found to have acute thrombosis of his right ICA. Color flow imaging showed the characteristic "*blue cap*" of the reversed flow at the site of the occlusion. Doppler velocity tracings demonstrated a low amplitude flow with absence of end-diastolic flow in the distal CCA and a reversed flow in the bulb (**b**)

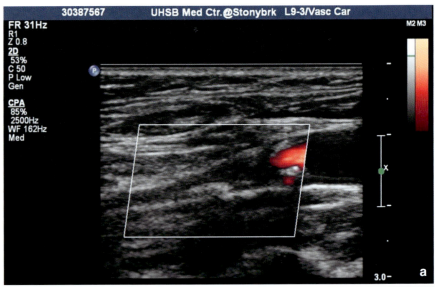

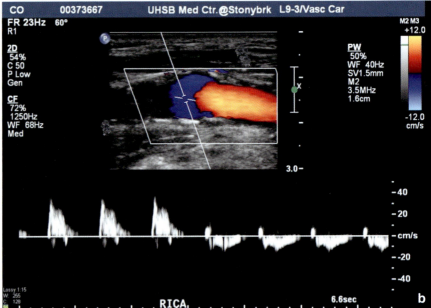

Fig. 30.8 Planimetric evaluation of stenosis. he carotid artery diameter is measured in three different planes, and the average diameter is taken, as shown in the schematic drawing (**a**). Three different views and diameter measurements are shown in the left ICA using the power Doppler imaging (**b–d**). The cross-sectional area and the velocity measurements correspond with the average diameter (**e**)

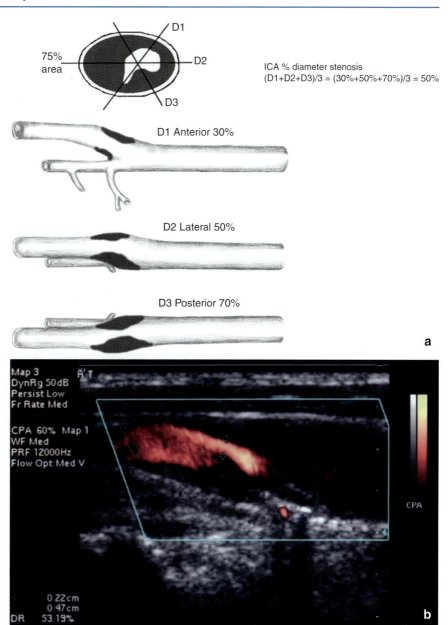

Fig. 30.8 (continued)

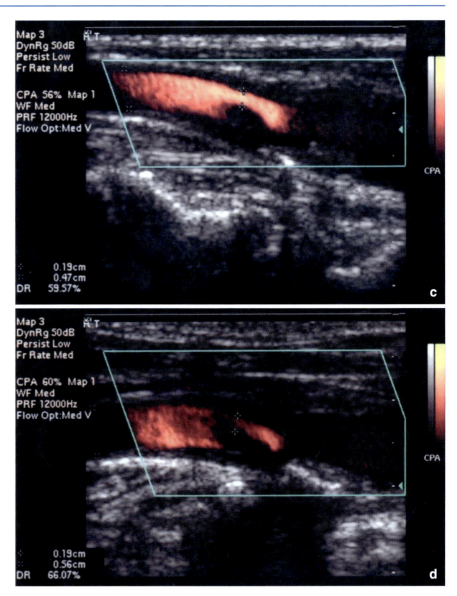

Fig. 30.8 (continued)

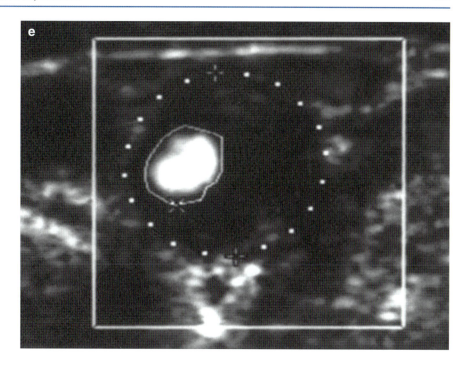

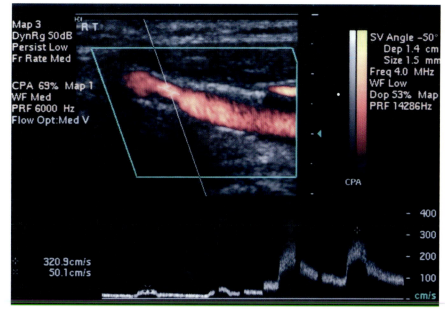

Fig. 30.9 ICA in-stent stenosis. A female patient with greater than 80% symptomatic left ICA stenosis underwent stent placement. At 9 months, the patient developed a greater than 80% in-stent restenosis. Velocity measurements were taken throughout the stent. The PSV was obtained before and after the stenosis. The PSV ratio within the stent was 6.4 (320/50). The power Doppler flow was not optimize for the stenosis but rather to show flow throughout the stent. Therefore, the stenosis does not look as severe on the two-dimensional (2D) image

References

1. Gelabert HA, Moore WJ. Carotid endarterectomy without angiography. *Surg Clin North Am.* 1990;70:213–223.
2. Farmilo RW, Scott DJA, Cole SE, Jeans WD, Horrocks M. Role of duplex scanning in the selection of patients for carotid endarterectomy. *Br J Surg.* 1990;77:388–390.
3. Polak JF. Noninvasive carotid evaluation: Carpe diem. *Radiology.* 1993;186:329–331.
4. Executive Committee for the Asymptomatic Carotid Atherosclerosis Study. Endarterectomy for asymptomatic carotid artery stenosis. *JAMA.* 1995;73:1421–1428.
5. North American Symptomatic Carotid Endarterectomy Trial Collaborators. Beneficial effect of carotid endarterectomy in symptomatic patients with high-grade carotid stenosis. *N Engl J Med.* 1991;325:445–453.
6. European Carotid Surgery Trialists Collaborative Group. MRC European carotid surgery trial: Interim results for symptomatic patients with severe (70–99%) or with mild (0–29%) carotid stenosis. *Lancet.* 1991;337:1235–1243.
7. MRC Asymptomatic Carotid Surgery Trial (ACST) Collaborative Group. Prevention of disabling and fatal strokes by successful carotid endarterectomy in patients without recent neurological symptoms: randomized controlled trial. *Lancet.* 2004;363:1491–1502.
8. Nicolaides AN et al. Angiographic and duplex grading of internal carotid stenosis: can we overcome the confusion? *J Endovasc Surg.* 1996;3:158–165.
9. Williams MA, Nicolaides AN. Predicting the normal dimensions of the internal and external carotid arteries from the diameter of the common carotid. *Eur J Vasc Surg.* 1987;1:91–96.
10. Bladin CF, Alexandrov AV, Murphy J. Carotid stenosis index: a new method of measuring internal carotid artery stenosis. *Stroke.* 1995;26:230–234.
11. Norris JW, Alexandrov AV, Bladin CF. Progress in evaluating carotid artery stenosis. *J Vasc Surg.* 1995;22: 637–638.
12. Bluth EI et al. Carotid duplex sonography: a multicenter recommendation for standardized imaging and Doppler criteria. *Radiographics.* 1988;8:487–506.
13. Grant EG et al. Ability to use duplex US to quantify internal carotid arterial stenoses: fact or fiction? *Radiology.* 2000;214(1):247–252.
14. Grant EG et al. Carotid artery stenosis: gray-scale and Doppler US diagnosis – Society of Radiologists in ultrasound consensus conference. *Radiology.* 2003;229: 340–346.
15. Langlois Y et al. Evaluating carotid artery diseases: the concordance between pulsed Doppler spectrum analysis and angiography. *Ultrasound Med Biol.* 1983;9:51–63.
16. Roederer GO. A simple spectral parameter for accurate classification of severe carotid disease. *Bruit.* 1984;8:174–178.
17. Taylor DC, Strandness DE. Carotid artery duplex scanning. *J Clin Ultrasound.* 1987;15:635–644.
18. Zweibel WJ. Spectrum analysis in carotid sonography. *Ultrasound Med Biol.* 1987;13:625–636.
19. Nicolaides A et al. Asymptomatic internal carotid artery stenosis and cerebrovascular risk stratification. *J Vasc Surg.* 2010;52:1486–1496.
20. Steinke W, Hennerici M, Rautenberg W, Mohr JP. Symptomatic and asymptomatic high grade carotid stenosis in Doppler color flow imaging. *Neurology.* 1992;42:131–137.
21. Sitzer M et al. Between-method correlation in quantifying internal carotid stenosis. *Stroke.* 1993;24:1513–1518.
22. Bray JM et al. Color Doppler imaging duplex sonography and angiography of carotid bifurcations. Prospective and double blind study. *Neuroradiology.* 1995;37:219–224.
23. Hetzel A et al. Colour-coded duplex sonography of preocclusive carotid stenoses. *Eur J Ultrasound.* 1998;8 (3):183–191.
24. Berman SS, Devine JJ, Erdoes LS, Hunter GC. Distinguishing carotid artery pseudo-occlusion with color-flow Doppler. *Stroke.* 1995;26(3):434–438.
25. Mansour MA et al. Detection of total occlusion, string sign, and preocclusive stenosis of the internal carotid artery by color-flow duplex scanning. *Am J Surg.* 1995;170 (2):154–158.
26. AbuRahma AF, Pollack JA, Robinson PA, Mullins D. The reliability of color duplex ultrasound in diagnosing total carotid artery occlusion. *Am J Surg.* 1997;174(2):185–187.
27. Sitzer M, Fürst G, Siebler M, Steinmetz H. Usefulness of an intravenous contrast medium in the characterization of high-grade internal carotid stenosis with color Doppler-assisted duplex imaging. *Stroke.* 1994;25(2):385–389.
28. Ferrer JM et al. Use of ultrasound contrast in the diagnosis of carotid artery occlusion. *J Vasc Surg.* 2000;31(4):736–741.
29. Holden A, Hope JK, Osborne M, Moriarty M, Lee K. Value of a contrast agent in equivocal carotid ultrasound studies: pictorial essay. *Australas Radiol.* 2000;44(3): 253–260.
30. Hansberg T, Wong KS, Droste DW, Ringelstein EB, Kay R. Effects of the ultrasound contrast-enhancing agent Levovist on the detection of intracranial arteries and stenoses in chinese by transcranial Doppler ultrasound. *Cerebrovasc Dis.* 2002;14(2):105–108.
31. Tateishi Y et al. Contrast-enhanced transcranial color-coded duplex sonography criteria for basilar artery stenosis. *J Neuroimaging.* 2008;18(4):407–410.
32. Mittl RL Jr et al. Blinded-reader comparison of magnetic resonance angiography and duplex ultrasonography for carotid artery bifurcation stenosis. *Stroke.* 1994;25:4–10.
33. Robinson ML, Sacks D, Perlmutter GS, Marinelli DL. Diagnostic criteria for carotid duplex sonography. *AJR Am J Roentgenol.* 1988;151(5):1045–1049.
34. Moneta GL et al. Correlation of North American Symptomatic Carotid Endarterectomy Trial (NASCET) angiographic definition of 70% to 99% internal carotid artery stenosis with duplex scanning. *J Vasc Surg.* 1993;17:152–159.
35. Moneta GL et al. Screening for asymptomatic internal carotid artery stenosis: duplex criteria for discriminating 60% to 99% stenosis. *J Vasc Surg.* 1995;21(6):989–994.
36. Williams MA et al. Duplex scanning in detection and grading of internal carotid artery stenosis improved criteria. In: Nicolaides AN, Salmasi MA, eds. *Cardiovascular Applications of Doppler Ultrasound.* New York: Churchill-Livingstone; 1989:247–260.
37. Knox RA et al. Computer based classification of carotid arterial disease: a prospective assessment. *Stroke.* 1982;13:589–594.

38. Faught WE et al. Color-flow duplex scanning of carotid arteries: new velocity criteria based on receiver operator characteristic analysis for threshold stenoses used in the symptomatic and asymptomatic carotid trials. *J Vasc Surg.* 1994;19(5):818–827.
39. Hood DB et al. Prospective evaluation of new duplex criteria to identify 70% internal carotid artery stenosis. *J Vasc Surg.* 1996;23(2):254–261.
40. Hunink MG, Polak JF, Barlan MM, O'Leary DH. Detection and quantification of carotid artery stenosis: efficacy of various Doppler velocity parameters. *AJR Am J Roentgenol.* 1992;160(3):619–625.
41. Jahromi AS, Cinà CS, Liu Y, Clase CM. Sensitivity and specificity of color duplex ultrasound measurement in the estimation of internal carotid artery stenosis: a systematic review and meta-analysis. *J Vasc Surg.* 2005;41(6):962–972.
42. El-Saden SM et al. Imaging of the internal carotid artery: the dilemma of total versus near total occlusion. *Radiology.* 2001;221:301–308.
43. Pan XM et al. Assessment of carotid artery stenosis by ultrasonography, conventional angiography, and magnetic resonance angiography: correlation with ex vivo measurement of plaque stenosis. *J Vasc Surg.* 1995;82(8):88–89.
44. Oates CP et al. Joint recommendations for reporting carotid ultrasound investigation in the United Kingdom. *Eur J Vasc Endovasc Surg.* 2009;37(3):251–261.
45. Jmor S et al. Grading internal carotid artery stenosis using B-mode ultrasound (in vivo study). *Eur J Vasc Endovasc Surg.* 1999;18(4):315–322.
46. Tola M, Yurdakul M. Effect of Doppler angle in diagnosis of internal carotid artery stenosis. *J Ultrasound Med.* 2006;25(9):1187–1192.
47. Arbeille P, Desombre C, Aesh B, Philippot M, Lapierre F. Quantification and assessment of carotid artery lesions: degree of stenosis and plaque volume. *J Clin Ultrasound.* 1995;23(2):113–124.
48. Londrey GL et al. Does color-flow imaging improve the accuracy of duplex carotid evaluation? *J Vasc Surg.* 1992;13(5):659–663.
49. Eckstein HH, Post K, Hoffman E, Hupp T, Allenberg JR. Determination of the degree of stenosis of the internal carotid artery in the surgical specimen after eversion TEA: comparison with angiography and c-w-Doppler ultrasound. *Vasa.* 1995;24(2):176–183.
50. Eckstein HH et al. Grading of internal carotid artery stenosis: validation of Doppler/duplex ultrasound criteria and angiography against endarterectomy specimen. *Eur J Vasc Endovasc Surg.* 2001;21(4):301–310.
51. Beebe HG et al. Carotid arterial ultrasound scan imaging: a direct approach to stenosis measurement. *J Vasc Surg.* 1999;29(5):838–844.
52. Wardlaw JM, Lewis S. Carotid stenosis measurement on colour Doppler ultrasound: agreement of ECST, NASCET and CCA methods applied to ultrasound with intra-arterial angiographic stenosis measurement. *Eur J Radiol.* 2005;56(2):205–211.
53. Nederkoorn PJ, van der Graaf Y, Hunink MG. Duplex ultrasound and magnetic resonance angiography compared with digital subtraction angiography in carotid artery stenosis: a systematic review. *Stroke.* 2003;34(3):1324–1332.
54. Ray SA, Lockhart SJ, Dourado R, Irvine AT, Burnand KG. Effect of contralateral disease on duplex measurements of internal carotid artery stenosis. *Br J Surg.* 2000;87(8):1057–1062.
55. Hayes AC et al. The effect of contralateral disease on carotid Doppler frequency. *Surgery.* 1988;103(1):19–23.
56. Spadone DP, Barkmeier LD, Hodgson KJ, Ramsey DE, Sumner DS. Contralateral internal carotid artery stenosis or occlusion: pitfall of correct ipsilateral classification – a study performed with color-flow imaging. *J Vasc Surg.* 1990;11(5):642–649.
57. Fujitani RM, Mills JL, Wang LM, Taylor SM. The effect of unilateral internal carotid arterial occlusion upon contralateral duplex study: criteria for accurate interpretation. *J Vasc Surg.* 1992;16(3):459–467.
58. AbuRahma AF et al. Effect of contralateral severe stenosis or carotid occlusion on duplex criteria of ipsilateral stenoses: comparative study of various duplex parameters. *J Vasc Surg.* 1995;22(6):751–761.
59. Busuttil SJ, Franklin DP, Youkey JR, Elmore JR. Carotid duplex overestimation of stenosis due to severe contralateral disease. *Am J Surg.* 1996;172(2):144–147.
60. van Everdingen KJ, van der Grond J, Kappelle LJ. Overestimation of a stenosis in the internal carotid artery by duplex sonography caused by an increase in volume flow. *J Vasc Surg.* 1998;27(3):479–485.
61. Lal BK et al. Duplex ultrasound velocity criteria for the stented carotid artery. *J Vasc Surg.* 2008;47(1):63–73.
62. Lal BK, Hobson RW II, Goldstein J, Chakhtoura EY, Durán WN. Carotid artery stenting: is there a need to revise ultrasound velocity criteria? *J Vasc Surg.* 2004;39(1):58–66.
63. Lal BK, Hobson RW II. Management of carotid restenosis. *J Cardiovasc Surg (Torino).* 2006;47(2):153–160.
64. Hobson RW II. CREST (Carotid Revascularization Endarterectomy versus Stent Trial): background, design, and current status. *Semin Vasc Surg.* 2000;13(2):139–143.
65. Yadav JS et al. Protected carotid-artery stenting versus endarterectomy in high-risk patients. *N Engl J Med.* 2004;351(15):1493–1501.
66. Gray WA et al. Protected carotid stenting in high-surgical-risk patients: the ARCHeR results. *J Vasc Surg.* 2006;44(2):258–268.
67. Gray WA et al. The CAPTURE registry: predictors of outcomes in carotid artery stenting with embolic protection for high surgical risk patients in the early post-approval setting. *Catheter Cardiovasc Interv.* 2007;70(7):1025–1033.
68. Leung WH, Lau CP. Effects of severity of the residual stenosis of the infarct-related coronary artery on left ventricular dilation and function after acute myocardial infarction. *J Am Coll Cardiol.* 1992;20(2):307–313.
69. Miyazaki S et al. Correlation of residual stenosis immediately after coronary angioplasty with long term prognosis. *Catheter Cardio Diag.* 1998;43(3):262–270.
70. Stanziale SF, Wholey MH, Boules TN, Selzer F, Makaroun MS. Determining in-stent stenosis of carotid arteries by duplex ultrasound criteria. *J Endovasc Ther.* 2005;12(3):346–353.

71. Peterson BG et al. Duplex ultrasound remains a reliable test even after carotid stenting. *Ann Vasc Surg*. 2005;19(6): 793–797.
72. Chahwan S et al. Carotid artery velocity characteristics after carotid artery angioplasty and stenting. *J Vasc Surg*. 2007; 45(3):523–526.
73. Chi YW, White CJ, Woods TC, Goldman CK. Ultrasound velocity criteria for carotid in-stent restenosis. *Catheter Cardio Diag*. 2007;69(3):349–354.
74. Armstrong PA et al. Duplex scan surveillance after carotid angioplasty and stenting: a rational definition of stent stenosis. *J Vasc Surg*. 2007;46(3):460–465.
75. AbuRahma AF et al. Optimal carotid duplex velocity criteria for defining the severity of carotid in-stent restenosis. *J Vasc Surg*. 2008;48(3):589–594.
76. Zhou W et al. Ultrasound criteria for severe in-stent restenosis following carotid artery stenting. *J Vasc Surg*. 2008; 47(1):74–80.

The Significance of Echolucent Plaques: Past and Future Perspectives

31

Martin Græbe and Henrik Sillesen

31.1 Introduction

Like most other scientific discoveries of significance, assessment of plaque pathohistological features using ultrasonographic morphology was first described in scattered and scarce single observations. In the beginning of the 1980s, visual assessment of echolucency was linked to the histology of symptomatic carotid plaques (at that time mainly considered to be intraplaque hemorrhage) and the first prospective studies considering risk of stroke within different gradings of echolucency were published. Since then, several prospective studies have addressed the association between carotid plaque morphology and histology, risk of stroke, and also cardiovascular risk in general. Plaque morphology assessed by B-mode ultrasonography has achieved a large impact on clinical research and, as outlined in this chapter, echogenicity can be implemented in several areas of clinical risk assessment of cardiovascular disease. In this chapter, the existing literature will be discussed in order to provide the reader with an evaluation of where, within these different topics, the echolucent carotid plaque is of significance. Finally, the future of ultrasonic plaque characterization will be assessed.

31.2 What Is the Echolucent Plaque?

An echolucent (often called hypoechoic or anechoic) plaque, as opposed to an echogenic (often called hyperechoic or echorich) plaque, consists of tissue that poorly reflects ultrasound waves. Blood echoreflectivity which is near zero (i.e., appears black on the ultrasound image) can be used as the reference for echolucent plaques in visual assessment, muscle (sternocleid or platysma) as an intermediate reference and vessel wall adventitia or bone as reference for the echorich plaque (Fig. 31.1). The evidence for a link between echolucent ultrasound morphology and both histological and molecular features of the vulnerable plaque is growing. The vulnerable or unstable atherosclerotic plaque exhibits a thin fibrous cap, a high degree of inflammation, a large lipid or necrotic core, hemorrhage, and most important, a high risk of fissuring or rupturing, thereby causing symptoms (Chaps. 1 and 2). Visual assessment of echolucency has substantiated that plaque echolucency represents either the large homogenous core of lipid, intraplaque hemorrhage, or both.[1–4] Different parts of the plaque might exhibit different degrees of echolucency and visual assessment of plaque texture, or heterogeneity, has also been found by several studies to support the association between echolucency and vulnerability.[5–8] Visual classification of plaque echogenicity has been thoroughly investigated (Chap. 12), and throughout the years, many times adjusted to improve intraobserver and interobserver reproducibility.[2,3,8,9] Image normalization using linear scaling with blood and adventitia as reference points has improved reproducibility of computer-assisted quantification using gray scale median (GSM) measurements[10] and more

M. Græbe • H. Sillesen (✉)
Department of Vascular Surgery, Rigshospitalet, University of Copenhagen, Copenhagen, Denmark

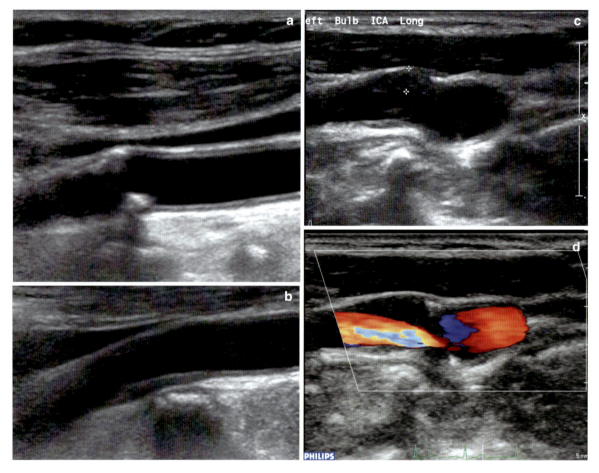

Fig. 31.1 (a) Echogenic plaque at the distal common carotid artery. (b) Small mainly echolucent plaque in proximal internal carotid artery. (c) Uniformly echolucent plaque in the proximal internal carotid artery (*between markers*). (d) Same plaque as in (c) using color-coded ultrasound

recently integrated backscatter analyses.[11] Thus, standardized methods for quantification of echogenicity (though averaging heterogeneity) have been introduced (Chap. 12) and histological features of vulnerable plaques have been shown to be associated with quantification of echolucency.[11–14]

The histological findings of the echolucent plaque, taken together with the repeated findings of an association between echolucency and symptomatology as well as future risk of stroke described below, strongly indicate that an echolucent plaque represents the vulnerable plaque.

Two major areas of research implementing plaque echolucency can be identified: (a) population-based observations using echogenicity as a surrogate marker for vulnerable plaques and (b) individual plaque assessment for stratifying patients into different levels of risk for stroke to identify those who might benefit from carotid endarterectomy in addition to medical preventive treatment. The latter can be divided into research regarding primary prevention in patients with asymptomatic plaques and secondary prevention in patients with symptomatic plaques.

31.3 The Asymptomatic Echolucent Plaque

Worldwide incidence rate of ischemic stroke is 70/100,000 person-years,[15] and a considerable part is believed to be related to carotid bifurcation atherosclerotic plaques.[16,17] Although asymptomatic carotid bifurcation plaques are relatively common, the incidence of stroke amongst patients with such plaques is low. Thus, the need for identification of risk factors that differentiate high- from low-risk subjects is crucial in order to improve stratification of asymptomatic patient selection for carotid endarterectomy. Annual stroke incidence rate in patients with asymptomatic internal carotid artery stenosis greater than 60% in relation to the distal normal internal carotid has been reported to be 2%,[18,19] and recent studies seem to find lower rates in agreement with improvements in medical therapy.[20–22]

In 1985, the first prospective study considering risk of stroke and transient ischemic attack (TIA) within different grades of echolucency was published. Johnson et al. showed that asymptomatic patients with "soft" plaques (anechoic with greater than 75% stenosis) were more likely to become symptomatic than patients with dense or calcified plaques with similar stenosis within a follow-up of 3 years.[23] Several studies have confirmed this finding using both visual grading of plaque morphology[8,24–27] and GSM analysis.[28,29] In these studies of the natural history of asymptomatic carotid stenosis, the use of echolucency as an independent risk marker (corrected for degree of stenosis, age, and other known risk factors) identified high-risk patient subgroups with higher annual risk of stroke or TIA. However, two studies were unable to identify significantly different risk between echolucent and echorich plaques when only considering risk of ipsilateral stroke in asymptomatic patients with carotid stenosis.[19,30] The Asymptomatic Carotid Stenosis and Risk of Stroke Study (ACSRS) demonstrated that prior to image normalization, which changed echogenicity classification of 50% of the plaques, no difference in the ipsilateral cerebral event rate was found (Chap. 12). However, after image normalization and plaque reclassification, event rates, including stroke, were high in patients with echolucent plaques and low in echogenic plaques. The authors pointed out that in the absence of image normalization, especially in multicentre studies, the results of plaque echolucency or plaque classification should be viewed with caution.[8]

Two major randomized trials have assessed the benefit of carotid endarterectomy in asymptomatic patients: In the Asymptomatic Carotid Atherosclerosis Study (ACAS) published in 1995, the 5-year risk of ipsilateral stroke in subjects with greater than 60% stenosis randomized to best medical treatment alone was 11%. This was approximately double the risk of that in patients undergoing endarterectomy, including any perioperative stroke or death (5-year risk of 5.1%). With an absolute risk reduction of 5.9%, 17 patients should be operated to prevent one cerebrovascular event in 5 years (of whom 16 would never get a stroke on medical therapy alone – numbers needed to treat = 17)[18] (Chap. 4). Similar results were found in the Asymptomatic Carotid Surgery Trial (ACST) in 2004: A 5-year event rate of stroke (any; not confined to ipsilateral) of 11% vs. 5.8% in patients referred to CEA.[19] ACST implemented plaque echolucency (visual assessment without image normalization) but found no significant effect on risk reduction in subgroup analyses using this for stratification.

Although tempting, there is no strong evidence to support the use of visually assessed echolucency with or without image normalization to be implemented in the clinical decision making concerning asymptomatic carotid stenosis. To meet significance in stratification for carotid endarterectomy, quantification of echogenicity after image normalization needs to be evaluated in trials of surgery in patients also receiving best medical treatment. Based on the risk reduction observed in patients with asymptomatic carotid stenosis undergoing endarterectomy (which has been shown to reduce the annual risk of stroke from 2% to 1%), and the currently believed risk of 1%, it can even be argued that asymptomatic operative intervention should be avoided, an argument not surprisingly presented more often by neurologists than surgeons.[21,22,31] On the other hand, when considering that the current selection criterion for surgery, degree of stenosis, is only able to identify such low-risk patients, the need for improved selection criteria seems obvious.

31.4 The Symptomatic Echolucent Plaque

In 20% of all patients presenting with stroke, the event is preceded by TIA or minor stroke.[32] If a carotid artery plaque is present – ipsilateral to the affected hemisphere – the plaque is considered symptomatic, and prophylactic treatment is indicated based on the following. The North American Symptomatic Carotid Endarterectomy Trial (NASCET)[33] and the European Carotid Surgery Trial (ECST)[34] conducted in the 1990s randomized symptomatic patients to either carotid endarterectomy or best medical treatment alone. Pooled data from these trials showed that surgery was of some benefit in patients with moderate (50–69%) stenosis and of greater benefit in high (>70%) degree of stenosis. The 5-year risk of ipsilateral stroke in symptomatic patients with more that 70% stenosis treated with medical treatment alone was 21.2% and an absolute risk reduction of 16% (numbers needed to treat = 6) was observed in the group undergoing surgery. Subsequent meticulous analyses of the data identified subgroups of patients that would benefit the most, and current guidelines for operation are based on these analyses. Plaque echogenicity assessed ultrasonographically was not part of these studies. As with asymptomatic plaques, echolucency as a stratifying tool for patient selection is of course tempting, but again the evidence is scarce. In 2001, Grønholdt et al.[30] showed in 135 patients that symptomatic echolucent plaques had a 3.1-fold (relative risk) increase of ipsilateral ischemic stroke compared to echorich plaques during a follow-up of 4.4 years. GSM analyses without image normalization were used to differentiate plaque echogenicity. There were no significant differences between risk in moderate and severe degree of stenosis. The authors concluded that computer-assisted ultrasound imaging could improve patient selection for CEA, but no trial has randomized symptomatic patients and used echolucency of plaques for stratification into best medical treatment or surgery. The experienced surgeon might use ultrasonographic assessment of echolucency in individual risk assessment; in cases where the conventional indicators for intervention might be borderline, e.g., where time since last symptom or degree of stenosis is just within or below consensus, echolucency weighted with other risk markers (e.g., age and gender) may flip the coin. In order to implement plaque morphology in a more significant stratification for CEA, new randomized trials are warranted where benefit of CEA in patients with echolucent plaques is investigated.

31.5 Perioperative Risk and Echolucency

An alternative to endarterectomy is endovascular carotid artery stenting. Current European guidelines do not recommend stenting whenever carotid endarterectomy is possible due to the increased perioperative risk of stroke and death.[35] Although originally introduced as a minimally invasive surgical procedure, perioperative complications remain the Achilles heel of carotid stenting. Increasingly advanced protection devices and procedures have been introduced and efforts to identify the "vulnerable" carotid stenting patient have emerged. Preprocedural assessment of plaque echolucency has been investigated in this context with different results.[36–39] It should meet the reader's attention that if echolucency could be considered as a risk factor for iatrogenic events, the need for randomized trials of surgical benefit when stratifying patients by plaque morphology is obvious; if echolucent plaques indeed do impair perioperative complication rates, having extrapolated results from prospective studies of future events to benefit of treatment could be deleterious. Perioperative complications of carotid endarterectomy have not been investigated with regard to echolucency, but it has been shown that perioperative and 30-day postoperative risk of stroke or death after carotid endarterectomy is significantly lower (OR 0.61) in asymptomatic than symptomatic subjects.[40]

31.6 Echolucent Plaques in Population-Based Research

The natural history studies of patients with carotid bifurcation atherosclerosis have provided evidence for a significant potential use of echolucent plaques as independent markers of not just cerebral events, but cardiovascular events in general[8,26,27,41] (Chap. 24). This association is believed to represent the systemic inflammatory nature of atherosclerosis, and carotid plaque echolucency has been widely and increasingly used to identify groups of vulnerable patients. It is also used for evaluation of circulating biomarkers of inflammation to access further insight to the pathogenesis of the vulnerable plaque.[42–45]

Finally, plaque echolucency can be used in monitoring of plaque stabilizing drug therapies as an adjunct to other risk markers (e.g., lipid profile). For example, it has been shown that treatment with lipid-lowering drugs may reduce carotid plaque echolucency over time[46–48] (Chap. 35).

31.7 Future Applications

Recent studies have shown a tremendous effect of urgent medical treatment in reducing recurrent stroke in patients with TIA or minor stroke[49] and the decrease in overall incidence of ischemic stroke is probably due to increased efficacy of best medical treatment.[50–52] Since perioperative risk of stroke or death remains stable for carotid endarterectomy,[53] imaging for risk stratification and identification of patients at high risk, eligible for operation, meets increasing demands of high sensitivity in order to improve absolute risk reduction further.

Although less available and much more expensive, novel imaging modalities such as magnetic resonance imaging (MRI) for morphological plaque assessment may prove superior to ultrasound in such stratification.[54,55] Recent implementation of molecular imaging using positron emission tomography also seems promising for this purpose.[56–58] In the "Asymptomatic Carotid Stenosis and Risk of Stroke" (ACSRS) prospective study, semiquantitative assessment of echolucency (visual evaluation after image normalization) enabled the authors to identify two subgroups in 905 asymptomatic patients with internal carotid artery stenosis greater than 75%. In one group of 724 patients with echolucent plaques, the annual risk of ipsilateral ischemic cerebral events (any) was 2%. In the other group of 181 patients with echogenic plaques, the annual risk was 0.14%.[8] Thus, echolucency could be used to identify patients at low risk, and ultrasound may serve as method for stratification and selection of patients for more advanced imaging.[56]

In the most recent publication of the ACSRS data, plaque area, GSM, and the presence of discrete white areas indicating heterogeneity were independent predictors of ipsilateral ischemic cerebral and retinal events. When these ultrasonic features were combined with stenosis and history of contralateral TIAs or stroke, they could stratify patients into different levels of risk. Of the 923 patients with greater than 70% stenosis, estimated risk of stroke within 5 years was less than 5% in 495, 5–9.9% in 202, 10–19.9% in 142, and more than 20% in 84 patients. The authors concluded that "cerebrovascular risk stratification is possible using a combination of clinical and ultrasonic plaque features, but these findings need to be validated in additional prospective studies in patients having current medical intervention."[59]

All the data evaluating the prognostic value of plaque morphology has been generated using conventional two-dimensional ultrasound imaging with the well-known limitations with respect to reproducibility due to differences in scanning angle. Technological advances may improve the diagnostic accuracy in ultrasound imaging, and the recent introduction of three-dimensional ultrasound imaging (Chaps. 16–18) may bring plaque morphology to a new stage.

31.8 Conclusion

Identification of an echolucent plaque provides insight to the patient's risk profile, and due to the systemic inflammatory nature of atherosclerosis, it provides a readily accessible surrogate marker for vulnerability. The latter is of pivotal importance in current research in screening other possible risk markers – both of chemical, physical, and biological nature. In clinical practice, carotid plaque morphology is still not implemented. Risk stratification still lacks trials evaluating benefit in assessing echolucency with modern computer-assisted and standardized settings in both asymptomatic and symptomatic patients undergoing carotid endarterectomy in conjunction with modern medical intervention.

References

1. European Carotid Plaque Study Group. Carotid artery plaque composition – relationship to clinical presentation and ultrasound B-mode imaging. *Eur J Vasc Endovasc Surg*. 1995;10(1):23–30.
2. Gray-Weale AC, Graham JC, Burnett JR, Byrne K, Lusby RJ. Carotid artery atheroma: comparison of preoperative B-mode ultrasound appearance with carotid endarterectomy specimen pathology. *J Cardiovasc Surg (Torino)*. 1988;29(6):676–681.
3. Belcaro G et al. Ultrasonic classification of carotid plaques causing less than 60% stenosis according to ultrasound morphology and events. *J Cardiovasc Surg (Torino)*. 1993;34(4):287–294.
4. Gronholdt ML et al. Macrophages are associated with lipid-rich carotid artery plaques, echolucency on B-mode imaging, and elevated plasma lipid levels. *J Vasc Surg*. 2002;35(1):137–145.
5. Reilly LM et al. Carotid plaque histology using real-time ultrasonography. Clinical and therapeutic implications. *Am J Surg*. 1983;146(2):188–193.
6. AbuRahma AF, Kyer PD III, Robinson PA, Hannay RS. The correlation of ultrasonic carotid plaque morphology and carotid plaque hemorrhage: clinical implications. *Surgery*. 1998;124(4):721–726, discussion 726–728.
7. Gronholdt ML et al. Lipid-rich carotid artery plaques appear echolucent on ultrasound B-mode images and may be associated with intraplaque haemorrhage. *Eur J Vasc Endovasc Surg*. 1997;14(6):439–445.
8. Nicolaides AN et al. Effect of image normalization on carotid plaque classification and the risk of ipsilateral hemispheric ischemic events: results from the asymptomatic

carotid stenosis and risk of stroke study. *Vascular*. 2005; 13(4):211–221.
9. Polak JF, Dobkin GR, O'Leary DH, Wang AM, Cutler SS. Internal carotid artery stenosis: accuracy and reproducibility of color-doppler-assisted duplex imaging. *Radiology*. 1989; 173(3):793–798.
10. Elatrozy T et al. The effect of B-mode ultrasonic image standardisation on the echodensity of symptomatic and asymptomatic carotid bifurcation plaques. *Int Angiol*. 1998;17(3):179–186.
11. Nagano K et al. Quantitative evaluation of carotid plaque echogenicity by integrated backscatter analysis: correlation with symptomatic history and histologic findings. *Cerebrovasc Dis*. 2008;26(6):578–583.
12. Denzel C et al. Relative value of normalized sonographic in vitro analysis of arteriosclerotic plaques of internal carotid artery. *Stroke*. 2003;34(8):1901–1906.
13. Tegos TJ et al. Echomorphologic and histopathologic characteristics of unstable carotid plaques. *AJNR Am J Neuroradiol*. 2000;21(10):1937–1944.
14. Grogan JK et al. B-mode ultrasonographic characterization of carotid atherosclerotic plaques in symptomatic and asymptomatic patients. *J Vasc Surg*. 2005;42(3):435–441.
15. Feigin VL, Lawes CM, Bennett DA, Barker-Collo SL, Parag V. Worldwide stroke incidence and early case fatality reported in 56 population-based studies: a systematic review. *Lancet Neurol*. 2009;8(4):355–369.
16. Pessin MS, Duncan GW, Mohr JP, Poskanzer DC. Clinical and angiographic features of carotid transient ischemic attacks. *N Engl J Med*. 1977;296(7):358–362.
17. Sacco RL et al. American heart association prevention conference.IV. Prevention and rehabilitation of stroke. Risk factors. *Stroke*. 1997;28(7):1507–1517.
18. Executive Committee for the asymptomatic Carotid Atherosclerosis Study. Endarterectomy for asymptomatic carotid artery stenosis. *JAMA*. 1995;273(18):1421–1428.
19. Halliday A et al. Prevention of disabling and fatal strokes by successful carotid endarterectomy in patients without recent neurological symptoms: randomised controlled trial. *Lancet*. 2004;363(9420):1491–1502.
20. Naylor AR, Bell PR. Treatment of asymptomatic carotid disease with stenting: con. *Semin Vasc Surg*. 2008;21(2): 100–107.
21. Abbott AL. Medical (nonsurgical) intervention alone is now best for prevention of stroke associated with asymptomatic severe carotid stenosis: results of a systematic review and analysis. *Stroke*. 2009;40(10):e573–e583.
22. Marquardt L, Geraghty OC, Mehta Z, Rothwell PM. Low risk of ipsilateral stroke in patients with asymptomatic carotid stenosis on best medical treatment: a prospective, population-based study. *Stroke*. 2010;41(1):e11–e17.
23. Johnson JM, Kennelly MM, Decesare D, Morgan S, Sparrow A. Natural history of asymptomatic carotid plaque. *Arch Surg*. 1985;120(9):1010–1012.
24. Langsfeld M, Gray-Weale AC, Lusby RJ. The role of plaque morphology and diameter reduction in the development of new symptoms in asymptomatic carotid arteries. *J Vasc Surg*. 1989;9(4):548–557.
25. O'Holleran LW, Kennelly MM, McClurken M, Johnson JM. Natural history of asymptomatic carotid plaque. Five year follow-up study. *Am J Surg*. 1987;154(6):659–662.
26. Polak JF et al. Hypoechoic plaque at us of the carotid artery: an independent risk factor for incident stroke in adults aged 65 years or older. Cardiovascular health study. *Radiology*. 1998;208(3):649–654.
27. Mathiesen EB, Bonaa KH, Joakimsen O. Echolucent plaques are associated with high risk of ischemic cerebrovascular events in carotid stenosis: the Tromsø study. *Circulation*. 2001;103(17):2171–2175.
28. El-Barghouty N, Geroulakos G, Nicolaides A, Androulakis A, Bahal V. Computer-assisted carotid plaque characterisation. *Eur J Vasc Endovasc Surg*. 1995;9(4):389–393.
29. Biasi GM et al. Computer analysis of ultrasonic plaque echolucency in identifying high risk carotid bifurcation lesions. *Eur J Vasc Endovasc Surg*. 1999;17(6):476–479.
30. Gronholdt ML, Nordestgaard BG, Schroeder TV, Vorstrup S, Sillesen H. Ultrasonic echolucent carotid plaques predict future strokes. *Circulation*. 2001;104(1):68–73.
31. Naylor AR, Gaines PA, Rothwell PM. Who benefits most from intervention for asymptomatic carotid stenosis: patients or professionals? *Eur J Vasc Endovasc Surg*. 2009;37(6): 625–632.
32. Rothwell PM, Buchan A, Johnston SC. Recent advances in management of transient ischaemic attacks and minor ischaemic strokes. *Lancet Neurol*. 2006;5(4):323–331.
33. North American Symptomatic Carotid Endarterectomy Trial Collaborators. Beneficial effect of carotid endarterectomy in symptomatic patients with high-grade carotid stenosis. *N Engl J Med*. 1991;325(7):445–453.
34. Randomised trial of endarterectomy for recently symptomatic carotid stenosis: Final results of the MRC European Carotid Surgery Trial (ECST). *Lancet*. 1998;351(9113): 1379–1387.
35. Liapis CD et al. ESVS guidelines. Invasive treatment for carotid stenosis: indications, techniques. *Eur J Vasc Endovasc Surg*. 2009;37(4 Suppl):1–19.
36. Ohki T et al. Ex vivo human carotid artery bifurcation stenting: correlation of lesion characteristics with embolic potential. *J Vasc Surg*. 1998;27(3):463–471.
37. Biasi GM et al. Carotid plaque echolucency increases the risk of stroke in carotid stenting: the Imaging in Carotid Angioplasty and Risk of Stroke (ICAROS) study. *Circulation*. 2004;110(6):756–762.
38. Reiter M et al. Plaque echolucency is not associated with the risk of stroke in carotid stenting. *Stroke*. 2006;37(9): 2378–2380.
39. Rosenkranz M et al. Cerebral embolism during carotid artery stenting: role of carotid plaque echolucency. *Cerebrovasc Dis*. 2009;27(5):443–449.
40. Rothwell PM, Slattery J, Warlow CP. A systematic comparison of the risks of stroke and death due to carotid endarterectomy for symptomatic and asymptomatic stenosis. *Stroke*. 1996;27(2):266–269.
41. Reiter M et al. Increasing carotid plaque echolucency is predictive of cardiovascular events in high-risk patients. *Radiology*. 2008;248(3):1050–1055.
42. Russell DA, Wijeyaratne SM, Gough MJ. Changes in carotid plaque echomorphology with time since a neurologic event. *J Vasc Surg*. 2007;45(2):367–372.
43. Skjelland M et al. Plasma levels of granzyme B are increased in patients with lipid-rich carotid plaques as determined by echogenicity. *Atherosclerosis*. 2007;195(2):e142–e146.

44. Ostling G, Hedblad B, Berglund G, Goncalves I. Increased echolucency of carotid plaques in patients with type 2 - diabetes. *Stroke*. 2007;38(7):2074–2078.
45. Eldrup N, Gronholdt ML, Sillesen H, Nordestgaard BG. Elevated matrix metalloproteinase-9 associated with stroke or cardiovascular death in patients with carotid stenosis. *Circulation*. 2006;114(17):1847–1854.
46. Watanabe K et al. Stabilization of carotid atheroma assessed by quantitative ultrasound analysis in nonhypercholesterolemic patients with coronary artery disease. *J Am Coll Cardiol*. 2005;46(11):2022–2030.
47. Hirano M et al. Rapid improvement of carotid plaque echogenicity within 1 month of pioglitazone treatment in patients with acute coronary syndrome. *Atherosclerosis*. 2009;203(2):483–488.
48. Nakamura T et al. Rapid stabilization of vulnerable carotid plaque within 1 month of pitavastatin treatment in patients with acute coronary syndrome. *J Cardiovasc Pharmacol*. 2008;51(4):365–371.
49. Rothwell PM et al. Effect of urgent treatment of transient ischaemic attack and minor stroke on early recurrent stroke (express study): a prospective population-based sequential comparison. *Lancet*. 2007;370(9596):1432–1442.
50. Sillesen H et al. Atorvastatin reduces the risk of cardiovascular events in patients with carotid atherosclerosis: a secondary analysis of the Stroke Prevention by Aggressive Reduction in Cholesterol Levels (SPARCL) trial. *Stroke*. 2008;39(12):3297–3302.
51. Sillesen H. What does 'best medical therapy' really mean? *Eur J Vasc Endovasc Surg*. 2008;35(2):139–144.
52. Goessens BM, Visseren FL, Kappelle LJ, Algra A, van der Graaf Y. Asymptomatic carotid artery stenosis and the risk of new vascular events in patients with manifest arterial disease: the SMART study. *Stroke*. 2007;38(5):1470–1475.
53. Rerkasem K, Rothwell PM. Temporal trends in the risks of stroke and death due to endarterectomy for symptomatic carotid stenosis: an updated systematic review. *Eur J Vasc Endovasc Surg*. 2009;37(5):504–511.
54. Takaya N et al. Association between carotid plaque characteristics and subsequent ischemic cerebrovascular events: a prospective assessment with MRI – initial results. *Stroke*. 2006;37(3):818–823.
55. U-King-Im JM et al. Characterisation of carotid atheroma in symptomatic and asymptomatic patients using high resolution MRI. *J Neurol Neurosurg Psychiatry*. 2008;79(8):905–912.
56. Graebe M, Pedersen SF, Hojgaard L, Kjaer A, Sillesen H. (18)FDG PET and ultrasound echolucency in carotid artery plaques. *JACC Cardiovasc Imaging*. 2010;3(3):289–295.
57. Graebe M et al. Molecular pathology in vulnerable carotid plaques: Correlation with [18]-fluorodeoxyglucose positron emission tomography (FDG-PET). *Eur J Vasc Endovasc Surg*. 2009;37(6):714–721.
58. Rudd JH et al. Imaging atherosclerotic plaque inflammation with [18f]-fluorodeoxyglucose positron emission tomography. *Circulation*. 2002;105(23):2708–2711.
59. Nicolaides AN et al. Asymptomatic internal carotid artery stenosis and cerebrovascular risk stratification. *J Vasc Surg*. 2010;52(6):1486–1496.

Intravascular Ultrasound: Plaque Characterization

32

Donald B. Reid, Carol Watson, Barun Majumder, and Khalid Irshad

32.1 Introduction

For many years, vascular surgeons have respected the uncertain nature of carotid bifurcation plaque because of the unpredictable complications of disabling and fatal stroke during carotid endarterectomy. Early investigators noted that the composition of carotid artery plaque had an important role in the development of subsequent cerebral ischemic events, while others tried to correlate the preoperative ultrasound images with the pathology of the endarterectomy specimen.[1,2] In the 1990s, the movement away from invasive open surgery to less invasive vascular interventions culminated in the introduction of carotid angioplasty and stenting.[3,4] This endovascular treatment quickly gained momentum for both symptomatic and asymptomatic patients with carotid bifurcation. However, the realization that cerebral complication rates were as common as in carotid endarterectomy cases spurred further and more sophisticated investigation into the assessment of carotid plaque.[5–8] One of these techniques, intravascular ultrasound (IVUS), is performed during the carotid stenting procedure and provides the operator with magnified and detailed ultrasound images of the carotid plaque from within the carotid artery lumen.[9] Such close proximity to the plaque not only allows accurate cross-sectional diameter measurements but also morphological evaluation of the lesion.[10]

The most recent technological advance in IVUS is virtual histology (VH-IVUS), which for the first time provides the ability to accurately identify the type of carotid plaque being treated and creates a color-coded map of the different histological components.[11] This morphological information requires considerable experience to interpret, but it has the enticing potential to identify how the plaque is likely to behave at the moment of treatment: Will it resist complete stent expansion or will it break up and embolize debris to the brain? This chapter outlines the clinical role of carotid IVUS imaging with particular regard to plaque characterization.

32.2 Technical Aspects of IVUS

Conventional grayscale IVUS images are created from a transducer at the tip of the IVUS probe (Fig. 32.1). The transducer uses phased-array imaging whereby an electric current rotates around the transducer tip to send ultrasound signals in a circular sweep of the vessel in the same principle as a ship's radar. Reflected ultrasound signals from the tissues then return and a cross-sectional circular brightness mode (B-mode) image is created. The image is dependent on the intensity (amplitude) of the returning signal. The vessel wall is either brightly reflective (echogenic, white), dark (echolucent), or in-between (gray), and can be seen in anatomical detail since the different wall layers reflect ultrasound at different intensities of brightness. Calcified plaque also reflects grayscale ultrasound brightly, typically creating an acoustic shadow beyond the calcification (Fig. 32.2). The luminal blood flow is identified using color flow IVUS, and real-time

D.B. Reid (✉) • C. Watson • B. Majumder • K. Irshad
Department of Vascular Surgery, Wishaw General Surgery, Wishaw, Lanarkshire, UK

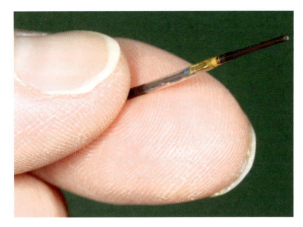

Fig. 32.1 Intravascular ultrasound probe. The gold chip transducer is approximately 1 cm from the tip

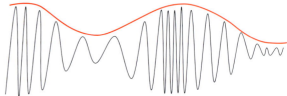

Fig. 32.3 VH-IVUS collects different frequency signals as well as the amplitude of the returning ultrasound from the tissues

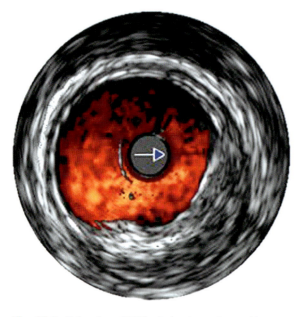

Fig. 32.2 Color flow IVUS of the internal carotid artery showing a brightly reflective intima, dark media, and a white adventitia. A crescent of plaque with some calcification is also identified

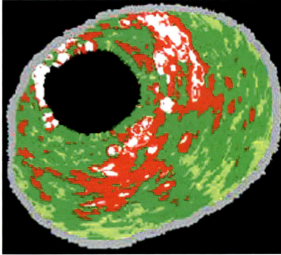

Fig. 32.4 VH-IVUS produces a color-coded map of the four histological components of plaque (*dark green*: fibrous, *yellow/green*: fibrofatty, *white*: calcified, and *red*: necrotic lipid core) with the lumen appearing *black* and the media border *gray*

images are immediately available in the operating room during the procedure.[10]

VH-IVUS creates an image using the frequency as well as the amplitude of the returning signal: different tissues reflect ultrasound at different frequencies [12] (Fig. 32.3). Meticulous correlation of IVUS frequency data from diseased coronary arteries with subsequent tissue histopathological sections of the explanted vessels has enabled VH data to be classified into four histological components: fibrous, fibrofatty, calcified, and necrotic lipid core.[13] A color-coded map is then produced by the VH-IVUS software (dark green: fibrous; yellow/green: fibrofatty; white: calcified; red: necrotic lipid core plaque) (Fig. 32.4).

32.2.1 Performing a Pullback

For VH-IVUS assessment of carotid bifurcation disease, the authors use a 2.9 Fr 20-MHz "Eagle Eye" probe (Volcano Therapeutics, Rancho Cordova, California, USA). This low profile probe is ideally suited for carotid plaque evaluation as it tracks over the 0.014″ wire of most cerebral protection devices.

The relatively high-frequency signal produces high-resolution images in the relatively small caliber artery.

Following selective arteriography and immediately following placement of a cerebral protection device in the distal internal carotid artery, the 135-cm-long IVUS catheter is placed just cephalad to the lesion. Here, diameter measurements to guide balloon and stent sizes are taken. A motorized pullback device can be used but the authors prefer a manual pullback at approximately 1–2 mm/s, remembering that VH-IVUS imaging is electrocardiographically gated to one frame per heartbeat. Real-time imaging is available during the pullback for live IVUS interrogation. The authors prefer to sample one IVUS frame at the narrowest point of the stenosis which is the largest cross-sectional area of the plaque: assessment needs to be made rapidly in order not to delay the carotid stenting procedure. Color flow IVUS is inactivated during a VH pullback.

The borders of the intima and the external elastic lamina are automatically selected by the computer software to isolate and then color the plaque in the arterial wall. The vessel lumen is colored black. In practice, these borders usually require some manual correction, hence, the authors' preference for choosing a single frame to evaluate the carotid lesion rapidly during the case. The VH image shows the four histological components of plaque and their proportions per frame together with cross-sectional and diameter measurements. Balloon and stent type and sizing are confirmed at this time, and the balloon inflation pressure to create a satisfactory channel is guided by the morphological understanding of the lesion.

Following stent deployment, the authors then routinely perform color flow IVUS to assess the completeness of treatment. VH-IVUS is of limited value following stenting. Any residual stenosis or untreated disease is corrected, balanced with the knowledge that overzealous treatment risks neurological complications.[14] Good clinical judgment is required.

32.3 Clinical Illustrative Examples

One of the authors' earliest clinical experiences with VH-IVUS impressed them with its ability to correctly predict plaque behavior. An elderly patient who was asymptomatic and referred for carotid stenting prior to coronary artery bypass operation had a focal, tight stenosis at the origin of his right internal carotid artery (Fig. 32.5). VH-IVUS examination was performed following placement of a cerebral protection device. It showed predominantly dark green fibrous tissue and calcified white areas. As anticipated, following stenting, there was incomplete stent expansion despite reballooning at high inflation pressures. Fibrous collagen fragments found in the filter correlated with the fibrous plaque composition seen on VH-IVUS (Fig. 32.6).

Another patient who had undergone previous carotid endarterectomy presented with restenosis at the site of surgery. VH-IVUS examination was performed following selective carotid arteriography and placement of a cerebral protection device in the distal internal carotid artery. This showed almost exclusively dark green fibrous material which also resisted complete stent expansion despite high balloon inflation pressures (Fig. 32.7).

These two early case examples demonstrated to the authors the potential for VH-IVUS to predict the physical properties of plaque during carotid stenting. However, the authors' interpretation of the VH images at this time was, in retrospect, primitive. It took them a further period of time and experience together with an appreciation of the histopathology of plaque progression for their understanding and interpretation to become more sophisticated.

32.4 Plaque Progression and Virtual Histology

Histopathologists have investigated the development of atherosclerotic plaque for many years.[15,16] It is postulated that, initially, plaque starts when lipids penetrate the subintimal space, stimulating smooth muscle cells to proliferate and deposit collagen (Chaps. 1 and 2) (Fig. 32.8). Macrophages move in to digest the lipid. The oxidized lipids cause local cell destruction and development of a necrotic lipid core which enlarges and eventually ruptures through the thin fibrous cap. Blood enters the necrotic core, and this highly thrombogenic surface causes thrombosis.[17–19]

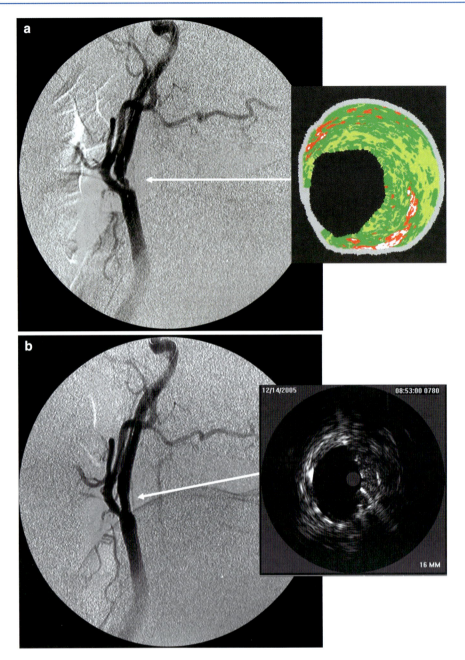

Fig. 32.5 (**a**) Angiography and IVUS demonstrate a focal stenosis at the origin of the right ICA in an asymptomatic 70-year-old man. At the narrowest point of the stenosis, the VH-IVUS shows predominantly fibrous (*dark green*) and calcified (*white*) areas. (**b**) As anticipated, following stenting, there was incomplete stent expansion with mid-stent "waisting" despite redilation at high pressures (Reprinted from Irshad et al.[11] © International Society of Endovascular Specialists)

This process of atherosclerotic plaque progression causes luminal narrowing and ultimately, thrombosis of the vessel. Indeed, clinical association between stroke and carotid artery plaque rupture, and mural thrombosis has been demonstrated in a large histopathology study.[17] Such ruptured plaques may remain clinically unstable following initial rupture, and this "vulnerable plaque" state may give rise to further

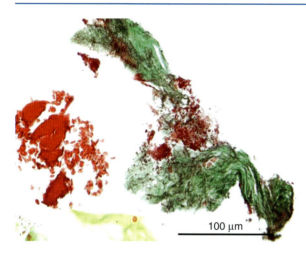

Fig. 32.6 Light microscopy of fibrous collagen fragments and blood clot from particles collected in the cerebral protection filter following treatment (Reprinted from Irshad et al.[11] © International Society of Endovascular Specialists)

cerebral events. Histopathologists have classified the different stages of plaque progression into different histopathological plaque types.[20] This classification is based on the proportion of the same histological components that VH-IVUS identifies. Since VH-IVUS produces a proportional map of these histological components, criteria to classify different plaque types using VH-IVUS have been established[21] (Table 32.1).

The diagnostic accuracy of VH-IVUS to correctly identify plaque types was investigated and validated in the Carotid Artery Plaque Virtual Histology Evaluation (CAPITAL) Study where VH-IVUS interpretation was compared with the true histopathology of carotid plaque.[21] In a Food and Drug Administration (FDA)–approved study and with institutional review board (IRB) ethical approval, patients undergoing carotid endarterectomy had an antegrade puncture of the common carotid artery after surgical exposure of the carotid artery bifurcation. An access sheath was placed and VH-IVUS was performed using a cerebral protection filter device. Carotid endarterectomy was then completed, and the endarterectomy specimen sent to histopathology. In this double-blinded study, 153 VH-IVUS images were compared with the true histopathology sections from the endarterectomy specimens. The predictive accuracy of VH-IVUS to agree with true histology in the different carotid plaque types was: 99.4% for thin-cap fibroatheroma, 96.1% for calcified thin-cap fibroatheroma, 85.9% for fibroatheroma, 85.5% for fibrocalcific, 83.4% for pathological intimal thickening, and 72.4% for calcified fibroatheroma (see Table 32.2 and Fig. 32.9). This study found that VH-IVUS accurately diagnoses the different carotid artery plaque types. It was most accurate in "vulnerable plaque" types (thin-cap fibroatheroma and calcified thin-cap fibroatheroma).

32.5 Discussion

Intravascular ultrasound is a specialized guidance system which is used in a wide variety of endovascular interventions.[22–24] In patients undergoing carotid angioplasty and stenting, its main role has hitherto been to assess the completeness of stent deployment, given that carotid bifurcation disease is frequently composed of hard calcified plaque.[9,14] In a study of 50 consecutive patients undergoing carotid stenting, the authors have found that IVUS could detect incomplete stent deployment in 40% of cases.[14] All these patients required reballooning, improving the cross-sectional area by 42%.

VH-IVUS provides the operator with morphological information on carotid artery plaque immediately before stenting. Currently, only a minority of endovascular specialists use IVUS in carotid endoluminal repair. However, if VH-IVUS is subsequently shown to identify patients with plaques at high risk of neurological complication, then its wide spread use could be anticipated.

While the authors' own early experience of carotid artery VH-IVUS was initially simplistic (looking for resistant plaque or plaque with a high content of necrotic core), their progressive understanding of plaque histopathology and the results of the CAPITAL study have given them more confidence in its clinical role. The authors are now able to identify the six different plaque types in the operating room, immediately before stenting and have become familiar with these plaque type appearances. This extra information allows us to tailor their procedures based upon the nature of the bifurcation disease. Indeed, a retrospective analysis of a patient who suffered a procedural stroke gave them insight into the potential for VH-IVUS to identify high-risk plaque (Fig. 32.10).

Fig. 32.7 (**a**) Multidetector (64 slice) CTA shows a tight restenosis of the left ICA. (**b**) The angiogram and VH-IVUS of the restenosis following carotid endarterectomy. VH shows predominantly dark green fibrous tissue. (**c**) Completion angiogram and IVUS after dilation and stent placement (Reprinted from Irshad et al.[11] © International Society of Endovascular Specialists)

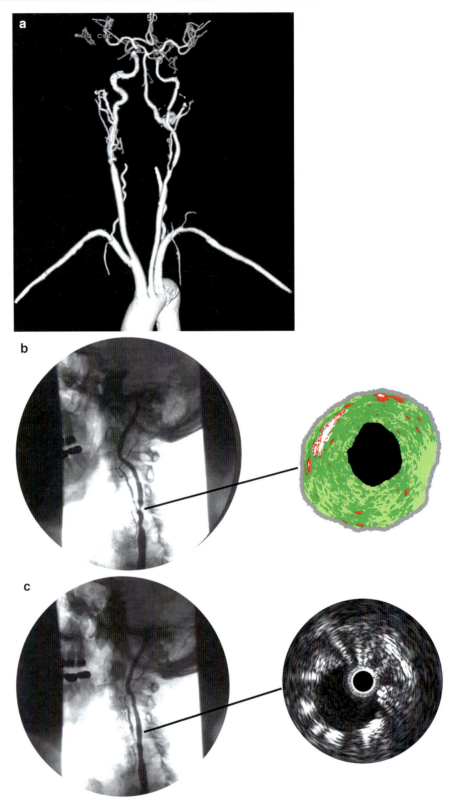

32 Intravascular Ultrasound: Plaque Characterization

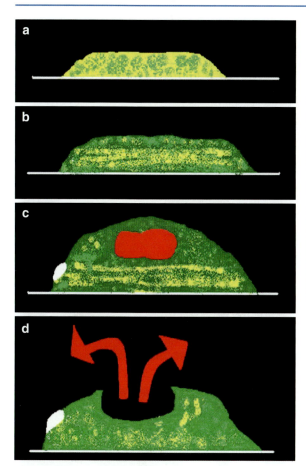

Fig. 32.8 (a) Plaque progression begins with intimal thickening. (b) Smooth muscle cell proliferation and collagen deposition. (c) Macrophages digest lipid causing cell destruction and the development of a necrotic lipid core. (d) Plaque rupture through the thin fibrous cap

Table 32.1 VH-IVUS criteria for classifying different plaque types

Pathological intimal thickening	Intimal media thickness >600 micron
Fibroatheroma	Confluent necrotic core or calcium <10% of the total plaque cross-sectional area
Calcified fibroatheroma	Fibroatheroma plaque with a confluent area of calcium
Thin-cap fibroatheroma	Necrotic core > 10% of the total plaque cross-sectional area and necrotic core confluent against the lumen
Calcified thin-cap fibroatheroma	Thin-cap fibroatheroma plaque with a confluent area of calcium
Fibrocalcific	Confluent area of calcium > 10%, with necrotic core < 10% of the total plaque cross-sectional area, and fibrofatty plaque < 10% of the total plaque cross section area.

Immediately following stenting, this patient developed a pronounced hemiparesis and dysphasia. Subsequent postoperative analysis of the VH-IVUS identified a small vulnerable plaque near the luminal surface which the authors had not noticed. This may have produced embolic material.[25] Since that time, the authors have used the VH-IVUS findings to determine balloon inflation pressures, and where there is an obvious vulnerable plaque, they now use covered stents to try to prevent embolic complications.[11]

During carotid stenting, VH-IVUS does have some limitations. The computer software does not always choose the borders which delineate the plaque accurately. This often requires time consuming manual correction before processing the image. Furthermore, it would be advantageous to be able to assess carotid plaque noninvasively before any interventional treatment. Unfortunately, transcutaneous two-dimensional (2D) B-mode ultrasound examination is too remote from the plaque and provides limited information (one plane only) to be able to provide VH data for the whole plaque. The contribution of transcutaneous 3D high-resolution ultrasound (Chaps. 16–18) in this area remains to be seen.

An interesting finding relating to plaque characterization in the CAPITAL study was that proportionally less necrotic core plaque was found in patients on aspirin (this was statistically significant, $p < 0.05$). Similarly, the finding that nodules projecting into the lumen was statistically significantly associated with previous neurological symptoms gives an indication of the clinical importance of these different morphological characteristics of carotid plaque (Fig. 32.11).

As surgeons, the authors have long recognized that some patients' plaque may be "biologically" more active and symptomatic while others are "structurally" tightly stenosed but stable and asymptomatic (Chap. 36). If the information gained from VH-IVUS assessment could be used to determine what stage the carotid plaque has progressed to and whether it is stable or likely to rupture, then we could choose to treat the lesion not just based on the degree of arterial stenosis. Work in the field of plaque progression

Table 32.2 VH-IVUS accuracy by plaque types

Plaque type by VH-IVUS	Predictive accuracy (%)	Sensitivity (%)	Specificity (%)
Thin-cap fibroatheroma	99.4	75.0	100
Calcified thin-cap fibroatheroma	96.1	90.0	97.1
Fibroatheroma	85.9	54.1	96.9
Fibrocalcific	85.5	87.1	84.5
Pathological intimal thickening	83.4	88.5	82.0
Calcified fibroatheroma	72.4	32.5	93.0

Fig. 32.9 The six different plaque types. VH compared with true histopathology sections (Reprinted from Diethrich et al.[21] © International Society of Endovascular Specialists)

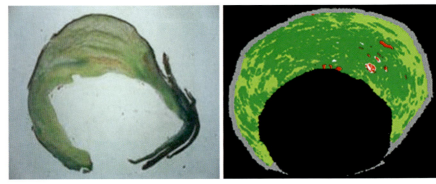

Intimal thickening

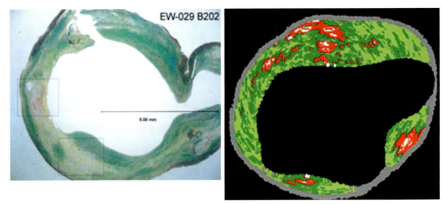

Fibroatheroma

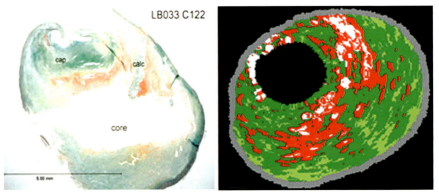

Calcified fibroatheroma

Fig. 32.9 (continued)

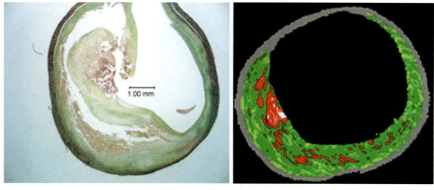

Thin cap fibroatheroma

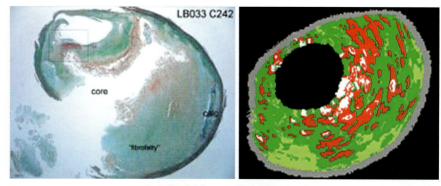

Calcified thin cap fibroatheroma

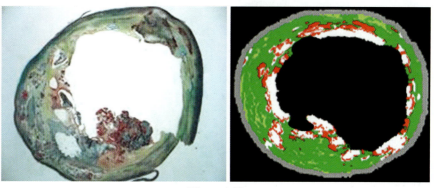

Fibrocalcific

together with proposed medical and interventional treatments is accelerating.[17,26,27]

In summary, the authors have found IVUS to be highly beneficial in patients undergoing carotid stenting, particularly in providing luminal measurements and assessing the completeness of stent deployment. VH-IVUS is a promising technique for carotid interventionalists to accurately diagnose plaque types. However, further studies need to be performed to see whether VH-IVUS can accurately predict which lesions are safe, or at increased risk of neurological complications.

Fig. 32.10 VH-IVUS of a carotid artery plaque in a patient who suffered a stroke immediately after ballooning the self-expanding stent. A small calcified thin-capped fibroatheromatous plaque is identified

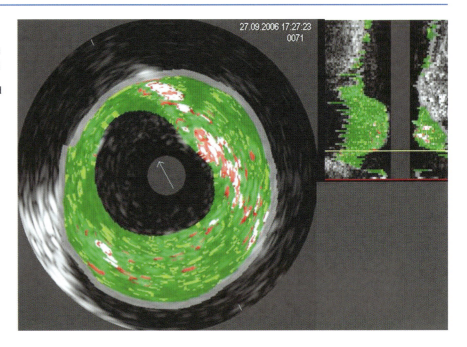

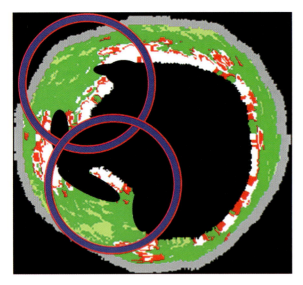

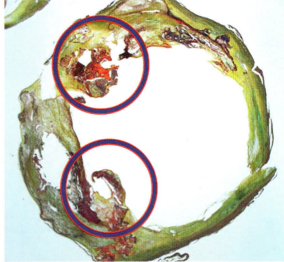

Fig. 32.11 VH-IVUS and true histopathology section of carotid artery plaque show calcified projections (*circled*). The presence of such calcified projections were statistically associated with previous neurological symptoms (Reprinted from Diethrich et al.[21] © International Society of Endovascular Specialists)

References

1. Gray-Weale AC, Graham JC, Burnett JR, Byrne K, Lusby RJ. Carotid artery atheroma: comparison of preoperative B-mode ultrasound appearance with carotid endarterectomy specimen pathology. *J Cardiovasc Surg (Torino)*. 1988;29: 676–681.
2. Lusby RJ. Lesions: dynamic and pathogenic mechanisms responsible for ischaemic events in the brain. In: Moore WS, ed. *Surgery for Cerebrovascular Disease*. New York: Churchill Livingstone; 1987:51–76.
3. Diethrich EB, Ndiaye M, Reid DB. Stenting in carotid surgery: initial experience in 110 patients. *J Endovasc Surg*. 1996;2:42–62.

4. Diethrich EB, Marx P, Wrasper P, Reid DB. Percutaneous techniques for endoluminal carotid interventions. *J Endovasc Surg*. 1996;3:182–202.
5. Reid DB. Carotid plaque characterization: helpful to endarterectomy and endovascular surgeons. *J Endovasc Surg*. 1998;5:247–250.
6. Biasi GM et al. Carotid plaque echolucency increases the risk of stroke in carotid stenting: the Imaging in Carotid Angioplasty and Risk of Stroke (ICAROS) study. *Circulation*. 2004;110:756–762.
7. Ohki T et al. Ex vivo human carotid artery bifurcation stenting: correlation of the lesion characteristics with embolic potential. *J Vasc Surg*. 1998;27:463–471.
8. Irshad K et al. The role of intravascular ultrasound in carotid angioplasty and stenting. In: Henry M, ed. *Angioplasty and Stenting of the Carotid and Supra-Aortic Trunks*. London: Martin Dunitz; 2004:127–133.
9. Reid DB, Diethrich EB, Marx P, Wrasper R. Intravascular ultrasound assessment in carotid interventions. *J Endovasc Surg*. 1996;3:203–210.
10. Diethrich EB, Irshad K, Reid DB. Virtual histology and color flow intravascular ultrasound in peripheral interventions. *Semin Vasc Surg*. 2006;19:155–162.
11. Irshad K et al. Virtual histology intravascular ultrasound in carotid interventions. *J Endovasc Ther*. 2007;14:198–207.
12. Vince DG, Davies SC. Peripheral application of intravascular ultrasound virtual histology. *Semin Vasc Surg*. 2004;17:119–125.
13. Nair A, Kuban BD, Obuchowski N, Vince DG. Assessing spectral algorithms to predict atherosclerotic plaque composition with normalized and raw intravascular ultrasound data. *Ultrasound Med Biol*. 2001;27(10):1319–1331.
14. Reid DB, Diethrich EB, Marx P, Wrasper R. Clinical applications of intravascular ultrasound in peripheral vascular disease. In: Siegel RJ, ed. *Intravascular Ultrasound Imaging in Coronary Artery Disease*. New York: Marcel Dekker; 1998:309–341.
15. von Rokitansky C. *A Manual of Pathological Anatomy*, vol. IV. London: Sydenham Society; 1852:271–273.
16. Virchow R. *Phlogose und thrombose in gefassystem, gesammehe abhandlungen zu wissenschaftlichen medicin*. Frankfurt-am-Main: MeidingerSohn; 1856:458.
17. Spagnoli LG et al. Extracranial thrombotically active carotid plaque as a risk factor for ischaemic stroke. *JAMA*. 2004;292:1845–1852.
18. Virmani R et al. Atherosclerotic plaque progression and vulnerability to rupture: angiogenesis as a source of intraplaque haemorrhage. *Arterioscler Thromb Vasc Biol*. 2005;25:2054–2061.
19. Virmani R, Burke AP, Kolodgie FD, Farb A. Pathology of the thin-cap fibro atheroma. *J Interv Cardiol*. 2003;16:267–272.
20. Stary HC et al. A definition of advanced types of atherosclerotic lesions and a histological classification of atherosclerosis. A report from the Committee on Vascular Lesions of the Council on Arteriosclerosis, American Heart Association. *Circulation*. 1995;92:1355–1374.
21. Diethrich EB et al. Virtual histology intravascular ultrasound assessment of carotid artery disease: The Carotid Artery Plaque Virtual Histology Evaluation (CAPITAL) study. *J Endovasc Ther*. 2007;14:676–686.
22. Irshad K et al. Early clinical experience with color three-dimensional intravascular ultrasound in peripheral interventions. *J Endovasc Ther*. 2001;8:329–338.
23. Irshad K et al. The role of intravascular ultrasound and peripheral endovascular interventions. In: Heuser RR, Henry M, eds. *Textbook of Peripheral Vascular Interventions*. London: Martin Dunitz; 2004:25–34.
24. White RA, Scoccianti M, Back M, Kopchok G, Donayre C. Innovation in vascular imaging: arteriography, three-dimensional CT scans, and two- and three-dimensional intravascular ultrasound of an abdominal aortic aneurysm. *Ann Vasc Surg*. 1994;8:285–289.
25. Naghavi M et al. From vulnerable plaque to vulnerable patient: a call for new definitions and risk assessment strategies: part I. *Circulation*. 2003;108:1664–1672.
26. Kuchulakanti P et al. Identification of "vulnerable plaque" using virtual histology in angiographically benign looking lesion of proximal left anterior descending artery. *Cardiovasc Radiat Med*. 2003;4(4):225–227.
27. Fujii K et al. Intravascular ultrasound assessment of ulcerated ruptured plaque: a comparison of culprit and non-culprit lesions of patients with acute coronary syndrome and lesions in patients without acute coronary syndromes. *Circulation*. 2003;108:2473–2478.

Grayscale-Based Stratified Color Mapping of Carotid Plaque

Roman Felix Sztajzel

33.1 Introduction

Besides degree of stenosis, plaque morphology, defined by its structure and surface characteristics, is thought to play an important role in the pathogenesis of stroke. An unstable carotid plaque is associated with a thinning of the fibrous cap, infiltration of inflammatory cells leading to surface ulceration, and plaque rupture[1-4] (Chap. 2). The fibrous cap is composed of connective tissue embedded with smooth cells overlying a core of lipid and necrotic debris. Rupture of the fibrous cap with the resultant exposure of thrombogenic subendothelial plaque constituents is believed to be the critical event that leads to thromboembolic complications.[2,3] Furthermore, detailed histological examinations have demonstrated that in atherosclerotic plaques removed from symptomatic patients, the necrotic core is placed nearer the fibrous cap, and the minimum cap thickness is less. In one study recently published by Bassiouny et al., the necrotic core was twice as close to the lumen in symptomatic plaques when compared with asymptomatic ones (0.27 ± 0.3 mm vs 0.5 ± 0.5 mm; $p < 0.01$).[4,5] They concluded that the topography of individual plaque components in relation to the fibrous cap and the lumen may determine symptomatic outcome. Therefore, imaging techniques that allow a precise characterization of the fibrous cap and resolve the position of the necrotic core to this fibrous cap should help to identify high-risk stenosis before disruption and development of symptomatic carotid disease.

Several noninvasive imaging techniques have emerged in recent years for the assessment of arterial wall pathology. Among these, high resolution ultrasound studies have shown that hypo-anechoic plaques carry a higher risk of cerebrovascular events than echogenic (hyperechoic) ones.[6-9] Similarly, heterogeneous plaques presenting a complex pattern of echogenicity have also been more frequently associated with the occurrence of neurological symptoms than homogenous lesions.[10,11] Further, most studies determining the surface characteristics in ultrasound have found that ulceration also predicts increased risk of subsequent stroke.[12-16] However, most of the studies performed so far, based on a visual analysis, have used very different classification systems and yielded a poor inter- and intraobserver agreement.[17] A more operator-independent approach is the quantification of the echogenicity of the plaque by means of a computer-assisted analysis of the grayscale values after image normalization (Chap. 12). Various studies using this approach demonstrated that plaques yielding low grayscale median (GSM) values were more frequently encountered among symptomatic than asymptomatic patients. However, although characterization of the plaque's internal structure by computer-assisted image analysis correlated in most of the studies closely with clinical symptoms,[18-23] there were conflicting results between this computerized analysis of the plaque and the corresponding histopathological findings.[24-28] In fact, GSM analysis represents a median value of the whole atherosclerotic area and therefore may not necessarily reflect the ultrasonographic characteristics of regional components, in particular of the surface of the plaque.

R.F. Sztajzel
Department of Neurology, University Hospital Geneva/
Switzerland, Geneva, Switzerland

The author's decided to evaluate whether a stratified approach of the carotid plaque, analyzing each millimeter from the surface till the bottom of the lesion, combined with a color mapping could in fact be more accurate than a whole plaque measurement. Different aspects were studied, including correlation with plaque histology, with presence of cerebrovascular symptoms and microembolic signals. Furthermore, the author's team performed a comparison between visual analysis and semi-automated grayscale-based color mapping of the carotid plaque.

33.2 Semi-automated Grayscale-Based Color Mapping of the Plaque

All the images stored on the hard disc of the ultrasound device (Acuson Sequoia Apparatus, 7.5 MHz probe, Siemens AG, Munich, Germany) were first transferred to a personal computer (bitmap image) and then analyzed by an in-house written program in MATLAB 7.9 (MathWorks, Natick, Massachusetts, USA) with image processing toolbox including graphical user interface (GUI). The frequency distribution of grayscale values of the pixels within the whole plaque or a region of it was used as the measurement of the echogenicity. The following steps were performed: the plaque was outlined automatically at its surface on its longitudinal section. For this, an algorithm was used in order to delineate the boundary between the color flow and the surface of the plaque. At the adventitial border, the plaque was outlined manually (Fig. 33.1). All carotid plaques were then normalized by linear scaling with the use of the reference values of 0 for blood and 190 for adventitia (Chap. 12). The plaque pixels were further mapped into three different colors: red, yellow, and green according to their grayscale value.

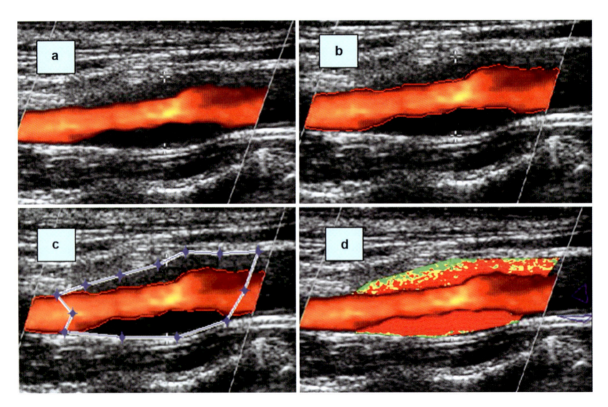

Fig. 33.1 Ultrasound image of the carotid plaque in an asymptomatic patient. (**a**) Note the different echogenic characteristics of the plaque (anechoic in the far wall and more echogenic in the near wall region). (**b**) The color flow is automatically outlined (see *red lines*); the limit represents the border zone between the surface of the plaque and the color flow. (**c**) Manual delineation of the adventitia. (**d**) Color mapping of the plaque according to the threshold <60 *red*, 60–90 *yellow*, and >90 *green*. The surface is delineated automatically between 0 and 0.5 mm, 0 and 1 mm, 0 and 1.5 mm, and 0 and 2 mm. Also note the normalization of the plaque (selection of the darkest and the brightest regions 0–190 with *blue triangles*)

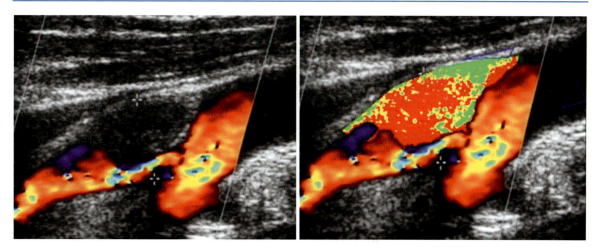

Fig. 33.2 Plaque image from an 87-year-old patient with an asymptomatic left carotid stenosis of 80%. The proportion of the *red color* at the surface is of 68% within the 0–0.5 mm, 60% within the 0–1 mm, 57% within the 0–1.5 mm, and 57% within the 0–2 mm regions. The proportion of *red color* for the whole plaque is of 59%. These findings suggest a plaque with low risk

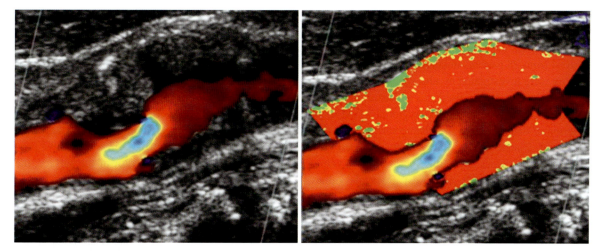

Fig. 33.3 Plaque image from a 72-year-old man with a symptomatic right carotid stenosis of 70%. The proportion of *red color* at the surface of the plaque is of is 95% within the 0–0.5 mm, 95% within the 0–1 mm, 94% within the 0–1.5 mm, and 93% within the 0–2 mm region. The proportion of *red color* for the whole plaque is of 89%. These findings suggest a plaque with high risk

Five different threshold values had been evaluated for each color: lowest grayscale values less than 60, 50, 40, 30, and 20 were mapped in red, corresponding intermediate values between 60 and 90, 50 and 80, 40 and 70, 30 and 60, and 20 and 50 were mapped in yellow, and highest corresponding values greater than 90, 80, 70, 60, and 50 were mapped in green. For each plaque, the proportion of each color present on the whole plaque and on its surface was then calculated automatically (Figs. 33.2 and 33.3). Several different levels were considered for the surface of the plaque: the proportion of each color was evaluated at the surface automatically between 0 and 0.5 mm, 0 and 1 mm, 0 and 1.5 mm, and 0 and 2 mm.[29]

In a cohort of 89 patients with 50–99% carotid stenosis, the author's team found that the predominance of the red color on the surface of the plaque and, in particular, at the level 0–0.5 mm ($p < 0.04$) was the best predictor, besides degree of stenosis of the presence of symptoms [stroke/transient ischemic attack (TIA)] and of ischemic brain lesions on magnetic resonance imaging (MRI) (silent or not).

Interobserver agreement (color mapping performed by two experienced sonographers) reached a very good score with this method; in particular, the results obtained with the semi-automated color mapping of the surface were quite similar to those of the whole plaque analysis and suggested a good reproducibility of the method (evaluation of the whole plaque, correlation coefficient 0.87 and for the surface of the plaque 0.90).

33.2.1 Correlation with Plaque Histology with the Presence of Cerebrovascular Symptoms and Microembolic Signals

The author's team sought to determine whether a stratified grayscale analysis of the carotid plaque combined with a color mapping could predict plaque histology better than a whole plaque measurement.[30] Thirty-one carotid plaques producing 60–90% stenosis in relation to the distal internal carotid diameter derived from 28 patients undergoing carotid endarterectomy were investigated by ultrasound. GSMs of the whole plaque were used as measurement of echogenicity. A profile of the regional GSM as a function of distance from the plaque surface was also generated. Plaque pixels were further mapped into three different colors depending on their GSM value. Thresholds were chosen as: lowest grayscale values (<50 mapped in red), intermediate values (between 50 and 80 mapped in yellow), and highest values (>80 mapped in green). The author's team determined for each plaque the predominant color present on the surface, which was defined as the upper third part of the lesion, and the predominant color of the whole plaque or plaque segment.

The following parameters were determined on plaque histology: fibrosis, hemorrhage, calcification or necrotic/lipid core, and were respectively expressed as large or small if they occupied more or less than 50% of the total area of the plaque. The fibrous cap was measured using an ocular micrometer: a value of less than 80 μm corresponded to a thin and more than 80 to a thick fibrous cap. The necrotic/lipid core was considered near the surface in a juxtalumenal position (not covered by the fibrous cap) or distant from the surface of the plaque (covered by the fibrous cap whatever its thickness).

Plaques with large calcifications presented the highest grayscale values; those with large hemorrhagic areas or with a predominant necrotic core exhibited the lowest ones. Fibrous plaques had intermediate values. A necrotic core located in a juxtalumenal position was associated with significantly lower grayscale values ($p = 0.009$) and with a predominant red color (GS <50) at the surface ($p = 0.0019$) (Table 33.1). With respect to the thickness of the fibrous cap and the position of the necrotic core, the sensitivity and specificity of the predominant red color of the whole plaque was respectively 45% and 67%, 53% and 75%; considering the predominant red color of the surface, the sensitivity and specificity increased to 73% and 67%, 84% and 75%, respectively. In this study, the stratified grayscale measurement combined with color mapping showed a good correlation with the different

Table 33.1 Grayscale-based color mapping of the carotid plaque: Comparison between surface characteristics and whole plaque measurement: Correlation between stratified grayscale analysis and color mapping of 31 plaques and two determinants of plaque instability on histology

$N = 31$	Thick fibrous cap $N = 9/31$ (29%)	Thin fibrous cap $N = 22/31$ (71%)	Lipid necrotic core distant from surface $N = 12/31$ (39%)	Lipid necrotic core in juxtalumenal position $N = 19/31$ (61%)
Predominant color of whole plaque	Red 3/9 (33%) Green and yellow 6/9 (67%)	Red 10/22 (45%) Green and yellow 12/22 (54%) $p = 0.5$	Red 3/12 (25%) Green and yellow 9/12 (75%)	Red 10/19 (53%) Green and yellow 9/19 (47%) $p = 0.12$
Predominant color of the plaque surface	Red 3/9 (33%) Green and yellow 6/9 (67%)	Red 16/22 (73%) Green and yellow 6/22 (27%) $p = 0.0019$	Red 3/12 (25%) Green and yellow 9/12 (75%)	Red 16/19 (84%) Green and yellow 3/19 (16%) $p = 0.056$

histopathological components and further allowed one to identify with a good accuracy determinants of plaque instability.

In a subsequent study, the author's team evaluated whether a stratified grayscale analysis of the carotid plaque combined with color mapping correlated better with the presence of neurological symptoms and microembolic signals (MES) than a whole plaque measurement.[31]

One hundred and thirty-one patients presenting with 167 carotid stenoses between 30% and 99% were analyzed by ultrasound. Microembolic detection was performed by transcranial Doppler. For each plaque, the grayscale values at depth 0 mm (surface) and at one third and one half of the plaque thickness were compared with the values obtained for the whole plaque. The plaque pixels were mapped into three colors: red, yellow, and green, depending on their grayscale value as described above. Mean grayscale values were lower among symptomatic plaques, but a statistically significant difference between values of the whole plaque and those of the surface was obtained only for microembolic signal positive (MES+) stenoses ($p < 0.01$). In a logistic regression model based on four subgroups with an increasing clinical risk (MES−/symptoms−, MES−/symptoms+, MES+/symptoms−, MES+/symptoms+), low mean grayscale values and the predominant red color at the surface were independent factors associated with the presence of symptoms and/or MES ($p < 0.0005$). Furthermore, in comparison with a whole plaque measurement, analysis of the surface values predicted systematically with a greater sensitivity and specificity for (receiver operator characteristic [ROC] curves) each one of these four subgroups. Thus, low mean grayscale values and predominance of the red color at the surface correlated with most of the symptomatic and/or MES+ stenoses.

MES may represent plaque instability as demonstrated in a study performed by Sitzer and colleagues who found, in asymptomatic and recently symptomatic patients undergoing carotid endarterectomy, a strong association between plaque ulceration, intraluminal thrombosis and downstream cerebral microembolic signals.[32] In several studies, the presence of MES has been associated with an increased risk of further cerebrovascular events in symptomatic as well as in asymptomatic patients.[33–37] However, it should be noted that MES are frequently found among recently symptomatic patients, but much more rarely among asymptomatic ones.[38] Therefore, our findings suggest that low grayscale values assessed by color mapping were associated with the presence of MES and, thereby, may contribute to discriminate between low- (MES−) and high-risk (MES+) asymptomatic stenoses. However, whether the surface grayscale values per se may identify high-risk asymptomatic stenoses independently of the presence of MES should be further investigated.

A recent study by Griffin et al. attempted to determine the diagnostic value of a juxtaluminal black (hypoechoic) area without a visible echogenic cap (JBA) in ultrasonic images of internal carotid artery plaques. Ultrasonic images of plaques from 324 patients with asymptomatic ($n = 139$) and symptomatic ($n = 185$) internal carotid 50–99% stenosis in relation to the bulb referred for duplex scanning were studied. The JBA in square millimeter and the grayscale median (GSM) were obtained after image normalization. Cut off points for GSM and JBA (combined highest sensitivity with highest specificity) were determined from ROC curves.

In this study, JBA greater than 8 mm^2 was associated with a high prevalence of symptomatic plaques in all grades of stenosis. In a multiple logistic regression model, increasing stenosis (mild, moderate, severe), GSM less than 15, and JBA equal or greater than 8 mm^2 were associated with hemispheric symptoms. This model could identify a high-risk group of 188 plaques which contained 142 (77%) of the 185 symptomatic plaques (OR 6.7, 95% CI 4.08–10.91), ($p < 0.001$), (Sensitivity: 77%, specificity 66%, PPV 75%, NPV 68%).[39]

33.2.2 A Comparison Between Visual Analysis and Semi-automated Grayscale-Based Color Mapping of the Carotid Plaque

The correlation between plaque echo structure and the presence of cerebrovascular events and/or lesions on MRI was assessed by two different ultrasonographic methods in patients with moderate or high grade carotid stenosis.[29] Visual analysis of plaque echogenicity using a five-type classification was performed.[40] Further, a semi-automated grayscale-based color mapping of the whole plaque and of its

Table 33.2 Grayscale-based color mapping of the carotid plaque: Comparison between surface characteristics and whole plaque measurement: Main differences observed between symptomatic and asymptomatic and between MRI+ and MRI− stenoses

$N = 89$	SYMPT+ $N = 31$	SYMPT− $N = 58$	[b]MRI+ $N = 27$	MRI− $N = 45$
[a]Type I/II N (%)	24 (77%)	24 (41%)	18 (67%)	20 (44%)
Type III/IV N (%)	7 (23%)	34 (59%)	9 (33%)	25 (56%)
p value	$p \leq 0.01$		$p \leq 0.10$	
Predominant red color in whole plaque N (%)	17 (55%)	17 (29%)	16 (59%)	11 (24%)
Not predominant red color in whole plaque N (%)	14 (45%)	41 (71%)	11 (41%)	34 (76%)
p value	$p < 0.02$		$p < 0.01$	
Predominant red color on surface (0 mm) N (%)	30 (97%)	36 (62%)	25 (93%)	30 (66%)
Not predominant red color on surface (0 mm) N (%)	1 (3%)	22 (38%)	2 (7%)	15 (33%)
p value	$p < 0.001$		$p < 0.02$	

[a]The plaques were classified according to the five-type classification proposed by Geroulakos et al.[40]
[b]MRI+ was considered if presence of a lesion located in the ipsilateral cortical or subcortical area with an embolic aspect or in a watershed area. Lesions were considered as silent whenever not associated to neurological symptoms but still in the territory of the carotid artery

surface was achieved. There were 31 (35%) symptomatic (23 strokes and 8 TIAs) and 58 (65%) asymptomatic carotid stenoses. MRI lesions were present in 27 cases (30%). In a multivariate logistic regression model, degree of stenosis ($p = 0.03$) and a predominant red color adjacent to the surface ($p = 0.04$) were independent factors associated with the presence of cerebrovascular events and/or lesions on MRI. No correlation was observed with any particular type of plaque based on visual analysis alone (Table 33.2).

33.3 Conclusions

The different studies showed a strong correlation between determinants of carotid plaque instability (thickness of the fibrous cap, position of the necrotic core, presence of microembolic signals) and the echogenic characteristics of plaque surface assessed by a grayscale-based color mapping method. A very fair score was further achieved for the interobserver agreement. The main limitation relies on the fact that all studies performed so far have been cross-sectional and therefore limited in their prognostic value. A prospective trial is needed in order to confirm the present results.

References

1. Golledge J, Greenhalgh RM, Davies AH. The symptomatic carotid plaque. *Stroke*. 2000;31:774–781.
2. Ross R. Atherosclerosis-an inflammatory disease. *N Engl J Med*. 1999;340:115–126.
3. Lusis AJ. Atherosclerosis. *Nature*. 2000;407:233–241.
4. Bassiouny HS et al. Critical carotid stenoses: morphologic and chemical similarity between symptomatic and asymptomatic plaques. *J Vasc Surg*. 1989;9:202–212.
5. Bassiouny HS et al. Juxtalumenal location of plaque necrosis and neoformation in symptomatic carotid stenosis. *J Vasc Surg*. 1997;26:585–594.
6. Langsfeld M, Gray-Weale AC, Lusby RJ. The role of plaque morphology and diameter reduction in the development of new symptoms in asymptomatic carotid arteries. *J Vasc Surg*. 1989;9:548–557.
7. O'Holleran LW, Kennelly MM, McClurken M, Johnson JM. Natural history of asymptomatic carotid plaque. Five year follow-up study. *Am J Surg*. 1987;154:659–662.
8. Bock W, Lusby RJ. Carotid plaque morphology and interpretation of the echolucent lesion. In: Labs KH, Jäger KA, Fitzgerald DE, Woodcock JP, Neuerburg-Heusler D, eds. *Diagnostic Vascular Imaging*. London: Arnold; 1992: 225–236.
9. Mathiesen EB, Bonaa KH, Joakimsen O. Echolucent plaques are associated with high risk of ischemic cerebrovascular events in carotid stenosis: the Tromsø study. *Circulation*. 2001;103:2171–2175.
10. AbuRahma AF, Wulu JT Jr, Crotty B. Carotid plaque ultrasonic heterogeneity and severity of stenosis. *Stroke*. 2002;33:1772–1775.
11. Aburahma AF, Thiele SP, Wulu JT. Prospective study of the natural history of asymptomatic 60% to 69% carotid stenosis according to ultrasonic plaque morphology. *J Vasc Surg*. 2002;36:437–442.
12. Steinke W, Hennerici M, Rautenberg W, Mohr JP. Symptomatic and asymptomatic high-grade carotid stenoses in Doppler color-flow imaging. *Neurology*. 1992;42: 131–138.
13. Rothwell PM. Carotid artery disease and the risk of ischemic stroke and coronary vascular events. *Cerebrovasc Dis*. 2000;10:21–33.

14. Eliassziw M et al. Significance of plaque ulceration in symptomatic patients with high-grade carotid stenosis. *Stroke*. 1994;25:304–308.
15. Streifler JY et al. Angiographic detection of carotid plaque ulceration: comparison with surgical observations in a multicenter study. *Stroke*. 1994;25:1130–1132.
16. Rothwell PM, Gibson R, Warlow CP, on behalf of the European Carotid Surgery Trialist Collaborative Group. Interrelation between plaque surface morphology and degree of stenosis on carotid angiograms and the risk of ischemic stroke in patients with symptomatic carotid stenosis. *Stroke*. 2000;31:615–621.
17. Mayor I, Momjian S, Lalive P, Sztajzel R. Carotid plaque: comparison between visual and grey-scale median analysis. *Ultrasound Med Biol*. 2003;29:961–966.
18. Gronholdt ML, Nordestgaard BG, Schroeder TV, Vorstrup S, Sillesen H. Ultrasonic echolucent carotid plaques predict future strokes. *Circulation*. 2001;104:68–73.
19. El-Atrozy T et al. The effect of B-mode ultrasonic image standardisation on the echodensity of symptomatic and asymptomatic carotid bifurcation plaques. *Int Angiol*. 1998;17:179–186.
20. Tegos TJ et al. Echomorphologic and histopathologic characteristics of unstable carotid plaques. *Am J Neuroradiol*. 2000;21:1937–1944.
21. Tegos TJ et al. Patterns of brain computed tomography infarction and carotid plaque echogenicity. *J Vasc Surg*. 2001;33:334–339.
22. Sabetai MM et al. Carotid plaque echogenicity and types of silent CT-brain infarcts. Is there an association in patients with asymptomatic carotid stenosis? *Int Angiol*. 2001;20:51–57.
23. El-Barghouty N, Nicolaides AN, Tegos T, Geroulakos G. The relative effect of carotid plaque heterogeneity and echogenicity on ipsilateral cerebral infarction and symptoms of cerebrovascular disease. *Int Angiol*. 1996;15:300–306.
24. El-Barghouty N, Levine T, Ladva S, Flanagan A, Nicolaides A. Histological verification of computerized carotid plaque characterisation. *Eur J Vasc Endovasc Surg*. 1996;11:414–416.
25. Lal BK et al. Pixel distribution analysis of B-mode ultrasound scan images predicts histologic features of atherosclerotic carotid plaques. *J Vasc Surg*. 2002;35:1210–1217.
26. Matsagas MI et al. Computer-assisted ultrasonographic analysis of carotid plaques in relation to cerebrovascular symptoms, cerebral infarction, and histology. *Ann Vasc Surg*. 2000;14:130–137.
27. El-Barghouty N, Geroulakos G, Nicolaides A, Androulakis A, Bahal V. Computer-assisted carotid plaque characteristaion. *Eur J Vasc Endovasc Surg*. 1995;9:389–393.
28. Sabetai MM et al. Reproducibility of computer-quantified carotid plaque echogenicity: can we overcome the subjectivity? *Stroke*. 2000;13:2189–2196.
29. Momjian-Mayor I et al. Visual analysis or semi-automated grey-scale based colour mapping of the carotid plaque: which method correlates the best with the presence of cerebrovascular symptoms and/or lesions on MRI? *J Neuroimaging*. 2009;19:119–126.
30. Sztajzel R et al. Stratified GSM analysis and colour mapping of the carotid plaque: correlation with endarterectomy specimen histology of 28 patients. *Stroke*. 2005;36:741–745.
31. Sztajzel R, Momjian-Mayor I, Comelli M, Momjian S. Correlation of cerebrovascular symptoms and microembolic signals with the stratified grey-scale and colour mapping of the carotid plaque. *Stroke*. 2006;37:824–829.
32. Sitzer M et al. Plaque ulceration and lumen thrombus are the main sources of cerebral microemboli in high-grade internal carotid artery stenosis. *Stroke*. 1995;26:1231–1233.
33. Sliwka U et al. Prevalence and time course of microembolic signals in patients with acute stroke. A prospective study. *Stroke*. 1997;28:358–363.
34. Goertler M et al. Rapid decline of cerebral microemboli of arterial origin after intravenous acetylsalicylic acid. *Stroke*. 1999;30:66–69.
35. Markus HS, Thomson ND, Brown MM. Asymptomatic cerebral embolic signals in symptomatic and asymptomatic carotid artery disease. *Brain*. 1995;118:1005–1011.
36. Siebler M, Sitzer M, Rose G. Cerebral microembolism and the risk of ischemia in asymptomatic high grade internal carotid artery stenosis. *Stroke*. 1995;26:2184–2186.
37. Siebler M, Sitzer M, Steinmetz H. Detection of intracranial emboli in patients with symptomatic extracranial carotid artery disease. *Stroke*. 1992;23:1652–1654.
38. Spence JD, Tamayo A, Lownie SP, Ng WP, Ferguson GG. Absence of microemboli on transcranial Doppler identifies low-risk patients with asymptomatic carotid stenosis. *Stroke*. 2005;36:2373–2378.
39. Griffin MB et al. Juxtaluminal hypoechoic area in ultrasonic images of carotid plaques and hemispheric symptoms. *J Vasc Surg*. 2010;52:69–76.
40. Geroulakos G, Ramaswami G, Nicolaides A. Characterisation of symptomatic and asymptomatic carotid plaques using high resolution real time ultrasound. *Br J Surg*. 1993;80:1274–1277.

34 Transcranial Doppler and Cerebrovascular Risk Stratification in Patients with Internal Carotid Artery Atherosclerosis

Anne L. Abbott

34.1 Introduction

The instrumentation and principles of duplex scanning, which combines brightness mode (B-mode) imaging with gated Doppler, has been described in detail in Chap. 5. Transcranial Doppler (TCD) uses 2-MHz probes that allow transmission of ultrasound through the scull. Velocity recordings of the intracranial arteries can be made by positioning the Doppler sample volume on the desired artery seen on the screen by color flow. For continuous monitoring special headgear is used that holds the probe in a fixed position.

TCD was introduced into clinical practice in the early 1990s to record blood flow velocity in the basal cerebral arteries.[1] The equipment currently used for continuous monitoring does not use B-mode imaging and has advantages of being portable, noninvasive, reproducible, giving results in "real time" and is relatively inexpensive. TCD has become an excellent tool for the diagnosis, management and better understanding of cerebral ischemia, bleeding and disordered autoregulation. Accordingly, much progress has been made in relation to better understanding atherosclerotic disease of the proximal internal carotid artery (ICA), a site predisposed to such arterial disease.[2]

This chapter provides an outline of TCD techniques, current research and clinical applications with respect to risk stratification of proximal ICA atherosclerotic disease states.

34.2 Intracranial Arterial Examination

34.2.1 TCD Acoustic Windows

The skull consists of three layers of bone influencing the ultrasound in different ways.[3] The inner and outer tables of ivory bone are important for refraction, while the inner table follows the windings of the brain acting as a lens. The middle layer (dipole) contains bony spicules that attenuate and scatter ultrasound. These spicules are absent in the temporal region (where the skull is thinnest) and can be avoided with insonation via the orbit, the frontal sinus, submandibular region and foramen magnum.[3] These areas, allowing relatively easy ultrasound passage, are known as TCD acoustic windows.[4] The ophthalmic artery is evaluated via the orbit with minimal error due to the favorable insonation angle (<15°).[5] However, if an examination is necessary, it is extremely important to reduce acoustic energy to a minimum (10–15%) and minimize study duration to avoid damage to the eye lens.[6]

34.2.2 General Normal Arterial Findings

There are three main sources of information for artery identification[3]:
1. The spatial relations between intracranial signals, including sample volume depth and probe angle
2. The direction of flow relative to the transducer and spectral distribution
3. Signal response to compression or vibration maneuvers

A.L. Abbott
Department of Preventative Health, Baker IDI Heart and Diabetes Institute, Melbourne, VIC, Australia

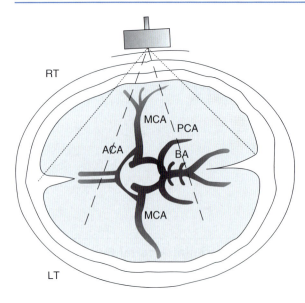

Fig. 34.1 Orientation of major intracerebral arteries using TCD and the temporal window. Flow direction in the middle cerebral artery (*MCA*) is toward the probe whereas it is away from the probe in the anterior cerebral artery (*ACA*). Flow direction in the proximal posterior cerebral artery is toward the probe and away from the probe distally (Reprinted with permission from Bartels[6])

Middle cerebral artery (MCA) identification is of particular importance for diagnosis and risk stratification of proximal ICA arterial disease. The MCA runs laterally and slightly anteriorly as a continuation of the intracranial ICA. It is usually the only artery arising from the circle of Willis traveling laterally toward the temporal window (Fig. 34.1). It is usually the only artery seen between the depth of 50 and 25 mm from the temporal window and usually has the highest flow volume and signal intensity of all circle of Willis branches. An anterior temple window allows almost zero degree angle of insonation, whereas the angle from the posterior temporal window is somewhat blunter.

The criteria for MCA identification are[3]:
1. The Doppler signal can be followed laterally with only slight probe movements from the termination of the ICA out of to a depth of about 30 mm.
2. The flow is toward the transducer. The spectrum obtained from the proximal segment of the MCA is smooth with relatively high intensity in the upper frequency region. A broader spectrum and lower frequency shifts are found at 40–25 mm where the artery divides into a trifurcation or bifurcation and further branches.
3. The signal responds to ipsilateral vibration of the lower common carotid artery (if latter is patent).

An important landmark is the bifurcation of the intracranial ICA into the MCA and anterior cerebral artery (ACA), usually at a depth of 55–60 mm. The MCA should be differentiated from the P1 segment of posterior cerebral artery cerebral (PCA) which also produces flow toward the temporally placed transducer. However, the P1 segment is found more posteriorly and returns lower frequencies. The proximal PCA can be scanned inward to the basilar tip where the contralateral PCA flows in the opposite direction (Fig. 34.1).

With 2-MHz probes, an adequate transtemporal signal can be obtained in about 80–95% of older Caucasian patients.[7–13] Success depends on the experience of the sonographer and the qualities of the bony windows. The latter tend to be poorer in older patients, especially women.[7]

Normal velocity profiles for the proximal basal cerebral arteries have been described by Aaslid et al.[1,3] and others.[14] Such measurements facilitate intercenter comparisons of both normal and abnormal vasculature. Information obtained by TCD spectral analysis can be supplemented by the use of B-mode imaging. Again, a pulsed-echo technique is used, and echoes are received back from a number of interfaces at variable distances over a single orientation to produce a "scan line." A two dimensional black and white image is created using juxtaposed scan lines.[6] Color-coded Doppler may be superimposed to give flow directional information. This also allows the determination of the angle of insonation on screen so more exact (angle corrected) measurements of flow velocity can be made. Intravenous "contrast agents," made up of stabilized microbubbles which increase the ultrasound backscatter, can be used to amplify received signals.[15,16] Contrast agents allow more detailed artery identification, especially in those with poor bony windows.[17,18] Other techniques to improve vascular image quality include Power Doppler[19] and 3-dimensional TCD.[20] Further details regarding general TCD vascular examination are available elsewhere.[1,3,21,22]

34.2.3 General Arterial Findings with ICA Disease

34.2.3.1 ICA Stenosis/Occlusion

Determining the presence or absence of atherosclerotic disease of the proximal ICA is the first step in vascular risk stratification. While cervical imaging is useful in diagnosing ICA stenosis or occlusion, TCD may be used for this purpose and also for assessment of the net cerebral hemodynamic effect of these conditions.[23] Special tests of the autoregulatory effects of ICA stenosis/occlusion will be discussed in the next section. Meanwhile, most general TCD findings indicating the presence of significant ICA stenosis or occlusion fall into two groups: dampened or absent velocity spectrum from downstream arteries and those due to collateral blood flow. The prevalence of any single TCD marker of ICA obstruction increases with the degree of stenosis, becoming statistically significant when the stenosis is greater than 80% in relation to the normal internal carotid diameter as defined by duplex and is maximal with occlusion.[24] Sensitivity in detecting significant stenosis/occlusion increases if a battery of markers is used, approximating 45–80%, while specificities in the order of 86–99% are achievable.[24,25]

34.2.3.2 Dampened or Absent Velocity Spectra in ICA Stenosis/Occlusion

Reduced flow velocities in ipsilateral MCA compared to the contralateral side or normal subjects can be seen if the collateral supply is insufficient, and velocities may rise following carotid endarterectomy (CEA).[5,26-28] However, MCA mean velocities vary widely with different grades of carotid stenosis and overlap with control values. Therefore, the hemodynamic effect of ICA stenosis cannot be satisfactorily assessed from the MCA velocity alone, even when an MCA with normal inflow conditions is available for comparison.[23]

Other indicators of flow include the "pulsatility index" (PI), a measure of the steepness of the down stroke of the Doppler velocity waveform.[24] PI is the difference between the maximal and minimal velocities divided by the mean flow velocity over the cardiac cycle.[21] It tends to fall in association with ipsilateral ICA stenosis or occlusion.[5] However, the PI is strongly influenced by systemic hemodynamic factors, such as blood pressure, heart rate, arterial pCO_2, and vascular compliance, and it varies greatly between individuals. The pulsatility transmission index (PTI) corrects for this individual variability in PI. It is the PI measured in the study MCA expressed as a percentage of the PI of another basal artery with presumed unimpeded flow.[23] The PTI probably reflects both the pressure drop across the stenosis and the cerebral autoregulatory response with a reduction due to reduced MCA inflow pressure and lowered cerebrovascular resistance. An MCA PTI of less than 92 is usually found in patients with ipsilateral ICA stenosis in excess of 75% (sensitivity 96%, specificity 100%).[23]

Low flow acceleration of the ipsilateral MCA is another indicator of high-grade carotid stenosis or occlusion. It is the difference in flow velocity from the start of the Doppler waveform to the peak divided by the time differential in seconds. It is a measure of the steepness of the up stroke of the Doppler waveform.[24] There is a linear inverse relationship between degree of ICA stenosis and flow acceleration values. A flow acceleration of about 350 cm/s or less is indicative of 70–100% ICA stenosis with a sensitivity of 82% and positive predictive value of about 80%.[29] Finally, systolic ophthalmic artery blood velocity may be reduced ipsilateral to ICA occlusion compared to contralateral velocities,[5] and there may be absent flow in the ipsilateral ophthalmic, periorbital arteries, or carotid siphon.[30]

34.2.3.3 Collateral Flow in ICA Stenosis/Occlusion

There are three sources of collateral flow for each cerebral hemisphere. TCD can be used to detect the first two:

1. Circle of Willis from the contralateral carotid or vertebrobasilar system (Fig. 34.2),
2. Ipsilateral external carotid artery via anastomoses, especially with the ophthalmic, frontal, and supraorbital arteries (Fig. 34.3), and
3. Any major intracranial cerebral vessel via brain surface pial anastomoses.

Indicators of collateral supply are particular patterns of increased velocity and reversed direction of blood flow. These need to be differentiated from changes associated with other local sites of cerebrovascular disease and/or systemic conditions. In patients with significant ICA stenosis/occlusion, collateral supply to the MCA from the contralateral carotid system

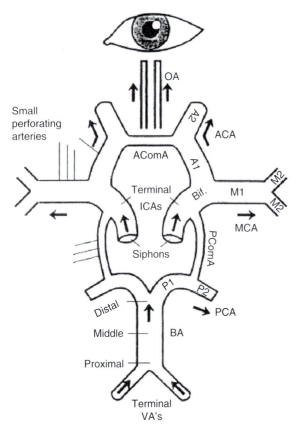

Fig. 34.2 Anatomical basis of circle of Willis collateral flow. *OA* ophthalmic artery, *ICA* internal carotid artery, *ACA* anterior cerebral artery (with A1 and A2 segments), *AComA* anterior communicating artery, *MCA* middle cerebral artery (with M1, M2 segments), *PCA* posterior cerebral artery (with P1 and P2 segments), *PComA* posterior communicating artery (Reprinted with permission from Alexandrov[4])

via the circle of Willis is indicated by reversed flow in the origin of anterior cerebral artery (ACA) ipsilateral to high-grade carotid stenosis/occlusion (recipient side). This is found in about 17% of patients with ipsilateral critical (80–99%) ICA stenosis and about 42% of patients with ipsilateral ICA occlusion. There may also be increased flow in the contralateral ACA (supplying side), found in about 7% of patients with ipsilateral critical (80–99%) ICA stenosis and about 11% with ICA occlusion.[24] Increased blood flow in the vertebral arteries, including particularly the proximal PCA,[23] may indicate collateral supply from the vertebrobasilar system. The presence of these TCD findings may vary from day to day in the same patients (Abbott et al, unpublished data) and correlate well with angiographic findings.[23]

Another important source of collateral supply to vascular territory distal to a compromised ICA is the external carotid artery via the periorbital arteries (Fig. 34.3). Normally the periorbital arteries are supplied by the ophthalmic artery (first branch of the ICA) so that flow direction is toward the transducer placed over the closed eye. Collateral flow via terminal ophthalmic and external carotid artery branch anastomoses produce reversal of normal flow direction in the recipient periorbital arteries. Reversed ophthalmic artery flow is one of the most sensitive, single TCD markers of ipsilateral significant ICA obstruction,[24] being found in about 50% of cases of occlusion and about 28% of cases of severe (80–99%) stenosis.[24] Its presence is unlikely when collateral flow is supplied by the circle of Willis, for example, if the ipsilateral ECA is also occluded. Detection of reversed flow in the frontal artery above the eye has the same significance and can be examined without risking eye damage.

34.2.3.4 Intracranial Stenosis/Occlusion

Tandem lesions, like MCA obstruction, are being more commonly recognized with more widespread use of noninvasive intracranial imaging. This should lead to more accurate measurements of stroke risk and better risk stratification methods in patients with and without proximal ICA stenosis, whether or not such obstructions are due to local disease or embolic material. Recognition and grading of MCA stenosis using TCD is an evolving area.[31] Criteria vary between sonographers and centers. As a general guide, intracranial stenoses are diagnosed using TCD on the basis of the following criteria and results compare favorably with conventional angiography.[6,32–34]

1. Local flow acceleration
2. Disturbed flow with spectral broadening in the region of the stenosis due to the increase in low-frequency and retrograde flow components
3. Reduced maximum and mean flow velocities distal to the stenosis

Published TCD criteria for middle cerebral artery (MCA) stenosis include a peak MCA systolic flow velocity higher than 150–160 cm/s, a mean MCA flow velocity greater than 80–90 cm/s, a side to side difference in MCA velocity of at least 30 cm/s or greater than 50% increase in velocity compared to the contralateral side or normal reference values.[6,7,33,35] However, wide ranging normal MCA peak (and to a

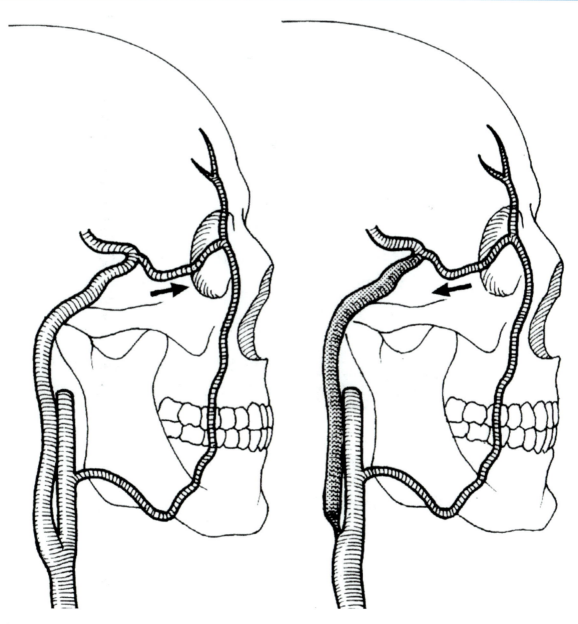

Fig. 34.3 Collateral connections between the internal and external carotid arteries. Normal physiological flow direction in the ophthalmic artery and its terminal branches is intra- to extracranial. This direction is often reversed in high-grade obstruction to flow in the ipsilateral ICA proximal to the origin of the ophthalmic artery (Reprinted with permission from Bartels[6])

lesser extent mean) systolic velocities have been published, and normal values fall with age.[1,3,36–39] False positive and negative results, respectively, can occur in association with severe extracranial stenosis and collateral flow or poor inflow.[35] In addition, care must be taken in interpretation of results because the exact angle of insonation is often unknown, allowing for underestimations in flow velocity.[40]

Transcranial findings from normal and diseased cerebral arteries (especially the MCA) when compared with those of digital subtraction angiography are similar.[32,33,35,41–44] One must be wary of comparing results of different techniques as each may have different limitations. For example, MCA stenosis may be detected or quantitated using TCD yet missed using angiography which provides only one anterior-posterior

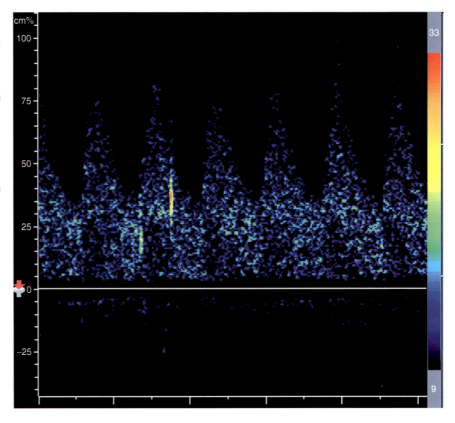

Fig. 34.4 An embolic signal in the MCA Doppler spectrum. Time is represented by the *x*-axis and velocity (in cm/s) by the *y*-axis. The intensity scale is indicated by the color bar on the right. High signal intensities are represented by *yellow-orange shades*. This patient had ipsilateral recently symptomatic (>3 months) >50%. ICA stenosis (Photo courtesy of Alice King, Centre for Clinical Neuroscience, St. Georges University, London. Printed with permission)

projection plane.[45] The intracranial circulation, in particular, may be suboptimally imaged using intravenous digital subtraction angiography (DSA) compared to conventional angiography.[46] Further, different modalities, if temporally separated, may show different findings due to the dynamic pathophysiology of stroke.

34.2.4 Detection of Emboli

The Doppler shift from blood flowing in arteries is not a single pure frequency derived from one moving reflector. The signal received is a mixture of different frequency components coming from reflectors moving at different velocities. In addition, the intensity of the reflected Doppler signal depends on several factors, including the size and surface of the reflecting particles and their acoustic impedance (resistance to sound propagation). Detection of emboli is based on the principle that embolic materials reflect and scatter more of the incident ultrasound than the surrounding blood cells because their size, shape, and acoustic impedance differ. This effect results in the appearance of short duration high-intensity signals in the Doppler spectrum, each with an accompanying crisp sound (Fig. 34.4).

The method of ultrasonic detection of embolic signals (ES) developed from observations in the 1960s when ultrasound was used to detect air embolism in vascular lines during cardiopulmonary bypass surgery.[47–49] Later, a high prevalence of similar, yet apparently asymptomatic signals, was noted in patients with mechanical prosthetic heart valves.[50,51] These cardiac derived signals could be suppressed by the administration of inspired supplemental oxygen indicating that these were too predominantly gaseous in nature.[52–55] The detection of signals of atheromatous microemboli started in the field of CEA much later.[56,57] Emboli likely to be gaseous (occurring upon release of the common carotid artery cross-clamps) were differentiated from other identical signals which were likely to be solid, occurring (for instance) during carotid artery dissection and wound closure.[57]

The technical validity of TCD detection of microemboli has been established in a number of animal and benchtop models.[58,59] Basic identification criteria for ES detection have been published based on recordings from a single sample volume.[60]

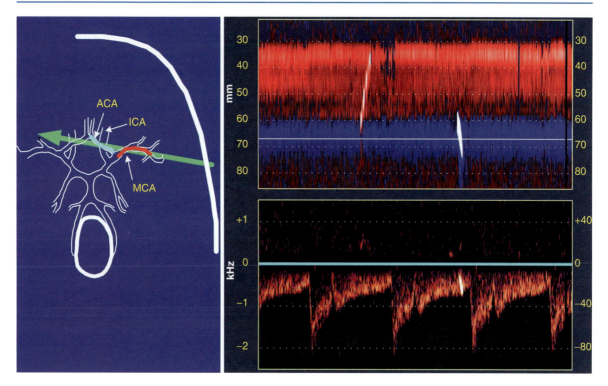

Fig. 34.5 Power M-mode and embolus detection. An example of a spectrogram of the middle cerebral artery (*MCA, in red*) and anterior cerebral artery (*ACA, in blue*) obtained from a Power M-mode Doppler device. The *oblique white lines* each represent a microembolus tracking through each cerebral artery (Image courtesy of Dr. Mark A. Moehring of Spencer Technologies)

Later technology, multigated[61] or Power motion mode (M-mode) Doppler,[62] has allowed simultaneous recording from multiple sample volumes at different depths. This has permitted tracking of emboli as they move (and even stop momentarily) along vessels, providing new diagnostic criteria (Fig. 34.5).[63] Good reproducibility of TCD detection of emboli can be achieved and is facilitated by standardization of study methods.[64,65] In most clinical contexts, humans are still superior to electronic methods of identifying emboli,[66] particularly when ES are relatively infrequent and of low signal intensity, as with asymptomatic carotid stenosis (see below).[67]

The clinical significance of TCD detected embolism is thought to depend on such variables as the composition, number and size of the microemboli (embolic load), microembolic vascular distribution, adequacy of cerebral blood flow (including collateral), and the presence or absence of previous cerebrovascular insults.[68–71] Damage may be caused by obstruction and/or inflammation.[72,73] Although, technologies are developing to differentiate gaseous from solid emboli,[74,75] currently the composition of TCD detected embolic material is still usually assumed from the clinical context. Although gaseous embolism may be responsible for stroke symptoms,[76–78] it appears that, in general, the brain tolerates gaseous better than solid microembolism. Usually, however, even most solid emboli detected with TCD are asymptomatic, being much more prevalent than stroke symptoms. Doppler detection of emboli has permitted a more complete pathophysiologic understanding of adverse outcomes in a variety of settings, including orthopedic[79] and cardiac[80] surgery, and ICA disease. This has allowed improved patient risk stratification and testing and implementation of preventive measures, as discussed below.

34.2.5 Testing Intracranial Arterial Autoregulation

Cerebral autoregulation is a process by which cerebral blood flow is maintained despite fluctuations in cerebral perfusion pressure.[81] Autoregulation is essential in avoiding the catastrophic consequences of cerebral hypoperfusion (as may occur with severe ICA stenosis or occlusion) or hyperperfusion (as may occur after CEA).

Understanding cerebral autoregulation requires an understanding of cerebral perfusion pressure, directly determined by systemic blood pressure, and various intracranial factors.[81] Methods of measuring cerebral autoregulation have led to the definition of two main types.[81] Autoregulation in steady state is associated with the concept of static autoregulation. This can be studied by various techniques which do not provide continuous measurements, such as xenon-133 clearance. Increasing interest in the continuous variations of cerebral blood flow led to the concept of dynamic autoregulation which requires real-time recordings of cerebral blood flow, as can be provided by TCD.[82]

In cerebrovascular risk stratification studies, terms associated with measuring cerebral autoregulation include "hemodynamics," a general reference to the study of blood flow, and "cerebral arterial vascular reactivity." The latter refers to arterial blood flow changes in response to a stimulus, often a dilatory one. It reflects the compensatory capacity of cerebral arterioles, an important component of cerebral autoregulation, and a marker of vascular reserve. In patients with occlusive ICA disease (especially ≥80% stenosis or occlusion), TCD has demonstrated reduced compensatory increases to ipsilateral MCA flow in response to hypercapnea (induced with inspired carbon dioxide or breath-holding)[83–85] and acetazolamide[85] compared to patients without such ICA disease. These markers of low cerebrovascular reserve are more common with symptomatic compared to asymptomatic carotid disease and may improve after carotid endarterectomy.[83] TCD tests of cerebrovascular reserve are relatively inexpensive and easy to perform, although they may be less sensitive in detecting patients with higher stroke risk than other methods.[86] Contrast agents may improve reliability.[87] TCD tests of arterial vascular reactivity as predictors of cerebrovascular risk in ICA occlusive disease will be discussed below.

34.3 Cerebrovascular Risk Stratification in Different ICA Disease States

34.3.1 Proximal ICA Stenosis

Atherosclerosis of the proximal ICA is usually described with reference to the presence or absence of luminal narrowing (stenosis) greater or less than about 50–75% stenosis (severe vs. nonsevere stenosis), presence or absence of previous symptoms of stroke or transient ischemic attack (TIA) in the distribution of the artery (symptomatic vs. asymptomatic), and presence or absence of any flow (occluded vs. nonoccluded). This terminology has developed with a focus on selecting patients for carotid surgery (endarterectomy or CEA), a practice supported by previous randomized trials showing a stroke prevention benefit, particularly for patients with symptomatic severe carotid stenosis.[88,89]

However, categories of stenosis based on symptoms and stenosis severity represent different spectra of disease and precise separation of patients into these groups is not possible. This is because stroke/TIA symptoms are not always recognized or reported, and one cannot be certain of the mechanism of stroke in particular patients (i.e., extent of hemodynamic, embolic, or a combination). Nor can one identify every embolic source or be certain that a recognized embolic source (such as proximal ICA stenosis) is responsible for particular stroke symptoms.[90] Further, methods of measuring stenosis have limitations.[91] It comes down to spectra of disease states and probabilities of risk. It is important to recognize these limitations when assessing new strategies for estimating risk, which may otherwise seem to provide information which is inconsistent with our previous thinking. ES detection and tests of autoregulation in risk stratification of ICA stenosis will be discussed separately, reflecting the way these topics have been studied so far.

34.3.1.1 Detection of Emboli in Risk Stratification of ICA Stenosis

The two most established and familiar markers of elevated stroke risk in relation to proximal ICA stenosis are the presence of previous ipsilateral symptoms of stroke or TIA and greater than about 50–75% stenosis in relation to the distal internal carotid diameter in both asymptomatic[92] and symptomatic patients.[93] It is also well recognized that the risk of recurrent stroke symptoms among patients with ipsilateral carotid stenosis[94,95] or general stroke/TIA patients[96] is inversely related to the time since stroke symptoms. Emboli detection studies of patients with carotid stenosis have usually been performed for about 30–60 min from a single sample volume depth and results are consistent with these clinical markers of risk.

Such observations support the thromboembolic basis of many strokes caused by carotid atherosclerosis.

Embolic signals are more commonly detected ipsilateral to the cerebral deficit in general stroke/TIA patients[97–99] and more often ipsilateral to presumed large artery caused infarcts (cortical or territorial) compared to lacunes.[98,99] More specifically, the proportion of patients from whom any emboli can be detected with TCD of the ipsilateral MCA is higher with symptomatic compared to asymptomatic carotid stenosis[13,100–106] or healthy volunteers.[104,107–109] This applies across any degree of stenosis (0–99%+/−occlusion) and the moderate-severe (>50%) range. Where given, rates of ipsilateral MCA emboli detected per hour of monitoring are also higher with symptomatic compared to asymptomatic carotid stenosis.[105,106,108] Where bilateral TCD monitoring has been performed in patients with carotid stenosis, ES are more often detected ipsilateral to the symptomatic hemisphere[11] or symptomatic stenosis.[10] The proportion of ES-positive patients with at least one ES detected rises with the duration and frequency of monitoring.[110,111] As expected from clinical observations, an inverse relationship between time since stroke/TIA symptoms and embolus detection has been reported in patients with ipsilateral symptomatic carotid stenosis. This applies across any degree of stenosis (0–99%+/−occlusion) and the moderate-severe (>50%) range.[13,103,105,112–117] An inverse relationship between time since stroke/TIA symptoms and detection of emboli has also been reported in more general stroke/TIA patients.[10,98]

The likelihood of detecting any ES using TCD also rises with the degree of stenosis, at least in samples of patients mixed with respect to symptomatic status and degree of stenosis (symptomatic and asymptomatic, 0–99% stenosis +/−occlusion).[101,109,112,114,118] Among symptomatic patients, the likelihood of detecting any ES rises with degree of stenosis within the 0–99% range[11] and mild-severe (≥20/30%) range.[105,119] Among asymptomatic patients with 20–99% stenosis[105] or >60% stenosis,[120] the likelihood of detecting any ES and/or number detected increases with increasing stenosis. In addition, Abbott et al. in a study of 202 patients with baseline 60–99% asymptomatic carotid stenosis[111] found a statistically significant association between the detection of at least one ES and maximal degree of stenosis during follow-up period (Abbott et al. unpublished data). A reduction in ES rates has also been found once stenosis becomes critical (>90–95%),[13] particularly in the presence of reduced poststenotic velocities.[119] This is in keeping with observed decreased incidence in stroke in both symptomatic[121] and asymptomatic patients[92] with severe stenosis and distal lumen collapse. ES are unlikely to be found in association with normal or occluded carotid arteries.[112]

The carotid plaque appears to be particularly embologenic compared to some other potential sources of cerebral embolism, particularly cardiac disorders.[11,122] Also consistent with the thromboembolic mechanism of stroke caused by carotid stenosis are consistent observations that ES detection ipsilateral to symptomatic carotid stenosis is less likely soon after ipsilateral CEA,[103,104,108,112,123,124] although ES detection may not cease completely in all patients.[125] This is perhaps because of a persisting embologenic carotid lesion or persistent generation of emboli from other sites.[123] Other observations consistent with the embologenic potential of stenosing carotid lesions include the simultaneous detection of ipsilateral emboli with TCD and new symptoms of stroke during carotid duplex examination.[126]

ES detection has also been linked to the presence of plaque surface ulceration or irregularity (determined angiographically[13,118,127,128] or with duplex[102]) and luminal carotid thrombus seen at carotid surgery.[129] A limitation of testing ES detection in relation to plaque surface features is that surface irregularities become more common with increasing severity of stenosis and reliable identification of plaque ulceration has been difficult in vivo.[89] Studies of ES detection and cross-sectional ultrasonic plaque features have differed with respect to patient baseline risk and plaque characterization methods. Some researchers have found that ES detection is more likely with low echogenicity plaque after image normalization in one study,[99] while others have not.[106,117]

Several prospective observational cohort studies have been performed to test the stroke/TIA risk stratification potential of TCD ES detection in patients specifically with moderate-severe carotid stenosis. These have generally been motivated by efforts to identify patients who may particularly benefit from CEA or stenting. Studies outlined in Tables 34.1 and 34.2, respectively, are listed by publication year and are all those identified in relation to symptomatic[13,110,115,116] or asymptomatic[13,111,130–133] carotid stenosis. Baseline degree of stenosis was ≥50%, 60%, or 70% (except in one study in which it was 70–90%[130]) and measured using carotid duplex,[13,110,111,116,130,132,133] conventional angiography,[131] or a combination.[115] Patients with recognized noncarotid sources of cerebral embolism were excluded from some studies.[13,110,111,115,116,130,131] In some studies of "asymptomatic" carotid stenosis, a proportion of patients with remote (>18–24 months) ipsilateral stroke/TIA were included.[132,133] One study of symptomatic patients included patients with carotid or MCA stenosis.[110] The study by Markus and MacKinnon[116] was a continuation of an earlier study.[13] It was stated that ES analysis was performed blinded to clinical data in most studies.[13,110,111,116,130,133]

Patients in studies of symptomatic carotid stenosis were recruited within the first 1–12 months of symptom onset (Table 34.1). ES-positive was defined in all as the detection of at least one ipsilateral ES during monitoring which consisted of one 1 h baseline TCD study in all accept in one study (where monitoring was performed for at "least 30 min"[115]). With this protocol, 30–45% of patients were ES-positive with a median rate, where stated, of 4 ES/h. The primary outcome event in all studies was recurrent ipsilateral stroke/TIA (cerebral +/− retinal), except in one where it was "recurrent stroke or TIA".[110] Follow-up duration was relatively brief, over a few weeks, and 8–16% of each cohort had recurrent ipsilateral events. In all studies, a significantly higher risk of recurrent stroke/TIA was measured in ES-positive compared to ES-negative patients. These results remained significant after adjustment for other vascular risk factors in the last two studies, with odds ratio (OR) 37 (95% confidence interval [CI] 3.5–333.4; $P = 0.003$)[110] and OR 4.7 (95% CI 2.0–11.0, $P < 0.0001$[116]), respectively. ES detection was a stronger predictor of increased risk than time since symptoms in the largest study.[116] Markus and MacKinnon also found a significantly higher risk of recurrent stroke alone in ES-positive patients, although the number of strokes was too small for multivariate analysis.[116] Markus et al. found no significant predictive value of different hourly rates of ES detection with respect to recurrent stroke/TIA risk, acknowledging that their study may have been underpowered for this purpose. One hour of ES detection is relatively brief in the dynamic setting of emboli shedding.[116] The identification of the elevated risk among patients with ES-positive and recently symptomatic severe carotid stenosis raises the possibility of improving methods of selecting patients for medical and surgical interventions to reduce their stroke risk and has helped fuel the use of ES detection as a surrogate endpoint in pharmacological studies (see below).

By contrast, testing the stroke predictive value of ES detection in relation to asymptomatic moderate-severe carotid stenosis has required much more work and has so far been less than conclusive. This is because this lesion carries a much smaller risk of stroke, and accordingly, the prevalence and average rates of ES detection are much lower. In addition, clinical risk is strongly dependent on the nature of the medical (nonsurgical) intervention received by patients.[120,134]

Among the six relevant published studies of asymptomatic carotid stenosis, definition of ES-positive was the detection of at least one[13,111,131,133] or at least two[130,132] ES during one to ten 60 min TCD recordings performed at various time intervals (Table 34.2). The prevalence of ES-positive arteries using these definitions was usually about 10–12% (with about 1 h of baseline monitoring) rising to about 42% with six to eight 1-h 6-monthly monitoring sessions. Where stated, the overall average hourly rate of ES detection was 0.16/h[111] and 0.26/h (H.S. Markus, personal communication, 2010). This is about 15–25 times lower than the average rate of ES detected with symptomatic carotid stenosis. Also, in contrast to studies of symptomatic patients, asymptomatic patients were followed up for many months or years rather than days and average event rates were described as annual rather than daily.

In each study of asymptomatic patients, the primary outcome was ipsilateral stroke/TIA except in one study where it was any territory stroke.[132] In the two earliest studies of asymptomatic carotid stenosis, which involved small samples, patients defined as ES-positive had a significantly higher risk of subsequent ipsilateral stroke/TIA than those defined as ES-negative. In the larger study by Abbott et al., ES-positive patients had more ipsilateral stroke/TIA symptoms during follow-up. However, this was not statistically significant. Spence et al. found a significant correlation between ES detection and risk of any territory stroke, although this was not significant after adjustment for other vascular risk factors. The recently published international Asymptomatic Carotid Emboli

Table 34.1 TCD ES detection and prediction of ipsilateral stroke/TIA in patients with symptomatic carotid artery stenosis

Study	n	Monitoring protocol for primary analysis	Primary outcome event	Follow up duration (years)	Primary outcome event (% total patient rate/ daily patient rate)	Prevalence ES + Arteries (%)	Overall ES rate/h	Correlation of ES and primary outcome event
Molloy et al. (1999)[13]	69	1 h	Recurrent ipsilateral carotid stroke/TIA	Mean 22.6 days	13[c]/0.6[c]	42	–	Significant[a]
Censori et al. (2000)[115]	50	>30 min	Recurrent ipsilateral cerebral + retinal ischaemic symptoms	Median 19 days	14[c]/0.7[c]	40	4 median (range 1–60)	Significant[a]
Blaser et al. (2004)[110]	86	1 h	Recurrent TIA/stroke	Mean 28 days	8[c]/0.3[c]	29	–	Significant[b]
Markus et al. (2005)[116]	200	1 h	i. Recurrent ipsilateral stroke/TIA ii. Recurrent ipsilateral stroke	FU < 90 days Mean not given	i. 16[c]/0.2[c] ii. 3.5[c]/0.04[c]	45	4 median (range 1–57)	Significant for ipsilateral stroke[a] Significant for ipsilateral stroke/TIA[b]

[a]Statistically significant with univariate analysis only
[b]Statistically significant after multivariate analysis
[c]Calculated using raw data; number of events, number of patients, duration of follow up (mean followup if given, otherwise median or maximum followup duration per patient).

Table 34.2 TCD ES detection and prediction of ipsilateral stroke/TIA in patients with asymptomatic carotid artery stenosis

Study	n	Monitoring protocol for primary analysis	Primary outcome event	Follow up duration (years)	Average annual primary outcome event rate/patient (%)	Prevalence ES + arteries (%)	Overall ES rate/h	Correlation of ES and primary outcome event
Siebler et al. (1995)[130]	64	1 h (at baseline + 6 months)	First ipsilateral carotid stroke or TIA/patient	1.4	5.6[d]	12.5	–	Significant[a]
Molloy et al. (1999)[13]	42	1 h at baseline only	First ipsilateral carotid stroke or TIA/patient	0.7	6.7[d]	29	–	Significant[a]
Orlandi et al. (2002)[131]	21	1 h (baseline + 6, 12, 18, 24 months)	Ipsilateral carotid stroke/TIA	–/–	–	28	–	–
Abbott et al. (2005)[111]	202	1 h baseline + 6 monthly (1–10, mean 4 studies/artery)	First ipsilateral carotid stroke or TIA/patient	2.8	3.2[d] (1.2 for first ipsilateral stroke without prior ipsilateral TIA[d])	12% after 1 h baseline study, rising to 42% by 8–10 1 h follow-up studies	0.16 (range 0–11)	Not significant
Spence et al. (2005)[132]	319	Up to 1 h at baseline + 2 weeks later	Any territory stroke	1	2.5 for any territory stroke[d] (5.0 for any territory stroke/TIA[d])	10% at baseline	–	Significant[a]
Markus et al. (2010)[133]	467	1 h twice (1 week apart) at baseline	Ipsilateral stroke/TIA	Up to 2	3.4 for all ipsilateral stroke/TIA[d] (1.1 for all ipsilateral stroke[d] 0.6 for first ipsilateral stroke without prior ipsilateral TIA)[d]	10% after a single 1 h baseline study	0.26[c]	Significant[b]

[a]Statistically significant with univariate analysis only
[b]Statistically significant with multivariate analysis
[c]Personal communication from Prof Markus, 2010
[d]Calculated using raw data; number of events, number of patients, duration of follow up (mean followup if given, otherwise median or maximum followup duration per patient).

Study (ACES) was the largest study.[133] In the primary analysis of 477 patients, ES detected at baseline was found to be predictive of subsequent ipsilateral stroke or TIA (hazards ratio 2.5, 95%CI 1.2–5.4, $p = 0.015$) and subsequent ipsilateral stroke alone (hazards ratio 5.6, 95%CI 1.6–19.3, $p = 0.007$) during the following 2 years. These results, compared to ES-negative patients, remained statistically significant after adjusting for baseline degree of stenosis, age, sex, hypertension, smoking, diabetes, and antiplatelet therapy. In addition, ACES patients underwent 1 h of ES detection at 6, 12, and 18 months. A statistically significant correlation was also found between ipsilateral stroke or TIA or ipsilateral stroke alone and ES detected in the preceding 6 months, even after adjustment for antiplatelet therapy and other risk factors.

These statistically significant associations for asymptomatic severe carotid stenosis are the strongest published so far, and they again support the thromboembolic basis of stroke associated with carotid atherosclerosis. However, there is not sufficient evidence yet that ES detection is ready to be used to select patients for carotid surgery or stenting for stroke prevention. There are several reasons for this, some of which help to explain interstudy variability in results. Firstly, methods of event rate calculations may not be clearly explained or, where explained, differ significantly. This is especially important where stroke symptom event rates are relatively low, as in association with asymptomatic carotid stenosis. For example, in some cases, only the first ipsilateral stroke symptoms (stroke or TIA) were included in correlations with ES detection,[111] and in others, recurrent stroke symptoms were included (ipsilateral stroke after ipsilateral TIA). From the ACES results published so far,[133] in ES-positive patients, the absolute annual risk of ipsilateral stroke/TIA between baseline and 2 years was 7.1% (3.0% in ES-negative patients) and 3.6% for ipsilateral stroke alone (0.70% in ES-negative patients). However, four of the ten ipsilateral strokes included in correlations with ES detection occurred in patients after ipsilateral TIA. If such strokes in "newly symptomatic" patients were excluded, the stroke rate would have been almost halved, and a statistically significant association may not have been found.

Secondly, as noted above, stroke symptom and ES detection rates are highly dependent on patient risk factor load and the nature of the arterial disease medical intervention given.[120,134] Further, average annual stroke rates among medically managed hospital-referred patients with asymptomatic severe carotid stenosis have fallen significantly over the last 25–30 years to 0.5-1.0%, Abbott, 2010 Veithsymposium paper, available online,[135] indicating that surgery is no longer advisable.[134] All published studies of ES detection and stroke symptom risk associated with asymptomatic carotid stenosis so far lack documentation of risk factor load and medical intervention given leading up to and during the entire study period. Stroke symptom risk stratification of ES detection in the context of current best practice medical intervention alone has not been documented.

Thirdly, ES detection in this setting is still best done manually and is too time consuming and tedious for routine practice.[111,133] Further clinical study and clinical application is impractical unless reliable prolonged automated ES detection systems become available. Finally, if ES detection is one day shown to be a reliable method of identifying patients with asymptomatic carotid stenosis at sufficiently higher risk of ipsilateral stroke, despite current best medical intervention alone, such patients will probably also be at higher risk of stroke or death from carotid surgery or stenting. Therefore, randomized trials of additional surgery or stenting will be required for these high risk subgroups, and clinical practice will need to become organized to replicate the randomized trial methods, as minimum standards, when the preferred course of action is declared.

A shared finding of the larger studies of asymptomatic severe carotid stenosis is a low positive predictive value and a high negative predictive value with respect to the detection of at least one or two ES and subsequent ipsilateral or any territory stroke or TIA.[111,132,133] This suggests that ES-negativity is more strongly predictive of cerebral outcome than ES-positivity as most patients remain asymptomatic with the ES loads tested so far. In any future risk stratification studies of asymptomatic carotid stenosis, methods of event rate calculations should be clearly stated and raw data provided (number of events, number of patients, and mean follow-up). Further, only the first event of interest per patient should be used in primary outcome analyses. Patient risk factor load and interventions given leading up to and during the entire study period should be fully documented, and different rates of ES detection should be tested. Such studies should test the best medical intervention available and would benefit from larger sample sizes, inclusion of nonstroke/TIA complications of atherosclerosis, longer and more frequent ES monitoring, longer patient follow-up, and assured blinding of clinical from ES data.

34.3.1.2 Tests of Cerebral Autoregulation in Risk Stratification in ICA Stenosis

TCD tests indicating poor cerebrovascular reserve in patients with asymptomatic carotid stenosis[136,137] or occlusion[137] identify those with elevated future ipsilateral stroke (+/−TIA) risk.[137] This has been demonstrated after allowances for other general baseline risk factors such as age, gender, diabetes, smoking, and brain imaging apparent cerebral infarct.[136,137] Such "high risk" patients have not yet been shown to benefit from interventions such as carotid surgery or stenting. Further, studies of the risk stratification potential of these TCD markers of cerebrovascular reserve have not been performed in the context of current, intensive vascular disease medical intervention alone. Nor have studies been performed in relation to carotid stenosis to test the combined risk stratification of TCD indicators of poor cerebrovascular reserve and other specialized markers of risk, such as detection of emboli.

34.3.2 Carotid Dissection

Carotid dissection may present with impaired consciousness, focal neurological signs or incidentally. TCD may suggest its presence because of the typical flow findings associated with carotid stenosis or occlusion described above[138–142] or reveal ipsilateral MCA occlusion if ACA and PCA signals are detected, and MCA signals are not.[138] In addition, TCD reveals embolization in about 45–60% of patients monitored for 20–60 min on one or several occasions.[138,140,141] Rates of ES detection of 1–60/h have been reported.[140,142] Sometimes, TCD signs of carotid obstruction may be very important in raising suspicion that a dissection is present, particularly with traumatic dissections which are often located close to the skull base beyond the range of carotid duplex.[139] Spontaneous dissections, by contrast, tend to be more proximal in the ICA.

Stroke in these patients may be caused by uncompensated ICA occlusion and/or perhaps more commonly, distal embolization.[143] Therefore, TCD may be useful in cerebrovascular risk stratification. Srinivasan et al. in a nonblinded study of 17 patients with traumatic or spontaneous carotid dissection found that ES were more frequent in patients who had presented with stroke than those who did not.[140] The only identified prospective TCD risk stratification study of carotid dissection was published by Molina et al.[141] In a study of 28 patients with carotid dissection associated with ipsilateral stroke/TIA, those with embolic signals were more likely to experience recurrent stroke symptoms. The best treatment to reduce risk of stroke caused by carotid dissection is unknown. Although anticoagulants and antithrombotic agents have been used, no randomized studies have been conducted to make clear if/how effective these are.[144] TCD may prove helpful in the assessment of such interventions. TCD may also be used to follow resolution.[138–140]

34.3.3 Carotid Territory Stroke

Acute ICA territory stroke and TIA are other parts of the spectrum of proximal ICA atherosclerotic disease. Moderate to severe proximal ICA stenosis is estimated to cause about 7–12% of all strokes and 12–21% of all anterior circulation ischemic strokes.[89] TCD techniques compare favorably with other modalities, such as computed tomography (CT) angiography in diagnosing acute occlusions of proximal basal cerebral arteries,[145] sometimes caused by embolism or extended thrombus generated from proximal carotid atherosclerosis. Characteristic information can be derived from residual flow (velocity measurements, flow waveforms), presence of flow diversion (collaterals), and ES generation at the site of obstruction.[146–148] Grading residual flow using the TCD TIBI (thrombolysis in brain ischemia) system correlates with baseline and 24-hour National Institutes of Health Stroke Scale (NIHSS) scores, recanalization and in-hospital mortality (lower TIBI implies poor recanalization and poorer clinical outcome).[148,149] TCD monitoring can be used to follow the process of recanalization in real time. Information like degree of and time to recanalization can be used to predict clinical outcome[150] and help guide therapeutic decisions.

Further, transcranial application of readily available diagnostic TCD technology (with 2-MHz probes) is showing promise in assisting clot lysis and improving outcome for those with acute ischemic symptoms and circle of Willis occlusions with evidence from in vitro[151] and in vivo studies.[152] Larger clinical trials are required to confirm the clinical effectiveness.[151] There is also evidence that microbubbles could be used to enhance the effect of ultrasound on thrombolysis,[153] and a further study is underway.[151]

34.3.4 Carotid Endarterectomy, Angioplasty, and Stenting

34.3.4.1 Carotid Endarterectomy

Stroke is a serious complication of CEA occurring in approximately 2.3–7.0% of patients in large randomized trials.[88,89] Most strokes occur during or immediately after the procedure.[154,155] Of concern, perioperative stroke is often not anticipated at the time of surgical closure.[156] Depending to some extent on the stage of surgery, carotid thrombosis and embolism is thought to be the dominant mechanism, followed by hypo and hyperperfusion.[157,158] TCD has been used to identify risk of cerebral complications caused by these mechanisms, leading to improvements in surgical outcomes.[9,157,159–163]

Most emboli detected during carotid dissection and during or after arterial closure are thought to be solid,[157,164] consistent with these emboli being highly predictive of perioperative cerebrovascular ischemic symptoms.[165] Embolic signals are often detected during CEA.[9,157,166–168] Using multifrequency TCD, Skjelland et al. estimated that about 20% of emboli detected during CEA are solid and 80% gaseous.[167] Most solid emboli were noted during establishment of shunt flow and carotid clamp release, times when total ES counts are high.[166] In their series of 91 patients (comprising 30 who underwent angioplasty, and 60 who underwent CEA), Skjelland et al. found that total gaseous and solid emboli counts during CEA were both predictive of procedure related ipsilateral ischemic stroke and new ipsilateral cerebral diffusion weighted lesions on magnetic resonance imaging.

Earlier work established that ES (particularly ≥10 or ≥10–15/h) detected intraoperatively (particularly during carotid dissection or wound closure) correlate with the appearance of new magnetic resonance imaging (MRI) ischemic cerebral lesions,[9,166,168,169] deterioration in postoperative cognitive function[8] and perioperative cerebral ischemic symptoms.[9,164,168,170,171] Golledge et al. found a higher risk of operative stroke among those with more than 10 ES detected specifically during carotid artery closure.[165]

High rates of ES detected immediately after CEA (generally ≥8–30 ES/h) also correlate well with elevated risk of postoperative stroke/TIA and new lesions on brain imaging.[170,172–174] The first postoperative hour is the most important time to detect postoperative embolism. The proportion of ES-positive patients and total ES counts fall progressively during the first 24–36 h after CEA,[125,175,176] in keeping with falling stroke symptom risk. Women, those having a left CEA or CEA for symptomatic carotid stenosis and those without preoperative antiplatelet agents, are more likely to have *any* ES detected during or soon after carotid surgery.[165,170,171,177] This is in keeping with higher risk of stroke symptoms in these subgroups undergoing CEA.[89] TCD identification of high risk patients using ES detection in this setting can be easily performed manually with a single sample volume and some centers are using automated programs of ES detection to facilitate routine identification of high risk patients.[178]

Perfusion extremes are the other major cause of cerebral injury associated with CEA. During the dissection phase of carotid surgery, a relatively low MCA mean blood flow velocity (≥28–35 cm/s) has been found predictive of new postoperative diffusion weighted MR lesions and new neurological deficits.[168,179] This is perhaps an even stronger marker of elevated risk than the detection of more than 10 ES.[168] Ogasawara et al. noted that the combination of these findings was additive in risk stratification,[168] supporting the concept that low flow velocities may impair clearance of the embolic load.[180] A decrease in MCA peak systolic velocity of more than 90% at cross clamping has also been shown to be independently predictive of operative stroke.[164]

Hyperperfusion syndrome is a form of hyperemia and disordered autoregulation which may complicate procedures to improve flow to a chronically ischemic hemisphere. Pathology shows features consistent with malignant hypertension.[181,182] It is characterized by severe headache, nausea, vomiting, photophobia, dizziness, sometimes hypertension, seizures and focal neurological signs with/without intracranial edema or hemorrhage.[160,183–185] Symptoms occur in 0.5–6% of post-CEA patients usually in the first 1–2 postoperative weeks and may last hours to days. Although most patients have mild symptoms, hyperperfusion accounts for a significant proportion of perioperative strokes and deaths.[184] TCD markers of increased risk and/or diagnosis include reduced preoperative blood flow velocity and pulsatility,[186] preoperative "exhausted vasomotor reactivity,"[187] a greater than 100–175% increase over baseline MCA mean blood flow velocity or pulsatility index immediately after declamping of the ICA or postoperatively.[157,160,162,183,188–192] Postoperative monitoring may also show reassuring normalization of cerebral blood flow velocities, redirectioning of normal collateral blood flow, and increasing carbon dioxide reactivity in the immediate postoperative period or some months later.[160,193–195]

34.3.4.2 Carotid Angioplasty/Stenting

Embolic signals are also often detected during or soon after carotid angioplasty.[78,167] Skjelland et al. estimated that about 17% of emboli detected during carotid angioplasty are solid and 80% gaseous.[167] Most solid emboli occurred during stent delivery and dilatation. Most gaseous emboli occurred during catheter flushing and angiography, times when total ES counts are high.[78,196] Multiple showers of microemboli (>5) postdilatation after stent deployment, particulate macroemboli, massive air embolism, angioplasty induced asystole, and prolonged hypotension with greater than 70% reduction of MCA blood flow velocities are independent predictors of cerebral deficits.[78] As with CEA, it has been proposed that reduced MCA blood flow and embolism are additive in elevating risk during angioplasty/stenting.[179] Higher embolic counts and higher rates of perioperative cerebral/retinal cerebrovascular complications have been reported in patients undergoing stenting compared to CEA.[78,197] Although these studies were not designed to compare risk of clinical complications of the two interventions, it is expected that rates of embolization will be proportional to clinical risk.

34.3.5 Medical (Noninvasive) Interventions for Vascular Disease

In patients at risk of embolic stroke, including those with carotid stenosis, the likelihood of detecting embolic signals and rates of ES detection fall under the influence of vascular protective drugs, in keeping with composition of emboli[198] and the fall in stroke symptom risk with these drugs. In some cases, the effect of particular drugs (usually antiplatelet agents) on ES detection has been measured in relative isolation. For this purpose, the most commonly studied patient groups are those with relatively high rates of ES detection and relatively high risk of stroke symptoms, such as those with recently symptomatic severe carotid stenosis and those undergoing CEA.

In patients with recently symptomatic moderate/severe (>50%) carotid stenosis, oral combination therapy with clopidogrel and aspirin is more effective than aspirin alone in reducing the likelihood of detecting emboli.[199] Intravenous acetylsalicylic acid and intravenous tirofiban (glycoprotein IIb/IIIa inhibitor) reduce rates of ES detection in patients with symptomatic carotid stenosis[200] or those awaiting CEA.[201] Other researchers have found that tirofiban reduces ES rates in stroke/TIA patients, many with carotid disease, and have also noted reversibility of antiplatelet effect.[202] Among patients undergoing CEA, the absence of perioperative aspirin is associated with a higher risk of detecting emboli with TCD,[177,203] just as it is associated with a higher risk of perioperative stroke.[89] Preoperative clopidogrel, in addition to aspirin, reduces embolization further.[204] Intravenous administration of antiplatelet agents can quickly reduce rates of ES detection in ES-positive patients soon after CEA. These include tirofiban,[201] Dextran 40,[175] L-arginine,[205] and S-nitrosoglutathione.[205–207]

In other situations, the combined effect of drugs and other strategies on ES detection has been measured. For instance, Spence et al. in a study of 468 patients with asymptomatic severe carotid stenosis reported a marked decline in the proportion of ES-positive patients, slower plaque progression, and lower risk of vascular disease symptoms coinciding with more aggressive medical (nonsurgical) intervention, including better control of plasma lipids and hypertension.[120] This important observation is consistent with the lower rate of stroke and ES detection among more recently treated patients with acute coronary syndromes whose intervention now commonly includes new medical (noninvasive) interventions and coronary angioplasty rather than intravenous thrombolytics.[208] Risk stratification studies are performed in the context of the interventions available at the time. It is now clear that medical intervention alone, which includes risk factor identification, public education, healthy lifestyle practices, and appropriate use of drugs, has become highly effective in reducing the risk of both cerebral[134,209] and cardiac[210] complications of vascular disease.

34.4 Summary

There is now sufficient evidence that embolism, thrombosis, and hemodynamic limitations are responsible for most stroke symptoms in relation to atherosclerotic disease of the proximal ICA. While not a substitute for other imaging modalities, TCD is unique in detecting these phenomena because it allows prolonged, direct observation of these dynamic pathophysiologic processes, giving new information in real time. This allows better, more immediate risk stratification and intervention. Other advantages of TCD are it is safe, relatively inexpensive and space efficient. It is likely that combinations of risk markers will be most important in identifying those at greatest stroke risk. For the best results, as with other modalities, TCD requires special expertise. The discipline will benefit from ongoing collaborative research, training, standardization, and routine use in clinical practice. Better adaptation of TCD to individual patient circumstances will come with the development of less expensive, even more effective contrast agents and more reliable automated systems of emboli detection which better differentiate embolus composition. Also helpful would be easier monitoring of multiple sites to better localize the embolic source and efforts to extend the duration of comfortable monitoring.

It is also clear from current evidence that embolism, thrombosis, and hemodynamic disturbances in relation to ICA disease will be detected by TCD in proportion to clinical risk of stroke symptoms, reflecting pathophysiology. Accordingly, it has been easier to establish TCD as a useful risk stratification tool in patients with stroke or TIA or symptomatic carotid stenosis and those undergoing CEA than for those with asymptomatic carotid stenosis.[211] Risk of stroke symptoms will be highly dependent on the average inherent risk of the patients studied and the nature of the vascular disease medical intervention received. The latter has become very effective over the last 30 years. Therefore, it is crucial that the risk stratification potential of modalities such as TCD be interpreted in the context of the patients studied and the medical intervention given. Finally, risk stratification strategies should only be tested in the context of the most effective medical intervention available, particularly if relatively invasive and expensive interventions (like CEA, angioplasty, or stenting) are being considered for prevention of stroke symptoms.

References

1. Aaslid R, Markwalder TM, Nornes H. Noninvasive transcranial Doppler ultrasound recording of flow velocity in basal cerebral arteries. *J Neurosurg*. 1982;57:769–774.
2. Abbott AL. *The Natural History of High Grade Asymptomatic Carotid Stenosis and Identification of High Ipsilateral Stroke or TIA Risk Using Microembolus Detection* [Ph.D. thesis]. Melbourne: University of Melbourne (Medicine); 2003:439.
3. Aaslid R. *Transcranial Doppler Sonography*. Berlin, Germany: Springer/Wien; 1986.
4. Alexandrov AV. *Cerebrovascular Ultrasound in Stroke Prevention and Treatment*. Oxford: Futura (Blackwell); 2004.
5. Schneider PA, Rossman ME, Bernstein EF, Ringelstein EB, Otis SM. Noninvasive assessment of cerebral collateral blood supply through the ophthalmic artery. *Stroke*. 1991;22:31–36.
6. Bartels E. *Colour-Coded Duplex Ultrasonography of the Cerebral Vessels: Atlas and Manual*. Stuttgart: Schattauer; 1999.
7. Niederkorn K, Myers LG, Nunn CL, Ball MR, McKinney WM. Three-dimensional transcranial Doppler blood flow mapping in patients with cerebrovascular disorders. *Stroke*. 1988;19:1335–1344.
8. Gaunt ME et al. Clinical relevance of intraoperative embolization detected by transcranial Doppler ultrasonography during carotid endarterectomy: a prospective study of 100 patients. *Br J Surg*. 1994;81:1435–1439.
9. Ackerstaff RG et al. The significance of microemboli detection by means of transcranial Doppler ultrasonography monitoring in carotid endarterectomy. *J Vasc Surg*. 1995;21:963–969.
10. Sliwka U et al. Prevalence and time course of microembolic signals in patients with acute stroke. A prospective study. *Stroke*. 1997;28:358–363.
11. Koennecke HC et al. Frequency and determinants of microembolic signals on transcranial Doppler in unselected

patients with acute carotid territory ischemia. A prospective study. *Cerebrovasc Dis.* 1998;8:107–112.
12. Kaposzta Z, Young E, Bath PM, Markus HS. Clinical application of asymptomatic embolic signal detection in acute stroke: a prospective study. *Stroke.* 1999;30:1814–1818.
13. Molloy J, Markus HS. Asymptomatic embolization predicts stroke and TIA risk in patients with carotid artery stenosis. *Stroke.* 1999;30:1440–1443.
14. Ringelstein EB, Kahlscheuer B, Niggemeyer E, Otis SM. Transcranial Doppler sonography: anatomical landmarks and normal velocity values. *Ultrasound Med Biol.* 1990;16:745–761.
15. Nabavi DG et al. Potential and limitations of echocontrast-enhanced ultrasonography in acute stroke patients: a pilot study. *Stroke.* 1998;29:949–954.
16. Postert T et al. Contrast-enhanced transcranial color-coded sonography in acute hemispheric brain infarction. *Stroke.* 1999;30:1819–1826.
17. Otis S, Rush M, Boyajian R. Contrast-enhanced transcranial imaging. Results of an American phase-two study. *Stroke.* 1995;26:203–209.
18. Postert T, Federlein J, Przuntek H, Büttner T. Comparison of transcranial power Doppler and contrast-enhanced color-coded sonography in the identification of intracranial arteries. *J Ultrasound Med.* 1998;17:91–96.
19. Kenton AR, Martin PJ, Evans DH. Power Doppler: an advance over colour Doppler for transcranial imaging? *Ultrasound Med Biol.* 1996;22:313–317.
20. Lyden PD, Nelson TR. Visualization of the cerebral circulation using three-dimensional transcranial power Doppler ultrasound imaging. *J Neuroimaging.* 1997;7:35–39.
21. Newell D, Aaslid R. *Transcranial Doppler.* New York: Raven; 1992.
22. Alexandrov AV et al. Practice standards for transcranial Doppler ultrasound: part I – test performance. *J Neuroimaging.* 2007;17:11–18.
23. Lindegaard KF et al. Assessment of intracranial hemodynamics in carotid artery disease by transcranial Doppler ultrasound. *J Neurosurg.* 1985;63:890–898.
24. Wilterdink JL, Feldmann E, Furie KL, Bragoni M, Benavides JG. Transcranial Doppler ultrasound battery reliably identifies severe internal carotid artery stenosis. *Stroke.* 1997;28:133–136.
25. Christou I et al. A broad diagnostic battery for bedside transcranial Doppler to detect flow changes with internal carotid artery stenosis or occlusion. *J Neuroimaging.* 2001;11:236–242.
26. Wechsler LR, Ropper AH, Kistler JP. Transcranial Doppler in cerebrovascular disease. *Stroke.* 1986;17:905–912.
27. Schneider PA et al. Effect of internal carotid artery occlusion on intracranial hemodynamics. Transcranial Doppler evaluation and clinical correlation. *Stroke.* 1988;19:589–593.
28. Kelley RE, Namon RA, Juang SH, Lee SC, Chang JY. Transcranial Doppler ultrasonography of the middle cerebral artery in the hemodynamic assessment of internal carotid artery stenosis. *Arch Neurol.* 1990;47:960–964.
29. Kelley RE, Namon RA, Mantelle LL, Chang JY. Sensitivity and specificity of transcranial Doppler ultrasonography in the detection of high-grade carotid stenosis. *Neurology.* 1993;43:1187–1191.
30. Wilterdink JL, Feldmann E, Bragoni M, Brooks JM, Benavides JG. An absent ophthalmic artery or carotid siphon signal on transcranial Doppler confirms the presence of severe ipsilateral internal carotid artery disease. *J Neuroimaging.* 1994;4:196–199.
31. Hao Q et al. Pilot study of new diagnostic criteria for middle cerebral artery stenosis by transcranial Doppler. *J Neuroimaging.* 2010;20(2):122–129.
32. Lindegaard KF, Bakke SJ, Aaslid R, Nornes H. Doppler diagnosis of intracranial artery occlusive disorders. *J Neurol Neurosurg Psychiatry.* 1986;49:510–518.
33. Ley-Pozo J, Ringelstein EB. Noninvasive detection of occlusive disease of the carotid siphon and middle cerebral artery. *Ann Neurol.* 1990;28:640–647.
34. Wechsler L. Cerebrovascular disease. In: Babikian VL, Weschler LR, eds. *Transcranial Doppler Sonography.* 2nd ed. Boston: Butterworth-Heinemann; 1999:91–108.
35. Rorick MB, Nichols FT, Adams RJ. Transcranial Doppler correlation with angiography in detection of intracranial stenosis. *Stroke.* 1994;25:1931–1934.
36. Bishop CC, Powell S, Rutt D, Browse NL. Transcranial Doppler measurement of middle cerebral artery blood flow velocity: a validation study. *Stroke.* 1986;17:913–915.
37. Arnolds BJ, von Reutern GM. Transcranial Doppler sonography. Examination technique and normal reference values. *Ultrasound Med Biol.* 1986;12:115–123.
38. Hennerici M, Rautenberg W, Schwartz A. Transcranial Doppler ultrasound for the assessment of intracranial arterial flow velocity – part 2. Evaluation of intracranial arterial disease. *Surg Neurol.* 1987;27:523–532.
39. Mattle H, Grolimund P, Huber P, Sturzenegger M, Zurbrügg HR. Transcranial Doppler sonographic findings in middle cerebral artery disease. *Arch Neurol.* 1988;45:289–295.
40. Thiele BL et al. Standards in noninvasive cerebrovascular testing. Report from the Committee on Standards for Noninvasive Vascular Testing of the Joint Council of the Society for Vascular Surgery and the North American Chapter of the International Society for Cardiovascular Surgery. *J Vasc Surg.* 1992;15:495–503.
41. Zanette EM et al. Comparison of cerebral angiography and transcranial Doppler sonography in acute stroke. *Stroke.* 1989;20:899–903.
42. Zanette EM et al. Spontaneous middle cerebral artery reperfusion in ischemic stroke. A follow-up study with transcranial Doppler. *Stroke.* 1995;26:430–443.
43. Kushner MJ et al. Transcranial Doppler in acute hemispheric brain infarction. *Neurology.* 1991;41:109–113.
44. Lyrer PA, Engelter S, Radü EW, Steck AJ. Cerebral infarcts related to isolated middle cerebral artery stenosis. *Stroke.* 1997;28:1022–1027.
45. Röther J, Schwartz A, Wentz KU, Rautenberg W, Hennerici M. Middle cerebral artery stenoses: assessment by magnetic resonance angiography and transcranial Doppler ultrasound. *Cerebrovasc Dis.* 1994;4:273–279.
46. Earnest F et al. The accuracy and limitations of intravenous digital subtraction angiography in the evaluation of

46. atherosclerotic cerebrovascular disease: angiographic and surgical correlation. *Mayo Clin Proc.* 1983;58:735–746.
47. Austen WG, Howry DH. Ultrasound as a method to detect bubbles or particulate matter in the arterial line during cardiopulmonary bypass. *J Surg Res.* 1965;5:283–284.
48. Spencer MP, Lawrence GH, Thomas GI, Sauvage LR. The use of ultrasonics in the determination of arterial aeroembolism during open-heart surgery. *Ann Thorac Surg.* 1969;8:489–497.
49. Padayachee TS et al. The detection of microemboli in the middle cerebral artery during cardiopulmonary bypass: a transcranial Doppler ultrasound investigation using membrane and bubble oxygenators. *Ann Thorac Surg.* 1987;44:298–302.
50. Georgiadis D, Grosset DG, Kelman A, Faichney A, Lees KR. Prevalence and characteristics of intracranial microemboli signals in patients with different types of prosthetic cardiac valves. *Stroke.* 1994;25:587–592.
51. Markus HS, Droste DW, Brown MM. Detection of asymptomatic cerebral embolic signals with Doppler ultrasound. *Lancet.* 1994;343:1011–1012.
52. Droste DW et al. Oxygen inhalation can differentiate gaseous from nongaseous microemboli detected by transcranial Doppler ultrasound. *Stroke.* 1997;28:2453–2456.
53. Georgiadis D et al. Influence of oxygen ventilation on Doppler microemboli signals in patients with artificial heart valves. *Stroke.* 1997;28:2189–2194.
54. Kaps M et al. Clinically silent microemboli in patients with artificial prosthetic aortic valves are predominantly gaseous and not solid. *Stroke.* 1997;28:322–325.
55. Skjelland M et al. Solid cerebral microemboli and cerebrovascular symptoms in patients with prosthetic heart valves. *Stroke.* 2008;39:1159–1164.
56. Padayachee TS, Gosling RG, Bishop CC, Burnand K, Browse NL. Monitoring middle cerebral artery blood velocity during carotid endarterectomy. *Br J Surg.* 1986;73:98–100.
57. Spencer MP, Thomas GI, Nicholls SC, Sauvage LR. Detection of middle cerebral artery emboli during carotid endarterectomy using transcranial Doppler ultrasonography. *Stroke.* 1990;21:415–423.
58. Russell D, Madden KP, Clark WM, Sandset PM, Zivin JA. Detection of arterial emboli using Doppler ultrasound in rabbits. *Stroke.* 1991;22:253–258.
59. Markus H, Loh A, Brown MM. Detection of circulating cerebral emboli using Doppler ultrasound in a sheep model. *J Neurol Sci.* 1994;122:117–124.
60. Consensus Committee NICHS. Basic identification criteria of Doppler microembolic signals. *Stroke.* 1995;26:1123.
61. Molloy J, Markus HS. Multigated Doppler ultrasound in the detection of emboli in a flow model and embolic signals in patients. *Stroke.* 1996;27:1548–1552.
62. Moehring MA, Spencer MP. Power M-mode Doppler (PMD) for observing cerebral blood flow and tracking emboli. *Ultrasound Med Biol.* 2002;28:49–57.
63. Saqqur M et al. Improved detection of microbubble signals using power M-mode Doppler. *Stroke.* 2004;35:e14–e17.
64. Markus HS, Molloy J. Use of a decibel threshold in detecting Doppler embolic signals. *Stroke.* 1997;28:692–695.
65. Markus HS et al. Intercenter agreement in reading Doppler embolic signals. A multicenter international study. *Stroke.* 1997;28:1307–1310.
66. Van Zuilen EV et al. Automatic embolus detection compared with human experts. A Doppler ultrasound study. *Stroke.* 1996;27:1840–1843.
67. Cullinane M, Kaposzta Z, Reihill S, Markus HS. Online automated detection of cerebral embolic signals from a variety of embolic sources. *Ultrasound Med Biol.* 2002;28:1271–1277.
68. Steegmann AT, De La Fuente J. Experimental cerebral embolism. II. Microembolism of the rabbit brain with seran polymer resin. *J Neuropathol Exp Neurol.* 1959;18:537–558.
69. Luessenhop AJ, Gibbs M, Velasquez AC. Cerebrovascular response to emboli. Observations in patients with arteriovenous malformations. *Arch Neurol.* 1962;7:264–274.
70. Winding O. Cerebral microembolization following carotid injection of dextran microspheres in rabbits. *Neuroradiology.* 1981;21:123–126.
71. Gaunt ME, Naylor AR, Bell PR. Preventing strokes associated with carotid endarterectomy: detection of embolisation by transcranial Doppler monitoring. *Eur J Vasc Endovasc Surg.* 1997;14:1–3.
72. Muth CM, Shank ES. Gas embolism. *N Engl J Med.* 2000;342:476–482.
73. Rapp JH et al. Microemboli composed of cholesterol crystals disrupt the blood-brain barrier and reduce cognition. *Stroke.* 2008;39:2354–2361.
74. Smith JL, Evans DH, Bell PR, Naylor AR. A comparison of four methods for distinguishing Doppler signals from gaseous and particulate emboli. *Stroke.* 1998;29:1133–1138.
75. Russell D, Brucher R. Online automatic discrimination between solid and gaseous cerebral microemboli with the first multifrequency transcranial Doppler. *Stroke.* 2002;33:1975–1980.
76. Murphy BP, Harford FJ, Cramer FS. Cerebral air embolism resulting from invasive medical procedures. Treatment with hyperbaric oxygen. *Ann Surg.* 1985;201:242–245.
77. Wijman CA, Kase CS, Jacobs AK, Whitehead RE. Cerebral air embolism as a cause of stroke during cardiac catheterization. *Neurology.* 1998;51:318–319.
78. Ackerstaff RG et al. Prediction of early cerebral outcome by transcranial Doppler monitoring in carotid bifurcation angioplasty and stenting. *J Vasc Surg.* 2005;41:618–624.
79. Kelly GL, Dodi G, Eiseman B. Ultrasound detection of fat emboli. *Surg Forum.* 1972;23:459–461.
80. Sylivris S et al. Pattern and significance of cerebral microemboli during coronary artery bypass grafting. *Ann Thorac Surg.* 1998;66:1674–1678.
81. Bellapart J, Fraser JF. Transcranial Doppler assessment of cerebral autoregulation. *Ultrasound Med Biol.* 2009;35:883–893.
82. Aaslid R, Lindegaard KF, Sorteberg W, Nornes H. Cerebral autoregulation dynamics in humans. *Stroke.* 1989;20:45–52.
83. Widder B, Paulat K, Hackspacher J, Mayr E. Transcranial Doppler CO_2 test for the detection of hemodynamically critical carotid artery stenoses and occlusions. *Eur Arch Psychiatry Neurol Sci.* 1986;236:162–168.

84. Hartl WH, Furst H. Application of transcranial Doppler sonography to evaluate cerebral hemodynamics in carotid artery disease. Comparative analysis of different hemodynamic variables. *Stroke*. 1995;26:2293–2297.
85. Muller M, Voges M, Piepgras U, Schimrigk K. Assessment of cerebral vasomotor reactivity by transcranial Doppler ultrasound and breath-holding. A comparison with acetazolamide as vasodilatory stimulus. *Stroke*. 1995;26:96–100.
86. Rohrberg M, Brodhun R. Measurement of vasomotor reserve in the transcranial Doppler-CO(2) test using an ultrasound contrast agent (Levovist). *Stroke*. 2001;32:1298–1303.
87. Pindzola RR, Balzer JR, Nemoto EM, Goldstein S, Yonas H. Cerebrovascular reserve in patients with carotid occlusive disease assessed by stable xenon-enhanced ct cerebral blood flow and transcranial Doppler. *Stroke*. 2001;32:1811–1817.
88. Rothwell PM et al. Analysis of pooled data from the randomised controlled trials of endarterectomy for symptomatic carotid stenosis. *Lancet*. 2003;361:107–116.
89. Abbott A, Bladin C, Levi C, Chambers BR. What should we do with asymptomatic carotid stenosis? *Int J Stroke*. 2007;2:27–39.
90. Caplan L. Clinical diagnosis of brain embolism. *Cerebrovasc Dis*. 1995;5:79–88.
91. Nicolaides AN et al. Angiographic and duplex grading of internal carotid stenosis: can we overcome the confusion? *J Endovasc Surg*. 1996;3:158–165.
92. Inzitari D et al. The causes and risk of stroke in patients with asymptomatic internal-carotid-artery stenosis. North American Symptomatic Carotid Endarterectomy Trial Collaborators. *N Engl J Med*. 2000;342:1693–1700.
93. MRC European Carotid Surgery Trial. Interim results for symptomatic patients with severe (70–99%) or with mild (0–29%) carotid stenosis. European Carotid Surgery Trialists' Collaborative Group. *Lancet*. 1991;337:1235–1243.
94. Johnston SC, Gress DR, Browner WS, Browner WS, Sidney S. Short-term prognosis after emergency department diagnosis of TIA. *JAMA*. 2000;284:2901–2906.
95. Rothwell PM et al. Endarterectomy for symptomatic carotid stenosis in relation to clinical subgroups and timing of surgery. *Lancet*. 2004;363:915–924.
96. Coull AJ, Lovett JK, Rothwell PM. Population based study of early risk of stroke after transient ischaemic attack or minor stroke: implications for public education and organisation of services. *BMJ*. 2004;328:326.
97. Valton L, Larrue V, le Traon AP, Massabuau P, Géraud G. Microembolic signals and risk of early recurrence in patients with stroke or transient ischemic attack. *Stroke*. 1998;29:2125–2128.
98. Gucuyener D, Uzuner N, Ozkan S, Ozdemir O, Ozdemir G. Micro embolic signals in patients with cerebral ischaemic events. *Neurol India*. 2001;49:225–230.
99. Tegos TJ et al. Correlates of embolic events detected by means of transcranial Doppler in patients with carotid atheroma. *J Vasc Surg*. 2001;33:131–138.
100. Siebler M, Kleinschmidt A, Sitzer M, Steinmetz H, Freund HJ. Cerebral microembolism in symptomatic and asymptomatic high-grade internal carotid artery stenosis. *Neurology*. 1994;44:615–618.
101. Babikian VL, Hyde C, Pochay V, Winter MR. Clinical correlates of high-intensity transient signals detected on transcranial Doppler sonography in patients with cerebrovascular disease. *Stroke*. 1994;25:1570–1573.
102. Ries S, Schminke U, Daffertshofer M, Schindlmayr C, Hennerici M. High intensity transient signals and carotid artery disease. *Cerebrovasc Dis*. 1995;5:124–127.
103. Sitzer M, Siebler M, Steinmetz H. Silent emboli and their relation to clinical symptoms in extracranial carotid artery disease. *Cerebrovasc Dis*. 1995;5:121–123.
104. Markus HS, Thomson ND, Brown MM. Asymptomatic cerebral embolic signals in symptomatic and asymptomatic carotid artery disease. *Brain*. 1995;118(pt 4):1005–1011.
105. Droste DW, Dittrich R, Kemény V, Schulte-Altedorneburg G, Ringelstein EB. Prevalence and frequency of microembolic signals in 105 patients with extracranial carotid artery occlusive disease. *J Neurol Neurosurg Psychiatry*. 1999;67:525–528.
106. Telman G et al. Determinants of micro-embolic signals in patients with atherosclerotic plaques of the internal carotid artery. *Eur J Vasc Endovasc Surg*. 2009;38:143–147.
107. Siebler M, Sitzer M, Steinmetz H. Detection of intracranial emboli in patients with symptomatic extracranial carotid artery disease. *Stroke*. 1992;23:1652–1654.
108. Georgiadis D et al. Detection of intracranial emboli in patients with carotid disease. *Eur J Vasc Surg*. 1994;8:309–314.
109. Eicke BM, von Lorentz J, Paulus W. Embolus detection in different degrees of carotid disease. *Neurol Res*. 1995;17:181–184.
110. Blaser T et al. Time period required for transcranial Doppler monitoring of embolic signals to predict recurrent risk of embolic transient ischemic attack and stroke from arterial stenosis. *Stroke*. 2004;35:2155–2159.
111. Abbott AL et al. Embolic signals and prediction of ipsilateral stroke or transient ischemic attack in asymptomatic carotid stenosis: a multicenter prospective cohort study. *Stroke*. 2005;36:1128–1133.
112. Orlandi G, Parenti G, Bertolucci A, Murri L. Silent cerebral microembolism in asymptomatic and symptomatic carotid artery stenoses of low and high degree. *Eur Neurol*. 1997;38:39–43.
113. Forteza AM, Babikian VL, Hyde C, Winter M, Pochay V. Effect of time and cerebrovascular symptoms of the prevalence of microembolic signals in patients with cervical carotid stenosis. *Stroke*. 1996;27:687–690.
114. Wijman CA et al. Cerebral microembolism in patients with retinal ischemia. *Stroke*. 1998;29:1139–1143.
115. Censori B, Partziguian T, Casto L, Camerlingo M, Mamoli A. Doppler microembolic signals predict ischemic recurrences in symptomatic carotid stenosis. *Acta Neurol Scand*. 2000;101:327–331.
116. Markus HS, MacKinnon A. Asymptomatic embolization detected by Doppler ultrasound predicts stroke risk in symptomatic carotid artery stenosis. *Stroke*. 2005;36:971–975.
117. Zuromskis T et al. Prevalence of micro-emboli in symptomatic high grade carotid artery disease: a transcranial

Doppler study. *Eur J Vasc Endovasc Surg.* 2008;35: 534–540.
118. Orlandi G et al. Carotid plaque features on angiography and asymptomatic cerebral microembolism. *Acta Neurol Scand.* 1997;96:183–186.
119. Goertler M et al. Reduced frequency of embolic signals in severe carotid stenosis with poststenotic flow velocity reduction. *Cerebrovasc Dis.* 2005;19:229–233.
120. Spence JD et al. Effects of intensive medical therapy on microemboli and cardiovascular risk in asymptomatic carotid stenosis. *Arch Neurol.* 2010;67(2):180–186.
121. Rothwell PM, Warlow CP. Low risk of ischemic stroke in patients with reduced internal carotid artery lumen diameter distal to severe symptomatic carotid stenosis: cerebral protection due to low poststenotic flow? On behalf of the European carotid surgery trialists' collaborative group. *Stroke.* 2000;31:622–630.
122. Georgiadis D et al. Intracranial microembolic signals in 500 patients with potential cardiac or carotid embolic source and in normal controls. *Stroke.* 1997;28:1203–1207.
123. Siebler M, Sitzer M, Rose G, Bendfeldt D, Steinmetz H. Silent cerebral embolism caused by neurologically symptomatic high-grade carotid stenosis. Event rates before and after carotid endarterectomy. *Brain.* 1993;116(pt 5): 1005–1015.
124. van Zuilen EV et al. Detection of cerebral microemboli by means of transcranial Doppler monitoring before and after carotid endarterectomy. *Stroke.* 1995;26:210–213.
125. Kimura K et al. High intensity transient signals in patients with carotid stenosis may persist after carotid endarterectomy. *Cerebrovasc Dis.* 2004;17:123–127.
126. Khaffaf N, Karnik R, Winkler WB, Valentin A, Slany J. Embolic stroke by compression maneuver during transcranial Doppler sonography. *Stroke.* 1994;25:1056–1057.
127. Valton L, Larrue V, Arrué P, Géraud G, Bès A. Asymptomatic cerebral embolic signals in patients with carotid stenosis. Correlation with appearance of plaque ulceration on angiography. *Stroke.* 1995;26:813–815.
128. Rothwell PM, Gibson R, Warlow CP. Interrelation between plaque surface morphology and degree of stenosis on carotid angiograms and the risk of ischemic stroke in patients with symptomatic carotid stenosis. On behalf of the European Carotid Surgery Trialists' Collaborative Group. *Stroke.* 2000;31:615–621.
129. Sitzer M et al. Plaque ulceration and lumen thrombus are the main sources of cerebral microemboli in high-grade internal carotid artery stenosis. *Stroke.* 1995;26: 1231–1233.
130. Siebler M et al. Cerebral microembolism and the risk of ischemia in asymptomatic high-grade internal carotid artery stenosis. *Stroke.* 1995;26:2184–2186.
131. Orlandi G, Fanucchi S, Sartucci F, Murri L. Can microembolic signals identify unstable plaques affecting symptomatology in carotid stenosis? *Stroke.* 2002;33: 1744–1746, author reply 1744–1746.
132. Spence JD, Tamayo A, Lownie SP, Ng WP, Ferguson GG. Absence of microemboli on transcranial Doppler identifies low-risk patients with asymptomatic carotid stenosis. *Stroke.* 2005;36:2373–2378.
133. Markus HS et al. Asymptomatic embolisation for prediction of stroke in the asymptomatic carotid emboli study (ACES): a prospective observational study. *Lancet Neurol.* 2010;9:663–671.
134. Abbott AL. Medical (nonsurgical) intervention alone is now best for prevention of stroke associated with asymptomatic severe carotid stenosis: results of a systematic review and analysis. *Stroke.* 2009;40:e573-e583.
135. Marquardt L, Geraghty OC, Mehta Z, Rothwell PM. Low risk of ipsilateral stroke in patients with asymptomatic carotid stenosis on best medical treatment. A prospective, population-based study. *Stroke.* 2010;41(1):e11-e17.
136. Silvestrini M et al. Impaired cerebral vasoreactivity and risk of stroke in patients with asymptomatic carotid artery stenosis. *JAMA.* 2000;283:2122–2127.
137. Markus H, Cullinane M. Severely impaired cerebrovascular reactivity predicts stroke and TIA risk in patients with carotid artery stenosis and occlusion. *Brain.* 2001;124:457–467.
138. Kaps M, Dorndorf W, Damian MS, Agnoli L. Intracranial haemodynamics in patients with spontaneous carotid dissection. Transcranial Doppler ultrasound follow-up studies. *Eur Arch Psychiatry Neurol Sci.* 1990;239:246–256.
139. Achtereekte HA, van der Kruijk RA, Hekster RE, Keunen RW. Diagnosis of traumatic carotid artery dissection by transcranial Doppler ultrasound: case report and review of the literature. *Surg Neurol.* 1994;42:240–244.
140. Srinivasan J, Newell DW, Sturzenegger M, Mayberg MR, Winn HR. Transcranial Doppler in the evaluation of internal carotid artery dissection. *Stroke.* 1996;27:1226–1230.
141. Molina CA et al. Cerebral microembolism in acute spontaneous internal carotid artery dissection. *Neurology.* 2000;55:1738–1740.
142. Roy J, Akhtar N, Watson T, Demchuk AM, Saqqur M. Transcranial Doppler microembolic signal monitoring is useful in diagnosis and treatment of carotid artery dissection: two case reports. *J Neuroimaging.* 2007;17: 350–352.
143. Lucas C, Moulin T, Deplanque D, Tatu L, Chavot D. Stroke patterns of internal carotid artery dissection in 40 patients [see comments]. *Stroke.* 1998;29:2646–2648.
144. Lyrer P, Engelter S. Antithrombotic drugs for carotid artery dissection. *Cochrane Database Syst Rev.* 2003; CD000255.
145. Brunser AM et al. Accuracy of transcranial Doppler compared with ct angiography in diagnosing arterial obstructions in acute ischemic strokes. *Stroke.* 2009;40:2037–2041.
146. Demchuk AM et al. Accuracy and criteria for localizing arterial occlusion with transcranial Doppler. *J Neuroimaging.* 2000;10:1–12.
147. Alexandrov AV, Demchuk AM, Burgin WS. Insonation method and diagnostic flow signatures for transcranial power motion (M-mode) Doppler. *J Neuroimaging.* 2002;12:236–244.
148. Mikulik R, Alexandrov AV. Acute stroke: therapeutic transcranial Doppler sonography. *Front Neurol Neurosci.* 2006;21:150–161.
149. Demchuk AM et al. Thrombolysis in brain ischemia (TIBI) transcranial Doppler flow grades predict clinical severity, early recovery, and mortality in patients treated with intravenous tissue plasminogen activator. *Stroke.* 2001;32:89–93.

150. Molina CA et al. Improving the predictive accuracy of recanalization on stroke outcome in patients treated with tissue plasminogen activator. *Stroke*. 2004;35:151–156.
151. Barreto AD et al. Safety and dose-escalation study design of transcranial ultrasound in clinical sonolysis for acute ischemic stroke: the TUCSON trial. *Int J Stroke*. 2009;4:42–48.
152. Alexandrov AV et al. Ultrasound-enhanced systemic thrombolysis for acute ischemic stroke. *N Engl J Med*. 2004;351:2170–2178.
153. Molina CA et al. Microbubble administration accelerates clot lysis during continuous 2-MHz ultrasound monitoring in stroke patients treated with intravenous tissue plasminogen activator. *Stroke*. 2006;37:425–429.
154. Ferguson GG et al. The North American Symptomatic Carotid Endarterectomy Trial: surgical results in 1415 patients. *Stroke*. 1999;30:1751–1758.
155. Riles TS et al. The cause of perioperative stroke after carotid endarterectomy. *J Vasc Surg*. 1994;19:206–214, discussion 215–206.
156. Lennard N et al. Prevention of postoperative thrombotic stroke after carotid endarterectomy: the role of transcranial Doppler ultrasound. *J Vasc Surg*. 1997;26:579–584.
157. Spencer MP. Transcranial Doppler monitoring and causes of stroke from carotid endarterectomy. *Stroke*. 1997;28:685–691.
158. de Borst GJ et al. Stroke from carotid endarterectomy: when and how to reduce perioperative stroke rate? *Eur J Vasc Endovasc Surg*. 2001;21:484–489.
159. Gaunt ME. Diagnosis of early postoperative carotid artery thrombosis determined by transcranial Doppler scanning. *J Vasc Surg*. 1994;20:1004–1006.
160. Gossetti B, Martinelli O, Guerricchio R, Irace L, Benedetti-Valentini F. Transcranial Doppler in 178 patients before, during, and after carotid endarterectomy. *J Neuroimaging*. 1997;7:213–216.
161. Feuerstein G, Wang X, Barone FC. Cytokines in brain ischemia – the role of TNF alpha. *Cell Mol Neurobiol*. 1998;18:695–701.
162. Dalman JE, Beenakkers IC, Moll FL, Leusink JA, Ackerstaff RG. Transcranial Doppler monitoring during carotid endarterectomy helps to identify patients at risk of postoperative hyperperfusion. *Eur J Vasc Endovasc Surg*. 1999;18:222–227.
163. Naylor AR et al. Reducing the risk of carotid surgery: a 7-year audit of the role of monitoring and quality control assessment. *J Vasc Surg*. 2000;32:750–759.
164. Ackerstaff RG et al. Association of intraoperative transcranial Doppler monitoring variables with stroke from carotid endarterectomy. *Stroke*. 2000;31:1817–1823.
165. Golledge J et al. Determinants of carotid microembolization. *J Vasc Surg*. 2001;34:1060–1064.
166. Wolf O et al. Microembolic signals detected by transcranial Doppler sonography during carotid endarterectomy and correlation with serial diffusion-weighted imaging. *Stroke*. 2004;35:e373-e375.
167. Skjelland M et al. Cerebral microemboli and brain injury during carotid artery endarterectomy and stenting. *Stroke*. 2009;40:230–234.
168. Ogasawara K et al. Intraoperative microemboli and low middle cerebral artery blood flow velocity are additive in predicting development of cerebral ischemic events after carotid endarterectomy. *Stroke*. 2008;39:3088–3091.
169. Jansen C et al. Impact of microembolism and hemodynamic changes in the brain during carotid endarterectomy. *Stroke*. 1994;25:992–997.
170. Laman DM, Wieneke GH, van Duijn H, van Huffelen AC. High embolic rate early after carotid endarterectomy is associated with early cerebrovascular complications, especially in women. *J Vasc Surg*. 2002;36:278–284.
171. Müller M, Behnke S, Walter P, Omlor G, Schimrigk K. Microembolic signals and intraoperative stroke in carotid endarterectomy. *Acta Neurol Scand*. 1998;97:110–117.
172. Cantelmo NL et al. Cerebral microembolism and ischemic changes associated with carotid endarterectomy. *J Vasc Surg*. 1998;27:1024–1030, discussion 1030–1021.
173. Horn J et al. Identification of patients at risk for ischaemic cerebral complications after carotid endarterectomy with TCD monitoring. *Eur J Vasc Endovasc Surg*. 2005;30:270–274.
174. Abbott AL, Levi CR, Stork JL, Donnan GA, Chambers BR. Timing of clinically significant microembolism after carotid endarterectomy. *Cerebrovasc Dis*. 2007;23:362–367.
175. Levi CR et al. Dextran reduces embolic signals after carotid endarterectomy. *Ann Neurol*. 2001;50:544–547.
176. van der Schaaf IC, Horn J, Moll FL, Ackerstaff RG, Antonius Carotid Endarterectomy Angioplasty and Stenting Study Group. Transcranial Doppler monitoring after carotid endarterectomy. *Ann Vasc Surg*. 2005;19:19–24.
177. Stork JL, Levi CR, Chambers BR, Abbott AL, Donnan GA. Possible determinants of early microembolism after carotid endarterectomy. *Stroke*. 2002;33:2082–2085.
178. Munts AG, Mess WH, Bruggemans EF, Walda L, Ackerstaff RG. Feasibility and reliability of on-line automated microemboli detection after carotid endarterectomy. A transcranial Doppler study. *Eur J Vasc Endovasc Surg*. 2003;25:262–266.
179. Orlandi G et al. Impaired clearance of microemboli and cerebrovascular symptoms during carotid stenting procedures. *Arch Neurol*. 2005;62:1208–1211.
180. Caplan LR, Hennerici M. Impaired clearance of emboli (washout) is an important link between hypoperfusion, embolism, and ischemic stroke. *Arch Neurol*. 1998;55:1475–1482.
181. Bernstein M, Fleming JF, Deck JH. Cerebral hyperperfusion after carotid endarterectomy: a cause of cerebral hemorrhage. *Neurosurgery*. 1984;15:50–56.
182. Mansoor GA, White WB, Grunnet M, Ruby ST. Intracerebral hemorrhage after carotid endarterectomy associated with ipsilateral fibrinoid necrosis: a consequence of the hyperperfusion syndrome? *J Vasc Surg*. 1996;23:147–151.
183. van Mook WN et al. Cerebral hyperperfusion syndrome. *Lancet Neurol*. 2005;4:877–888.
184. Wagner WH, Cossman DV, Farber A, Levin PM, Cohen JL. Hyperperfusion syndrome after carotid endarterectomy. *Ann Vasc Surg*. 2005;19:479–486.
185. Nyamekye IK, Begum S, Slaney PL. Post-carotid endarterectomy cerebral hyperperfusion syndrome. *J R Soc Med*. 2005;98:472–474.

186. Keunen R et al. An observational study of pre-operative transcranial Doppler examinations to predict cerebral hyperperfusion following carotid endarterectomies. *Neurol Res.* 2001;23:593–598.
187. Naylor AR et al. Factors influencing the hyperaemic response after carotid endarterectomy. *Br J Surg.* 1993;80:1523–1527.
188. Powers AD, Smith RR. Hyperperfusion syndrome after carotid endarterectomy: a transcranial Doppler evaluation. *Neurosurgery.* 1990;26:56–59, discussion 59–60.
189. Jorgensen LG, Schroeder TV. Defective cerebrovascular autoregulation after carotid endarterectomy. *Eur J Vasc Surg.* 1993;7:370–379.
190. Jansen C et al. Prediction of intracerebral haemorrhage after carotid endarterectomy by clinical criteria and intraoperative transcranial Doppler monitoring. *Eur J Vasc Surg.* 1994;8:303–308.
191. Fujimoto S et al. Diagnostic impact of transcranial color-coded real-time sonography with echo contrast agents for hyperperfusion syndrome after carotid endarterectomy. *Stroke.* 2004;35:1852–1856.
192. Ogasawara K et al. Cerebral hyperperfusion following carotid endarterectomy: diagnostic utility of intra-operative transcranial Doppler ultrasonography compared with single-photon emission computed tomography study. *AJNR Am J Neuroradiol.* 2005;26:252–257.
193. Markus HS, Harrison MJ, Adiseshiah M. Carotid endarterectomy improves haemodynamics on the contralateral side: implications for operating contralateral to an occluded carotid artery. *Br J Surg.* 1993;80:170–172.
194. Hartl WH, Janssen I, Furst H. Effect of carotid endarterectomy on patterns of cerebrovascular reactivity in patients with unilateral carotid artery stenosis. *Stroke.* 1994;25:1952–1957.
195. Vriens EM et al. Flow redistribution in the major cerebral arteries after carotid endarterectomy: a study with transcranial Doppler scan. *J Vasc Surg.* 2001;33:139–147.
196. Markus HS, Clifton A, Buckenham T, Brown MM. Carotid angioplasty. Detection of embolic signals during and after the procedure. *Stroke.* 1994;25:2403–2406.
197. Jordan WD Jr et al. Microemboli detected by transcranial Doppler monitoring in patients during carotid angioplasty versus carotid endarterectomy. *Cardiovasc Surg.* 1999;7:33–38.
198. Marder VJ et al. Analysis of thrombi retrieved from cerebral arteries of patients with acute ischemic stroke. *Stroke.* 2006;37:2086–2093.
199. Markus HS et al. Dual antiplatelet therapy with clopidogrel and aspirin in symptomatic carotid stenosis evaluated using Doppler embolic signal detection: the Clopidogrel and Aspirin for Reduction of Emboli in Symptomatic Carotid Stenosis (CARESS) trial. *Circulation.* 2005;111:2233–2240.
200. Goertler M et al. Rapid decline of cerebral microemboli of arterial origin after intravenous acetylsalicylic acid. *Stroke.* 1999;30:66–69.
201. van Dellen D et al. Transcranial Doppler ultrasonography-directed intravenous glycoprotein IIb/IIIa receptor antagonist therapy to control transient cerebral microemboli before and after carotid endarterectomy. *Br J Surg.* 2008;95:709–713.
202. Junghans U, Siebler M. Cerebral microembolism is blocked by tirofiban, a selective nonpeptide platelet glycoprotein IIb/IIIa receptor antagonist. *Circulation.* 2003;107:2717–2721.
203. Goertler M, Blaser T, Krueger S, Lutze G, Wallesch CW. Acetylsalicylic acid and microembolic events detected by transcranial Doppler in symptomatic arterial stenoses. *Cerebrovasc Dis.* 2001;11:324–329.
204. Payne DA et al. Beneficial effects of clopidogrel combined with aspirin in reducing cerebral emboli in patients undergoing carotid endarterectomy. *Circulation.* 2004;109:1476–1481.
205. Kaposzta Z et al. L-arginine and S-nitrosoglutathione reduce embolization in humans. *Circulation.* 2001;103:2371–2375.
206. Molloy J, Martin JF, Baskerville PA, Fraser SC, Markus HS. S-nitrosoglutathione reduces the rate of embolization in humans. *Circulation.* 1998;98:1372–1375.
207. Kaposzta Z, Clifton A, Molloy J, Martin JF, Markus HS. S-nitrosoglutathione reduces asymptomatic embolization after carotid angioplasty. *Circulation.* 2002;106:3057–3062.
208. Meseguer E et al. Prevalence of embolic signals in acute coronary syndromes. *Stroke.* 2010;41:261–266.
209. Rothwell PM et al. Change in stroke incidence, mortality, case-fatality, severity, and risk factors in Oxfordshire, UK from 1981 to 2004 (Oxford Vascular Study). *Lancet.* 2004;363:1925–1933.
210. Unal B, Critchley JA, Fidan D, Capewell S. Life-years gained from modern cardiological treatments and population risk factor changes in England and Wales, 1981–2000. *Am J Public Health.* 2005;95:103–108.
211. King A, Markus HS. Doppler embolic signals in cerebrovascular disease and prediction of stroke risk: a systematic review and meta-analysis. *Stroke.* 2009;40:3711–3717.

Effect of Statin Therapy on Carotid Plaque Morphology

Gregory C. Makris, Andrew Nicolaides, Anthi Lavida, and George Geroulakos

35.1 Introduction

The predictive ability of intima-media thickness (IMT) and plaque measurements for future cardiovascular events has been discussed in Chaps. 22–26. It has been demonstrated that carotid plaque size (thickness, area, volume) is a stronger predictor of cardiovascular risk than IMT when the latter is measured in the common carotid artery (IMTcc). It has also been shown that the presence of plaque is the main component associated with clinical cardiovascular disease[1] and cardiovascular risk in measurements of IMT (mean or maximum) (Chaps. 23–25). This is because measurements of IMT (mean or maximum) are performed at multiple sites of the carotid bifurcation that involves the carotid bulb and internal carotid artery where atherosclerotic plaques often occur.

Changes in plaque size during progression (or regression in response to therapy) are much larger than changes in IMT and therfore studies using plaque measurements require a smaller number of patients than studies which use IMT measurements (Chaps. 23–25). In an attempt to overcome this problem of small changes, some studies investigating the effect of statins on IMT have excluded patients or individuals with normal IMT (IMT < 1.2 mm in the Measuring Effects on intima media Thickness: an Evaluation of Rosuvastatin (METEOR) trials[2] and IMT < 1.3 mm in the Pravastatin, Lipids, and Atherosclerosis in the Carotid arteries (PLAC-II) trials).[3] This is because it was unlikely to be able to detect the small changes of regression, if any, that may occur in a normal IMT as a result of therapy but more likely to detect changes in a thick IMT which implies the presence of plaque. The different response of IMT and plaques to different medical therapies is not surprising because IMT and plaque have different biological determinants (Chaps. 23, 25, and 28).

Hypoechoic (echolucent) plaques which are considered to be unstable (Chaps. 12, 23, 24, and 31) tend to grow faster (Chap. 24) and have a stronger association with future coronary events[4,5] than hyperechoic (echogenic) plaques (Chaps. 23 and 24) which have a high collagen or calcium content and a small lipid core. Increasing echolucency of carotid artery plaques within a 6–9-month interval is also predictive of clinical cardiovascular events.[6]

The effect of statin therapy on carotid IMT has been demonstrated in a large number of randomized, placebo-controlled studies [Asymptomatic Carotid Atherosclerosis Progression Study (ACAPS),[7] Kuopio Atherosclerosis Prevention Study (KAPS),[8] PLAC-2[3], Carotid Atherosclerosis Italian Ultrasound Study (CAIUS),[9] Regression Growth Evaluation Statin Study (REGRESS),[10] Beta-Blocker Cholesterol-Lowering Asymptomatic Plaque Study (BCAPS),[11] Fukuoka Atherosclerosis Trial (FAST),[12] METEOR[2]].

G.C. Makris
Division of Vascular Surgery, Imperial College of London, London, UK

A. Nicolaides (✉)
Imperial College and Vascular Screening and Diagnostic Centre, London, UK

A. Lavida
Department of Vascular Surgery, Ealing Hospital/Imperial College London, Southall, Middlesex, UK

G. Geroulakos
Department of Surgery, Charing Cross Hospital, London, UK

A meta-analysis of seven such studies involving 3,034 individuals published in 2005[13] has demonstrated that statins reduce IMT by 0.012 mm/year (95% confidence interval [CI] 0.016–0.007) with an associated reduction in clinical cardiovascular events (odds ratio [OR] 0.48; 95% CI 0.30–0.78).

The effect of statin therapy on coronary artery atherosclerotic plaque volume has been demonstrated by several studies using intravascular ultrasound (IVUS).[14] The more intensive the therapy, the greater was the plaque volume reduction. In the ASTEROID (A Study to Evaluate the Effect of Rosuvastatin on Intravascular Ultrasound-Derived Coronary Atheroma Burden) trial which involved 349 patients[15] and in which low-density lipoprotein (LDL) cholesterol decreased from baseline 130.4 ± 34.3 to 60.8 ± 20.0 mg/dL using rosuvastatin 40 mg daily, the mean atheroma volume change in the most diseased 10-mm segment at 24 months was -6.1 (± 10.1) mm^3 with a median of -5.6 mm^3 (97.5% CI -6.8 to -4.0) ($P < 0.001$).

In one study, patients with stable angina were randomized to pravastatin (20 mg/day), atorvastatin (20 mg/day) or diet.[16] Integrated backscatter values from coronary plaques using IVUS were color-coded, and a three-dimensional (3D) reconstruction of the color-coded map was performed by computer software as a means of quantitative tissue characterization of plaque composition (virtual histology). Statin therapy reduced the lipid component and increased fibrous volume without reducing the degree of stenosis.

A number of studies using repeat magnetic resonance imaging (MRI) have demonstrated reduced rates of carotid plaque progression,[17,18] regression in plaque volume[19] or reduction in lipid core volume.[20–22] Useful information on atherosclerotic plaque composition and behavior has been provided by MRI. However, MRI is relatively expensive and time consuming with a limitation on the number of patients that can be studied in a day. The question therefore is whether ultrasound can provide similar information. The aim of this chapter is to review the available studies investigating the effect of statin therapy on carotid plaque size and texture using ultrasound.

35.2 Effect of Statins on Plaque Size

35.2.1 Plaque Thickness

Two studies using ultrasound have demonstrated the reduction in plaque thickness.

One of the early studies performed in 2001 by Kurata et al.[23] showed that cerivastatin administered to five patients for 12 months produced a reduction in mean maximum carotid plaque thickness from baseline 3.7 ± 0.9 mm to 3.0 ± 0.7 mm. It was also observed that the fibrous matrix of the plaque increased significantly.

In a more recent study by Yamagami et al.,[24] 81 hypercholesterolemic patients with carotid plaques were randomized to statin therapy (simvastatin 10 mg/day, $n = 24$ or atorvastatin 5 mg/day, $n = 16$ depending on physician choice) or diet only ($n = 41$). All patients underwent dietary modification. In the statin group, at 12 months, there was a reduction in plaque thickness of -0.22 ± 0.34 mm vs 0.02 ± 0.44 mm in the diet only group ($P = 0.008$). There was an associated increase in plaque echogenicity in the statin group as measured by integrated backscatter (IBS) (see below).

35.2.2 Plaque Area

In a cohort of 468 patients with asymptomatic carotid stenosis, 199 were enrolled in the years 2000–2002 and 269 during 2003–2007. The authors compared (a) the proportion of patients who had microemboli on transcranial Doppler (TCD), (b) clinical cardiovascular events, (c) the rate of carotid plaque progression, and (d) baseline medical therapy, before and since 2003.[25] Before 2003, microemboli were present in 12.6% of patients, and 17.6% of patients had stroke, myocardial infarction, carotid endarterectomy for symptoms or died. After 2003, microemboli were present in only 3.7% of patients, and only 5.6% of patients had stroke, myocardial infarction, carotid endarterectomy for symptoms or died. The rate of plaque progression in the first year of follow-up was 69 ± 96 mm^2 in those recruited before 2003 and 23 ± 86 mm^2 in those recruited after 2003 ($P < 0.001$). The decline in microemboli coincided with better control of plasma lipids and slower progression of carotid plaque area.

35.2.3 Plaque Volume Changes Using 3D Ultrasound

Two studies have assessed plaque progression with 3D ultrasound under statin therapy.

The first was a study in 23 patients with 31 carotid plaques followed up for 15.1 ± 4.5 months.[26] Sixteen of the patients were treated with statins. Quantitative measurements of carotid artery plaque volumes were performed after 3D reconstruction of parallel transverse duplex ultrasound scans (slice distance = 0.1 mm) into volumetric 3D data sets and segmentation of voxels representing the carotid plaque. In the treatment group, plaques progressed less frequently (11%, $n = 9$ vs 64%, $n = 14$; $P = 0.016$) if they were hypoechoic or if the baseline total cholesterol was higher than 8.0 mmol/L (9%, $n = 11$ vs 75%, $n = 12$; $P = 0.002$). This study established the feasibility of 3D volume changes in assessing the effect of statin therapy on plaque progression.

The second study was a double-blind, randomized, placebo-controlled pilot study in 38 patients with greater than 60% internal carotid stenosis.[27] It was designed to determine the magnitude of quantitative changes and thus calculate the sample size needed to detect the effects of treatment using 3D ultrasound. Seventeen patients were assigned to atorvastatin 80 mg daily and 21 to placebo. 3D plaque volume was measured at baseline and after 3 months. The method of 3D reconstruction and volume measurements has been described in detail in Chap. 16, and the study has been summarized in Chap. 25. The mean rate of progression was 16.8 ± 74.1 mm^3 in the placebo group and −90.2 ± 85.1 mm^3 (regression) in the treatment group ($P < 0.0001$). The authors concluded that in view of the magnitude of the observed changes, sample sizes of 22 per group would be sufficient to show an effect change of 25% in 6 months. These numbers compare very favorably with the larger numbers needed when plaque thickness or area was measured and the extremely large numbers needed when IMT was measured.

35.3 Effect of Statins on Plaque Echogenicity

35.3.1 Grayscale Median

Three recent publications from the same group[28–30] have explored the effect and intensity of statin therapy on carotid plaque echogenicity using grayscale median (GSM) after image normalization.

The aim of the first study[28] was to assess whether intensive lipid-lowering treatment with atorvastatin improved GSM score and inhibited cardiovascular biomarkers including vascular calcification inhibitors such as osteopontin (OPN) and osteoprotegerin (OPG). Ninety-seven patients with carotid stenosis greater than 40% in relation to the distal internal carotid artery were treated to a target LDL cholesterol of less than 100 mg/dL for 6 months. Atorvastatin treatment improved lipid profile and reduced high sensitivity C-reactive protein (hsCRP) ($P = 0.002$), WBC count ($P = 0.041$), OPN ($P < 0.001$), and OPG levels ($P < 0.001$). Mean GSM increased from 58.3 ± 24.4 at baseline to 79.3 ± 22.3 ($P < 0.001$) at 6 months. GSM increase was related to OPN, OPG, and LDL reduction.

The second study[29] consisted of two groups of symptomatic patients. Patients in group A ($n = 46$) had a greater than 70% stenosis in relation to the distal internal carotid diameter and had ipsilateral carotid stenting but had a contralateral stenosis of 30–69%. Patients in group B ($n = 67$) had bilateral stenosis of 30–69%. Similar to the previous report,[27] all patients were treated to a target LDL cholesterol of less than 100 mg/dL for 6 months. GSM improved from baseline in both groups ($P < 0.01$), but the increase was more pronounced in group A ($P = 0.041$). There was an inverse linear relationship between GSM and serum changes in OPN, OPG, and LDL cholesterol.

The aim of the third study[30] was to test the hypothesis that 12-month aggressive lipid-lowering therapy with atorvastatin is more effective than moderate lipid lowering in increasing plaque echogenicity in patients with moderate carotid stenosis. One hundred and forty patients with 30–60% symptomatic and 30–70% asymptomatic stenosis were enrolled. Patients were randomized to moderate lipid-lowering therapy of atorvastatin 10–20 mg daily to target LDL cholesterol of less than 100 mg/dL (group A) or aggressive lipid-lowering therapy of atorvastatin 80 mg daily to target LDL cholesterol of less than 70 mg/dL (group B). GSM improved from baseline in both groups, but the increase was greater in group B (from 66.4 ± 23.7 to 100.4 ± 25.3) than in group A (from 64.4 ± 23.6 to 85.4 ± 20.2) ($P = 0.024$). There was no change in the degree of carotid stenosis in both treatment arms. The changes in serum biomarkers OPN and OPG were also more pronounced in group B.

These studies indicate that plaque stabilization by statins as previously known to occur in atherosclerotic animal models can now be demonstrated in patients with relatively simple and inexpensive technology. In addition, they demonstrate that such studies can be performed in humans with a relatively small number of subjects and a short follow-up time.

Thus, a potentially new surrogate ultrasonic biomarker of the effect of medical therapy on plaque stabilization is available.

35.3.2 Integrated Backscatter

As discussed in Chap. 12, integrated backscatter (IBS) is another method of measuring plaque echogenicity. It differs from GSM only in the way the echogenicity score is determined from the digitized ultrasound values. With both methods, the echogenicity score is normalized in relation to blood and adventitia. IBS has become popular in Japan because it is available in ultrasound equipment marketed there.

Four studies from different centers have investigated the effect of statins on plaque echogenicity.[24,31–33]

In the first study by Watanabe et al.,[31] 60 consecutive nonhypercholesterolemic patients with coronary artery disease and carotid plaques were randomized to "Adult Treatment Panel III" diet therapy or pravastatin. At 6 months, there was a significant increase in plaque echogenicity in the pravastatin group from -18.5 ± 4.1 dB to -15.9 ± 3.7 dB ($P < 0.001$). The change in the diet group from -18.5 ± 4.0 to -18.9 ± 3.5 dB was not significant ($P = 0.13$). There were no changes in plaque thickness.

Another study by Nakamura et al.[32] tested the effect of pitavastatin 4 mg/day in patients with acute coronary syndrome. Thirty-three patients were randomized to the pitavastatin group and 32 in the placebo group. All patients had echolucent carotid plaques. IBS changed at 1 month in both groups, but the improvement was greater in the pitavastatin group (-18.7 ± 3.3 dB to -12.7 ± 2.3 dB; $P < 0.001$) than in the placebo group (-19.0 ± 3.5 dB to -16.9 ± 3.2 dB; $P < 0.05$). The difference between the groups at 1 month was significant ($P < 0.01$). Levels of biomarkers CRP, vascular endothelial growth factor (VEGF), and tumor necrosis factor alpha (TNF alpha) at 1 month were significantly lower in the pitavastatin than the placebo group.

A third study by Yamagami et al.[24] investigated the effect of 12-month statin therapy on carotid plaque echogenicity and plaque thickness in hypercholesterolemic patients with carotid plaques. Eighty-one hypercholesterolemic patients with carotid plaques were randomized to statin therapy (simvastatin 10 mg/day, $n = 24$ or atorvastatin 5 mg/day, $n = 16$ depending on physician choice) or diet only ($n = 41$). All patients underwent dietary modification. In the statin group, at 12 months, there was a significant increase in echogenicity in the statin group but not in the diet group (4.7 ± 12.0 dB vs -1.7 ± 13.6 dB; $P = 0.028$). As indicated above in this study, there was also a reduction in plaque thickness in the statin but not in the diet group (-0.22 ± 0.34 mm vs 0.02 ± 0.44 mm; $P = 0.008$).

In the most recent study by Yamada et al.,[33] 40 non- or slightly hypercholesterolemic patients with moderate carotid artery stenosis were randomized to diet ($n = 20$) or atorvastatin ($n = 20$). Three-dimentional imaging with IBS measurements at baseline and at 6 months demonstrated that there was a significant decrease in relative lipid volume of plaques in the statin group from 58.4 ± 25.6 mm^3 to 47.8 ± 23.5 mm^3 ($P < 0.01$) but not in the diet group (52.6 ± 23.8 mm^3 to 56.9 ± 20.2 mm^3; $P > 0.05$). The overall plaque IBS, volume, and thickness changes between the two groups were not significant. This is the first study that has combined 3D ultrasound with IBS to study changes in individual plaque components.

35.4 Conclusion

The results of the studies presented in this chapter indicate that ultrasound can be used to study changes in plaque size and texture. Plaque volume is promising to become the gold standard for longitudinal studies. Plaque stabilization by increasing plaque collagen and decreasing lipid core can also be visualized and measured. What is needed is the ability to combine 3D volume and texture measurements in a practical way[33] (Chap. 18).

A great benefit of current methodology is that it has provided new surrogate phenotypes which are available for the initial study of novel therapies. For example, a recent study by Hirano et al.[34] investigated the effect of pioglitazone, an agonist of peroxisome proliferator-activated receptor gamma, on plaque stabilization in patients with acute coronary syndrome and type 2 diabetes mellitus and echolucent carotid plaques. Five days after the acute coronary symptoms, 61 patients were randomized to pioglitazone (15 or 30 mg/day; $n = 31$) or placebo ($n = 30$). At 1 month after treatment, plaque echolucency as measured by calibrated IBS increased significantly in the pioglitazone but not in the placebo group. Thus, novel therapies and their dose effect can be studied in a human model prior to large prospective trials with clinical endpoints.

References

1. Ebrahim S et al. Carotid plaque, intima media thickness, cardiovascular risk factors, and prevalent cardiovascular disease in men and women: the British Regional Heart Study. *Stroke*. 1999;30:841–850.
2. Crouse JR III et al. Effect of rosuvastatin on progression of carotid intima-media thickness in low-risk individuals with subclinical atherosclerosis: the METEOR trial. *J Am Med Assoc*. 2007;297(12):1344–1353.
3. Crouse JR III et al. Pravastatin, lipids and atherosclerosis in the carotid arteries (PLAC II). *Am J Cardiol*. 1995;75(7): 455–459.
4. Honda O et al. Echolucent carotid plaques predict future coronary events in patients with coronary artery disease. *J Am Coll Cardiol*. 2004;43:1177–1184.
5. Seo Y et al. Echolucent carotid plaques as a feature in patients with acute coronary syndrome. *Circ J*. 2006;70: 1629–1634.
6. Reiter M et al. Increasing carotid plaque echolucency is predictive of cardiovascular events in high risk patients. *Radiology*. 2008;248:1050–1055.
7. Furberg CD et al. Effect of lovastatin on early carotid atherosclerosis and cardiovascular events. Asymptomatic Carotid Artery Progression Study (ACAPS) Research Group. *Circulation*. 1994;90:1679–1687.
8. Salonen R et al. Kuopio Atherosclerosis Prevention Study (KAPS). A population-based primary preventive trial of the effect of LDL lowering on atherosclerotic progression in carotid and femoral arteries. *Circulation*. 1995;92: 1758–1764.
9. Mercuri M et al. Pravastatin reduces carotid intima-media thickness progression in an asymptomatic hypercholesterolemic Mediterranean population: the Carotid Atherosclerosis Italian Ultrasound Study. *Am J Med*. 1996;101:627–634.
10. de Groot E et al. B-mode ultrasound assessment of pravastatin treatment effect on carotid and femoral artery walls and its correlations with coronary arteriographic findings: a report of the Regression Growth Evaluation Statin Study (REGRESS). *J Am Coll Cardiol*. 1998;31:1561–1567.
11. Hedblad B, Wikstrand J, Janzon L, Wedel H, Berglund G. Low-dose metoprolol CR/XL and fluvastatin slow progression of carotid intima-media thickness: main results from the Beta-Blocker Cholesterol-Lowering Asymptomatic Plaque Study (BCAPS). *Circulation*. 2001;103:1721–1726.
12. Sawayama Y et al. Effects of probucol and pravastatin on common carotid atherosclerosis in patients with asymptomatic hypercholesterolemia. Fukuoka Atherosclerosis Trial (FAST). *J Am Coll Cardiol*. 2002;39:610–616.
13. Espeland MA et al. Carotid intimal-media thickness as a surrogate for cardiovascular disease events in trials of HMG-CoA reductase inhibitors. *Curr Control Trials Cardiovasc Med*. 2005;6(1):3.
14. Rodriguez-Granillo GA et al. Meta-analysis of the studies assessing temporal changes in coronary plaque volume using intravascular ultrasound. *Am J Cardiol*. 2007;99:5–10.
15. Nissen SE et al. ASTEROID Investigators. Effect of very high-intensity statin therapy on regression of coronary atherosclerosis: the ASTEROID trial. *JAMA*. 2006;295:1556–1565.
16. Kawasaki M et al. Volumetric quantitative analysis of tissue characteristics of coronary plaques after statin therapy using three-dimensional integrated backscatter intravascular ultrasound. *J Am Coll Cardiol*. 2005;45(12):1946–1953.
17. Saam T et al. Predictors of carotid atherosclerotic plaque progression as measured by noninvasive magnetic resonance imaging. *Atherosclerosis*. 2007;194:e34-e42.
18. Boussel L et al. MAPP Investigators. Atherosclerotic plaque progression in carotid arteries: monitoring with high-spatial-resolution MR imaging – multicenter trial. *Radiology*. 2009;252:789–796.
19. Corti R et al. Effects of aggressive versus conventional lipid-lowering therapy by simvastatin on human atherosclerotic lesions: a prospective, randomized, double-blind trial with high-resolution magnetic resonance imaging. *J Am Coll Cardiol*. 2005;46:106–112.
20. Zhao XQ et al. Effects of prolonged intensive lipid-lowering therapy on the characteristics of carotid atherosclerotic plaques in vivo by MRI: a case-control study. *Arterioscler Thromb Vasc Biol*. 2001;21:1623–1629.
21. Phan BA et al. Association of high-density lipoprotein levels and carotid atherosclerotic plaque characteristics by magnetic resonance imaging. *Int J Cardiovasc Imaging*. 2007;23:337–342.
22. Underhill HR et al. Effect of rosuvastatin therapy on carotid plaque morphology and composition in moderately hypercholesterolemic patients: a high-resolution magnetic resonance imaging trial. *Am Heart J*. 2008;155:584. e1–584.e8.
23. Kurata T, Kurata M, Okada T. Cerivastatin induces carotid artery plaque stabilization independently of cholesterol lowering in patients with hypercholesterolaemia. *J Int Med Res*. 2001;29:329–334.
24. Yamagami H et al. Statin therapy increases carotid plaque echogenicity in hypercholesterolemic patients. *Ultrasound Med Biol*. 2008;34:1353–1359.
25. Spence JD et al. Effects of intensive medical therapy on microemboli and cardiovascular risk in asymptomatic carotid stenosis. *Arch Neurol*. 2010;67:180–186.
26. Schminke U, Hilker L, Motsch L, Griewing B, Kessler C. Volumetric assessment of plaque progression with 3-dimensional ultrasonography under statin therapy. *J Neuroimaging*. 2002;12:245–251.
27. Ainsworth CD et al. 3D ultrasound measurement of change in carotid plaque volume: a tool for rapid evaluation of new therapies. *Stroke*. 2005;36:1904–1909.
28. Kadoglou NP et al. Intensive lipid-lowering therapy ameliorates novel calcification markers and GSM score in patients with carotid stenosis. *Eur J Vasc Endovasc Surg*. 2008;35:661–668.
29. Kadoglou NP et al. Beneficial changes of serum calcification markers and contralateral carotid plaques echogenicity after combined carotid artery stenting plus intensive lipid-lowering therapy in patients with bilateral carotid stenosis. *Eur J Vasc Endovasc Surg*. 2010;39:258–265.

30. Kadoglou NP et al. Aggressive lipid-lowering is more effective than moderate lipid-lowering treatment in carotid plaque stabilization. *J Vasc Surg*. 2010;51:114–121.
31. Watanabe K et al. Stabilization of carotid atheroma assessed by quantitative ultrasound analysis in non-hypercholesterolemic patients with coronary artery disease. *J Am Coll Cardiol*. 2005;46:2022–2030.
32. Nakamura T et al. Rapid stabilization of vulnerable carotid plaque within 1 month of pitavastatin treatment in patients with acute coronary syndrome. *J Cardiovasc Pharmacol*. 2008;51:365–371.
33. Yamada K et al. Effects of atorvastatin on carotid atherosclerotic plaques: a randomized trial for quantitative tissue characterization of carotid atherosclerotic plaques with integrated backscatter ultrasound. *Cerebrovasc Dis*. 2009;28:417–424.
34. Hirano M et al. Rapid improvement of carotid plaque echogenicity within 1 month of pioglitazone treatment in patients with acute coronary syndrome. *Atherosclerosis*. 2009;203:483–488.

36 Image Analysis of Carotid Plaques and Risk Stratification

Andrew Nicolaides, Efthyvoulos Kyriacou, Maura Griffin, Stavros K. Kakkos, and George Geroulakos

36.1 Introduction

The multidisciplinary approach combining angiography, high-resolution ultrasound imaging, transcranial Doppler studies of embolic signals, plaque pathology, histochemistry, coagulation studies, and, more recently, molecular biology has led to a better understanding of the mechanism of carotid plaque rupture, the key mechanism underlying the development of cerebrovascular events[1-3] (Chap. 1).

Plaques with a large extracellular lipid-rich core, thin fibrous cap, reduced smooth muscle cell density, and increased numbers of activated macrophages and mast cells appear to be most vulnerable to rupture[3,4] (Chaps. 1 and 2). Fibrous caps may rupture because of decreased collagen synthesis as well as increased matrix degradation or in response to extrinsic mechanical or hemodynamic stresses.[5] Plaques at the carotid bifurcation coincide with points at which stresses produced by biomechanical and hemodynamic forces are maximal.[6]

Histological studies on the vascular biology of symptomatic and asymptomatic carotid plaques have been reviewed by Golledge et al.[7] They showed that the features of unstable plaques removed from symptomatic patients were surface ulceration and plaque rupture, thinning of the fibrous cap, and infiltration of the cap by a greater number of macrophages and T-lymphocytes.

The identification of unstable plaques in vivo and subsequent plaque stabilization by medical intervention may prove to be an important modality for a reduction in the lethal consequences of atherosclerosis.[8,9] This putative concept of plaque stabilization, although attractive, had not yet been rigorously validated in humans until recently. Initially, indirect data from clinical trials involving lipid lowering/modification and lifestyle/risk factor modification provided strong support for this new approach.[10] In recent years, ultrasound has played an important role because it has provided a new noninvasive method of assessing plaque progression or regression and measurements of texture features associated with plaque stabilization. (Chaps. 16, 23, 25, and 35).

Ultrasonic characteristics of unstable (vulnerable) plaques have been determined[11-13] (Chaps. 12, 23, 24, 33, and 35) and populations or individuals at increased risk for cardiovascular events have been identified[14] (Chaps. 24 and 29).

The aim of this chapter is to summarize the advances in ultrasonic plaque characterization and highlight their potential applications in clinical practice.

A. Nicolaides (✉)
Imperial College and Vascular Screening and Diagnostic Centre, London, UK

E. Kyriacou
Department of Computer Science and Engineering, Frederick University Cyprus, Lemesos, Cyprus

M. Griffin
Vascular Screening and Diagnostic Centre, London, UK

S.K. Kakkos
Department of Vascular Surgery, University of Patras Medical School, Patras, Achaia, Greece

G. Geroulakos
Department of Surgery, Charing Cross Hospital, London, UK

36.2 Ultrasonic Plaque Classification

36.2.1 Historical Aspects

Several studies in the 1980s have shown that "complicated" carotid plaques are often associated with ipsilateral neurological symptoms and share common ultrasonic characteristics, being more echolucent (weak reflection of ultrasound and therefore containing echo-poor structures) and heterogenous (having both echolucent and echogenic areas). In contrast, "uncomplicated" plaques, which are often asymptomatic, tend to be of uniform consistency (uniformly hypoechoic or uniformly hyperechoic) without evidence of ulceration.[11,15,16]

A number of different classifications of plaque ultrasonic appearance have been proposed. In 1983, Reilly et al. classified carotid plaques as homogenous and heterogenous,[15] defining as homogenous plaques those with "uniformly bright echoes" that are now known as uniformly hyperechoic (type 4) (see below). Johnson et al. classified plaques as dense and soft,[17,18] Widder et al. as echolucent and echogenic based on their overall level of echo patterns,[19] while Gray-Weale et al. described 4 types: type 1, predominantly echolucent lesions; type 2, echogenic lesions with substantial (>75%) components of echolucency; type 3, predominately echogenic with small area(s) of echolucency, occupying less than a quarter of the plaque; and type 4, uniformly dense echogenic lesions.[20] Geroulakos et al. subsequently modified the Gray-Weale classification by using a 50% area cutoff point instead of 75%, and by adding type 5, for plaques that as a result of heavy calcification on their surface cannot be correctly classified.[11]

In an effort to improve the reproducibility of visual (subjective) classification, a consensus conference in 1997 suggested that echodensity should reflect the overall brightness of the plaque with the term hyperechoic referring to echogenic (white) and the term hypoechoic referring to echolucent (black) plaques.[21] The reference structure, to which plaque echodensity should be compared with, should be blood for hypoechoic, the sternomastoid muscle for isoechoic, and bone for hyperechoic plaques. Subsequently, a similar method has been used by Polak et al.[22]

In the past a number of workers had confused echogenicity with homogeneity.[15] It is now realized that measurements of texture which depend on the distribution of pixels are different from measurements of echogenicity. The observation that two different atherosclerotic plaques may have the same overall echogenicity but frequently have variations of texture within different regions of the plaque has been made as early as 1983.[23] The term homogenous should therefore refer to plaques of uniform consistency irrespective of whether they are predominantly hypoechoic or hyperechoic. The term heterogenous should be used for plaques of nonuniform consistency, i.e., having both hypoechoic and hyperechoic components (Gray-Weale types 2 and 3).[20] Although O'Donnnell et al. had proposed this otherwise simple classification in 1985[16] and Aldoori et al. in 1987,[24] there has been considerable diversity in terminology used by others, as shown in Table 36.1.[18,22,25-34] Because of this confusion, frequently, plaques having intermediate echogenicity or being complex are inadequately described. For example, echolucent plaques have been considered as heterogenous.[26] A reflection of this confusion is a report from the committee on standards for noninvasive vascular testing of the Joint Council of the Society for Vascular Surgery and the North American Chapter of the International Society for Cardiovascular Surgery proposing in 1992 that carotid plaques should be classified as homogeneous or heterogenous.[35] This oversimplification did not allow for the fact that a proportion of homogenous plaques are uniformly hypoechoic and "unstable," while the majority are uniformly hyperechoic and "stable."

36.2.2 Correlation with Histology

Reilly et al. demonstrated for the first time in 1983 that carotid-plaque characteristics on brightness-mode (B-mode) ultrasound performed before operation correlated with carotid-plaque histology.[15] However, at that time, color flow was not available and uniformly hypoechoic plaques were not easily visualized. By visually evaluating the sonographic characteristics of carotid plaques, two main patterns could be identified: a homogeneous pattern containing uniform hyperechoic echoes corresponding to dense fibrous tissue and a heterogenous pattern containing a mixture of hyperechoic areas (white) representing fibrous tissue and anechoic areas (black) that represent intraplaque hemorrhage or lipid.[35]

Table 36.1 Design of published studies on carotid plaque characterization in relation to risk for neurologic events

Authors year (ref.)	Carotid bifurcations n	Follow-up in years	Type of patients	Plaque characteristics studied
O'Holleran et al., 1987[18]	296	3.8	A	Calcified, dense, soft
Sterpetti et al., 1988[25]	238	2.8	A and S	Homogenous, heterogenous
Langsfeld et al., 1989[26]	419	1.8	A	Plaque types 1–4
Bock et al., 1993[27]	242	2.3	A	Echolucent, echogenic
Polak et al., 1998[22]	270	3.3	A	Hypo-, iso-, hyperechoic
Mathiesen et al., 2001[28]	223	3.0	A	Plaque types 1–4
Grønholdt et al., 2001[29]	111	4.4	A	Gray scale median
	135	4.4	S	Gray scale median
Liapis et al., 2001[30]	442	3.7	A and S	Plaque types 1–4
AbuRahma et al., 1998[31]	391	3.1	A	Homogenous, heterogenous
Carra et al., 2003[32]	291	2.7	A	Homogenous, heterogenous
Hashimoto et al., 2009[33]	297	1.8	A	% area of lipid like echogenicity
Nicolaides et al., 2010[34]	1,121	4.0	A	Plaque types 1–4
				Gray scale median
				Plaque area
				Presence of discrete white areas

A asymptomatic, *S* symptomatic

Thus, it was realized early that ultrasound could not distinguish between hemorrhage and lipid. Because most heterogenous lesions contained intraplaque hemorrhage and ulcerated lesions, it was thought at the time that the presence of a plaque hemorrhage reflected the potential for plaque rupture and development of symptoms. However, it was subsequently realized that plaque hemorrhage was very common and was found in equal frequency in both symptomatic and asymptomatic plaques,[36] and that ultrasound was highly sensitive (93%) in demonstrating plaque hemorrhage, as well as specific (84%).[16,31,37] It was also both sensitive and specific in demonstrating calcification in carotid endarterectomy specimens.[38]

Aldoori et al. reported that plaque hemorrhage was seen histologically in 21 patients, 19 (78%) of whom were diagnosed preoperatively as having predominently echolucent heterogenous plaques on ultrasound imaging.[24] Gray-Weale et al.[20] also validated his plaque classification by demonstrating a statistically significant relationship ($p < 0.001$) between ultrasound appearance of types 1 and 2 plaques (echolucent appearance) and the presence of either intraplaque hemorrhage or ulceration in the endarterectomy specimen. It is now apparent from those ultrasound-histology correlations that Reilly's heterogenous plaques correspond closely to Gray-Weale's echolucent (types 1 and 2) plaques.

The above findings were confirmed by studies performed in the 1990s using the new generation of ultrasound scanners with their improved resolution. Van Damme et al.[39] reported that fibrous plaques ("dense," homogenous hyperechoic lesions) were detected with a specificity of 87% and a sensitivity of 56%. Recent intraplaque hemorrhage was echographically apparent as a hypoechoic area in 88% of cases, corresponding to a specificity of 79% and a sensitivity of 75%. Kardoulas et al.,[40] in another study, confirmed Van Damme's results on fibrous plaques, with fibrous tissue being significantly greater in plaques with an echogenic character compared with those with an echolucent morphology.

The European Carotid Plaque Study Group that performed a multi-center study confirmed that plaque echogenicity was inversely related to hemorrhage and lipid, ($p = 0.005$) and directly related to collagen content and calcification ($p < 0.0001$).[41]

Plaque shape (mural vs nodular) on ultrasound has been shown to be associated with histology features characteristic of unstable plaques. Weinberger et al.[42] demonstrated that mural plaques propagating along the carotid wall had a 72% frequency of recent organizing hemorrhage. In contrast, nodular plaques causing local narrowing of the vessel had only a 23% incidence of organizing hemorrhage ($p < 0.01$).

As indicated at the beginning of this chapter, it is now known that stable atherosclerotic plaques have on histological examination a thick fibrous cap, a small lipid core, are rich in smooth muscle cells (SMC) which produce collagen and have a poor content of macrophages. In contrast, unstable plaques that are prone to rupture and development of symptoms have a thin fibrous cap, a large lipid core, have few SMC, and are rich in macrophages.[3] Macrophages are responsible for the production of enzymes, matrix metaloproteinases (stromelysins, gelatinases, and collagenases) that play an important role in remodeling the plaque matrix and erosion of the fibrous cap.[43] Lammie et al.[44] reported a highly significant association between a thin fibrous cap and a large necrotic core ($p < 0.002$) in carotid endarterectomy specimens and a good agreement between ultrasound and pathological measurements of fibrous cap thickness (thick vs thin fibrous cap, kappa = 0.53).

There is considerable debate on the question of whether thrombosis on the surface of the plaque, being an otherwise significant feature of complicated plaques, can discriminate between symptomatic and asymptomatic plaques. In one study, acute thrombosis on ultrasound appeared as a completely echolucent defect adjacent to the lumen,[45] and it was almost certain that by the time the operation was performed (usually several weeks after the event), the thrombus had undergone remodeling.

36.3 Natural History Studies

36.3.1 Early Studies Without Image Normalization (Table 36.2)

Johnson et al. did the first study, which showed the value of ultrasonic characterization of carotid bifurcation plaques in asymptomatic patients in the early 1980s.[17,18] In that study, hypoechoic carotid plaques in comparison to hyperechoic or calcified ones, increased the risk of stroke during a follow-up period of 3 years; this effect was prominent in patients with carotid stenosis more than 75% (estimated by cross-sectional area calculations and spectral analysis), as stroke occurred in 19% of them. None of the patients with calcified plaques developed a stroke.

A second study performed in the 1980s by Sterpetti et al.[25] has shown that the severity of stenosis (lumen-diameter reduction greater than 50%) and the presence of a heterogenous plaque were both independent risk factors for the development of new neurological deficits [transient ischemic attack (TIA) and stroke]. Twenty seven percent of the patients with heterogenous plaques and hemodynamically significant stenosis developed new symptoms. Unfortunately, their study had mixed cases with 37% of the patients having a history of previous neurological cerebral hemispheric symptoms. History of neurological symptoms was a risk factor for the development of new neurological

Table 36.2 Results of prospective studies of plaque characterization in relation to risk for neurologic events

Authors year (ref.)	Endpoint	Stenosis (%)	Findings
O'Holleran et al., 1987[18]	Stroke, TIA	>75	Cumulative 5-year stroke risk was: 80% for soft (echolucent plaques), 10% for dense (echogenic and calcified plaques)
Sterpetti et al., 1988[25]	Stroke, TIA	>50	Events: 27% for heterogenous plaques, 9% for homogenous plaques
Langsfeld et al., 1989[26]	Neurological symptoms	>75	Events: 15% for echolucent plaques, 9% for echogenic plaques
Bock et al., 1993[27]	Stroke, TIA	–	Annual event rate: 5.7% for echolucent plaques, 2.4% for echogenic plaques
Polak et al., 1998[22]	Stroke	>50	RR for ipsilateral stroke was 2.78 in hypoechoic plaques
Mathiesen et al., 2001[28]	Neurological	>35	RR for cerebrovascular events was 4.6 in subjects with echolucent plaques
Grønholdt et al., 2001[29]	Ipsilat. stroke	>80	RR for ischemic stroke was 7.9 in subjects with echolucent plaques
Liapis et al., 2001[30]	Stroke, TIA	>70	RR was 2.96 for stroke and 2.02 for TIA in echolucent plaques
AbuRahma et al., 1998[31]	Stroke, TIA	–	Ipsilateral stroke occurred in: 13.6% of heterogenous plaques, 3.1% of homogenous plaques
Carra et al., 2003[32]	Stroke, TIA	>70	Ipsilateral event occurred in: 5% of heterogenous plaques, 1.3% of homogenous plaques

RR relative risk

symptoms during the follow-up period, although this was found only in the univariate analysis. Because no subgroup analysis was performed, no conclusion could be drawn regarding asymptomatic or symptomatic patients.

In a similar study of patients with asymptomatic carotid stenosis, AbuRahma et al.[31] reported that the incidence of ipsilateral strokes during follow-up was significantly higher in patients having heterogenous than in those having homogenous plaques: 13.6% versus 3.1% ($p = 0.0001$; odds ratio: 5.0). Similarly, the incidence rate of all neurological events (stroke or TIA) was higher in patients with heterogenous than in those with homogenous plaques: 27.8% versus 6.6% ($p = 0.001$; odds ratio, 5.5). Heterogenous plaques were defined as those composed of a mixture of hypoechoic, isoechoic, and hyperechoic lesions, and homogenous plaques, those which consisted of only one of the three components. Similar results indicating an increased risk in patients with heterogenous plaques were reported by Carra et al.[32]

The study published in 1989 by Langsfeld et al.[26] confirmed that patients with *hypoechoic plaques* (type 1, predominantly echolucent raised lesions, with thin "egg shell" cap of echogenicity and type 2, echogenic lesions with substantial areas of echolucency) had a twofold risk of stroke: 15% in comparison to 7% in those having *hyperechoic plaques* (type 3, predominately echogenic with small area(s) of echolucency deeply localized and occupying less than a quarter of the plaque and type 4, uniformly dense echogenic lesions). A confounding factor was that patients with greater than 75% stenosis were also at increased risk. However, the overall incidence of new symptoms was low, in contrast to the previous studies, perhaps because only asymptomatic patients were included in that study. Based on their results, the authors proposed an aggressive approach in those patients with greater than 75% stenosis and heterogenous plaques. There was some confusion regarding the interchangeable use of the terms heterogenous and hypoechoic in that article. The authors raised the point that it is important for each laboratory to verify its ability to classify plaque types. The same group in another study published 4 years later reported a 5.7% annual vessel event rate (TIA and stroke) for echolucent carotid plaques versus 2.4% for the echogenic ones ($p = 0.03$).[27]

Given the fair interobserver reproducibility for type 1 plaques, as indicated above, the use of reference points was proposed: anechogenicity to be standardized against circulating blood, isoechogenicity against sternomastoid muscle, and hyperechogenicity against bone (cervical vertebrae). This method was used in the late 1990s by Polak et al.[22] who investigated the association between stroke and internal carotid artery plaque echodensity in 4886 asymptomatic individuals aged 65 years or older, who were followed-up prospectively for 48 months. Some 68% of those had carotid artery stenosis, which exceeded 50% in 270 patients. In this study, plaques were subjectively characterized as hypoechoic, isoechoic or hyperechoic in relation to the surrounding soft tissues. Out of the hypoechoic plaques causing 50–99% stenosis were associated with a significantly higher incidence of ipsilateral, non-fatal stroke than iso- or hyperechoic plaques of the same degree of stenosis (relative risk 2.78 and 3.08, respectively). The authors of this study suggested that quantitative methods of grading carotid plaque echomorphology such as computer-assisted plaque characterization might be more precise in determining the association between hypoechoic (echolucent) plaques and the incidence of stroke. Subsequent studies using computer-assisted measurements of gray scale median (GSM)[28–30] have supported the finding that hypoechoic plaques are associated with an increased risk when compared with hyperechoic plaques, as shown below. It is now known that echolucent and heterogenous plaques are not mutually exclusive, and the risk is increased in both. Type 2 plaques, which are associated with the highest incidence of neurological events, are, by definition, included in both echolucent and heterogenous groups (see section on plaque types below).

36.3.2 Recent Studies with Image Normalization and Measurements of GSM

The clinical importance of ultrasonic plaque characterization following image normalization has been focused on two main areas: first, cross-sectional studies aiming at better understanding of the pathophysiology of carotid disease and second, natural history studies seeking to identify high and low risk groups for stroke in order to refine the indications for selection of symptomatic or asymptomatic patients for carotid endarterectomy.

36.3.3 Cross-Sectional Studies Using GSM

The use of image normalization and computer measurements of GSM has resulted in the identification of differences in carotid plaque structure – in terms of echodensity and degree of stenosis – not only between symptomatic and asymptomatic plaques in general but also between plaques associated with retinal or hemispheric symptoms.[12,46–50] In a series of asymptomatic and symptomatic patients presenting with amaurosis fugax, TIAs and stroke with good recovery having 50–99% stenosis on the carotid duplex scan, plaques associated with symptoms were significantly more hypoechoic, with higher degrees of stenosis than those not associated with symptoms (mean GSM = 13.3 versus 30.5 and mean degree of stenosis = 80.5% versus 72.2%). Furthermore, plaques associated with amaurosis fugax were hypoechoic (mean GSM = 7.4) and severely stenotic (mean stenosis 85.6%). Plaques associated with TIAs and stroke had a similar echodensity and a similar degree of stenosis (mean GSM = 14.9 versus 15.8 and degree of stenosis = 79.3% versus 78.1%).[48] These findings confirmed previous reports, which had shown that hypoechoic plaques were more likely to be associated with symptoms. In addition, they supported the hypothesis that amaurosis fugax had a different pathophysiological mechanism to that of TIAs and stroke.

The authors' group has found that GSM separates echomorphologically the carotid plaques associated with silent nonlacunar computed tomography (CT) demonstrated brain infarcts from plaques that are not so associated. The mean GSM of plaques associated with ipsilateral nonlacunar silent CT-brain infarcts was 14, and that of plaques that were not so associated was 30 ($p = 0.003$).[48] Additionally, emboli counted on transcranial Doppler (TCD) in the ipsilateral middle cerebral artery were more frequent in the presence of low-plaque echodensity (low GSM), but not in the presence of a high degree of stenosis.[51] These data support the embolic nature of cerebrovascular symptomatology.

There are several biologic findings that can explain the association of hypoechoic plaques with symptoms. The authors' group has found that hypoechoic plaques with a low GSM have a large necrotic core volume.[52] In addition, hypoechoic plaques have increased macrophage infiltration on histological examination of the specimen after endarterectomy.[53]

The role of biomechanical forces in the induction of plaque fatigue and rupture has been emphasized.[54,55] In the authors' group of patients, carotid plaques associated with amaurosis fugax were hypoechoic and were associated with very high-grade stenoses. It may well be that the plaques that are hypoechoic and homogenous, undergo low internal stresses and therefore do not rupture but progress to tighter stenosis with post-stenotic dilatation, turbulance, and platelet adhesion in the post-stenotic area resulting in the eventual production of showers of small platelet emboli. Such small platelet emboli may be too small to produce hemispheric symptoms but are detected by the retina. In contrast, plaques associated with TIAs and stroke were less hypoechoic and less stenotic than those associated with amaurosis fugax. These plaques are hypoechoic but more heterogenous and may undergo stronger internal stresses. Therefore, they may tend to rupture at an earlier stage (lower degrees of stenosis), producing larger particle debris (plaque constituents or thrombi) that deprive large areas of the brain of adequate perfusion.

36.3.4 Prospective Studies

The Tromsø study conducted in Norway in 223 subjects with carotid stenosis greater than 35% has found that subjects with echolucent atherosclerotic plaques have increased risk of ischemic cerebrovascular events independent of degree of stenosis.[28] The adjusted relative risk for all cerebrovascular events in subjects with echolucent plaques was 4.6 (95% confidence interval [CI] 1.1–18.9), and there was a significant linear trend ($p = 0.015$) for higher risk with increasing plaque echolucency. Ipsilateral neurological events were also more frequent in patients with echolucent or predominantly echolucent plaques. The authors concluded that evaluation of plaque morphology in addition to the grade of stenosis might improve clinical decision-making and differentiate treatment for individual patients, and that computer-quantified plaque morphology assessment, being a more objective method of ultrasonic plaque characterization, may further improve this.

This method of measuring GSM has been also used by Grønholdt et al.[29] who found that echolucent plaques causing >50% diameter stenosis were associated with increased risk of future stroke in symptomatic ($n = 135$) but not asymptomatic ($n = 111$) individuals (Chap. 31). Echogenicity of carotid plaques was evaluated with high-resolution B-mode ultrasound and computer-assisted image processing, but without image normalization. The mean of the standardized median gray-scale values of the plaque was used to divide plaques into echolucent and echorich. Relative to symptomatic patients with echorich 50–79% stenotic plaques, those with echorich 80–99% stenotic plaques, echolucent 50–79% stenotic plaques, and echolucent 80–99% stenotic plaques had relative risks of ipsilateral ischemic stroke of 3.1 (95% CI, 0.7–14), 4.2 (95% CI, 1.2–15), and 7.9 (95% CI, 2.1–30), equivalent to absolute risk increase of 11%, 18%, and 28%, respectively. The authors suggested that measurement of echolucency, together with the degree of stenosis, might improve selection of patients for carotid endarterectomy. The relatively small number of events in the asymptomatic individuals and lack of image normalization were probably the reasons why plaque characterization was not helpful in predicting risk in the asymptomatic group.

More recently, Hashimoto and his colleagues[33] investigated whether plaque heterogeneity (i.e., the distribution of pixel intensities) could predict the instability of asymptomatic plaque. They first compared carotid endarterectomy specimens and the GSM values of known tissues on B-mode images, and the GSM values for blood, lipid, muscle/fibrous tissue, and calcification were determined. Then, they estimated the percent area of each tissue component for 297 asymptomatic plaques causing 40–99% carotid artery stenosis in 250 patients, and monitored the incidence of atherothrombotic cerebral infarction due to carotid stenosis during follow-up. Eight infarcts occurred during a follow-up period of 22 (± 15) months. Plaques in the top tertile for the percent area of lipid-like echogenicity and in the lowest tertile for calcification, showed an association with future infarction. This association remained significant after adjustment for the severity of carotid stenosis (hazard ratio 4.4 for lipid-like and 0.24 for calcification-like component, both $p < 0.05$). The authors concluded that the distribution of pixel intensities could be employed to predict instability of asymptomatic plaques and possibly to select patients for interventional procedures.

36.4 Ultrasonic Plaque Ulceration

Several studies have indicated a strong association between macroscopic plaque ulceration and the development of embolic symptoms (amaurosis fugax, TIAs, stroke) and signs such as silent infarcts on CT-brain scans.[56–60] However, the ability of conventional two-dimensional (2D) ultrasound to identify plaque ulceration is poor.[15,19,61–67] The sensitivity is low (41%) when the stenosis is greater than 50% and moderately high (77%) when the stenosis is less than 50%. This is because ulceration is much easier to detect in the presence of mild stenosis when the residual lumen and plaque surface are more easily seen, than with severe stenosis when the residual lumen and the surface of the plaque are not easily defined because they are not always in the plane of the ultrasound beam.

Two studies have investigated plaque surface characteristics and the type of plaque in relation to symptoms. The first one was a retrospective analysis of 578 symptomatic patients (242 with stroke and 336 with TIAs) recruited for the B-scan Ultrasound Imaging Assessment Program. A matched case-control study design was used to compare brain hemispheres with ischemic lesions to unaffected contralateral hemispheres with regard to the presence and characteristics of carotid artery plaques. Plaques were classified as smooth when the surface had a continuous boundary, irregular when there was an uneven or pitted boundary, and pocketed when there was a crater-like defect with sharp margins. The results demonstrated an odds ratio of 2.1 for the presence of an irregular surface and of 3.0 for hypoechoic plaques in carotids associated with TIAs and stroke.[68]

The second study included 258 symptomatic and 65 asymptomatic patients. Carotid plaque morphology was classified according to Gray-Weale et al.,[20] and plaque surface features were assessed. The results demonstrated that plaque types 1 and 2 were more common in symptomatic patients. The incidence of ulceration was 23% in the symptomatic and 14% in the asymptomatic group ($p = 0.04$).[69]

The detection of plaque ulceration with three-dimensional (3-D) ultrasound appears to be more accurate than with 2D ultrasound (Chap. 17). However, in the absence of any prospective natural history studies in which ultrasound has been used for identifying plaque ulceration, the finding of plaque ulceration cannot be used for making clinical decisions.

Table 36.3 Natural history studies of patients with asymptomatic internal carotid artery stenosis in which grades of stenosis up to 99% have been included

Publication	Grading of stenosis				Mean Follow-up (years)	Events				Event rate (annual)		
	Area	N%	E%	n		TIAs + AF	Stroke	TIAs + stroke		TIAs + AF (%)	Stroke (%)	TIAs + stroke (%)
Johnson et al., 1985[17]	<75	<50	<70	176	3	12	3	15		2.3	0.6	1.7
	>75	>50	>70	121		57	12	69		15.7	3.3	19
Chambers and Norris, 1986[70]	<75	<50	<70	387	2	8	6	14		1.0	0.1	1.8
	>75	>50	>70	113		16	6	22		7.0	2.6	9.7
Hennerici et al., 1987[71]		<80	<88	119	2.5	15	4	19		5.0	1.3	6.4
		>80	>88	36		2	3	5		2.2	3.3	5.5
Norris et al., 1991[72]		<50	<70	303	3.4	11	13	24		1.1	1.3	2.3
		50–75	**72–85**	216		28	5	33		3.8	0.6	4.5
		75–99	**85–99**	177		36	11	47		6.0	1.8	7.8
Zhu and Norris, 1991[73]		<50	<72	734[a]	4	12	10	22		0.4	0.3	0.7
		50–74	**72–85**	172[a]		12	2	14		1.7	0.3	2.0
		75–99	**85–99**	94[a]		23	6	29		6.1	1.6	7.7
Mackey et al., 1997[74]		<12	**<50**	358	3.6	5	5	10		0.4	0.4	0.8
		12–65	**50–79**	207		3	6	9		0.4	0.8	1.2
		65–99	**79–99**	113		12	7	19		2.9	1.7	4.7
Nadareishvili et al., 2002[75]		<50	<72	108	10	–	–	10		–	–	0.9
		50–99	72–99	73		–	–	12		–	–	7.7
ECST (Asymptomatic side), 1995[76]		<47	**0–69**	2,113	4.5	–	54	–		–	0.5	–
		47–99	**70–99**	127		–	13	–		–	2.3	–
NASCET (Asymptomatic side)		<50	<72	1,496	5	–	116	–		–	1.5	–
Inzitari et al., 2000[77]		**50–74**	**72–85**	172		–	31	–		–	2.8	–
		75–99	**85–99**	73		–	12	–		–	3.3	–
		<60	<77	1,604		–	128	–		–	1.6	–
		60–99	**77–99**	73		–	34	–		–	3.1	–
ACSRS Nicolaides et al., 2010[34]		12–49	**50–69**	194	4.0	11	5	12		0.2	0.6	1.5
		50–82	**70–89**	593		36	29	57		0.8	1.2	2.4
		82–99	**90–99**	328		24	25	40		0.5	1.9	3.1

The method used to grade the stenosis in each study (Area, N% = NASCET or E% = ECST) is shown in bold
[a] Indicates carotid arteries rather than patients

36.5 Stenosis: A Confounding Factor

Natural history studies have demonstrated that the risk of developing ipsilateral symptoms including stroke increases with increasing severity of internal carotid artery stenosis (Table 36.3).[17,34,70–76,78] In addition, a number of important messages have emerged recently. One is that the different methods used on either side of the Atlantic to express the degree of stenosis have a different relationship to risk. Another is the realization that a considerable number of events occur, even in patients with low-grade asymptomatic carotid stenosis. Also, the relationship between risk and degree of internal carotid stenosis depends on the methodology used.[78] Finally, both the severity of internal carotid stenosis and plaque characterization texture features are independent predictors of risk and can complement each other. Thus, one cannot consider plaque characterization independent of stenosis.

Two main methods are currently used to express percent diameter stenosis. The first one defines the residual lumen as a percentage of the normal distal internal carotid artery (ICA). It has been used in North America since the late 1960s and more recently the North American Symptomatic Carotid Endarterectomy Trial (NASCET)[79] and the Asymptomatic Carotid Atherosclerosis Study (ACAS).[80] It has become known as the North American, "NASCET" or "N" method.[81] The second method expresses the residual lumen as a percentage of the diameter of the carotid bulb and has been used in the European Carotid Surgery Trial (ECST)[82] to become known as the European or "ECST" or "E" method.[81] The relationship between both methods is shown in Table 30.1 in Chap. 30.

The NASCET-randomized controlled study has used angiography and a cutoff point of 70% stenosis in relation to the distal internal carotid which is equivalent to 83% stenosis in relation to the bulb (Table 30.1). The ECST randomized controlled study has used angiography also, but a cutoff point of 70% stenosis in relation to the bulb which is equivalent to 47% stenosis in relation to the distal internal carotid artery. Many vascular surgeons are under the impression that these cutoff points are similar! The only similarity is the value of 70%. In reality the difference in terms of plaque size or residual lumen is considerable. However, with increasing degrees of stenosis the values of the two methods converge and the discrepancy decreases (Table 30.1).

Several natural history studies[17,34,70–76,78] (Table 36.3) have indicated that the risk of stroke in asymptomatic patients is low (0.1–1.6% per year) for NASCET stenosis less than 75–80% and higher (2.0–3.3% per year) with greater degrees of stenosis (Table 36.3). Different cutoff points, ranges and methods of grading stenosis have been used in these natural history studies[17,34,70–75] and randomized controlled trials.[76,79,80,82,83] Universal agreement as to the best method for grading ICA stenosis and optimum cutoff points in relation to risk have not yet been established.

36.6 Conclusion

The material reviewed in this chapter suggests that several ultrasonic features could improve on the stroke-risk stratification as currently provided by the degree of carotid stenosis. It also indicates that of the plaque features and methodologies described in previous chapters, relatively few have been used in prospective clinical studies. The question whether a combination of the degree of stenosis and plaque texture features can produce a better stratification of risk than stenosis alone was the aim of the Asymptomatic Carotid Stenosis and Risk of Stroke (ACSRS) study presented in the next chapter.

References

1. Libby P. Molecular basis of acute coronary syndromes. *Circulation*. 1995;91:2844–2850.
2. Clinton S et al. Macrophage-colony stimulating factor gene expression in vascular cells and human atherosclerosis. *Am J Pathol*. 1992;140:301–316.
3. Davies MJ, Richardson PD, Woolf N, Katz DR, Mahn J. Risk of thrombosis in human atherosclerotic plaques: role of extracellular lipid, macrophage and smooth muscle cell content. *Br Heart J*. 1993;69:377–381.
4. Falk E. Why do plaques rupture. *Circulation*. 1992;86(6): 30–42.
5. Glagov S, Bassiouny HS, Sakaguchi Y, Goudet CA, Vito RP. Mechanical determinants of plaque modeling, remodeling and disruption. *Atherosclerosis*. 1997;131:3–4.
6. Shah PK. Role of inflammation and metalloproteinases in plaque disruption and thrombosis. *Vasc Med*. 1998;3: 199–206.

7. Golledge J, Greenhalgh RM, Davies AH. The symptomatic carotid plaque. *Stroke*. 2000;31(3):774–781.
8. Shah PK. Pathophysiology of plaque rupture and the concept of plaque stabilization. *Cardiol Clin*. 1996;14(1):17–29.
9. Muller WD, Faust M, Kotzka J, Krone W. Mechanisms of plaque stabilization. *Herz*. 1999;24:26–31.
10. Rabbani R, Topol EJ. Strategies to achieve coronary arterial plaque stabilization. *Cardiovasc Res*. 1999;41:402–417.
11. Geroulakos G et al. Characterisation of symptomatic and asymptomatic carotid plaques using high-resolution real time ultrasonography. *Br J Surg*. 1993;80:1274–1277.
12. Sabetai MM et al. Hemispheric symptoms and carotid plaque echomorphology. *J Vasc Surg*. 2000;31:39–49.
13. Tegos TJ et al. Patterns of brain computed tomography infarction and carotid plaque echogenicity. *J Vasc Surg*. 2001;33:334–339.
14. Belcaro G et al. Ultrasound morphology classification of the arterial wall and cardiovascular events in a 6-year follow-up study. *Arterioscler Thromb Vasc Biol*. 1996;16:851–856.
15. Reilly LM et al. Carotid plaque histology using real-time ultrasonography: clinical and therapeutic implications. *Am J Surg*. 1983;146:188–193.
16. O'Donnell TF Jr et al. Correlation of B-mode ultrasound imaging and arteriography with pathologic findings at carotid endarterectomy. *Arch Surg*. 1985;120:443–449.
17. Johnson JM, Kennelly MM, Decesare D, Morgan S, Sparrow A. Natural history of asymptomatic carotid plaque. *Arch Surg*. 1985;120:1010–1012.
18. O'Holleran LW, Kennelly MM, Decesare D, McClurken M, Johnson JM. Natural history of asymptomatic carotid plaque. Five year follow-up study. *Am J Surg*. 1987;154:659–662.
19. Widder B et al. Morphological characterization of carotid artery stenoses by ultrasound duplex scanning. *Ultrasound Med Biol*. 1990;16:349–354.
20. Gray-Weale AC, Graham JC, Burnett JR, Burne K, Lusby RJ. Carotid artery atheroma: comparison of preoperative B-mode ultrasound appearance with carotid endarterectomy specimen pathology. *J Cardiovasc Surg*. 1988;29:676–681.
21. deBray JM, Baud JM, Dauzat M, for the Consensus Conference. Concensus on the morphology of carotid plaques. *Cerebrovasc Dis*. 1997;7:289–296.
22. Polak JF et al. Hypoechoic plaque at US of the carotid artery: an independent risk factor for incident stroke in adults aged 65 years or older. *Radiology*. 1998;208:649–654.
23. Wolverson MK, Bashiti HM, Peterson GJ. Ultrasonic tissue characterization of atheromatous plaques using a high resolution real time scanner. *Ultrasound Med Biol*. 1983;9:599–609.
24. Aldoori MI et al. Duplex scanning and plaque histology in cerebral ischaemia. *Eur J Vasc Surg*. 1987;1:159–164.
25. Sterpetti AV et al. Ultrasonographic features of carotid plaque and the risk of subsequent neurologic deficits. *Surgery*. 1988;104:652–660.
26. Langsfeld M, Gray-Weale AC, Lusby RJ. The role of plaque morphology and diameter reduction in the development of new symptoms in asymptomatic carotid arteries. *J Vasc Surg*. 1989;9:548–557.
27. Bock RW et al. The natural history of asymptomatic carotid artery disease. *J Vasc Surg*. 1993;17:160–171.
28. Mathiesen EB, Bønaa KH, Joakimsen O. Echolucent plaques are associated with high risk of ischemic cerebrovascular events in carotid stenosis. The Tromsø study. *Circulation*. 2001;103:2171–2175.
29. Grønholdt M-LM, Nordestgaard BG, Schroeder TV, Vorstrup S, Sillesen H. Ultrasonic echolucent carotid plaques predict future strokes. *Circulation*. 2001;104:68–73.
30. Liapis CD, Kakisis JD, Kostakis AG. Carotid stenosis factors affecting symptomatology. *Stroke*. 2001;32:2782–2786.
31. AbuRahma AF, Kyer PD III, Robinson PA, Hannay RS. The correlation of ultrasonic carotid plaque morphology and carotid plaque hemmorhage: clinical implications. *Surgery*. 1998;124:721–728.
32. Carra G et al. Carotid plaque morphology and cerebrovascular events. *Int Angiol*. 2003;22:284–289.
33. Hashimoto H, Takaya M, Niki H, Etani H. Computer-assisted analysis of heterogeneity on B-mode imaging predicts instability of asymptomatic carotid plaque. *Cerebrovasc Dis*. 2009;28:357–364.
34. Nicolaides A et al. Asymptomatic internal carotid artery stenosis and cerebrovascular risk stratification. *J Vasc Surg*. 2010;52(6):1486–1496.
35. Thiele BL et al. Standards in non-invasive cerebrovascular testing. Report from the committee on standards for non-invasive vascular testing of the Joint Council of the Society for Vascular Surgery and the North American Chapter of the International Society for cardiovascular surgery. *J Vasc Surg*. 1992;15:995–1003.
36. Fisher CM, Ojemann RG. A clinicopathologic study of carotid endarterectomy plaques. *Rev Neurol (Paris)*. 1986;142:573–576.
37. Bluth EI et al. Sonographic characterization of carotid plaque: detection of hemorrhage. *AJR Am J Roentgenol*. 1986;146:1061–1065.
38. Bendick PJ et al. Carotid plaque morphology: correlation of duplex sonography with histology. *Ann Vasc Surg*. 1988;2:6–13.
39. Van Damme H, Trotteur G, Vivario M, Limet R. Echographic characterization of carotid plaques. *Acta Chir Belg*. 1993;93:233–238.
40. Kardoulas DG et al. Ultrasonographic and histologic characteristics of symptom-free and symptomatic carotid plaque. *Cardiovasc Surg*. 1996;4:580–590.
41. European Carotid Plaque Study Group. Carotid artery plaque composition – relationship to clinical presentation and ultrasound B-mode imaging. *Eur J Vasc Endovasc Surg*. 1995;10:23–30.
42. Weinberger J et al. Atherosclerotic plaque at the carotid artery bifurcation. Correlation of ultrasonographic imaging with morphology. *J Ultrasound Med*. 1987;6:363–366.
43. Shah PK et al. Human monocyte–derived macrophages induce collagen breakdown in fibrous caps of atherosclerotic plaques. Potential role of matrix degrting metaloproteinases and implications for plaque rapture. *Circulation*. 1995;92:1565–1569.
44. Lammie GA et al. What pathological components indicate carotid atheroma activity and can these be identified reliably using ultrasound? *Eur J Ultrasound*. 2000;11:77–86.

45. Urbano LA et al. Thrombus in the internal carotid artery complicating an "unstable" atheromatous plaque. *Circulation*. 2003;107:e19-e20.
46. El-Barghouty NM, Nicolaides A, Bahal V, Geroulakos G, Androulakis A. The identification of high risk carotid plaque. *Eur J Vasc Surg*. 1996;11:470–478.
47. Biasi GM et al. Computer analysis of ultrasonic plaque echolucency in identifying high risk carotid bifurcation lesions. *Eur J Vasc Endovasc Surg*. 1999;17:476–479.
48. El-Atrozy T et al. The effect of B-mode image standardisation on the echodensity of symptomatic and asymptomatic carotid bifurcation plaques. *Int Angiol*. 1998;17:179-186.
49. Tegos TJ et al. Comparability of the ultrasonic tissue characteristics of carotid plaques. *J Ultrasound Med*. 2000; 14:399–407.
50. Sabetai MM et al. Reproducibility of computer-quantified carotid plaque echogenicity. *Stroke*. 2000;31:2189–2196.
51. Tegos TJ et al. Correlates of embolic events detected by means of transcranial Doppler in patients with carotid atheroma. *J Vasc Surg*. 2001;33:131–138.
52. Sabetai MS et al. The association of carotid plaque necrotic core volume and echogenicity with ipsilateral hemispheric symptoms. *Circulation*. 2001;104(suppl 2):671 (abst).
53. Gronholdt M-LM et al. Macrophages are associated with lipid-rich carotid artery plaques, echolucency on B-mode imaging, and elevated plasma lipid levels. *J Vasc Surg*. 2002;35:137–145.
54. Ku DN, McCord BN. Cyclic stress causes rupture of the atherosclerotic plaque cap. *Circulation*. 1993;88(suppl 1): 1362 (abst).
55. Glagov S, Bassiouny HS, Sakaguchi Y, Goudet CA, Vito RP. Mechanical determinants of plaque modeling, remodeling and disruption. *Atherosclerosis*. 1997;131(suppl):S13-S14.
56. Zukowski AJ et al. The correlation between carotid plaque ulceration and cerebral infarction seen on CT scan. *J Vasc Surg*. 1984;1:782–786.
57. Persson AV, Robichaux WT, Silverman M. The natural history of carotid plaque development. *Arch Surg*. 1983; 118:1048–1052.
58. Seager JM, Klingman N. The relationship between carotid plaque composition and neurological symptoms. *J Surg Res*. 1987;43:78–85.
59. Sterpetti AV, Hunter WJ, Schulz RD. Importance of ulceration of carotid plaque. *J Cardiovasc Surg*. 1991;32:154–158.
60. Eliasziw M, Streifler JY, Fox JA. Significance of plaque ulceration in symptomatic patients with high-grade stenosis. *Stroke*. 1994;25:305–308.
61. Fisher GG, Anderson DC, Farber R, Lebow S. Prediction of carotid disease by ultrasound and digital subtraction angiography. *Arch Neurol*. 1985;42:224–227.
62. O'Leary DH, Holen J, Ricotta JJ, Roe S, Schenk EA. Carotid bifurcation disease: prediction of ulceration with B-mode ultrasound. *Radiology*. 1987;162:523–525.
63. Comerota AJ, Katz ML, White JV, Grosh JD. The preoperative diagnosis of the ulcerated carotid atheroma. *J Vasc Surg*. 1990;11:505–510.
64. Farber R et al. B-mode real-time ultrasonic carotid imaging: impact on decision-making and prediction of surgical findings. *Neurology*. 1984;34:541–544.
65. Ricotta JJ. Plaque characterization by B-mode scan. *Surg Clin North Am*. 1990;70:191–199.
66. Goodson SF et al. Can carotid duplex scanning supplant arteriography in patients with focal carotid territory symptoms? *J Vasc Surg*. 1987;5:551–557.
67. Rubin JR, Bondi JA, Rhodes RS. Duplex scanning versus conventional arteriography for the evaluation of carotid artery plaque morphology. *Surgery*. 1987;102:749–755.
68. Iannuzzi A et al. Ultrasonographic correlates of carotid atherosclerosis in transient ischemic attack and stroke. *Stroke*. 1995;26:614–619.
69. Golledge J, Cuming R, Ellis M, Davies AH, Greenhalgh RM. Carotid plaque characteristics and presenting symptom. *Brit J Surg*. 1997;84:1697–1701.
70. Chambers BR, Norris JW. Outcome in patients with asymptomatic neck bruits. *N Engl J Med*. 1986;315:860–865.
71. Hennericci M, Hulsbomer HB, Hefter H, Lammerts D, Rautenberg W. Natural history of asymptomatic extracranial arterial disease. Results of a long-term prospective study. *Brain*. 1987;110:777–791.
72. Norris JW, Zhu CZ, Bornstein NM, Chambers BR. Vascular risks of asymptomatic carotid stenosis. *Stroke*. 1991; 22:1485–1490.
73. Zhu CZ, Norris JW. A therapeutic window for carotid endarterectomy in patients with asymptomatic carotid stenosis. *Can J Surg*. 1991;34:437–440.
74. Mackey AE et al. Outcome of asymptomatic patients with carotid disease. *Neurology*. 1997;48:896–903.
75. Nadareishvili ZG, Rothwell PM, Beletsky V, Pagniello A, Norris JW. Long-term risk of stroke and other vascular events in patients with asymptomatic carotid artery stenosis. *Arch Neurol*. 2002;59:1162–1166.
76. The European Carotid Surgery Trialists Collaborative Group. Risk of stroke in the distribution of an asymptomatic carotid artery. *Lancet*. 1995;345:209–212.
77. Inzitari D et al. The causes and risk of stroke in patients with asymptomatic internal-carotid-artery stenosis. North American Symptomatic Carotid Endarterectomy Trial Collaborators. *N Engl J Med*. 2000;342:1693–1700.
78. Nicolaides AN et al. Severity of asymptomatic carotid stenosis and risk of ipsilateral hemispheric ischaemic events: results from the ACSRS study. *Eur J Vasc Endovas Surg*. 2005;30:275–284.
79. North American Symptomatic Carotid Endarterectomy Trial Collaborators. Beneficial effect of carotid endarterectomy in symptomatic patients with high-grade carotid stenosis. *N Engl J Med*. 1991;325:445–453.
80. Executive Committee for the Asymptomatic Carotid Atherosclerosis Study. Endarterectomy for asymptomatic carotid artery stenosis. *J Am Med Assoc*. 1995;273:1421–1428.
81. Nicolaides AN et al. Angiographic and duplex grading of internal carotid stenosis: can we overcome the confusion? *J Endovasc Surg*. 1996;3:158–165.
82. European Carotid Surgery Trialists Collaborative Group. MRC European carotid surgery trial: Interim results for symptomatic patients with severe (70–99%) or with mild (0–29%) carotid stenosis. *Lancet*. 1991;337: 1235–1243.
83. MRC Asymptomatic Carotid Surgery Trial (ACST) Collaborative Group. Prevention of disabling and fatal strokes by successful carotid endarterectomy in patients without recent neurological symptoms: randomized controlled trial. *Lancet*. 2004;363:1491–1502.

37 Ultrasonic Plaque Characterization: Results from the Asymptomatic Carotid Stenosis and Risk of Stroke (ACSRS) Study

Andrew Nicolaides, Stavros K. Kakkos, Efthyvoulos Kyriacou, Maura Griffin, George Geroulakos, and Constantinos S. Pattichis

37.1 Introduction

The Asymptomatic Carotid Stenosis and Risk of Stroke (ACSRS) study was a multicenter natural history study. Its primary aim was to identify clinical, biochemical, and plaque features that, when used in combination, would allow risk stratification for ipsilateral carotid territory hemispheric ischemic events, especially stroke. It was planned in 1996, soon after the publication of the Asymptomatic Carotid Atherosclerosis Study (ACAS),[1] and recruitment started in 1998. The ACSRS is the largest natural history study of patients with asymptomatic carotid stenosis performed to date with 1,121 patients followed for 6–96 months (mean 48 months). Results of different aspects such as quality control, stenosis and risk, factors associated with cardiovascular mortality, effect of image normalization on carotid plaque classification, silent ipsilateral cerebral embolic infarcts on computed tomography (CT) brain scans and stroke risk, and stroke risk stratification using baseline plaque texture features have already been published.[2–8] The aim of this chapter is to present the main messages that have come out of this study in relation to ultrasonic plaque characterization and highlight potential clinical applications.

37.2 Methodology Used

37.2.1 Participating Centers

Participating centers had an active noninvasive vascular laboratory with color duplex facility, a volume of patients of at least 500 per year, and staff experienced in the investigation of patients with extracranial cerebrovascular disease: a neurologist, a vascular physician or surgeon, and a radiologist. Also, they were able to identify on average 15 individuals or patients with asymptomatic atherosclerotic carotid bifurcation disease that could be recruited to the study by screening new attendees to their practice.

37.2.2 Quality Control

The ultrasound methodology in the ACSRS study included a set of procedures designed to control quality and monitor key components of measurements. These included instrumentation settings, method of recording data, standardization of the method of scanning as reported in Chap. 12, standardization of

---

A. Nicolaides (✉)
Imperial College and Vascular Screening and Diagnostic Centre, London, UK

S.K. Kakkos
Department of Vascular Surgery, University of Patras Medical School, Patras, Achaia, Greece

E. Kyriacou
Department of Computer Science and Engineering Frederick University Cyprus, Lemesos, Cyprus

M. Griffin
Vascular Screening and Diagnostic Centre, London, UK

G. Geroulakos
Department of Surgery, Charing Cross Hospital, London, UK

C.S. Pattichis
Department of Computer Science, University of Cyprus, Nicosia, Cyprus

criteria for grading internal carotid artery stenosis, and personnel training at the coordinating center. Throughout the study, performance was compared to the set standards. Results of the quality control already published[2] indicated that the goal of prospectively controlling quality in the ACSRS study had been achieved.

37.2.3 Patient Recruitment

Newly referred (<3 months) patients with 50–99% internal carotid artery (ICA) stenosis in relation to the carotid bulb diameter [European Carotid Surgery Trial (ECST) method] without previous ipsilateral cerebral or retinal ischemic (CORI) symptoms and without neurological abnormality were recruited to the study. Patients who had had contralateral cerebral hemispheric/retinal or vertebrobasilar symptoms were included if asymptomatic for at least 6 months prior to recruitment. For patients with bilateral asymptomatic carotid atherosclerosis, the side with the more severe stenosis was considered ipsilateral (the study artery). During the planning of the study, it was argued that selection of patients from the records of a department or a vascular laboratory was likely to introduce bias toward the selection of patients with stable plaques because some patients with unstable plaques could have had developed symptoms in the meantime. Thus, only newly referred patients were admitted to the study.

37.2.4 Duplex Examination

Bilateral carotid duplex scanning was performed on admission to the study. Ultrasonographers from all centers were trained at the coordinating center in grading internal carotid stenosis and plaque image capture.[2] The entire duplex examination, recorded on S-VHS videotape, was sent to the coordinating center for quality control.

37.2.4.1 Grading of Internal Carotid Stenosis

Velocities were obtained at the point of maximum stenosis in the internal carotid artery and at the center of the common carotid artery lumen, with the beam of ultrasound at 60° to the direction of flow. Because absolute velocity measurements could underestimate stenosis (e.g., in the presence of cardiac arrhythmia) or overestimate stenosis (e.g., in the presence of severe contralateral disease), ultrasonographers at each center were trained to use a combination of absolute velocity measurements and velocity ratios as shown in Table 37.1.[9] Based on the velocities and velocity ratios, the percent diameter stenosis could be expressed in relation to the distal normal internal carotid [North American Symptomatic Carotid Endarterectomy Trial (NASCET) or "N" method] and bulb diameter (ECST or "E" method). Emphasis has been placed on the ratio of the peak systolic velocity in the internal carotid (site of highest velocity) (PSVic) over the end diastolic velocity in the common carotid (EDVcc)[9] (Fig. 37.1). The accuracy of this ratio has been validated in our department

Table 37.1 Duplex velocity criteria selected for highest accuracy

Angiographic diameter stenosis		Duplex velocity criteria				
N%	E%	PSV_{IC}	EDV_{IC}	PSV_{IC}/PSV_{CC}	PSV_{IC}/EDV_{CC}	EDV_{IC}/EDV_{CC}
12	50	<120	<40	<1.5	<7	
30	60					<2.6
47	70	120–150	40–80	1.5–2	7–10	
60	77		80–130	2–3.2		
65	80	150–250				
70	83		>130	3.2–4	10–20	2.6–5.5
82	90	>250		>4	20–30	
90	95				>30	>5.5
99	99			Trickle flow		

Source: Reprinted with permission from Nicolaides et al.[9] © International Society of Endovascular Specialists
N NASCET, *E* ECST, *PSV* peak systolic velocity, *EDV* end-diastolic velocity, *IC* internal carotid, *CC* common carotid

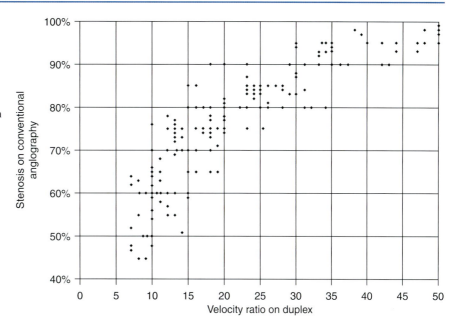

Fig. 37.1 The ratio of the peak systolic velocity of the internal carotid artery to the end-diastolic velocity of the common carotid artery (PSV_{IC}/EDV_{CC}) plotted against the angiographic percentage stenosis in relation to the distal internal carotid (Reprinted with permission from Nicolaides et al.[9] © International Society of Endovascular Specialists)

against digital subtraction angiography in the late 1980s and early 1990s. In plaques that were not calcified, anatomical criteria using color flow or power Doppler imaging of the artery in transverse section (percent diameter stenosis from measurements of vessel and residual lumen diameter at the site of maximum stenosis) were used to supplement velocity criteria also described in Chap. 30.[10–12] As indicated above, the entire duplex examination was recorded on S-VHS videotape and sent to the coordinating center. Contralateral ICA occlusion was noted. Bilateral vertebral artery flow was reported as cephalad, reversed, or not visualized.

37.2.4.2 Recording of Plaque Images

A high-frequency linear array transducer was used, and the technical ultrasound settings as described in Chap. 12[13] were observed to ensure optimum image quality for plaque type classification and texture analyses:

1. Maximum dynamic range was used which ensured the greatest possible display of gray scale values.
2. Persistence was set on low and frame rate on high, the latter ensuring good temporal scale values.
3. The time gain compensation curve (TGC) was sloping through the tissues but was positioned vertically through the lumen of the vessel because there was little attenuation of the ultrasound beam as it passed through blood. This ensured that the brightness of the adventitia of the anterior and posterior walls was similar.
4. The overall gain was adjusted to give optimum image quality. This was achieved by adjustment of the gain control to minimize but not abolish noise.
5. The most linear post-processing available curve was used.
6. The ultrasound beam was at 90° to the arterial wall.
7. The minimum depth was used so that the plaque occupied a large part of the image.

The above settings were essential prerequisites for plaque texture analysis, which was performed at the coordinating center. Ultrasonographers from participating centers attended for 2 days training at the coordinating center. They were instructed not only on equipment settings and method of image recording but also on the method of image normalization. Although they were not expected to perform image analysis, it was felt that knowledge of how it was done would ensure that all prerequisites for image analysis described above would be included. A specially prepared video recording with instructions how to perform the examination was provided. Video recordings of the examination and frozen images of plaques were sent to the coordinating center for image analysis.

37.2.4.3 Image Normalization and Analysis

Images that were recorded on video tapes were digitized off-line on a PC using a video grabber card (Videologic, TV Snap version 1.0.3 c 1994) at a resolution of 640 × 480 pixels at the coordinating center by two members of the team who were experienced in carotid scanning. Image normalization, standardization, and analysis were performed by the same members of the team as described in Chap. 12 using the "Plaque Texture Analysis" software version 3.2 (Iconsoft International Ltd, PO Box 172, Greenford, London UB6 9ZN, UK).[13]

37.2.5 Definitions and Reproducibility of Texture Features Used in the ACSRS

1. *Gray scale median (GSM)*. This was the median of the gray values of all the pixels in the plaque image. In a reproducibility study of 35 plaques measured by two observers, the interobserver mean difference of GSM was 3.6, the within-subject standard deviation was 13.6, and the intraclass correlation coefficient was 0.93.[13]
2. *Plaque type*. Plaques were classified automatically by the software into the following types according to a modified Geroulakos classification[14] as defined below:
   Type 1. Uniformly echolucent (black): <15% of the pixels in the plaque area were occupied by pixels with gray scale values >25.
   Type 2. Mainly echolucent: pixels with gray scale values >25 occupy 15–50% of the plaque area.
   Type 3. Mainly echogenic: pixels with gray scale values >25 occupy 50–85% of the plaque area.
   Type 4 or 5. Uniformly echogenic: pixels with gray scale values >25 occupy >85% of the plaque area. Examples of type 1–4 plaques are shown in Fig. 12.8.
   A reproducibility study involving 1,062 plaques classified visually by one observer after image normalization and automatically by the software had a kappa statistic of 0.61 ($p < 0.001$). Because of the low event rate in plaque types 4 and 5 as previously demonstrated[5] and because the software cannot distinguish between them, these plaque types have been grouped together.
3. *Plaque area*. This was calculated by the software using the distance scale on the side of the image frame for calibration and the plaque area outlined by the operator. It was expressed in mm^2.[2,13,15] In a reproducibility study involving 50 plaques, the interobserver intraclass correlation coefficient was 0.73.
4. *Discrete White Areas (DWA)*. The presence of DWA defined as areas with pixels having gray scale values >124 (colored red by the software for easy visual identification) not producing acoustic shadowing in plaque types 1–3 was noted (Fig. 12.8). A reproducibility study involving 80 plaques classified visually after image normalization by two observers for presence or absence of DWA had a kappa statistic of 0.83 ($P < 0.01$).
5. *Plaque ulceration*. This was defined as a defect $>2 \times 2$ mm on the surface of the plaque shown by color flow or power Doppler to be communicating with the vessel lumen. It was reported by the ultrasonographers from each partner center.[16]
6. *Juxtaluminal black area without a visible echogenic cap (JBA)*. This was measured as described in Chap. 12. When the JBA (range 0–110 mm^2) of 324 plaques was measured by two observers using the "Plaque Texture Analysis" software, the interobserver mean difference between repeat measurements was 2.5 mm^2, the within-subject standard deviation was 6.9 mm^2, and the intraclass correlation coefficient was 0.94.
7. *Other texture features*. A total of 84 additional texture features were automatically extracted by the software as described in Chaps. 12, 14, and 15. They consisted of First Order Statistics (FOS), Spatial Gray Level Dependence Matrix (SGLDM), Gray Level Difference Statistics (GLDS), Gray Level Run Length Statistics (RUNL), and other features as described in Chap. 12.

37.2.6 Clinical and Biochemical Characteristics

At baseline all patients had a history taken and a physical examination by the local neurologist, electrocardiographic (ECG) examination, and collection of fasting blood for determination of the following:
- Age, gender, body mass index (BMI), systolic and diastolic blood pressure, smoking history, and accrued pack-years.

- Medication usage including antiplatelet, anti-hypertensive, and lipid-lowering agents.
- Presence of hypertension (antihypertensive medication or BP $\geq$ 140 mmHg systolic or $\geq$90 mmHg diastolic); coronary artery disease (documented myocardial infarction/angina, coronary artery bypass, or stenting); diabetes (antihyperglycemic therapy or fasting blood glucose >120 mg/dL); and previous contralateral stroke/transient ischemic attack (TIA) or vertebrobasilar symptoms.
- ECG evidence of atrial fibrillation, previous myocardial infarction (MI), myocardial ischemia, and left ventricular hypertrophy (LVH) on baseline ECG. ECGs were reported at the coordinating center by two cardiologists.
- Fibrinogen, fasting lipids [total cholesterol, high-density lipoprotein (HDL) cholesterol, low-density lipoprotein (LDL) cholesterol, triglycerides], serum creatinine, and hematocrit.

37.2.7 Outcome Measures

Primary outcome measures were (a) ipsilateral CORI events, i.e., cerebral or retinal ischemic events which included stroke, and (b) ipsilateral cerebral ischemic stroke (fatal or non-fatal). Stroke and TIA were defined as cerebral deficits most likely of vascular origin lasting >24 h or <24 h, respectively. For each stroke, details recorded by the local neurologist, a 6-month modified Rankin score, and CT or magnetic resonance imaging (MRI) brain scan results were requested. Two coordinating center members, including a neurologist, made the final classification of ipsilateral strokes. Local team members diagnosed amaurosis fugax TIAs and vertebrobasilar strokes.

Secondary outcome measures were all other strokes and TIAs, contralateral retinal vascular events, and all other deaths. Cause of death was determined by local team members using death certificates, hospital records, and family doctor information.

37.2.8 Study Exit Points

Follow-up ceased with the first occurrence of any of the following: the first primary outcome measure, carotid endarterectomy/angioplasty or stenting for the still asymptomatic study artery, death from causes other than ipsilateral stroke, or loss to follow-up. Stroke, TIA, or death associated with carotid endarterectomy/angioplasty or stenting for the still asymptomatic study artery were not included in event rate calculations.

37.3 Results and Key Messages

37.3.1 Numbers Recruited

1,121 patients aged 39–89 years (mean age 70.0, standard deviation [SD] 7.7, 61% male) were recruited during 1998–2002, with a follow-up of 6–96 months (mean 48 months). 66% of patients were recruited from medical services (vascular internists: 8%, neurologists: 16%, cardiologists: 10%, hypertension clinics: 5%, metabolic units: 3%, and screening programs: 4%). 34% of patients were recruited from surgical services (vascular: 32%, cardiac surgery: 2%).

37.3.2 Ipsilateral Cerebrovascular Events

A total of 130 first ipsilateral CORI events occurred (59 strokes of which 12 were fatal, 49 TIAs, and 22 amaurosis fugax). For ischemic stroke, the modified Rankin scale at 6 months was zero in 4 cases, 1 in 9 cases, 2 in 6 cases, 3 in 8 cases, 4 in 18 cases, 5 in 2 cases, and 6 in 12 cases. There were two additional first ipsilateral fatal hemorrhagic strokes.

37.3.3 Other Outcome Measures

There were 49 first contralateral CORI events: 18 ischemic strokes of which 7 were fatal, 22 TIAs, and 9 amaurosis fugax. There were two vertebrobasilar strokes. Of the 18 contralateral strokes, 4 occurred in the 125 patients with plaques producing 90–99% stenosis, 1 in the 170 producing 70–89% stenosis, and the remaining 13 in the 826 producing less than 70% stenosis. Plaque characterization was not performed on the contralateral side. The only factor associated with contralateral stroke was the presence of atrial fibrillation (odds ratio [OR] 8.28; 95% confidence interval [CI] 2.26–30).

There were a total of 214 deaths (195 non-stroke deaths) of which 157 (73%) were due to vascular causes: myocardial infarction: 110, fatal stroke: 19 (12 ipsilateral and 7 contralateral, already mentioned above), heart failure: 17, pulmonary embolism: 3, lower limb ischemia/gangrene: 3, ruptured abdominal aortic aneurysm: 3, renal failure: 1, and mesenteric artery thrombosis: 1. There were 56 nonvascular deaths; malignancy: 37, pneumonia/respiratory failure: 12, gastrointestinal hemorrhage: 2, dementia: 2, road traffic accident: 2, and general surgical procedure: 1. Cause of death was unknown in one patient.

Ipsilateral carotid endarterectomy was performed in 129 patients for a still asymptomatic study artery (stenosis median: 85% ECST; interquartile range:75–90) because the clinician in charge or the patient requested it. This occurred soon after publication of the Asymptomatic Carotid Surgery Trial (ACST) results. Of these 129 patients, 11 (5.6%) were in the group of 198 with less than 70% stenosis, 77 (12.9%) in the group of 598 with 70–89% stenosis, and 40 (12.3%) in the group of 325 with 90–99% stenosis. Twenty-one patients were lost to follow-up. In these, contact was lost with 15, 5 declined to re-attend (too old to travel), and 1 emigrated. Thus, 150 patients (13.4%) have been "lost" from the study. They have been included in the analysis up to the last follow-up visit. The remaining 971 (86.6%) have been followed up to a primary event, death, or termination of the study in December 2006.

37.3.4 Effect of Stenosis on Risk

37.3.4.1 CORI Events

The ipsilateral cerebral or retinal ischemic (CORI) events [amaurosis fugax (AF), TIAs, and stroke] and ipsilateral ischemic cerebral stroke for all patients and subgroups according to ECST stenosis and NASCET stenosis for comparison with previous publications that have used these methods are shown in Table 37.2 and Figs. 37.2 and 37.3.

Ipsilateral% ECST stenosis was mild (50–69%) in 198 patients, moderate (70–89%) in 598 patients, and severe (90–99%) in 325 patients.

The cumulative 5-year ipsilateral CORI event rate for the three stenosis groups was 9%, 15%, and 20% (Log Rank test $P = 0.009$), giving an average annual event rate of 1.8%, 3.0%, and 4.0%, respectively. During the whole period of follow-up, there were 130 events of which 16 were in the mild, 65 in the moderate, and 49 in the severe stenosis group (Fig. 37.2a).

The cumulative 5-year stroke rate for the three stenosis groups was 4%, 7%, and 12% (Log Rank test $P = 0.011$), giving an average annual stroke rate of 0.8%, 1.4%, and 2.4%, respectively. During the whole period of follow-up, there were 59 strokes of which 5 were in the mild, 29 in the moderate, and 25 in the severe stenosis group (Fig. 37.2b). For stenosis greater than 70%, the cumulative 5-year stroke rate was 8%, giving an average annual stroke rate of 1.6%

The NASCET 60% cut-off point as used in the ACAS trial produced a mild stenosis group (<60%)

Table 37.2 Ipsilateral cerebral or retinal ischemic (CORI) events (AF, TIAs, and stroke) and ipsilateral ischemic cerebral stroke for all patients and subgroups according to ECST stenosis (*) as used in this chapter and NASCET stenosis (**) for comparison with publications that have used these methods. Follow-up 6 months to 8 years (mean: 48 months). P values were calculated using chi-square test for trend

ECST stenosis (%)	NASCET stenosis (%)	N	CORI events	Strokes
All patients		1,121	130 (11.6%)	59 (5.3%)
50–69*	<50	198	16 (8.1%)	5 (2.5%)
70–89*	50–79	598	65 (10.9%)	29 (4.8%)
90–99*	80–99	325	49 (15.1%)	25 (7.7%)
			$P = 0.01$	$P = 0.008$
<80	<70**	514	50 (9.7%)	21 (4.1%)
80–99	70–99**	607	80 (13.2%)	38 (6.3%)
			$P = 0.07$	$P = 0.10$

Reprinted from Nicolaides et al.[8] with permission from Elsevier

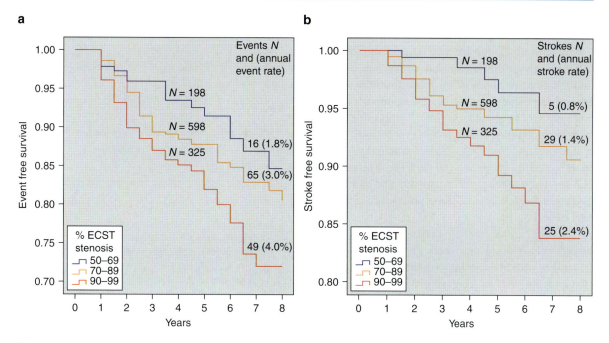

Fig. 37.2 (**a, b**) Kaplan–Meier plots showing (**a**) ipsilateral cerebrovascular or retinal ischemic (CORI) event free survival and (**b**) ipsilateral cerebral ischemic stroke-free survival stratified by European Carotid Surgery Trial (ECST) stenosis: log rank P for trend = 0.002

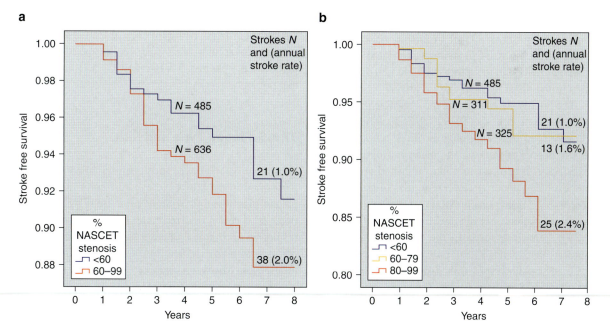

Fig. 37.3 (**a, b**) Kaplan–Meier plots showing ipsilateral cerebral ischemic stroke-free survival stratified by North American Symptomatic Carotid Endarterectomy Trial (NASCET) stenosis (**a**) of <60% or >60% as used in the ACAS trial: log rank P for trend = 0.126 and (**b**) of <60%, 60–79%, and 80–99% stenosis: P for trend = 0.042

with 485 patients and a moderate/severe stenosis group (≥60%) with 636 patients. The cumulative 5-year stroke rate for the two groups was 5% and 10%, giving an average annual stroke rate of 1.0% and 2.0%, respectively (Log Rank test $P = 0.126$). During the whole period of follow-up, 21 strokes were in the mild and 38 in the moderate/severe stenosis group (Fig. 37.3a).

Ipsilateral% NASCET stenosis was mild (<60%) in 485 patients, moderate (60–79%) in 311 patients, and severe (80–99%) in 325 patients. The cumulative 5-year stroke rate for the three groups was 5%, 8%, and 12% (Log Rank test $P = 0.042$), giving an average annual stroke rate of 1.0%, 1.6%, and 2.4%, respectively. During the whole period of follow-up, 21 strokes were in the mild, 13 in the moderate, and 25 in the severe stenosis group (Fig. 37.3b).

The results indicate that severity of stenosis is a relatively poor indicator of stroke risk with a receiver operator characteristic (ROC) area under the curve (AUC) of 0.603 (95% CI 0.525–0.682). Severity of stenosis cannot identify a high-risk group that contains the majority of strokes. As far as stratifying patients into low, moderate, and high risk, the ECST method performs better than the NASCET method. It has already been demonstrated that ECST% stenosis has a linear relationship to risk while NASCET% stenosis does not.[3] The reason for this is probably the fact that ECST% stenosis is related to plaque volume in the bulb, while NASCET% stenosis is related to lumen diameter reduction in relation to the lumen diameter of the normal distal internal carotid artery.

The inclusion criteria in the ACSRS provided a wide range of stenosis (50–99% ECST). This allowed classification into subgroups of mild, moderate, and severe degree of stenosis and better evaluation of this risk factor in contrast to other published studies that had excluded upper or lower extremes of the range of stenosis.[17–24] Only one previous prospective study has recruited patients within the full range of 50–99% ECST stenosis as used in the authors' study[23] and graded the stenosis as mild (<50%), moderate (50–79%), and severe (80–99%). This study which involved 678 patients with a mean follow-up of 3.6 years showed an increasing ipsilateral CORI event and stroke rate with increasing grades of stenosis (Table 36.3).

High-grade internal carotid stenosis (ECST 90–99%) was associated with a high cardiovascular mortality

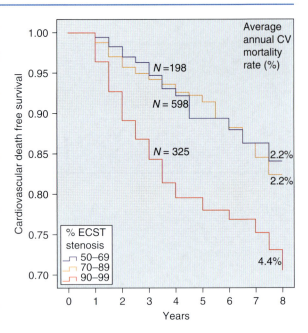

Fig. 37.4 Kaplan–Meier plots showing cardiovascular (CV) death free survival stratified by European Carotid Surgery Trial (ECST) grades of stenosis: log rank: P for trend <0.001

(Fig. 37.4). The cumulative 5-year cardiovascular mortality rate for the three ECST stenosis groups was 11%, 11%, and 22% (Log Rank test $P < 0.001$), giving an average annual rate of 2.2%, 2.2%, and 4.4%, respectively. This high cardiovascular mortality rate remained significant after adjusting for clinical factors associated with cardiovascular death (age, gender, cardiac failure, myocardial ischemia, LVH on ECG, and antiplatelet therapy).

37.3.5 Plaque Type and Risk

As pointed out above, most natural history studies performed in the past have used different methods of plaque classification without prior image normalization. It is now realized that image normalization results in a marked change in the appearance of plaques with reclassification of a large number. The relationship between plaque classification before image normalization and after image normalization in patients admitted to the ACSRS study has been presented in Chap. 12. The automated classification of plaques (Geroulakos classification) using the "Plaque Texture Analysis" software is also presented in the same chapter.

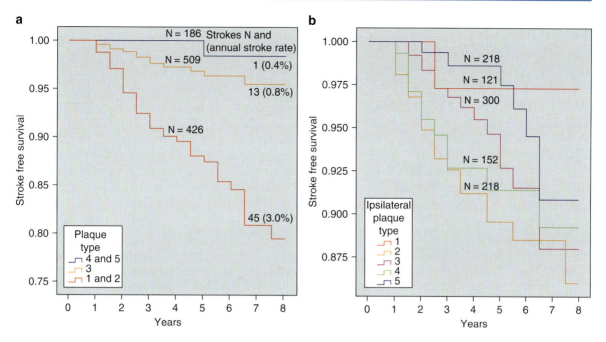

Fig. 37.5 (**a, b**) Kaplan–Meier plots showing ipsilateral cerebral ischemic stroke-free survival stratified by plaque type (**a**) after image normalization: log rank P for trend < 0.001 and (**b**) before image normalization: log rank P for trend $= 0.06$

During the follow-up period, one stroke occurred in the 186 patients with plaque types 4 and 5 (classified as type 4 by the software), 13 strokes in 509 patients with plaque type 3, and 45 strokes in the 426 patients with plaque types 1 and 2. The cumulative 5-year stroke rate for these three groups was 2%, 4%, and 15% (Log Rank test $P < 0.001$), giving an average annual stroke rate of 0.4%, 0.8%, and 3.0%, respectively (Fig. 37.5a). The plaque type was determined by the software after image normalization. Life table analysis for the plaque types classified visually by an experienced ultrasonographer prior to image normalization did not show a clear-cut separation of risk (Fig. 37.5b). These findings emphasize the importance of image normalization prior to image analysis and demonstrate the low stroke risk associated with type 4 and 5 plaques irrespective of the degree of stenosis. Of the 186 patients with type 4 and 5 plaques, 51 had mild, 99 moderate, and 36 severe stenosis. Most important is that 76% of the strokes (45 out of 59) occurred in the 38% of patients (426 out 1,121 patients studied) with type 1 and 2 plaques at baseline. Severe and fatal ipsilateral strokes ($n = 14$) (Rankin score 5 and 6) occurred exclusively in plaque types 1 and 2 (10 in type 2 and 4 in type 1).

Several research teams have indicated that the risk for stroke is higher with echolucent plaques (type 1 and 2) when compared with echogenic plaques (type 3 and 4). Others have claimed that heterogenous plaques are associated with a higher risk for stroke than homogenous plaques. As pointed out earlier, the results of the ACSRS study are compatible with both findings. This is because type 2 plaques that are associated with the highest stroke risk (Table 37.3) are included by most authors in both the echolucent (hypoechoic) and heterogenous groups (see below).

37.3.6 Gray Scale Median (GSM)

The measurement of GSM after image normalization has become an established reproducible measurement of overall plaque echodensity (Chaps. 12, 15, 24, and 31). The ACSRS study confirms the findings of other prospective studies[25,26] that a low GSM is a strong predictor of future ipsilateral CORI events including stroke. GSM was high, >30 in 609 patients; moderate, 15–30 in 269 patients; and low, <15 in 243 patients. These three ranges of GSM were associated with low, moderate, and high risk of stroke. The cumulative

Table 37.3 The average annual stroke rate in individual plaque types (1–4) and when reclassified as homogenous, heterogenous, hypoechoic, or hyperechoic

	Homogenous	Heterogenous	Total
Hypoechoic	Type 1 ($n = 85$) Prevalence 7.6% Strokes 9 Annual stroke rate 2.8%	Type 2 ($n = 341$) Prevalence 30.4% Strokes 36 Annual stroke rate 3.0%	Type 1 and 2 ($n = 426$) Prevalence 38.0% Strokes 45 Annual stroke rate 3.0%
Hyperechoic	Type 4 ($n = 186$) Prevalence 16.6% Strokes 1 Annual stroke rate 0.4%	Type 3 ($n = 509$) Prevalence 45.4% Strokes 13 Annual stroke rate 0.8%	Type 4 and 3 ($n = 695$) Prevalence 62% Strokes 14 Annual stroke rate 0.6%
Total	Type 1 and 4 ($n = 271$) Prevalence 24.1% Strokes 10 Annual stroke rate 1.2%	Type 2 and 3 ($n = 850$) Prevalence 75.8% Strokes 49 Annual stroke rate 1.6%	

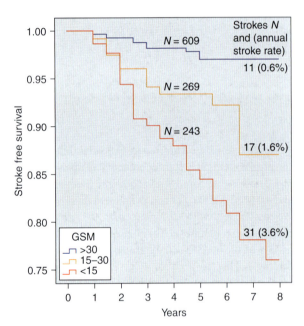

Fig. 37.6 Kaplan–Meier plots showing ipsilateral cerebral ischemic stroke–free survival stratified by gray scale median (GSM) after image normalization: log rank P for trend < 0.001

5-year stroke rate for these three groups was 2%, 4%, and 15% (Log Rank test $P < 0.001$), giving an average annual stroke rate of 0.6%, 1.6%, and 3.6%, respectively (Fig. 37.6). During the whole period of follow-up, 11 strokes occurred in the high, 17 in the intermediate, and 31 in the low-GSM group. Most important is that a GSM <15 could identify a high-risk group consisting of 22% of patients (243 out 1,121patients studied) that contained 52% of the strokes, (31 out of 59) that occurred during follow-up.

Severe and fatal ipsilateral strokes ($n = 14$) (Rank in score 5 and 6) occurred exclusively in plaques with GSM < 30 (4 in plaques with GSM 15–30 and 10 in plaques with GSM < 15).

37.3.7 Discrete White Areas

Plaque heterogeneity has already been shown to be associated with symptomatic plaques.[27] With the exception of calcified plaques, it is the result of the presence of discrete white areas (DWA) without acoustic shadow in hypoechoic areas. These DWA are often hyperperfused as shown by ultrasonic contrast perfusion agents and correspond to areas of neovascularization and increased numbers of macrophages on histology.[28] Whether the presence of these areas are responsible for the development of intraplaque hemorrhage, non-uniform plaque stresses promoting plaque rupture or erosion of the fibrous cap by the macrophages merits further investigation.

The presence of DWA (more than one) was associated with increased ipsilateral CORI events ($P < 0.001$) (Fig. 37.7a). However, there was a non-significant ($P = 0.124$) trend for an increased stroke rate after the first 3 years (Fig. 37.7b).

37.3.8 Plaque Ulceration

Ultrasonic plaque ulceration as detected by ultrasound had promising results in two prospective studies[29,30] (Chap. 36). In the ACSRS study, ultrasonic ulcer was

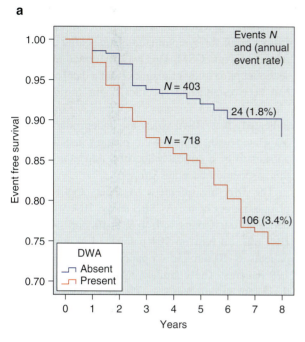

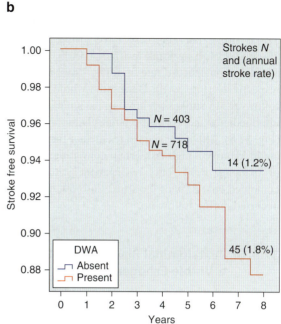

Fig. 37.7 (**a**, **b**) Kaplan–Meier plots showing (**a**) ipsilateral cerebrovascular or retinal ischemic (CORI) event free survival stratified by presence or absence of discrete white areas (DWA): log rank P for trend <0.001 and (**b**) ipsilateral cerebral ischemic stroke-free survival stratified by presence or absence of discrete white areas (DWA): log rank P for trend $= 0.124$

visible in 101 plaques. However, ulceration was not associated with ipsilateral CORI events or stroke. The ultrasound scanners used in the ACSRS for the baseline images obtained mainly in the late 1990s were bought by most centers in the early or mid 1990s when the resolution and the ability to visualize ulcers were inferior to that of current instruments. It remains to be seen whether ulceration as detected by modern instruments can contribute to risk stratification.

37.3.9 Plaque Area

Carotid plaque area has already been reported to be a strong predictor of myocardial infarction and stroke[15] in patients with mild degrees of stenosis. The results from the ACSRS study show that plaque area can be used to stratify cerebrovascular risk in patients with plaques producing greater than 50% stenosis (Fig. 37.8). Plaque area was small, <40 mm^2 in 518 patients; intermediate, 40–80 mm^2 in 489 patients; and large, >80 mm^2 in 114 patients. These three

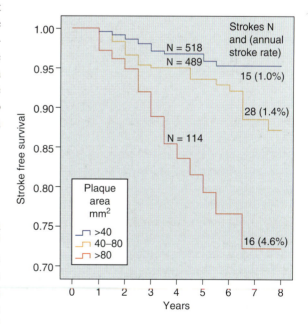

Fig. 37.8 Kaplan–Meier plots showing ipsilateral cerebral ischemic stroke-free survival stratified by plaque area: log rank P for trend < 0.001

ranges of plaque area were associated with low, moderate, and high risk of stroke. The cumulative 5-year stroke rate for these three groups was 5%, 7%, and 23% (Log Rank test $P < 0.001$), giving an average annual stroke rate of 1.0%, 1.4%, and 4.6%, respectively (Fig. 37.8). During the whole period of follow-up, 15 strokes occurred in the small, 28 in the intermediate, and 16 in the large plaque area group (Fig. 37.8). Although plaque area greater than 80 mm^2 could identify a high-risk group consisting of 10.2% of patients (114 out 1,121 patients studied), it contained only 27% of the strokes (16 out of 59) that occurred during follow-up.

37.3.10 Juxtaluminal Black Area Without a Visible Echogenic Cup

The presence of a juxtaluminal black (hypoechoic) area (JBA) without a visible echogenic cap has been reported to be associated with symptomatic plaques (Chap. 12).[31] However, cut-off points for the size of such an area have not been reported. The authors performed a pilot study to determine (a) an appropriate cut-off point for JBA without a visible echogenic cap in ultrasonic images of internal carotid artery plaques and (b) to determine the diagnostic value of this cut-off point for symptomatic plaques after adjusting for stenosis and GSM. This was performed in a cross-sectional pilot study of plaques from a database which had been established specifically for testing newly identified texture features[32] (Chap. 12). The results indicated that JBA was an independent factor associated with symptomatic plaques and that there appears to be a critical value of 8 mm^2 above which this association becomes strong.

The JBA measurement has been applied to the plaque images of the ACSRS study. JBA was classified into four groups: <4, 4–8, 8–10, and >10 mm^2. JBA was <4 mm^2 in 704 patients, 4–8 mm^2 in 171 patients, 8–10 mm^2 in 46 patients, and >10 mm^2 in 198 patients. The cumulative 5-year stroke rate for these four groups was 2%, 7%, 16%, and 23% (Log Rank test $P < 0.001$), giving an average annual stroke rate of 0.4%, 1.4%, 3.2%, and 5.0%, respectively (Fig. 37.9a). During the whole period of follow-up, 8 strokes occurred in the <4 mm^2 group, 9 in the 4–8 mm^2 group, 6 in the 8–10 mm^2 group, and 36 in the 8–10 mm^2 group. The results indicate that a high-risk group can be identified, which contains the

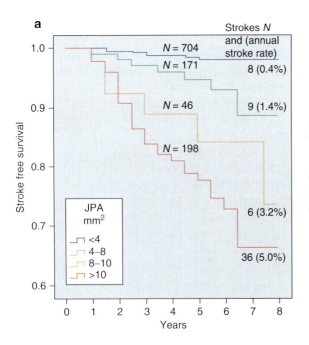
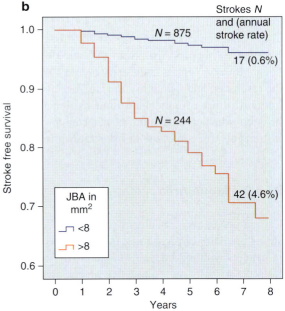

Fig. 37.9 (**a, b**) Kaplan–Meier plots showing ipsilateral cerebral ischemic stroke-free survival stratified by (**a**) size of juxtaluminal plaque area: log rank P for trend < 0.001 and (**b**) by juxtaluminal plaque area less than 8 mm^2 or more than 8 mm^2: log rank P for trend <0.001

majority of the strokes and confirms the previous finding that 8 mm² is a critical cut-off point.

The stroke-free survival time of the two groups of patients based on the 8-mm² cut-off point is shown in Fig. 37.9b. The resulting two groups of 875 patients with JBA < 8 mm² and 244 patients with JBA > 8 mm² were associated with low and high risk of stroke. The cumulative 5-year stroke rate for the group with JBA < 8 mm² was 3% and for the group with JBA > 8 mm² was 23% (Log Rank test $P < 0.001$), giving an average annual stroke rate of 0.6% and 4.6%, respectively (Fig. 37.9b). During the whole period of follow-up, 17 strokes occurred in the low- and 42 in the high-risk group (Fig. 37.9b).

The design of the ACSRS did not foresee such a measurement, and the ultrasonographers were not trained to provide images of confirmed presence of JBA using multiple color flow images in addition to the gray scale image. It may well be that some of the JBAs were an artifact by poor color filling of the lumen, as often seen just distal to severely stenotic plaques. Thus, the results should be interpreted with caution and need to be validated in another prospective study. Ideally three-dimensional (3D) imaging should be used for such a validation. If this finding can be validated, then the presence of a JBA could prove a powerful diagnostic tool. The presence of such an area would indicate a thin fibrous cap not detected by ultrasound, overlying a large lipid core or an intraplaque hemorrhage close to the lumen; an alternative would be a fresh thrombus on the plaque surface.

Schulte-Altedorneburg et al. reported that thrombosis at the plaque surface was often seen in "completely echolucent" plaques ($P < 0.001$).[33] It is likely that the echolucent plaque component represents the thrombus or its combination with the lipid core. A recent study has demonstrated a strong association between symptomatic plaques and intraluminal thrombus attached to the plaque.[34] It may well be that the presence of a black area adjacent to the lumen identifies plaques, many of which are associated with thrombus formation. This needs to be tested in future studies.

37.3.11 Clinical and Biochemical Features Associated with Increased Risk

Age, systolic blood pressure, plasma creatinine, smoking (more than ten pack-years) showed an association with ipsilateral CORI events or stroke, but when combined with stenosis and other plaque features in Cox proportional hazards models, they were no longer significant.[8] The only clinical factor that had a strong association with future CORI events and stroke and remained significant in all the Cox models was the presence of a history of contralateral TIAs or stroke.

The stroke-free survival in the patients without and those with a history of contralateral TIAs or stroke is shown in Fig. 37.10. The cumulative 5-year stroke rate for the group of 948 patients without such a history was 6% and for the group of 173 patients with such a history was 17% (Log Rank test $P < 0.001$), giving an average annual stroke rate of 1.2% and 3.4%, respectively (Fig. 37.10). During the whole period of follow-up, 39 strokes occurred in the low- and 20 in the high-risk group. In the Cox regression models, this risk factor was associated with approximately double the risk of developing a stroke. The key message is that the presence of a history of contralateral TIA or stroke, although present in a minority of patients (15%), is a risk factor that should be combined with plaque features in calculations of risk and taken into consideration in future studies.

An interesting finding is that 5 of the 14 severe and fatal ipsilateral strokes (Rankin score 5 and 6) occurred in the 173 with a history of contralateral

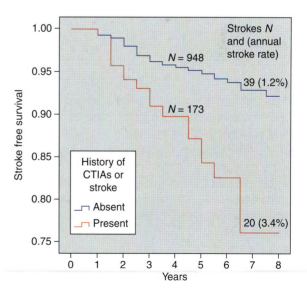

Fig. 37.10 Kaplan–Meier plots showing ipsilateral cerebral ischemic stroke-free survival stratified by presence or absence of history of contralateral TIA (CTIA) or stroke: log rank P for trend < 0.001

TIA or stroke ($P = 0.035$; OR 3.10 95% CI 1.03–9.38). Also, 7 of the 14 severe and fatal ipsilateral strokes (Rankin score 5 and 6) occurred in the 231 patients with diabetes, with the other 7 in the remaining 890 patients ($P = 0.006$; OR 3.94 95% CI 1.37–11.35).

37.3.12 Computer-Generated Texture Features

With the exception of GSM, very few studies have investigated the association between texture features of carotid plaque ultrasonic images and patient symptoms[35–37] (Chaps. 15 and 16). Thus, it has been suggested that the additional use of texture features, which provide information on the spatial distribution of the pixels of different shades, might improve the identification of high-risk plaques.[38,39] Ultrasonic texture characterization using computer algorithms has been successfully applied to liver images.[40,41]

Some of the texture features offered by the fifth module of the "Plaque Texture Analysis software" version 3.2 (Iconsoft International Ltd, PO Box 172, Greenford, London UB6 9ZN, UK)[13] have been found to be associated with symptomatic plaques while others did not (Figs. 37.11 and 37.12).

A two-stage project was undertaken. First, the value of texture features in identifying plaques associated with symptoms has been tested on the images of a database obtained from a cross-sectional study of symptomatic and asymptomatic carotid plaque images. This database was established for the initial testing of diagnostic algorithms[32] as described in Chap. 12. The same features were subsequently applied to the images of the ACSRS study.

The images ($n = 324$) of the database from the cross-sectional study were collected prospectively from patients referred to the authors' vascular laboratory for diagnostic carotid ultrasound in order to detect the presence and severity of internal carotid stenosis. Of these 324 patients, 140 were asymptomatic, 37 had presented with AF, 59 with TIA, and 88 with stroke

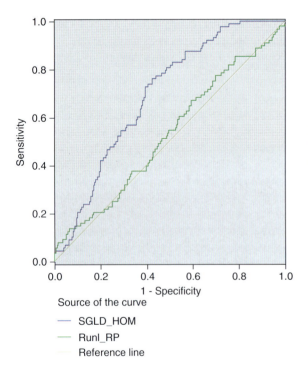

Fig. 37.11 Receiver operating characteristic (ROC) curves for stroke using SGLDM-HOM and RUNL-Run Percentage (RUNL-RP) as continuous variables in the cross-sectional study of 324 patients

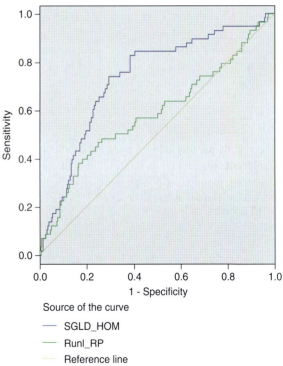

Fig. 37.12 Receiver operating characteristic (ROC) curves for stroke using SGLDM-HOM and RUNL-RP as continuous variables in the ACSRS study

and good recovery. Asymptomatic patients were referred because of hyperlipidemia, the presence of a cervical bruit, or for screening prior to cardiac surgery. Symptomatic patients presented with amaurosis fugax, ipsilateral hemispheric TIAs, or stroke as diagnosed by referring physicians or surgeons and subsequently confirmed by a neurologist. Duplex scanning was performed on an ATL HDI 3000 ultrasound unit and a high-frequency linear array transducer (4–7 MHz) (Philips/Advanced Technologies Laboratories, Bothel, Washington, USA). Images were stored on magneto-optical disks. At the end of the routine clinical examination for the grading of internal carotid stenosis, plaques with ECST stenosis greater than 50% were imaged and recorded with the view to creating a database for future studies on the diagnostic value of plaque texture features. The equipment presets and method described under "image acquisition of carotid plaques" above were used. The plaque images were collected consecutively with elimination of plaques that produced less than 50% (ECST) stenosis and emergency cases scanned after normal working hours. As a result, a database was created consisting of images of symptomatic and asymptomatic plaques. The ultrasonographers that performed the examinations and obtained the plaque images knew the reason for referral since they were performing routine diagnostic testing for the presence and grading of stenosis. However, for the purpose of testing new diagnostic algorithms, the images of the database were anonymized, and the persons who subsequently did the image normalization and image analysis did not know whether the plaques were symptomatic or asymptomatic.

This database of images is now being used as a testing ground for the potential clinical value of different texture features and appropriate cut-off points prior to testing the latter in prospective studies. Thus, for prospective studies, cut-off points would be predetermined and not data derived.

An example of how texture features perform in both the cross-sectional study and the ACSRS is given below. Four SGLDM features (SGLDM-Homogeneity or SGLDM-HOM, SGLDM-Sum Average or SGLDM-SAV, SGLDM-Sum Variance or SGLDM-SVA, SGLDM-Difference Entropy or SGLDM-DEN) and RUNL-Gray Level Distribution (RUNL-GLD) were selected because they had an ROC area under the curve (AUC) greater than 0.6 when stroke was used as the end-point in the cross-sectional study (see Chap. 14 for their description). For each feature, the cut-off point that produced the highest sensitivity with the highest specificity was obtained (Table 37.4). These cut-off points provided a high- and a low-risk group. The odds ratio for stroke was calculated when the high-risk group was compared with the low-risk group. The same features with the same cut-off points obtained from the cross-sectional study were subsequently applied to the images of the ACSRS. It can be seen from Table 37.4 that the odds ratios were similar, but the proportion of the population included in the high-risk groups was different.

When a Cox proportional hazards model was used with these five features as categorical variables (cut-off points from the cross-sectional study) in the ACSRS, only SGLDM-SAV and RUNL-GLD were significant. These two categorical variables could identify a low-risk group with 698 patients (average

Table 37.4 Performance of five texture features in the cross-sectional study and ACSRS in terms of ROC areas under the curve (ROC) and odds ratios for stroke

Texture feature	Cross-sectional study						ACSRS				
	ROC	Cut-off	OR	95% CI	P	N	ROC	OR	95% CI	P	N
SGLDM-SVA	0.601	2,169	1.87	1.14–3.08	0.009	151 (47%)	0.552	1.89	1.07–3.34	0.026	236 (21%)
SGLDM-HOM	0.691	0.467	2.80	1.69–4.65	0.001	143 (44%)	0.734	3.20	1.07–9.54	0.028	28(25%)
SGLDM-SAV	0.677	38	3.00	1.80–4.98	0.001	143 (44%)	0.705	3.02	1.67–4.98	0.001	145 (13%)
SGLDM-DEN	0.653	2.05	2.45	1.46–4.11	0.001	170 (52%)	0.644	2.14	1.44–4.02	0.001	151 (13%)
RUNL-GLD	0.653	217	1.98	1.13–3.49	0.016	217 (67%)	0.653	2.53	1.48–4.33	0.006	396 (35%)

annual stroke rate of 0.8%), two intermediate groups of 284 and 33 patients (average annual stroke rate of 1.4% and 1.8%, respectively), and a high-risk group of 112 patients (average annual stroke rate of 3.4%) (Table 37.5). However, only 13 (22%) of the 59 strokes occurred in the 112 patients in the high-risk group. The remaining 46 strokes occurred in the rest of the population. Such a result is unlikely to be of clinical value. It appears that although the texture features perform reasonably well in both the cross-sectional study and the ACSRS, a recalibration is needed when applied to the ACSRS. This is related to the fact that in the cross-sectional study, approximately half the population was symptomatic, while in the ACSRS, only 11% became symptomatic.

In addition to developing methods of recalibration, future research should concentrate on identifying computer-generated texture features that are "robust," i.e., do not vary when different equipment is used. This is particularly important now when image post-processing and manipulation such as dispeckling or XRES have been introduced. It is expected that some features will be associated with unstable plaques (good predictors of future events) but not reproducible on different equipment, while some may be highly reproducible but poor predictors of risk. What is needed is a group of features that are both reproducible, i.e., independent of equipment variability, and highly predictive of risk.

37.3.13 Calculation of Stroke Risk in Individual Patients

For this exercise, a number of features shown by several previous cross-sectional and/or prospective studies using different duplex scanners to be associated with symptomatic plaques were selected and applied to image analysis of the ACSRS study. This selection ensured at least a moderate inter-center reproducibility. Stenosis, history of contralateral TIAs or stroke, GSM, plaque area, and presence of DWA proved to be not only associated with the development of future CORI events including stroke in a univariate but also in a multivariate analysis.[8] In a Cox proportional hazards model, they were shown to be independent predictors of future events (Table 37.6). On the basis of this model, the risk of any patient could be calculated (see "On Line Data Supplement" of reference [8]). Alternatively it can be obtained from specially constructed tables (Figs. 37.13 and 37.14) derived from this model.

On the basis of the Cox model, the predicted cumulative 5-year rates for ipsilateral cerebral stroke were

Table 37.5 Identification of low- and high-risk groups in the ACSRS study by run length gray level distribution (RUNL-GLD) and spatial gray level dependence matrices sum average (SGLDM-SAV) texture features as categorical variables using the cut-off points from the cross-sectional study

	RUNL-GLD < 217	RUNL-GLD > 217
SGLDM-SAV < 38	$N = 689$	$N = 284$
	21 strokes	20 strokes
	Annual stroke rate 0.8%	Annual stroke rate 1.4%
SGLDM-SAV > 38	$N = 33$	$N = 112$
	4 strokes	13 strokes
	Average annual stroke rate 1.8%	Annual stroke rate 3.4%

Table 37.6 Clinical factors with plaque features with transformations as used in the Cox model. Ipsilateral CORI events as the dependent variable

Variable	β	HR	95% CI	P
Stenosis (% ECST)	0.01641	1.02	1.00–1.03	0.03
Log(GSM + 40)	−2.4574	0.09	0.04–0.17	<0.001
Plaque area1/3 (mm²)	0.6543	1.92	1.51–2.46	<0.001
DWA (Present vs. absent)	0.7533	2.12	1.33–3.39	0.002
History of contralateral TIAs and/or stroke (Yes vs No)	0.6706	1.96	1.33–2.87	0.001

β regression coefficient, HR hazard ratio

Fig. 37.13 Estimated percent risk of annual ipsilateral ischemic cerebral stroke for patients with 50–79% ECST stenosis

Stenosis 50–79% NASCET (n = 598)
6 months to 8 year follow-up

		No history of contralateral TIAs or stroke				History of contralateral TIAs or stroke			Annual stroke rate %
	>80	1.0%	2.2%	4.4%	>80	2.2%	5.2%	8.7%	≥4
Plaque area (mm^2)	40–80	0.5%	1.0%	2.1%	40–80	1.0%	2.5%	5.0%	3.0–3.9
									2.0–2.9
	<40	0.2%	0.7%	1.5%	<40	0.9%	1.7%	3.5%	
									1.0–1.9
		≥30	15–29	<15		≥30	15–29	<15	<1.0
			GSM				GSM		

Fig. 37.14 Estimated percent risk of annual ipsilateral ischemic cerebral stroke for patients with 80–99% ECST stenosis

Stenosis 80–99% NASCET (n = 325)
6 months to 8 year follow-up

		No history of contralateral TIAs or stroke				History of contralateral TIAs or stroke			Annual stroke rate %
	>80	1.2%	3.4%	5.9%	>80	2.7%	4.0%	10.0%	≥4
Plaque area (mm^2)	40–80	0.6%	1.5%	3.0%	40–80	1.5%	3.5%	6.5%	3.0–3.9
									2.0–2.9
	<40	0.5%	1.0%	2.1%	<40	1.0%	2.5%	4.7%	
									1.0–1.9
		≥30	15–29	<15		≥30	15–29	<15	<1.0
			GSM				GSM		

estimated for different combinations of risk factor subgroups. Figure 37.15 shows calibration for the model. At low predicted probabilities, the model seems to slightly over-predict. At higher predicted probabilities, the model predicts very nicely, with estimates close to the line of agreement and confidence intervals overlapping. The predicted 5 year percentage stroke rate (observed; 95% CI) was <5% (very low risk) in 654 (1%; 0.2 to 2), 5–9.9% (low risk) in 225 (8%; 5–13), 10–19.9% (moderate risk) in 156 (12%; 7–18), and ≥20% (high risk) in 86 patients (29%; 14–33). Of the 923 patients with ≥70% stenosis, 495 were included in the very low, 202 in the low, 142 in the moderate, and 84 in the high-risk group.

37.3.14 Semi-automated Method of Image Analysis and Stroke Risk Prediction

The "Plaque Texture Analysis Software" version 3.4 (Iconsoft International Ltd, PO Box 172, Greenford,

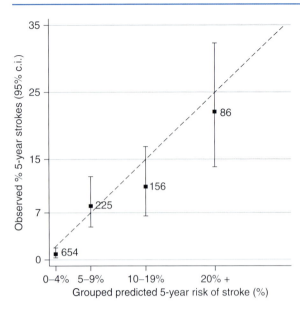

Fig. 37.15 Calibration plot for Cox model shown in Table 37.6 based on all 1,121 patients in the ACSRS study (*dashed line* shows the line of perfect agreement between predicted and observed 5-year stroke risk) (Reprinted from the Nicolaides et al.[8] with permission from Elsevier)

London UB6 9ZN, UK) has now incorporated the calculation of risk for an individual patient based on the Cox model in the ACSRS study.[8] It provides a report of the measurement of key texture features including the predicted annual stroke risk (Fig. 37.16). The software is powerful yet user friendly so that it can be used in all vascular laboratories or vascular departments. It has overcome the difficulties of image analysis and associated time-consuming procedures. The difficulty has now shifted to image capture and the essential training of ultrasonographers (see below).

This software is now being validated by applying it to both symptomatic and asymptomatic plaques "blind," i.e., the operator is not aware of the presenting symptomatology. The authors' hypothesis is that the majority of plaques identified as high risk will be symptomatic. Next, it should be validated in future prospective natural history studies or the medical arm of randomized studies.

37.3.15 General Remarks and Conclusions

The ACSRS is the largest prospective study of patients with asymptomatic carotid artery stenosis undergoing medical intervention alone. The results demonstrate that a number of baseline clinical characteristics and ultrasonic plaque features are independent predictors of subsequent ipsilateral CORI events.

This study is unique not only because of the relatively large number of patients studied but also because, in contrast to previous studies that had concentrated on one feature only, it shows how plaque characteristics can add significantly to the improvement of risk stratification. It also provides a method that allows estimation of risk for any patient.

Ultrasonic imaging is to a certain extent operator dependent. This can be overcome by training ultrasonographers in equipment presets and image capture; also, by performing image normalization with computerized analysis. The importance of training vascular ultrasonographers in equipment settings and plaque imaging for optimal results cannot be overemphasized.

A limitation of the ACSRS study was that the medical management of patients was according to what was considered best medical therapy at each center at the time. At each center, the clinician-in-charge was free to change therapy according to changing indications. At the beginning of the study, only 84% of patients were on antiplatelet therapy and only 25% on lipid-lowering therapy. Toward the end of the study, these percentages were 95% and 85%, respectively. However, the intensity of the treatment varied, and unlike current guidelines, very few patients were treated to target cholesterol level. In addition, this "freedom" in management resulted in 129 (11.5%) patients having a carotid endarterectomy in the absence of symptoms soon after the results of the ACST were published. Despite this, follow-up to a CORI event, death, or to the end of the study was achieved in 87% of patients.

The clinical implication of the ACSRS study is that clinical and ultrasonic plaque features can be used to stratify risk and may lead to refinement of the indications for carotid endarterectomy. The availability of user-friendly software for image analysis and automatic calculation of risk can make the method part of routine practice in the vascular laboratory.

Validation of predicted risk in this study was limited since this was done internally, that is for the same group of patients on whom the score was developed. The findings need to be validated in additional prospective observational studies using current medical intervention

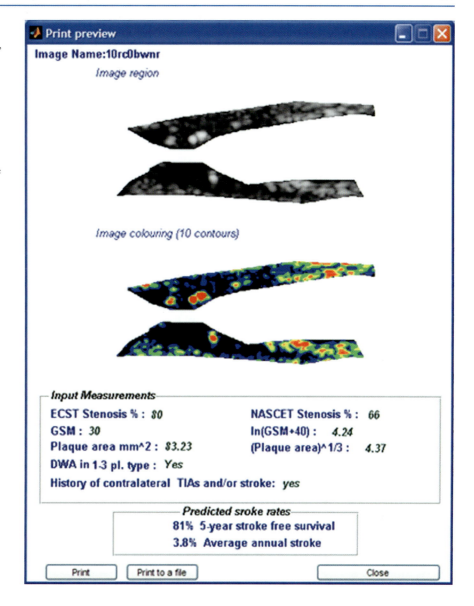

Fig. 37.16 Report produced by the "Plaque Texture Analysis Software" version 3.4. It includes the normalized plaque image, the color-contoured plaque image, the texture features and their transformations as used in the Cox model of Table 37.6, and the predicted annual stroke rate

or in the medical arm of randomized controlled trials comparing carotid endarterectomy plus medical intervention against medical intervention alone.

The databases of plaque images from both the cross-sectional study and the ACSRS are a valuable source for exploring and testing new methods of image analysis and new algorithms for calculation of risk. The experience of the authors is available to all who wish to embark on future studies. Training courses for image capture and analysis are now established.

References

1. Executive Committee for the Asymptomatic Carotid Atherosclerosis Study. Endarterectomy for asymptomatic carotid artery stenosis. *J Am Med Assoc*. 1995;273:1421–1428.
2. Nicolaiders A et al. The Asymptomatic Carotid Stenosis and Risk of Stroke (ACSRS) study. Aims and results of quality control. *Int Angiol*. 2003;22:263–272.
3. Nicolaides A et al. Severity of asymptomatic carotid stenosis and risk of ipsilateral hemispheric ischemic events: results from the ACSRS study. *Eur J Vasc Endovasc Surg*. 2005;30:275–284.

4. Kakkos SK et al. Factors associated with mortality in patients with asymptomatic carotid stenosis: results from the ACSRS study. *Int Angiol*. 2005;24:221–230.
5. Nicolaides A et al. Effect of image normalization on carotid plaque classification and the risk of ipsilateral hemispheric ischemic events: results from the asymptomatic carotid stenosis and risk of stroke study. *Vascular*. 2005;13:211–221.
6. Nicolaides AN, Kakkos S, Griffin M, Geroulakos G, Ioannidou E. Severity of asymptomatic carotid stenosis and risk of ipsilateral hemispheric ischaemic events: results from the ACSRS study. *Eur J Vasc Endovasc Surg*. 2006;31:336.
7. Kakkos SK et al. Silent embolic infarcts on computed tomography brain scans and risk of ipsilateral hemispheric events in patients with asymptomatic internal carotid artery stenosis. *J Vasc Surg*. 2009;49:902–909.
8. Nicolaides AN et al. Asymptomatic internal carotid artery stenosis and cerebrovascular risk stratification. *J Vasc Surg*. 2010;52:1486–1496.
9. Nicolaides AN et al. Angiographic and duplex grading of internal carotid stenosis: can we overcome the confusion? *J Endovasc Surg*. 1996;3:158–165.
10. Steinke W, Hennericci M, Rautenberg W, Mohr JP. Symptomatic and asymptomatic high grade carotid stenosis in Doppler color flow imaging. *Neurology*. 1992;42:131–137.
11. Sitzer M et al. Between method correlation in quantifying internal carotid stenosis. *Stroke*. 1993;24:1513–1518.
12. De Bray JM et al. Color Doppler imaging duplex sonography and angiography of carotid bifurcations. Prospective and double blind study. *Neuroradiology*. 1995;37:219–224.
13. Griffin M, Nicolaides AN, Kyriacou E. Normalisation of ultrasonic images of atherosclerotic plaques and reproducibility of grey scale median using dedicated software. *Int Angiol*. 2007;26:372–377.
14. Geroulakos G et al. Characterisation of symptomatic and asymptomatic carotid plaques using high-resolution real time ultrasonography. *Br J Surg*. 1993;80:1274–1277.
15. Spence JD et al. A tool for targeting and evaluating vascular preventive therapy. *Stroke*. 2002;33:2916–2922.
16. Ricotta JJ. Plaque characterization by B-mode scan. *Surg Clin North Am*. 1990;70:191–199.
17. Johnson JM, Kennelly MM, Decesare D, Morgan S, Sparrow A. Natural history of asymptomatic carotid plaque. *Arch Surg*. 1985;120:1010–1012.
18. Bock RW et al. The natural history of asymptomatic carotid artery disease. *J Vasc Surg*. 1993;17:160–171.
19. Chambers BR, Norris JW. Outcome in patients with asymptomatic neck bruits. *N Engl J Med*. 1986;315:860–865.
20. Hennericci M, Hulsbomer HB, Hefter H, Lammerts D, Rautenberg W. Natural history of asymptomatic extracranial arterial disease. Results of a long-term prospective study. *Brain*. 1987;110:777–791.
21. Norris JW, Zhu CZ, Bornstein NM, Chambers BR. Vascular risks of asymptomatic carotid stenosis. *Stroke*. 1991;22:1485–1490.
22. Zhu CZ, Norris JW. A therapeutic window for carotid endarterectomy in patients with asymptomatic carotid stenosis. *Can J Surg*. 1991;34:437–440.
23. Mackey AE et al. Outcome of asymptomatic patients with carotid disease. *Neurology*. 1997;48:896–903.
24. Nadareishvili ZG, Rothwell PM, Beletsky V, Pagniello A, Norris JW. Long-term risk of stroke and other vascular events in patients with asymptomatic carotid artery stenosis. *Arch Neurol*. 2002;59:1162–1166.
25. Mathiesen EB, Bønaa KH, Joakimsen O. Echolucent plaques are associated with high risk of ischemic cerebrovascular events in carotid stenosis. The Tromsø study. *Circulation*. 2001;103:2171–2175.
26. Hashimoto H, Takaya M, Niki H, Etani H. Computer-assisted analysis of heterogeneity on B-mode imaging predicts instability of asymptomatic carotid plaque. *Cerebrovasc Dis*. 2009;28:357–364.
27. Carra G et al. Carotid plaque morphology and cerebrovascular events. *Int Angiol*. 2003;22:284–289.
28. Shah F et al. Contrast-enhanced ultrasound imaging of atherosclerotic carotid plaque neovascularization: a new surrogate marker of atherosclerosis? *Vasc Med*. 2007;12(4):291–297.
29. Iannuzzi A et al. Ultrasonographic correlates of carotid atherosclerosis in transient ischemic attack and stroke. *Stroke*. 1995;26:614–619.
30. Golledge J, Cuming R, Ellis M, Davies AH, Greenhalgh RM. Carotid plaque characteristics and presenting symptom. *Br J Surg*. 1997;84:1697–1701.
31. Pedro LM et al. Ultrasonographic risk score of carotid plaques. *Eur J Vasc Endovasc*. 2002;24:492–498.
32. Griffin M et al. Juxtaluminal hypoechoic area in ultrasonic images of carotid plaques and hemispheric symptoms. *J Vasc Surg*. 2010;52:69–76.
33. Schulte-Altedorneburg G et al. Preoperative B-mode ultrasound plaque appearance compared with carotid endarterectomy specimen histology. *Acta Neurol Scand*. 2000;101:188–194.
34. Fisher M et al. Carotid plaque pathology. Thrombosis, ulceration and stroke pathogenesis. *Stroke*. 2005;36:253–257.
35. Mazzone AM et al. In vivo ultrasonic parametric imaging of carotid atherosclerotic plaque by videodensitometric technique. *Angiology*. 1995;46:663–672.
36. Elatrozy T, Nicolaides A, Tegos T, Griffin M. The objective characterisation of ultrasonic carotid plaque features. *Eur J Vasc Endovasc Surg*. 1998;16:223–230.
37. Tegos TJ et al. Types of neurovascular symptoms and carotid plaque ultrasonic textural characteristics. *J Ultras Med*. 2001;20:113–121.
38. Christodoulou CI, Pattichis CS, Pantziaris M, Nicolaides A. Texture based classification of atherosclerotic carotid plaques. *IEEE Trans Med Imaging*. 2003;22:902–912.
39. Kyriacou E et al. Classification of atherosclerotic carotid plaques using morphological analysis on ultrasound images. *Appl Intell*. 2009;30:3–23.
40. Wu Q. *Automatic Tumor Detection for MRI Liver Images* [Ph.D. thesis]. London: Imperial College; 1996:48–59
41. Jirák D, Dezortová M, Tamir P, Hájek M. Texture analysis of human liver. *J Magn Reson Imaging*. 2002;15:68–74.

Index

A

Acoustic densitometry, 205
Acoustic radiation force imaging (ARFI), 336–337
ACSRS study. *See* Asymptomatic Carotid Stenosis and Risk of Stroke
Albumin-to-creatinine ratio (ACR), 424
Amplitude modulation-frequency modulation (AM-FM) motion estimation model
    asymptomatic and symptomatic plaques, 231
    combined energy functional, 363
    FM components, 363
    iterative computational scheme, 363–364
Angina Prognosis Study in Stockholm (APSIS), 404
Ankle-brachial index (ABI), 511
Arterial Biology for the Investigation of the Treatment Effects of Reducing Cholesterol (ARBITER), 415
Arterial mechanics
    pulse
        peaks, wave intensity, 328, 329
        wave intensity plot, CCA, 328
    structure
        elastin and collagen, 328
        intima, media and adventitia, 327–328
Arteriography, 32
Asymmetric dimethylarginine (ADMA), 466–467
Asymptomatic Carotid Atherosclerosis Study (ACAS)
    BMT, 59
    ipsilateral stroke, 547
    outcomes, 54
    temporal changes, 60
Asymptomatic carotid stenosis
    AHA guidelines, 55
    carotid screening, 54
    CAS, asymptomatic patients, 54
    CEA "appropriateness", 53
    clinical governance
        ACAS and ACST, 55
        death/stroke rate, 56
    data, registry, 58–59
    financial burden, 57
    inability, risk stratification, 57–58
    "ipsilateral" and "any" stroke, 59–60
    medical therapy, 55
    NEJM, 55
    patients prioritization, failure, 56–57
    polarized opinion, 55
    randomized trials, 53, 55
    severity, 58
    surgeon's beliefs, 56
Asymptomatic Carotid Stenosis and Risk of Stroke (ACSRS) study
    clinical and biochemical
        characteristics, 618–619
        features, 627–628
    computer-generated texture features, 628–630
    CORI events, 620–622
    description, 615
    discrete white areas (DWA), 624
    duplex examination
        grading, internal carotid stenosis, 616–617
        image normalization and analysis, 618
        recording, plaque images, 617
    exit points, 619
    GSM
        ipsilateral CORI events, 623
        Kaplan-Meier plots, 624
        severe and fatal ipsilateral strokes, 624
    ipsilateral cerebrovascular events, 619
    JBA
        without visible echogenic cup, 626–627
    outcome measures, 619–620
    participating centers, 615
    patient recruitment, 616
    plaque area, 625–626
    "Plaque Texture Analysis Software" report, 633
    plaque type and risk
        echolucent plaques, 623
        image normalization, 622
        ipsilateral cerebral ischemic stroke-free survival, 623
        stroke, 623
    plaque ulceration, 624–625
    quality control, 615–616
    recruited numbers, 619
    semi-automated method, image analysis, 631–632
    semiquantitative assessment, echolucency, 549
    stroke risk, individual patients, 630–631
    texture features
        DWA and JBA, 618
        GSM, 618
        plaque type and area, 618
        plaque ulceration, 618
Atherogenesis, carotid atherosclerosis
    anatomy, arterial wall
        ability, endothelial monolayer, 28

hemodynamic stress, 28
matrix, elastic fibers, 28
mural structure, artery, 27, 28
nonthrombogenic conduit, blood flow, 27
endothelial damage and plaque
  balloon-injury model, 28–29
  description, 28
  immune response, propagation, 29
  macrophages, 29
  MMPs, 29
  organization, cells and matrix fibers, 29
  smooth muscle cell proliferation, 29
Atherosclerosis
  atheromatous degeneration, 489
  blood flow, endothelial layer, 45
  Bruneck study (*see* Bruneck study)
  cell senescence, 508, 509
  definite plaques, 508
  endothelial activation, 489
  genetics, systemic inflammation
    gene–environment interactions, 493
    noxes, 493–494
    pathways and mechanisms, 494
  geometric parameters, disturbed flow, 47–48
  hemodynamic
    factors, 489
    interactions, 45
    parameters, arterial disease, 46–47
  inflammation and early vessel pathology
    frequency and risk conditions, 505
    immunity, heat-shock proteins, 507–508
    IMT assessment, 505–507
  inflammation sources
    autoimmune disorders, 492
    cardiovascular risk factors, 492–493
    chronic infections, 492
    chronic inflammatory and allergic diseases, 492
  intra-plaque hemorrhage, 491
  lesions and properties, 45
  monkey models, 435
  oscillatory shear *vs.* intimal thickness, 46
  progression
    auto-catalytic component, 498
    inflammation and dysimmunity, 499
    vascular risk factors, 498, 500
  stable atheroma, 490
  stages, 497
  T-cells, 489, 490
  time-averaged shear stress, 46
  tissue factor, 491
  transition, 490
  ultrasound phenotypes
    genetics, 433
    plaque and stenosis, 434
    stages, 434
    therapies, 435
  unexplained, 444
  vascular calcification, 491
  vascular remodeling
    Bruneck study, 498, 499
    common and internal carotid arteries, 498
  efficacy, 499
  plaque growth, 498
Atherosclerosis in insulin resistance (AIR) study
  apolipoproteinB/apolipoproteinA-I ratio (apoB/apoA-I), 456
  re-examinations, 452
  stratified sampling, 452
  subclinical carotid atherosclerosis, 451
Atherosclerosis Progression in Familial Hypercholesterolemia study (ASAP), 414
Atherosclerotic plaque motion analysis
  motion estimation (ME) algorithms, 369
  ultrasound videos, carotid artery plaques, 369–370
Audio video interleave (AVI) format, 302
AVI format. *See* Audio video interleave format

B

Bidimensional histogram (2DH), 183
Biomarkers and subclinical atherosclerosis
  ACE I/D polymorphism
    DD genotype, 465
    genetic variants, 464
    meta-analysis, Caucasians, 465
  ADMA (*see* Asymmetric dimethylarginine)
  apoB/apoA1
    PIVUS and Cyprus study, 467
    proatherogenic *vs.* antiatherogenic particles, 467
  apoE E2/E3/E4 polymorphism, 467–468
  CD40 ligand (CD40L)
    description, 468
    inflammation and atorvastatin effect, 468
    sCD40L, 468
  CETP (*see* Cholesterylester transfer protein)
  cross-reactive protein (CRP)
    description, 470
    elevated serum levels, 470
  endothelium nitric oxide synthase (eNOS), 470–471
  fibrinogen, 471
  gene expression
    atherosclerotic plaque, 477–478
    description, 476–477
    plaques, pathological grades, 478–480
    primary *vs.* restenotic plaques, 478
    symptomatic *vs.* asymptomatic patients/plaques, 477
  genetic marker, defined, 463
  heritability, ultrasonic features
    intermediate phenotypes, 464
    plaques presence, 464
    twin pairs, 464
  homocysteine
    association, 471, 472
    hyperhomocysteinemia, 471
    metabolism, vascular cells, 471
    5,10-methylenetetrahydrofolate reductase (MTHFR), 472
  interleukin–6 (IL6), 472
  lipoprotein(a), 473
  MCP–1, 475
  metalloproteinases (MMPs), 474–475
  MetS (*see* Metabolic syndrome)
  Ox-LDL, 475–476
  risk factor, 463

Index 635

TNF-α, 476
ultrasonographically assessment
    carotid and femoral plaques, 466
    CIMT, 465
β-Blocker Cholesterol-lowering Asymptomatic Plaque Study (BCAPS), 414
B-mode imaging
    identification, stents and sutures
        carotid arteries, 84, 87
    plaque echodensity
        2D brightness mode and color Doppler image, 84, 86
        echogenicity, carotid plaque, 83, 85
        intraluminal echoes, 83, 85
    processing
        coherent speckle, 82–83
        damping, tissue, 82
        description, 82
        2-D method, 83, 84
        formation, 82, 83
British Regional Heart Study (BRHS) scoring systems, 399
Bruneck study
    incidence, carotid atherosclerosis, 496
    population recruitment and follow-up
        baseline examination, 494
        extrapolation, cross-sectional data, 496
    risk profiles, 496–497
    scanning protocol
        atherosclerotic lesions, 496
        CCA and ICA, 496
        peak systolic velocities, 496

C
CACS. *See* Coronary artery calcium score
Cardiovascular risk assessment, carotid plaques. *See* Carotid plaques
Carotid anatomy, ultrasonic imaging
    atherosclerotic plaques, 68
    frequency, wavelength and resolution
        anisotropic, 69
        arteries, 68
        cross-sectional image, artery, 69, 71
        2-D Fourier transforms, 69, 70
        echo amplitude range, 68
        impedence change, 69
    IMT, 67
    resolution, 70
Carotid artery IMT and lumen diameter
    advantages, 173
    atherosclerosis and complication, 167
    axial resolution, 173
    B-mode ultrasound, 167
    and coronary atherosclerosis, 174–175
    echo interfaces, 173
    far-wall IMT, 172
    leading and far edge, definition, 167, 168
    lumen diameter, measurements, 172
    near-wall
        adventitia, 171
        and adventitia thickness, 172
        intima/lumen interface, 172
        issue, 176–177
    noninvasive recordings, 167
    Pignoli and coworkers, 168, 169
    plaque area, 174
    precision, 173–174
    ultrasound measurement, 175
    ultrasound studies, precaution, 175
    visibility, below-resolution structures, 168
    Wendelhag and coworkers
        air bubbles, 169–171
        arterial wall, anatomy, 168
        B-mode 2D image, 169
        interpretation, ultrasound image, 169
        leading and far edge, definition, 168
        trepanation experiment, 169, 170
        ultrasound recording, 168
    Wong and coworkers, 168, 170–171
Carotid artery IMT measurement
    atherosclerosis, 179
    B-mode ultrasound image, 180
    boundary tracings
        CGB, 190–192
        description, 190
        metrological note, 192–193
        PST, 192
    dynamic programming techniques
        advantage, 189
        description, 188
        echo interface, 188–189
    edge-based and gradient approaches
        cropped B-mode image, 186, 187
        FOAM operator, 186–187
        LI/MA, 186
        noise, 186
    GA, 189–190
    guidance zone
        B-mode image, 181
        CGB, 181
        HT, 183–185
        integrated approach, 182
        statistics and signal analysis, 182–184
        template matching, 184–185
    IMT, 179
    morphological representations, 180–181
    snake-based LI/MA
        forces, 187
        output, 188
        parameters, 188
    ultrasound, 179
Carotid atherosclerosis
    atherogenesis
        anatomy, arterial wall, 27–28
        endothelial damage and plaque, 28–29
    carotid bifurcation (*see* Carotid bifurcation)
    3D carotid imaging
        cube view approach, 267–269
        mechanical linear, 266–267
        reconstruction, 267
        TPV measurement, 268
        ultrasound method, 266
        vessel wall measurement, 269

Carotid atherosclerosis (*cont.*)
    defined, stroke, 27
    noninvasive imaging modality, 27
    quantification
        TPV, 269
        VWV, 270
    regression monitoring
        3D and 2D carotid maps, 274
        mapping spatial and temporal changes, 274–276
        TPA measurements, 270
        VWV measurements, 270, 272–274
    vulnerable asymptomatic plaque
        calcification, 36
        defined, echolucency, 35
        echolucency/gray scale median, 35
        intraplaque hemorrhage, 36
Carotid Atherosclerosis Italian Ultrasound Study (CAIUS), 413
Carotid Atherosclerosis Progression Study (CAPS), 386
Carotid bifurcation
    atherosclerosis
        arteriography, 32
        CT, 32–33
        duplex ultrasound, 32
        histopathology, 34
        inflammation, 31
        modeling, stress distribution and magnitude, 31
        MRI, 33–34
        plaque structural components, 31
    hemodynamic force localization, plaque, 30–31
    stroke (*see* Stroke)
    vascular hemodynamics (*see* Vascular hemodynamics, carotid bifurcation)
Carotid endarterectomy (CEA)
    ACAS and ACST trials, 54
    asymptomatic patients, 54–56
    description, 53
    randomized trials, 53
Carotid plaques. *See also* Image analysis, carotid plaques
    area, cardiovascular event predictor
        arterial wall, 409
        risk assessment tool, 410
    color mapping (*see* Grayscale-based stratified color mapping)
    echogenicity and cardiovascular risks
        calcified plaque, 410
        echolucent plaques, 410
        hypoechoic plaque, 410
        predictive power, 411
    genes
        candidate, 443
        GWAS, 443
    statin therapy (*see* Statin therapy, carotid plaque morphology)
Carotid plaque surface irregularity
    area-preserving flattened map, 285
    computer-aided analysis methods, 281
    curvatures smoothing
        algorithm, 284
        vertex weight, 285
    discrete Gaussian curvature
        Gauss–Bonnet theorem, 283
        Gaussian curvature, 284
    discrete mean curvature
        surface partitioning schemes, 282, 284
        vertex, algorithm, 283
    3D ultrasound image acquisition, 286
    fissures and size quantification, 282
    Gauss–Bonnet theorem, 287
    images, 3D, 286
    luminal surfaces, 294
    maps, curvature
        2D Gaussian and mean, 288, 290, 291
        3D image, 288, 290, 291
        transverse views, 291
    mean and Gaussian curvature computation, 287, 293
    phantom, ulcers, 290, 293
    proposed automatic algorithm, 297
    segmentation and surface reconstruction, 287
    surface curvature estimation
        categories, 282
        shapes, Gaussian and mean, 282, 283
    synthetic tori, parameters, 285
    types, synthetic surfaces, 285
    ulcer detection algorithm, 295
    vascular phantom, 285–290
    x-ray angiography and ultrasound imaging, 281
Carotid plaque texture analysis
    ACSRS, 322
    B-mode images, 299
    3D image capture
        carotid bifurcation, 302
        color flow, 303
        DICOM files, 302
        equipment, 301–302
        presets, 302
    image analysis
        3D visualization and orientation, 304
        QLAB settings, 305
        segmentation, 3D images, 305–307
        volume and texture measurement, 307–308
    IVUS virtual histology
        B-mode grayscale image, 300
        carotid endarterectomy plaques, 300
        CT brain scan, 299
        Haralick's texture features, 300
        JBA, 300
        texture analysis, 3D reconstruction, 301
    principles, 299
    symptomatic and asymptomatic plaque
        2D image, 309–310, 314–316, 318
        3D image, 310, 312, 316, 317, 319–320
        hypoechoic areas, 309
        JBV, 308
        severity, stenosis, 313
        stenotic plaque, 312
        texture features, 320–321
Carotid stenosis
    arteriography, 32
    CT, 32–33
    duplex ultrasound, 32
    histopathology, 34
    MRIs, 33–34
    prevalence and risk factors, 425

Carotid ultrasound
    atherosclerosis (*see* Atherosclerosis)
    genetic research
        IMT and plaque thickness, 442–443
        plaque volume and vessel wall volume, 444–445
        total plaque area, 444
    response, therapy
        IMT and plaque thickness, 445
        plaque volume and vessel wall volume, 445–446
        total plaque area, 445
    risk stratification
        IMT and plaque thickness, 435–437
        plaque volume and vessel wall volume, 440
        total plaque area, 436–440
    vascular risk factors evaluation
        IMT and plaque thickness, 440–442
        plaque volume and vessel wall volume, 442
        total plaque area, 442
CBM. *See* Constant brightness model
CCA. *See* Common carotid artery
cdfs. *See* Cumulative density functions
CEA. *See* Carotid endarterectomy
Cerebrovascular risk stratification
    carotid angioplasty/stenting, 588
    carotid dissection
        stroke, 586
        TCD, 586
    carotid endarterectomy
        embolic signals, 587
        gaseous and solid emboli counts, 587
        hyperperfusion syndrome, 587–588
        MRI, 587
        perfusion extremes, 587
        postoperative monitoring, 588
        stroke, 587
    carotid territory stroke
        acute condition, 586
        grading residual flow, 586
        microbubbles, 587
        TCD monitoring, 586
    medical/noninvasive interventions, vascular disease, 588–589
    proximal ICA stenosis
        atherosclerosis, 580
        cerebral autoregulation, risk stratification, 586
        emboli detection, 580–586
        stroke/transient ischemic attack, 580
CETP. *See* Cholesterylester transfer protein
CGB. *See* Computer-generated boundaries
Cholesteryl ester transfer protein (CETP)
    animal studies, 469
    atherosclerosis progression, 415, 416
    description, 468
    gene polymorphisms
        homogeneity, 469
        I405V, 469
        TaqIB, 469
    mediated transfer, cholesteryl esters, 469
    meta-analysis, 469
Common carotid artery (CCA)
    carotid bifurcation, 42

3D images, 287
    noise ratio regions, 44
    planarity angle, 48
Computed tomography (CT)
    description, 32
    noncalcified components, 33
    strandness and Zweibel duplex, ICA stenosis, 33
Computer-generated boundaries (CGB)
    GT, 190
    HDM, 190–191
    MAD, 190, 191
    PDM, 191–192
Constant brightness model (CBM)
    Euler-Lagrange equations, 361
    numerical differentiation, 361
    oriented smoothness constraint
        Gauss-Seidel iterations, 362
        variation, motion field, 361
    quantization error and noise, 361
Coronary artery calcium score (CACS)
    disadvantage, 513
    NCEP III guidelines, 513
    relative risks and confidence interval, 512
    screening, 512
CT. *See* Computed tomography
Cumulative density functions *(cdfs)*
    asymptomatic, 261
    grayscale morphological, 261
    plaques, 257
    symptomatic, 256–258
Cyprus epidemiological study
    carotid and femoral bifurcations, 513
    low FRS, 515
    NICE, 515
    Odds ratios (OR), 514, 515
    total plaque area (TPA), 514
    total plaque thickness (TPT), defined, 513

D

Despeckle filtering algorithms
    defined, ultrasound imaging system, 101
    diffusion, 103
    geometric (*see* Geometric filtering)
    homomorphic (*see* Homomorphic filtering)
    local statistical
        first order (DsFlsmv, DsFwiener), 101–102
        homogenous mask area (DsFlsminsc), 102
        subregion calculation, 101
    logarithmic compression, 101
    median (*see* Median filtering)
    pixel neighborhood (*see* Pixel neighborhood filtering)
Despeckling
    defined, speckle, 97
    distance measures, 105
    filtering
        algorithm (*see* Despeckle filtering algorithms)
        diffusion, 103
        homomorphic, 98
        logarithmic, ultrasound images, 104
    image processing technique, 97

Despeckling (cont.)
    image quality evaluation metrics
        algorithms, 111
        asymptomatic and symptomatic images, 113
        atherosclerotic carotid plaques, 106
        defined, 105
        measures, 106
        percentage, kNN classifier, 112
    kNN classifier, 105
    limitations, 100–101
    linear filtering, 99
    MMSE, 98
    normalization and plaque segmentation, image, 104
    techniques, 97–98
    texture analysis
        distance measures, 108–111
        kNN classifier, 111
        ultrasound images, 104
    ultrasound images
        material and recording, 103–104
        real carotid, 107–108
    univariate statistical analysis, 105
    visual evaluation, experts
        description, 106
        percentage score, 114
    wavelet shrinkage approach, 100
2DH. See Bidimensional histogram
Diabetes, Impaired Glucose Tolerance in Women, and Atherosclerosis (DIWA) Study, 452
DICOM. See Digital imaging and communications in medicine
Digital imaging and communications in medicine (DICOM), 302
Discrete dynamic contour (DDC), 287
Discrete white areas (DWA), 618
Doppler, ultrasonic imaging
    angle
        description, 92
        examination, 92–93
        image and waveform, carotid artery, 93, 95
        magnitude and waveforms, vector, 93, 96
        vs. systole, carotid artery, 93, 95
        test, carotid artery, 92, 94
    arterial wall tissue
        diametric strain and wall strain, carotid artery, 89, 90
        tissue motions, 90
        unidirectional plaque strain, 89
    frequency measurement
        FFT spectral waveforms, 91
        post-stenotic flow, 91, 93
        "turbulence", 91
    identification, stenosis
        calcified carotid plaque, 88
    reprise
        advantages and applications, 94
        atherosclerotic stenosis and embolic stroke, relationship, 93
        cardiac factors, 94
    superimposed data
        B-mode image formation, 83, 86
        2-D B-mode, 84, 86
        2-D B-mode and color Doppler, 86, 88
    tissue vibrometry
        cross-axis Doppler measurement, 91, 92
        description, 90
        vibration signature, spectral waveforms, 90–91
DsFgf4d. See Geometric filtering
DsFhomo. See Homomorphic filtering
DsFhomog. See Pixel neighborhood filtering
DsFmedian. See Median filtering
Duplex ultrasound, 32, 532
3D visualization and image orientation, 304

E
Echolucent plaques
    ACSRS, 549
    asymptomatic
        ACAS and ACST, 547
        ACSRS, 547
        risk reduction, 547
        "soft" plaques, 547
        stroke, incidence rate, 546–547
    cerebrovascular risk stratification, 549
    description, 545
    distal and proximal carotid artery, 546
    MRI, 549
    perioperative risk, 548
    population-based
        and individual plaque assessment, 546
        research, 548
    symptomatic
        ipsilateral stroke, 548
        NASCET and ECST, 547
    visual classification, 545
    vulnerable plaque, 545
Elastic modulus
    brachial systolic and diastolic pressures, 333
    Moens–Korteweg equation, 338
    pressure-strain, 333, 338
    stiffness index, 333
Emboli detection, ICA stenosis
    ACES, 585
    asymptomatic and symptomatic carotid stenosis, 582
    carotid plaque, 581
    ES-negativity and ES-positivity, 585
    limitation, 581
    recurrent stroke, 580, 582
    signals, 581
    stroke predictive value, 582
    TCD
        monitoring, 581
        TCD ES and ipsilateral stroke/TIA prediction, 581, 583, 584

F
FDTA. See Fractal dimension texture analysis
FFT. See Fourier transform
Finite wall thickness, 338
Firefighters and their endothelium (FATE) study, 468
First-order absolute moment edge operator (FOAM), 186
First order statistics (FOS), 207

FOAM. *See* First-order absolute moment edge operator
FOS. *See* First order statistics
Fourier power spectrum (FPS), 104, 242
Fourier transform (FFT)
   defined, 103
   homomorphic filtering, 98
FPS. *See* Fourier power spectrum
Fractal dimension texture analysis (FDTA), 104, 241–242
Framingham stroke risk score (FSRS), 427

G
GA. *See* Greedy algorithm
Gauss–Bonnet theorem, 282, 283, 287
GDIM. *See* Generalized dynamic image model
Gene expression
   atherosclerotic plaque
      fibrous cap, 478
      plaque instability, 477
   defined, 476–477
   plaques, pathological grades
      coronary artery segments, 478
      cytoskeleton organization and cell-growth genes, 479
      ECM-receptor interaction pathway, 481
      leukocyte transendothelial migration pathway, 480
      pathway analysis, 478–479
   primary *vs.* restenotic plaques
      microarrays, 478
      microscopic tissue, 478
      neointimal thickening, 478
   quantitative reverse transcription polymerase chain
         reaction (qRT-PCR), 477
   symptomatic *vs.* asymptomatic patients/plaques
      endarterectomy plaques, 477
      Helsinki Carotid Endarterectomy Study, 477
Generalized dynamic image model (GDIM)
   errors, 362
   Euler-Lagrange differential equations, 362
   expression, 360
   Gauss-Seidel iteration scheme, 363
   Laplacian approximation, velocities, 363
   minimization problem, 362
Geometric filtering (DsFgf4d), 102
GLDS. *See* Gray level difference statistics
Gothenburg studies
   AIR study (*see* Atherosclerosis in insulin resistance
         (AIR) study)
   arterial wall
      apoB, apoA-I ratio and metabolic syndrome, 455
      HDL and LDL levels, 456
      oxidized LDL and metabolic syndrome, 457
      small LDL particles, and metabolic syndrome, 456–457
   arterial wall, inflammation and metabolic syndrome
      adiponectin, 459
      cell adhesion molecules, 458
      circulating CD44, 459
      high-sensitivity C-reactive protein (hsCRP), 458
      LDL autoantibodies, 457–458
      metalloproteinase 9, 458–459
      oxidation, 457
   DIWA, 452
   impaired glucose tolerance
      cardiovascular risk, 455
      meta-analysis, 455
      OGTT, 455
   IMT, plaque occurrence, intervention effects and CVD
      AIR study, 453
      cardiovascular risk factor intervention, 454
      plaque burden, 453
      RIS study, 453
   insulin resistance
      defined, 454
      hyperinsulinemia, 454–455
      proinsulin, 455
      sensitivity, 454
   metabolic syndrome, 455
   RIS, 452
   type 2 diabetes, 455
   ultrasound methods, 452–453
Grading, internal carotid artery stenosis
   angiography
      disadvantage, 524
      ECST, 524
      "N" and "E" methods, 524
      residual lumen, 523
   clinical cases
      acute and chronic occlusion, 538
      amaurosis fugax, 534
      asymptomatic bruit, 534
      hemodynamic conditions, 533
      planimetric evaluation, 539–541
      stent placement, 541
      string sign, 536–537
      transient ischemic attack, 535
   contralateral disease, duplex measurements, 532
   CT and MRI, 523
   end-diastolic velocity in the internal carotid (EDVic), 527
   guidelines, "N" method, 528–529
   joint recommendations, United Kingdom, 529–530
   meta-analysis, 527
   peak systolic velocity in the internal carotid (PSVic), 527
   ratio, PSVic and EDVcc, 528
   restenosis, stented carotid arteries (*see* Restenosis)
   stratification
      brighter reflectors injection, 527
      color flow Doppler, 527
      positive and negative predictive value, 527
      residual lumen, 526
      "trickle flow", 526
      ultrasound identifiers, 526
   ultrasound methods
      B-mode image measurement, 530
      color Doppler, 530–531
      guidelines, Society of Radiologists in Ultrasound, 531
      vs. MRA and CTA, 531
      multiplanar anatomical measurements, 530
      planimetric evaluation, 531
   University of Washington, Duplex criteria
      "E" and "N" methods, 525
      limitations, 529
   velocities
      degree, stenosis, 524

duplex scanning, 524
stenotic strata, 524
velocity ratios
accrediting bodies, 526
criteria, highest accuracy, 525, 526
sensitivity, 525
ultrasound, 525, 526
Gray level difference statistics (GLDS), 104, 208, 239
Grayscale-based stratified color mapping
fibrous cap, 565
GSM analysis, 565
noninvasive imaging techniques, 565
semi-automated
asymptomatic left carotid stenosis, 567
cerebrovascular symptoms and microembolic signals, 568–569
interobserver agreement, 568
MATLAB 7.9, 566
MRI, 567
plaque pixels, 566–567
right carotid stenosis, asymptomatic, 567
threshold values, 567
ultrasound image, 566
and visual analysis, 569–570
Gray scale median (GSM). *See also* Asymptomatic Carotid Stenosis and Risk of Stroke (ACSRS) study
adobe photoshop *vs.* plaque texture analysis software
Bland–Altman plot, 199, 203
description, 198
echogenicity, 199
MG and AN, 199, 204
analysis, 205
vs. IBS
ROI, 204
usage, 203–204
ipsilateral hemispheric symptoms, 230
measurements, 218
plaque
echogenicity, 597–598
geometrical studies, 231
SAMEE, 221
single ROI studies, 226
ultrasound plaque image, 235
Greedy algorithm (GA)
ground truth (GT), 189
merging, profiles, 190
representation, 189
GSM. *See* Gray scale median

H
Harmonic IVUS
in vivo
bolus, transducer agent, 141
CD31 staining, endothelial cells, 144
decanted Definity™, atherosclerotic rabbit aorta, 142, 143
fundamental and imaging modes, 141–142
hematoxylin/eosin stained section, 144
post-injection, 143

phantom experiments
coronary images, 141, 142
feasibility and performance, 140
imaging agent, 140, 141
tissue, 144
Hausdorff distance metric (HDM)
computation, 190–191
limitation, 191
usage, 191
HDM. *See* Hausdorff distance metric
Heat-shock proteins immunity, 507–508
High pulse repetition frequency (PRF), 76
Homomorphic filtering (DsFhomo), 103
Hough transform (HT)
CA recognition, 183, 185
validation, 184
wall segmentation, 183–184
HT. *See* Hough transform

I
IBS. *See* Integrated backscatter
ICA. *See* Internal carotid artery
Image analysis, carotid plaques
cross-sectional studies, GSM
amaurosis fugax, 608
asymptomatic and symptomatic patients, 608
biomechanical forces, 608
CT and CTD, 608
hypoechoic plaques, 608
echogenicity, 609
fibrous caps, 603
with image normalization, 607
plaque heterogeneity, 609
rupture, 603
stenosis
asymptomatic internal carotid artery, 610
NASCET and ECST, 611
risk, stroke, 611
Tromsø study, Norway, 608
ulceration, ultrasonic, 609
ultrasonic classification
"complicated" and "uncomplicated" plaques, 604
correlation, histology, 604–606
echodensity, 604
echolucent and echogenic, 604
homogenous and heterogenous, 604
"unstable" and "stable", 604
unstable plaques, 603
without image normalization
GSM, 607
heterogenous plaques, defined, 607
hyperechoic/calcified plaques, 606, 607
interobserver reproducibility, 607
ipsilateral strokes, 607
neurological symptoms, 606–607
stroke, 607
Image-based beam steering and compounding
axial and radial strains, 351, 353
in vivo B-mode image, 353

radial strain imaging, 351, 352
theoretical radial and circumferential strain
images, 352, 353
Image-based computational fluid dynamics modeling
comparison, in-plane velocity vectors, 44–45
description, 44
MRI *vs.* CFD, 44
OSI and WSS, 45
Image normalization
acquisition, 194–195
description, 193
development, 193–194
effect
description, 200
echolucent and heterogenous plaques, 202–203
ipsilateral neurological events, 202, 205
plaque classification, 201–202, 204
GSM, 193
plaque texture analysis software
anterior and posterior, 197, 198
calcified visible bright areas, 198, 202
extraction module, 197, 199
features, 197, 200
Geroulakos classification, 198
GSM, 198, 199, 203–205
image crop, 197
module, 196–197
types, 198, 201–202
technique, 195–196
Impaired glucose tolerance, 455
IMT. *See* Intima-media thickness
Inflammation and oxidative stress markers
chemokine receptors and impaired fibrinolysis
atherothrombosis, 504
32-bp frameshift deletion mutation, 503
Bruneck study, 503
CCR5, 503
CCR5-del32 association, 504
cumulative hazard curves, 503
FSAP Marburg I polymorphism, 504
CRP
acute-phase reactants, 499
levels, 499
iron overload
lipid-induced atherogenesis, 501
micro-hemorrhages, 501
tissue and macrophage iron, 500
validity, 501
Lp-PLA$_2$ (*see* Lipoprotein-associated phospholipase A$_2$)
OPG–RANK–RANKL system, 502–503
oxidized phospholipids
pro-atherogenic, 500
reactive oxygen species, 500
Integrated backscatter (IBS)
index measurements, 203–204
plaque echogenicity
12-month statin therapy, 598
nonhypercholesterolemic patients, 598
pitavastatin, 598
three-dimensional imaging, 598
usage, 219

Internal carotid artery (ICA)
acute and chronic occlusion, 538
atherosclerosis (*see* Internal carotid artery
atherosclerosis)
carotid bifurcation, 42
geometric parameters, 48
stenosis, 44
stenosis/occlusion
collateral flow, 575–576
dampened/absent velocity spectra, 575
description, 575
stent stenosis, 541
Internal carotid artery atherosclerosis
cerebrovascular risk stratification
angioplasty/stenting, carotid, 588
carotid dissection, 586
carotid territory stroke, 586–587
CEA (*see* Carotid endarterectomy)
noninvasive interventions, vascular disease, 588–589
proximal ICA stenosis, 580–586
TCD (*see* Transcranial Doppler)
Intima-media thickness (IMT). *See also* Carotid artery
IMT and lumen diameter
assessment
ARFY study, 505
ARMY study, 505–506
young individuals, 506–507
atherosclerosis severity
ARIC study, 383, 386
calcification, abdominal aorta, 386
coronary angiography, 386
biomarker
description, 381
"validated," 382
CAD prevalence, 404
change, time
annual rate of change, 390
AtheroGene Study, 389
IMTcc, 389
Rotterdam study, 389
coronary artery disease
APSIS, 404
bypass graft surgery, 403
IMTmax value evaluation, 404
cross-sectional image, carotid, 69, 71
defined, 453
gold standard and reproducibility
atherosclerosis, 383
biomarker, 382
"far wall" and "near wall" measurement, 382
intraclass correlation coefficient (ICC), 383
HDL elevation
ARBITER 2 and 3, 415
CETP, 415
CLAS, 415
RADIANCE 2 study, 416
horizontal arrows, 84
interventions, time
antihypertensive treatment, 392
blood-pressure-lowering treatment, 391
HMG-CoA reductase inhibitors, trials, 391

lipid lowering trials, 389
modification, risk factors, 389
KIHD study, 386
level and risk change, 391
parameters and location, measurement
arterial wall thickness, 400
extracranial carotid anatomical sites, 400
normal carotid segment, 401
older populations, 400
vs. plaque
development mechanism, 405
evaluation studies, 406–409
pathophysiology, 404–405
predictive value, 405–406
risk factor association, 404
plaque thickness
genetic research, 442–443
risk stratification, 435–436
vascular risk factors, 440–442
primary risk stratification
Cardiovascular Health Study, 401
KIHD, 400
meta-analysis, 401
prognostic indicator, 401, 402
stroke and acute myocardial infarction, 402
Tromsø study, 402
prognosis determinants, 381
publications, 382
risk factors and prevalent disease
cardiovascular, 384–385
C-reactive protein (CRP), elevated levels, 383
diastolic blood pressure, 383
SMART study, 386
specular reflection, 69
surrogate endpoint, 381
utility, youth
children, hypercholesterolemia and diabetes, 402
obese children, 403
premature cardiovascular disease (PFHPCD), 402–403
vascular events, 387–388
Intravascular ultrasound (IVUS)
advantage, 207
contrast behavior
frequency and microbubble sizes, 138–139
nonlinear microbubble, 139–140
defined, preclinical context, 150
description, 137
harmonic
*in vi*vo, 141–144
phantom experiments, 140–141
tissue, 144
invasiveness, 160–161
mechanisms, vasa vasorum, 150–151
molecular imaging
description, 147
nonlinear, 148–151
neovascular vasa vasorum, 137
non-culprit lesions, 137
nonlinear (*see* Nonlinear contrast IVUS)
plaque characterization (*see* Plaque characterization, IVUS)

role and limitations, 151
sensitivity and robustness, 138
strain imaging
drawback, 346–347
palpogram, 345
principle, elastography, 345, 347
vulnerable plaques, 346
subharmonic
*in vi*vo, 145–147
phantom experiments, 145
technical aspects
calcified plaque, 553, 554
"Eagle Eye" probe, 554–555
gold chip transducer, 554
grayscale images, 553, 554
luminal blood flow, 553–554
selective arteriography, 555
stent deployment, 555
VH-IVUS, 554
IVUS. *See* Intravascular ultrasound

K
Kaplan-Meier analysis, 227, 230
k-nearest-neighbor (kNN) classifier
description, 105
percentage, classification, 112, 115
texture analysis, 101, 111, 117
use, 105
Kuopio Ischemic Heart Disease Risk Factor (KIHD) study, 386, 400
Kyoto Encyclopedia of Genes and Genomes (KEGG), 479, 480

L
Lagrangian speckle motion estimator
functions, 349
measures, 349–350
rf data, 349
Laws texture energy measures (TEMs), 104
Law's texture energy method (LTE), 208
LDL. *See* Low-density lipoprotein
Lipid-lowering therapy
IMT progression and cardiovascular events
clinical studies, 412–413
statin therapy, 411
surrogate endpoint, 411
therapeutic agents and cholesterol composition, 411
LDL reduction therapies and IMT
ASAP, 414
atorvastatin, 414
beta-blocker and statin, 414
fluvastatin, 414
KAPS, 413
lovastatin, 414
MARS, 413
PLACII trial, 411
REGRESS, 411
rosuvastatin, 414–415
statin therapy, 413

Lipoprotein-associated phospholipase A_2 (Lp-PLA_2), 501–502
Long-term Intervention with Pravastatin in Ischemic Disease (LIPID) study, 413
Low-density lipoprotein (LDL)
   activating effect, infiltration, 7
   and metabolic syndrome, 456–457
   oxidized (*see* Oxidized LDL)
   phases, 5
   similarity, chemical composition, 4
LTE. *See* Law's texture energy method (LTE)

M

MAD. *See* Mean Absolute point-by-point distance
Magnetic resonance imaging (MRI)
   brain scans, 206
   carotid artery hemodynamics
      flow quantification, 42–43
      Fourier velocity encoding, 43
      ICA stenosis, 44
      MIP image, bifurcation, 43
      nuclear magnetic resonance, 42
      techniques, angiography, 42
      TOF and echo phase contrast angiography, 43
   cerebrovascular events/lesions, 569, 570
   description, 33
   human atherosclerotic lesions, pathology, 34
   long scanning time, 34
   stress, plaque, 336
Matrix metalloproteinases (MMPs)
   classification, 13
   components, extracellular matrix, 13
   description, 12
   dilation, arterial segment, 29
   media remodeling, 17
Maximum intensity projection (MIP)
   carotid artery bifurcation, 42, 43
   ICA stenosis, 44
Mean Absolute point-by-point distance (MAD), 190
Mean-square error (MSE), 100, 106
Mechanical index (MI), 80
Median filtering (DsFmedian), 102
Metabolic syndrome (MetS), 473–474
MI. *See* Mechanical index
Microbubble imaging
   contrast side-by-side display, 126–127
   disruption
      blood flow, capillary bed, 123
      defined, MI, 123
      ECG, 123–124
   low mechanical index, 124
   nonlinear (*see* Nonlinear imaging methods)
   nonlinearity
      description, 122
      ultrasonic waves, bubbles and echoes, 123
Minimum-mean-square error (MMSE), 98
MIP. *See* Maximum intensity projection
MMPs. *See* Matrix metalloproteinases
MMSE. *See* Minimum-mean-square error
Molecular imaging, carotid plaque
   atherosclerotic plaque markers
      antibodies *vs.* ICAM–1, 159
      GP IIbIIIa, 160
      parallel plate chamber flow studies, 159
      preclinical animal studies, 160
      receptors, 158
      ultrasound contrast molecular, murine vasculature, 159
   bifurcation, 160
   invassiveness, IVUS, 161
   markers, vascular endothelium, 155
   microbubble contrast
      construction, 156
      dwell time, 155
      latter agent approach, 156
      radioactive probes, 155–156
   phosphatidylserine microbubbles, 158
   signal-to-background ratio
      concentration, microbubbles, 157–158
      contrast imaging modality, 157
      detection, microbubbles, 156
      ligand target, 156
      multipulse technique, 156
      murine vascular inflammation model, 157
      ultrasound, 156, 157
   target, VEGF receptors, 160
   ultrasound contrast agents, defined, 155
   ultrasound molecular, atherosclerotic murine vasculature, 160, 161
Motion estimation, carotid artery plaques
   atherosclerotic plaque motion analysis
      algorithms, 369
      mean squared error (MSE), 369
      ultrasound videos, 369–370
   global and local optical flow solutions, 366
   and optical flow
      AM-FM model, 358, 363–364
      CBM, 358, 360–362
      digital video, 358
      GDIM, 362–363
      image intensity, 358
      least squares (LS), 364–365
      model assumptions and energy functionals, 359
      motion parameters, 359
      nonconstant brightness intensity optical flow model, 360
      optimization theory, 357
      quantitative comparisons, 358
   optimization, parameter
      relative error, 371, 372
      speckle simulation results, 371
      stenosis, 371
      ultrasound videos, 371, 373
      velocity estimation error, 373
   parameter selection
      data-driven approach, 366–367
      Horn and Schunck method, 371
      maximum likelihood/maximum a posteriori (MML/MAP), 367–368
      ME algorithms, 370–371
      velocity magnitudes, 371
   techniques, 368

MRI. *See* Magnetic resonance imaging
MSE. *See* Mean-square error
Multi-Ethnic Study of Atherosclerosis (MESA), 468
Multi-line methods, ultrasound beam
    PWV and TDI, 329
    wall-motion patterns, 329, 331

N
National Cholesterol Education Program III (NCEP III), 513
Neighborhood gray tone difference matrix (NGTDM), 104, 239–240
NGTDM. *See* Neighborhood gray tone difference matrix
Nonconstant brightness intensity optical flow model, 360
Noninvasive carotid elastography
    IVUS strain imaging, 345–347
    principles, ultrasound strain imaging
        displacements and strains calculation, 344, 346
        soft and hard tissues, 344, 345
    stable and vulnerable plaques, 343
    ultrasound
        imaging planes, 348
        intravascular *vs.* transcutaneous approach, 347
        strain imaging (*see* Strain imaging)
    vulnerable plaque detection, 343
Nonlinear contrast IVUS
    description, 140
    harmonic and sub-harmonic signals, 140
    prototype system, 140
    transducers, 140
Nonlinear imaging methods
    description, 124
    harmonic, 124
    PI, 124, 125
    PM, 124–125
    PMPI, 125–127

O
OFC. *See* Optical flow constraint
OGTT. *See* Oral glucose tolerance test
Optical flow and motion estimation
    digital video, 358
    energy functionals, 359
    models
        AM-FM image, 358
        constant brightness optical flow, 358, 360
    motion parameters, 359
    nonconstant brightness intensity, 360
    oriented smoothness constraint, 358
Optical flow constraint (OFC)
    smoothness constraint, 361
    spatial intensity gradient estimation, 360
    weighted version, 364
Oral glucose tolerance test (OGTT), 455
Osteoprotegerin (OPG), 424–425
Oxidized LDL (Ox-LDL)
    atherosclerosis, 457–458
    circulating, 459
    LDL cholesterol, 457
    plasma concentrations, 457

P
PCA. *See* Principal component analysis
pdfs. *See* Probability density functions
PDM. *See* Polyline distance metric
Percent statistic test (PST), 192
PI. *See* Pulse inversion
Pixel distribution analysis (PDA)
    carotid plaques, 206
    endarterectomy, 205–206
    GSM, 205
    IVUS, 207
    JBA, 206
Pixel neighborhood filtering (DsFhomog), 102
Planimetric evaluation, ICA, 531, 539–541
Plaque characterization, IVUS
    CAPITAL study, 559
    carotid bifurcation plaque, 553
    carotid stenting, 559
    clinical cases
        angiography, 556
        light microscopy, fibrous collagen fragments, 557
        multidetector CTA, 558
        plaque behavior prediction, 555
    intravascular ultrasound, 557
    progression and virtual histology
        atherosclerotic plaque, 555, 556
        diagnostic accuracy, VH-IVUS, 557
        macrophages, 555
        ruptured plaques, 556–557
        types, plaques, 557, 560–561
    VH-IVUS
        accuracy, 560
        calcified projections, 562
        carotid artery plaque, 562
        criteria, classification, 559
        lesion safety, 561
        neurological complication, 557
Plaque classification
    atherosclerosis
        heterogeneity and clinical implications, 250
        ultrasound, 249
    automatic
        image acquisition, 254
        material, 254
        PCA, 254–255
        PNN, 254
        segmentation, 254
        SVM, 254
        tests, 255
    carotid, ultrasound, 251, 252
    description, 249
    grayscale morphological analysis
        pdfs and *cdfs*, 258, 261–262
        SVM and PNN, 261, 263
    multilevel binary morphological analysis
        pdfs and *cdfs*, 256–258
        PNN and SVM, 257
        ROC analysis, 258–261
    texture analysis
        PNN and SVM, 255–256
        SGLDM, 255

ultrasound image analysis
    GSM, 250
    histogram features, 251
    morphological features, 252
    semiautomated method, 253
    standard texture features, 251–252
    TIA, 252
Plaque feature extraction
    carotid atherosclerotic, dataset, 233, 234
    3D plaque studies, 225, 229, 232
    FDTA, 241–242
    FPS, 242
    GLDS, 239
    interpretation and significance
        CT-brain scans, 234–235
        morphology and stroke risk, 234
        ultrasound images, carotid plaques, 234, 236
    morphology features
        application, atherosclerotic carotid plaques, 245
        gray scale, analysis, 245
        multilevel binary, analysis, 243–244
        pattern spectra, 243
    multivariate selection, 232–233
    NGTDM, 239–240
    pattern classification system, 225
    PCA, 233
    SF, 237
    SFM, 240–241
    SGLDM, 237–239
    single point based statistical, studies
        carotid endarterectomy, 230
        GSM, 230
        image normalization, 230
        single and multi-ROIs, 226–228
    spatial-based, studies
        geometrical, early texture features and multi-scale, 228–229, 231
        morphology feature, 231
    spatiotemporal
        block motion, 2D and 3D velocity, 229, 231
        B-mode ultrasound, 232
    symptomatic and asymptomatic examples, 225, 226
    TEM, 241
    two-dimensional scatter plots, asymptomatic and symptomatic plaques, 233, 235
    univariate selection, 232
    verbal interpretation, arithmetical values, 233, 235
Plaques automated classification
    backscattered ultrasound
        echogenicity and texture, 218
        GSM, 218
        IBS, 219
    boundary detection
        2D representation, 218
        performance, 217–218
        tissue, segmentation, 217
    carotid artery, 215
    classification
        model, 216
        training, 216
        validation, 216–217

images preprocessing, 217
method
    SAMEE algorithm, 219–221
    software solution, 219
ultrasound, 215–216
PM. *See* Power modulation
PMPI. *See* Power modulated pulse inversion
PNN. *See* Probabilistic neural network
Polyline distance metric (PDM)
    CGB and GT, 191–192
    IMT, 191
Polyvinylidene fluoride (PVDF), 72
Power modulated pulse inversion (PMPI), 125–127
Power modulation (PM), 124–125
Pravastatin, lipids and atherosclerosis in the carotid arteries (PLACII trial), 411
Principal component analysis (PCA), 233, 254
Probabilistic neural network (PNN)
    advantage, 254
    SVM, 249
Probability density functions *(pdfs)*, 256, 257, 261
Prospective Cardiovascular Münster (PROCAM) Score, 433
PST. *See* Percent statistic test
Pulsatility transmission index (PTI), 575
Pulse inversion (PI), 124, 125
Pulse wave velocity (PWV)
    Bramwell-Hill equation, 338
    distension coefficient DC 337
    Poisson's ratio inclusion, 338
    pressure–velocity loop, 334
    "water hammer" equation, 333
PVDF. *See* Polyvinylidene fluoride
PWV. *See* Pulse wave velocity

Q
Quick Like A Bunny (QLAB), 305

R
Radiofrequency (RF)
    accuracy, 328
    analysis, 335
    echo tracking, 334
Rating Athero-sclerotic Disease Change by Imaging with a New CETP Inhibitor 1 (RADIANCE 1) study, 415
Regression Growth Evaluation Statin Study (REGRESS), 411
Restenosis, 532–533
RF. *See* Radiofrequency
Risk Factor Intervention (RIS) Study, 452
Root-mean-square error (RMSE), 287, 293

S
Screening, cardiovascular risk
    ABI (*see* Ankle-brachial index (ABI))
    CACS, 512–513
    individuals and FRS
        high, 516
        intermediate, 515–516
        low, 515

Screening (cont.)
    individuals, low FRS, 515
    methods, 511
    ultrasound
        Cyprus epidemiological study, 513–515
        femoral bifurcations, 513
        IMT, 513
        plaque echolucency, 513
        Tromsø study, 513
Second Manifestations of Arterial Disease (SMART) study, 386
Semi-automated grayscale-based stratified color mapping
    asymptomatic left carotid stenosis, 567
    cerebrovascular symptoms and microembolic signals
        fibrous plaques, 568
        GSM, 568
        juxtaluminal black area, diagnostic value, 569
        microembolic detection and signals, 569
        multiple logistic regression model, 569
        neurological symptoms, 569
        parameters, 568
        predominant color, 568
    interobserver agreement, 568
    MATLAB 7.9, 566
    MRI, 567
    plaque pixels, 566–567
    right carotid stenosis, asymptomatic, 567
    threshold values, 567
    ultrasound image, 566
    and visual analysis
        MRI, 569, 570
        symptomatic and asymptomatic, 570
Semi-automated method to evaluate echogenicity (SAMEE)
    GSM, 221
    method, 220
    program, 220
    PW, 219
SFM. *See* Statistical feature matrix
SFs. *See* Statistical features
SGLDM. *See* Spatial gray level dependence matrix
Single-line methods, ultrasound beam
    RF data, 328–329
    wall motion, CCA, 329, 330
SMC. *See* Smooth muscle cells
Smooth muscle cells (SMC)
    apoptosis/programmed cell death, 14
    description, 3
    fibrous cap, 11, 13
    layers, elastic lamellae, 3–4
    stimulation, osteopontin, 8
Spatial gray level dependence matrix (SGLDM)
    correlation, 207–208
    energy and entropy, 207–208
    homogeneity and contrast, 207
    and SF, 231
    texture measures, 238
    unnormalized probability density functions, 237
Stable and vulnerable atherosclerotic plaques
    acute coronary syndromes
        calcified nodules, 11
        fatal infarctions, 11
        human carotid endarterectomy specimens, 9
        lesions, luminal thrombi, 10
        link, rupture and onset, 9
        mechanism, thrombosis, 9
        rupture, defined, 10
        thin-cap atheromas, 10
        thromboxane A2, pateints, 10
    atheromatous/lipid core
        breakdown, macrophage foam cells, 11–12
        lipids, 12
        physicochemical studies, 12
        popcorn plaque, 11
        postmortem analysis, 12
        TF, 12
    bone morphogenic proteins, 8
    calcification, 18
    cell death and formation, necrotic core, 7
    definitions, 8
    description, 3
    early lesions, 4–5
    effect, LDL infiltration, 7
    endothelial dysfunction, 3
    fibrous cap
        description, 13
        factors, platelets degranulation, 13
        MMPs, 13
    formation, 4
    healed rupture, 19
    histological and imaging studies, 18
    histological examples, 6
    histological structure, humans artery
        layers, 3
        SMC, 3–4
        structure, large artery, 4
    idendification, stenosis, 19
    media and adventitia change, 17–18
    neovascularization and intraplaque hemorrhage
        A-I and B, apolipoproteins, 14
        description, 16
        histologic examination, vulnerable lesions, 15
        neovessels, 14
        oxygen diffusion, 14
        pathways, erythrocytes, 15
    preatheroma/intermediate lesions, 5
    "response-to-injury" hypothesis, 3
    role, macrophage inflammation, 7
    type Va, plaques/fibroatheromas, 8
    vascular remodeling
        constrictive and expansive arterial, 16–17
        description, 16
        in vitro, human coronary arteries and mouse model, 17
        luminal narrowing, 16
        x-ray angiography, 16
Statin therapy, carotid plaque morphology
    ASTEROID, 596
    echogenicity
        GSM, 597–598
        IBS, 598
    hypoechoic plaques, 595
    IMT measurements, 595
    MRI, 596
    pioglitazone, 598–599

placebo-controlled studies, 595
stable angina, 596
thickness and area, plaque, 596
volume changes, 3D ultrasound, 596–597
Statistical feature matrix (SFM), 104, 240–241
Statistical features (SFs), 104, 237
Statistics and signal analysis, carotid artery recognition
    characteristics, 182–183
    cropped B-mode image, 183
    2DH, 183
Stiffness index, 338–339
Strain imaging
    longitudinal cross-sections
        cross-correlation-based methods, 350
        Doppler-based method, 348–349
        LSME, 349–350
    transverse cross-sections
        image-based beam steering and compounding, 351–353
        line-based beam steering, 351
        radial and circumferential, 350–351
Stroke
    ACSRS (*see* Asymptomatic carotid stenosis and risk of stroke study)
    annual risk, 58
    asymptomatic carotid stenosis, 59–60
    carotid bifurcation
        description, transient hemispheric and monocular vision loss, 35
        left carotid artery occlusion, patient, 34
        reconstruction, 35
    disability, 121
    embolic, 93, 94
    Framingham stroke risk score (FSRS), 427
    "ipsilateral" and "any", 59–60
    ischemic, 121
    rate, 56
    symptomatic, 301
Subharmonic IVUS
    in vivo
        "BSci40" images, atherosclerotic plaque, 145
        3D BSci40 IVUS image, longitudinal section, 147, 148, 150, 151
        F30 and SH15 imaging, atherosclerotic rabbit aorta, 149–151
        vessel phantom images, small bubble agent, 145, 146
    phantom experiments, 145
Support vector machine (SVM)
    PNN, 255
    RBF, 253
SVM. *See* Support vector machine

T
Tagged Image File Format (TIFF), 307
TDI. *See* Tissue doppler imaging
TEMs. *See* Laws texture energy measures
Texture energy measures (TEM), 241
Texture features
    clinical value, 210
    correlation, SGLDM, 208

    ESCT, 209
    FOS, 207
    GLDS, 208
    RUNL, 208
    SFM and LTE, 208
    SGLDM, 207–208
    SGLDM *vs.* RUNL, 208–209
TF. *See* Tissue factor
Thermal index (TI), 80
TI. *See* Thermal index
Tissue Doppler imaging (TDI)
    multi-line methods, 329
    techniques, 329
Tissue factor (TF), 12
Total plaque volume (TPV), 269
Transcranial Doppler (TCD)
    acoustic windows, 573
    advantages, 573
    arterial findings
        bifurcation, intracranial ICA, 574
        contrast agents, 574
        identification, 573
        2-MHz probes, 574
        middle cerebral artery (MCA) identification, 574
        pulsed-echo technique, 574
    emboli detection
        gaseous and solid embolism, 579
        power M-mode, 579
        principle, 578
        ultrasonic, 578
    ICA stenosis/occlusion
        cervical imaging, 575
        collateral flow, 575–576
        dampened/absent velocity spectra, 575
        diagnosis criteria, 576
        digital subtraction angiography (DSA), 578
        MCA, 576–577
        sensitivity, 575
        tandem lesions, 576
    intracranial arterial autoregulation
        cerebrovascular reserve, 580
        description, 579
        "hemodynamics" and "cerebral arterial vascular reactivity", 580
    risk stratification tool, 589
Tromsø study
    cardiovascular disease and mortality
        carotid plaque burden, measurement, 425
        ischemic stroke, 426
        multivariable-adjusted HR, 425–426
        myocardial infarction proportion, 426
        randomized controlled trials, 427
        Rotterdam Study, 427
    carotid plaques prevalence
        defined, 421
        men and women, 422
        stroke, risk of, 422
    carotid stenosis, 425
    plaque echogenicity and cardiovascular risk
        atherosclerosis and osteoporosis, 428
        Gray-Weale classification, 427

ischemic cerebrovascular events proportion, 427
men and women, 428
risk factors
  carotid artery intima-media thickness (CIMT), 422
  echogenicity, 423
  high-density lipoprotein (HDL) levels, 423
  inflammation markers, 424
  low plasma lipoprotein lipase activity, 423
  LPL mobilization, 423
  microalbuminuria, 424
  OPG, 424–425
  plaque size progression, 422–423
  predictors, novel plaque formation, 422
  proinsulin, 424
  sex hormones, 424
  TAT and F1 + 2, 424
  testosterone levels, 424
  VLDL particles, 423
ultrasonography, 421
Tumor necrosis factor-α (TNF-α), 476
Type 2 diabetes
  DIWA study, 455
  meta-analysis, 455

U

Ultrasonic imaging
  advantages and limitations, pulse-echo ultrasound examination, 67
  beam patterns
    description, 75
    Doppler examination angle, 75
    dual Doppler signals, 76, 78
    and grating lobes, 75, 77
    PRF, 76
    reflection, 76–77
    sidelobe, image thickness direction, 76
    zero and first-order element sidelobe, 75
  bifurcations, longitudinal view, 67, 68
  B-mode (see B-mode imaging)
  carotid anatomy (see Carotid anatomy, ultrasonic imaging)
  demodulation
    architecture, ultrasound, 79, 81
    B-mode, 81
    parameters, 80–81
    pulse-echo cycle, 80
    RF, voltage vs. fast time, 81, 82
  Doppler (see Doppler, ultrasonic imaging)
  electronic beam former
    2-D B-mode image, 77–78
    pulse-echo cycle, 77, 79
    single-line Doppler examination, 78
    ultrasound system architecture, 77, 79
  intraplaque tissue type, 67
  phase processing
    adjacent line echoes, 86
    2D lateral coherence, carotid artery, 84, 87
  safety
    description, 78
    effects, MI, 80
    TI, theoretical computation, 80
    ultrasound–transmit burst, 78–79
  transducers
    alignment, 74
    aperture and cross-sectional beam profile, 72, 74
    array and receiver signal path, 73
    array vs. patient's skin, 71
    "backing ghost", defined, 74
    channel vs. beam former, 75
    compression/decompression waves, 74
    coupling and damping, transducer, 72
    description, 70
    piezoelectric property, crystal, 70–71
    scanhead construction, 72
Ultrasonic plaque characterization
  ACSRS (see Asymptomatic Carotid Stenosis and Risk of Stroke study)
  computer-quantified plaque morphology assessment, 608

V

Vascular endothelial growth factor (VEGF)
  endothelial vasa vasorum neovasculature, 160
  receptor, 158
Vascular hemodynamics, carotid bifurcation
  and atherosclerosis (see Atherosclerosis)
  description, 41
  flow parameters, 41
  image-based computational fluid dynamics modeling, 44–45
  influence, posture change
    3D surface reconstruction image, 49
    geometric difference, 48
    ICA, graphical representation, 49
    morphological changes, 48
    optimization and implantation, design, 50
    stimulations, 49
  inhibition, NO, 41
  MRI, 42–44
  ultrasound measurements, 42
  WSS, 42
Vascular phantom
  curvature computation algorithm, 285
  3D ultrasound image, 285, 286
  Gaussian curvature, 289, 297
  mean curvature and flattened maps, 287, 294–296
Vascular ultrasound imaging, contrast agents
  cardiovascular disease, 121
  CT and MR, 121
  Doppler-based techniques, 121
  markers, 122
  microbubble
    contrast side-by-side display, 126–127
    disruption, 123–124
    low mechanical index, 124
    nonlinear (see Nonlinear imaging methods)
    nonlinearity, 122–123
  quantification, microcirculation
    demonstration, time-intensity curve, 131
    indication dilution, 131

indicator dilution models, 131
nonlinear bubbly fluid, 132–133
results, 132
quantification results and clinical importance
CEUS, 134
ECST criteria, 133
pixels, ROI, 134
TICs and lognormal function, 133
WIT and MTT, 134
signal intensity *vs.* time curve, 122
ultrasound examination
B-image, carotid plaque, 128
clinical example, 129
description, 127
EMEA, 128–129
hyperplastic vasa vasorum, 130
nonlinear pulsing scheme, 128
plaque neovascularization, 129
VEGF. *See* Vascular endothelial growth factor
Vessel wall volume (VWV), 270

W

Wall motion analysis
applications
atherosclerosis, 334
diabetes and blood glucose, 334
diseases and risk factors, 334
healthy arteries, 334
arterial mechanics
pulse, 328
structure, 327–328
cardiac cycle, 327
2D motion
atherosclerotic plaque, 331
surface motion calculation, 332
elastic modulus and stress estimation, plaque, 336
finite wall thickness, 338
healthy arteries, 334
and induced vibration

B-mode and ARFI strain image, 336, 337
clinical medicine, 336
PWV, 337–338
radial motion
blood pressure, 333
distension, 332–333
elastic moduli, 333
PWV, 333–334
stiffness index, 338–339
strain measurement
2D strain images, 335, 336
techniques, heart, 335
stress estimation, non-diseased arteries, 335
transverse, beam, 331
ultrasound beam
multi-line methods, 329–331
single-line methods, 328–329
Wall shear stress (WSS)
arterial wall
friction, 30
hemodynamic forces, carotid bifurcation, 30
pulsatile flow, defined, 30
atherosclerosis, 48
atherosclerotic lesions, 45
carotid bifurcation, 41, 42
defined, mean shear direction, 47
3D velocity flow field, 44
endothelial function and remodeling
boundary layer separation, 30
functional alterations, monolayer, 31
mapping, 31
nitric oxide, atheroprotective effect, 31
physiologic variations, 30
hemodynamic
indices, 47
parameter, 43, 49
PDGF-β chain expression, 41
temporal and spatial gradients, 46
WSS. *See* Wall shear stress